Diagnostic Pediatric Hematopathology

Diagnostic Pediatric Hematopathology

Edited by

Maria A. Proytcheva MD

Northwestern University Feinberg School of Medicine,
Department of Pathology and Laboratory Medicine,
Children's Memorial Hospital, Chicago, IL, USA

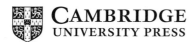

CAMBRIDGE
UNIVERSITY PRESS

CAMBRIDGE UNIVERSITY PRESS
Cambridge, New York, Melbourne, Madrid, Cape Town, Singapore,
São Paulo, Delhi, Dubai, Tokyo, Mexico City

Cambridge University Press
The Edinburg Building, Cambridge CB2 8RU, UK

Published in the United States of America by
Cambridge University Press, New York

www.cambridge.org
Information on this title: www.cambridge.org/9780521881609

First published 2011

Printed in the United Kingdom at the University Press, Cambridge

A catalog record for this publication is available from the British Library

ISBN 978-0-521-88160-9 Hardback

To Glauco Frizzera, and all of my teachers, for the inspiration they have given me.

Contents

Contributors

Barbara J. Bain MBBS FRACP FRCPath
Professor of Diagnostic Haematology, St Mary's Hospital
Campus of Imperial College Faculty of Medicine, London;
Honorary Consultant Haematologist, St Mary's Hospital,
London, UK

Stanley Chaleff MD
Attending Physician, Maine Children's Cancer Program,
Scarborough, ME; Assistant Professor of Pediatrics, University
of Vermont School of Medicine, Burlington, VT; Assistant
Professor of Pediatrics, Tufts School of Medicine, Boston, MA,
USA

Kenneth Chang MD
University of Toronto, The Hospital for Sick Children,
Toronto, Ontario, Canada

John Kim Choi MD PhD
Associate Professor and Director of Pediatric
Hematopathology, Department of Pathology and Laboratory
Medicine, Children's Hospital of Philadelphia, University of
Pennsylvania School of Medicine, Philadelphia, PA, USA

Chiang-Ching Huang PhD
Feinberg School of Medicine at Northwestern University,
Chicago, IL, USA

Ronald Jaffe MBBCh
Professor of Pathology, University of Pittsburgh School of
Medicine; Department of Pathology, Children's Hospital of
Pittsburgh, Pittsburgh, PA, USA

Lawrence Jennings MD PhD
Assistant Professor of Pathology, Northwestern University
Feinberg School of Medicine; Director, Molecular Pathology,
Department of Pathology and Laboratory Medicine,
Children's Memorial Hospital, Chicago, IL, USA

Jeffrey Jhang MD
Director, Special Hematology and Coagulation Laboratory,
New York Presbyterian Hospital; Assistant Professor of
Clinical Pathology, Columbia University Medical Center, New
York, NY, USA

Alexander Kratz MD PhD
Associate Professor of Pathology and Cell Biology, Columbia
University College of Physicians and Surgeons; Director of the
Core Laboratory, New York Presbyterian Hospital, New York,
NY, USA

Katrin Carlson Leuer PhD
Assistant Professor of Pathology, Northwestern University
Feinberg School of Medicine; Scientific Director, Cytogenetics
Laboratory, Department of Pathology and Laboratory
Medicine, Children's Memorial Hospital, Chicago, IL, USA

Robert B. Lorsbach MD PhD
Associate Professor of Pathology and Director of
Hematopathology, University of Arkansas for Medical
Sciences, Little Rock, AR, USA

Mihaela Onciu MD
Director, Hematology and Special Hematology Laboratories,
Department of Pathology; Associate Member, St. Jude Faculty,
St. Jude Children's Research Hospital, Memphis, TN, USA

Sherrie L. Perkins MD PhD
Professor, University of Utah Health Sciences Center; Director,
Hematopathology and Chief Medical Officer, ARUP
Laboratories, Salt Lake City, UT, USA

Elena Pope MD MSc FRCPC
Associate Professor, University of Toronto; Head, Section of
Dermatology, Division of Paediatric Medicine, The Hospital
for Sick Children, Toronto, Ontario, Canada

Maria A. Proytcheva MD
Assistant Professor of Pathology, Northwestern University
Feinberg School of Medicine, Department of Pathology and
Laboratory Medicine, Children's Memorial Hospital, Chicago,
IL, USA

Andrea M. Sheehan MD
Director of Hematology and Flow Cytometry,
Hematopathology, Texas Children's Hospital; Assistant
Professor of Pathology and Immunology, Baylor College of
Medicine, Houston, TX, USA

Suresh G. Shelat MD PhD

Medical Director, Hematology Laboratory and Central Laboratory Services; Attending Physician, Apheresis and Transfusion Medicine, Children's Hospital of Philadelphia; Assistant Professor, Department of Pathology and Laboratory Medicine, University of Pennsylvania School of Medicine, Philadelphia, PA, USA

Glenn Taylor MD FRCPC

Head, Division of Pathology, Paediatric Laboratory Medicine, The Hospital for Sick Children, Toronto, Ontario, Canada

Angela E. Thomas MBBS PhD FRCPE FRCPath FRCPCH

Consultant Paediatric Haematologist, Royal Hospital for Sick Children, Edinburgh, UK

J. Han van Krieken MD

Professor, Department of Pathology, Radboud University Nijmegen Medical Centre, Nijmegen, The Netherlands

Sa A. Wang MD PhD

Assistant Professor and Associate Director of Flow Cytometry Laboratory, Department of Hematopathology, The University of Texas M.D. Anderson Cancer Center, Houston, TX, USA

Victor Zota MD

Pathologist, Oncology Translational Laboratories, Novartis Institutes for BioMedical Research, Inc., Cambridge, MA, USA

Acknowledgements

Many people, directly or indirectly, have made this project possible. At the start, I want to thank Madeleine Kraus, who was the first to envision this project and who helped me establish contact with Cambridge University Press. Marc Strauss, then the Publishing Director of the Scientific, Technical, and Medical Division of the Press' North American Branch, was crucial at the initial stage of the project. I am grateful as well to Cambridge University Press, and particularly Nicholas Dunton, Senior Commissioning Editor, Medicine, and his team for committing to a Pediatric Hematopathology text and for standing behind the project until its completion. During the editing and copy-editing stages, Dr. Clare Lendrem was invaluable to me. The effects of her considerable skills are evident throughout the book and I am very thankful to her.

I owe an enormous debt to my mentor, Elizabeth Perlman, for many things. Among them is the encouragement she gave me to take this opportunity and the constant support she gave me the entire way. I want to thank the Hematology Laboratories staff, particularly Deborah Runnels, as well as my colleagues at Children's Memorial Hospital for the exceptional job they do that has enriched my understanding of the hematologic diseases in children. And, much appreciation goes to Marian Stevenson for her wonderful technical support and to Loren Lott for his excellent assistance with the flow cytometric analysis.

I express special thanks to all the contributors for the outstanding work they did while they were also taking care of sick children.

On a personal note, I give thanks to my family – to Snejana, Mihail, Silvia, and Irina – both for who they are and for their unconditional love and support. I am also profoundly indebted to James L. German, III, a teacher and dear friend, and his wife Margaret. Together they gave me a hand and supported me over the years while I was beginning my journey in the world of human genetics that ultimately led me to hematopathology. They did so much to help me make a new life in a land so different from my native Bulgaria. I greatly appreciate Professor Robert Gundlach, Program Director, Writing Program at the Northwestern University, for helping me to see that writing, as every craft, can be learned. My largest debt is to John Schwarz. Without him, this project would neither have been started nor ever completed. Words cannot express the gratitude I feel. John, thank you from the bottom of my heart!

Maria A. Proytcheva

Introduction

Maria A. Proytcheva

Pediatric hematopathology is a special and highly challenging field. Despite its importance, however, and despite the sea of publications that exist in the field of hematopathology, few texts focus on the diagnosis of benign and malignant hematologic disorders found in children. As a result, even though the uniqueness of developmental factors and pathology in children is well recognized and appreciated, the specifics are not widely known or understood, which poses great difficulties for the diagnosis of hematologic diseases in children.

Diagnostic Pediatric Hematopathology presents an accurate and up-to-date examination of such diseases in children – both non-neoplastic and neoplastic. One goal is to provide knowledge about how the hematopoietic and lymphoid systems develop and how this development affects what can be considered normal and abnormal findings in children at various ages. A second key goal is to focus on the morphologic, immunophenotypic, cytogenetic, and molecular genetic characteristics of most pediatric-specific hematologic diseases so as to provide a resource that can be helpful in reaching a proper diagnosis when evaluating pediatric peripheral blood, bone marrow, and lymph nodes. The text addresses these goals through a team of experienced pediatric hematopathologists and clinical scientists drawn from major academic children's hospitals in the United States, Canada, and Europe, and this text is a result of our collaborative efforts.

Several major differences between pediatric and adult hematopathology are especially important and create the need for a separate text such as this book.

First, the hematopoietic system is not fully developed at birth. Instead, it continues to evolve during childhood to reach its maturity during the teenage years. As a result, both the peripheral blood and the bone marrow findings will be related to the developmental stage, such that what should be considered normal will depend upon the age of the child. These differences – both between children of various ages and between children and adults – can be substantial and have great clinical relevance. They are explored in the chapters on hematologic values in the healthy fetus, neonate, and child and normal bone marrow.

Age, along with underlying genetic abnormalities, has been recognized as integral to the diagnosis of certain hematologic malignancies. The latest *WHO Classification of Tumours of Haematopoietic and Lymphoid Tissues*,[1] for example, includes several disorders, such as juvenile myelomonocytic leukemia, childhood myelodysplastic syndrome, and myeloid proliferations related to Down syndrome, as conditions with unique morphologic features, underlying genetic mechanisms, and different treatment outcomes in children as compared to the adult counterparts. It also identifies disorders that are exclusively seen in children, such as systemic EBV+ T-cell lymphoproliferative diseases of childhood. The unique features of these hematologic malignancies are explored in the appropriate chapters.

Second, there are differences in the type and prevalence of hematologic diseases in children as compared to adults. For instance, acute leukemias, particularly lymphoblastic leukemias, are frequent in children, and lymphomas are rare. This is in contrast to adults, where mature B-cell lymphomas/leukemias are much more frequent, and acute leukemias are relatively rare. The pediatric leukemias have specific morphologic features and underlying genetic mechanisms that are explored in the chapters on precursor B- and T-lymphoblastic leukemias, acute myeloid leukemias, chromosomal abnormalities, and expression profiling in pediatric hematologic malignancies.

Third, the treatment for pediatric leukemia differs and the outcomes themselves are far superior than is the case for adults. The better outcomes are due in part to the unique pathogenetic mechanisms causing these diseases in children, but they are also due to the unusual speed with which advances have taken place in the treatment of the diseases in children. Those advances are based upon standardized protocols that have been developed for the treatment of children through randomized clinical trials. The trials have been conducted through the pediatric

---

[1] **Swerdlow SH, Campo E, Harris NL**, *et al.* (eds.). *WHO Classification of Tumours of Haematopoietic and Lymphoid Tissues* (4th edn.). Lyon: IARC Press; 2008.

---

cooperative groups, such as the Children's Oncology Group (COG) and St. Jude Children's Research Hospital in the United States, Berlin–Frankfurt–Münster ALL protocol in Germany, European Organization for Research and Treatment of Cancer – Children's Leukemia Group, and the Medical Research Council in the United Kingdom. In contrast with adults, most children with leukemia under the age of 15 in the United States, Canada, Europe, Australia, and New Zealand are currently treated on such protocols.

These protocols set specific requirements for a standardized approach to the diagnosis and follow-up evaluation of the bone marrow of children with leukemias. Accordingly, bone marrow studies are performed at specific time points to determine responses to therapy and detect minimal residual disease. However, the iatrogenic changes that occur following chemotherapy, along with the unique regeneration patterns of the bone marrow in children, may mimic residual disease, which makes the detection of minimal residual disease challenging. The dynamics of these changes are explored in the chapter covering the effects of therapy and hematopoietic stem cell transplants.

Information resulting from a child's particular response to therapy and the presence or absence of minimal residual leukemia is an important guide for the therapeutic management of children with leukemia. Given its importance, the hematopathologist is brought into the clinical oncology team to collaborate, not simply regarding initial diagnoses, but also for follow-up treatments. For that reason, the text includes an examination, coming from a clinician's perspective, of the advances in diagnosis, prognostication, and treatment of pediatric acute leukemia. The aim is to help broaden the pathologist's understanding of the likely clinical expectations of the oncology team during the management of such diseases.

As leukemias affect children and adults differently, the incidence of reactive lymphadenopathies and lymphomas differs as well. There is a higher prevalence of reactive lymphadenopathies early in life and a relative paucity of lymphomas. Most of the enlarged lymph nodes in children are reactive and frequently arise as part of the normal immunologic response to various antigens. However, the reaction can be so exuberant that it can resemble lymphoma, or children may present with constitutional and laboratory abnormalities suggesting malignancy in the settings of reactive lymphoid hyperplasia. Thus, it is crucial in making a proper diagnosis to avoid the considerable possibilities for misinterpreting lymph node

changes of children. These types of issues, as well as the most common lymphadenopathies in children, are examined in the chapter on reactive lymphadenopathies. It also provides a comprehensive review of the development of lymph nodes and the normal immune reaction, which is important to appreciate in the morphologic examination of lymph nodes. A chapter on immunodeficiency associated with lymphoproliferative disorders is included as well, since many of these diagnostically challenging conditions occur mainly during childhood.

Unlike adults, too, nearly all lymphomas in children are high grade, such as Burkitt lymphoma, diffuse large B-cell lymphoma, and ALK1+ anaplastic large cell lymphoma. The unique characteristics of the pediatric mature B- and T-cell lymphomas as well as Hodgkin lymphoma are covered in the respective chapters on them and, as with the rest of the text, the discussions are current with the latest WHO classification.

Small blue cell tumors metastatic to the bone marrow represent one more set of conditions for which the pathology is unique to children. These tumors have various propensities to metastasize to the marrow and can manifest with different patterns that may resemble leukemia. The characteristic morphologic patterns and how to avoid pitfalls in their diagnosis are discussed in the chapter on bone marrow metastasis.

Finally, the text also includes chapters on the disorders of erythrocyte production, hemoglobin synthesis, hemolytic anemia, bone marrow failure syndromes, and storage diseases that most frequently are seen in children, but where the differences between children and adults are not always so clear. In addition, some very infrequent diseases, such as cutaneous and subcutaneous lymphomas in children and histiocytic proliferations in childhood that are rarely systematically covered in the literature, are included here.

The *Diagnostic Pediatric Hematopathology* text focuses on the diagnostic aspects of benign and neoplastic hematologic diseases in children and discusses a wide range of key problems and issues that must be addressed in reaching a proper diagnosis. The text is intended as a helpful instrument in the everyday practice of pathologists, pediatric pathologists, and hematopathologists, along with fellows, pathology residents and medical students, and clinical scientists in the field. Since many pediatric hematologists/oncologists are involved in the diagnosis of childhood hematologic diseases as well, this book can be valuable for them, too.

Section 1

General and non-neoplastic hematopathology

General and non-neoplastic hematopathology

1

Hematologic values in the healthy fetus, neonate, and child

Maria A. Proytcheva

The hematopoietic system is not fully developed at birth, and the normal hematologic values of newborns and infants differ as compared to older children and adults. The differences are a manifestation of the unique characteristics of the embryonal and fetal development of the hematopoietic system that continues to evolve after birth. Furthermore, preanalytical and analytical factors unique for neonates and young children also contribute to these differences. This chapter will explore these factors and discuss how they define the normal hematologic values for different age groups.

Developmental hematopoiesis: a general view

The hematopoietic development, unlike any other organ system, occurs in successive anatomic sites where the hematopoietic stem cells (HSCs) are generated, maintained, and differentiate into various cell types [1]. The hematopoiesis begins in the yolk sac with the generation of angioblastic foci or "blood islands" that contain primitive erythroblasts. It then progresses further in several waves involving multiple anatomic sites: the aorta–gonadal–mesonephros (AGM) region, fetal liver, and bone marrow (BM) [2, 3]. Depending on the site of major hematopoietic activity, the hematopoiesis has been divided into three stages: the mesenchymal, hepatic, and myeloid stages with the yolk sac, liver, and bone marrow as major hematopoietic sites where hematopoietic cells with characteristic features are generated [4] (Fig. 1.1). There is a considerable temporal overlap between different stages. At birth and thereafter, the hematopoiesis is restricted to the bone marrow and continues to evolve in order to adapt to the new oxygen-rich environment and the needs of the growing organism.

It is currently accepted that the HSCs develop from hemangioblasts, which are mesodermal multipotent progenitors that give rise to hematopoietic as well as endothelial and vascular smooth muscle cells (Fig. 1.2A) [2, 5]. The first blood islands consisting of primitive erythroblasts surrounded by endothelial cells are formed in the *yolk sac* between days 16 and 19 of gestation [6]. During this stage, the hematopoiesis generates mostly

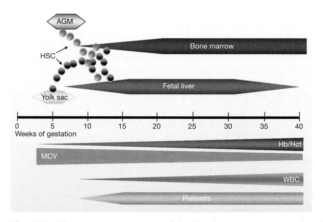

Fig. 1.1. Schematic representation of the developmental time windows for shifting sites of hematopoiesis in humans. The hematopoiesis occurs in successive anatomic sites – yolk sac, fetal liver, and bone marrow. It is currently believed that hematopoietic cells (HSCs) from extraembryonic (yolk sac) and intraembryonic (aorta, genital ridge, and mesonephros (AGM) region) sites seed the fetal liver and bone marrow where the HSCs are maintained and differentiate into various cell types. The blood generated during each phase has a different composition. With the advancing of the gestational age, the mean corpuscular volume (MCV) of the erythrocytes decreases and the hemoglobin, hematocrit, white blood cell, and platelet counts increase.

primitive and only a few definitive erythroblasts, as well as a few megakaryocytes at the sixth and seventh weeks of gestation. The primitive erythroblasts differ from the definitive erythroblasts in several aspects (Table 1.1). They are macrocytic [mean corpuscular volume (MCV) of 250 fL/cell]. They differentiate within the vascular network and remain nucleated for their entire lifespan. These cells have an increased sensitivity to erythropoietin (EPO) and a shorter lifespan as compared to the later fetal, definitive erythroblasts and adult counterparts. The hallmark of the primitive erythroid cells is the expression of embryonic hemoglobins such as Gower 1 ($\zeta_2\varepsilon_2$), Gower 2 ($\alpha_2\varepsilon_2$), and Portland ($\zeta_2\gamma_2$). The yolk sac hematopoiesis declines after the eighth week of gestation.

The *ventral aspect of the aorta* is another site of erythropoietic activity in the human embryo from 20 to 40 days of gestation [6]. This region corresponds to the aorta, genital ridge,

Diagnostic Pediatric Hematopathology, ed. Maria A. Proytcheva. Published by Cambridge University Press.
© Cambridge University Press 2011.

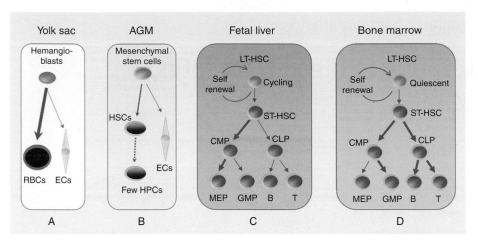

Fig. 1.2. Schematic representation of the hematopoiesis in each anatomic site with the production of specific blood lineages depending on each location. (A) The yolk sac favors the generation of primitive erythroblasts. (B) The AGM is mostly involved in the generation of hematopoietic progenitors which, along with the hematopoietic progenitors generated in the yolk sac, seed the fetal liver and bone marrow. (C) The fetal liver generates mostly definitive erythroid progenitors and to a lesser degree granulocytes, monocytes, and lymphocytes. (D) The fetal bone marrow generates multilineage hematopoiesis which in the early stages is mostly granulocytic. Abbreviations: AGM, aorta–gonadal–mesonephros region; EC, endothelial cell; RBC, red blood cell; HPC, hematopoietic progenitor cell; LT-HSC, long-term hematopoietic cell; ST-HSC, short-term hematopoietic cell; CMP, common myeloid progenitor; CLP, common lymphoid progenitor; MEP, megakaryocyte/erythroid progenitor; GMP, granulocyte/macrophage progenitor. (Redrawn with modifications from Orkin, Zon [4], with permission.)

Table 1.1. Characteristic features of the primitive and definitive erythropoiesis during ontogeny.

	Primitive hematopoiesis	Definitive hematopoiesis
Hematopoietic site	Yolk sac Vascular endothelium	Fetal liver and fetal bone marrow Hematopoietic niches
Type of hematopoiesis	Mostly erythroid	Multilineage hematopoiesis
RBC characteristics		
Nucleated	Remain nucleated during their entire lifespan	Enucleated RBCs
Cell size	Macrocytic (MCV 250 fL)	MCV decreases with gestational age
Sensitivity to EPO	Increased	Lower sensitivity
Lifespan	Short	Increases with gestation
Hemoglobins	Embryonic: Gower 1 ($\zeta_2\varepsilon_2$), Gower 2 ($\alpha_2\varepsilon_2$), and Portland ($\zeta_2\gamma_2$)	Fetal: Hb F ($\alpha_2\gamma_2$) and adult: Hb A ($\alpha_2\beta_2$)

Abbreviations: RBC, red blood cell; MCV, mean corpuscular volume; EPO, erythropoietin; Hb, hemoglobin.

and mesonephros (AGM) region in various vertebrate species. Most of the cells generated in this region are multipotent HSCs, and their number is highest around the 23rd day of gestation (Fig. 1.2B).

The HSCs from AGM (intraembryonic site) as well as cells from the yolk sac (extraembryonic site) colonize the fetal liver and bone marrow, where they are maintained, expanded, and differentiated into definitive blood cells [4, 6–8]. The definitive hematopoietic precursors develop in the hematopoietic niche, which provides a complex microenvironment generated by the stromal elements of the fetal liver, bone marrow, and the microvasculature endothelium; it plays a seminal role in the regulation of the hematopoiesis.

The *fetal liver* is the major site of hematopoiesis between 11 and 24 weeks of gestation (Fig. 1.2C). The hepatic hematopoiesis is mostly erythroid, and in the second trimester of pregnancy about half of the nucleated cells in the liver are erythroid progenitors. However, other cell lineages such as megakaryocytic, myeloid, and lymphoid progenitors are also generated in the fetal liver. Unlike the yolk sac erythropoiesis, the hepatic erythropoiesis occurs extravascularly within the complex cellular milieu of the fetal liver. The fetal erythropoiesis is definitive and resembles that found in postnatal life. It generates enucleated red blood cells that are seen in the circulation by eight weeks of gestation. The MCV of the definitive erythroblasts is lower than the MCV of the primitive erythroblasts. These cells contain predominantly Hb F ($\alpha_2\gamma_2$).

The *fetal bone marrow* hematopoiesis is initiated at about 6–8.5 weeks of gestation and occurs in several morphologically distinctive stages described in detail in Chapter 2 [9]. The process is completed by the 16th week of gestation, but the BM does not become a major site for hematopoiesis until the 25th week of gestation. The fetal BM hematopoiesis is multilineal and generates definitive enucleated RBCs containing Hb F and Hb A ($\alpha_2\beta_2$) as well as myeloid and lymphoid progenitors (Fig. 1.2D).

Between the 14th and 24th week of gestation, both the fetal liver and bone marrow are hematopoietic organs concomitantly, yet each supports a somewhat distinctive set of hematopoietic lineages [10]. The liver is the major site for erythropoiesis (Fig. 1.3) whereas, in the BM, the hematopoiesis is shifted to granulopoiesis and lymphopoiesis and the erythropoiesis is only a minor component (Fig. 1.4) [11]. These differences are a result of different stimulatory and/or inhibitory

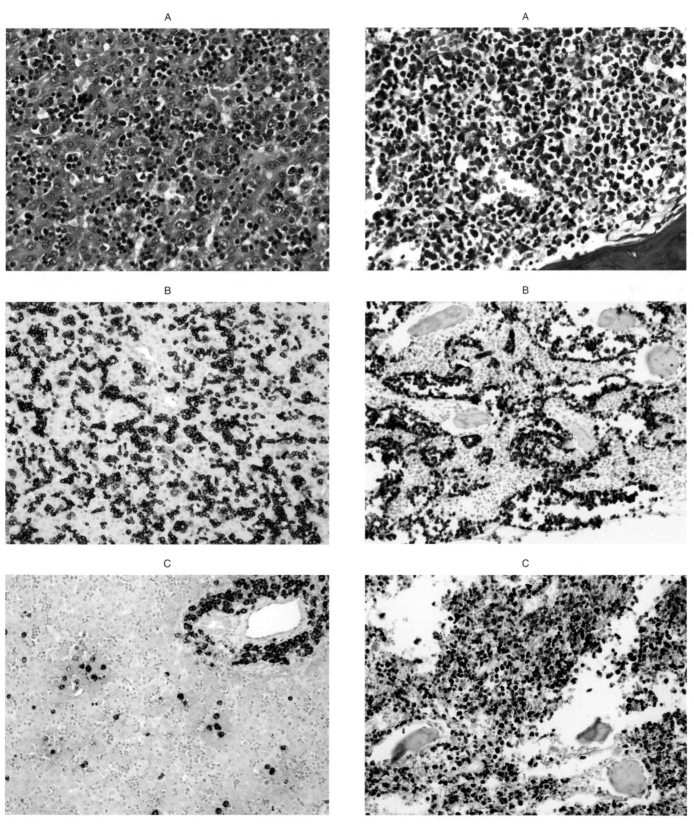

Fig. 1.3. Fetal liver, 21 weeks of gestation. (A) Numerous hematopoietic progenitors and hepatocytes [hematoxylin and eosin (H&E) stain]. (B) Predominance of glycophorin A-positive erythroid progenitors (immunoperoxidase stain). (C) Paucity of myeloid progenitors in the fetal liver parenchyma and higher number of myeloid precursors in the periportal spaces (immunoperoxidase stain, myeloperoxidase). (Courtesy of Dr. Linda Ernst.)

Fig. 1.4. Fetal bone marrow, 21 weeks of gestation. (A) Cellular bone marrow with numerous hematopoietic progenitors (H&E stain). (B) There is a paucity of erythroid progenitors; most of the positive cells are erythrocytes filling the dilated sinuses (immunoperoxidase stain for glycophorin A). (C) Predominance of myeloid progenitors in the fetal bone marrow (immunoperoxidase stain for myeloperoxidase). (Courtesy of Dr. Linda Ernst.)

signals from the microenvironment of the liver and BM that determine the fate of the HSC and their differentiation into erythroid or myeloid pathways. A quantitative analysis of the leukocyte content along with the percentage of CD34+ cells, lymphocytes, granulocytes, and monocytes in fetal liver, BM, and spleen, revealed a comparable absolute number of CD34+ cells in the liver and marrow throughout the second trimester of gestation but different proportions of maturing hematopoietic cells [12]. While the liver in the second trimester appears to be responsible for sustaining erythropoiesis, and to a lesser degree for the myelopoiesis and megakaryopoiesis, the BM is mainly involved in granulopoiesis and B-cell lymphogenesis. The *fetal spleen* in mid gestation, however, does not normally function as an active erythropoietic organ, and along with the thymus is involved in the B-cell and T-cell lineage development [12–14].

There are significant differences between the fetal hematopoietic stem cells and adult bone marrow progenitors. The fetal hematopoietic progenitors are notable for a rapid cycling rate resulting in constant expansion of the pool size, higher sensitivity to EPO, and a low sensitivity to granulocyte/monocyte colony stimulating factor (GM-CSF). As a result, during fetal development the hematopoietic cells mature mostly along the erythroid pathway. *In vitro* studies show that the fetal hematopoietic progenitors form threefold more burst-forming units – erythrocytes (BFU-Es) at mid trimester than at birth [15].

The EPO plays a central role and is the most important cytokine regulator of mammalian erythropoiesis. Targeted disruption of either EPO or its receptor leads to almost complete block of fetal liver erythropoiesis, resulting in fetal death. During mid and late gestation, EPO mRNA has been detected in the liver and to a lesser degree in the spleen, bone marrow, and kidney [16]. This is in contrast to adults where the kidney is the major site for EPO synthesis. The precise EPO signaling of prenatal erythropoiesis is still not completely understood. It is known that between 13 and 23 weeks of gestation the erythroid progenitors are more sensitive to growth factors: colony forming units – erythrocytes (CFU-Es), EPO, BFU-Es [17]. In adults, the EPO provides both a proliferative signal to early erythroid progenitors and a differentiation signal to late erythroid progenitors such as to prevent apoptosis of early progenitors.

Growth factors and cytokines, such as a granulocyte colony stimulating factor (G-CSF), interleukin (IL)-6, IL-1, IL-4, IL-9, and insulin growth factor-1, also regulate the rate of the proliferation and differentiation of the hematopoietic precursors [4, 18]. During the second trimester, the hematopoietic stem cells are less sensitive to GM-CSF and G-CSF. The total white blood cell (WBC) count is very low and gradually increases prior to birth. The monocytes are the first and the neutrophils are the last white blood cells to appear in the fetal blood. The neutrophil count is very low and gradually increases from the 20th to the 30th week of gestation. During the second and third trimester, the lymphocytes comprise the largest white blood cell population.

Composition of fetal blood

Blood samples obtained fetoscopically from live fetuses early in the second and third trimester of pregnancy have demonstrated the marked changes that occur in the composition of fetal blood during this stage of development [15, 19–21]. The results from two major studies, involving almost 3000 fetal blood samples, are presented in Table 1.2. They point out that, with the advance of gestation, the mean hemoglobin (Hb) progressively increases from 10.9 ± 0.7 g/dL at age 10 weeks to 16.6 ± 4 g/dL at age 39 weeks, while the MCV, mean corpuscular hemoglobin (MCH), and reticulocyte counts gradually decrease (Fig. 1.5). In addition to these quantitative characteristics, fetal erythrocytes have different membrane properties, unique metabolic profiles, and contain fetal hemoglobin (Hb F).

The *white blood cell count* is very low and gradually increases from 1.6 ± 0.7 at the 15th week of gestation to reach 6.40 ± 2.99 at the 30th week of gestation [15, 19]. Immunophenotyping of fetal blood in the second and third trimester by flow cytometry reveals that the lymphocytes are the major white blood cell population of the fetal blood and that their absolute numbers are similar to those in adults [20, 22, 23]. The majority of lymphocytes in fetal blood are naïve and express CD45RA, a marker of "virgin" cells. These fetal lymphocytes remain almost entirely unprimed prior to birth, and only a minority express CD45RO, a marker of primed lymphocytes [22].

Most of the fetal lymphocytes express T- or B-cell surface differentiation antigens. During the second and third trimester, the percentage and absolute number of T-cells is lower as compared to adults [20, 24] (Table 1.3). The CD4+ T-cell subset predominates and the proportion of CD8+ T-cells is low. In addition, $\gamma\delta$ T-cell and NK-cell counts are lower in fetal blood than in neonates and adults. In contrast, the proportion of B-cells in fetal blood is higher than in adults.

There are also functional differences between the fetal and postnatal lymphocytes. While fetal lymphocytes have been shown to proliferate spontaneously *in vitro*, they fail to respond to mitogen phytohemagglutinin (PHA) or allogeneic stimulations *in vitro*. Fetal mononuclear cells are unable to produce IL-2, IL-4, and IFN-γ (interferon gamma) *in vitro* but do secrete IL-10, IL-6, and TNF-α (tumor necrosis factor alpha) *in vitro* [24].

The first morphologically recognizable *platelets* appear in the fetal circulation at 8 to 9 weeks of gestation, and the number of platelets reaches adult levels before 18 weeks of gestation. Intrauterine thrombocytopenia can be reliably diagnosed through fetal blood sampling after 18 weeks of gestation.

Hematologic values in term neonates and infants

After birth, the marked improvement in tissue oxygenation results in a dramatic drop in EPO levels, leading to a significant decline in the red cell production by a factor of 2 to 3 during the first few days of life, and by a factor of about

Table 1.2. Hematologic values of normal fetuses between 15 and >30 weeks of gestation.

Weeks of gestation (Number of subjects)	RBC count (×10¹²/L)	Hb (g/dL)	Hct (%)	MCV (fL)	WBC and NRBC[a] count (×10⁹/L)	WBC corrected[b] count (×10⁹/L)	PLT count (×10⁹/L)
Data from Millar DS, Davis LR, Rodeck CH, *et al.* Normal blood cell values in the early mid-trimester fetus. *Prenatal Diagnosis.* 1985;5:367–373							
15 (N = 6)	2.43 ±0.26	10.9 ±0.7	34.6 ±3.6	143 ±8	–	1.6 ±0.7	190 ±31
16 (N = 5)	2.68 ±0.21	12.5 ±0.8	38.1 ±2.1	143 ±12	–	2.4 ±1.7	208 ±57
17 (N = 16)	2.74 ±0.23	12.4 ±0.9	37.4 ±2.8	137 ±8	–	2.0 ±0.8	202 ±25
18 (N = 18)	2.77 ±0.33	12.4 ±1.2	37.3 ±4.2	135 ±9	–	2.4 ±0.9	192 ±45
19 (N = 29)	2.92 ±0.27	12.3 ±1.2	37.5 ±3.1	129 ±6	–	2.5 ±0.8	211 ±48
20 (N = 12)	3.12 ±0.36	13.0 ±1.1	39.3 ±4.1	126 ±6	–	2.6 ±1.2	170 ±60
21 (N = 13)	3.07 ±0.42	12.30 ±0.8	37.3 ±3.5	123 ±8	–	2.7 ±0.7	223 ±61
Data from Forestier F, Daffos F, Catherine N, *et al.* Developmental hematopoiesis in normal human fetal blood. *Blood.* 1991;77:2360–2363							
18–21 (N = 760)	2.8 ±0.42	11.69 ±1.27	37.3 ±4.32	131.1 ±10.97	4.68 ±2.96	2.57 ±0.42	234 ±57
22–25 (N = 1 200)	3.09 ±0.34	12.20 ±1.60	38.59 ±3.94	125.1 ±7.84	4.72 ±2.82	3.73 ±2.17	247 ±59
26–29 (N = 460)	3.46 ±0.41	12.91 ±1.38	40.88 ±4.40	118.5 ±7.96	5.16 ±2.53	4.08 ±0.84	242 ±69
>30 (N = 440)	3.82 ±0.64	13.64 ±2.21	43.55 ±7.20	114.4 ±9.34	7.71 ±4.99	6.40 ±2.99	232 ±87

[a] Total nucleated blood cell count includes WBCs and nucleated red blood cells.
[b] WBC count after correction for the nucleated red blood cells.
Values are given as mean ± standard deviation (SD). The blood samples were analyzed with *Coulter "S" Plus* and *Coulter "S" Plus II* (Coulter, Hialeah, FL) instruments. Abbreviations: RBC, red blood cell; Hb, hemoglobin; Hct, hematocrit; MCV, mean corpuscular volume; WBC, white blood cell; NRBC, nucleated red blood cell; PLT, platelet.

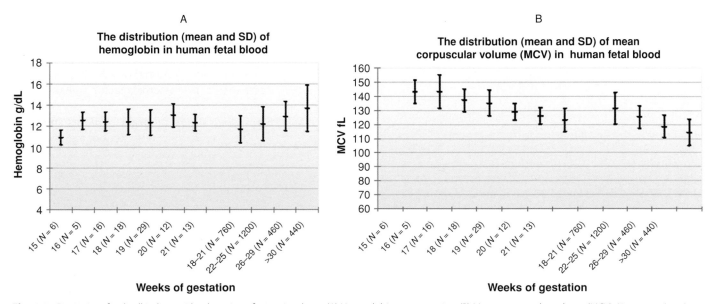

Fig. 1.5. Dynamics of red cell indices with advancing of gestational age. (A) Hemoglobin concentration. (B) Mean corpuscular volume (MCV). (Data reanalyzed from Millar *et al.* [19] and Forestier *et al.* [15].)

Table 1.3. Lymphocyte subsets in fetal blood as compared to full-term neonates and adults.

	Week 16–20 fetus (N = 10)	Week 20–27 fetus (N = 7)	Full-term neonate (N = 15)	Adult (N = 10)
Absolute lymphocyte count[a] ($\times 10^9$/L)	1.9 ± 0.7	2.6 ± 0.7	5.6 ± 1.0	2.1 ± 0.7
CD3+ [b] T-lymphocytes	68.2 ± 10.3	71.1 ± 8.7	73.2 ± 6.4	76.9 ± 5.6
CD4+ T-lymphocytes	47.7 ± 6.0	50.2 ± 7.2	51.3 ± 4.8	46.1 ± 4.2
CD8+ T-lymphocytes	18.2 ± 6.9	23.1 ± 7.6	24.3 ± 4.5	27.8 ± 4.8
CD4 : CD8 ratio	2.95 ± 1.1	2.41 ± 0.9	2.17 ± 0.5	1.65 ± 0.35
CD19+ B-lymphocytes	15.6 ± 8.7	22 ± 8.1	163 ± 7.9	9.4 ± 5.5
Leu7+ NK-cells	0.3 ± 0.6	1.4 ± 2.2	0.6 ± 0.7	6.4 ± 4.2

[a] Blood samples were obtained by ultrasound-guided aspiration from the umbilical vein at the placental cord insertion.
[b] The lymphocyte subsets were determined by immunogold-silver staining with OKT3 (CD3), OKT4 (CD4), OKT8 (CD8), Leu12 (CD19), and Leu7 (an NK-cell marker) antibodies.
Data from De Waele et al. [20].

Table 1.4. Postnatal changes in some red cell parameters of capillary blood in the first 12 weeks of life in healthy full-term infants according to Matoth et al. [25].

Age	No. of cases	RBC count ($\times 10^{12}$/L)	Hb (g/dL)	Hct (%)	MCV (fL)	MCHC (%)	Retic count (%)
Days							
1	19	5.14 ± 0.7	19.3 ± 2.2	61 ± 7.4	119 ± 9.4	31.6 ± 1.9	3.2 ± 1.4
2	19	5.15 ± 0.8	19.0 ± 1.9	60 ± 6.4	115 ± 7.0	31.6 ± 1.4	3.2 ± 1.3
3	19	5.11 ± 0.7	18.8 ± 2.0	62 ± 9.3	116 ± 5.3	31.1 ± 2.8	2.8 ± 1.7
4	10	5.00 ± 0.6	18.6 ± 2.1	57 ± 8.1	114 ± 7.5	32.6 ± 1.5	1.8 ± 1.1
5	12	4.97 ± 0.4	17.6 ± 1.1	57 ± 7.3	114 ± 8.9	30.9 ± 2.2	1.2 ± 0.2
6	15	5.00 ± 0.7	17.4 ± 2.2	54 ± 7.2	113 ± 10.0	32.2 ± 1.6	0.6 ± 0.2
7	12	4.86 ± 0.6	17.9 ± 2.5	56 ± 9.4	118 ± 11.2	32.0 ± 1.6	0.5 ± 0.4
Weeks							
1–2	32	4.80 ± 0.8	17.3 ± 2.3	54 ± 8.3	112 ± 19.0	32.1 ± 2.9	0.5 ± 0.3
2–3	11	4.20 ± 0.6	15.6 ± 2.6	54 ± 8.3	111 ± 8.2	33.9 ± 1.9	0.8 ± 0.6
3–4	17	4.00 ± 0.6	14.2 ± 2.1	43 ± 5.7	105 ± 7.5	33.5 ± 1.6	0.6 ± 0.3
4–5	15	3.60 ± 0.4	12.7 ± 1.6	36 ± 4.8	101 ± 8.1	34.9 ± 1.6	0.9 ± 0.8
5–6	10	3.55 ± 0.2	11.9 ± 1.5	36 ± 6.2	102 ± 10.2	34.1 ± 2.9	1.0 ± 0.7
6–7	10	3.40 ± 0.4	12.0 ± 1.5	36 ± 4.8	105 ± 12.0	33.8 ± 2.3	1.2 ± 0.7
7–8	17	3.40 ± 0.4	11.1 ± 1.1	33 ± 3.7	100 ± 13.0	33.7 ± 2.6	1.5 ± 0.7
8–9	13	3.40 ± 0.5	10.7 ± 0.9	31 ± 2.5	93 ± 12.0	34.1 ± 2.2	1.8 ± 1.0
9–10	12	3.60 ± 0.3	11.2 ± 0.9	32 ± 2.7	91 ± 9.3	34.3 ± 2.9	1.2 ± 0.6
10–11	11	3.70 ± 0.4	11.4 ± 0.9	34 ± 2.1	91 ± 7.7	33.2 ± 2.4	1.2 ± 0.7
11–12	13	3.70 ± 0.3	11.3 ± 0.9	33 ± 3.3	88 ± 7.9	34.8 ± 2.2	0.7 ± 0.3

Abbreviations: RBC, red blood cell; Hb, hemoglobin; Hct, hematocrit; MCV, mean corpuscular volume; MCHC, mean corpuscular hemoglobin concentration; Retic, reticulocyte.

10 during the first week of life [17]. This results in dramatic changes in the blood composition after birth. The blood of newborns and neonates has been subject to detailed studies for several decades [25–28]. At birth, there is polycythemia and macrocytosis followed by a gradual decrease in the red blood cell (RBC) count, Hb concentration, and the MCV in the first several months of life (Table 1.4). The mean RBC count drops steadily, reaching its lowest point in the 7th week, but the hemoglobin concentration lags and reaches its lowest level during the 9th week. This delay in the drop of hemoglobin is explained by the relatively high MCV that gradually decreases and reaches adult levels by the 11th week. While the RBC counts, Hb, and MCV levels are higher in newborns, the mean corpuscular hemoglobin concentration (MCHC) is relatively

low by adult standards. The MCHC increases significantly in the first five to six weeks and remains constant thereafter. Thus, while the neonatal erythrocytes are bigger and contain more hemoglobin relative to their increased size, the hemoglobin within the cells is neither more nor less concentrated than for adults. The red cell distribution width (RDW) in newborns and neonates is increased as compared to adults and reflects a significant variability in the size of the neonatal red cells. The reticulocyte count is relatively high immediately after birth and through the first several days, indicating the persistence of considerable erythropoietic activity. After the initial drop at the end of the first week, the reticulocyte count thereafter remains low: in the 0.5–1% range. It slowly increases and reaches its peak during the ninth week.

There is considerable morphologic heterogeneity in the erythrocytes of the newborn. Newborns have a higher number of irregularly shaped erythrocytes as compared to adults. Using scanning electron microscopy, Zipursky et al. found a markedly increased number of stomatocytes (bowl-shaped red blood cells) as compared to adults' erythrocytes (40% vs. 18%) [29]. In neonates, the number of normal, disc-shaped red cells (discocytes) was significantly lower than in adults (43% vs. 78%). Interference-contrast microscopy reveals a significantly higher number of erythrocytes with pits or craters in term neonates as compared to adults (24.3% vs. 2.6%) [30]. In this study, the mean pit count reached near-adult levels at two months of age. The significance of pitted erythrocytes is still unknown; it is suspected that the pits are cytoplasmic vacuoles and represent hypofunction of the spleen and/or other reticuloendothelial cell-rich sites in trapping and eliminating pitted erythrocytes from the circulation. Pits like this have been observed with such high frequency, so far, only in asplenic patients.

Nucleated red blood cells (NRBCs) are present in the blood of healthy newborns in the first day of life. Finding 0–10 NRBCs/100 WBCs is typical, although these values are highly dependent on the total WBC count. In a term neonate, NRBCs are rapidly cleared from the circulation after birth, and in a healthy neonate virtually no NRBCs are found after the third or fourth day of life, although they may persist in small numbers up to one week in preterm newborns [31].

In full-term neonates, 50–80% of the hemoglobin is Hb F and 15–50% is Hb A. After birth, the majority of the newly produced red blood cells contain Hb A, which has a lower affinity for oxygen as compared to Hb F. As a consequence, there is an improvement in tissue oxygenation after birth, along with a resultant decline of EPO production. After birth, the EPO synthesis shifts from the liver and bone marrow to the kidney [17].

Newborns have a high WBC count and a high percentage of neutrophils at birth. Two major studies performed almost 40 years apart demonstrate that the total WBC and neutrophil counts are dynamic and change in the first five days of life [27, 28]. The high neutrophil count at birth continues to rise in the first 8–12 hours, when it reaches a peak and then gradually decreases to its nadir observed around 72 hours after birth. After that time, the neutrophil count gradually increases again

to reach a stable level by day five, and remains unchanged to the end of the neonatal period.

The cause of the leukocytosis and neutrophilia at birth and shortly thereafter is still not entirely understood. Most likely, the increased neutrophil count is a result of bone marrow mobilization of the preexisting neutrophil pool due to stress during labor, and less likely it is due to an increase in white blood cell production [17]. Multiple factors play a role. Epinephrine stimulation of the neutrophil demargination may be one such factor. However, the level of epinephrine and its relatively short action cannot explain the slow return to normal, taking several days, which suggests other mechanisms. Perinatal factors, such as the mode of delivery, maternal hypertension, maternal fever prior to delivery, hemolytic disease, and hemorrhage, have also been suggested [28]. In a recent study, gender was found to be a statistically significant factor in blood neutrophil concentration, with females averaging concentrations 2.0×10^9/L higher than males [27].

At birth, along with the neutrophilia, there is a granulocytic shift to immaturity with an increased number of metamyelocytes, myelocytes, and even circulating blasts [32]. In the early neonatal period, rare circulating micromegakaryocytes may also be present, and such a finding should not be considered pathologic.

While at birth the lymphocytes comprise a smaller population relative to the granulocytes, they become the major white blood cell population shortly after birth. The absolute number of CD19+ B-cells increases twofold after birth, remains stable until two years of age, and then subsequently gradually decreases sixfold from two years to adult age [33]. CD3+ T-cells increase 1.5-fold immediately after birth and decrease threefold from two years to adult age. The absolute CD3+/CD4+ pattern follows the T-cells. CD3+/CD8+ cells remain stable until two years of age and then decrease three- to fourfold until adulthood. NK-cells decrease two- to threefold after birth and remain stable thereafter (Table 1.5).

A detailed longitudinal analysis of the changes in lymphocyte subpopulations in 11 healthy infants followed from birth to one year of age defines these trends more specifically, though the sample is a small one [34]. It shows that the total lymphocyte count and T-lymphocytes increase at one week of age, the B-lymphocytes increase at six weeks of age, and the number of natural killer (NK) cells is highest at birth and sharply declines thereafter. In addition, it shows that most of the T-cells express T-cell receptor (TCR) $\alpha\beta$, and most of the T-lymphocytes are CD45RA+ naïve T-cells. In contrast to adults, the relative frequency of CD45RO+ memory T-cells is lower in infants. The CD4+ helper T-cells follow the pattern of total T-lymphocyte count with an increase at one week of age. The CD4 : CD8 ratio during the first year of life is higher than in adults.

With respect to the normal B-cell progenitors, also known as hematogones, hardly any such early B-cells are present in the blood of infants and adults. Moreover, there is no indication that in infants these cells leave the bone marrow at an earlier stage

Table 1.5. Absolute lymphocyte subpopulation count in peripheral blood of children compared to adults.

	Neonates (N = 20)	1 week–2 months (N = 13)	2–5 months (N = 46)	5–9 months (N = 105)	9–15 months (N = 70)	15–24 months (N = 33)	2–5 years (N = 33)	5–10 years (N = 35)	10–16 years (N = 23)	Adults (N = 51)
Total lymphocytes[a]	4.8 (0.7–7.3)	6.7 (3.5–13.1)	5.9 (3.7–9.6)	6.0 (3.8–9.6)	5.5 (2.6–10.4)	5.6 (2.7–11.9)	3.3 (1.7–6.9)	2.8 (1.1–6.9)	2.2 (1.0–5.3)	1.8 (1.0–2.8)
CD19+ B-cells	0.6 (0.04–1.1)	1.0 (0.6–1.9)	1.3 (0.6–3.0)	1.3 (0.7–2.5)	1.4 (0.6–2.7)	1.3 (0.6–3.1)	0.8 (0.2–2.1)	0.5 (0.2–1.6)	0.3 (0.2–0.6)	0.2 (0.1–0.5)
CD3+ T-cells	2.8 (0.6–5.0)	4.6 (2.3–7.0)	3.6 (2.3–6.5)	3.8 (2.4–6.9)	3.4 (1.6–6.7)	3.5 (1.4–8.0)	2.3 (0.9–4.5)	1.9 (0.7–4.2)	1.5 (0.8–3.5)	1.2 (0.7–2.1)
CD3+/CD4+ T-cells	1.9 (0.4–3.5)	3.5 (1.7–5.3)	2.5 (1.5–5.0)	2.8 (1.4–5.1)	2.3 (1.0–4.6)	2.2 (0.9–5.5)	1.3 (0.5–2.4)	1.0 (0.3–2.0)	0.8 (0.4–2.1)	0.7 (0.3–1.4)
CD3+/CD8+ T-cells	1.1 (0.2–1.9)	1.0 (0.4–1.7)	1.0 (0.5–1.6)	1.1 (0.6–2.2)	1.1 (0.4–2.1)	1.2 (0.4–2.3)	0.8 (0.3–1.6)	0.8 (0.3–1.8)	0.4 (0.2–1.2)	0.4 (0.2–0.9)
CD3+/HLA-DR+ T-cells	0.09 (0.03–0.4)	0.3 (0.03–3.4)	0.2 (0.07–0.5)	0.2 (0.07–0.5)	0.2 (0.1–0.6)	0.3 (0.1–0.7)	0.2 (0.08–0.4)	0.2 (0.05–0.7)	0.06 (0.02–0.2)	0.09 (0.03–0.2)
CD3− (CD16,56)+ NK-cells	1.0 (0.1–1.9)	0.5 (0.2–1.4)	0.3 (0.1–1.3)	0.3 (0.1–1.0)	0.4 (0.2–1.2)	0.4 (0.1–1.4)	0.4 (0.1–1.0)	0.3 (0.09–0.9)	0.3 (0.07–1.2)	1.9 (1.0–3.6)

[a] Absolute lymphocyte counts ($\times 10^9$/L).
Values are given as median values of lymphocyte subsets and the 5th to 95th percentile range.
Data from Comans-Bitter et al. [33].

Table 1.6. Percentage of double-positive lymphocyte subsets in the peripheral blood of healthy newborns and adults.

Lymphocyte subsets	1–3-day-old newborns (N = 42)	Adults (N = 38)
CD10/CD19	1.5 (1.0–4.0)[a]	0
CD20/CD5	13.0 (5.0–18.0)[a]	6.0 (2.0–9.7)
CD3/HLA-DR	2.0 (1.0–3.0)[a]	6.0 (3.0–13.0)
CD3/CD25	7.0 (5.9–8.0)[a]	10.0 (8.6–22.2)
CD8/HLA-DR	2.0 (0–3.0)[a]	5.0 (2.0–11.7)
CD8/CD57	0 (0–1.0)[a]	8.0 (4.0–12.0)
CD8/CD28	19.0 (13.2–27.0)	19.0 (15.0–23.7)
CD8/CD38	21.0 (16.7–29.0)	19.0 (11.3–25.7)

[a] Statistically significant differences between newborns and adults measured by the Mann–Whitney U test.
Values are presented as median and range (10th to 90th percentiles).
Data from O'Gorman et al. [36].

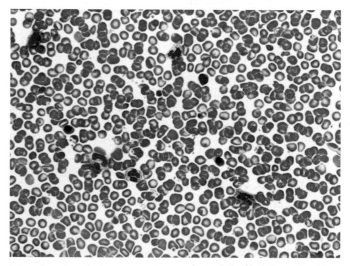

Fig. 1.6. Peripheral blood smear from a term newborn shows relative polycythemia, macrocytosis, moderate anisopoikilocytosis, marked polychromasia with rare nucleated red blood cells, high white blood cell count with relative neutrophilia, and adequate platelet count (Wright stain).

of their development, either [35]. Throughout the first year, the number of B-lymphocytes is high and the relative frequency of CD5+ B-lymphocytes is higher in infants than in older children and adults. The percentage of double-positive lymphocyte subsets in the peripheral blood of healthy newborns and adults is shown in Table 1.6 [36].

Of the three major components of the blood, platelets are the only ones that have completed their development prior to birth. As a result, their count and morphology at birth are similar to the platelets in adults [37].

Examination of a peripheral blood smear of a normal term newborn shows polycythemia, leukocytosis with a shift to immaturity, and an adequate platelet count, as shown in Figure 1.6. Due to the polycythemia, the red cell morphology may be difficult to appreciate since the blood films of newborns may have a short feather-edge as compared to blood films of older children and adults.

Hematologic values in small-for-gestational-age (SGA) term newborns

Babies with birth weight below the 10th percentile are considered small for gestational age (SGA), and their hematologic parameters at birth differ from full-term, appropriate-for-gestational-age (AGA) newborns. Several studies show higher hemoglobin, hematocrit, and RBC and NRBC counts at day one

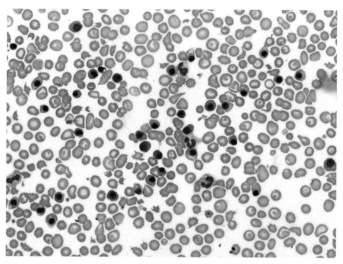

Fig. 1.7. Peripheral blood smear from a neonate born at 25 weeks of gestation. Note the marked anisopoikilocytosis of the red cells, polychromasia, and numerous nucleated red blood cells that obscure the white blood cells. The platelet count is mildly decreased (Wright stain).

in the SGA neonates when compared to AGA [37, 38]. The SGA newborns have lower WBC count and a more pronounced shift to immaturity manifested by a higher number of metamyelocytes as compared to the AGA term newborns. While platelet counts are below 150×10^9/L in 34.4% of the SGA group as compared to only 4.4% in the AGA term group, they return to normal by the end of the first week of life [38]. Small babies, presumably due to intrauterine hypoxia, have higher erythropoietin levels as compared to babies with appropriate birth weight. This results in relative polycythemia and elevated RBC indices in SGA as compared to AGA newborns.

Hematologic values in preterm neonates

The normal developmental sequences of hematopoiesis are disrupted by a premature birth and, as a result, the preterm newborns have hematologic parameters that are appropriate for their gestational age rather than for their postnatal age. Multiple studies over the years show that premature babies have a lower RBC count, Hb, and hematocrit (Hct) levels, higher MCV, and a high number of nucleated red blood cells as compared to term newborns (Fig. 1.7) [17, 21, 26, 39–41]. While all studies found this to be true, there is a great variability and considerable inconsistency between the reported values. For example, the Hct of infants born at 29 to 31 weeks of gestation ranged from 43.5% as reported by Forestier *et al.* to 60% as reported by Zaizov *et al.* [21, 40]. While these differences are due in part to the degree of immaturity and the developmental factors affecting the fetal hematopoiesis, they may also be affected by preanalytical factors such as the blood sampling site, limited blood availability, delay in the umbilical cord clamping, and time of sampling after birth, along with others. Such factors are not standardized between different studies, which makes the comparison of their conclusions difficult. We return to the subject of preanalytical factors further below.

The maturation of the hematopoietic system follows its natural course and does not accelerate due to birth. For this reason, the hematologic differences will continue during the neonatal period and early infancy as more pronounced anemia of prematurity develops, because factors contributing to such anemia include the shorter red blood cell lifespan, rapid body growth resulting in hemodilution, poor iron stores, and an initial reliance on the liver as the primary site of erythropoietin production [42]. As a result, the Hb concentration in premature infants continues to decline after birth for a longer period of time (8–12 weeks) and exhibits a lower nadir as compared to the physiologic anemia of term newborns [17].

Premature neonates also have significantly lower absolute neutrophil counts as compared to larger full-term neonates, due to the effects of development on neutrophil dynamics [39, 43]. Mouzinho and colleagues [39] studied the absolute neutrophil counts in healthy very-low-birth-weight neonates, and found boundaries starting at 0.5×10^9/L and rising to 2.2×10^9/L at 18 to 20 hours after birth, and 1.1×10^9/L to 6.0×10^9/L between 61 hours and 28 days, respectively. These low boundaries of normal absolute neutrophil counts are significantly beneath the low boundaries of larger, term newborns. Thus, if the gestational age is not taken into account, a significant proportion of premature newborns might be considered neutropenic.

There are only a few studies of the lymphocyte profiles of preterm infants. In a comparison of the lymphocyte subsets of 28 preterm infants (<32 weeks of gestation) with 39 term infants, Berrington and colleagues found significant differences in the lymphocyte profiles of the preterm infants [44]. Premature babies had lower counts for absolute lymphocytes, B-cells, T-cells, and T-helper cells, and they had a lower CD4/CD8 ratio as compared to term babies. The T-cell subset shows, in addition, a larger proportion of T-cells that express CD25, an activation marker, and a smaller proportion of all T-cells that express the naïve (CD45RA) phenotype. These differences may represent the ongoing development of the immune repertoire, or stress attendant upon exhaustion of the neonatal pool of lymphocytes that is associated with premature birth. Differences such as this merit further studies with regard to the increased risk of infection in premature babies.

Hematologic values during early childhood and in older children

During early childhood, the hemoglobin concentration and MCV are lower and the total white blood cell count is higher as compared to older children and adults [45]. Furthermore, early in life, the lymphocytic component is higher than the proportion of neutrophils. During that time, the immune system encounters many antigens and induces massive proliferation, activation, and maturation until sufficient levels of specific immune surveillance and memory cells are reached. The results of a large-scale cross-sectional study of lymphocyte subsets in healthy children of various ethnic backgrounds aged from birth through 18 years are shown in Table 1.7 [46]. Children

Table 1.7. Absolute counts of peripheral blood lymphocyte subsets in healthy children; distribution by age.

Subset	N	0–3 months	3–6 months	6–12 months	1–2 years	2–6 years	6–12 years	12–18 years
Total WBC	800	10.6 (7.2–18.0)	9.2 (6.7–14.0)	9.1 (6.4–13.0)	8.8 (6.4–12.0)	7.1 (5.2–11.0)	6.5 (4.4–9.5)	6.0 (4.4–8.1)
Lymphocytes	800	5.4 (3.4–7.6)	6.3 (3.9–9.0)	5.9 (3.4–9.0)	5.5 (3.6–8.9)	3.6 (2.3–5.4)	2.7 (1.9–3.7)	2.2 (1.4–3.3)
CD3 (Total T-cells)	699	3.7 (2.5–5.5)	3.9 (2.5–5.6)	3.9 (1.9–5.9)	3.5 (2.1–6.2)	2.4 (1.4–3.7)	1.8 (1.2–2.6)	1.5 (1.0–2.2)
CD19 (Total B-cells)	699	0.73 (0.30–4.00)	1.55 (0.43–3.00)	1.52 (0.61–2.60)	1.31 (0.72–2.60)	0.75 (0.39–2.60)	0.48 (0.27–0.86)	0.30 (0.11–0.57)
CD16/CD56 (NK-cells)	770	0.42 (0.17–1.10)	0.42 (0.17–0.83)	0.40 (0.16–0.83)	0.36 (0.18–0.92)	0.30 (0.13–0.72)	0.23 (0.10–0.48)	0.19 (0.07–0.48)
CD4 (Helper T-cells)	699	2.61 (1.6–4.0)	2.85 (1.8–4.0)	2.67 (1.4–4.3)	2.16 (1.3–3.4)	1.38 (0.7–2.2)	0.98 (0.7–1.5)	0.84 (0.5–1.3)
CD8 (Cytotoxic T-cells)	699	0.98 (0.56–1.70)	1.05 (0.59–1.60)	1.04 (0.50–1.70)	1.04 (0.62–2.00)	0.84 (0.49–1.30)	0.68 (0.37–1.10)	0.53 (0.33–0.92)

Subset counts presented as number of cells $\times 10^9$/L.
Values are presented as median and range (10th to 90th percentiles).
Data from Shearer et al. [46].

experience a gradual decrease in the percentage of CD4+ T-cells and increase in the percentages of CD8+ T-lymphocytes and B-lymphocytes. The CD8+ T-cell levels are low early in life and increase to reach a maximum at 12–18 years of age. The number of naïve helper T-cells (CD4CD45RACD62L) gradually decreases and the number of antigen-committed memory T-cells (CD3CD4CD45RO) increases at 12–18 years. The CD19+ B-cells reach a plateau from 3 months to 2 years of life, before returning to lower levels at 12–18 years. In this study, the most significant variables affecting the lymphocyte populations were age and the laboratory variations, while the sex and race of the individuals produce only infrequent differences.

Preanalytical issues related to pediatric blood samples

Preanalytical factors are well known to affect test results, but some of these considerations are special to children. With respect to young children, the most important factors include limited blood availability, location of the blood sampling site, and the effect of exertion and violent crying [47]. A more extensive review of these and other issues important in the neonatal cellular analysis can be found elsewhere [48].

Limited blood availability

As a general rule, blood drawn for laboratory testing should not exceed 5% of the total blood volume per draw [49]. However, the amount of blood needed for testing in newborns and neonates, in whom the total blood volume ranges from 80 to 115 mL/kg, may comprise a substantial proportion of a child's blood and exceed 5%. This is particularly true for low-birth-weight term and preterm neonates, where the amount of blood required for a laboratory testing may approach 10% (Fig. 1.8). As a result,

drawing blood from small babies, even for routine testing, may cause iatrogenic anemia.

To account for the limited blood availability and diminish the risk of excessive blood drawing in young children, several microtainer tubes are currently available on the market (Fig. 1.9). These microtainer tubes, while solving some of the problems, pose their own challenges, such as the quality not being sufficient (QNS) for testing; hemolysis; or frequent clotting if the blood is not properly mixed with the anticoagulant. In our hematology laboratories, as high as 3–5% of the microtainer tubes are QNS, thus requiring an additional blood draw with all the consequences. Furthermore, the presence of an excess of anticoagulant (ethylenediaminetetraacetic acid, EDTA), due to insufficient filling of the microtainer with blood, may result in the formation of WBC or platelet aggregates or fibrin precipitates, which can lead to a spurious reduction in the WBC and/or platelet counts. This can be further complicated by the fact that abnormal test results in such children may not be able to be confirmed by a repeat testing due to the limited blood available for sampling.

Effect of blood sampling site on the hematology test results

In young children, blood is frequently obtained from multiple sources – venous, arterial, and/or capillary. However, the blood obtained from these sources, and particularly capillary blood, has different composition and cannot be considered equivalent. For example, blood obtained from skin puncture contains a mixture of undetermined proportion of blood from arterioles, venules, and interstitial and intracellular fluids, and its composition is different from venous and arterial blood. Warming the baby's heel to improve arterial circulation does not

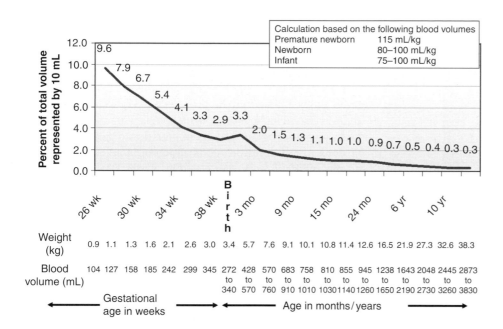

Calculation based on the following blood volumes	
Premature newborn	115 mL/kg
Newborn	80–100 mL/kg
Infant	75–100 mL/kg

Fig. 1.8. Relationship of 10 mL blood sample volume to total blood volume, body weight, and age of infants and children. (Redrawn from Werner [50]. With permission.)

	26 wk	30 wk	34 wk	38 wk	Birth	3 mo		9 mo	15 mo	24 mo		6 yr	10 yr	
Weight (kg)	0.9 1.1 1.3	1.6	2.1 2.6 3.0	3.4	5.7 7.6 9.1	10.1 10.8	11.4 12.6	16.5	21.9 27.3	32.6 38.3				
Blood volume (mL)	104 127 158	185	242 299 345	272 to 340	428 to 570	570 to 760	683 to 910	758 to 1010	810 to 1030	855 to 1140	945 to 1260	1238 to 1650	1643 to 2190	2048 to 2730	2445 to 3260	2873 to 3830

Gestational age in weeks ← → Age in months/years →

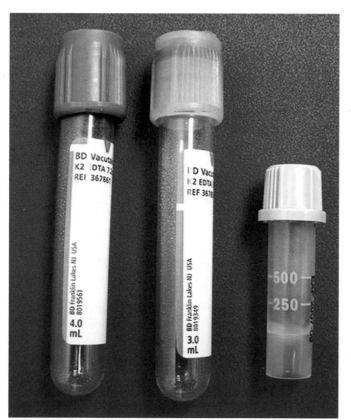

Fig. 1.9. Blood collection tubes.

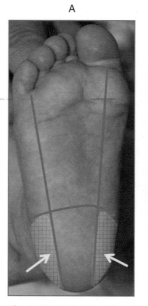

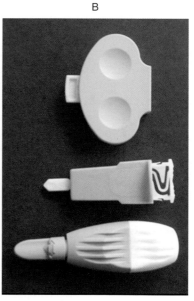

Fig. 1.10. (A) In infants less than one year of age, heal puncture to the lateral or medial plantar surface of the heel is usually performed. The skin puncture must be no deeper than 2.0 mm and should be applied in the shaded areas indicated by arrows. (Photograph contributed by Dr. Laurie S. Glezer.) (B) Automated devices for obtaining capillary blood.

diminish these differences [51]. The differences between arterial and venous blood are less pronounced.

In children, capillary blood is a preferred source and, in neonates and infants, the heel is the most preferred site (Fig. 1.10). Sufficient blood for laboratory testing can be collected by applying a standard incision with a safe depth of penetration on the heel [49]. Capillary blood, however, shows consis-

tently higher Hb, Hct, RBC count, and lower MCV as compared to blood obtained from other sources [52–54]. Hemoconcentration of the capillary blood, decreased perfusion, metabolic state, and other factors affecting the microcirculation might be contributing to these differences and result in higher capillary hematocrit than venous hematocrit [54].

The sampling site affects the leukocyte count as well. Simultaneous sampling of arterial, venous, and capillary blood of neonates shows significant differences in the WBC and differential counts [53] (Fig. 1.11). The magnitude of these differences appears to be unrelated to the time elapsed since

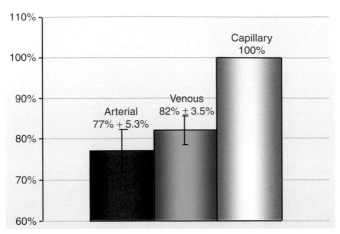

Fig. 1.11. Effect of sampling site on the white blood cell (WBC) count – a comparison of the WBC counts obtained simultaneously from capillary, venous, and arterial blood. (Data reanalyzed from from Christensen *et al.* [53].)

delivery and other clinical conditions, and is mostly due to the sampling site.

In premature babies, the differences in hemoglobin and neutrophil counts of capillary blood as compared to arterial blood are even more pronounced. For instance, Thurlbeck *et al.* found that every capillary hemoglobin value in premature babies was higher than its corresponding arterial value, with a mean difference of 2.3 g/dL (range 0.6–4.9 g/dL). Similarly, the capillary WBC count was significantly higher than the arterial sample by an average of 1.8×10^9/L (range 0.4–5.9 $\times 10^9$/L) [55]. The differences between the hematologic values obtained from capillary as opposed to either venous or arterial blood in premature babies are clinically relevant. Thus, if a clinical decision is made on the basis of results from specimens obtained from different sources, or without knowledge of the source, there is a risk of unnecessary interventions such as blood transfusion, or of extensive workups for infection.

The effect of sampling site on the platelet count is unclear. Some studies have found no differences in platelet counts whether drawn from arterial line, venipuncture, or heel stick [37, 55]. However, others found significantly lower platelet counts obtained from skin puncture as compared to the corresponding venous values [52]. The lower platelet count in this latter study might be due to the increased platelet activation, aggregation, and local consumption resulting from the heel puncture and applied pressure. Such a finding is supported by the fact that capillary platelets have a higher mean platelet volume (MPV) relative to venous platelets. It is known that activated platelets have higher MPV than resting platelets.

Effect of exertion and violent crying on the white blood cell count

Exertion causes significant leukocytosis and neutrophilia, with or without a shift to immaturity, as a result of the mobilization of leukocytes from the marginal to the circulating granulocyte pool [56]. In babies, similar changes in the leukocyte

count are seen after violent crying or a physical therapy to the chest. Christensen and colleagues compared the total leukocyte counts of blood samples obtained pre- and post-circumcision and physical therapy, and found an increase in the total leukocyte count of up to 146% ± 6% and the neutrophil count of up to 148% ± 7% after the procedures [53]. While both procedures caused leukocytosis, neutrophilia with a shift to immaturity was observed only after circumcision. This indicates that noxious stimuli result in mobilization of bone marrow stores, whereas milder exercise generated by physical therapy seems to cause only demargination of an already existing granulocytic pool. Exercise-induced leukocytosis, if not recognized as such, may lead to misunderstanding of the actual clinical condition during the neonatal period.

Other preanalytical factors affecting hematologic test results in neonates

The time of *umbilical cord clamping* also affects the hemoglobin levels in neonates. Meta-analysis of 15 controlled trials demonstrates that delayed clamping for two minutes or more after birth is beneficial to the Hb levels of the newborn, although it may cause asymptomatic polycythemia [57]. This beneficial effect extends into early infancy, with the result that children whose umbilical cord clamping was delayed develop less severe physiologic anemia [58]. The *mode of delivery* affects the WBC count as well. Babies born though vaginal delivery have higher WBC and band counts when compared to babies delivered by cesarean section [59]. Factors related to a patient's ethnicity are well known to affect the hematologic parameters, as well. New studies show that low white blood cell and neutrophil counts are, in part, *genetically determined* [60, 61]. *High altitude* has also been shown to increase the neutrophil counts of newborns [62].

Analytical issues related to pediatric blood samples

Pediatric samples are routinely analyzed on various hematology platforms. Despite the difference in methodology, however, there is so far no clearly superior instrument in terms of utility in children. Many of the fetal and neonatal blood counts data in the literature are obtained using various instruments. They include Coulter instruments: Coulter S, Coulter STKS, or Beckman Coulter LH750 [15, 19, 26–28, 53, 63], and to a lesser degree Sysmex (TM NE 8000 and SE-9500) [39, 64] or Abbott (Cell-Dyn 3700) [38] instruments. Yet, most of the above-mentioned publications are focused on the biological variables and lack discussion of the strengths and limitations of the instrumentation when used in evaluation of neonatal blood samples.

In the neonatal period, the most important interferences occur due to the resistance of neonatal red blood cells to lysis, the presence of a high number of nucleated red blood cells, hyperbilirubinemia, and in neonates on total parenteral nutrition, the presence of lipidemia. The resistance of neonatal RBCs to lysis and the presence of NRBCs can result in a spurious increase of the white blood cell count. Some hematology analyzers (Abbott Cell-Dyn 4000) generate messages indicating the occurrence of RBCs resistant to lysis, and give access to an extended mode with longer lysis. Hematology analyzers with a dedicated channel for counting of WBC nuclei after lysis with a strong lysing solution and a channel for total WBC count will demonstrate a discrepancy between the two WBC counts. Software that will automatically adjust the WBC count and determine the number of nucleated RBCs is available on some hematology analyzers [65].

The presence of hyperlipidemia in neonates on total parenteral nutrition, hyperbilirubinemia, or elevated WBC count may result in increased turbidity of the sample and lead to a spurious elevation of hemoglobin levels as well as levels of the calculated hemoglobin derivatives, such as hematocrit, MCH, and MCHC. In such cases, an abnormally high MCHC (>36 g/dL) corresponding to the high Hb is observed.

Lastly, the small non-standard size of the microtainer tubes requires manual processing of such samples, since none of the current laboratory automated robotic systems or hematology analyzers are adapted to process microtainer tubes. The manual handling of these samples results in a longer turnaround time.

Interpretation of hematologic test results in children

As has already been shown, the hematologic test results in children are affected by many factors: biological variables and pre-analytical factors, as well as analytical interferences. Such considerations should be taken into account when interpreting hematologic test results in children, particularly in the cases of neonates and infants. They also need to be considered when developing age-specific reference intervals.

While developing reference intervals is the responsibility of each laboratory, when it comes to children, due to limited blood availability, many hematology laboratories turn toward published reference intervals. For instance, in the United States, a College of American Pathologists (CAP) Q-Probes study of normal ranges used by 163 clinical laboratories found that only 10% of the facilities conducted internal studies to establish hematology reference ranges, and most laboratories relied on external sources to establish reference intervals for pediatric patients [66]. However, while easily accessible, the published reference intervals for neonates and young children can bring their own problems. Many of them, including ones cited in the most respected recent publications, such as the *Nathan and Oski's Hematology of Infancy and Childhood*, seventh edition, 2009 [67], were developed more than 30 years ago and are not directly applicable to the current practice. It is known that the reference intervals are method (technology) dependent, and dated guidelines cannot be applied directly to individual patients.

An example of the challenges associated with using published data for reference intervals is two major studies of absolute neutrophil count in newborns – Schmutz *et al.* and Manroe *et al.* – that we discussed earlier [27, 28]. These studies were performed almost 40 years apart and both found the same dynamics in the neutrophil count from birth to 72 hours of age, yet quite different absolute neutrophil counts. While Manroe found the upper limit of the absolute neutrophil count to be 6.0×10^9/L, and the lower limit 1.8×10^9/L, Schmutz *et al.* reported an upper limit of the neutrophil count at delivery of 18.0×10^9/L and a lower limit of 3.5×10^9/L. Such differences also exist in the later time points at the peak (8–12 hours) and nadir (120 hours). Thus, while the two studies show the same dynamic of the neutrophil counts from birth to five days of life, the absolute values are clinically different, so that the data cannot be used as reference intervals. The reasons for the differences between the two studies are not clear. Perhaps the studies were performed using different instrumentation – Coulter S vs. Beckman Coulter LH750 – or are affected by different altitude – for example, Dallas vs. Salt Lake City – or other variables might help explain these discrepancies as well. Therefore, such studies should be used cautiously. They should not be applied directly as a reference interval, in order to avoid an erroneous diagnosis of absolute neutropenia or neutrophilia.

To overcome the constraints of limited blood availability in developing reference intervals for young children, many turn to the use of statistical analysis of hematologic values of hospitalized children who have health problems that do not significantly affect the hematologic values [45]. However, if such references do not provide information on the gestational age, sampling site, or race of the subjects included in the study, they are also limited and should be used cautiously.

In addition, all published reference intervals need to be verified and made compatible with the patient population of a particular laboratory before being applied as clinical reference intervals. There are racial and ethnic differences that are not well incorporated into current reference intervals. The hemoglobin, Hct, and MCV values are all higher in Caucasian than in black infants [41]. Similarly, applying term reference intervals to premature neonates may also lead to an erroneous diagnosis of anemia, leukopenia, or thrombocytopenia, with unnecessary workups and additional blood draw that will contribute further to development of anemia. Reference intervals for premature neonates are badly needed and should be established using similar approaches as for term neonates.

Other factors affecting neonatal testing

With the advance of information technology and increasing complexity of clinical laboratory operations, the center of attention has shifted in emphasis from the analytical phase to the preanalytical and post-analytical operations of clinical laboratories [68]. The drive is to have not simply accurate laboratory testing, but also for the testing to be fast and efficient, so that test results can be delivered to clinicians in a timely manner needed for decision making, rather than after the fact. This is particularly important for blood samples from newborns and infants, since the clinical history for them may be unreliable, the physical examination may underestimate the severity of the disease, and the disease may progress unusually rapidly. The limited blood availability in small children and other preanalytical and analytical interferences can result in the delay of specimen processing and reporting of results. Thus, knowledge about these factors, both for term and preterm infants, is imperative in order to achieve fast and efficient testing and provide accurate test results in conjunction with meaningful reference intervals.

Data release and delta check are particularly challenging for pediatric samples, precisely because there are significant differences between normal hematologic test results at birth, after the first week of life, at the end of the neonatal period, and so on. For this reason, the delta check for young children cannot be used reliably to uncover and identify errors in specimen collection, handling, and labeling.

To conclude, understanding developmental hematopoiesis and how it affects both term and preterm hematologic values of neonates is essential for the proper interpretation of hematologic test results. Information about the most important preanalytical and analytical factors is also critical and needs to be included in the regular practice and when developing reference intervals in children.

Acknowledgments: I extend my gratitude to Dr. Frederic A. Smith for his help in reanalyzing of some of the published data.

References

1. **Palis J**. Ontogeny of erythropoiesis. *Current Opinion in Hematology.* 2008;**15**:155–161.

2. **Mikkola HKA, Orkin SH**. The journey of developing hematopoietic stem cells. *Development.* 2006;**133**:3733–3744.

3. **Dame C, Juul SE**. The switch from fetal to adult erythropoiesis. *Clinics in Perinatology.* 2000;**27**:507–526.

4. **Orkin SH, Zon LI**. Hematopoiesis: an evolving paradigm for stem cell biology. *Cell.* 2008;**132**:631–644.

5. **Kennedy M, D'Souza SL, Lynch-Kattman M, Schwantz S, Keller G**. Development of the hemangioblast defines the onset of hematopoiesis in human ES cell differentiation cultures. *Blood.* 2007;**109**:2679–2687.

6. **Tavian M, Hallais MF, Peault B**. Emergence of intraembryonic hematopoietic precursors in the pre-liver human embryo. *Development.* 1999;**126**:793–803.

7. **Cumano A, Godin I**. Ontogeny of the hematopoietic system. *Annual Review of Immunology.* 2007;**25**:745–785.

8. **Heissig B, Ohki Y, Sato Y**, *et al.* A role for niches in hematopoietic cell development. *Hematology.* 2005;**10**:247–253.

9. **Charbord P, Tavian M, Humeau L, Péault B**. Early ontogeny of the human marrow from long bones: an immunohistochemical study of hematopoiesis and its microenvironment. *Blood.* 1996;**87**:4109–4119.

10. **Slayton WB, Juul SE, Calhoun DA**, *et al.* Hematopoiesis in the liver and marrow of human fetuses at 5 to 16 weeks postconception: quantitative assessment of macrophage and neutrophil populations. *Pediatric Research.* 1998;**43**:774–782.

11. **Muench MO, Namikawa R**. Disparate regulation of human fetal erythropoiesis by the microenvironments of the liver and bone marrow. *Blood Cells, Molecules, and Diseases.* 2001;**27**:377–390.

12. **Wilpshaar J, Joekes EC, Lim FTH**, *et al.* Magnetic resonance imaging of fetal bone marrow for quantitative definition of the human fetal stem cell compartment. *Blood.* 2002;**100**:451–457.

13. **Calhoun DA, Li Y, Braylan RC**. Assessment of the contribution of the spleen to granulocytopoiesis and erythropoiesis of the mid-gestation human fetus. *Early Human Development.* 1996;**46**:217–227.

14. **Ishikawa H**. Differentiation of red pulp and evaluation of hemopoietic role of human prenatal spleen. *Archivum Histologicum Japonicum – Nippon Soshikigaku Kiroku.* 1985;**48**:183–197.

15. **Forestier F, Daffos F, Catherine N**, *et al.* Developmental hematopoiesis in normal human fetal blood. *Blood.* 1991;**77**:2360–2363.

16. **Dame C, Fahnenstich H, Freitag P**, *et al.* Erythropoietin mRNA expression in human fetal and neonatal tissue. *Blood.* 1998;**92**:3218–3225.

17. **Palis J, Segel GB**. Developmental biology of erythropoiesis. *Blood Reviews.* 1998;**12**:106–114.

18. **Fisher JW**. Erythropoietin: physiology and pharmacology update. *Experimental Biology and Medicine.* 2003;**228**:1–14.

19. **Millar DS, Davis LR, Rodeck CH**, *et al.* Normal blood cell values in the early mid-trimester fetus. *Prenatal Diagnosis.* 1985;**5**:367–373.

20. **De Waele M, Foulon W, Renmans W**, *et al.* Hematologic values and lymphocyte subsets in fetal blood. *American Journal of Clinical Pathology.* 1988;**89**:742–746.

21. **Forestier F, Daffos F, Galacteros F**, *et al.* Hematological values of 163 normal fetuses between 18 and 30 weeks of gestation. *Pediatric Research.* 1986;**20**:342–346.

22. **Peakman M, Buggins AG, Nicolaides KH, Layton DM, Vergani D**. Analysis of lymphocyte phenotypes in cord blood from early gestation fetuses. *Clinical and Experimental Immunology.* 1992;**90**:345–350.

23. **Berry SM, Fine N, Bichalski JA**, *et al.* Circulating lymphocyte subsets in second- and third-trimester fetuses: comparison with newborns and adults. *American Journal of Obstetrics and Gynecology.* 1992;**167**:895–900. Erratum appears in *American Journal of Obstetrics and Gynecology.* 1992;**167**:1898.

24. **Zhao Y, Day ZP, Lv P, Gao XM**. Phenotypic and functional analysis of human T lymphocytes in early second- and third-trimester fetuses. *Clinical and Experimental Immunology.* 2002;**129**:302–308.

25. **Matoth Y, Zaizov R, Varsano I**. Postnatal changes in some red cell parameters. *Acta Paediatrica Scandinavica.* 1971;**60**:317–323.

26. **Christensen RD, Jopling J, Henry E, Wiedmeier SE**. The erythrocyte indices of neonates, defined using data from over 12,000 patients in a multihospital

health care system. *Journal of Perinatology.* 2008;**28**:24–28.

27. **Schmutz N, Henry E, Jopling J, Christensen RD.** Expected ranges for blood neutrophil concentrations of neonates: the Manroe and Mouzinho charts revisited. *Journal of Perinatology.* 2008;**28**:275–281.

28. **Manroe BL, Weinberg AG, Rosenfeld CR, Browne R.** The neonatal blood count in health and disease. I. Reference values for neutrophilic cells. *Journal of Pediatrics.* 1979;**95**:89–98.

29. **Zipursky A, Brown E, Palko J, Brown EJ.** The erythrocyte differential count in newborn infants. *American Journal of Pediatric Hematology/Oncology.* 1983;**5**: 45–51.

30. **Holroyde CP, Oski FA, Gardner FH.** The "pocked" erythrocyte. Red-cell surface alterations in reticuloendothelial immaturity of the neonate. *New England Journal of Medicine.* 1969;**281**:516–520.

31. **Hermansen MC.** Nucleated red blood cells in the fetus and newborn. *Archives of Disease in Childhood Fetal and Neonatal Edition.* 2001;**84**:F211–F215.

32. **Christensen RD.** Circulating pluripotent hematopoietic progenitor cells in neonates. *Journal of Pediatrics.* 1987;**110**:623–625.

33. **Comans-Bitter WM, de Groot R, Van Den Beemd R,** *et al.* Immunophenotyping of blood lymphocytes in childhood. Reference values for lymphocyte subpopulations. *Journal of Pediatrics.* 1997;**130**:388–393.

34. **de Vries E, de Bruin-Versteeg S, Comans-Bitter WM,** *et al.* Longitudinal survey of lymphocyte subpopulations in the first year of life. *Pediatric Research.* 2000;**47**:528–537.

35. **de Vries E, de Groot R, de Bruin-Versteeg S, Comans-Bitter WM, van Dongen JJM.** Analysing the developing lymphocyte system of neonates and infants. *European Journal of Pediatrics.* 1999;**158**:611–617.

36. **O'Gorman MR, Millard DD, Lowder JN, Yogev R.** Lymphocyte subpopulations in healthy 1–3-day-old infants. *Cytometry.* 1998;**34**:235–241.

37. Christensen RD (ed.). *Hematologic Problems of the Neonate.* Philadelphia, PA: WB Saunders; 2000.

38. **Ozyurek E, Cetinta S, Ceylan T,** *et al.* Complete blood count parameters for healthy, small-for-gestational-age, full-term newborns. *Clinical and Laboratory Haematology.* 2006;**28**: 97–104.

39. **Mouzinho A, Rosenfeld CR, Sanchez PJ, Risser R.** Revised reference ranges for circulating neutrophils in very-low-birth-weight neonates. *Pediatrics.* 1994;**94**:76–82.

40. **Zaizov R, Matoth Y.** Red cell values on the first postnatal day during the last 16 weeks of gestation. *American Journal of Hematology.* 1976;**1**:275–278.

41. **Alur P, Devapatla SS, Super DM,** *et al.* Impact of race and gestational age on red blood cell indices in very low birth weight infants. *Pediatrics.* 2000;**106**: 306–310.

42. **Salsbury DC.** Anemia of prematurity. *Neonatal Network: NN.* 2001;**20**:13–20.

43. **Coulombel L, Dehan M, Tchernia G, Hill C, Vial M.** The number of polymorphonuclear leukocytes in relation to gestational age in the newborn. *Acta Paediatrica Scandinavica.* 1979;**68**:709–711.

44. **Berrington JE, Barge D, Fenton AC, Cant AJ, Spickett GP.** Lymphocyte subsets in term and significantly preterm UK infants in the first year of life analysed by single platform flow cytometry. *Clinical and Experimental Immunology.* 2005;**140**:289–292.

45. **Soldin SJ, Brugnara C, Wong EC.** *Pediatric Reference Intervals* (6th edn.). Washington, DC: AACC Press; 2007.

46. **Shearer WT, Rosenblatt HM, Gelman RS,** *et al.* Lymphocyte subsets in healthy children from birth through 18 years of age: the pediatric AIDS clinical trials group P1009 study. *Journal of Allergy and Clinical Immunology.* 2003;**112**: 973–980.

47. **Coffin CM, Hamilton MS, Pysher TJ,** *et al.* Pediatric laboratory medicine: current challenges and future opportunities. *American Journal of Clinical Pathology.* 2002;**117**:683–690.

48. **Proytcheva MA.** Issues in neonatal cellular analysis. *American Journal of Clinical Pathology.* 2009;**131**:560–573.

49. **Ernst DJ, Ballance LO, Calam RR,** *et al. Procedures and Devices for the Collection of Diagnostic Capillary Blood Specimens: Approved Standard* (6th edn.). Wayne, PA: Clinical and Laboratory Standards Institute; 2008.

50. **Werner M.** Clinical applications of microchemistry. In *Microtechniques for the Clinical Laboratory: Concepts and Applications.* New York: John Wiley and Sons, Inc. 1976, 1–15.

51. **Janes M, Pinelli J, Landry S,** *et al.* Comparison of capillary blood sampling using an automated incision device with and without warming the heel. *Journal of Perinatology.* 2002;**22**: 154–158.

52. **Kayiran SM, Ozbek N, Turan M,** *et al.* Significant differences between capillary and venous complete blood counts in the neonatal period. *Clinical and Laboratory Haematology.* 2003;**25**: 9–16.

53. **Christensen RD, Rothstein G.** Pitfalls in the interpretation of leukocyte counts of newborn infants. *American Journal of Clinical Pathology.* 1979;**72**: 608–611.

54. **Linderkamp O, Versmold HT, Strohhacker I,** *et al.* Capillary-venous hematocrit differences in newborn infants. I. Relationship to blood volume, peripheral blood flow, and acid base parameters. *European Journal of Pediatrics.* 1977;**127**:9–14.

55. **Thurlbeck SM, McIntosh N.** Preterm blood counts vary with sampling site. *Archives of Disease in Childhood.* 1987;**62**:74–75.

56. McPherson RA, Pincus MR, Henry JB (eds.). *Henry's Clinical Diagnosis and Management by Laboratory Methods* (21st edn.). Philadelphia, PA: Saunders Elsevier; 2007.

57. **Hutton EK, Hassan ES.** Late vs early clamping of the umbilical cord in full-term neonates: systematic review and meta-analysis of controlled trials. *JAMA.* 2007;**297**:1241–1252.

58. **Ceriani Cernadas JM, Carroli G, Pellegrini L,** *et al.* The effect of timing of cord clamping on neonatal venous hematocrit values and clinical outcome at term: a randomized, controlled trial. *Pediatrics.* 2006;**117**:e779–e786.

59. **Hasan R, Inoue S, Banerjee A.** Higher white blood cell counts and band forms in newborns delivered vaginally compared with those delivered by cesarean section. *American Journal of Clinical Pathology.* 1993;**100**:116–118.

60. **Nalls MA, Wilson JG, Patterson NJ,** *et al.* Admixture mapping of white cell count: genetic locus responsible for

lower white blood cell count in the Health ABC and Jackson Heart studies. *American Journal of Human Genetics.* 2008;**82**:81–87. Erratum appears in *American Journal of Human Genetics.* 2008;**82**:532.

61. **Reich D, Nalls MA, Kao WHL**, *et al.* Reduced neutrophil count in people of African descent is due to a regulatory variant in the Duffy antigen receptor for chemokines gene. *PLoS Genetics.* 2009;**5**:e1000360.

62. **Carballo C, Foucar K, Swanson P, Papile LA, Watterberg KL**. Effect of high altitude on neutrophil counts in newborn infants. *Journal of Pediatrics.* 1991;**119**:464–466.

63. **Schelonka RL, Yoder BA, desJardins SE**, *et al.* Peripheral leukocyte count and leukocyte indexes in healthy newborn term infants. *Journal of Pediatrics.* 1994;**125**:603–606.

64. **Maconi M, Rolfo A, Cardaropoli S**, *et al.* Hematologic values in healthy and small for gestational age newborns. *Laboratory Hematology.* 2005;**11**:152–156.

65. **Rolfo A, Maconi M, Cardaropoli S**, *et al.* Nucleated red blood cells in term fetuses: reference values using an automated analyzer. *Neonatology.* 2007;**92**:205–208.

66. **Friedberg RC, Souers R, Wagar EA**, *et al.* The origin of reference intervals. *Archives of Pathology and Laboratory Medicine.* 2007;**131**:348–357.

67. Orkin SH, Nathan DG, **Ginsburg D**, *et al.* (eds.). *Nathan and Oski's Hematology Of Infancy and Childhood* (7th edn.). Philadelphia, PA: Saunders/Elsevier; 2009.

68. **Bossuyt X, Verweire K, Blanckaert N**. Laboratory medicine: challenges and opportunities. *Clinical Chemistry.* 2007;**53**:1730–1733.

Normal bone marrow

Maria A. Proytcheva

The hematopoietic system is unique in comparison to other organ systems because its anatomic location shifts during the embryogenesis and fetal development from the yolk sac to the fetal liver and finally to the bone marrow (BM). At birth and thereafter, the hematopoiesis is restricted to the BM, which continues to evolve in order to accommodate the changing oxygenation needs of the growing child. As a result, the composition of the BM depends on the child's age – particularly early in life – as well as on the demands of the growing child, and so differs from the BM of adults. Knowledge of these differences needs to be considered when evaluating a child's BM in order to distinguish between normal development and pathologic processes.

Ontogeny of the hematopoietic system

Until definitive (adult) hematopoietic organs are fully developed, hematopoiesis occurs in successive anatomic sites where hematopoietic stem cells (HSCs) are generated, maintained, and expended to differentiate into blood cells [1, 2]. The HSCs develop from the hemangioblast, a mesoderm-derived multipotent precursor that gives rise to hematopoietic as well as endothelial and vascular smooth muscle cells [3, 4]. This process is initiated in the yolk sac between days 16 and 19 of gestation, with the formation of angioblastic foci or "blood islands" that contain primitive erythroblasts surrounded by endothelial cells. The yolk sac hematopoiesis is transient and generates HSCs that differentiate in the vasculature into primitive and definitive erythroblasts and rare macrophages.

Currently it is believed that the HSCs from extraembryonic (yolk sac) and intraembryonic (aorto–gonadal–mesonephros region, AGM) sites colonize the fetal liver and bone marrow, where they are maintained, expanded, and differentiated into definitive blood cells [1, 2, 5]. Unlike the primitive erythroid progenitors generated in the vasculature spaces of the yolk sac, the definitive hematopoietic precursors develop in the hematopoietic niche, a complex microenvironment generated by stromal elements of the fetal liver and bone marrow [6, 7]. The vascular endothelium, particularly microvasculature endothelium within the hematopoietic microenvironment of the fetal liver and bone marrow, plays a seminal role in the regulation of the hematopoiesis and the fate of the hematopoietic stem cells.

The bone marrow is the last blood-forming tissue that develops in ontogenesis, when hematopoiesis already exists in the yolk sac and transiently proceeds in the liver. Studies of the early ontogeny of human marrow show that the hematopoiesis development begins in the long bones as early as 6–8.5 weeks of gestation. It is completed by 16 weeks of gestation with a final organization of the bones into areas of dense hematopoiesis surrounded by areas of fully calcified bone [8, 9]. This process occurs in several morphologically distinctive stages involving cartilage regression and angiogenesis, followed by the development of hematopoiesis as will be described here.

Initially, the bones consist entirely of cartilaginous rudiment, and the marrow formation begins with vascularization and development of capillaries with CD34+ endothelial cells. These cells are essential for the development of local hematopoiesis. The second stage is characterized by a significant chondrolysis/cell invasion and remodeling resulting in appearance of marrow spaces lined by newly immigrated cells. These include osteoblasts, which closely surround the cartilage islands, and numerous CD68+ cells, some of them multinucleated, suggesting that they are osteoclastic in nature. At the end of this stage, except for the CD68+ cells, no other hematopoietic cells are present.

During the third stage, there is a continuous vascular proliferation and angiogenesis in the absence of hematopoiesis. Stage four is characterized by the onset of hematopoiesis which is primarily granulocytic and develops in distinct solid structures called primary logettes. The logettes appear as early as week 9 of gestation, but up to week 10.5 they are devoid of hematopoietic cells. During the last stage (week 16 onward), there is a final organization of the long bones into areas of fully calcified bone and areas of dense hematopoiesis. The logettes are no longer visible. The BM hematopoiesis is predominantly granulocytic, unlike the fetal liver hematopoiesis, which is a predominantly erythropoietic site during the second trimester [8]. While the hematopoietic ontogeny progresses in the same order and shows similar steps in the long bones and thoracic vertebrae, there is a delay in its initiation in the vertebrae. At this site, hematopoietic cells are recognizable at week 13.9 and beyond [9].

Studies of fetal BM between the 12th and 24th week of gestation show that during the early stages of the establishment of hematopoiesis, the fetal BM shows morphologic evidence of modulation and transformation of the endosteal and endothelial cells into stromal cells such as stellate, reticular, and fibroblast-like cells [10]. During this time, the marrow is entirely hematopoietic, such that no fat cells are seen at this stage. At 20–24 weeks of gestation, the BM is hematopoietically active with the predominance of the hematopoiesis in the epiphyseal end of the long bones. Up to 22 weeks of gestation, the hematopoiesis is detected in all bones except the calvarian bones (skull) [11]. The lack of hematopoiesis in the calvarian bones most likely is due to the fact that the skull bone osteogenesis does not develop from cartilage but takes place through intramembranous ossification instead of endochondral osteogenesis.

Between the 11th and 24th week of gestation, both the fetal liver and bone marrow are hematopoietic organs concomitantly, yet each supports a somewhat distinctive set of hematopoietic lineages [12]. While the liver is the major site for erythropoiesis, the BM hematopoiesis is shifted to granulopoiesis and lymphopoiesis, and the erythropoiesis is only a minor component [13]. The main difference between the hematopoiesis of the liver and BM is not in the number of stem cells but in the presence of erythropoietic regulatory factors, as well as other factors with burst-promoting activity in the microenvironment of the liver. They determine the fate of the HSCs and their differentiation in the erythroid pathway. A quantitative analysis of the leukocyte content and the percentage of CD34+ cells, lymphocytes, granulocytes, and monocytes in fetal liver, BM, and spleen revealed comparable absolute numbers of CD34+ cells in the marrow and liver throughout the second trimester of gestation [11].

The hematopoietic shift from the liver to the BM occurs after the 24th week of gestation. While the number of CD34+ stem cells does not shift, a changing microenvironment during development is most likely responsible for different signals to the differentiating precursor cells resulting in lineage-specific development. The total bone marrow volume markedly increases during the second trimester. Studies using magnetic resonance imaging (MRI) of intact fetuses during that period show a volume of 934 µL at 17–18 weeks that increases to 4563 µL at 22–23 weeks of gestation [11]. The vertebral bodies of the spine make the largest contribution (26.4% ± 2.7%) to the total BM volume.

Postnatal bone marrow

From birth onwards, the BM is the major hematopoietic site. At birth, all marrow cavities of the skeleton contain red, hematopoietic marrow and almost no fat. With age, the number of fat cells increases and the red hematopoietic marrow diminishes. By age 25, active hematopoiesis is confined to the proximal quarters of the shafts of the femur and humerus and the axial skeleton (skull bones, ribs, sternum, scapulae, clavicles, vertebrae, pelvis, and upper half of the sacrum) [14]. Even though young children are significantly smaller than adults, due to the relatively high percentage of red, hematopoietic marrow the absolute amount of active BM they have is approximately the same as in adults.

The bone marrow is a functionally dynamic structure such that, if the needs for erythrocyte, leukocyte, or megakaryocyte production increase, the hematopoiesis expands and the fat is replaced by active marrow. In children, of course, that particular expansion is limited since the number of fat cells is low. Instead, the increased hematopoiesis is accommodated by a reduction in the proportions of marrow sinusoids. In severe congenital anemias, when the demand for red cells increases, the marrow cavities expand, leading to bony deformities.

The BM is located between the trabeculae of the cancellous bones and has a highly complex three-dimensional structure composed of capillary venous sinus, surrounding an extracellular matrix, and stromal cells including osteoblasts [6, 15]. This highly organized matrix provides a milieu for the HSCs to reside, proliferate, and differentiate into various blood cell types. The interaction between the various stimulatory or inhibitory factors with the stem and progenitor cells is what determines their fate. The spaces between the small vessels contain a few reticular fibers and a variety of cell types. The sinusoids of the marrow have thin walls lined by endothelial cells with little or no underlying basement membrane and outer incomplete layer of adventitial cells. The endothelial cells produce an extracellular matrix as well as c-kit ligand or stem cell factor, IL-6, GM-CSF, IL-1a, IL-11, and G-CSF which are intimately involved in the regulation of hematopoiesis [14].

At least two distinct hematopoietic niches – osteoblastic and vascular – play an important role in regulating mobilization of the HSCs [5, 6, 16]. These niches have different functions. While the osteoblastic niche is associated with HSC homing, the vascular niche is important in HSC mobilization. Whether these niches are separate structures or part of a bigger complex is still to be determined, but the HSCs are found in close proximity to both osteoblasts and endothelial cells.

The extracellular matrix of the normal marrow consists of a scanty, incomplete network of fine branching fibers between the parenchymal cells. The BM stroma is a three-dimensional meshwork of reticular fibroblastoid cells that form the adventitial surface of the vascular sinuses and extend cytoplasmic processes to create a lattice on which blood cells are found. It contains collagen, type I–III, fibronectin, laminin, and proteoglycans. The meshwork of reticulin is highlighted by reticulin stain. The cellular elements of the stroma include cells of mesenchymal origin such as osteoblasts, adiposities, nonphagocytic reticular cells, hematopoietic cells such as osteoclasts, macrophages, and mast cells, and endothelial cells.

Table 2.1. Key transcription factors in the hematopoietic development.

Stem cell class transcription factors	
SCL/TAL-1	
LMO2	
MLL	Required for the production, survival, or
RUNX1	self-renewal of hematopoietic stem cells (HSCs)
GATA2	
TEL/ETV6	
Transcription factors required for multilineage gene expression	
GATA1	Stimulates common myeloid progenitors (CMPs) to differentiate into megakaryocytic/erythroid progenitors (MEPs).
PU.1	Stimulates CMPs to differentiate into granulocyte/monocyte progenitors (GMPs)
C/EBPα	Granulocyte/monocyte progenitors (GMPs)
Ikaros	Required for lymphocyte development
PAX-5	Required for proper B-cell development
Notch signaling	T-cell development
GATA3	T-cell specific in the context of Notch signaling

Furthermore, there are reticular fibroblastoid cells that serve as an adhesive framework for the marrow and produce essential hematopoietic colony stimulating factors (CSFs) that have important functions in cell–cell interactions and secretion of extracellular matrix proteins.

A number of transcription factors, including virtually all classes of DNA-binding proteins, are critical for hematopoiesis [5] (Table 2.1). It is fascinating that a majority of the these factors are involved in either chromosomal translocations or somatic mutations in human hematopoietic malignancies (Table 2.2). Examples of such factors include MLL, RUNX1, TEL/ETV6, SCL/TAL-1, and LMO1, which account for the majority of known leukemia-associated translocations. In broader terms, the leukemogenic effect is due to translocations resulting in locus deregulation. That is the case for *SCL/TAL1* and *LMO2* in T-lymphoblastic leukemias or in the generation of a chimeric fusion protein in translocations involving *MLL*, *RUNX1*, and *TEL/ETV6* in myeloid and lymphoid leukemias that are frequently seen in children. Detailed exploration of these transcription factors and the mechanisms of action and interactions between various factors is beyond this text and can be found elsewhere [1, 5, 17].

A simplified view of important transcription factors in hematopoiesis, depicted in the "classical" hierarchy diagram, is shown in Fig. 2.1. Currently the HSCs are viewed as a group of cells with varying developmental potentials based on intrinsic networks that are driven by transcription factors and inputs from the cellular niches in which they reside. This is a highly coordinated process in which hematopoietic progenitors differentiate into common myeloid progenitors (CMPs) and common lymphoid progenitors (CLPs) with subsequent cellular differentiation into specific lineages.

Several key transcription factors are responsible for further differentiation of the CMPs and CLPs. *GATA1* and *FOG1* promote CMPs to differentiate further to megakaryocytic/erythroid progenitors, giving rise to platelets and erythro-

cytes. *PU.1* promotes CMP to differentiate into granulocyte/macrophage progenitors, generating neutrophils, eosinophils, mast cells, and monocytes. *PAX5* is required for proper B-cell development, and in its absence and under the appropriate growth factor conditions the progenitors differentiate to T-, NK-, or dendritic cells, macrophages, neutrophils, or erythroid precursors instead. NOTCH signaling is essential in T-cell development.

Myeloid hematopoiesis, in the first year of life, occurs in both the axial and appendicular skeletons. Thereafter, there is a gradual decrease in the hematopoiesis in the long bones until about age 15. At that age, the flat bones of the axial skeleton are the exclusive sites of the production of myeloid cells. In histologic sections, the cells with proliferative activity are preferentially located near the bony trabeculae; by contrast, the differentiated elements are observed in the central, intratrabecular spaces [10].

Location of the various hematopoietic cells is also nonrandom (Fig. 2.2). Megakaryocytes are found adjacent to marrow sinuses, which allows easy shedding of platelets directly into the lumen. The erythroid progenitors differentiate and mature in erythroblastic islands that comprise niches of erythropoiesis [18]. The erythroblastic islands are found in the bone marrow and fetal liver, and consist of developing erythroblasts surrounding a central macrophage, which is a key component of erythroid differentiation. As their erythroblasts become more differentiated, the erythroid islands migrate toward sinusoids, since they are mobile structures. The early myeloid progenitors are localized in the paratrabecular areas close to the adventitia of the small arteries. With maturation, the cells migrate to the intertrabecular spaces. Normally, the layer of immature granulocytes does not exceed two to three rows of maturing cells.

Age-specific differences in the bone marrow

At birth and in young children, the bone marrow cellularity and composition differs from that of older children and adults (Table 2.3). This is due not only to the relative immaturity of the hematopoietic system at birth, but also to the nature of the hematopoiesis and its dynamic response to the needs for oxygenation and the immune response of the growing organism. Although the presence of age-related differences is generally recognized, their specific variations are not well known. In addition, important misperceptions exist, particularly in terms of bone marrow cellularity.

Several studies attempting to define the normal BM cellularity and composition of children have been hampered by the difficulties in obtaining bone marrow from *normal* children, as well as a lack of standard sampling sites or methodology in defining BM cellularity. Furthermore, the cell classification, definition, and nomenclature of the hematopoietic progenitors have evolved with the years, which limits to some extent the applicability of data from older studies. For these reasons, as

Table 2.2. Regulatory transcription factors involved in hematopoiesis and leukemogenesis.

Transcription factor/official name	Alternative names	Function	Gene locus
RUNX1 (Runt-related transcription factor 1)	AML1; CBFA2; EVI-1; AMLCR1; PEBP2aB; AML1-EVI-1	Heterodimeric transcription factor; chromosomal translocations involving *RUNX1* result in several types of leukemia Point mutations identified in MDS and familial thrombocytopenia with propensity to myeloid malignancies	21q22.3
STIL (SCL/TAL-1 interrupting locus)	SIL; MCPH7; DKFZp686O09161; STIL	Cytoplasmic protein implicated in the regulation of the mitotic spindle checkpoint Chromosomal deletions that result in fusion of STIL with the adjacent locus commonly occur in T-cell leukemias	1p32
LMO1	TTG1; RBTN1; RHOM1	Encodes a cysteine-rich, two LIM domain transcriptional regulator T-cell leukemia development	11p15
LMO2 (LIM domain only 2)	TTG2; RBTN2; RHOM2; RBTNL1	Required for yolk sac erythropoiesis Critical role in hematopoietic development T-cell acute lymphoblastic leukemia	11p13
MLL (Myeloid/ lymphoid or mixed-lineage leukemia)	HRX; TRX1; ALL-1; CXXC7; HTRX1; KMT2A; MLL1A; FLJ11783; MLL/GAS7; TET1-MLL; MLL	Encodes DNA binding protein that methylates histone H3 Frequent target for recurrent translocation in acute myeloid leukemia (AML) and acute lymphoblastic leukemia (ALL) in infants Leukemogenic translocations of *MLL* result in fusion proteins that have lost H3K4 methyltransferase activity. A key feature of MLL fusion proteins is their ability to efficiently transform hematopoietic cells into leukemia stem cells	11q23
ETV6	TEL; TEL/ABL	Encodes ETS family transcription factor. Knockout studies in mice show it is required for hematopoiesis and maintenance of the developing vascular network Involved in large number of chromosomal translocations associated with leukemia and congenital fibrosarcoma	12p13
GFI1 (Growth factor independent 1 transcription repressor)	SCN2; GFI-1; ZNF163; FLJ94509	Encodes nuclear zinc finger protein that functions as transcriptional repressor. Plays a role in diverse developmental contexts – hematopoiesis and oncogenesis *GFI1* mutations cause autosomal dominant severe congenital neutropenia, and also dominant non-immune chronic idiopathic neutropenia of adults, resulting in predispositions to leukemias and infections	1p22
GATA1 (GATA binding protein 1)	ERYF1; GF-1; GF1; NFE1; XLTT	Member of the GATA family of transcription factors. The protein plays an important role in erythroid development by regulating the switch of fetal hemoglobin to adult hemoglobin Mutations have been associated with X-linked dyserythropoietic anemia and thrombocytopenia, as well as with myeloid proliferations related to Down syndrome	Xp11.23

Abbreviation: MDS, myelodysplastic syndrome.

of now, no well-defined normal reference intervals exist for the cellularity and composition of BM in children.

The largest and most relevant study for routine pathology practice determined the BM cellularity by direct visualization in the posterior iliac crest core biopsies or clot sections of 448 healthy BM donors and children with non-neoplastic hematologic disorders or non-hematologic malignancies [19]. The children's age ranged from less than 1 year to 18 years. The study found that the average cellularity in the first two decades of life is lower than previously thought (Table 2.4). The highest BM cellularity (79.8%) was observed in children younger than two years of age. In older children, the cellularity declined to 68.6% for children between the ages of two to four years, and to 59.1% for children from five to nine years old. The study demonstrated a progressive decline of the BM cellularity, down to roughly 60% during the first five years of life, and relatively constant BM cellularity comparable to other age groups after that. There were no significant differences between the BM cellularities of boys and girls. However, some disease-related differences were observed, suggesting that other factors affect the BM cellularity and should be considered. Children with hematologic non-malignant diseases had higher cellularity as compared to healthy donors and to children with non-hematologic malignancies.

These findings are in general agreement with other smaller studies, despite differences in the methodologies that were used.

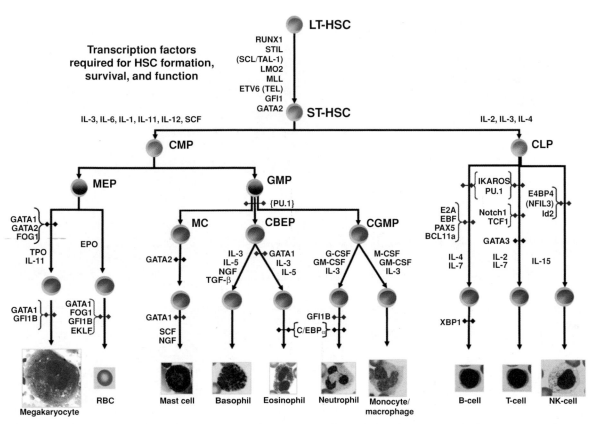

Fig. 2.1. A schematic model of hematopoiesis depicting key transcription factors and cytokines required for the generation and maturation of hematopoietic cells. The bars indicate the stages at which hematopoietic development is blocked in the absence of transcription factors, as determined through conventional gene knockouts. The transcription factors in red have been involved in translocations or mutated in human/mouse hematologic malignancies. Key cytokines required for proper development are shown in blue. Abbreviations: LT-HSC, long-term hematopoietic stem cell; ST-HSC, short-term hematopoietic stem cell; CMP, common myeloid progenitor; CLP, common lymphocytic progenitor; MEP, megakaryocyte/erythroid progenitor; GMP, granulocyte/macrophage progenitor; CBEP, common basophil/eosinophil progenitor; CGMP, common granulocyte/monocyte progenitor; MC, mast cell; RBC, red blood cell; M-CSF, monocyte colony stimulating factor. (Redrawn based on data from Orkin, Zon [5], and Foucar et al. [15].)

For example, using volumetric and microscopic patterns of BM from normal infants and children, Sturgeon found that in normal infants – 3 months of age or younger – BM particles show 80% or more hematopoietic tissues [20]. Particles that were histologically free of fat (100% cellularity) were found only in three children younger than 2 months of age. The study found differences between different sampling sites. Particles obtained from the sternum and iliac crest of normal individuals aged 18 months through 11 years had comparable cellularity, ranging from 50 to 70%. Aspirates obtained from the tibia, however, had lower cellularity as compared to samples from the sternum or iliac crest. Furthermore, an image-analyzing system used by Ogawa also found 60.0% ± 20.0% cellularity in the BM of children aged from 0 to 9 years, declining to 56.5% ± 4.4% for ages 10 to 19 years [21–26]. While these and other studies examine only a small numbers of subjects, they provide a general impression regarding the overall normal cellularity and histologic pattern in infants and children.

The reasons for the general misperception that the BM cellularity in children is much higher than it actually is are still unclear. Perhaps it results from some older studies using a vol-

umetric technique, or bone marrow crit, which is now known to be insensitive and to underestimate the percentage of fat in the marrow. Or perhaps the misperception is due to the rarely recognized observation that subcortical bone in children, unlike adults, is more cellular, thus giving a wrong impression of the BM cellularity in small pediatric biopsies (Fig. 2.3). Since bone marrow biopsies in children are frequently small and fragmented and contain mostly subcortical bone marrow, perhaps this observed increase in cellularity may be the source of the misperceptions and overestimation. Estimation of bone marrow cellularity using a "100% minus patient's age" formula will significantly overestimate the cellularity in young children and should not be applied.

There are few systematic studies focused on the cellular composition of the bone marrow in normal infants and children [20–23]. While the studies include a high number of normal children, their results are limited by outdated methodologies, use of old terminology and classification of hematopoietic progenitors, and by the lack of modern techniques such as immunophenotyping or genetic studies.

Notwithstanding these limitations, however, several important differences between the cellular composition of the BM

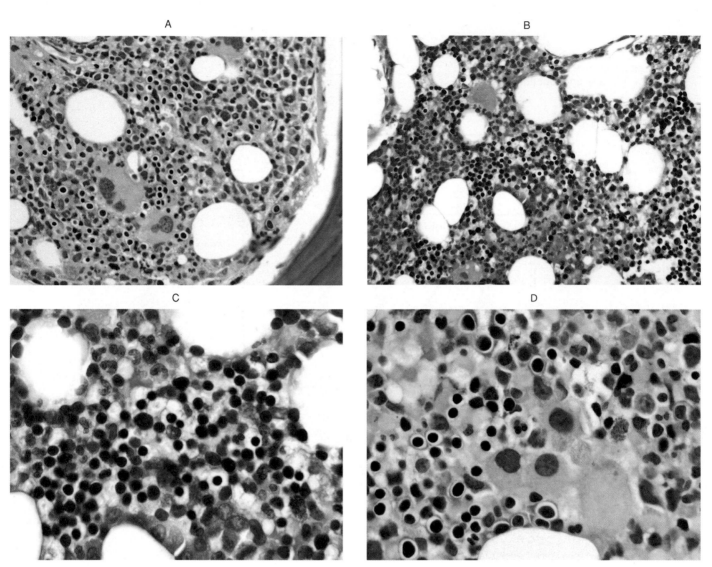

Fig. 2.2. Bone marrow biopsies from an 11-month-old infant show spatial organization of the maturing progenitors (H&E stain). (A) Immature myeloid progenitors are present along the bony trabeculae. Erythroid progenitors are evident in the intertrabecular areas. Megakaryocytes are situated along marrow sinusoids, where they shed mature platelets. (B) Erythroid progenitors surrounding central macrophage, a key component of erythroid islands. (C) Notice the central macrophage seen at high magnification. (D) In young children, the megakaryocytes may be small, monolobated, and may form clusters.

in children and adults emerge. As with the bone marrow's cellularity, the composition of the bone marrow is also age dependent. This is supported by the most well-controlled prospective study, which examines the BM of 88 clinically healthy children with normal peripheral blood counts, serum proteins, and transferrin saturations of at least 16% in the first 18 months of life (Table 2.5) [22]. This study shows that the most significant changes take place during the first month of life and are manifested by a decrease in the percentage of myeloid progenitors and erythroblasts and an increase in the number of lymphocytes (Fig. 2.4). At birth, the bone marrow has a predominance of myeloid progenitors, and the number of erythroid progenitors and lymphocytes is low. The percentage of total myeloid progenitors exhibits an initial decrease during the

first two weeks of life, followed by a sharp drop around the third week, and then reaches a steady level of around 30–35% after the first month. The marrow eosinophils range between 2 and 3%, and the basophils at all times remain below 1%. The monocytes too, remain below 2% during the first 18 months, and the megakaryocytes, plasma cells, and other marrow cells comprise only a small fraction of the total cellularity.

The number of erythroid progenitors also decreases significantly during the first month of life. A transient peak follows at the end of the second month, followed by a more gradual but significant secondary decrease through months three and four, to stabilize at an incidence of total erythroblasts of between 7 and 9%. These changes are broadly followed by the peripheral blood reticulocyte count.

Table 2.3. Age-related normal histology of bone marrow.

Age groups	Cellularity (%)	Cellular composition	Bony trabeculae
Newborn	90–100	Relative myeloid hyperplasia with a shift to immaturity. Blasts less than 5%	
Neonate (birth to 28 days)	90	Marked increase in the number of lymphocytes, mostly B-cells, at the end of the first month	
Infant (1 month to 1 year)	80–90	Diffuse interstitial lymphocytosis Predominance of normal B-cell progenitors (hematogones) T-cells and NK-cells minor components Plasma cells – rare, polytypic, frequently associated with various diseases Lymphoid aggregates not normally present Myeloid progenitors – initial drop in the first 2 weeks of life to reach a steady state level ~30–35% after the first month Erythroid progenitors – relative erythroid hypoplasia most pronounced during the physiologic nadir Iron stores – absent in young children Myeloid to erythroid ratio 5–12 : 1 L : M : E ratio[a] ~ 6 : 5 : 1	Very active bone remodeling Incomplete ossification Prominent osteoblastic rimming
2 to 5 years	60–80	Gradual decrease in the number of B-cells and hematogones and slight increase in the number of T-cells Iron stores gradually increase – detectable stainable iron after age 4–5 years	Active bone remodeling
Children older than 6 years	50–70	Similar to adults	Bone remodeling may be evident, particularly boys
Adults	40–60	Myeloid to erythroid ratio 3–4 : 1 Lymphocytes usually inconspicuous, but may range up to 20% T-cells ≪ B-cells Lymphogranuloma and lymphoid aggregates may be present	Inconspicuous osteoblasts and osteoclasts Bone remodeling absent Bony trabeculae may be thinned (osteopenia, especially women)

Data from references [15, 19–25].

[a] L : M : E ratio – the relative proportions of lymphocytes, myeloid, and erythroid progenitors. Based on data from Rosse *et al.* [22].

Table 2.4. Mean bone marrow cellularity of 448 children according to age.

Age	Mean bone marrow cellularity ± SD (%)
<2 years	79.8 ± 15.7
2 to 4 years	68.6 ± 16.5
5 to 9 years	59.1 ± 20.1
10 to 14 years	60.0 ± 17.9
>15 years	61.1 ± 14.9

Data from Friebert *et al.* [19].

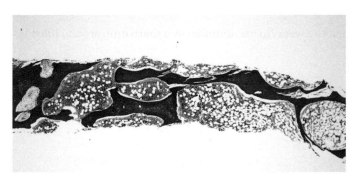

Fig. 2.3. Bone marrow biopsy from an 11-year-old girl shows extreme variation in the marrow cellularity. While the subcortical marrow is hypercellular, the deeper marrow is markedly hypocellular. A small bone marrow biopsy containing subcortical marrow will significantly overestimate the marrow cellularity (H&E stain).

A significant difference between the BM composition of young children and adults is the presence of a high number of lymphocytes early in life. Lymphocytes increase significantly in the immediate neonatal period to become the largest population in the marrow (47.2 ± 9.2%) by the end of the first month. The overall number of lymphocytes is stable in the first 18 months, whereupon they begin to decrease gradually [22].

Except for the natural killer (NK) cells, the distribution of all lymphoid subsets in the BM of infants, children, and adults differs significantly between different age groups. In a study of the lymphocyte subsets of BM biopsies of the sternum of 44 children aged 2 weeks to 15 years and 12 adults aged 15–64 years undergoing cardiovascular surgery, Rego *et al.* found that the B-lymphocytes represented more than 65% of the total lymphocytic population during the first 4 years of life, and the T-lymphocytes were a minor population at this age, in contrast to older children and adults (Table 2.6) [24]. Most of the B-cells were normal B-cell progenitors, hematogones, that express CD10, CD19, PAX5, and TdT (Fig. 2.5). The rest were naïve B-lymphocytes expressing CD20 and surface immunoglobulins. The proportion of CD20+ B-cells increased gradually with age. Plasma cells were virtually absent in the bone marrow in the newborn period and their number was low in normal bone marrow of the children. The lymphocytes infiltrate the intertrabecular spaces diffusely and, unlike adults, lymphoid aggregates are not normally present in the BM of young children [20].

Table 2.5. Percentages of cell types (mean ± standard deviation) in tibial bone marrow of infants from birth to 18 months of age.

	Month										
Cell type	0 (N = 57)	1 (N = 71)	2 (N = 48)	3 (N = 24)	4 (N = 19)	5 (N = 22)	6 (N = 22)	9 (N = 16)	12 (N = 18)	15 (N = 12)	18 (N = 19)
Small lymphocytes	14.42 ± 5.54	47.05 ± 9.24	42.68 ± 7.90	43.63 ± 11.83	47.06 ± 8.77	47.19 ± 9.93	47.55 ± 7.88	48.76 ± 8.11	47.11 ± 11.32	42.77 ± 8.94	43.55 ± 8.56
Transitional cells[a]	1.18 ± 1.13	1.95 ± 0.94	2.38 ± 1.35	2.17 ± 1.64	1.64 ± 1.01	1.83 ± 0.89	2.31 ± 1.16	1.92 ± 1.39	2.32 ± 1.90	1.70 ± 0.82	1.99 ± 1.00
Proerythroblasts	0.02 ± 0.06	0.10 ± 0.14	0.13 ± 0.19	0.10 ± 0.13	0.05 ± 0.10	0.07 ± 0.10	0.09 ± 0.12	0.07 ± 0.09	0.02 ± 0.04	0.07 ± 0.12	0.08 ± 0.13
Basophilic erythroblasts	0.24 ± 0.25	0.34 ± 0.33	0.57 ± 0.41	0.40 ± 0.33	0.24 ± 0.24	0.47 ± 0.33	0.32 ± 0.24	0.31 ± 0.24	0.30 ± 0.25	0.38 ± 0.37	0.50 ± 0.34
Early erythroblasts	0.27 ± 0.26	0.44 ± 0.42	0.71 ± 0.51	0.50 ± 0.38	0.28 ± 0.30	0.55 ± 0.36	0.41 ± 0.30	0.39 ± 0.28	0.39 ± 0.27	0.46 ± 0.36	0.59 ± 0.34
Polychromatic erythroblasts	13.06 ± 6.78	6.90 ± 4.45	13.06 ± 3.48	10.51 ± 3.39	6.84 ± 2.58	7.55 ± 2.35	7.30 ± 3.60	7.73 ± 3.39	6.83 ± 3.75	6.04 ± 1.56	6.97 ± 3.56
Orthochromatic erythroblasts	0.69 ± 0.73	0.54 ± 1.88	0.66 ± 0.82	0.70 ± 0.87	0.34 ± 0.30	0.46 ± 0.51	0.38 ± 0.56	0.39 ± 0.48	0.37 ± 0.51	0.50 ± 0.65	0.44 ± 0.49
Extruded nuclei	0.47 ± 0.46	0.16 ± 0.17	0.26 ± 0.22	0.19 ± 0.12	0.16 ± 0.17	0.14 ± 0.11	0.16 ± 0.22	0.22 ± 0.25	0.23 ± 0.25	0.17 ± 0.12	0.21 ± 0.19
Late erythroblasts	14.22 ± 7.14	7.60 ± 4.84	13.99 ± 3.82	11.40 ± 3.43	7.34 ± 2.54	8.16 ± 2.58	7.85 ± 4.11	8.34 ± 3.31	7.42 ± 4.11	6.72 ± 1.80	7.62 ± 3.63
Early/late ratio	1:50	1:15	1:18	1:22	1:23	1:15	1:17	1:19	1:17	1:15	1:10
Fetal erythroblasts	14.48 ± 7.24	8.04 ± 5.00	14.70 ± 3.86	11.90 ± 3.52	7.62 ± 2.56	8.70 ± 2.69	8.25 ± 4.31	8.72 ± 3.34	7.81 ± 4.26	7.18 ± 1.95	8.21 ± 3.71
Blood reticulocytes	4.18 ± 1.46	1.06 ± 1.13	3.39 ± 1.22	2.90 ± 0.91	1.65 ± 0.73	1.38 ± 0.65	1.74 ± 0.80	1.67 ± 0.52	1.79 ± 0.79	2.10 ± 0.91	1.84 ± 0.46
Neutrophils											
Promyelocytes	0.79 ± 0.91	0.76 ± 0.65	0.78 ± 0.68	0.76 ± 0.80	0.59 ± 0.51	0.87 ± 0.80	0.67 ± 0.66	0.41 ± 0.34	0.69 ± 0.71	0.67 ± 0.58	0.64 ± 0.59
Myelocytes	3.95 ± 2.93	2.50 ± 1.48	2.03 ± 1.14	2.24 ± 1.70	2.32 ± 1.59	2.73 ± 1.82	2.22 ± 1.25	2.07 ± 1.20	2.32 ± 1.14	2.48 ± 0.94	2.49 ± 1.39
Total early neutrophils	4.74 ± 3.43	3.27 ± 1.94	2.81 ± 1.62	3.00 ± 2.18	2.91 ± 2.01	3.60 ± 2.50	2.89 ± 1.71	2.48 ± 1.46	3.02 ± 1.52	3.16 ± 1.19	3.14 ± 1.75
Metamyelocytes	19.37 ± 4.84	11.34 ± 3.59	11.27 ± 3.38	11.93 ± 13.09	6.04 ± 3.63	11.89 ± 3.24	11.02 ± 3.12	11.80 ± 3.90	11.10 ± 3.82	12.48 ± 7.45	12.42 ± 4.15
Bands	28.89 ± 7.56	14.10 ± 4.63	13.15 ± 4.71	14.60 ± 7.54	13.93 ± 6.13	14.07 ± 5.48	14.00 ± 4.58	14.08 ± 4.53	14.02 ± 4.88	15.17 ± 4.20	14.20 ± 5.23
Mature neutrophils	7.37 ± 4.64	3.64 ± 2.97	3.07 ± 2.45	3.48 ± 1.62	4.27 ± 2.69	3.77 ± 2.44	4.85 ± 2.69	3.97 ± 2.29	5.65 ± 3.92	6.94 ± 3.88	6.31 ± 3.91
Late neutrophils	55.63 ± 7.98	29.08 ± 6.79	27.50 ± 6.88	31.00 ± 11.17	31.30 ± 7.80	29.73 ± 7.19	29.86 ± 6.74	29.86 ± 7.36	30.77 ± 8.69	34.60 ± 7.35	32.93 ± 7.01

Early/late neutrophil ratio	1:12	1:9	1:9	1:9	1:11	1:8	1:10	1:12	1:10	1:10	1:10
Total neutrophils	60.37 ± 8.66	32.35 ± 7.68	30.31 ± 7.27	34.01 ± 11.95	34.21 ± 8.61	33.12 ± 8.34	32.75 ± 7.03	32.33 ± 7.75	33.79 ± 8.76	37.76 ± 7.32	36.06 ± 7.40
Total eosinophils	2.70 ± 1.27	2.61 ± 1.40	2.50 ± 1.22	2.54 ± 1.46	2.37 ± 4.13	1.98 ± 0.86	2.08 ± 1.16	1.74 ± 1.08	1.92 ± 1.09	3.39 ± 1.93	2.70 ± 2.16
Total basophils	0.12 ± 0.20	0.07 ± 0.16	0.08 ± 0.10	0.09 ± 0.09	0.11 ± 0.14	0.09 ± 0.13	0.10 ± 0.13	0.11 ± 0.13	0.13 ± 0.15	0.27 ± 0.37	0.10 ± 0.12
Total myeloid cells	63.19 ± 9.10	35.03 ± 8.09	32.90 ± 7.85	36.64 ± 2.26	36.69 ± 8.91	35.40 ± 8.54	34.93 ± 7.52	34.18 ± 8.13	35.83 ± 8.84	41.42 ± 7.43	38.86 ± 7.92
Monocytes	0.88 ± 0.85	1.01 ± 0.89	0.91 ± 0.83	0.68 ± 0.56	0.75 ± 0.75	1.29 ± 1.06	1.21 ± 1.01	1.17 ± 0.97	1.46 ± 1.52	1.68 ± 1.09	2.12 ± 1.59
Miscellaneous cells											
Megakaryocytes	0.06 ± 0.15	0.05 ± 0.09	0.10 ± 0.13	0.06 ± 0.09	0.06 ± 0.06	0.08 ± 0.09	0.04 ± 0.07	0.09 ± 0.12	0.05 ± 0.08	0.00 ± 0.00	0.07 ± 0.12
Plasma cells	0.00 ± 0.02	0.02 ± 0.06	0.02 ± 0.05	0.00 ± 0.02	0.01 ± 0.03	0.05 ± 0.11	0.03 ± 0.07	0.01 ± 0.03	0.03 ± 0.07	0.07 ± 0.12	0.06 ± 0.08
Unknown blasts[b]	0.31 ± 0.31	0.62 ± 0.50	0.58 ± 0.50	0.63 ± 0.60	0.56 ± 0.53	0.5 ± 0.37	0.56 ± 0.48	0.42 ± 0.50	0.37 ± 0.33	0.46 ± 0.32	0.43 ± 0.45
Unknown cells	0.22 ± 0.34	0.21 ± 0.25	0.16 ± 0.24	0.19 ± 0.21	0.23 ± 0.25	0.17 ± 0.22	0.10 ± 0.15	0.14 ± 0.17	0.11 ± 0.14	0.13 ± 0.18	0.20 ± 0.23
Damaged cells	5.79 ± 2.78	5.50 ± 2.46	5.09 ± 1.78	4.75 ± 2.30	4.80 ± 2.29	4.86 ± 1.25	5.04 ± 1.08	4.89 ± 1.60	5.34 ± 2.19	4.99 ± 1.96	5.05 ± 2.15
Total	6.38 ± 2.84	6.39 ± 2.63	5.94 ± 1.94	5.63 ± 2.36	5.66 ± 2.30	5.66 ± 1.41	5.78 ± 1.74	5.55 ± 1.74	5.90 ± 2.03	5.65 ± 2.02	5.81 ± 2.16

[a] Transitional cells are defined as cells that range in size between small lymphocyte and blast cells and have finely dispersed nuclear chromatin, inconspicuous nucleoli, and a small amount of cytoplasm.
[b] Unknown blasts – cells with nucleoli and visible cytoplasm expanding all the way around the nucleus.
From Rosse et al. [22].

Table 2.6. Age-related changes of bone marrow lymphocyte subsets.

Markers	N	Less than 1 year of age (%)	N	1 to 4 years of age (%)	N	5 to 15 years of age (%)	N	Older than 15 years of age (%)
CD3+	11	11.3 (5.3–24.8)	20	11.4 (6.8–17.5)	13	19.3 (16.6–25.2)	11	34.8 (22.6–50.6)
CD4+	11	3.8 (2.0–9.3)	20	3.6 (2.1–5.2)	13	4.9 (4.2–7.3)	11	11.7 (8.0–13.9)
CD8+	11	7.2 (2.3–11.4)	20	7.2 (4.1–10.1)	13	13.8 (10.0–18.5)	11	24.1 (20.3–37.2)
CD4/CD8 ratio	11	0.9 (0.5–1.2)	20	0.5 (0.4–0.6)	13	0.4 (0.3–0.6)	11	0.4 (0.3–0.5)
CD7+	10	9.3 (5.0–24.4)	18	10.7 (6.2–16.7)	10	17.0 (13.4–20.8)	12	24.0 (20.6–39.9)
CD2+	10	9.4 (4.6–23.7)	17	13.0 (8.5–16.9)	11	20.0 (15.3–23.6)	12	34.1 (26.1–51.5)
CD19+	11	66.5 (44.1–70.4)	20	67.8 (53.5–78.1)	13	52.5 (41.6–58.4)	12	33.6 (16.5–40.3)
CD19+/CD10+	11	53.5 (23.1–64.7)	20	60.8 (39.8–67.2)	13	45.1 (32.7–53.1)	12	13.0 (6.0–19.1)
CD19+/CD20+	9	17.8 (6.0–30.2)	9	34.0 (25.8–38.6)	9	25.0 (24.2–32.0)	9	16.2 (12.3–22.7)
CD3− (CD16,56)+	11	4.8 (2.3–7.5)	20	3.4 (1.6–5.3)	13	2.7 (1.1–4.6)	11	4.4 (3.2–7.1)
CD33+/CD34+	11	4.4 (2.0–9.7)	20	4.0 (2.2–9.0)	13	4.8 (3.0–9.5)	11	6.0 (5.4–6.8)
CD14+	11	3.0 (0.0–4.7)	20	4.1 (0.7–5.0)	13	3.5 (0.4–4.5)	11	4.9 (1.0–7.0)
CD33-/CD34+	11	6.9 (2.3–9.8)	20	5.5 (2.8–8.7)	13	6.0 (2.0–9.5)	11	7.8 (5.3–9.5)
Male/Female		4/7		8/12		5/8		9/3

Distribution of the cellular subsets (%) in the lymphoid window exclude contamination by nucleated erythroid precursors.
Results are presented as median and range (25th to 75th percentiles).
Note: the samples are small and further confirmation of the results is warranted.
Adapted from Rego *et al.* [24].

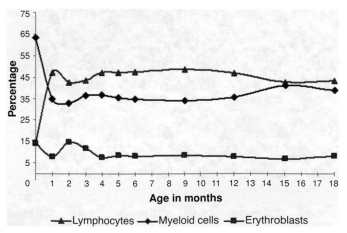

Fig. 2.4. Changes in the mean percentages of lymphocytes, myeloid cells, and erythroblasts in bone marrow from birth to 18 months of age. (Redrawn from Rosse *et al.* [22].)

The number of normal B-cell progenitors is increased in children with congenital or acquired cytopenias, anemia, non-hematologic diseases, or solid tumors, as well as in recovering BM after myeloablative chemotherapy and bone marrow transplantation (Fig. 2.6) [25, 27]. In terms of degree of maturation, the normal B-cell progenitors constitute a heterogeneous group of cells with a variable expression of CD10 and CD20 that can be demonstrated by flow cytometry (Fig. 2.7). Only the very immature, stage I progenitors are CD34 positive, and most of these cells are CD34 negative (Fig. 2.8). The hematogones need to be distinguished from leukemic B-lymphoblasts that show more uniform expression of CD34, CD10, or CD20 resulting from a maturation arrest as part of the pathogenesis of the disease.

After the fourth year of life, the number of B-cells declines progressively, and this decline is accompanied by an increase in the number of CD3+ T-lymphocytes. Regardless of age, all

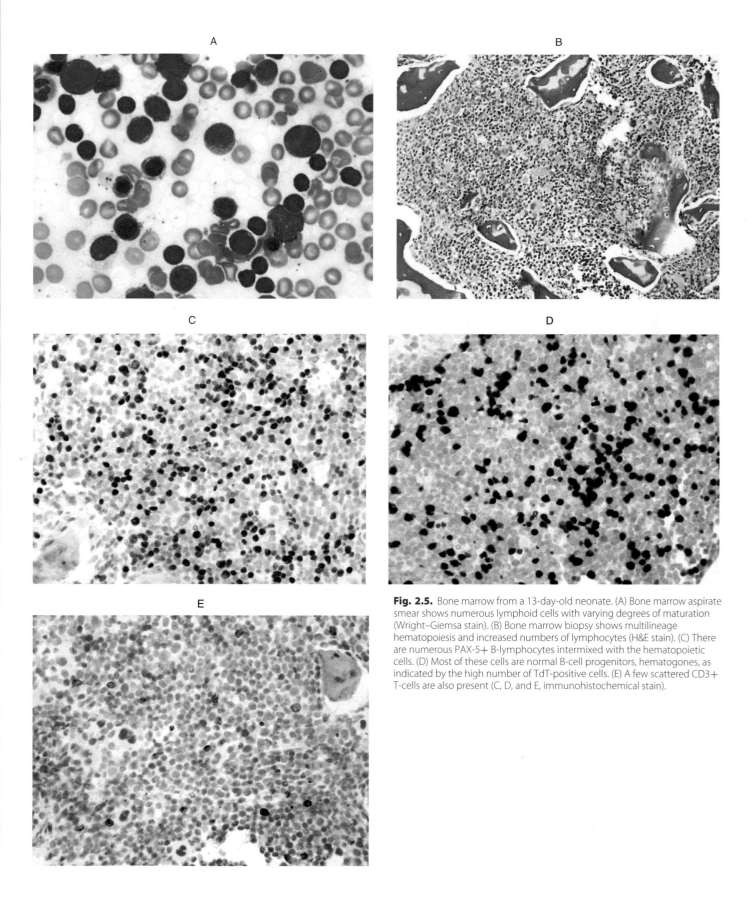

Fig. 2.5. Bone marrow from a 13-day-old neonate. (A) Bone marrow aspirate smear shows numerous lymphoid cells with varying degrees of maturation (Wright–Giemsa stain). (B) Bone marrow biopsy shows multilineage hematopoiesis and increased numbers of lymphocytes (H&E stain). (C) There are numerous PAX-5+ B-lymphocytes intermixed with the hematopoietic cells. (D) Most of these cells are normal B-cell progenitors, hematogones, as indicated by the high number of TdT-positive cells. (E) A few scattered CD3+ T-cells are also present (C, D, and E, immunohistochemical stain).

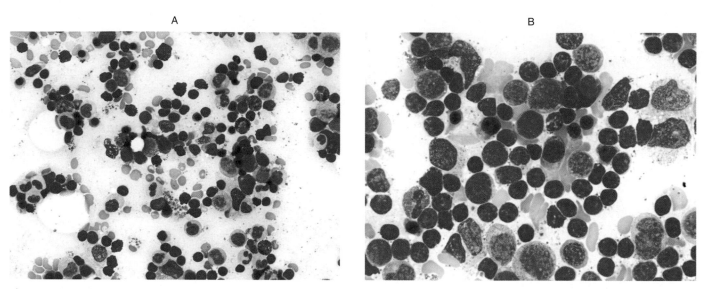

Fig. 2.6. Bone marrow from a 10-month-old infant with congenital cytopenias shows increased numbers of hematogones (Wright–Giemsa stain). (A) The marrow aspirate smear shows a heterogeneous population of lymphoid cells of variable size and degree of maturation. (B) These cells have round to oval to irregular nuclear contours, homogeneous chromatin, and very scant excentric cytoplasm. The least mature forms are larger and may have nucleoli. Some immature hematogones have irregular nuclear contours.

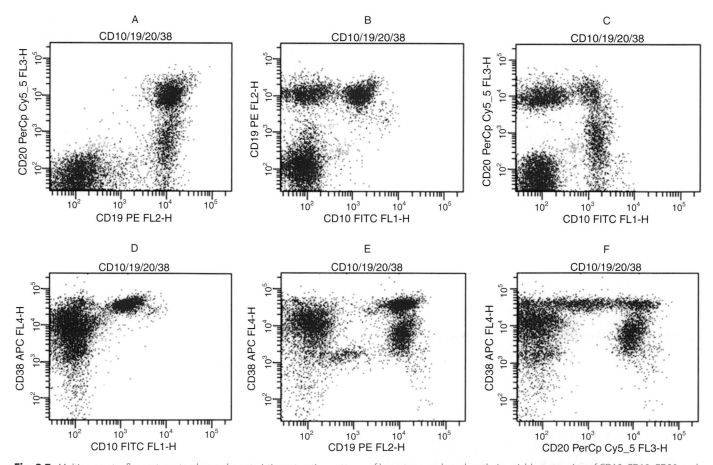

Fig. 2.7. Multiparameter flow cytometry shows characteristic maturation patterns of hematogones based on their variable expression of CD10, CD19, CD20, and CD38. (A) While most hematogones express the early B-cell marker CD19, CD20, a late B-cell marker, is negative in a subset of cells. (B) CD10 helps to characterize these cells further. The less-mature B-cells are CD10+, while the more-mature forms are CD10 negative. (C) This is the characteristic inverted "J" pattern resulting from a variable expression of CD10 and CD20. There are three populations of B-cells: mature B-cells (CD20+/CD10−), upper left; immature B-cells (CD20−/CD10+), lower right; and intermediate forms (CD20+/CD10+), upper right. In this case, the more-mature forms predominate. (D) Hematogones have a characteristic bright expression of CD38. (E) The intensity of CD38 decreases with maturation. (F) The CD20/CD38 shows the maturation pattern as well. These antibody combinations are particularly helpful in distinguishing the normal B-cell progenitors from leukemic blasts.

A

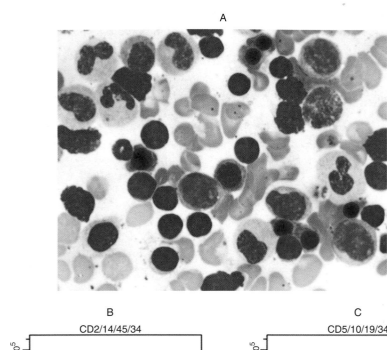

Fig. 2.8. Bone marrow aspirate from a four-month-old infant. (A) Aspirate smear shows increased number of a heterogeneous population of lymphoid cells. The least-mature form resembles leukemic blasts or other non-hematopoietic small blue cell tumors, and the mature forms are easily recognizable as small lymphocytes (Wright–Giemsa stain). (B–E) Multiparameter flow cytometry confirms the antigenic heterogeneity of these cells: (B) CD45 is variably expressed, from dim to bright; (C) While most of the these cells are CD34 negative, a small subset is CD34 positive; (D) Based on the expression of CD10 and CD34, the hematogones can be divided into stage I, least-mature forms (CD34+/CD10−); stage II, intermediate forms (CD34+/CD10+); and, stage III, most mature forms (CD34−/CD10+). (E) Characteristic CD10/CD20 expression pattern. Note, in this case, unlike the case in Figure 2.7, there is a predominance of stage I and II hematogones and lower number of stage III forms.

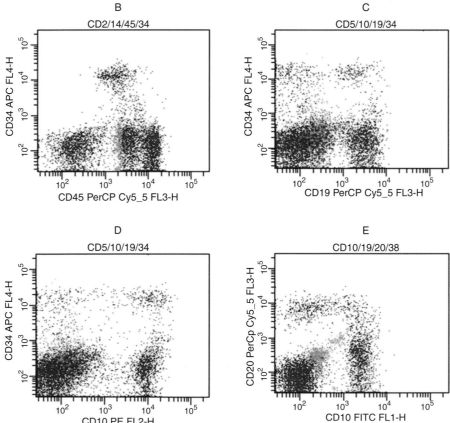

T-cells in the marrow are mature and express either CD4 or CD8. The percentage of CD8-positive cells is at least twice the percentage of CD4-positive cells. The number of NK-cells in the BM is low and is not age dependent.

Some studies have suggested that the proliferative capacity of BM in children and young adults determined by Ki-67+ cells is higher, while the apoptotic rate of children and young adults is lower as compared to older people [26].

While there are well-documented race-related differences in the peripheral blood of Caucasian and African-American children, the racial differences in the bone marrow composition are negligible. The only difference that has been demonstrated is a slight relative erythroid hyperplasia in African-American infants as compared to Caucasian infants [28]. Otherwise, in terms of bone marrow composition, no significant differences are known.

A

B

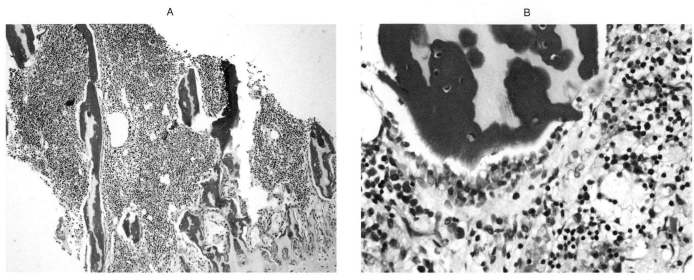

Fig. 2.9. Bone marrow biopsy from a four-month-old infant (H&E stain). (A) Incomplete ossification of the bony trabeculae. (B) There is prominent osteoblastic rimming.

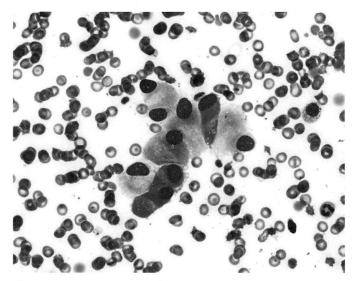

Fig. 2.10. Bone marrow aspirate from a 15-month-old child shows a cluster of osteoblasts (Wright–Giemsa stain).

Table 2.7. Most frequent indications for bone marrow examination in children.

Investigation of abnormal complete blood cell counts and peripheral blood smear morphology suggestive of bone marrow pathology
Unexplained organomegaly in children with mass lesions inaccessible for biopsy
Following the response to therapy in children with acute leukemia, and detection of minimal residual disease
Suspected bone marrow relapse
Staging of patients with non-Hodgkin and Hodgkin lymphomas and solid tumors
Unexplained focal bony lesions on imaging studies
For microbiological cultures
Evaluation of iron stores. Note: not an indication in young children
Evaluation of bone marrow engraftment after hematopoietic stem cell transplant

Active bone remodeling is normal for children and is expected, unlike for adults where it may signify pathology. Prominent osteoblastic rimming, osteoid seams, and incomplete ossification are frequently seen in pediatric BM biopsies (Fig. 2.9). Single or clusters of osteoblasts are frequently found in aspirate smears (Fig. 2.10).

Bone marrow examination in children

Bone marrow examination is essential for diagnosis and follow-up of bone marrow disorders. As with adults, the diagnosis in children is based on the integration of data from various diagnostic approaches, including peripheral blood counts and smear, BM aspirate smears, particle clot sections, BM trephine biopsy and imprint morphology, along with the results of other relevant studies – cytochemistry, immunophenotypic analysis, cytogenetic, and molecular studies [29–31].

The marrow cellularity is best determined through bone marrow biopsies or marrow clot sections. In children, however, BM aspirates are more frequently performed and BM biopsies may not be performed routinely. Yet, the BM aspirates alone may not provide a reliable estimate of the BM cellularity and composition since they contain a mixture of bone marrow with sinusoidal blood. For example, comparing the cellularity in BM biopsies, aspirate smears, and volumetric measurements of buffy coat of 53 children with leukemia or aplastic anemia, Gruppo found discrepancies in 39% of the cases where BM was estimated to be normo- or hypercellular by biopsy but was considered moderately or severely hypocellular when aspirate smears were evaluated [32]. In this study, the volumetric measurements of buffy coat provided the least-acceptable results.

The most frequent *indications* for bone marrow examination in children are summarized in Tables 2.7 and 2.8. In children,

Table 2.8. Indications for bone marrow biopsy in children.

Bone marrow aspirate dry tap in a patient with acute leukemia
Workup of a child with peripheral cytopenias and suspected occult neoplasm
Suspected bone marrow failure syndrome
Staging for non-Hodgkin and Hodgkin lymphoma or metastatic neuroblastoma or rhabdomyosarcoma
Follow-up of the response to therapy in children with metastatic disease
Prior to hematopoietic stem cell transplantation
– Determine presence/absence of residual disease
– Assess cellularity and degree of stromal damage and iron overload
After hematopoietic stem cell transplant
– Determine engraftment, graft failure, residual disease

BM studies are undertaken for the diagnosis of suspected primary bone marrow pathology or metastatic disease, to follow the patient's response to therapy, or for evaluation of the marrow prior to and following a hematopoietic stem cell transplant. However, in the case of young children, unlike adults, BM aspirates along with peripheral blood may be sufficient for the establishment of the diagnosis of acute leukemia. Thus, the indications for a BM biopsy in young children are limited to those instances when the BM aspirate and PB (peripheral blood) are insufficient to provide the necessary information to establish a diagnosis.

In children with acute leukemia, the response to therapy and detection of minimal residual disease (MRD) is a standard of care. Since the presence of MRD is an important predictor of relapse, BM studies are routinely performed after the first week of induction (day 8), the end of induction (day 29), and the end of consolidation in children with precursor B-cell acute lymphoblastic leukemia. The presence of MRD at day 29 is associated with a shorter event-free survival in all risk groups [33]. By contrast, a lack of MRD is associated with a favorable outcome [34].

BM studies are helpful and may be the initial workup for a child with peripheral cytopenias and suspected occult malignancy or the presence of a mass that is not easily accessible for sampling. In such cases, both marrow aspirates and biopsies have a higher yield in reaching the proper diagnosis than either of these techniques alone [35]. Bilateral bone marrow studies are a part of the staging of children with neuroblastoma and rhabdomyosarcoma. For the rest of the pediatric small round blue cell tumors, BM studies are performed only in rare instances of a widespread disease. BM is seldom aspirated for microbiological cultures.

In young children, BM studies are not indicated for the determination of iron stores, since stainable iron is absent from the marrow during the first year of life and the storage of iron progressively increases and reaches adult levels only by the fifth to sixth year [36]. Similarly, BM studies are not required in the initial evaluation of children with thrombocytopenia prior to initiation of steroid therapy, since such studies have been shown to contribute little and not to change significantly the quality-adjusted life years of such children [37].

The posterior iliac crest, anterior iliac crest, and the tibia are the most frequent sites of BM sampling in children. In newborns and neonates, conventional BM biopsies are difficult to perform and alternative techniques, such as obtaining marrow clot sections, can be successfully utilized [38]. Clot sections with marrow particles contain preserved BM architecture so that they provide information on the bone marrow cellularity and the number of megakaryocytes. Such sections can also be used for immunohistochemical stains or other special stains. In older children, the iliac crest is most frequently sampled.

The requirements for an adult BM biopsy of bone marrow of at least 1.5–2 cm in length [29, 30] may not be achievable in most young children. While there are no well-established requirements for the length of bone marrow biopsies in children, the general rule is that if the biopsy does provide information relevant to the main question prompting the BM studies, it can be considered adequate.

In the absence of particles or megakaryocytes, or other hematopoietic precursors, the sample should be reported as "dry tap" or peripheral blood [30]. However, BM aspirate smears at day 8 and 15 of induction chemotherapy are usually paucicellular and do not contain hematopoietic elements since the marrow has not regenerated after the initial cytoreduction following induction chemotherapy. In such instances, BM biopsies along with flow cytometry of aspirate smears will provide more valuable information to determine the presence of minimal residual disease and the degree of BM regeneration.

The BM aspirates should be reviewed first at low-power magnification to determine the number and cellularity of marrow particles and the number of megakaryocytes, and also scanned for clumps of tumor or abnormal cells of low incidence. The morphological assessment of the hematopoiesis at higher magnification provides valuable information on the composition of marrow particles, cytological details, and cell inclusions. Both quantitative and qualitative evaluation of the erythroid, myeloid, and lymphoid components as well as of the megakaryocytes are important in generating a differential diagnosis. Similarly to adults, the nucleated differential count (NDC) in children assesses the hematopoietic activity and compares proportions of the different cell lineages. The myeloid to erythroid ratio should also be documented. The cellularity of BM particles can be evaluated by assessing several particles in smears. However, it is best assessed on trephine biopsies.

Bone marrow reporting in children should follow the established guidelines that are applicable to adults [30, 31]. This includes quantitative and qualitative comments on all cell lineages – myeloid and erythroid progenitors with M : E ratio, megakaryocytes, lymphocytes, and plasma cells – and any abnormal cells such as blasts, increased number or abnormal mast cells, histiocytes displaying hemophagocytosis, and the presence of cells extrinsic to the bone marrow. The BM cellularity can be described as acellular, reduced, normal, increased, or markedly increased. The appearance of the particles as well as the presence of stromal damage, chemotherapy effect, or other stromal changes should be noted.

The final BM interpretation should be made in the context of the clinical and preliminary diagnostic findings. The bone marrow diagnosis or differential diagnosis, when applicable, should be in accord with the international consensus guidelines [29]. The findings of the smear aspirate and the trephine biopsy should always be correlated, and if there are major discrepancies, the reasons need to be explained. Flow cytometric findings, cytogenetics, and molecular studies should be incorporated in the pathology report and should correlate with the BM morphologic findings. Lastly, the findings should be correlated with the previous results if the studies are performed to monitor the disease progression or response to therapy.

References

1. **Cumano A, Godin I.** Ontogeny of the hematopoietic system. *Annual Review of Immunology.* 2007;**25**:745–785.

2. **Palis J.** Ontogeny of erythropoiesis. *Current Opinion in Hematology.* 2008;**15**:155–161.

3. **Mikkola HKA, Orkin SH.** The journey of developing hematopoietic stem cells. *Development.* 2006;**133**:3733–3744.

4. **Kennedy M, D'Souza SL, Lynch-Kattman M, Schwantz S, Keller G.** Development of the hemangioblast defines the onset of hematopoiesis in human ES cell differentiation cultures. *Blood.* 2007;**109**:2679–2687.

5. **Orkin SH, Zon LI.** Hematopoiesis: an evolving paradigm for stem cell biology. *Cell.* 2008;**132**:631–644.

6. **Heissig B, Ohki Y, Sato Y,** *et al.* A role for niches in hematopoietic cell development. *Hematology.* 2005;**10**:247–253.

7. **Rafii S, Mohle R, Shapiro F, Frey BM, Moore MA.** Regulation of hematopoiesis by microvascular endothelium. *Leukemia and Lymphoma.* 1997;**27**:375–386.

8. **Charbord P, Tavian M, Humeau L, Peault B.** Early ontogeny of the human marrow from long bones: an immunohistochemical study of hematopoiesis and its microenvironment. *Blood.* 1996;**87**:4109–4119.

9. **Chen LT, Weiss L.** The development of vertebral bone marrow of human fetuses. *Blood.* 1975;**46**:389–408.

10. **Islam A, Glomski C, Henderson ES.** Endothelial cells and hematopoiesis: a light microscopic study of fetal, normal, and pathologic human bone marrow in plastic-embedded sections. *Anatomical Record.* 1992;**233**:440–452.

11. **Wilpshaar J, Joekes EC, Lim FTH,** *et al.* Magnetic resonance imaging of fetal bone marrow for quantitative definition of the human fetal stem cell compartment. *Blood.* 2002;**100**:451–457.

12. **Slayton WB, Juul SE, Calhoun DA,** *et al.* Hematopoiesis in the liver and marrow of human fetuses at 5 to 16 weeks postconception: quantitative assessment of macrophage and neutrophil populations. *Pediatric Research.* 1998;**43**:774–782.

13. **Muench MO, Namikawa R.** Disparate regulation of human fetal erythropoiesis by the microenvironments of the liver and bone marrow. *Blood Cells, Molecules, and Diseases.* 2001;**27**:377–390.

14. **Wickramasinghe SN.** Bone marrow. In: Mills SE, ed. *Histology for Pathologists.* 3rd edn. Philadelphia: Lippincott Williams & Wilkins; 2007:800–36.

15. **Foucar K, Viswanatha DS, Wilson CS.** Normal anatomy and histology of bone marrow. In Foucar K, Viswanatha DS, Wilson CS, eds. *Non-Neoplastic Disorders of Bone Marrow.* Atlas of Nontumor Pathology, Series I. Washington, DC: American Registry of Pathology in collaboration with the Armed Forces Institute of Pathology; 2008, 1–40.

16. **Yin T, Li L.** The stem cell niches in bone. *The Journal of Clinical Investigation.* 2006;**116**:1195–1201.

17. **Cantor AB, Orkin SH.** Transcriptional regulation of erythropoiesis: an affair involving multiple partners. *Oncogene.* 2002;**21**:3368–3376.

18. **Chasis JA, Mohandas N.** Erythroblastic islands: niches for erythropoiesis. *Blood.* 2008;**112**:470–478.

19. **Friebert SE, Shepardson LB, Shurin SB, Rosenthal GE, Rosenthal NS.** Pediatric bone marrow cellularity: Are we expecting too much? *Journal of Pediatric Hematology/Oncology.* 1998;**20**(5): 439–443.

20. **Sturgeon P.** Volumetric and microscopic pattern of bone marrow in normal infants and children: III. Histologic pattern. *Pediatrics.* 1951;**7**: 774–781.

21. **Glaser K, Limarzi LR, Poncher HG.** Special Reviews: Cellular composition of the bone marrow in normal infants and children. *Pediatrics.* 1950;**6**:789–824.

22. **Rosse C, Kraemer MJ, Dillon TL, McFarland R, Smith NJ.** Bone marrow cell populations of normal infants; the predominance of lymphocytes. *Journal of Laboratory and Clinical Medicine.* 1977;**89**:1225–1240.

23. **Sturgeon P.** Volumetric and microscopic pattern of bone marrow in normal infants and children. II. Cytologic pattern. *Pediatrics.* 1951;**7**: 642–650.

24. **Rego EM, Garcia AB, Viana SR, Falcão RP.** Age-related changes of lymphocyte subsets in normal bone marrow biopsies. *Cytometry.* 1998;**34**:22–29.

25. **Longacre TA, Foucar K, Crago S,** *et al.* Hematogones: a multiparameter analysis of bone marrow precursor cells. *Blood.* 1989;**73**:543–552.

26. **Ogawa T, Kitagawa M, Hirokawa K.** Age-related changes of human bone marrow: a histometric estimation of proliferative cells, apoptotic cells, T cells, B cells and macrophages. *Mechanisms of Ageing and Development.* 2000;**117**:57–68.

27. **McKenna RW, Washington LT, Aquino DB, Picker LJ, Kroft SH.** Immunophenotypic analysis of hematogones (B-lymphocyte precursors) in 662 consecutive bone marrow specimens by 4-color flow cytometry. *Blood.* 2001;**98**:2498–2507.

28. **Kraemer MJ, Hunter R, Rosse C, Smith NJ.** Race-related differences in peripheral blood and in bone marrow cell populations of American black and American white infants. *Journal of the National Medical Association.* 1977;**69**: 327–331.

29. **Swerdlow SH, Campo E, Harris NL,** *et al.* (eds.). *WHO Classification of Tumours of Haematopoietic and Lymphoid Tissues* (4th edn.). Lyon: IARC Press; 2008.

30. **Lee S-H, Erber WN, Porwit A, Tomonaga M, Peterson LC.** ICSH guidelines for the standardization of bone marrow specimens and reports. *International Journal of Laboratory Hematology.* 2008;**30**:349–364.

31. **Peterson LC, Agosti SJ, Hoyer JD, Hematology clinical Microscopy Resource Committee, Members of the Cancer Committee CoAP.** Protocol for the examination of specimens from patients with hematopoietic neoplasms of the bone marrow: a basis for checklists. *Archives of Pathology &* *Laboratory Medicine.* 2002;**126**:1050–1056.

32. **Gruppo RA, Lampkin BC, Granger S.** Bone marrow cellularity determination: comparison of the biopsy, aspirate, and buffy coat. *Blood.* 1977;**49**:29–31.

33. **Borowitz MJ, Devidas M, Hunger SP,** *et al.* Clinical significance of minimal residual disease in childhood acute lymphoblastic leukemia and its relationship to other prognostic factors: a Children's Oncology Group study. *Blood.* 2008;**111**:5477–5485.

34. **Campana D.** Minimal residual disease in acute lymphoblastic leukemia. *Seminars in Hematology.* 2009;**46**:100–106.

35. **Aronica PA, Pirrotta VT, Yunis EJ, Penchansky L.** Detection of neuroblastoma in the bone marrow: biopsy versus aspiration. *Journal of Pediatric Hematology/Oncology.* 1998; **20**:330–334.

36. **Penchansky L.** *Pediatric Bone Marrow.* Berlin: Springer-Verlag; 2004.

37. **Klaassen RJ, Doyle JJ, Krahn MD, Blanchette VS, Naglie G.** Initial bone marrow aspiration in childhood idiopathic thrombocytopenia: decision analysis. *Journal of Pediatric Hematology/Oncology.* 2001;**23**:511–518.

38. **Sola MC, Rimsza LM, Christensen RD.** A bone marrow biopsy technique suitable for use in neonates. *British Journal of Haematology.* 1999;**107**: 458–460.

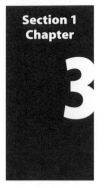

Disorders of erythrocyte production

Nutritional deficiencies, iron deficient, and sideroblastic anemia

Angela E. Thomas and Barbara J. Bain

Introduction

Defects in hemoglobin synthesis and erythroid nuclear maturation both give rise to disorders of erythrocyte production. Defects of hemoglobin synthesis can result from impaired heme synthesis, as seen in iron deficiency and sideroblastic anemia, or from impaired globin chain synthesis, which occurs in the thalassemia syndromes. Defects in erythroid nuclear maturation are seen in cobalamin (vitamin B_{12}) and folate deficiency and also in the rare hereditary abnormalities of cobalamin or folate metabolism, and result in defective erythrocyte production. Abnormal nuclear maturation is also present in other metabolic defects associated with megaloblastic anemia, such as Lesch–Nyhan syndrome, orotic aciduria, and thiamine-responsive megaloblastic anemia. In the anemia of chronic disorder, iron regulation is maladjusted so that iron is "locked away" and unavailable for erythropoiesis. Markedly ineffective erythropoiesis is seen where there are defects of nuclear maturation, in sideroblastic anemia, and in the thalassemia syndromes; iron deficiency and the anemia of chronic disorder are associated with decreased erythropoiesis. Of the nutritional deficiencies causing anemia, the commonest is iron deficiency. This is so for both children and adults in all parts of the world. The deficiency may be caused by insufficient iron in the diet, lack of absorption of iron, or increased losses primarily due to bleeding. Deficiency of vitamin B_{12} is rare in children; in neonates it is usually secondary to occult vitamin B_{12} deficiency in the mother, but when diagnosed in infancy or childhood is more often due to an inborn error of metabolism. Study of such abnormalities has helped elucidate the absorptive mechanisms and metabolic pathways of vitamin B_{12}. Folate deficiency too may occur in neonates due to maternal deficiency, but in the infant or child can be secondary to lack of intake, although this is less often seen now in countries where common foodstuffs are fortified with folate. Folate deficiency can be secondary to impaired absorption which is seen, for example, in inflammatory bowel disease and celiac disease, or to increased requirement as occurs in chronic hemolytic anemias. Some drugs such as methotrexate and anti-epileptic medications have an anti-folate action.

Iron

Iron is one of the most common elements on earth and makes up about 5% of the Earth's crust. It is essential to nearly all living organisms, but free iron is toxic and can cause significant tissue damage due to its role in the generation of free oxygen radicals. Perhaps because of this and the abundance of iron, the body has developed regulatory pathways to limit iron absorption, rather than enhance it, and has also developed methods of transportation and storage to allow iron to move between tissues and cells safely and efficiently.

Functional iron within cells in animals, plants, and fungi may be stored as heme, the prosthetic subunit (that is the non-protein component of a conjugated protein) of the hemoprotein family of metalloproteins. Heme consists of an atom of iron at the center of a porphyrin ring, and is an essential component of cytochrome proteins which mediate redox reactions and are involved in steroidogenesis and detoxification (cytochrome P450) and of oxygen-carrying proteins such as hemoglobin and myoglobin. Non-heme iron-dependent enzymes include ribonucleotide reductase, important in DNA synthesis, and aconitase, important in the tricarboxylic acid cycle which is of central significance in all living cells that use oxygen as part of cellular respiration.

Iron homeostasis is achieved through a fine balance between absorption of iron, utilization, storage, and loss. There is no controlled mechanism for iron excretion, iron being lost through shedding of cells, which accounts for only 1–2 mg iron per day in adults, and blood loss, which is variable, may be pathological and clearly differs between men and women during childbearing years. Under physiological conditions, iron enters the body through absorption of dietary iron, and this absorption is precisely regulated to balance the small losses. Disruption to this balance will result in either deficiency or overload of iron. Iron deficiency results from excess losses which occur mainly due to bleeding but also from the physiological loss in pregnancy where iron is transported across the placenta from the mother to the fetus. Inadequate intake, commonly due to dietary insufficiency but also to lack of absorption, will result in iron

Diagnostic Pediatric Hematopathology, ed. Maria A. Proytcheva. Published by Cambridge University Press.
© Cambridge University Press 2011.

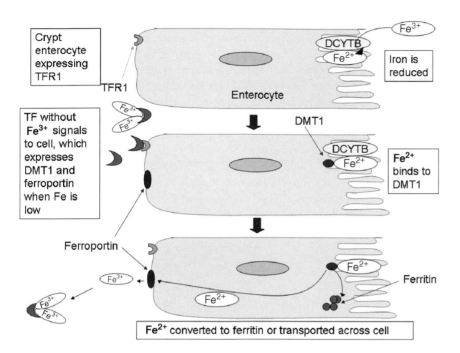

Fig. 3.1. Ferric iron is reduced to ferrous iron before passing through the apical border of the enterocyte into the cell where it is either stored as ferritin or transported across the cell to the non-enteral surface. Ferrous iron is oxidized to ferric iron as it is exported and then binds to transferrin for transport in the blood stream. Fe^{3+}, ferric iron; Fe^{2+}, ferrous iron; DCYTB, duodenal cytochrome b; TFR1, transferrin receptor 1; DMT1, divalent metal transporter 1; TF, transferrin.

deficiency. Iron overload is seen when there is failure of regulation, due to genetic defects in the regulatory proteins or to repeated blood transfusions allowing iron to bypass the absorptive control mechanisms.

Dietary iron

Iron in the diet comes from both heme and non-heme iron; of the two, heme iron is more easily absorbed. Non-heme iron in the diet is almost exclusively in its ferric (Fe^{3+}) form and needs to be reduced to the ferrous (Fe^{2+}) form before passing through the apical border of the enterocytes. Enhancers of non-heme iron absorption include acids such as hydrochloric acid, produced by the stomach, amino acids from the digestion of meat, and vitamin C [1]. Breast milk also enhances iron absorption from foodstuffs [2], and although low in total iron content, the iron is in a highly bioavailable form. Absorption of non-heme iron is reduced by phytates (organic polyphosphates) found in cereal grains, legumes, and nuts, and by tannins found in tea [1]. Drugs that reduce gastric acid secretion such as H_2 antagonists and acid pump blockers reduce iron absorption, but these are not commonly prescribed for children. It follows that a meal of vegetables eaten with meat and foods or drinks containing vitamin C will provide more iron than a vegetable- and cereal-based meal, particularly if taken with tea [3].

Iron transport

The pathway for the absorption of heme iron is not known, although heme carrier protein 1 (HCP1) has recently been found in duodenal enterocytes [4]. Its absorption is independent of gastric pH and increases with increased erythropoietic activity. In contrast, the pathways for the absorption of non-heme iron have been well characterized [5–7]. The mechanism of iron uptake depends on the cell type, and at least three mechanisms have been described. Direct transport of iron across the cell membrane occurs in intestinal cells and hepatocytes; cells such as the erythron and probably the hepatocyte have modified the transport mechanism to include an iron concentration step within subcellular compartments, and macrophages ingest senescent red cells and, through lysis of the cells, recycle the iron from the hemoglobin after breakdown by heme oxygenase.

Iron uptake from the intestine

Iron absorption takes place in the acidic environment of the proximal small intestine, with the absorptive capacity decreasing distally. The majority of non-heme iron is in the ferric form (Fe^{3+}) and needs to be reduced to the ferrous form (Fe^{2+}) by a ferrireductase which has recently been identified as duodenal cytochrome b (DCYTB) [8]. The ferrous iron accompanied by H^+ ions passes through the apical bilayer of the enterocytes by means of the membrane protein divalent metal transporter 1 (DMT1), into the cytoplasm of the cell [9]. Here, some of the iron is retained but then lost from the body when the enterocytes are shed after around two days.

The remaining iron leaves the cell via another membrane transporter, ferroportin, in the basolateral membrane [10]. Hephaestin, a transmembrane, copper-dependent ferroxidase [11–13], facilitates this process, probably by oxidizing the ferrous iron to ferric iron. Ferric iron is insoluble in the neutral pH of plasma and is therefore bound to the transport protein transferrin for which it has a high affinity. This protein has three main functions: to bind the iron so that it is soluble in plasma, to allow it to circulate in a non-toxic form, and to transport it to cells bearing transferrin receptors. A diagram of intestinal non-heme iron absorption is shown in Figure 3.1.

Iron uptake from the plasma

The majority of the transferrin-bound iron is taken up by the developing erythroid cells which express transferrin receptors, shedding them as they mature. Transferrin, with its two molecules of ferric iron, binds to the transferrin receptor and is then internalized, forming an endosome. The pH within the endosome is lowered by a proton pump, allowing the iron to be released from the transferrin and transported across the endosomal membrane into the cytoplasm, probably by DMT1. Once within the cytoplasm, iron is either stored or utilized to form heme. The transferrin, as apotransferrin, returns with the transferrin receptor to the cell surface where, at a neutral pH, the latter dissociates so that both the transferrin receptor and the transferrin can be reused. The expression of transferrin receptors is linked to intracellular iron stores and erythropoietic activity, with increased expression when iron is needed; it is not affected by inflammation. As the red cells mature, the number of transferrin receptors decreases, and cleaved fragments of the transmembrane receptor are found in plasma; these are derived primarily from reticulocytes [14]. Levels are raised in iron deficiency and ineffective erythropoiesis, but are unaffected by inflammation [15].

Other cells that express transferrin receptors include tumor cells and activated lymphocytes. This is presumably to optimize iron uptake to support rapid cell proliferation. Transferrin receptors are also present on the microvilli of the placenta [16], and aid iron transfer from the maternal to the fetal circulation.

Hepatocytes express transferrin receptors and probably take up iron using this mechanism. However, they also have the capability to take up iron that is not bound to transferrin. This occurs in pathological states where the capacity of transferrin, which is usually only about one-third bound, is exceeded, and is seen where repeated blood transfusions have been given or in hemochromatosis where there is disruption to iron homeostasis due to mutations in the genes of regulatory proteins.

The macrophages of the reticuloendothelial system recycle iron by ingesting senescent red cells as described. The recycled iron is either stored or released into the plasma depending on need. The concentration of plasma iron and thus transferrin saturation is dependent on macrophage iron release and utilization of iron by erythroid cells.

Iron storage

Iron is stored in cells either as heme within hemoproteins or as ferritin. The hemoproteins include the cytochromes and oxygen-carrying proteins such as hemoglobin and myoglobin. Ferritin is the main intracellular iron-storage protein, keeping it in a soluble, non-toxic form and allowing its release when needed. Ferritin is a globular protein consisting of 24 subunits, and can store several thousand iron atoms. The iron in ferritin can sometimes be deposited in the tissues in an insoluble form, hemosiderin; deposition, although often asymptomatic,

can lead to organ damage. Ferritin and hemosiderin are both increased in iron overload syndromes. If the capacity of ferritin to store iron is exceeded, iron is stored in parenchymal cells such as hepatocytes, which can take up non-transferrin-bound iron from the plasma, and other tissues including the myocardium and pancreas, causing significant damage. Iron from senescent red cells is stored in macrophages, and thus these cells become overloaded before parenchymal cells in iron overload due to repeated transfusions.

Although most ferritin is found within cells, some is secreted into the plasma, and it is likely that some escapes from necrotic cells. Levels reflect total body stores, falling with iron depletion and rising with iron loading. However, ferritin is an acute phase protein and increases with inflammation and infection, especially if chronic, and also in liver disease. It is regulated by the protein hepcidin (see below).

Iron regulation

Iron absorption must be balanced against iron loss while allowing circulation of iron between storage pools, developing erythrocytes and iron-containing enzymes. The regulatory mechanism must be responsive to the body's need for iron, for instance reducing iron absorption when stores are replete and increasing absorption and release from storage pools in response to increased erythropoietic activity or hypoxia. Inflammatory states also have a regulatory effect on iron, resulting in reduced availability of iron which may be protective in certain circumstances (see below). It appears that responses to storage iron, erythropoietic activity, hypoxia, and inflammation are mediated through the same pathway. Hepcidin is a systemic iron-regulatory hormone, which controls the absorption of iron from the gut and export of iron from the tissues to the plasma where it is accessible to developing erythrocytes [17]. Hepcidin binds and degrades ferroportin, and through this mechanism has a negative regulatory effect on iron absorption and mobilization. Thus, when hepcidin levels are decreased, more iron is available from the diet and from storage in macrophages and hepatocytes. Hepcidin synthesis is regulated in several ways: it is induced by dietary iron, it decreases in response to increased erythropoiesis and hypoxia, and increases in response to iron-loading and inflammation [18]. This last response, mediated by interleukin (IL)-6, is thought to contribute to the anemia of chronic disease where the iron is "locked" in the macrophages and unavailable for erythropoiesis. Due to lack of release of iron from macrophages, plasma iron falls rapidly by about 30%, reflecting the high turnover of iron through the transferrin compartment. It is possible that low serum iron has a role in host defense, as the growth of some microbes is enhanced by iron. Erythropoietic activity, however, is the most potent suppressor of hepcidin, predominating over the iron signal, as is seen in untransfused patients with thalassemia intermedia, where erythropoietic activity is increased but ineffective and hepcidin levels are low despite high plasma transferrin and ferritin levels [19, 20].

Hemoglobin synthesis

Hemoglobin synthesis requires the coordinated production of heme and globin. Lack of globin production is discussed in the chapter on thalassemias and will not be discussed here. Heme production starts and finishes in the mitochondria of the cells, with the intermediate steps taking place in the cytosol. The initial and rate-limiting step involves the enzyme δ-aminolevulinic acid synthetase (ALAS) in the production of δ-aminolevulinic acid from succinyl-CoA (succinyl coenzyme A) and glycine; δ-aminolevulinic acid is then transported to the cytosol to produce a coproprotoporphyrin ring. This molecule re-enters the mitochondrion and a protoporphyrin IX ring is produced, into which iron is inserted by the enzyme ferrochelatase. This process can be disrupted through loss of function of the enzymes involved but also with lack of iron. If iron is not available, trace amounts of zinc will be incorporated instead, resulting in a measurable increase in zinc protoporphyrin (ZPP). In sideroblastic anemias where enzymes are absent or reduced, erythrocyte protoporphyrin levels can rise, as they can with certain drugs and toxins, including ethanol and lead, which inhibit heme synthesis [21–23].

Age and iron needs

The need for iron varies during infancy and childhood depending on initial stores at birth and growth rate during different periods of childhood. Most iron deficiency occurs in toddlers and adolescents because the increase in hemoglobin iron per unit of body weight is greatest at these ages. In addition, as children enter puberty, boys in particular require increased iron for increase in body muscle mass and thus myoglobin, and girls require increased iron to replace that lost with menstruation. The increased requirements due to changes in body composition in males lessen, but increased requirements continue in girls following menarche.

Iron in the first year

Two-thirds of total fetal iron is transferred to the growing fetus in the third trimester of pregnancy by an active process; transferrin receptors are present on placental villi. The iron is used for synthesis of hemoglobin and iron-containing enzymes and proteins; excess iron is stored as ferritin [24]. Fetal hemoglobin has a higher oxygen affinity than adult hemoglobin, and to compensate for this and ensure adequate oxygen delivery to tissues, the hemoglobin level rises from week 20 to term. In full-term infants, the hemoglobin is higher than in children or adults and represents a storage pool of iron that can be easily utilized as blood volume expands and rapid growth takes place in the first six months of infancy [25]. At birth, the change from a relatively hypoxic to an oxygen-rich environment switches erythropoiesis off, and hemoglobin falls. The iron thus released is stored and later utilized as erythropoiesis becomes more active around the second month. There is synthesis of adult hemoglobin which, having a lower oxygen affinity, releases oxygen more easily, thus allowing a lower hemoglobin level and effectively making more efficient use of iron. There is little increase, therefore, in total body iron in the first four months of life, but, between four and twelve months, total body iron increases by about 130 mg, and thus iron intake needs to increase. Babies of mothers who are iron deficient during pregnancy are rarely anemic at birth, but do have lower iron stores and are at risk of iron deficiency later on [26]. It is not clear whether this reflects poor iron stores at birth or the same iron-deficient intake common to the mother and her baby.

Preterm babies are at risk of iron deficiency because the majority of iron is transferred from the mother to the fetus in the third trimester and they have a lower hemoglobin concentration and thus a diminished storage pool of iron at birth [27]. In addition, some may suffer intrauterine growth restriction (IUGR), which is seen with smoking and gestational conditions such as hypertension, all being associated with impaired placental function [28]. Although this can result in a raised hemoglobin level at birth reflecting intrauterine hypoxia, the increased demand for iron to support both increased erythropoiesis and organ development cannot be met, resulting in more iron directed to production of higher hemoglobin levels at the expense of tissue iron, for instance in the brain and liver [27]. Not only do preterm babies and babies with IUGR have lower iron stores, but they also have periods of rapid "catch-up" growth which full-term babies do not. In a normal term baby, the total hemoglobin mass doubles during the first year of life (from 180 mg at birth to 340 mg at one year); in a 2 kg baby born at term, the increase is threefold (110 to 330 mg), but in a preterm (1kg) baby, the increase is sixfold (50 to 300 mg).

Iron in the diet

Total fetal iron is a significant determinant of risk of developing iron deficiency in infancy, and recognition of this risk is important since iron deficiency is easily treatable. Other factors influencing risk are dietary iron content and gastrointestinal blood loss. The availability of iron from the milk given to the infant varies with the type of milk: iron in breast milk has high bioavailability, but it is important that the mother is not iron deficient; the infant's diet generally requires supplementation with iron-containing foods from six months onwards. Most formula milk is supplemented with adequate iron, but cow's milk is not, and may also cause chronic, occult blood loss from the gut. Severely iron-deficient infants or toddlers are frequently found to drink only cow's milk, and changing dietary habits is crucial, in addition to iron supplements (Fig. 3.2).

In developing countries, iron deficiency may affect up to one-third of children. Inadequate intake of iron-containing foods, poor bioavailability of iron from cereal-based diets, and chronic infection such as hookworm infestation causing intestinal blood loss are the major causes of anemia [29, 30]. In developed countries, children of immigrants or refugees have a higher incidence of iron deficiency due to socioeconomic deprivation and being unable to find foods with which they are

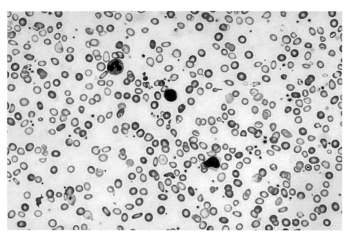

Fig. 3.2. Peripheral blood film from a patient with severe iron deficiency, whose diet consisted solely of cow's milk. The film shows a marked hypochromic microcytic picture (May–Grünwald–Giemsa stain).

familiar to provide a balanced diet. Provision of adequate iron from a meat-free diet requires iron sources such as pulses, and enhancers of absorption such as vitamin C and fish or poultry, if acceptable. Inexperienced dieting or vegetarianism may well result in inadequate iron intake; adolescent girls may be particularly susceptible in this regard.

Assessment of iron status

Iron deficiency anemia is characterized initially by a normocytic, normochromic anemia with an increase in the red cell distribution width, a non-specific finding that is indicative of anisocytosis. As deficiency becomes more severe, there is a falling mean corpuscular volume (MCV) and mean corpuscular hemoglobin (MCH), a reduction in red cell number and a microcytic, hypochromic anemia. When deficiency is severe, the mean cell hemoglobin concentration (MCHC) is also reduced. A microcytic, hypochromic anemia therefore represents a late stage of iron deficiency. Iron deficiency can be present before anemia becomes apparent, since stores will be exhausted first before the production of iron-deficient red cells. Other useful indicators of iron deficiency allowing detection at an earlier stage include serum ferritin [31], serum iron and transferrin (iron binding capacity), and newer variables such as soluble transferrin receptor (sTfR) levels [14, 15] and zinc protoporphyrin levels [32]. The gold standard for assessment of iron status is a bone marrow aspirate stained for iron, but this is neither practical nor justifiable in children.

Ferritin

Serum ferritin reflects total body ferritin, with levels rising as iron accumulates in the body and falling in iron deficiency [33]. However, apoferritin is increased by inflammatory cytokines as part of the acute phase reaction, and thus serum ferritin levels are determined both by iron stores and by severity of inflammation [34]. Iron deficiency can be present in the presence of inflammation with a ferritin level up to about 60 μg/L.

Serum iron and transferrin

Serum iron alone is not a helpful parameter and, if measured, transferrin (which correlates with iron-binding capacity) should also be determined. Serum iron, and thus transferrin saturation, is dependent on macrophage iron release and utilization of iron by erythroid cells; these parameters reflect the transport pool of iron. In iron deficiency, serum iron falls, transferrin rises, and thus transferrin saturation falls [35]. Low serum iron and transferrin saturation are also seen in the anemia of chronic disease, however transferrin levels are often reduced or at the lower limit of normal.

Zinc protoporphyrin

Zinc protoporphyrin (ZPP) is raised in defective heme synthesis, as zinc instead of iron is inserted into the protoporphyrin ring [32]. Production of heme can be disrupted through lack of iron, but also through loss of function of the enzymes involved in the reaction, which is seen in sideroblastic anemia (see below), increasing lead levels, and with ethanol, which inhibits heme synthesis. Lead absorption is enhanced by iron deficiency, since the same absorptive mechanisms are used for both metals, and iron deficiency is often seen in patients with high levels of lead [36].

Soluble transferrin receptor

Soluble transferrin receptor level is a useful parameter for distinguishing between different causes of microcytic anemias. Transferrin receptor expression and thus soluble transferrin receptor (sTfR) level is increased in iron deficiency and in conditions with increased erythropoietic activity, but to a lesser extent in the latter; sTfR levels are not affected by inflammation. Using the sTfR level and ferritin level together is a sensitive way to distinguish between iron deficiency anemia and the anemia of chronic disease [15]. The ratio of sTfR : ferritin (or the log of the ferritin level) is raised in iron deficiency and reduced in the anemia of chronic disease [37].

Assessing iron status in neonates and infants, especially in premature infants, is difficult due to lack of appropriate reference ranges, particularly for the new biomarkers, and the effects of therapy such as blood transfusion and erythropoietin on the parameters measured [38]. However, premature infants, especially those of diabetic mothers or those who have suffered IUGR, are particularly susceptible to iron deficiency both due to lack of iron reserves at birth and to the increased growth rate needed to catch up in the first year of life. Many neonatal units give iron supplements routinely to neonates born at less than 35 weeks' gestation.

Biomarkers of iron status need to be assessed together and in conjunction with the clinical status of the patient, a dietary and drug history, and birth history in infants. Apart from a low ferritin, which almost invariably indicates iron deficiency, other markers must be interpreted together and in the light of clinical information. Characteristics of iron deficiency anemia with a comparison to anemia of chronic disease are shown in Table 3.1.

Table 3.1. Biomarkers in iron deficiency anemia and anemia of chronic disease.

Biomarker	Iron deficiency anemia	Anemia of chronic disease
MCV	Reduced (normal only when anemia is mild)	Normal or reduced
MCH	Reduced (normal only when anemia is mild)	Normal or reduced
Serum ferritin	Reduced[a]	Increased or normal
Serum iron	Reduced	Reduced or normal
Serum transferrin	Increased	Reduced or normal
Transferrin saturation	Reduced	Reduced or normal
Zinc protoporphyrin	Increased	Normal
Soluble transferrin receptor	Increased	Normal

[a] Can be normal (20–60 μg/L) when iron deficiency is associated with chronic inflammation or infection.
Abbreviations: MCV, mean cell volume; MCH, mean cell hemoglobin.

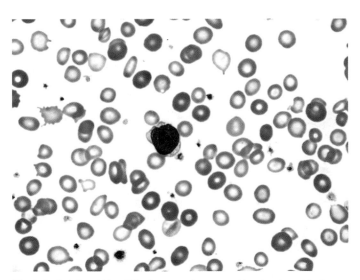

Fig. 3.3. Peripheral blood film from a patient on oral iron treatment for iron deficiency anemia. A dimorphic picture is seen with hypochromic, microcytic cells and normochromic, normocytic cells; polychromasia is also noted (May–Grünwald–Giemsa stain).

Treatment of iron deficiency

In children with iron deficiency secondary to a poor diet, dietary advice and encouragement to introduce iron-containing foods should be given. Changing dietary habit can be particularly difficult in young children who drink several pints of cow's milk a day in preference to solid food. Replacement iron is therefore usually needed and should be given orally unless there are good reasons for using another route. If oral preparations are taken reliably and are absorbed, the rise in hemoglobin is not significantly slower than with the parenteral route (Fig. 3.3). The hemoglobin should rise by 1–2 g/L per day over three to four weeks; a rise in reticulocyte count should be apparent from day three and can be used as a measure of response or compliance. Once the hemoglobin is within the normal range, treatment should be continued for at least a further three months to replenish stores. Overall, treatment is often needed for four to six months. Failure of response may be due to the wrong diagnosis, or poor absorption such as occurs in celiac disease, or continued iron loss through bleeding. In this last scenario, the reticulocyte count may be raised, whereas in the first two, it will be low. Inflammatory bowel disease may be complicated by continued bleeding, poor absorption and poor utilization of iron due to chronic inflammation. In chronic renal failure, when exogenous erythropoietin is given, erythropoietic drive is so great that the iron supply for erythropoiesis is inadequate and parenteral iron is required [39]. Gastrointestinal side effects are common with oral preparations and are often dose related. Although iron salts are best absorbed in the fasting state, side effects may be reduced by taking them after meals. If intolerance continues, the dose can be reduced in the first instance or an alternative preparation prescribed.

Vitamin B$_{12}$

Vitamin B$_{12}$ refers to a group of compounds known as cobalamins which contain a central cobalt ion and a corrin ring. The cobalt ion is bound to the corrin ring at four sites, and a fifth site is bound to a dimethylbenzimidazole group, whereas binding to the sixth site is variable, the ligand being a methyl, adenosyl, cyano, or hydroxyl group. Chemically, the term vitamin B$_{12}$ refers to hydroxocobalamin and cyanocobalamin, although in general use this term applies to all cobalamin forms. The two naturally occurring cobalamins in the body are methylcobalamin, the predominant form in serum, and adenosylcobalamin, the predominant form in the cytosol; hydroxocobalamin is a natural analog and cyanocobalamin is formed during the commercial production of vitamin B$_{12}$ from bacteria. In the body, one form of vitamin B$_{12}$ can be converted to another enzymatically [40].

Role in the body

Vitamin B$_{12}$ is involved in reactions of DNA synthesis, fatty acid synthesis, and energy production. In the body, there are two enzymes for which vitamin B$_{12}$ is a coenzyme: methylmalonyl coenzyme A mutase (MUT) and methionine synthase, also known as 5-methyltetrahydrofolate-homocysteine methyl transferase (MTR). Methylmalonyl coenzyme A mutase catalyzes the conversion of methylmalonyl-CoA to succinyl-CoA, and requires adenosylcobalamin as a coenzyme. Succinyl-CoA is a key molecule in the tricarboxylic acid cycle, and is important in the extraction of energy from proteins and fats. In a second reaction also dependent on MUT and adenosylcobalamin, methionine is converted to S-adenosyl methionine, which is needed for the myelination of myelin sheath phospholipids [41]. Vitamin B$_{12}$ deficiency results in raised methylmalonic acid levels, which prevent normal fatty acid synthesis, again compromising production of the myelin

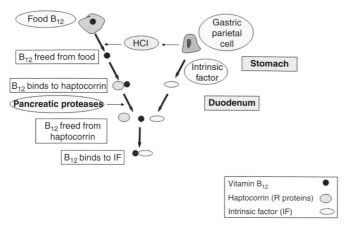

Fig. 3.4. Vitamin B$_{12}$ absorption in the stomach and duodenum.

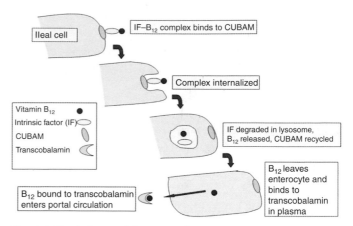

Fig. 3.5. The ileal stage of absorption of vitamin B$_{12}$.

sheath. The resultant defects give rise to demyelination, leading to neuropathies and subacute combined degeneration of the spinal cord. In the MTR reaction, methyltetrahydrofolate donates its methyl group to cobalamin which then, as methylcobalamin, transfers the methyl group to homocysteine to form methionine while regenerating cobalamin. Tetrahydrofolate is also generated in this reaction [41]. In vitamin B$_{12}$ deficiency, failure of this reaction leads to increased homocysteine levels but more importantly to reduced availability of 5–10-methylene tetrahydrofolate, which is essential for thymine synthesis and ultimately DNA synthesis. This leads to ineffective production of cells with a rapid turnover, such as blood cells and intestinal cells, leading to megaloblastic anemia and impaired intestinal absorption. These effects can be overcome if sufficient folate is given, in contrast to the loss of function of the MUT reaction, which has an absolute requirement for vitamin B$_{12}$. Thus, the neurologic effects of vitamin B$_{12}$ deficiency such as subacute combined degeneration of the cord can be arrested, and to some extent reversed, only by vitamin B$_{12}$ supplementation.

Dietary vitamin B$_{12}$

Vitamin B$_{12}$ cannot be made by plants or animals, only by bacteria and algae having the enzymes necessary for its synthesis. Animals, however, obtain vitamin B$_{12}$ either directly or indirectly from bacteria, for example from bacteria in the gut, and thus meat and dairy products are both sources of the vitamin. Plants are a source of vitamin B$_{12}$ only due to contamination by bacteria, from the soil and from bacteria in over-ripe damaged fruit and vegetables; therefore, undamaged, washed fruit and vegetables provide no vitamin B$_{12}$. Eggs are a good source of the vitamin despite poor bioavailability [42] due to vitamin B$_{12}$-binding proteins present in the white and the yolk [43]. Liver and shellfish are particularly rich in the vitamin.

Vitamin B$_{12}$ absorption and metabolism

The process for absorption of vitamin B$_{12}$ from food begins in the stomach, where it is released by pepsin digestion in an acid environment. The chief cells secrete pepsin, and the gastric parietal cells, hydrochloric acid. The parietal cells also secrete intrinsic factor, but this cannot bind the free vitamin B$_{12}$ as the environment is too acidic. The vitamin B$_{12}$ binds to haptocorrin (previously known as transcobalamin I), which is an R binder and secreted by the salivary glands, for transportation to the duodenum [44] (Fig. 3.4). There pancreatic proteases cleave the vitamin B$_{12}$ from the haptocorrin, allowing the former to bind to intrinsic factor in the higher pH of the duodenum. The vitamin B$_{12}$–intrinsic factor (IF) complex is transported to the ileum, where it binds to the CUBAM receptor, a complex of the proteins cubilin and amnionless which is present on the apical surface of the ileal cell [45, 46]. Once the CUBAM receptor has bound the vitamin B$_{12}$–IF complex, it is internalized, the intrinsic factor is degraded within the lysosome, vitamin B$_{12}$ released, and CUBAM recycled to the cell surface. The vitamin B$_{12}$ then leaves the enterocyte and some 6–20% binds to transcobalamin (previously known as transcobalamin II) in the plasma, enters the portal circulation and is delivered to target tissues where it binds to specific receptors and is internalized (Fig. 3.5). Most vitamin B$_{12}$, however, binds to haptocorrin and is delivered to the liver for storage. It follows therefore that functional vitamin B$_{12}$ deficiency can occur with a normal serum vitamin B$_{12}$ level [47].

The adult requirement for vitamin B$_{12}$ is around 2–3 µg per day, and the majority is absorbed via the system described above. This system is saturable at about 1.5–2.0 µg per meal under physiologic conditions, and thus vitamin B$_{12}$ bioavailability decreases with increasing intake per meal [42]. However, vitamin B$_{12}$ is also absorbed by passive diffusion, independent of either intrinsic factor or the terminal ileum. This system is much less efficient, with only 1% of vitamin B$_{12}$ being absorbed by this route. However, it becomes quantitatively significant when pharmacological doses of vitamin B$_{12}$ are given orally. If a large oral dose (300–1000 µg) is given, absorption of 1% will exceed the daily requirement and is sufficient to meet daily needs. In cases of pernicious anemia, it has been shown that the higher the dose given, the more rapid the hematological response. Vitamin B$_{12}$ is stored in the liver, and in adults these stores when replete contain about 2000–3000 µg. With a daily

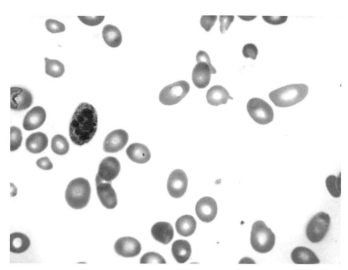

Fig. 3.6. Peripheral blood film from a patient with megaloblastic anemia showing a hypersegmented neutrophil, anisocytosis, macrocytosis, and poikilocytosis, with the poikilocytes including oval macrocytes (May–Grünwald–Giemsa stain).

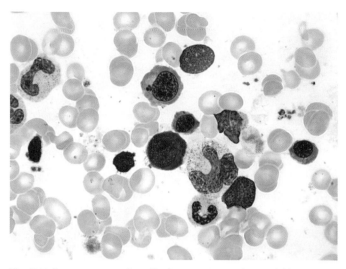

Fig. 3.7. Bone marrow aspirate film from a patient with megaloblastic anemia secondary to vitamin B_{12} deficiency. Megaloblastic maturation of the erythroid series is seen and also a giant metamyelocyte (May–Grünwald–Giemsa stain).

requirement of <3 μg, this provides enough vitamin B_{12} for at least two to three years assuming no absorption of vitamin B_{12}. Adequate daily intake of vitamin B_{12} for infants and children is less than for adults, being 0.4 μg/day up to the age of 6 months and 0.5–0.6 μg/day from 6 to 12 months, rising gradually over the years to 2.4 μg/day for 14–18-year-olds [47].

Vitamin B_{12} deficiency

Vitamin B_{12} deficiency in neonates is usually due to maternal deficiency [48], while causes in infants and older children include congenital or inherited defects of cobalamin absorption, transport, or metabolism, as well as acquired deficiencies [49]. Signs of deficiency result from the pancytopenia associated with megaloblastic anemia, and include pallor, bruising, and infection; in addition there are gastrointestinal symptoms such as anorexia, diarrhea, and failure to thrive, and neurologic dysfunction such as irritability and developmental delay or regression. In older children, a peripheral neuropathy manifesting as paresthesiae, predominantly in the legs, may occur with loss of proprioception and vibration sense (subacute combined degeneration of the cord), leading to a disturbance in gait. Epilepsy and psychiatric or ophthalmic symptoms may develop. Vitamin B_{12} deficiency is also seen secondary to poverty and malnutrition [30, 50, 51]. A full blood count may show a macrocytic anemia with neutropenia and thrombocytopenia; sometimes isolated cytopenias are seen. Morphological examination reveals oval macrocytes and hypersegmented neutrophils, the latter defined as $>5\%$ showing nuclei with five distinct lobes, or the presence of any neutrophils with six distinct lobes (Fig. 3.6). If a bone marrow aspiration has been performed, megaloblastic maturation is seen, characterized by asynchrony between nuclear and cytoplasmic maturation in the erythroid series and giant metamyelocytes in the myeloid series (Fig. 3.7). Due to the ineffective hematopoiesis, numbers of late precursors in the

bone marrow are reduced in relation to earlier forms, and serum bilirubin and lactate dehydrogenase are elevated.

Maternal vitamin B_{12} deficiency

Maternal vitamin B_{12} deficiency may be secondary to occult pernicious anemia, but is found too in mothers who have a strict vegetarian, vegan or macrobiotic diet [52]. Maternal deficiency is also seen in areas of the world where there is poverty and malnutrition. The neonate with vitamin B_{12} deficiency may present with irritability, failure to thrive, diarrhea and developmental regression. A macrocytic anemia with other cytopenias may follow with or without further neurologic signs. Infantile tremor syndrome is also seen in association with vitamin B_{12} deficiency, both prior to and during replacement therapy [52]. Magnetic resonance imaging has shown cerebellar and cerebral atrophy and defects in myelination. Therapy may not result in complete resolution of the neurologic defects [53].

Inherited disorders of transport and absorption of vitamin B_{12}

Inherited disorders of transport and absorption of vitamin B_{12} result from genetic defects in the key proteins involved in these processes (Table 3.2). Apart from haptocorrin deficiency, which is not clearly associated with clinical symptoms and signs of vitamin B_{12} deficiency (see below), these inherited disorders require lifelong pharmacologic doses of vitamin B_{12} [54].

In congenital pernicious anemia, there is a failure to secrete functional intrinsic factor, resulting in low serum vitamin B_{12} levels and megaloblastic anemia; developmental delay and myelopathy are also seen. It is an autosomal recessive disorder which has been identified in fewer than 100 patients; several different mutations have been identified in the *GIF* gene on chromosome 11 which encodes intrinsic factor. Presentation is usually between the ages of 1 and 5 years but may be later [55, 56].

Table 3.2. Disorders of vitamin B_{12} transport and absorption.

Disorder	N	Gene and gene map locus	Presentation	Cobalamin levels
Congenital pernicious anemia (absence of functional IF)	<100	GIF 11q13	1–5 years of age Symptoms of megaloblastic anemia Developmental delay Myelopathy	Very low
Defects in CUBAM receptor (Imerslund–Gräsbeck syndrome)	>250	CUBN (cubilin) 10p12.1 or AMN (amnionless) 14q32	<2 years of age Failure to thrive Fatigue and anorexia Proteinuria Symptoms of megaloblastic anemia	Very low
Transcobalamin deficiency	<50	TCN2 22q11.2-qter	Neonatal period Failure to thrive Anorexia and diarrhea Symptoms of megaloblastic anemia Isolated cytopenias Immune deficiency Later gait disturbance and epilepsy	Normal (occasionally low) Holotranscobalamin low or absent
Haptocorrin deficiency	Few	TCN1 11q11–q12	Has only rarely been associated with disease	Very low Holotranscobalamin normal

N = number of patients described.

Defects in the CUBAM receptor, necessary for absorption of intrinsic factor-bound vitamin B_{12}, result in congenital megaloblastic anemia with proteinuria – the Imerslund–Gräsbeck syndrome. Presentation is usually before the age of two years but may be later, and symptoms include failure to thrive, fatigue, and anorexia. Features of pancytopenia include pallor, bruising, and increased susceptibility to infection. Parenteral vitamin B_{12} corrects the anemia but not the proteinuria. More than 250 cases have been reported and inheritance is autosomal recessive. Genetic defects have been found in both the CUBN gene, encoding cubilin, and the AMN gene, encoding amnionless [45, 46]. Transcobalamin deficiency is also inherited in an autosomal recessive manner and results in severe vitamin B_{12} deficiency, although serum levels are usually normal [48]. This is because most of the serum vitamin B_{12} is bound to haptocorrin and is exclusively taken up by hepatocytes for storage in the liver; only about 20% is bound to transcobalamin and available to dividing cells. Some cases have been reported where serum vitamin B_{12} levels are low [57, 58]; measurement of transcobalamin-bound vitamin B_{12} (holotranscobalamin) reveals very low or absent levels. Presentation is in the neonatal period, again with failure to thrive and gastrointestinal symptoms followed by progressive symptoms and signs of megaloblastic anemia. Isolated cytopenias, in contrast to pancytopenia, have also been reported, as has immune deficiency. Neurological defects such as epilepsy and gait disturbance often present later and are not necessarily fully reversed by vitamin B_{12} replacement therapy, emphasizing the need to check vitamin B_{12} levels in infants with persistent, unexplained cytopenias or immune deficiency. Transcobalamin deficiency has been described in fewer than 50 patients and has been shown to be due to both absent and functionally abnormal transcobalamin. In families where one child has been diagnosed, subsequent children can be screened *in utero*, as transcobalamin is made by amniocytes and thus absent production can be detected from cultured amniotic fluid cells [59].

Haptocorrin deficiency has been described but it is not clear if it is associated with disease since, although serum levels of vitamin B_{12} are low, transcobalamin-bound vitamin B_{12} (holotranscobalamin) levels are normal.

Inborn errors of metabolism

Failure of the reactions for which vitamin B_{12} is coenzyme results in a clinical picture of deficiency but with metabolic disturbances dependent on where the defect occurs. As discussed, vitamin B_{12} is converted to adenosylcobalamin and, with methylmalonyl coenzyme A mutase (MUT), converts methylmalonyl-CoA to succinyl-CoA. Failure of this reaction can be due to a defect in MUT, a defect in adenosylcobalamin synthesis, or both. Such defects will result in raised blood levels of methylmalonic acid and thus a severe metabolic acidosis and methylmalonic aciduria. In the conversion of methyltetrahydrofolate to tetrahydrofolate, the methyl group is transferred to vitamin B_{12} which then donates it to homocysteine to form methionine. Failure of these reactions may be due to methionine synthase (MTR) deficiency or to deficiency of methionine synthase reductase, which reduces cobalamin to its functional form after transfer of its methyl group. Isolated defects of methylcobalamin synthesis will result in homocysteinemia. In some cases, abnormalities of both methylcobalamin and adenosylcobalamin are seen, resulting in raised levels of both methylmalonic acid and homocysteine. The defects of cobalamin metabolism have been classified from the results of somatic cell complementation studies; specific gene or protein abnormalities have not been identified in all. There are eight complementation groups, *cblA–cblH*, and various genetic mutations have been found in five of these groups: cblA, B, C, E, and G and are described in more detail in a review by Whitehead [49].

Methylmalonyl-CoA mutase deficiency

The gene for methylmalonyl-CoA mutase has been located to chromosome 6, and over 50 mutations have been described. These result in either absent or markedly reduced MUT activity, which may be due to absent or reduced protein production or the production of an unstable or dysfunctional protein. With severe deficiency, presentation is early, with failure to thrive, vomiting, lethargy, dehydration, and respiratory distress. Developmental delay occurs more commonly in those with severe deficiency compared to those with some residual MUT activity, and hepatomegaly is only seen in the former group [60]. Anemia and other cytopenias have been described. Metabolic derangements in addition to the acidosis and methylmalonic aciduria are also seen and include hypoglycemia and hyperammonemia. Glycine and ketones may be found in both blood and urine. The disorder is unresponsive to vitamin B_{12}, although a trial of therapy is justified once methylmalonic aciduria is suspected (see adenosylcobalamin deficiency below), and is managed by a protein restricted diet and avoidance of valine, isoleucine, methionine, and threonine, which will limit the amino acids using the propionate pathway [48]. Other therapeutic strategies have included carnitine, ascorbate, and metronidazole, the last to reduce propionate production by anaerobic bacteria in the gut [61, 62]. Even with therapy, renal dysfunction develops and brain infarcts have been reported [63].

Adenosylcobalamin deficiency

Adenosylcobalamin deficiency results in methylmalonic aciduria which is often vitamin B_{12} responsive. The complementation groups involved are cblA, where mutations in a gene functioning within the mitochondria have been found; cblB, where mutations in the cob(I)alamin adenosyl transferase gene have been identified; and cblH, where the causative protein abnormality has not been identified. Presentation is usually in infancy, and symptoms and signs are similar to those seen in MUT deficiency [60]. Importantly however, 90% of cblA patients respond to vitamin B_{12}, both hydroxo- and cyanocobalamin, whereas only 40% of those with cblB do. Initial protein restriction as for MUT deficiency is also necessary [48]. It follows, therefore, that if methylmalonic aciduria is suspected, it is appropriate to give intramuscular vitamin B_{12} as a therapeutic trial even though the patient may later be diagnosed as having MUT deficiency, as to withhold it would deny appropriate therapy to those who may respond.

Methylcobalamin deficiency

Methylcobalamin deficiency can result from defects in methionine synthase, complementation group cblG, or from defects in methionine synthase reductase, complementation group cblE, and is inherited in an autosomal recessive manner [64]. Patients commonly present in early infancy with lethargy, vomiting, and failure to thrive. Developmental delay, cerebral atrophy, and other neurologic defects, including blindness, may be seen. Features of megaloblastic anemia may also be present. Homocysteinemia is seen, but not methylmalonic aciduria. Mutations in the methionine synthase gene on chromosome 1 and the methionine synthase reductase gene on chromosome 5 have been identified. Treatment is with intramuscular vitamin B_{12}, which usually corrects the anemia and metabolic abnormalities, but the neurological abnormalities may only improve slowly [64].

Combined deficiencies

Combined adenosylcobalamin and methylcobalamin deficiencies result from defects in both MUT and methionine synthase, giving rise to methylmalonic aciduria, homocystinuria, and hypomethionemia. Complementation groups cblC, D, and F are involved, and recently the gene for the defect in cblD disease has been identified [65], but no other gene or protein abnormalities have been found. In cblC and cblD disease, vitamin B_{12} appears unable to enter the cell, whereas in cblF disease, excess vitamin B_{12} accumulates but is not metabolized and localizes to lysosomes. Patients with cblC disease usually present in early infancy with lethargy, failure to thrive, developmental delay, and microcephaly. Most will have megaloblastic anemia, but the metabolic abnormalities are variable, with some cases not having methylmalonic aciduria and others having normal homocysteine levels. There is a later-onset form of the disease in which neurologic features predominate and hematologic abnormalities are not always seen. Only a handful of patients with cblD and cblF have been described, and presentation is variable with a range of neurologic and hematologic symptoms and signs. Treatment is with high doses, up to 1 mg, of parenteral vitamin B_{12}, with some patients showing a better response to hydroxocobalamin than cyanocobalamin. Betaine has been used in some patients with additional benefit. Neurologic symptoms do not reverse completely and patients usually have moderate to severe developmental delay. Patients who present in the neonatal period often die [48].

Acquired vitamin B_{12} deficiency

Acquired disorders that affect absorption of vitamin B_{12} may also cause deficiency and generally involve diseases of the ileum as seen in severe, chronic celiac disease, or ileal resection for Crohn disease or necrotizing enterocolitis [66]. Infestations by fish tapeworm, or abnormal bowel flora due to blind loops of bowel are rarer causes of severe malabsorption. Lesser impairment of vitamin B_{12} absorption is seen in children with cystic fibrosis and pancreatic exocrine insufficiency due to lack of enzymes cleaving vitamin B_{12} from haptocorrin, and in those with less severe celiac or Crohn disease. In adults, in addition to the above, deficiency may arise due to reduced or absent gastric acid secretion, which can be secondary to drugs such as proton pump inhibitors, H_2 blockers, or the biguanides; atrophic gastritis which increases with aging; and total or partial gastrectomy. Pancreatic insufficiency secondary to chronic

Table 3.3. Diagnosis of vitamin B_{12} deficiency.

Vitamin B_{12} status	Influencing factors	Vitamin B_{12} level	MMA level	tHCy level	Holotranscobalamin level
Deficient	None	Low or equivocal	Increased	Increased	Reduced
	MPD/CGL/oral contraception	Normal or equivocal	Increased	Increased	Reduced
	Transcobalamin deficiency	Normal (rarely low)	Increased	Increased	Very low or absent
Normal	Renal failure/thyrotoxicosis	Normal	Increased	Increased	Normal
	Pregnancy	Normal or equivocal	Increased	Increased	Normal
	Haptocorrin deficiency	Low	Normal	Normal	Normal

Abbreviations: MMA, methylmalonic acid; tHCy, total homocysteine; MPD, myeloproliferative disorder; CGL, chronic granulocytic leukemia. Equivocal is defined as ≤25% below the lower limit of normal.

pancreatitis is also associated with decreased absorption. These are much less commonly seen in children, as are pernicious anemia secondary to intrinsic factor antibodies, and food vitamin B_{12} malabsorption. Nitrous oxide used in anesthetics can inactivate vitamin B_{12} causing both hematologic and neurologic symptoms if there is repeated exposure. Cases have been reported in infants and children.

Assessment

Vitamin B_{12} deficiency should be considered in any infant or child who presents with a macrocytic anemia or isolated cytopenia, gastrointestinal symptoms such as failure to thrive, anorexia, and diarrhea, or neurologic symptoms such as irritability, developmental regression or delay, epilepsy, or gait disturbance. Attention should be paid to children in high-risk groups for acquired deficiency, such as those with cystic fibrosis or intestinal disease. Serum vitamin B_{12} is the most commonly used test and has a sensitivity of 97% in those with clinical deficiency [67]. It is acknowledged, however, that deficiency can be present with low normal levels, and that the test is less reliable in subclinical deficiency. In addition, the lower limit of the normal range varies between methods and laboratories. Serum vitamin B_{12} radioimmunoassays may give falsely low results in those with folate deficiency or those who are pregnant or taking the oral contraceptive pill [68]. Conversely, levels can be within the normal range despite deficiency, in conditions such as chronic myeloid leukemia (CML) or other myeloproliferative disorder where there may be an increase in haptocorrin. Normal levels can also be seen in the severe deficiency associated with transcobalamin deficiency. In these circumstances, or if transcobalamin deficiency is suspected, measurement of transcobalamin-bound vitamin B_{12}, holotranscobalamin, will show low or absent levels. The use of holotranscobalamin in the routine diagnosis of vitamin B_{12} deficiency has not been established. Other biochemical markers such as serum methylmalonic acid and plasma total homocysteine levels can be used to help confirm deficiency, but although sensitive, are less specific and not always available routinely. High levels of total homocysteine in particular can be due to other causes and also to inappropriate sampling collection and processing [69]. A summary of investigations is shown in Table 3.3. Renal impairment can result in raised levels and thus false positives for tests of both methylmalonic acid and plasma total homocysteine. Levels of methylmalonic acid are raised in vitamin B_{12} deficiency, but plasma total homocysteine levels are raised in both vitamin B_{12} and folate deficiency [67]. A normal methylmalonic acid level tends to rule out vitamin B_{12} deficiency [69]. It is important to establish a diagnosis as neurologic manifestations may be irreversible if treatment is started too late. Neonates, infants, and older children who present due to an inborn error of metabolism have associated metabolic defects which should be sought if the deficiency cannot be otherwise explained. Methylmalonic aciduria and homocystinuria may be found alone or in combination, and plasma homocysteine and serum methylmalonic acid levels may be high and methionine levels low. In a neonate or infant with severe vitamin B_{12} deficiency secondary to defects causing methylmalonic aciduria, metabolic abnormalities such as acidosis, hypoglycemia, and hyperammonemia are also seen. Where there is a clear dietary cause or a medical history of significant gastrointestinal disease, no further investigation is necessary, but differentiating dietary causes is important from the point of view of treatment.

Treatment

In the UK, vitamin B_{12} deficiency, with the exception of inadequate dietary intake, is treated predominantly with parenteral hydroxocobalamin injections, 1 mg intramuscularly. In other countries such as the USA, parenteral cyanocobalamin is the treatment of choice. Daily oral administration of high doses of cyanocobalamin, 1 mg per day, has been shown to be effective in the treatment of vitamin B_{12} deficiency, including pernicious anemia, and is the preferred route in Sweden [70]. Most regimens for parenteral therapy include more frequent injections initially, from daily for five days in children with inborn errors of vitamin B_{12} metabolism, to up to three times weekly for two weeks in those with deficiency due to other causes. After this initial loading period, therapy is then reduced to a maintenance dose, usually 1 mg every three months. In those children with inborn errors of metabolism, response should be monitored, as not all will respond. Where methylmalonic aciduria is suspected or found, high dose, parenteral vitamin B_{12} should be given while confirming the precise defect. Patients may be maintained on oral therapy, but compliance may be a problem and, in those with inborn errors of metabolism, some only respond to parenteral therapy. Concomitant iron therapy may be needed, particularly for those with malabsorption, as iron deficiency may become apparent as hematopoiesis resumes. Oral cyanocobalamin in doses of 50–150 μg per day can be used in children with proven dietary deficiency after initial loading. Neonates born to mothers with vitamin B_{12} deficiency may themselves be vitamin B_{12} deficient, particularly if breast fed, and thus require initial replacement.

Folate

Folic acid and its anion form, folate, are water-soluble forms of vitamin B_9. Folate is the naturally occurring form found in foods, and folic acid is manufactured. The active folate coenzymes are polyglutamates with between four and six glutamate moieties attached by γ-peptide bonds, whereas the monoglutamates are the transport forms.

Role in the body

Since folate is essential for DNA synthesis, it is required by all dividing cells, deficiency having most effect on those cells with the highest turnover, such as hematopoietic cells. Folate deficiency causes a megaloblastic anemia which is characterized by macrocytic red cells in the peripheral blood, hypersegmented neutrophils, and usually an anemia and other cytopenias. Those who have ongoing hemolysis, such as patients with hereditary spherocytosis, will have an increased requirement for folate. Folate is also important during periods of rapid cell division such as pregnancy and fetal development, and infancy.

Dietary folate and folic acid

Rich sources of folate include legumes such as peas, lentils, and beans; yeast; liver; leafy vegetables such as spinach and lettuce; and other fruit and vegetables, particularly avocados, asparagus, and bananas. In some developed countries including the USA and Canada, folic acid is added to breakfast cereals and enriched cereal and grain products such as pasta, bread, and rice [71]. Folic acid is more easily absorbed than the naturally occurring folate in foods, which can also be destroyed by cooking, as well as by exposure to light and air; it is the form found in vitamin tablets.

Folate absorption and metabolism

Folate in the diet consists of both polyglutamate and monoglutamate forms, but only the latter are absorbed. Polyglutamates are therefore hydrolyzed to monoglutamates before absorption in the small intestine. This occurs by two mechanisms: specific transport mechanisms which allow absorption of low concentrations of folate and are saturable, and by a diffusion process for high concentrations of folate or folic acid. Specific mechanisms

include a transmembrane glycoprotein, reduced folate carrier (RFC), which transports reduced folates into mammalian cells and tissues, including tissues with specialized functions such as the intestinal epithelium and placenta. RFC has a low affinity for folate but a high capacity, and operates most efficiently at neutral pH. It has a twofold higher affinity for folinic acid than folic acid [64]. Another transporter which functions best at low pH and has a specificity for folate different from that of RFC has been recognized for several decades and has recently been characterized. The proton-coupled folate transporter or PCFT, a member of the super family of solute carriers, Solute Carrier family 46, member A1 (SLC46A1) (the gene for which has been mapped to chromosome 17), is responsible for transport of folate across the duodenal and jejunal mucosa and also into the central nervous system [72]. Its importance has been confirmed by demonstration of mutations in this gene resulting in the rare recessive disorder, hereditary folate malabsorption (see below) [73]. A third mechanism involves folate-binding proteins or folate receptors on cell membranes which are able to concentrate and internalize the folate. Folic acid is absorbed largely unchanged, especially if given in high doses, and is then converted to folate in the liver.

Folate is reduced in two steps by dihydrofolate reductase, first forming dihydrofolate, an inactive form of folate, and then tetrahydrofolate. Formaldehyde, serine and glycine act as single carbon donors and form methylene tetrahydrofolate, which can be reduced to methyltetrahydrofolate, or oxidized to formyltetrahydrofolate (folinic acid). These tetrahydrofolates serve as cofactors in one-carbon reactions for the *de novo* synthesis of purines, the remethylation of homocysteine to methionine, and the methylation of deoxyuridylate (dUMP) to thymidylate (dTMP), essential for thymine synthesis and ultimately nucleotide biosynthesis. Thymidylate is synthesized from dUMP and methylene tetrahydrofolate by thymidylate synthase, the rate-limiting step in DNA synthesis. Dihydrofolate reductase and serine hydroxymethyltransferase are required to regenerate methyl-tetrahydrofolate. Methyltetrahydrofolate, the major circulating form of folate, methylates homocysteine to form methionine by using cobalamin to transfer the methyl group while regenerating tetrahydrofolate, a reaction which is catalyzed by methionine synthase, also known as 5-methyltetrahydrofolate-homocysteine methyl transferase (MTR). Methionine is important in the regulation of methylated DNA, proteins, and lipids.

Folate deficiency

Folate deficiency reduces DNA synthesis through the inhibition of thymidylate synthesis, resulting in megaloblastic anemia, the clinical features of which are similar to those seen in vitamin B_{12} deficiency. In acquired folate deficiency, a severe neuropathy does not develop, although a mild peripheral neuropathy may be found in a minority of patients. Folate deficiency during fetal development and that resulting from inborn errors of metabolism however do have neurologic manifestations, which are described below.

Folate deficiency can result from an inadequate dietary intake of folate, malabsorption, increased utilization, liver disease, or drugs and substances such as alcohol which interfere directly or indirectly with folate absorption or metabolism.

Neonates and infants up to the age of six months require about 65 µg of folate per day, rising to 80 µg in the next six months. Daily requirements gradually increase from 150 µg for 1–3-year-olds to 200 µg from 4 to 8 years, and 300 µg from 9 to 13 years, reaching adult requirements of 400 µg from the age of 14 years. Stores of folate are generally sufficient for one to four months, but with inadequate intake, serum folate levels fall in two to three weeks. In pregnant women, requirement increases to 600–800 µg daily, falling to 500 µg during lactation [74].

Inadequate folate intake is seen where diet is poor and lacking in fresh fruit, vegetables, and meat. This is more common in under-developed countries but is also seen in the "tea and toast" diet and in alcoholics in whom diet, along with impaired folate absorption and altered metabolism, contributes to folate deficiency. Goat's milk has very low levels of folate (6 µg/L) compared to cow's milk (35–50 µg/L), giving rise to goat's milk anemia where it forms a major part of the diet. Both types of milk are low in iron.

Pregnancy

Maintenance of adequate folate levels during pregnancy requires increased intake and is important to reduce the risk of adverse events such as recurrent abortion, pregnancy-induced hypertension, and low birth weight [75]. The incidence of folate deficiency is increased in pregnant women, and this is more marked in under-developed countries where diet is poor. Maternal folate deficiency in the periconceptual period has been shown to cause more than 50% of cases of neural tube defects which include spina bifida, meningomyelocele, and anencephaly. The risk of neural tube defects is significantly reduced when supplemental folic acid is given, or foods rich in folate or enriched with folic acid are eaten [76, 77]. Enrichment of cereal and grain products with folic acid was introduced in the USA and Canada in 1998 and Chile in 2000, but this strategy has not been adopted in the UK, although some breakfast cereals and breads are fortified. Instead, it is currently recommended that women trying to become pregnant or who are pregnant should take 400 µg of supplementary folic acid daily. One argument for not adding folic acid to foods is that of masking vitamin B_{12} deficiency, where the megaloblastic anemia will respond to the increased folic acid intake but the neurologic manifestations will not [78]. This has not proved a problem in practice [79]. Neonates are not often folate deficient, despite maternal deficiency, as folate is preferentially transferred across the placenta. Neonatal serum and red cell folate levels are higher than in adults but fall rapidly in the first few weeks. The fall is most marked in the premature neonate, and folate deficiency and megaloblastic anemia may follow, particularly if there is concurrent infection, hemolysis, or poor feeding.

Malabsorption

Gluten-sensitive enteropathy, or celiac disease, commonly results in folate deficiency and anemia if untreated [80]. It is an autoimmune disease of the small bowel characterized by villous atrophy and crypt hyperplasia of the small intestine, causing malabsorption, and the finding of anti-endomysial and trans-glutaminase antibodies in the serum. Iron deficiency is also common, but vitamin B_{12} deficiency less so, as villous atrophy is more commonly seen in the proximal small bowel than the terminal ileum [81]. Gastrointestinal symptoms include diarrhea and steatorrhea, fatigue, mouth ulcers, bloating, weight loss, and growth retardation, but malabsorption can be present without any such symptoms. Children can present at any time from first exposure to gluten-containing foods. Younger children tend to present with gastrointestinal symptoms, whereas adults may present with just fatigue and anemia. Treatment is with a strict gluten-free diet. This is important not only from the nutritional point of view, but also because of the increased risk of lymphoma and adenocarcinoma of the small bowel in those who continue to eat gluten.

Tropical sprue, which is endemic to India, Southeast Asia, Central and South America, and the Caribbean, results in inflammation of the small intestine with subsequent intestinal villous atrophy and malabsorption. Gastrointestinal symptoms are seen with steatorrhea, weight loss, and malnutrition; megaloblastic anemia may develop due to malabsorption of folate and vitamin B_{12}, the latter being more commonly seen than in celiac disease [82]. The precise cause is not known, but is thought to be infective, and treatment with antibiotics such as sulfamethoxazole/trimethoprim or tetracyclines and supplements of folic acid and vitamin B_{12} for at least six months has been successful.

Other gastrointestinal causes of folate deficiency include resection of the small bowel, gastric bypass, and inflammatory bowel disease. Gastrointestinal bacterial overgrowth, although causing vitamin B_{12} deficiency, is rarely associated with folate deficiency, as the bacteria produce folate.

Increased utilization of folate

Folate requirements are increased where there is increased cell turnover. Such conditions where this is seen include pregnancy, which is discussed above, chronic hemolytic anemias, inflammatory conditions, widespread skin conditions, and malignancy. Infection such as HIV and systemic bacterial infections can also cause folate deficiency, and renal dialysis may cause excess losses.

Drugs

A number of drugs interfere with the biosynthesis of folate and tetrahydrofolate, including dihydrofolate reductase inhibitors such as trimethoprim and pyrimethamine, and methotrexate which inhibits both folate reductase and dihydrofolate reductase. Trimethoprim is only a weak inhibitor of human dihydrofolate reductase and is much more active against the bacterial enzyme, whereas pyrimethamine is most active against the malarial enzyme. Methotrexate is useful for treatment of certain cancers, including leukemia, because it inhibits the production of the active form of folate, tetrahydrofolate. It can cause megaloblastosis and significant gastrointestinal toxicity. This can be ameliorated by giving folinic but not folic acid. It is also used in lower doses in a variety of non-cancerous conditions including rheumatoid arthritis, psoriasis, primary biliary cirrhosis, and inflammatory bowel disease, and can deplete folate stores. Folic acid supplements or increasing dietary intake may help to reduce the toxic side effects without decreasing effectiveness. Other drugs such as phenytoin, carbamazepine, and sodium valproate may cause low folate levels. Folate replacement in those who are deficient in the case of phenytoin may lower phenytoin levels with seizure breakthrough, and therefore some advocate giving folic acid supplements at initiation of phenytoin therapy [83].

Inherited disorders of transport and metabolism

Inborn errors of folate metabolism are rare and include hereditary malabsorption of folate (also called congenital folate malabsorption), glutamate formiminotransferase deficiency, and severe methylene tetrahydrofolate reductase (MTHFR) deficiency. Polymorphisms of the *MTHFR* gene are, however, common and may have significant health implications in the older population. Homozygosity of the 677C to T polymorphism (TT) has shown 70% lower enzyme activity than the CC genotype and, when carried by the infant's mother or father, has been associated with an increased risk of neural tube defects in the infant [49, 84]. Functional methionine synthase (MTR) deficiency which involves both folate and vitamin B_{12} metabolism is discussed in the section on vitamin B_{12}.

Hereditary malabsorption of folate has been described in about 30 patients in a dozen or so families [85]. In some, this has been shown to be secondary to mutations in *SLC46A1*, the gene encoding PCFT. Mutation of both alleles leads to hereditary folate malabsorption [73]. Clinical features include anemia, hypoimmunoglobulinemia, susceptibility to opportunistic infections, chronic diarrhea, and neurological abnormalities. Both serum and cerebrospinal fluid (CSF) folate are low, with lowering of the normal CSF to serum folate ratio of 3 : 1 implying lack of transport across the blood–brain barrier. Parenteral treatment with folic acid has been given, and both high dose oral folate and folinic acid, the latter in doses ranging between 20 and 200 mg daily [73]. It is important to recognize and treat the disorder early since, if the treatment is delayed, the neurologic deficits can become permanent.

Other disorders of transport have been described in a handful of patients in which abnormalities of folate uptake into red blood cells and bone marrow cells with or without lymphocytes have been demonstrated. Hematological abnormalities such as aplastic anemia, pancytopenia, dyserythropoiesis, and leukemia have been described in probands and family members. Cerebral folate deficiency has been found in patients presenting with progressive neurological abnormalities in association with defects in the CNS-specific folate receptor protein FR1. Treatment with folinic acid has led to clinical improvement.

Methylene tetrahydrofolate reductase deficiency has been described in more than 100 patients, and many mutations in *MTHFR* have been identified. It is inherited in an autosomal recessive fashion. Presentation is variable in onset and severity, dependent on residual enzyme activity, and includes neurologic abnormalities such as developmental delay or retardation, epilepsy, and gait abnormalities, as well as thrombotic problems including stroke and retinal vein thrombosis. Hematologic abnormalities are not seen. Marked hyperhomocysteinemia and homocystinuria are found together with low or low normal plasma methionine; methylmalonic aciduria is absent. Treatment includes folic acid and methyltetrahydrofolate; betaine has improved prognosis, and other agents including methionine, vitamin B_{12}, and carnitine have been tried. Prognosis is poor but early diagnosis and treatment may attenuate neurological deterioration [64].

Glutamate formiminotransferase-cyclodeaminase (FTCD) deficiency is an autosomal recessive condition and has been described in about 20 patients. This enzyme catalyzes the transfer of a formimino group from histidine to tetrahydrofolate, followed by release of ammonia and the formation of methenyltetrahydrofolate. Defects result in increased formiminoglutamate (FIGLU), which is then excreted in the urine. A severe form of this disorder presents with severe developmental delay, megaloblastic anemia and high levels of FIGLU in the urine. A milder phenotype is characterized by mild developmental delay, no hematological abnormalities but again with high urinary FIGLU excretion, and mutations have been found in the FTCD gene in three such patients [86]. Serum folate and vitamin B_{12} levels are normal. Reduced FIGLU excretion has been shown in some patients treated with folic or folinic acid but not others. However, the relationship between FIGLU excretion and clinical outcome has not been elucidated.

Methionine synthase deficiency is discussed under methylcobalamin deficiency, above.

Assessment

Folate status can be assessed by measuring red cell and serum folate. Red cell folate is less influenced by recent changes in either diet or drug therapy. However, deficiency of vitamin B_{12} causes low red cell folate due to the effect on intracellular folate metabolism, but serum folate will be normal or raised in this situation. In combined deficiency, vitamin B_{12}, red cell folate, and serum folate levels will be low.

Plasma total homocysteine levels are raised in folate deficiency and can be used to help confirm the diagnosis, but although sensitive are less specific and not always available routinely. High levels of total homocysteine levels in particular can be due to other causes such as vitamin B_{12} deficiency, vitamin B_6 deficiency, renal failure, hypothyroidism, and some medications. Inappropriate sample collection and processing can lead to misleading results [69].

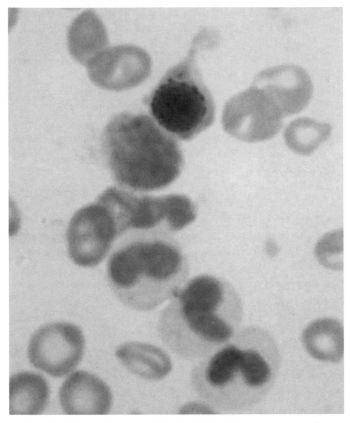

Fig. 3.8. Bone marrow aspirate film from a patient with acquired sideroblastic anemia showing a ring sideroblast (iron stain).

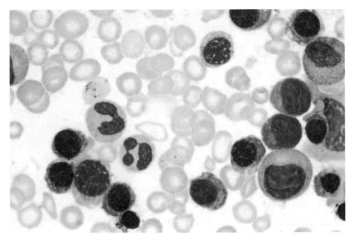

Fig. 3.10. Bone marrow aspirate film from a boy with congenital sideroblastic anemia, showing an erythrocyte with multiple Pappenheimer bodies and two abnormal erythroblasts, one with very scanty cytoplasm and one with vacuolated cytoplasm (May–Grünwald–Giemsa stain).

Treatment

Treatment of inborn errors of transport and metabolism has been outlined in the appropriate sections. In patients with megaloblastic anemia due to folate deficiency, replacement should be given daily for four months, with consideration of maintenance therapy dependent on the cause. Daily dose for neonates (birth to one month) is 1 mg, for infants (one month to

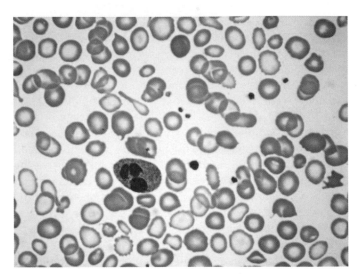

Fig. 3.9. Dimorphic blood film from a boy with congenital sideroblastic anemia (May–Grünwald–Giemsa stain).

a year), 500 µg/kg and for over one year, 5 mg. It is important that vitamin B_{12} deficiency is excluded as a cause, since high-dose folic acid will reverse the hematological aspects of the deficiency but will not treat the neurological aspects. For treatment of the folate-deficient state, including premature babies who are at high risk of folate deficiency, 250 µg/kg (up to 5 mg) should be given daily for six months, if a correctable cause, or lifelong if the cause is not correctable. In patients with chronic hemolysis, the benefit of supplementation with regard to development of megaloblastic anemia is not clear cut [87, 88], however supplementation is associated with reduced plasma homocysteine levels, which may be beneficial in the long term [89, 90]. Supplementation is recommended in those with a poor diet or severe hemolysis and in pregnancy; doses of folic acid of 2.5 mg/day up to the age of five years and 5 mg/day thereafter should be given [87]. For hemolysis due to ABO incompatibility, 50 µg/kg daily (rounded up to the nearest 50 µg) should be given for the first six weeks of life.

Sideroblastic anemia

Sideroblastic anemia arises when there is a defect in either heme biosynthesis or iron homeostasis within the mitochondria. The hallmark of this anemia is ineffective hemoglobin synthesis and erythropoiesis with ring sideroblasts present in the bone marrow. These are erythroblasts in which deposits of inorganic iron are found in the mitochondria, appearing as a ring around the nucleus when the cells are stained for iron (Fig. 3.8). These tend to appear in intermediate and late erythroblasts in both congenital and acquired sideroblastic anemia.

In most congenital forms of sideroblastic anemia, there is either a normoblastic, normocytic anemia or, more often, a microcytic and hypochromic anemia (Fig. 3.9). Often, there is a significant increase in body iron stores due to enhanced absorption secondary to the increased but ineffective erythropoietic activity (Fig. 3.10). Some patients have increases in free erythrocyte porphyrins [91], but the majority have normal levels and low protoporphyrins [92, 93]. This is in contrast to patients with idiopathic acquired sideroblastic anemia, where free erythrocyte porphyrin is almost always raised [93, 94, 95]. Sideroblastic anemia is usually X-linked, and thus is seen mainly in boys. Two X-linked proteins important in mitochondrial iron homeostasis are the enzyme erythroid δ-aminolevulinic acid synthetase (ALASE) and an ATP-binding cassette transporter protein, ABC7. Mutations in both genes have been identified in X-liked, sideroblastic anemia, resulting in functionally defective proteins [96–99]. Mutations in *ALASE*, the gene coding for the enzyme which catalyzes the rate-limiting, initial step in heme biosynthesis, result in impaired heme synthesis and thus hemoglobin production. This leads to a microcytic, hypochromic anemia, and unused iron accumulates in the mitochondria, giving rise to the ringed sideroblasts. The disorder can present in infancy or in later childhood, and may be associated with a progressive anemia requiring transfusion. This will exacerbate the iron loading secondary to continued ineffective erythropoiesis, and chelation therapy with drugs such as deferoxamine to remove the excess iron is required. Oral pyridoxine in pharmacologic doses can attenuate the clinical picture, probably due to its function as a cofactor of ALASE, although chelation therapy may be required first in some, to deplete the excess iron stores, before a response is seen [97, 98]. Mutations in *ABC7* result in a milder disorder which is associated with ataxia and may not require transfusion [96, 99].

Sideroblastic anemia is also seen as part of other syndromes where there is a mitochondrial cytopathy or other disturbances in cellular metabolism. An example of the former is Pearson syndrome, characterized by a sideroblastic anemia, neutropenia, and exocrine pancreatic dysfunction. Infants can present with variable cytopenias, cytoplasmic vacuolation of cells in both the peripheral blood and bone marrow, and a lactic acidosis [100] (Fig. 3.11). Hepatic, renal, and neurological dysfunction have also been described. A rare syndrome in which the main defect is one of thiamine transport is associated with sideroblasts in conjunction with a megaloblastic anemia, diabetes mellitus, and deafness. This disorder responds to pharmacological doses of thiamine and has been termed "thiamine-responsive megaloblastic anemia" [101].

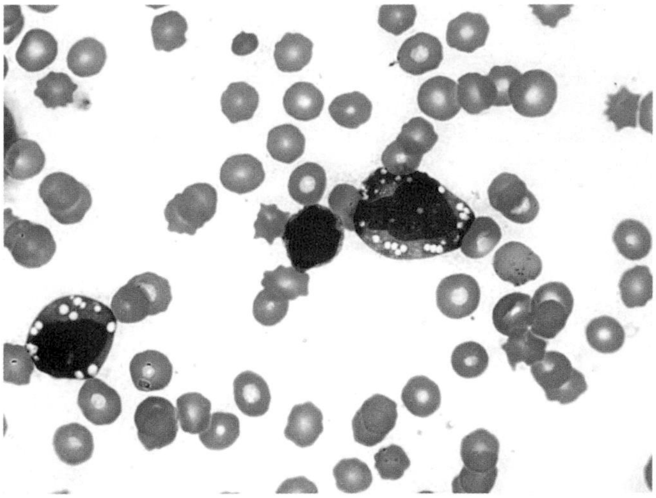

Fig. 3.11. Bone marrow aspirate film from an infant with Pearson syndrome, showing cytoplasmic vacuolation and an erythrocyte with multiple Pappenheimer bodies (May–Grünwald–Giemsa stain).

Acquired sideroblastic anemia is rarer in children than in adults, and, so far, screening some of the genes implicated in congenital sideroblastic anemia has not revealed any mutations [95]. The anemia can be secondary to drugs such as isoniazid or to toxins such as lead. Isoniazid inhibits ALASE activity, and it is standard to give pyridoxine when isoniazid is prescribed. Lead intoxication is an insidious cause of sideroblastic anemia and is more likely with iron deficiency, due to its utilization of the same absorptive pathway, which is enhanced in the deficiency state. Lead inhibits enzymes of the heme biosynthetic pathway in all cells, most importantly δ-aminolevulinic acid synthetase and the intramitochondrial enzyme ferrochelatase. Lead excess should be screened for in children presenting with sideroblastic anemia. Acquired sideroblastic anemia can also be a manifestation of a myelodysplastic process, sometimes associated with chromosomal abnormalities such as 5q− or 7q−. Neutropenia and thrombocytopenia may also be seen in such cases. In children, this form of sideroblastic anemia is rarely seen unless secondary to previous chemotherapy, particularly alkylating agents, for cancer [102]. Some patients with sideroblastic anemia will progress to acute myeloid leukemia, but the proportion in children is not known.

References

1. **Reddy MB, Cook JD.** Assessment of dietary determinants of nonheme-iron absorption in humans and rats. *American Journal of Clinical Nutrition.* 1991;**54**(4):723–728.

2. **Serfass RE, Reddy MB.** Breast milk fractions solubilize Fe(III) and enhance iron flux across Caco-2 cells. *Journal of Nutrition.* 2003;**133**(2):449–455.

3. **Engelmann MD, Davidsson L, Sandstrom B,** *et al.* The influence of meat on nonheme iron absorption in infants. *Pediatric Research.* 1998;**43**(6): 768–773.

4. **Shayeghi M, Latunde-Dada GO, Oakhill JS,** *et al.* Identification of an intestinal heme transporter. *Cell.* 2005; **122**(5):789–801.

5. **Anderson GJ, Frazer DM.** Recent advances in intestinal iron transport. *Current Gastroenterology Reports.* 2005; 7(5):365–372.

6. **Andrews NC.** The molecular basis of iron metabolism. In Provan D, Gribben J, eds. *Molecular Hematology* (2nd edn). Malden, MA: Blackwell; 2005, 150–157.

7. **Anderson GJ, Frazer DM, McKie AT, Vulpe CD, Smith A.** Mechanisms of haem and non-haem iron absorption: lessons from inherited disorders of iron metabolism. *Biometals.* 2005;**18**(4): 339–348.

8. **Latunde-Dada G, Van Der Westhuizen J, Vulpe C,** *et al.* Molecular and functional roles of duodenal cytochrome B (Dcytb) in iron metabolism. *Blood Cells, Molecules,*

and Diseases. 2002;**29**(3):356–360.

9. **Andrews NC**. The iron transporter DMT1. *International Journal of Biochemistry and Cell Biology.* 1999;**31**(10):991–994.

10. **Donovan A, Brownlie A, Zhou Y**, *et al.* Positional cloning of zebrafish ferroportin1 identifies a conserved vertebrate iron exporter. *Nature.* 2000;**403**(6771):776–781.

11. **Aisen P, Enns C, Wessling-Resnick M**. Chemistry and biology of eukaryotic iron metabolism. *International Journal of Biochemistry and Cell Biology.* 2001;**33**(10):940–959.

12. **Roy CN, Enns CA**. Iron homeostasis: new tales from the crypt. *Blood.* 2000;**96**(13):4020–4027.

13. **Vulpe CD, Kuo YM, Murphy TL**, *et al.* Hephaestin, a ceruloplasmin homologue implicated in intestinal iron transport, is defective in the sla mouse. *Nature Genetics.* 1999;**21**(2):195–199.

14. **Johnstone RM, Bianchini A, Teng K**. Reticulocyte maturation and exosome release: transferrin receptor containing exosomes shows multiple plasma membrane functions. *Blood.* 1989;**74**(5):1844–1851.

15. **Cook JD**. The measurement of serum transferrin receptor. *American Journal of the Medical Sciences.* 1999;**318**(4):269–276.

16. **Loh T, Higuchi D, van Bockxmeer F, Smith C, Brown E**. Transferrin receptors on the human placental microvillous membrane. *Journal of Clinical Investigation.* 1980;**65**(5):1182–1191.

17. **Ganz T**. Hepcidin and its role in regulating systemic iron metabolism. In Berliner N, Linker C, Schiffer C, eds. *American Society of Hematology Education Program Book.* Orlando, FL: American Society of Hematology; 2006, 29.

18. **Nicolas G, Chauvet C, Viatte L**, *et al.* The gene encoding the iron regulatory peptide hepcidin is regulated by anemia, hypoxia, and inflammation. *Journal of Clinical Investigation.* 2002;**110**(7):1037–1044.

19. **Papanikolaou G, Tzilianos M, Christakis JI**, *et al.* Hepcidin in iron overload disorders. *Blood.* 2005;**105**(10):4103–4105.

20. **Kearney SL, Nemeth E, Neufeld EJ**, *et al.* Urinary hepcidin in congenital chronic anemias. *Pediatric Blood and Cancer.* 2007;**48**(1):57–63.

21. **May A, Fitzsimons E**. Sideroblastic anaemia. *Baillière's Clinical Haematology.* 1994;**7**(4):851–879.

22. **Girdwood RH**. Drug-induced anaemias. *Drugs.* 1976;**11**(5):394–404.

23. **Tenner S, Rollhauser C, Butt F, Gonzalez P**. Sideroblastic anemia. A diagnosis to consider in alcoholic patients. *Postgraduate Medicine.* 1992;**92**(7):147–150.

24. **Oski FA**. Iron deficiency in infancy and childhood. *New England Journal of Medicine.* 1993;**329**(3):190–193.

25. **Georgieff MK, Wewerka SW, Nelson CA, Deregnier RA**. Iron status at 9 months of infants with low iron stores at birth. *Journal of Pediatrics.* 2002;**141**(3):405–409.

26. **Puolakka J, Janne O, Vihko R**. Evaluation by serum ferritin assay of the influence of maternal iron stores on the iron status of newborns and infants. *Acta Obstetricia et Gynecologica Scandinavica. Supplement.* 1980;**95**:53–56.

27. **Rao R, Georgieff MK**. Perinatal aspects of iron metabolism. *Acta Paediatrica (Oslo, Norway: 1992). Supplement.* 2002;**91**(438):124–129.

28. **Bada HS, Das A, Bauer CR**, *et al.* Low birth weight and preterm births: etiologic fraction attributable to prenatal drug exposure. *Journal of Perinatology.* 2005;**25**(10):631–637.

29. **Stoltzfus RJ, Chwaya HM, Montresor A**, *et al.* Malaria, hookworms and recent fever are related to anemia and iron status indicators in 0- to 5-y old Zanzibari children and these relationships change with age. *Journal of Nutrition.* 2000;**130**(7):1724–1733.

30. **Calis JC, Phiri KS, Faragher EB**, *et al.* Severe anemia in Malawian children. *New England Journal of Medicine.* 2008;**358**(9):888–899.

31. **Siimes MA, Addiego JE Jr., Dallman PR**. Ferritin in serum: diagnosis of iron deficiency and iron overload in infants and children. *Blood.* 1974;**43**(4):581–590.

32. **Labbe RF, Rettmer RL**. Zinc protoporphyrin: a product of iron-deficient erythropoiesis. *Seminars in Hematology.* 1989;**26**(1):40–46.

33. **Lipschitz DA, Cook JD, Finch CA**. A clinical evaluation of serum ferritin as an index of iron stores. *New England Journal of Medicine.* 1974;**290**(22):1213–1216.

34. **Elin RJ, Wolff SM, Finch CA**. Effect of induced fever on serum iron and ferritin concentrations in man. *Blood.* 1977;**49**(1):147–153.

35. **Morton AG, Tavill AS**. The role of iron in the regulation of hepatic transferrin synthesis. *British Journal of Haematology.* 1977;**36**(3):383–394.

36. **Piomelli S, Seaman C, Kapoor S**. Lead-induced abnormalities of porphyrin metabolism. The relationship with iron deficiency. *Annals of the New York Academy of Sciences.* 1987;**514**:278–288.

37. **Punnonen K, Irjala K, Rajamaki A**. Serum transferrin receptor and its ratio to serum ferritin in the diagnosis of iron deficiency. *Blood.* 1997;**89**(3):1052–1057.

38. **Beard J, Deregnier RA, Shaw MD, Rao R, Georgieff MK**. Diagnosis of iron deficiency in infants. *Laboratory Medicine.* 2007;**38**(2):103–108.

39. **Adamson JW**. The relationship of erythropoietin and iron metabolism to red blood cell production in humans. *Seminars in Oncology.* 1994;**21**(2 Suppl 3):9–15.

40. **Hogenkamp HPC**. The chemistry of cobalamins and related compounds. In Babior BM, ed. *Cobalamin: Biochemistry and Pathophysiology.* New York: John Wiley & Sons, Inc.; 1975, 21–74.

41. **Voet D, Voet JG**. *Biochemistry* (2nd edn.). New York: John Wiley & Sons, Inc.; 1995.

42. **Watanabe F**. Vitamin B12 sources and bioavailability. *Experimental Biology and Medicine (Maywood, NJ).* 2007;**232**(10):1266–1274.

43. **Levine AS, Doscherholmen A**. Vitamin B12 bioavailability from egg yolk and egg white: relationship to binding proteins. *American Journal of Clinical Nutrition.* 1983;**38**(3):436–439.

44. **Lee EY, Seetharam B, Alpers DH, DeSchryver-Kecskemeti K**. Immunohistochemical survey of cobalamin-binding proteins.

Gastroenterology. 1989;**97**(5):1171–1180.

45. **Aminoff M, Carter JE, Chadwick RB,** *et al.* Mutations in CUBN, encoding the intrinsic factor-vitamin B12 receptor, cubilin, cause hereditary megaloblastic anaemia 1. *Nature Genetics.* 1999;**21**(3):309–313.

46. **Kristiansen M, Aminoff M, Jacobsen C,** *et al.* Cubilin P1297L mutation associated with hereditary megaloblastic anemia 1 causes impaired recognition of intrinsic factor-vitamin B(12) by cubilin. *Blood.* 2000;**96**(2):405–409.

47. Institute of Medicine. Vitamin B12. In *Dietary Reference Intakes for Thiamin, Riboflavin, Niacin, Vitamin B6, Folate, Vitamin B12, Pantothenic Acid, Biotin, and Choline.* Washington DC: National Academic Press; 1998, 306–356.

48. **Rosenblatt DS, Whitehead VM.** Cobalamin and folate deficiency: acquired and hereditary disorders in children. *Seminars in Hematology.* 1999;**36**(1):19–34.

49. **Whitehead VM.** Acquired and inherited disorders of cobalamin and folate in children. *British Journal of Haematology.* 2006;**134**(2):125–136.

50. **Garcia-Casal MN, Osorio C, Landaeta M,** *et al.* High prevalence of folic acid and vitamin B12 deficiencies in infants, children, adolescents and pregnant women in Venezuela. *European Journal of Clinical Nutrition.* 2005;**59**(9):1064–1070.

51. **Rogers LM, Boy E, Miller JW,** *et al.* High prevalence of cobalamin deficiency in Guatemalan schoolchildren: associations with low plasma holotranscobalamin II and elevated serum methylmalonic acid and plasma homocysteine concentrations. *American Journal of Clinical Nutrition.* 2003;**77**(2):433–440.

52. **Emery ES, Homans AC, Colletti RB.** Vitamin B12 deficiency: a cause of abnormal movements in infants. *Pediatrics.* 1997;**99**(2):255–256.

53. **von Schenck U, Bender-Gotze C, Koletzko B.** Persistence of neurological damage induced by dietary vitamin B-12 deficiency in infancy. *Archives of Disease in Childhood.* 1997;**77**(2):137–139.

54. **Arlet JB, Varet B, Besson C.** Favorable long-term outcome of a patient with

transcobalamin II deficiency. *Annals of Internal Medicine.* 2002;**137**(8):704–705.

55. **Tanner SM, Li Z, Perko JD,** *et al.* Hereditary juvenile cobalamin deficiency caused by mutations in the intrinsic factor gene. *Proceedings of the National Academy of Sciences of the United States of America.* 2005;**102**(11):4130–4133.

56. **Gordon MM, Brada N, Remacha A,** *et al.* A genetic polymorphism in the coding region of the gastric intrinsic factor gene (GIF) is associated with congenital intrinsic factor deficiency. *Human Mutation.* 2004;**23**(1):85–91.

57. **Meyers PA, Carmel R.** Hereditary transcobalamin II deficiency with subnormal serum cobalamin levels. *Pediatrics.* 1984;**74**(5):866–871.

58. **Carmel R, Ravindranath Y.** Congenital transcobalamin II deficiency presenting atypically with a low serum cobalamin level: studies demonstrating the coexistence of a circulating transcobalamin I (R binder) complex. *Blood.* 1984;**63**(3):598–605.

59. **Mayes JS, Say F, Marcus F.** Prenatal studies in a family with transcobalamin II deficiency. *American Journal of Human Genetics.* 1987;**41**(4):686–687.

60. **Matsui SM, Mahoney MJ, Rosenberg LE.** The natural history of the inherited methylmalonic acidemias. *New England Journal of Medicine.* 1983;**308**(15):857–861.

61. **Linnell JC, Bhatt HR.** Inherited errors of cobalamin metabolism and their management. *Baillière's Clinical Haematology.* 1995;**8**(3):567–601.

62. **Thompson GN, Chalmers RA, Walter JH,** *et al.* The use of metronidazole in management of methylmalonic and propionic acidaemias. *European Journal of Pediatrics.* 1990;**149**(11):792–796.

63. **Mahoney MJ, Bick D.** Recent advances in the inherited methylmalonic acidemias. *Acta Paediatrica Scandinavica.* 1987;**76**(5):689–696.

64. **Rosenblatt DS, Fenton WA.** Inherited disorders of folate and cobalamin transport and metabolism. In Scriver CR, Beaudet AL, Sly WS, Valle D, eds. *The Metabolic and Molecular Bases of Inherited Metabolic Disease.* New York: McGraw-Hill; 2001, 3897–3933.

65. **Coelho D, Suormala T, Stucki M,** *et al.* Gene identification for the cblD defect

of vitamin B12 metabolism. *New England Journal of Medicine.* 2008;**358**(14):1454–1464.

66. **Davies BW, Abel G, Puntis JW,** *et al.* Limited ileal resection in infancy: the long-term consequences. *Journal of Pediatric Surgery.* 1999;**34**(4):583–587.

67. **Lindenbaum J, Savage DG, Stabler SP, Allen RH.** Diagnosis of cobalamin deficiency: II. Relative sensitivities of serum cobalamin, methylmalonic acid, and total homocysteine concentrations. *American Journal of Hematology.* 1990;**34**(2):99–107.

68. **Gardyn J, Mittelman M, Zlotnik J, Sela BA, Cohen AM.** Oral contraceptives can cause falsely low vitamin B(12) levels. *Acta Haematologica.* 2000;**104**(1):22–24.

69. **Rasmussen K, Moller J.** Methodologies of testing. In Carmel R, Jacobsen D, eds. *Homocysteine in Health and Disease.* Cambridge: Cambridge University Press; 2001, 199–211.

70. **Nilsson M, Norberg B, Hultdin J,** *et al.* Medical intelligence in Sweden. Vitamin B12: oral compared with parenteral? *Postgraduate Medical Journal.* 2005;**81**(953):191–193.

71. **Oakley GP Jr., Bell KN, Weber MB.** Recommendations for accelerating global action to prevent folic acid-preventable birth defects and other folate-deficiency diseases: meeting of experts on preventing folic acid-preventable neural tube defects. *Birth Defects Research. Part A, Clinical and Molecular Teratology.* 2004;**70**(11):835–837.

72. **Zhao R, Goldman ID.** The molecular identity and characterization of a Proton-coupled Folate Transporter—PCFT; biological ramifications and impact on the activity of pemetrexed. *Cancer Metastasis Reviews.* 2007;**26**(1):129–139.

73. **Zhao R, Min SH, Qiu A,** *et al.* The spectrum of mutations in the PCFT gene, coding for an intestinal folate transporter, that are the basis for hereditary folate malabsorption. *Blood.* 2007;**110**(4):1147–1152.

74. Institute of Medicine. Folate. In *Dietary Reference Intakes for Thiamin, Riboflavin, Vitamin B6, Folate, Vitamin B12, Pantothenic Acid, Biotin, and Choline.* Washington, DC: National Academies Press; 1998, 196–305.

75. **Gregory JF 3rd, Caudill MA, Opalko FJ, Bailey LB**. Kinetics of folate turnover in pregnant women (second trimester) and nonpregnant controls during folic acid supplementation: stable-isotopic labeling of plasma folate, urinary folate and folate catabolites shows subtle effects of pregnancy on turnover of folate pools. *Journal of Nutrition*. 2001;**131**(7):1928–1937.

76. **Czeizel AE, Dudas I**. Prevention of the first occurrence of neural-tube defects by periconceptional vitamin supplementation. *New England Journal of Medicine*. 1992;**327**(26): 1832–1835.

77. **Ray JG, Meier C, Vermeulen MJ**, *et al*. Association of neural tube defects and folic acid food fortification in Canada. *Lancet*. 2002;**360**(9350):2047–2048.

78. **Rothenberg SP**. Increasing the dietary intake of folate: pros and cons. *Seminars in Hematology*. 1999;**36**(1):65–74.

79. **Mills JL, Von Kohorn I, Conley MR**, *et al*. Low vitamin B-12 concentrations in patients without anemia: the effect of folic acid fortification of grain. *American Journal of Clinical Nutrition*. 2003;**77**(6):1474–1477.

80. **Hoffbrand AV**. Anaemia in adult coeliac disease. *Clinics in Gastroenterology*. 1974;**3**(1):71–89.

81. **Dickey W, Hughes DF**. Histology of the terminal ileum in coeliac disease. *Scandinavian Journal of Gastroenterology*. 2004;**39**(7):665–667.

82. **Lindenbaum J**. Aspects of vitamin B12 and folate metabolism in malabsorption syndromes. *The American Journal of Medicine*. 1979;**67**(6):1037–1048.

83. **Lewis DP, Van Dyke DC, Willhite LA, Stumbo PJ, Berg MJ**. Phenytoin-folic acid interaction. *The Annals of Pharmacotherapy*. 1995;**29**(7-8):726–735.

84. **Volsett SE, Botto LD**. Neural tube defects, other congenital malformations and single nucleotide polymorphisms in the 5,10-methylenetetrahydrofolate reductase (MTHFR) gene: a metanalysis. In Ueland PM, Rozen R, eds. *MTHFR Polymorphisms and Disease*. Georgetown, TX: Landes Bioscience; 2004, 126–144.

85. **Geller J, Kronn D, Jayabose S, Sandoval C**. Hereditary folate malabsorption: family report and review of the literature. *Medicine (Baltimore)*. 2002;**81**(1):51–68.

86. **Hilton JF, Christensen KE, Watkins D**, *et al*. The molecular basis of glutamate formiminotransferase deficiency. *Human Mutation*. 2003;**22**(1):67–73.

87. **Bolton-Maggs PH, Stevens RF, Dodd NJ**, *et al*. Guidelines for the diagnosis and management of hereditary spherocytosis. *British Journal of Haematology*. 2004;**126**(4):455–474.

88. **Rabb LM, Grandison Y, Mason K**, *et al*. A trial of folate supplementation in children with homozygous sickle cell disease. *British Journal of Haematology*. 1983;**54**(4):589–594.

89. **Lowenthal EA, Mayo MS, Cornwell PE, Thornley-Brown D**. Homocysteine elevation in sickle cell disease. *Journal of the American College of Nutrition*. 2000;**19**(5):608–612.

90. **Van Der Dijs FP, Fokkema MR, Dijck-Brouwer DA**, *et al*. Optimization of folic acid, vitamin B(12), and vitamin B(6) supplements in pediatric patients with sickle cell disease. *American Journal of Hematology*. 2002;**69**(4):239–246.

91. **Pagon RA, Bird TD, Detter JC, Pierce I**. Hereditary sideroblastic anaemia and ataxia: an X linked recessive disorder. *Journal of Medical Genetics*. 1985;**22**(4): 267–273.

92. **Pasanen AV, Salmi M, Tenhunen R, Vuopio P**. Haem synthesis during pyridoxine therapy in two families with different types of hereditary sideroblastic anaemia. *Annals of Clinical Research*. 1982;**14**(2):61–65.

93. **Takeda Y, Sawada H, Sawai H**, *et al*. Acquired hypochromic and microcytic sideroblastic anaemia responsive to pyridoxine with low value of free erythrocyte protoporphyrin: a possible subgroup of idiopathic acquired sideroblastic anaemia (IASA). *British Journal of Haematology*. 1995;**90**(1): 207–209.

94. **Romslo I, Brun A, Sandberg S**, *et al*. Sideroblastic anemia with markedly increased free erythrocyte protoporphyrin without dermal photosensitivity. *Blood*. 1982;**59**(3): 628–633.

95. **Steensma DP, Hecksel KA, Porcher JC, Lasho TL**. Candidate gene mutation analysis in idiopathic acquired sideroblastic anemia (refractory anemia with ringed sideroblasts). *Leukemia Research*. 2007;**31**(5):623–628.

96. **Buchanan GR, Bottomley SS, Nitschke R**. Bone marrow delta-aminolaevulinate synthase deficiency in a female with congenital sideroblastic anemia. *Blood*. 1980;**55**(1):109–115.

97. **Cotter PD, Rucknagel DL, Bishop DF**. X-linked sideroblastic anemia: identification of the mutation in the erythroid-specific delta-aminolevulinate synthase gene (ALAS2) in the original family described by Cooley. *Blood*. 1994; **84**(11):3915–3924.

98. **Cotter PD, May A, Li L**, *et al*. Four new mutations in the erythroid-specific 5-aminolevulinate synthase (ALAS2) gene causing X-linked sideroblastic anemia: increased pyridoxine responsiveness after removal of iron overload by phlebotomy and coinheritance of hereditary hemochromatosis. *Blood*. 1999;**93**(5): 1757–1769.

99. **Allikmets R, Raskind WH, Hutchinson A**, *et al*. Mutation of a putative mitochondrial iron transporter gene (ABC7) in X-linked sideroblastic anemia and ataxia (XLSA/A). *Human Molecular Genetics*. 1999;**8**(5):743–749.

100. **Rotig A, Cormier V, Blanche S**, *et al*. Pearson's marrow-pancreas syndrome. A multisystem mitochondrial disorder in infancy. *Journal of Clinical Investigation*. 1990;**86**(5):1601–1608.

101. **Porter FS, Rogers LE, Sidbury JB Jr**. Thiamine-responsive megaloblastic anemia. *Journal of Pediatrics*. 1969; **74**(4):494–504.

102. **Kitahara M, Cosgriff TM, Eyre HJ**. Sideroblastic anemia as a preleukemic event in patients treated for Hodgkin's disease. *Annals of Internal Medicine*. 1980;**92**(5): 625–627.

Disorders of hemoglobin synthesis
Thalassemias and structural hemoglobinopathies

Alexander Kratz and Jeffrey Jhang

Normal hemoglobins

Structure and function of hemoglobin

Hemoglobin consists of two alpha-like and two beta-like globin chains which combine to form a tetramer. The globin tetramer is hydrophilic on its surface, making the molecule water soluble. The center is hydrophobic, stabilizing the heme ring and the iron molecule in the ferrous state (Fe^{2+}). Located in the interior of each globin chain is a heme ring with an iron molecule in the center. It is in the heme ring that oxygen binding and release take place. In addition to oxygen transport, hemoglobin also plays a minor role in the transport of carbon dioxide, and as a scavenger of nitric oxide (NO).

As the partial pressure of oxygen is increased, hemoglobin becomes saturated with oxygen. The partial pressure at which 50% of hemoglobin is saturated is called the p50. Normal subjects have a p50 between 23 and 27 mmHg. Binding of an oxygen molecule in one heme changes the tetrameric structure so that additional oxygen molecules are bound with greater ease; this property of hemoglobin is called cooperativity, and is dependent on interactions between the globin chains ("heme–heme interaction"). The oxygen dissociation curve for hemoglobin A is sigmoid shaped because of this cooperativity (Fig. 4.1) [1, 2]. The sigmoid shape reflects how oxygen binding is favored at high oxygen tensions (lungs) and is rapidly released at low oxygen tensions (tissues). Physiologic conditions that have high oxygen demand, such as increased temperature and decreased pH, shift the oxygen dissociation curve to the right; this facilitates oxygen release to the tissues (increased p50). Conditions that increase oxygen affinity of hemoglobin, like decreased 2,3-diphosphoglycerate (2,3-DPG), shift the curve to the left and decrease oxygen delivery to the tissues (decreased p50).

Genetics and transcription control of hemoglobin

Globin genes are found throughout nature in invertebrates and vertebrates, suggesting that these genes have a common origin and that vertebrate α-like and β-like globin genes diverged from a common ancestor over 450 million years ago [3]. Globin

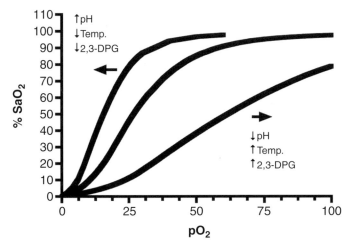

Fig. 4.1. Hemoglobin oxygen dissociation curve. The oxygen dissociation curve shows hemoglobin oxygen saturation (%SaO_2) versus the partial pressure of O_2 (pO_2). The middle curve represents the normal oxygen dissociation curve with a p50 of 26 mmHg. Decreased pH, increased temperature and increased 2,3-diphosphoglycerate (2,3-DPG) shift the curve to the right (increase the p50), which favors oxygen delivery to the tissues. The curve shifts to the left with increased pH and decreased temperature or 2,3-DPG. Graph plotted based on data in Adair [2].

gene duplications and other gene modifications have led to specialization of the globin chains, with the preservation of significant homology between species and between the duplicated genes. For example, the α-globin genes, $\alpha1$ and $\alpha2$, represent what is thought to be a duplication of a common ancestor. Each human α-like and β-like globin gene is composed of three exons and two introns (Fig. 4.2). The introns, also called intervening sequences 1 and 2 (IVS1 and IVS2) are located between exons 1 and 2 and exons 2 and 3, respectively. IVS2 is larger than IVS1 in both the α-like and β-like genes.

The human α-like and β-like globin genes are located on the short arm of chromosome 16 and chromosome 11, respectively, and are inherited as gene clusters (Fig. 4.2). The globin genes are ordered from 5' to 3', corresponding to the sequence in which they are expressed from embryogenesis to adulthood [4]. In the α-like globin cluster, the embryonic ζ-globin gene is expressed first, followed by the $\alpha2$- and $\alpha1$-globin genes during

Diagnostic Pediatric Hematopathology, ed. Maria A. Proytcheva. Published by Cambridge University Press.
© Cambridge University Press 2011.

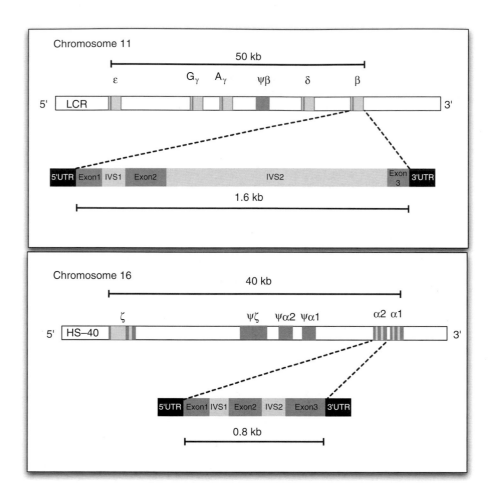

Fig. 4.2. The beta- and alpha-globin gene clusters; these are located on chromosomes 11 and 16, respectively. The beta- and alpha-like globins are arranged in the order in which they are expressed developmentally. The beta-globin cluster contains ε, $^{G}\gamma$, $^{A}\gamma$, δ, and β globin genes. The alpha-globin cluster consists of ζ, $\alpha2$, and $\alpha1$ genes. Both clusters also contain gene duplications with little or no known function. Upstream from the alpha and beta clusters are regulatory sequences known as HS-40 and the locus control region (LCR), respectively. Each globin gene contains three exons, two introns (IVS1, IVS2), and a 5' and 3' untranslated region (UTR).

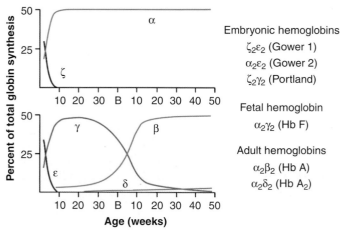

Fig. 4.3. Human hemoglobin switching: alpha- and beta-globin chain synthesis during human development. The relative percentages of alpha-like (top) and beta-like (bottom) globin chain synthesis during embryonic, fetal, and postnatal/adult life are shown. (Courtesy of Dr. David O'Neill, New York University, New York, NY.) The hemoglobins that are formed from these chains during each stage of development are indicated at the right (B = birth).

Embryonic hemoglobins
$\zeta_2\varepsilon_2$ (Gower 1)
$\alpha_2\varepsilon_2$ (Gower 2)
$\zeta_2\gamma_2$ (Portland)

Fetal hemoglobin
$\alpha_2\gamma_2$ (Hb F)

Adult hemoglobins
$\alpha_2\beta_2$ (Hb A)
$\alpha_2\delta_2$ (Hb A$_2$)

on the α-globin cluster. A recent report identified a novel transcript from this region (μ-globin) [5]. A regulatory sequence (HS-40) is located 5' to the α-globin cluster, and controls the level of expression of the genes in the α-globin cluster. During embryonic life, the ε-globin gene is the first β-like globin chain that is expressed; production ceases early after embryogenesis. During fetal life, the majority of the hemoglobin produced is hemoglobin F, which is encoded on the two homologous, duplicated γ genes denoted $^{G}\gamma$ and $^{A}\gamma$ that differ only by one amino acid (glycine in $^{G}\gamma$ and alanine in $^{A}\gamma$). $^{G}\gamma$ and $^{A}\gamma$ are expressed in a ratio of 3 : 1 during fetal life; after birth, this ratio changes to 3 : 2. Hemoglobin β and δ chains are produced later in development and into adulthood. The $\psi\beta$ pseudogene, which shares significant homology with its functional counterparts, does not produce any functional globin chains. The locus control region (LCR) is a region of regulatory sequences 5' to the β-globin cluster, and controls the expression of β-like globins.

During embryonic life, α-like and β-like globins combine to form tetramers to produce hemoglobin Gower 1 ($\zeta_2\varepsilon_2$), hemoglobin Gower 2 ($\alpha_2\varepsilon_2$), and hemoglobin Portland ($\zeta_2\gamma_2$) (Fig. 4.3). During fetal life, the majority of the hemoglobin produced is hemoglobin F ($\alpha_2\gamma_2$), while a small amount of hemoglobin A ($\alpha_2\beta_2$) is also produced. At birth, Hb A$_2$ is either not present or only present in minimal amounts. After birth, hemoglobin F production declines and hemoglobin A levels

fetal life, which continue to be expressed in adulthood. Protein production from the $\alpha2$ gene is approximately two-times higher than from the $\alpha1$ gene. The $\psi\zeta$, $\psi\alpha2$ and $\psi\alpha1$ genes, which were traditionally regarded as non-functioning duplicates of their functional counterparts (pseudogenes), are also located

increase rapidly; normal adult hemoglobin levels are usually present by the age of 12–18 months [4]. Hemoglobin F levels are higher in premature infants than in term newborns [6]. The majority of hemoglobin (95–98%) after the age of 12–18 months is Hb A. It is formed by two subunits of alpha-globin and two subunits of beta-globin ($\alpha_2\beta_2$). Hemoglobin A_2 ($\alpha_2\delta_2$; 2–3.5%) and fetal hemoglobin (Hb F; $\alpha_2\gamma_2$; less than 2%) are only minor fractions of the total hemoglobin.

Disorders of hemoglobin synthesis

Overview

Disorders of hemoglobin (Hb) synthesis can be divided into two major categories: structural hemoglobinopathies and thalassemias. *Structural hemoglobinopathies*, often simply referred to as hemoglobinopathies, are caused by mutations that lead to the transcription of structurally abnormal hemoglobins, such as Hb S, Hb C, Hb D-Punjab, and Hb O-Arab, while *thalassemias* are caused by mutations that lead to the reduced synthesis of normal globin chains. Certain structural hemoglobinopathies, such as Hb Constant Spring, Hb Lepore, and Hb E, share features of both structural hemoglobinopathies and thalassemias by producing structurally abnormal globin chains at a decreased rate or with reduced stability. A comprehensive relational database describing over 1200 genetic variants affecting hemoglobin synthesis and structure is available online at http://globin.cse.psu.edu [7]. The database lists the associated pathology, clinical and hematologic manifestations, electrophoretic mobility, methods of isolation, stability information, and ethnic occurrence, as well as references to the literature.

The majority of structural hemoglobinopathies are not clinically significant. Only a small number of mutations, such as Hb S, Hb C, Hb D-Punjab, Hb E, Hb O-Arab, Hb Chesapeake, or Hb Beth Israel are associated with clinical symptoms. Clinical manifestations frequently only occur in the homozygous (e.g., sickle cell disease) or compound heterozygous (e.g., SC disease) state. Unstable hemoglobins and hemoglobins with altered oxygen affinity are usually symptomatic in the heterozygous state. The majority of individuals who are carriers for mutations associated with thalassemias show only mild hematologic abnormalities without clinical symptoms. It is usually in the homozygous state that severe disease manifestations are observed. Thalassemias and hemoglobinopathies can be co-inherited, sometimes resulting in severe disease (e.g., compound heterozygous hemoglobin S/β°-thalassemia). The presence of a large number of genetic or environmental factors can also ameliorate or exacerbate these diseases, making it difficult to establish the prognosis.

Population genetics

Seven percent of the global population, or over 400 million individuals, are carriers of one or more mutations affecting the globin genes. With an annual birth rate globally for sickle cell disease and severe thalassemia of 300 000 to 500 000, hemoglobin disorders are the most common lethal single gene disorders [8, 9]. In the United States, sickle cell disease is the most common inherited blood disorder and affects 72 000 Americans [10]. One in 12 African-Americans and 1 in 100 Hispanic Americans are carriers of the sickle cell gene [11]. The geographic distribution of hemoglobin disorders follows the distribution of malaria, and it is widely accepted that this is a result of heterozygote protection from infection by *Plasmodium falciparum*. Hb S is more commonly found in Africa, α-thalassemia in Southeast Asia, and β-thalassemia is most frequent in people of Mediterranean and Southeast Asian descent. Knowledge of the ethnic origin of a patient can therefore be helpful in identifying a hemoglobin variant; however, many classical distribution patterns have been changed by migration.

In areas where hemoglobinopathies and thalassemias occur with high frequency, the associated morbidity and mortality have significant socioeconomic costs [12]. Prenatal screening programs have therefore been developed to provide either universal or targeted screening, with genetic counseling of couples at risk for having an infant with a hemoglobin disorder [13]. Some of these programs have been very successful; for example, carrier screening for β-thalassemia has been very successful in Sardinia and Cyprus and has led to a significant decrease in the number of affected births [14, 15]. The success of such programs is critically dependent on the education of the public and the availability of genetic counseling programs. For couples who do not wish to consider termination of a pregnancy, preimplantation genetic diagnosis of blastocysts conceived by *in vitro* fertilization may be an acceptable alternative.

In addition to the prenatal screening programs that have been implemented in many countries, neonatal screening programs for the early identification of sickle cell disease have been developed. In the United States, Congress passed the National Sickle Cell Anemia Control Act in 1972, which initiated grant support for sickle cell disease newborn screening. Universal screening for sickle cell disease is now mandated by law in all 50 states and the District of Columbia. The main impetus for universal newborn screening has been the demonstration that early education of parents and early medical intervention can markedly reduce morbidity and mortality caused by sickle cell disease in infancy and childhood. For example, prophylactic penicillin for newborns can reduce mortality due to sickle cell disease to 1.8% (vs. 8% in infants who are first diagnosed after the age of three months) [16]. The success of these approaches depends highly on the availability of programs that educate parents on the early detection of the signs and symptoms of possible complications of sickle cell disease and the availability of expert care.

Thalassemias

Thalassemias are quantitative deficiencies of structurally normal hemoglobins caused by genetic defects in the number of functional genes, DNA transcription, RNA splicing, translation

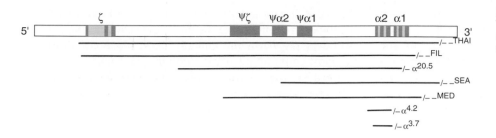

Fig. 4.4. Common alpha-globin gene deletions. The relative size and breakpoints of alpha gene deletions that cause α^+ and α°-thalassemia are shown (not to scale) below the alpha-globin cluster.

of hemoglobin genes, or stability of the final product. The thalassemias are classified according to the affected globin chain(s), with the majority of patients carrying alpha-thalassemia, beta-thalassemia, or delta-beta-thalassemia mutations [17, 18]. Many clinical manifestations of thalassemias are caused by an imbalance of the proportions of alpha- and beta-globin chains. This imbalance causes the formation of homotetramers, which precipitate in the red cells and cause hemolysis. Clinically, thalassemias are classified according to the severity of the symptoms as thalassemia minor (asymptomatic), thalassemia intermedia (non-transfusion-dependent anemia), and thalassemia major (transfusion-dependent, severe anemia). Patients with a thalassemic trait show an increased susceptibility to iron overload; it is therefore important to distinguish patients whose microcytosis and hypochromasia are due to thalassemic trait from patients with iron deficiency, in order to avoid the unnecessary and potentially harmful administration of iron [19].

Alpha-thalassemias

Alpha-thalassemias are most commonly caused by the deletion of one or more of the four α genes (Fig. 4.4); point mutations in upstream regulatory sequences or within the genes can also cause diminished alpha chain productions. The alteration in the rate of normal globin synthesis commonly leads to a microcytic, hypochromic anemia and, in contrast to iron deficiency anemia, a compensatory increase in the RBC count ("microcytosis with relative erythrocytosis"). Depending on the extent to which alpha chain production is reduced, γ-chain tetramers (Hb Bart) and β-chain tetramers (Hb H) can be formed in fetal and neonatal life and after birth, respectively. The lack of a single alpha gene ($-\alpha/\alpha\alpha$) is usually asymptomatic ("silent carrier"; α^+-thalassemia trait) or leads to mild microcytosis. Neonatal screening may show the presence of small amounts of Hb Bart. The absence of two alpha genes, also classified as alpha-thalassemia trait or alpha-thalassemia minor, can be caused by two different genotypes and often leads to a mild microcytic anemia. α°-thalassemia trait ($--/\alpha\alpha$), which is the lack of two alpha genes in cis, can be found in southern China, Southeast Asia, and the Mediterranean, while the $-\alpha/-\alpha$ genotype (homozygous α^+-thalassemia) is more common among people of African and southeast Indian descent; this genotype can be caused by compound heterozygosity for two different deletions on each chromosome.

Hemoglobin H disease ($--/-\alpha$; compound heterozygosity for α°-thalassemia and α^+-thalassemia) leads to the formation of β-chain tetramers (Hb H) that precipitate to cause a hemolytic anemia with splenomegaly. The formation of Heinz bodies by these precipitates can be visualized with a supravital stain, such as crystal violet. The complete absence of alpha chains ($--/--$; homozygous α°-thalassemia) leads to the formation of gamma tetramers *in utero* (Hb Bart). Hb Bart has a very high affinity for oxygen; the condition is not compatible with life, leading to hydrops fetalis or death shortly after birth.

Some individuals have three or even four copies of the alpha gene on the same chromosome. In patients with the genotype $--/\alpha\alpha\alpha$ or $-\alpha/\alpha\alpha\alpha$, the alpha chain excess from one chromosome balances the lack of genes on the other chromosome. This can be of importance in genetic counseling, since offspring who inherit the chromosome lacking the alpha gene(s) may show symptoms of thalassemia. In addition, coinheritance of beta-thalassemia trait and the genotype $\alpha\alpha/\alpha\alpha\alpha$ leads to an increased excess of alpha chains, with more severe hemolysis.

In extremely rare cases, alpha-thalassemia can be associated with mental retardation syndromes [17, 20]. Two types have been described: a deletional type involving chromosome 16 (ATR-16) and a non-deletional X-linked type (ATR-X) involving a transacting factor. These syndromes should be suspected in patients with mental retardation, dysmorphic facial features, and genitourinary abnormalities, who have mild hemoglobin H disease, yet do not have the ethnic or geographic background common for thalassemias (e.g., Northern Europeans).

Beta-thalassemias

Beta-thalassemias are mostly caused by a large number of different point mutations; only a minority are due to deletions or insertions [21]. Beta-thalassemias can be classified, according to the amount of beta chain production, into β°-thalassemia (total absence of beta chain production) or β^+-thalassemia (partial deficiency of beta chain production). Depending on the underlying mutation, the severity of clinical symptoms can range from laboratory abnormalities with no clinical manifestations (beta-thalassemia minor), to non-transfusion-dependent anemia (beta-thalassemia intermedia), and severe, transfusion-dependent anemia (beta-thalassemia major).

The majority of β-thalassemia heterozygotes are asymptomatic, but laboratory studies may show microcytosis in the absence of a structural hemoglobin variant and the presence of an elevated total Hb A_2. It is important to note that in patients with a structural delta chain variant (e.g., Hb A_2'), the total A_2 consists of the sum of the normal and the variant Hb A_2.

Approximately half of the patients may also show an elevation in Hb F, but usually not in excess of 5%. It should be noted that cases of beta-thalassemia trait with normal hemoglobin A_2 levels can be encountered, especially in the presence of concomitant conditions that reduce the percentage of hemoglobin A_2, such as alpha-thalassemia trait, delta-thalassemia, iron deficiency, anemia of chronic disease, myelodysplastic syndrome, and leukemias. Certain beta-thalassemia mutations are associated with a normal mean corpuscular volume (MCV).

Patients with homozygous or compound heterozygous beta-thalassemia develop severe anemia resulting from insufficient beta chain production, and hemolysis due to the formation of alpha-globin chain tetramers. They can develop skeletal changes due to ineffective erythropoiesis, hepatosplenomegaly, growth retardation, and infections. Since beta-globin chains are not significantly produced until several months after birth, neonates are generally asymptomatic at birth. With the lack of replacement of hemoglobin F with hemoglobin A, symptoms start to develop around the age of six months. The delay in the onset of symptoms until the age of six months in beta-thalassemia contrasts with alpha-thalassemia; the lack of alpha chains manifests itself already during fetal life or at birth, since alpha-globin is a component of hemoglobin F.

Delta-beta-thalassemias

Delta-beta-thalassemias are the consequence of the deletion of both the delta and beta genes. The only genes available for transcription on the affected chromosome are the gamma genes. Patients have a phenotype similar to beta-thalassemia trait, but without the increase in Hb A_2 (due to the lack of delta chain production). Therefore, it is important to exclude delta-beta-thalassemias in a patient with microcytosis and erythrocytosis but with a normal hemoglobin A_2 and elevated hemoglobin F. In heterozygotes, Hb F is elevated to 5–20%, with a heterocellular distribution of Hb F, while homozygotes express only Hb F. Elevation of hemoglobin F can also be found in *hereditary persistence of fetal hemoglobin* (HPFH). This is an asymptomatic condition characterized by the persistence of fetal hemoglobin into adult age, but with normal red cell indices.

Hemoglobin Lepore can be regarded as an unusual form of delta-beta-thalassemia. It arose by an unequal homologous recombination event which fused the 5′ end of the delta gene with the 3′ end of the beta gene. The resulting chromosome contains a fused $\delta\beta$ gene. Since the gene is under the control of the weak delta promoter, the resulting globin is poorly expressed. Heterozygotes have 6–10% Hb Lepore and show mild thalassemic features. Homozygotes have 90% Hb F and approximately 10% Hb Lepore.

Structural hemoglobinopathies

The first hemoglobin variants discovered were named with letters (e.g., Hb S); subsequently, the family name (e.g., Hb Lepore) or the place of residence (e.g., Hb Memphis) of the index case was used to name new hemoglobin variants. A systematic nomenclature identifies the chain, the location of the mutation, and the amino acid substitution on the affected globin chain (for example, the sickle cell mutation is designated as $\beta^{6Glu \rightarrow Val}$) [22].

The hemoglobin profiles of most patients who are heterozygous for both Hb A and a beta chain variant usually show approximately 55% Hb A, 40% variant hemoglobin, and small amounts of Hb F and Hb A_2. Patients who are heterozygous for a structural alpha gene mutation will generally have approximately 25% variant hemoglobin, since only one of the four alpha genes will carry the mutation. Since the $\alpha 1$ and $\alpha 2$ genes are transcribed at different rates, the exact ratio will depend on which alpha gene carries the structural mutation. Using high resolution methods, like high-performance liquid chromatography (HPLC), it can also be possible to demonstrate a split A_2 (or X_2) representing the tetramer formed by the delta chains and the variant alpha chain in patients with a structural alpha gene mutation.

Hemoglobin S

The *sickle cell mutation* is a single base substitution that results in the replacement of a hydrophilic glutamic acid with a hydrophobic valine in position six of the beta-globin polypeptide, with resultant polymerization of deoxygenated Hb S. The formation of Hb S polymers reduces red cell deformability and distorts the erythrocytes into the characteristic sickle-shaped cells. The sickled cells become entrapped in or adhere to the microvasculature, leading to the deleterious effects of vaso-occlusion. In general, conditions that increase the intracellular concentration of hemoglobin S or the interaction between hemoglobin S molecules increase the rate and extent of polymerization. In contrast, the presence of factors that decrease the interaction of hemoglobin molecules, such as increased concentration of hemoglobin F, interferes with Hb S polymerization and ameliorates the severity of the disease.

The *carrier state for Hb S* (Hb AS; sickle cell trait) is usually entirely asymptomatic, although patients who are exposed to extreme hypoxic or acidotic conditions such as anesthesia, respiratory infections, and high altitudes can in rare cases develop symptoms resembling sickle cell disease. Even in the absence of hypoxic conditions, patients with sickle trait can develop hematuria as a result of spontaneous sickling of red cells in the renal papillae.

The four most common types of *sickle cell disease* (SCD) are, in decreasing order of clinical severity, sickle cell anemia (Hb SS), Hb S/β°-thalassemia, Hb SC, and Hb S/β^+-thalassemia. Other compound heterozygous combinations with hemoglobin S, such as Hb SD-Punjab, Hb SO-Arab, and Hb SE, can also lead to clinically significant sickle syndromes [23]. Therefore, it is important to correctly identify these hemoglobins.

Neonates with sickle cell anemia (homozygosity for Hb S; Hb SS) usually appear well at birth because the majority of the total hemoglobin consists of Hb F. The hematologic manifestations of the disease become apparent at 10–12 weeks of age when the transcription of the abnormal beta chains becomes significant [24]. The first laboratory findings are usually anemia, polychromasia, and reticulocytosis. Initial clinical symptoms are usually sickle cell dactylitis or hand-foot syndrome, a painful, often symmetric swelling of the hand and feet [25, 26]. Presentation with bacterial sepsis is not uncommon. The disease course usually includes chronic hemolytic anemia and episodes of vaso-occlusive (e.g., acute chest, stroke), sequestration, hemolytic, or aplastic crisis.

Patients who are compound *heterozygous for Hb S and β°-thalassemia* (Hb S/β°-thalassemia) present with similar clinical and laboratory features to patients with sickle cell anemia. However, Hb S/β°-thalassemia can be distinguished from homozygous Hb SS by the presence of microcytosis and an elevated level of Hb A_2. Patients heterozygous for Hb S and β+-thalassemia (Hb S/β+-thalassemia) show variable clinical and laboratory features, which are similar, but usually milder, compared to patients with sickle cell anemia. Hemoglobin quantification demonstrates the presence of over 50% hemoglobin S, less than 50% Hb A, an increase in Hb A_2, and variable amounts of Hb F.

Hemoglobin C, hemoglobin D, and other rare hemoglobinopathies

Heterozygosity (*Hb C trait*) or homozygosity for Hb C (*Hb C disease*) is caused by a single base substitution that leads to replacement of glutamic acid by the positively charged lysine in the sixth amino acid of the hemoglobin β gene ($\alpha_2\beta_2^{6Glu \rightarrow Lys}$). Heterozygotes are usually clinically asymptomatic; homozygotes can show mild chronic hemolysis with splenomegaly and gallstones. The major importance of hemoglobin C is in the compound heterozygous state with hemoglobin S. The disease course of patients with SC disease is similar to patients with Hb SS, but symptoms are less severe and episodes of sickle cell crisis are less frequent in SC disease than in sickle cell anemia. Clinically significant hemoglobinopathies are also seen when hemoglobin S combines with Hb D-Punjab, Hb O-Arab, and Hb E.

Hemoglobin D-Punjab (also known as Hb D-Los Angeles) is a structural beta chain variant which is asymptomatic in both the heterozygote and homozygote states. The clinical significance of this hemoglobin lies in the fact that patients who are compound heterozygous for both Hb S and Hb D-Punjab do develop a sickling disorder. It is therefore important to correctly diagnose the presence of this hemoglobin. This can be difficult, because Hb D-Punjab migrates in the same position on both alkaline and acid electrophoresis as hemoglobin G-Philadelphia, an alpha chain variant with no clinical significance. They also elute with overlapping mean retention times on some HPLC systems [27]. The beta chain variant hemoglobin D-Punjab would be expected to comprise approximately 40%, and the alpha chain variant hemoglobin G-Philadelphia approximately 25% of the total hemoglobin. However, since Hb G-Philadelphia is frequently associated with alpha gene deletions, the percentages of these two variants overlap considerably in clinical practice, and can therefore frequently not be used to distinguish between these two variants. Since hemoglobin

G-Philadelphia is an alpha chain variant, it produces a second A_2 (G_2) band ($\alpha^G_2\delta_2$) on HPLC and electrophoresis, which will not be present in patients with hemoglobin D-Punjab. The two variants can be easily distinguished on isoelectric focusing (IEF).

Some structural hemoglobin variants are produced at a reduced rate or have reduced stability and therefore thalassemic features. An example is *Hemoglobin E*, a structural beta chain variant which is synthesized at a reduced rate. The percentage of hemoglobin E in heterozygotes (Hb AE) is therefore lower than the approximately 40% which is usually found in other beta chain variants. Heterozygotes for Hb E are asymptomatic; homozygotes have a reduced MCV and target cells on the peripheral blood smear. The clinical significance of hemoglobin E is cases of compound heterozygosity for Hb E and beta-thalassemia (Hb E/β°-thalassemia) or of Hb E and Hb S (Hb SE). Compound heterozygosity for Hb E and β°-thalassemia leads to a thalassemic syndrome, ranging in severity from thalassemia minor to major. Compound heterozygosity for Hb S and Hb E leads to hemoglobin SE disease, which is characterized by variable degrees of anemia and the development of sickling-related complications, including acute chest syndrome. Pediatric patients with hemoglobin SE disease usually have mild symptoms; more severe complications appear to be limited to patients older than 18 years [28].

An example of a thalassemic alpha chain variant is *hemoglobin Constant Spring*, an extension variant found in certain regions of Southeast Asia. A mutation in the last codon of the α2-globin gene changes a stop codon into a glutamine. This leads to a variant which is 31 amino acids longer than the normal alpha chain, but which is synthesized at a decreased rate. Heterozygotes for hemoglobin Constant Spring show few hematologic abnormalities; mild microcytosis and hypochromasia can be present. Homozygotes have normal-sized red cells, but develop a mild anemia due to hemolysis. The normal MCV in homozygotes is due to overhydration of erythrocytes containing Hb Constant Spring [29]. Patients who are compound heterozygotes for hemoglobin Constant Spring and a deletional alpha-thalassemia develop a variant of Hb H disease with severe anemia. The severity of the disease is not only due to the lack of alpha chain production, but also to increased red cell membrane rigidity caused by the association of oxidized $\alpha^{Constant\ Spring}$ with the erythrocyte membrane [29].

Interactions of structural hemoglobinopathies with thalassemias

These occur when an affected individual simultaneously carries a mutation leading to a structural hemoglobinopathy and a mutation causing thalassemia. This is not infrequent since the geographic and ethnic distributions of structural hemoglobinopathies and thalassemias overlap considerably. In the presence of fewer than four alpha genes, the percentage of the abnormal beta-globin variant will be significantly less than the 40% that would usually be observed. Therefore, the presence of a concomitant alpha-thalassemia trait with Hb S trait can lead to a decreased percentage of hemoglobin S (generally <35%), and also may be associated with microcytosis [30]. On the other hand, patients heterozygous for a structural beta chain variant and a mutation causing β^+-thalassemia will have a higher percentage of the abnormal hemoglobin. For example, a patient with Hb S/β^+-thalassemia can have 70% Hb S and 30% Hb A. If both a β°-thalassemia and a structural hemoglobinopathy are present, only the abnormal beta chain will be transcribed. For example, in a patient with Hb S/β°-thalassemia, almost all hemoglobin will be hemoglobin S, with a small fraction of hemoglobins F and A_2, and no hemoglobin A.

Certain hemoglobin mutations can *increase or decrease the oxygen affinity* of the hemoglobin molecule, leading to decreased oxygen delivery (high affinity) or increased oxygen delivery (low affinity) to the tissues, respectively. High affinity hemoglobins (e.g., Hb Chesapeake) have restricted release of oxygen to the tissues. The resulting tissue hypoxia causes increased erythropoietin production, leading to compensatory increase in the RBC count (polycythemia with increased red cell mass) and an elevated hematocrit. If oxygen affinity is decreased (low affinity hemoglobins, e.g., Hb Beth Israel), oxygen is released more easily to tissues, and erythropoietin production is consequently decreased. The patients have lower RBC counts and hematocrit levels are below the normal range; however, from a functional perspective, tissue oxygen delivery is not affected. Patients with high oxygen affinity are generally well compensated and asymptomatic, while patients with low oxygen affinity hemoglobins have increased concentration of deoxyhemoglobin and can have cyanosis.

Unstable hemoglobins are hemoglobin variants in which mutations, most commonly amino acid substitutions, weaken the binding forces that maintain the structure of the molecule, causing denaturation and precipitation of hemoglobin in red cells and ultimately hemolysis. The degree of *in vivo* hemolysis is variable; many patients are asymptomatic unless they are exposed to oxidative medications or are challenged by an infection. Other patients suffer the deleterious effects of severe, chronic hemolysis. The presence of an unstable hemoglobin can be confirmed with the isopropanol precipitation assay or the heat denaturation test. However, there is poor correlation between the *in vitro* stability of a variant hemoglobin and *in vivo* hemolysis. Many unstable hemoglobins are electrophoretically silent. Therefore, a normal electrophoretic pattern does not rule out the presence of an unstable hemoglobin. HPLC, isoelectric focusing, or molecular studies are often necessary for the diagnosis of an unstable hemoglobin. Some unstable hemoglobins have increased or decreased oxygen affinity.

While normal hemoglobins contain the ferrous form of iron (Fe^{2+}), *methemoglobin*s contain iron in the oxidized (ferric) form (Fe^{3+}). Methemoglobins do not transport oxygen to the tissues. The presence of a methemoglobin can be caused by amino acid substitutions in parts of the hemoglobin molecule adjacent to the heme moiety that stabilizes the iron in the ferric form; such variants are designated M-hemoglobins. Many affected patients will show a characteristic bluish-brown skin color resembling cyanosis, but are otherwise asymptomatic. If the mutation affects one of the alpha genes, cyanosis-like coloration is present from birth; patients with beta gene mutations will only begin to show the bluish color after the first few months of life, when hemoglobin F levels decline. It should be noted that deficiencies in NADH-diaphorase, as well as exposure to certain drugs and toxic substances, can also lead to methemoglobinemia. Assays for NADH-diaphorase levels are available in reference laboratories.

Laboratory evaluation

Introduction

Diagnostic testing for hemoglobin disorders has increased in importance and volume over the last few years due to the implementation of screening programs. In addition, prenatal and fetal testing, as well as preimplantation diagnosis, has been increasing. Testing of patients for hemoglobin disorders is also performed for many other reasons, including evaluation of anemia and microcytosis, pulmonary hypertension, and preoperative anesthesia evaluation.

Effects of hemoglobinopathies on general laboratory tests

Complete blood cell count

Abnormal red cell indices in a routinely ordered complete blood count (CBC) can be the first indication of the presence of a hemoglobinopathy, leading to further workup by specialized methods like HPLC or electrophoresis. Results of the CBC can also be essential for the diagnosis of thalassemias and for the assessment of the severity of a hemoglobinopathy. A CBC should therefore be ordered in all cases where a hemoglobin disorder is in the diagnostic differential. Additional automated testing available on most automated cell analyzers includes a reticulocyte count, which should be ordered if there is suspicion of hemolysis, frequently seen in sickle cell disease, thalassemia, or the presence of an unstable hemoglobin.

The reduced production of hemoglobin in thalassemias leads to microcytosis (reduced MCV) and hypochromasia (reduced MCH). The red cell count (RBC) is usually increased as a compensatory mechanism, and the red cell distribution width (RDW) is often normal. In contrast, in patients with iron deficiency, another frequent cause of microcytosis in children, the RBC is decreased and the RDW increased. The differential diagnosis of thalassemia and iron deficiency can nevertheless be challenging, and a variety of red cell indices have been proposed for this purpose. However, none of these indices appears to be superior to the MCV alone [31]. A cut off of 72 fL has been suggested as maximally sensitive and specific for the presumptive diagnosis of thalassemia in adults; it is imperative to use age-specific reference ranges in pediatric patients. It is also important to note that measurement of the MCV is

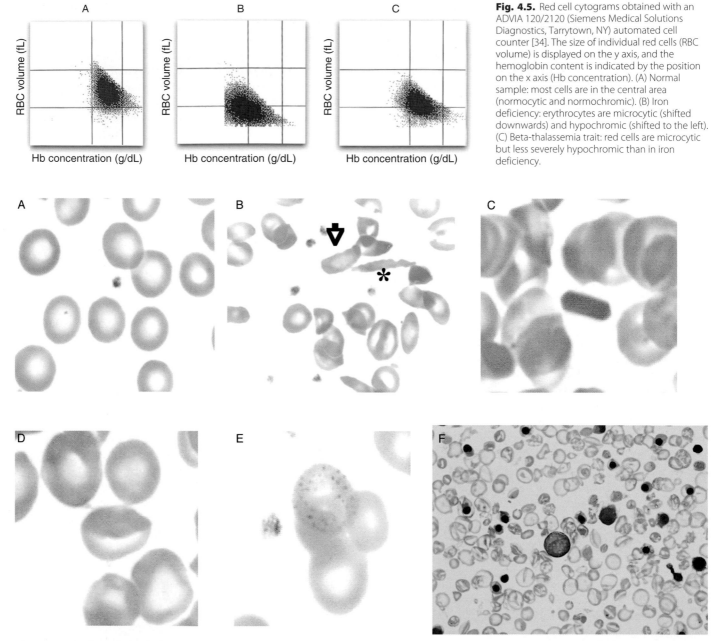

Fig. 4.5. Red cell cytograms obtained with an ADVIA 120/2120 (Siemens Medical Solutions Diagnostics, Tarrytown, NY) automated cell counter [34]. The size of individual red cells (RBC volume) is displayed on the y axis, and the hemoglobin content is indicated by the position on the x axis (Hb concentration). (A) Normal sample: most cells are in the central area (normocytic and normochromic). (B) Iron deficiency: erythrocytes are microcytic (shifted downwards) and hypochromic (shifted to the left). (C) Beta-thalassemia trait: red cells are microcytic but less severely hypochromic than in iron deficiency.

Fig. 4.6. Red cell morphology in hemoglobinopathies. (A) Normal red cell morphology in a patient with sickle cell trait; (B) Sickle cell (*) and boat cell (arrow) in a patient with sickle cell (SC) disease; (C) Hemoglobin C crystal in a patient homozygous for Hb C; (D) Folded cell in a patient with SC disease; (E) Basophilic stippling in a patient with beta-thalassemia trait; (F) Erythroblastosis and severe hypochromasia in a premature (30 weeks) newborn with Hb Bart hydrops fetalis. (Panel F courtesy of Dr. Monica Gallivan, Quest Diagnostics Nichols Institute, Chantilly, VA.)

method dependent; results from different automated cell counters can therefore not be directly compared. Blood samples that are not analyzed within eight hours of venipuncture should not be used because with storage the size of red cells will increase and obscure the presence of microcytosis.

Some automated cell counters can directly measure the volumes and hemoglobin concentrations of individual red cells. This allows the determination of chromasia and erythrocyte size on a cell-by-cell basis. This information can be presented in a red cell cytogram (Fig. 4.5), and can be used to determine the ratio of microcytic to hypochromic cells. This "M/H ratio" has been reported to be useful for the differentiation of iron deficiency and thalassemia [32, 33].

Peripheral blood film

Like an abnormal CBC, unusual findings on a routinely prepared blood smear can be the first indication of the presence of a hemoglobinopathy, and provide valuable information to direct the diagnostic evaluation. In many cases, the observations on the blood film serve to confirm the findings of other laboratory studies (Fig. 4.6). It is important to stress that blood smears from patients with sickle cell trait (Hb AS) are usually entirely normal; sometimes a small number of target cells can be observed, but the lack of target cells cannot be used to rule out sickle cell trait. In patients with sickle cell anemia, the blood film is usually normal at birth [35]. At approximately six months of age, blood smears usually show sickle cells (drepanocytes), target cells, anisocytosis, anisochromasia, polychromasia, basophilic stippling, and nucleated red cells [36]. Features of hyposplenism, such as Howell–Jolly bodies and more numerous target cells, can already be present at this age [35]. Sickle or crescent-shaped cells represent irreversibly sickled cells. Boat cells, also known as plump sickle cells or oat cells, are pointed at both ends, but wider than sickle cells.

The blood films of patients with hemoglobin C disease show a large number of target cells, microcytosis, and characteristic hemoglobin C crystals. These are dense octahedral structures, often compared to the Washington Monument, caused by the crystallization of hemoglobin C. Less classic forms are rhomboid, hexagonal, or rod-shaped. Since all hemoglobin in a cell is usually incorporated into the crystals, the cells appear empty ("ghost cells") except for the crystal. Hemoglobin crystals are more frequent (up to 10% of all circulating erythrocytes) in splenectomized patients.

In patients with SC disease, boat cells are more common than classical sickle cells and some cells can contain hemoglobin C crystals. Irregularly shaped cells, some of which appear to contain misshapen crystals ("folded cells" or "S/C poikilocytes"), often allow the preliminary diagnosis of SC disease by slide review alone. Target cells are more numerous in SC disease than in sickle cell anemia. Howell–Jolly bodies and other signs of hyposplenism are less frequent in patients with Hb SC than in patients with Hb SS [35].

Blood films from patients with thalassemia trait are characterized by the presence of target cells, elliptocytes, and basophilic stippling. Basophilic stippling is caused by the aggregation of ribosomes in reticulocytes. If the CBC does not support a diagnosis of thalassemia, other frequent causes of basophilic stippling in pediatric patients, including lead poisoning, should be explored.

When an unstable hemoglobin precipitates in circulating red cells, the resulting Heinz body is usually removed in the spleen, which leads to the presence of bite cells on the blood smear. However, bite cells are not specific for unstable hemoglobins, and can also be seen in other conditions associated with Heinz body formation, such as G6PD deficiency.

Target cells are caused by an increased surface membrane to volume ratio of red cells, and can be the result of a decrease in red cell content (e.g., thalassemias, iron deficiency) or increase in red cell membrane (e.g., post-splenectomy). The observation of target cells is therefore a very non-specific finding that can be seen in patients with a wide variety of hemoglobinopathies, including thalassemias, sickle cell disease, and hemoglobin C; they are also found in liver disease, disorders of lipid metabolism, and a large number of other diseases.

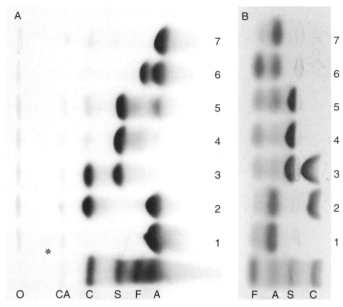

Fig. 4.7. Alkaline (cellulose acetate) and acid (citrate) hemoglobin electrophoresis for commonly encountered hemoglobinopathies. (A) Alkaline hemoglobin electrophoresis with origin at left and controls in bottom lane. From left to right are the O, origin; CA, carbonic anhydrase; C, position where hemoglobins C, E, O, and A_2 migrate; S, position where hemoglobins S, G, and D migrate; F, hemoglobin F; and A, hemoglobin A. Lane 1: Hemoglobin A_2' trait (delta chain variant) (*); Lane 2: hemoglobin C trait (AC); Lane 3: hemoglobin SC disease (compound heterozygous Hb S/C); Lane 4: sickle cell anemia (homozygous Hb SS); Lane 5: sickle cell/β^+-thalassemia with elevated hemoglobin A_2; Lane 6: normal level of hemoglobin F in a less-than-6-months-old infant; Lane 7: normal adult pattern (Hb AA with minor fraction Hb A_2 and Hb F). (B) Citrate agar (acid) hemoglobin electrophoresis with controls in bottom lane. From left to right are F, hemoglobin F; A, position where hemoglobins A, G, D, E, O, and A_2 migrate; S, hemoglobin S; and C, hemoglobin C. Lanes 1–7 contain samples from the same patients as in panel A.

Specialized laboratory tests for the diagnosis of hemoglobinopathies

Hemoglobin electrophoresis

In 1949, Linus Pauling first applied the principle of electrophoresis to hemoglobins. Electrophoresis is based on the movement of charged molecules in an electric field. It can be performed under alkaline (pH 8.0–8.6, usually on cellulose acetate) or acid (pH 6.0–6.2; performed on citrate agar or an appropriate agarose gel) conditions. A red cell hemolysate is applied to the carrier, and an electrical field is applied. Following sufficient migration of the fractions across the carriers, the strips are stained, and the distance the hemoglobins have migrated is compared to controls that are run simultaneously with the patient samples (Fig. 4.7). The various hemoglobins are usually quantified by scanning densitometry. Scanning densitometry is usually not sensitive enough to allow quantification of low-concentration hemoglobins, especially hemoglobin F and A_2. Elution of hemoglobin fractions after electrophoretic separation and measurement of the relative amounts by spectrophotometry is used less frequently than scanning densitometry, but is more sensitive.

The separation of the hemoglobins will largely be determined by their net electrical charge. For example, hemoglobin S, which has one net negative charge less than Hb A due to the replacement of glutamic acid by valine, migrates more slowly towards the anode. Under alkaline conditions, hemoglobin D and G migrate in the same position as Hb S, and Hb E and O-Arab migrate to the same position as Hb C [37]. Additional laboratory assays are therefore necessary to distinguish between these variants. Electrophoresis at acid pH is usually used for this purpose. However, electrophoresis does not allow a reliable distinction to be made between most types of hemoglobin D and G-Philadelphia, since these hemoglobins migrate in the same location under both alkaline and acidic conditions, and only very high quality gels allow the identification of the split A_2 band seen in Hb G trait. The distinction between hemoglobins D and G therefore is more easily made with other methods, like HPLC or IEF. This is important for prenatal counseling, because compound heterozygous Hb S/G is clinically similar to sickle cell trait, while compound heterozygous Hb S/D-Punjab can be a clinically significant sickling disorder.

Hemoglobin electrophoresis continues to be a sensitive and reliable technique for primary screening for structural hemoglobinopathies. Since different hemoglobins can migrate in the same location on electrophoresis, the technique often requires confirmation of abnormal findings with another method (e.g., rerun under acid conditions, sickle screen, isoelectric focusing, or HPLC). Hemoglobin electrophoresis is relatively labor intensive, and many laboratories have therefore replaced this assay with other, less manual methods, such as HPLC.

Isoelectric focusing

Isoelectric focusing (IEF) separates hemoglobins based on their isoelectric point. The method can be used as a primary screening test or as a confirmatory method for other screening assays. IEF is labor intensive and requires expert interpretation, but can be performed with small sample volumes, an important advantage in neonatal screening programs. IEF also allows differentiation of hemoglobin D and G, which can be very difficult to differentiate with electrophoresis or HPLC. Although Hb G-Philadelphia and hemoglobin Lepore migrate in the same location on IEF, they can usually be distinguished by the fact that Hb G-Philadelphia is usually present to a level of at least 25%, while Hb Lepore usually represents less than 10% of total hemoglobin.

Capillary electrophoresis

In capillary electrophoresis, narrow-bore fused-silica capillaries are used to separate hemoglobins. In the simplest form of capillary electrophoresis, *capillary zone electrophoresis*, charged molecules are separated according to their electrophoretic mobility in an alkaline buffer containing electrolytes that create an electro-osmotic flow [38]. The method can be automated and can be used for the quantification of normal as well as

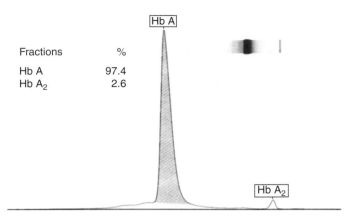

Fractions	%
Hb A	97.4
Hb A$_2$	2.6

Fig. 4.8. Capillary electrophoresis. Results from a normal subject on the Sebia Capillarys System (Sebia Electrophoresis, Norcross, GA). The hemoglobin fractionation pattern can be shown as peaks (similar to HPLC) or as a density pattern (upper right; resembling traditional electrophoresis). Normal hemoglobins (Hb A, A$_2$, and F), many hemoglobin variants (e.g., Hb S), and hemoglobin Bart and hemoglobin H can be clearly identified and quantified using this technique.

variant hemoglobins, including hemoglobin H and hemoglobin Bart (Fig. 4.8) [39]. Hemoglobin E can easily be differentiated from hemoglobin A_2. Since higher voltage can be used than in conventional electrophoresis, run times are shorter than with conventional electrophoresis. The small sample size required makes this assay especially well suited for pediatric samples. Some systems can be used for both hemoglobin and protein electrophoresis, and a large number of samples (5000–10 000) can be analyzed without the need to change capillaries. A disadvantage is the higher costs associated with the instrument procurement and reagents.

High-performance liquid chromatography (HPLC)

In many laboratories, cation-exchange HPLC has replaced electrophoresis as the method of choice for the fractionation, identification and quantification of normal and variant hemoglobins [22, 40, 41]. The significant advantages of HPLC over electrophoresis are lower labor costs due to full automation, the ability to identify and quantify a larger number of abnormal hemoglobins, the smaller sample size necessary for the method, and the ability to use samples such as dried spots of blood for neonatal testing. In addition, the ability to directly quantify Hb A_2 and Hb F by HPLC eliminates the need for additional tests in patients undergoing screening for beta-thalassemia. The main disadvantages of this method are higher capital and reagent costs and the additional training and expertise that are required.

Hemoglobins are adsorbed onto a negatively charged stationary phase in a chromatography column. A liquid mobile phase with a decreasing pH and an increasing concentration of cations is then injected; the cations in the mobile phase compete with the hemoglobins for the anionic binding sites in the column, and the hemoglobins are eluted at a rate related to their affinity for the stationary phase, detected and measured optically in the eluate, and identified by their elution times. HPLC allows the accurate quantification of all normal hemoglobins,

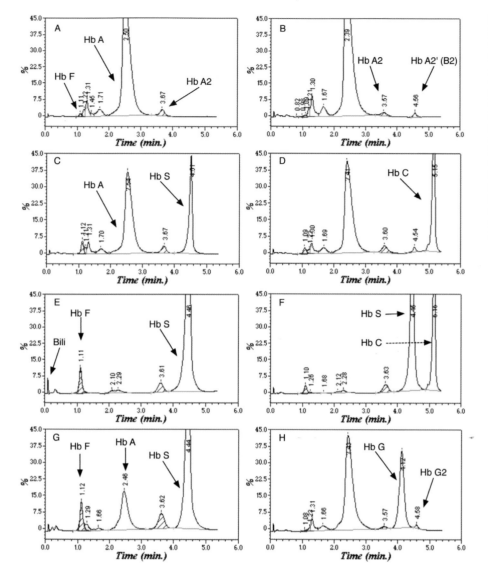

Fig. 4.9. High-performance liquid chromatography (HPLC) chromatograms for commonly encountered hemoglobinopathies. High-performance liquid chromatography (Bio-Rad Variant II; Bio-Rad Laboratories; Hercules, CA) chromatograms showing hemoglobin fractions for (A) Normal hemoglobin profile.
(B) Hemoglobin A_2' trait at 4.56 minutes. (C) Sickle cell trait (Hb AS). (D) Hemoglobin C trait (AC) with smaller peak of post-translationally modified Hb C at 4.54 minutes. (E) Sickle cell anemia (homozygous Hb SS) with elevation of hemoglobin F. In the presence of Hb S, Hb A_2 can be spuriously elevated on HPLC. Bili = bilirubin.
(F) Hemoglobin SC disease (compound heterozygous S/C). (G) Sickle cell/β^+-thalassemia with elevated Hb A_2 and Hb F. (H) Hemoglobin G-Philadelphia trait; note the presence of Hb G_2 ($\alpha_2^{\text{G-Philadelphia}}\delta_2$).

including Hb F and Hb A_2, as well as of a large number of variants (Fig. 4.9). Depending on the HPLC instrument and reagents used, most variant hemoglobins can be distinguished [37, 42]. However, many commercial systems do not allow the quantification of fast-eluting hemoglobins like Hb Bart and Hb H.

Some variant hemoglobins, like hemoglobin New York, co-elute with Hb A and will therefore yield a normal pattern on HPLC. In the presence of Hb S, Hb A_2 is spuriously increased on HPLC. The method should therefore not be used for the quantification of Hb A_2 in patients with Hb S. In addition, glycated hemoglobin S elutes in the hemoglobin A window, leading to samples from patients with Hb SS being misinterpreted as containing both Hb S and Hb A, and consequently an incorrect diagnosis of Hb S/β^+-thalassemia. Since Hb A_2 elutes very close to Hb E, these hemoglobins can not be distinguished from each other on HPLC. Hb E or another variant in the "A_2 window" should therefore be suspected when Hb A_2 exceeds 10%. In patients with elevated bilirubin levels, a spurious peak may

be confused with fast-eluting hemoglobins, such as hemoglobin Bart [43]. An elevation of the P2 elution peak, which can be seen with increases in Hb A1c, may interfere with the accurate quantification of hemoglobin F [44].

Many laboratories use HPLC-based assays to quantify hemoglobin A1c for the management of diabetes mellitus. The presence of variant hemoglobins can be observed in these assays. A hemoglobin A1c quantification is therefore sometimes the first indication that a patient is a carrier for a variant hemoglobin, leading to a referral from the diabetes laboratory to the hematology laboratory. It is also important to note that the presence of a variant hemoglobin, which may co-elute with hemoglobin A1c, can lead to spurious elevations in hemoglobin A1c on HPLC [44]. Alternative methods to measure glycated hemoglobin or other markers, such as fructosamine, may have to be used in such patients for the monitoring of the management of diabetes mellitus. It is therefore important that the diabetes laboratory is informed of the presence of a variant hemoglobin in a patient sample, so that non-HPLC-based

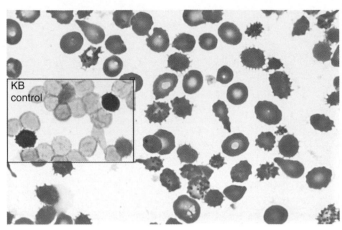

Fig. 4.10. Kleihauer–Betke stain of a sample from a patient with deletional hereditary persistence of fetal hemoglobin (HPFH). Note the homocellular distribution of hemoglobin F. (Courtesy of Dr. Monica Gallivan, Quest Diagnostics Nichols Institute, Chantilly, VA.)

assays are used for the quantification of hemoglobin A1c in these patients.

Microcolumn chromatography

Before the widespread use of cation-exchange HPLC, anion-exchange microcolumn chromatography was the method of choice for the quantification of Hb A_2. Standard columns for the measurement of Hb A_2 cannot be used in the presence of Hb S; modified columns are commercially available for this purpose [45].

Methods to measure Hb F

Alkaline denaturation can be used to determine the percentage of hemoglobin F. This technique is based on the ability of Hb F to resist denaturation in an alkaline solution. Sodium hydroxide, an alkaline reagent, is added to the hemolysate to denature all hemoglobins except for Hb F. Ammonium sulfate is then added to halt the denaturation process and precipitate the denatured hemoglobin. The solution is then filtered, and the amount of hemoglobin F is measured spectrophotometrically. Many laboratories have replaced this method with more automated assays, such as HPLC.

A *Kleihauer–Betke test* (KB) is performed to determine the cellular distribution of hemoglobin F. A blood smear is prepared and fixed with ethyl alcohol. Hemoglobin A is eluted from the erythrocytes using a citric acid–sodium buffer at a pH of 3.2 at 37°C; hemoglobin F precipitates and remains in the cells. The slide is stained with hematoxylin and eosin and examined microscopically. Cells devoid of Hb F appear as empty ghosts, while cells containing Hb F are stained. The number of cells containing Hb F and their distribution is determined (Fig. 4.10). The KB test is used when the percentage of hemoglobin F is elevated and the differential diagnosis is between hereditary persistence of fetal hemoglobin (HPFH) and beta or delta-beta-thalassemia. Deletional forms of HPFH will show a uniform (homocellular or pancellular) distribution of Hb F; in con-

trast, beta-thalassemia or delta-beta-thalassemia will show an unequal (heterocellular) distribution. The disadvantages of the assay include the subjectivity inherent to microscopic observation. In addition, technical variations, such as variations in the pH of the citric acid buffer, can lead to incorrect results.

Many laboratories have moved to flow-cytometry-based systems because of the poor reproducibility of the Kleihauer–Betke test. In these assays, red cells are fixed with glutaraldehyde and permeabilized by suspension in a non-ionic detergent. A monoclonal anti-hemoglobin F antibody is used for detection and quantification of red cells containing hemoglobin F [46, 47]. The method can be used to distinguish homocellular from heterocellular patterns and therefore to replace the Kleihauer–Betke test in differentiating HPFH from delta–beta-thalassemia.

Stain for inclusion bodies

Staining for red cell inclusions must be performed on a fresh blood sample within one hour of phlebotomy; otherwise, false-positive results will be obtained. Blood is incubated for 15 minutes, 30 minutes, or 1 hour at room temperature with a supravital stain such as crystal violet, and moist smear preparations of the mixture are examined microscopically for the presence of erythrocyte inclusions such as Heinz bodies and hemoglobin H inclusions. *Heinz bodies* are coarse inclusions, usually attached to the red cell membrane and appearing at the periphery of the cell. They represent denatured hemoglobins and can be found in individuals with unstable hemoglobins, in patients with defects of erythrocyte glycolytic enzymes, such as glucose 6-phosphate deficiency, or after exposure to oxidant drugs. Heinz bodies can also be observed in patients with severe alcoholic liver disease. Since the spleen normally removes Heinz bodies *in vivo* (causing the presence of bite cells on the blood smear), Heinz bodies are more easily detected after splenectomy. *Hemoglobin H* inclusions are small inclusions, evenly distributed through the red cells, similar to the dimples on a golf ball. The red cells are therefore often described as "golf ball cells." The inclusions represent beta chain tetrads which form in patients with deletion of three of the four alpha genes.

Tests for Hb S

The sickle cell test and the sickle solubility test are screening assays for the presence of sickling hemoglobins. These assays are not specific for Hb S, but will also be positive in the presence of other hemoglobins associated with sickling, such as Hb S-Travis and Hb C-Harlem (Table 4.1). In *the sickle cell test*, sodium metabisulfite ($Na_2S_2O_5$), a strong reducing agent, is used to deoxygenate red cells. Sickled red cells are then identified by microscopic examination of a blood smear. *Solubility tests* are based on the relative insolubility of Hb S in the presence of the reducing agent sodium dithionite (Fig. 4.11). Red cells are lysed with saponin, and hemoglobin S, if present, will form polymers. Visual inspection of the tube and comparison with a negative control allows rapid identification of samples containing Hb S. The commercially available tests will be positive if at least 20% Hb S is present; some systems are sensitive enough to

Table 4.1. Interpretation of sickle solubility test results.

True positive	False positive	False negative
Hemoglobin S Hemoglobin C-Harlem Hemoglobin S-Travis	Hyperglobulinemia Hemoglobin Bart Methemoglobin formation	Low percentage of hemoglobin S (e.g., infants with sickle cell disease <6 months of age) Elevated hemoglobin F Hematocrit <25%

detect down to 8% Hb S [37]. This method must not be used as a screening test for infants under the age of six months, because of the danger of false-negative results caused by the low levels of Hb S and high levels of hemoglobin F seen in this age group. In addition, this method cannot distinguish between Hb AS, Hb SS, or compound heterozygosity for Hb S and other abnormal hemoglobins. Additional caution is required when interpreting samples with a hematocrit less than 25% since such anemia can give false-negative results. All positive or equivocal results must be confirmed by a second, independent method such as electrophoresis, IEF, or HPLC.

Tests for unstable hemoglobin

Two types of test are available to confirm the presence of unstable hemoglobins. In the heat test, a buffered cyanmethemoglobin solution is incubated at 50 °C for one hour, or at 69.5 °C for six minutes, and examined for turbidity/flocculation. This test is more specific for unstable hemoglobins than examination for Heinz bodies. In the isopropanol precipitation assay, incubation of a hemolysate with buffered isopropanol at 37 °C breaks weak hydrophobic bonds in the unstable hemoglobin molecule, leading to precipitation of the dissociated globin chains.

Molecular genetic testing for hemoglobinopathies and thalassemias

Test selection

Although increased automation has made DNA-based testing accessible for routine clinical diagnosis, these tests are often still significantly more expensive than other assays. In addition, since many molecular assays are specific for certain mutations, diseases, or populations, they can only be applied to address extremely restricted questions. Expertise in both the underlying methodology and the distribution of mutations in the population are therefore prerequisites for the ordering of the appropriate assays and for the interpretation of test results. For example, gap-PCR for deletions in the alpha genes will only address the presence or absence of a very limited number of deletions (usually seven) in the alpha genes of a patient. The test should therefore only be ordered if other laboratory results (e.g., low MCV, high RBC, normal or low Hb A$_2$) indicate the possible presence of an alpha-thalassemia, and if the patient belongs to an ethnic group in which these specific deletions have been described. A negative result will only exclude the presence of certain specific deletions; other deletions or point mutations associated with an alpha-thalassemia may be present in

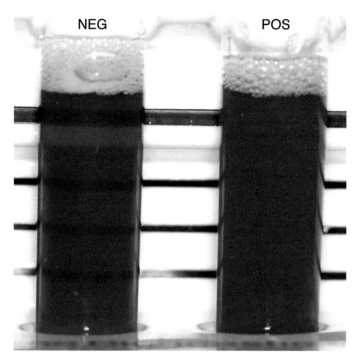

Fig. 4.11. Sickle solubility test. (NEG) Negative sickle solubility test from a normal donor; the black lines behind the sample remain clearly visible. (POS) Sample from a patient with sickle cell trait demonstrates a turbid solution that makes it impossible to see the lines behind the sample. It should be stressed that false-negative results can be obtained in patients less than six months old because the test is not sensitive enough to detect the low percentage of Hb S present at this age. Additional caution is required when interpreting samples with a hematocrit less than 25%, since such anemia can give false-negative results.

spite of a negative result. It is therefore often prudent to consult with experts in the field before ordering molecular assays for hemoglobinopathies. Such consultation will allow the most cost-effective ordering of the most appropriate assays for a patient based on the patient's clinical history, laboratory results, and ethnic background. Frequently, testing needs to be ordered in a stepwise manner, beginning with assays for high-incidence mutations and then proceeding to testing for lower probability variants. A database of laboratories performing genetic testing can be found online at www.genetests.org.

DNA sources for molecular testing

Genetic testing of newborns or adults is usually performed on peripheral blood samples, preferably anticoagulated with ethylenediaminetetraacetic acid (EDTA). Using standard phenol-chloroform extraction and cold ethanol or isopropyl alcohol precipitation, DNA can easily be isolated from the white blood cells in such samples. For prenatal testing, DNA is usually obtained from chorionic villi, amniocytes, or the blastocyst [48]. Although the isolation of fetal cells (e.g., nucleated fetal red cells) from the maternal circulation and the extraction of fetal DNA from maternal plasma have been shown to be feasible, these novel methods are presently only used in a research setting.

Table 4.2. Commonly used molecular methods for the diagnosis of structural hemoglobin variants and thalassemias.

Test method	Principle	Common use	Notes
DNA sequencing	Direct nucleotide sequencing	Detection of unknown mutations Confirmation of inconclusive results Definitive hemoglobin gene analysis	Information about the phenotype is essential for interpretation Large deletions may be missed
RFLP	Mutation alters restriction site; the mutant and wild-type fragments can be visualized on Southern blot	Hemoglobin S, D, G, E, and O Alpha-thalassemias Beta-thalassemia	More commonly used for structural hemoglobinopathies Cannot be used for diagnosis of Hb C
Gap-PCR	PCR amplification of mutant and wild-type allele depending on presence of large deletion	Alpha-thalassemias Beta-thalassemia (deletional) Hb Lepore $\delta\beta$-thalassemia $\gamma\delta\beta$-thalassemia	Limited to large deletional mutations with known breakpoints
Dot blot	Mutation specific, labeled oligonucleotide probes hybridized to patient DNA	Alpha-thalassemias Beta-thalassemia (non-deletional)	Large number of possible mutations requires tiered screening based on local prevalence Numerous probes must be hybridized to patient DNA
Reverse dot blot	Labeled patient DNA hybridized to a panel of mutation-specific oligonucleotide probes	Alpha-thalassemias Beta-thalassemia (non-deletional)	Large number of possible mutations requires tiered screening based on local prevalence
ARMS	Mutation-sequence-specific primers that amplify mutated allele	Hb S, C, D, E, O Alpha-thalassemias (non-deletional) Beta-thalassemias	Can be used to detect virtually any known point mutation

Chorionic villous sampling is performed at a gestational age of 10–12 weeks. Villi can be obtained either through the cervix or through the abdomen. In order to minimize the risk of contamination of the sample with maternal DNA, the decidua must be carefully dissected away from the villi. The risk of fetal loss caused by amniocentesis is approximately 2% [48].

Amniotic fluid sampling can be performed at a gestational age of 17–20 weeks. Small amounts of DNA can then be extracted directly from amniotic fluid. These amounts are usually only sufficient for polymerase chain reaction (PCR)-based tests. For other methods, amniocyte culture, a procedure which takes at least two weeks, is often necessary in order to obtain enough DNA. Disadvantages of amniocentesis include the risk of fetal loss (1.0–1.5%) and the fact that the results of the genetic testing may only be available at a time when the pregnancy can no longer be terminated.

It is important to minimize the possibility of incorrect results caused by maternal contamination in chorionic and amniotic samples. This can be achieved by amplifying DNA from the father, the mother, and the fetus with primers specific for highly polymorphic regions of the genome.

In preimplantation testing, a single cell is removed from the blastocyst stage of a fertilized egg (eight-cell stage) and the isolated DNA tested using PCR-based analysis. Only blastocysts which do not carry hemoglobin mutation(s) for which the parents are carriers are then implanted in the uterus. The method avoids the risk of contamination of the sample with maternal cells and the need for abortion of an established pregnancy.

Genetic tests

Gene sequencing and restriction fragment length polymorphism (RFLP) were historically the first methods applied to the analysis of mutations affecting the hemoglobin genes. These assays are still used in certain situations. For example, since a variety of point mutations in multiple different positions can cause beta-thalassemia, sequencing of the beta-globin gene is offered on a routine basis by reference laboratories. More recently developed assays for undefined mutations include single-strand conformational polymorphism (SSCP), denaturing gradient gel electrophoresis (DGGE), real-time PCR, and denaturing high-performance liquid chromatography (DHPLC) [49]. Assays for known mutations include amplification-created restriction site (ACRS) and multiplex ligation-dependent probe amplification (MLPA). The following discussion will concentrate on gap-PCR, sequence-specific oligonucleotides (allele-specific oligonucleotides), and amplification-refractory mutation analysis (ARMS) [49–51], methods which have become available only relatively recently, yet are already frequently used in the workup of hemoglobinopathies. The various assays and their applications are summarized in Table 4.2.

Gap-PCR is used to determine the presence or absence of large sequences of DNA. Three primers are used to form two primer pairs. One primer (5′ to 3′) is upstream from the breakpoint. The first reverse primer is designed to amplify a sequence of DNA located within the potentially deleted piece of DNA; the other reverse primer is downstream of the breakpoint (Fig. 4.12). In the wild-type allele (no deletion present), the PCR product will be the product of the upstream primer and the primer located within the potentially deleted DNA. Although the primer located downstream from the breakpoint hybridizes to the wild type, its distance from the upstream primer prevents the large-sized fragment from being produced. Only if the deletion is present will the primer located upstream and downstream from the breakpoint produce a product. The method is inexpensive and one of the easier molecular assays to perform.

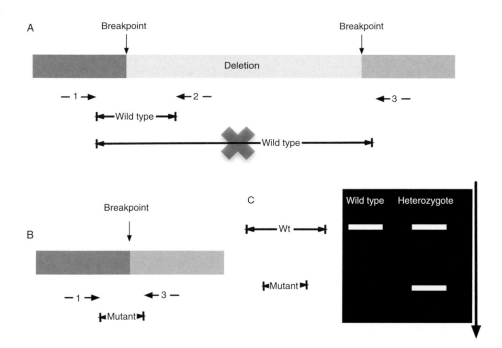

Fig. 4.12. Gap-PCR is used to detect the presence (or absence) of large deletions. Three primers are used: one primer (primer 1) is designed to adhere upstream from the 5′ breakpoint of the deletion. The other two primers are designed to amplify in the presence (primer 3) or absence (primer 2) of the deletion to produce different-sized fragments. A Southern blot is then performed and the results interpreted to determine hetero- or homozygosity. (A) Wild type: primers 1 and 2 produce a small amplification product; primer 3 adheres, but does not amplify, because it is too far from primer 1. (B) Deletion mutant: the DNA corresponding to primer 2 is deleted; there is therefore no amplification from primer 2. Primer 3 is now near enough to primer 1 to allow for amplification. (C) Southern blot showing the wild-type (left lane) and both wild-type and mutant (right lane) amplification products. Wt = wild type.

It is used to detect common deletions leading to α-thalassemia, δβ-thalassemia, and γδβ-thalassemia, as well as rearrangement mutations such as hemoglobin Lepore. The disadvantage of this technique is that the breakpoints of the deletion must be known. The assay will only detect large deletions, and will not identify point mutations.

Allele-specific oligonucleotides (ASOs) are DNA sequences 20 kb in length that correspond to specific mutations of interest. In dot blot assays, DNA from the patient is applied to a membrane and labeled allele-specific oligonucleotides are then hybridized to the membranes [52]. If the mutation is present, the dot blot will be positive with the oligonucleotides corresponding to the mutation. A disadvantage of the technique is that the patient sample must be hybridized to multiple membranes, once for every oligonucleotide probe used. This is avoided in reverse dot blotting. In this method, the oligonucleotide probes are applied to known areas of the membrane, and hybridized with labeled patient DNA. The method can be used for identification of specific mutations, as well as for screening programs.

Amplification-refractory mutation systems (ARMS) are PCR-based assays which can be used to identify any known point mutation [53–55]. Primers are designed to be specific for the wild-type and the mutant allele. Three primers are required for two reactions in two separate tubes. The first primer, a constant reverse primer, is added to both tubes. A primer specific for the wild-type allele is added to the first tube, and a primer specific for the mutant allele is added to the second tube. The presence of both the wild-type and the mutant allele can be detected at the same time, allowing a determination of homozygosity or heterozygosity. The limitation of the method is that only known point mutations can be assayed. Therefore, knowledge of the ethnic background of the patient population tested is essential.

This knowledge allows the design of a panel of primers specific for mutations which are commonly encountered in this population. If the results are not conclusive, additional panels with primers specific for less-common mutations can be used.

Screening algorithms and testing strategies

Neonatal screening

Neonatal screening programs for hemoglobinopathies have been established in many jurisdictions. Screening must be able to identify sickle cell trait, sickle cell anemia, Hb S/β$^+$-thalassemia, Hb S/β$^\circ$-thalassemia, and other clinically significant variants such as Hb C, Hb D-Punjab, Hb E, and Hb O-Arab. Possible results and their interpretations are shown in Table 4.3. Frequently, a dried bloodspot card used for biochemical screening for genetic disorders (e.g., phenylketonuria) is utilized to prepare an eluate. If cord blood is used, it is important to minimize the risk of contamination with maternal blood. Due to the small sample size required and the possibility for at least partial automation, HPLC or IEF are the screening methods of choice in many laboratories; they allow the detection of all clinically significant variants and of Hb A down to a concentration of 5% [37, 56]. It is important to stress that sickle solubility tests are not sufficiently sensitive to detect the small quantities of Hb S present in neonatal blood. Almost all laboratories will use a second method to confirm the presence of variant hemoglobins, including DNA analysis, and the identification of some hemoglobin variants may require the involvement of reference laboratories.

Pre- and post-analytical variables such as incorrect specimen labeling or specimen mix-ups, poor documentation of patient history, prolonged transport, and clerical reporting errors may lead to an inaccurate diagnosis. For example, if an

Table 4.3. Common neonatal screening results and their differential diagnosis.

Pattern	Differential diagnosis
FA	No structural hemoglobin abnormality present
FAS	Sickle cell trait Sickle cell disease s/p large transfusion
FSA	Hemoglobin S/β^+-thalassemia Sickle cell disease s/p transfusion Sickle cell disease with contamination with maternal blood
FS	Sickle cell anemia Hemoglobin S/β°-thalassemia Hemoglobin S/hereditary persistence of fetal hemoglobin Hemoglobin S/delta-beta-thalassemia
FSC	Hb SC disease
F	β°-thalassemia
Hb Bart	Alpha-thalassemia Hb Constant Spring
FAV	Heterozygosity for beta chain variant
FV	Homozygosity for beta chain variant Beta chain variant/β°-thalassemia

s/p = status post.
The pattern identified by primary screening methods is shown (left column): F, hemoglobin F; A, hemoglobin A; S, hemoglobin S; V, beta chain variant hemoglobin, e.g., hemoglobins C, E, D. The patterns are indicated in decreasing order of the hemoglobin percentage detected (e.g., FA denotes the presence of hemoglobin F and hemoglobin A with Hb F > Hb A). It must be stressed that the presence or absence of thalassemic traits cannot be addressed by neonatal screening.

intrauterine or postnatal transfusion was performed prior to the collection of the sample and this information is not provided to the pathologist, the interpretation will not be accurate. Interpretations therefore should include the caveat that the results are only valid if the infant has not been recently transfused. Reporting should be timely enough to provide time for counselors and physicians to inform and educate the family.

Testing after the neonatal period

Guidelines for the laboratory diagnosis of hemoglobinopathies [13, 37] and thalassemias [57] have been published. As mentioned, in many laboratories HPLC or capillary electrophoresis have replaced electrophoresis as the primary method for screening for structural hemoglobinopathies. Specialized methods, including sickle screens, assays for unstable hemoglobins, or special stains are then applied based upon the results of the first-line tests. A workup for thalassemia should minimally include a CBC (for the determination of the MCV, MCH, RBC, and RDW) and quantification of Hb A_2 and Hb F by HPLC or an equivalent method. It is important to note that α^+-thalassemia trait ($-\alpha/\alpha\alpha$) can be hematologically and clinically silent, with all CBC results within the reference range. Similarly, cases of beta-thalassemia trait with normal Hb A_2 have been described. CBC parameters and Hb A_2 levels within the normal range therefore do not fully exclude the presence of a thalassemic trait. In cases in which it is crucial to reliably exclude the presence of a thalassemic trait, for example for genetic counseling, additional studies may be necessary.

Special situations

Quantification of hemoglobin F in patients with sickle cell disease

Hemoglobin F has higher oxygen affinity than Hb A, and inhibits the polymerization of Hb S in patients with sickle cell disease. Patients with Hb F levels above 10% have significantly reduced organ damage, and the symptoms of sickle cell disease are almost completely eliminated if Hb F levels are higher than 25% [58]. Hydroxyurea has been shown to lead to a significant reduction of episodes of sickle cell crisis in patients with sickle cell disease; this is thought to be due to several mechanisms, including the increase in Hb F levels induced by the drug. Laboratories have to be aware that patients with sickle cell disease may be on long-term hydroxyurea regimens and that clinicians will request quantification of Hb F levels for these patients in order to assess the effectiveness of the therapy.

Juvenile myelomonocytic leukemia

The majority of patients with juvenile myelomonocytic leukemia (JMML) have increased levels of Hb F; in extreme cases the disease can mimic severe beta-thalassemia [59]. High Hb F levels at the time of diagnosis are associated with a poor prognosis in patients with pediatric myelodysplasia [60]. Laboratories may therefore be called upon to determine Hb F levels in these patients. It is important that clinicians understand that standard hemoglobin electrophoresis is not an adequate method for the quantification of Hb F, and that the optimal laboratory assays (HPLC, Hb F quantification) are performed.

Acknowledgements

The authors are indebted to Dr. Monica Gallivan and Dr. David O'Neill for careful reading of the manuscript and helpful advice.

References

1. **Hsia CC**. Respiratory function of hemoglobin. *New England Journal of Medicine*. 1998;**338**:239–247.

2. **Adair GS**. The hemoglobin system. *The Journal of Biological Chemistry*. 1925; **63**:529–545.

3. **Hardison R**. Hemoglobins from bacteria to man: evolution of different patterns of gene expression. *The Journal of Experimental Biology*. 1998;**201**: 1099–1117.

4. **Wood WG**. Haemoglobin synthesis during human fetal development.

   British Medical Bulletin. 1976;**32**: 282–287.

5. **Goh SH, Lee YT, Bhanu NV**, *et al*. A newly discovered human alpha-globin gene. *Blood*. 2005;**106**:1466–1472.

6. **Colombo B, Kim B, Atencio RP, Molina C, Terrenato L**. The pattern of

fetal haemoglobin disappearance after birth. *British Journal of Haematology.* 1976;**32**:79–87.

7. **Giardine B, van Baal S, Kaimakis P,** *et al.* HbVar database of human hemoglobin variants and thalassemia mutations: 2007 update. *Human Mutation.* 2007;**28**:206.

8. WHO. *Guidelines for the Control of Haemoglobin Disorders: Report of the Sixth Annual Meeting of the WHO Working Group on Haemoglobinopathies, Cagliari, Sardinia, 8–9 April 1989.* Geneva: WHO; 1994.

9. WHO. *Community Approaches to the Control of Hereditary Diseases: Report of a WHO Advisory Group.* Geneva: WHO; 1989.

10. **Ashley-Koch A, Yang Q, Olney RS.** Sickle hemoglobin (HbS) allele and sickle cell disease: a HuGE review. *American Journal of Epidemiology.* 2000;**151**:839–845.

11. **Bunn HF.** Pathogenesis and treatment of sickle cell disease. *New England Journal of Medicine.* 1997;**337**:762–769.

12. **Weatherall DJ, Clegg JB.** Inherited haemoglobin disorders: an increasing global health problem. *Bulletin of the World Health Organization.* 2001;**79**: 704–712.

13. ACOG Committee on Practice Bulletins. ACOG Practice Bulletin No. 78: hemoglobinopathies in pregnancy. *Obstetrics and Gynecology.* 2007;**109**: 229–237.

14. **Angastiniotis MA, Hadjiminas MG.** Prevention of thalassaemia in Cyprus. *Lancet.* 1981;**1**:369–371.

15. **Cao A, Furbetta M, Galanello R,** *et al.* Prevention of homozygous beta-thalassaemia by carrier screening and prenatal diagnosis in Sardinia. *American Journal of Human Genetics.* 1981;**33**:592–605.

16. **Vichinsky E, Hurst D, Earles A, Kleman K, Lubin B.** Newborn screening for sickle cell disease: effect on mortality. *Pediatrics.* 1988;**81**:749–755.

17. Steinberg MH, Forget BG, Higgs DR, Nagel RR (eds.). *Disorders of Hemoglobin. Genetics, Pathophysiology, and Clinical Management.* Cambridge: Cambridge University Press; 2001, 1268 pp.

18. **Weatherall DJ, Clegg JB.** *The Thalassemia Syndromes.* Oxford: Blackwell Science; 2001, 846 pp.

19. **Piperno A, Mariani R, Arosio C,** *et al.* Haemochromatosis in patients with beta-thalassaemia trait. *British Journal of Haematology.* 2000;**111**:908–914.

20. **Villard L, Fontes M.** Alpha-thalassaemia/mental retardation syndrome, X-Linked (ATR-X, MIM #301040, ATR-X/XNP/XH2 gene MIM #300032). *European Journal of Human Genetics: EJHG.* 2002;**10**:223–225.

21. **Rund D, Rachmilewitz E.** Beta-thalassemia. *New England Journal of Medicine.* 2005;**353**:1135–1146.

22. **Clarke GM, Higgins TN.** Laboratory investigation of hemoglobinopathies and thalassemias: review and update. *Clinical Chemistry.* 2000;**46**:1284–1290.

23. **Ohene-Frempong K.** Sickle cell diseases. In Rudolph CD, Rudolph AM, Hostetter MK, Lister G, Siegel NJ, eds. *Rudolph's Pediatrics.* New York: McGraw-Hill; 2003, 1531–1539.

24. **Brown AK, Sleeper LA, Miller ST,** *et al.* Reference values and hematologic changes from birth to 5 years in patients with sickle cell disease. Cooperative Study of Sickle Cell Disease. *Archives of Pediatrics and Adolescent Medicine.* 1994;**148**:796–804.

25. **Wethers DL.** Sickle cell disease in childhood: Part II. Diagnosis and treatment of major complications and recent advances in treatment. *American Family Physician.* 2000;**62**: 1309–1314.

26. **Wethers DL.** Sickle cell disease in childhood: Part I. Laboratory diagnosis, pathophysiology and health maintenance. *American Family Physician.* 2000;**62**:1013–1020, 1027–1028.

27. **Joutovsky A, Hadzi-Nesic J, Nardi MA.** HPLC retention time as a diagnostic tool for hemoglobin variants and hemoglobinopathies: a study of 60000 samples in a clinical diagnostic laboratory. *Clinical Chemistry.* 2004;**50**:1736–1747.

28. **Masiello D, Heeney MM, Adewoye AH,** *et al.* Hemoglobin SE disease: a concise review. *American Journal of Hematology.* 2007;**82**:643–649.

29. **Schrier SL, Bunyaratvej A, Khuhapinant A,** *et al.* The unusual pathobiology of hemoglobin Constant

Spring red blood cells. *Blood.* 1997;**89**: 1762–1769.

30. **Head CE, Conroy M, Jarvis M, Phelan L, Bain BJ.** Some observations on the measurement of haemoglobin A2 and S percentages by high performance liquid chromatography in the presence and absence of alpha thalassaemia. *Journal of Clinical Pathology.* 2004;**57**:276–280.

31. **Lafferty JD, Crowther MA, Ali MA, Levine M.** The evaluation of various mathematical RBC indices and their efficacy in discriminating between thalassemic and non-thalassemic microcytosis. *American Journal of Clinical Pathology.* 1996;**106**: 201–205.

32. **d'Onofrio G, Zini G, Ricerca BM, Mancini S, Mango G.** Automated measurement of red blood cell microcytosis and hypochromia in iron deficiency and beta-thalassemia trait. *Archives of Pathology and Laboratory Medicine.* 1992;**116**:84–89.

33. **Harris N, Kunicka J, Kratz A.** The ADVIA 2120 Hematology System: flow cytometry-based analysis of blood and body fluids in the routine hematology laboratory. *Laboratory Hematology.* 2005;**11**:47–61.

34. **Kotisaari S, Romppanen J, Penttila I, Punnonen K.** The Advia 120 red blood cells and reticulocyte indices are useful in diagnosis of iron-deficiency anemia. *European Journal of Haematology.* 2002;**68**:150–156.

35. **Bain BJ.** *Disorders of Red Cells and Platelets.* Oxford: Blackwell Science; 2002, 241–337.

36. **Bain BJ.** *Sickle Cell Haemoglobin and its Interactions with other Variant Haemoglobins and with Thalassemias.* Malden: Blackwell Publishing; 2006, 139–189.

37. **General Haematology Task Force of the British Committee for Standards in Haematology.** The laboratory diagnosis of haemoglobinopathies. *British Journal of Haematology.* 1998; **101**:783–792.

38. **Louahabi A, Philippe M, Lali S, Wallemacq P, Maisin D.** Evaluation of a new Sebia kit for analysis of hemoglobin fractions and variants on the Capillarys system. *Clinical Chemistry and Laboratory Medicine: CCLM/FESCC.* 2006;**44**:340–345.

39. **Cotton F, Lin C, Fontaine B,** *et al.* Evaluation of a capillary electrophoresis

method for routine determination of hemoglobins A2 and F. *Clinical Chemistry*. 1999;**45**:237–243.

40. **Wild BJ, Stephens AD.** The use of automated HPLC to detect and quantitate haemoglobins. *Clinical and Laboratory Haematology*. 1997;**19**: 171–176.

41. **Campbell M, Henthorn JS, Davies SC.** Evaluation of cation-exchange HPLC compared with isoelectric focusing for neonatal hemoglobinopathy screening. *Clinical Chemistry*. 1999;**45**:969–975.

42. **Fucharoen S, Winichagoon P, Wisedpanichkij R,** *et al.* Prenatal and postnatal diagnoses of thalassemias and hemoglobinopathies by HPLC. *Clinical Chemistry*. 1998;**44**:740–748.

43. **Howanitz PJ, Kozarski TB, Howanitz JH, Chauhan YS.** Spurious hemoglobin Barts caused by bilirubin: a common interference mimicking an uncommon hemoglobinopathy. *American Journal of Clinical Pathology*. 2006;**125**:608–614.

44. **Grey V, Wilkinson M, Phelan L, Hughes C, Bain BJ.** Inaccuracy of high-performance liquid chromatography estimation of haemoglobin F in the presence of increased haemoglobin A1c. *International Journal of Laboratory Hematology*. 2007;**29**:42–44.

45. **Baine RM, Brown HG.** Evaluation of a commercial kit for microchromatographic quantitation of hemoglobin A2 in the presence of hemoglobin S. *Clinical Chemistry*. 1981;**27**:1244–1247.

46. **Chen JC, Bigelow N, Davis BH.** Proposed flow cytometric reference method for the determination of erythroid F-cell counts. *Cytometry*. 2000;**42**:239–246.

47. **Davis BH, Olsen S, Bigelow NC, Chen JC.** Detection of fetal red cells in fetomaternal hemorrhage using a fetal hemoglobin monoclonal antibody by flow cytometry. *Transfusion*. 1998;**38**: 749–756.

48. **Scioscia AL.** Prenatal genetic diagnosis. In Creasy RK, Resnik R, eds. *Maternal-Fetal Medicine*. Philadelphia: WB Saunders; 1999, 40–62.

49. **Nagel RL.** *Hemoglobin Disorders: Molecular Methods and Protocols.* New York: Springer-Verlag; 2003, 322 pp.

50. **Clark BE, Thein SL.** Molecular diagnosis of haemoglobin disorders. *Clinical and Laboratory Haematology*. 2004;**26**:159–176.

51. **Patrinos GP, Kollia P, Papadakis MN.** Molecular diagnosis of inherited disorders: lessons from hemoglobinopathies. *Human Mutation*. 2005;**26**:399–412.

52. **Ristaldi MS, Pirastu M, Rosatelli C,** *et al.* Prenatal diagnosis of beta-thalassaemia in Mediterranean populations by dot blot analysis with DNA amplification and allele specific oligonucleotide probes. *Prenatal Diagnosis*. 1989;**9**:629–638.

53. **Newton CR, Graham A, Heptinstall LE,** *et al.* Analysis of any point mutation in DNA. The amplification refractory mutation system (ARMS). *Nucleic Acids Research*. 1989;**17**:2503–2516.

54. **Fischel-Ghodsian N, Hirsch PC, Bohlman MC.** Rapid detection of the hemoglobin C mutation by allele-specific polymerase chain reaction. *American Journal of Human Genetics*. 1990;**47**:1023–1024.

55. **Wu DY, Ugozzoli L, Pal BK, Wallace RB.** Allele-specific enzymatic amplification of beta-globin genomic DNA for diagnosis of sickle cell anemia. *Proceedings of the National Academy of Sciences of the United States of America*. 1989;**86**:2757–2760.

56. **Eastman JW, Wong R, Liao CL, Morales DR.** Automated HPLC screening of newborns for sickle cell anemia and other hemoglobinopathies. *Clinical Chemistry*. 1996;**42**:704–710.

57. **The Thalassaemia Working Party of the BCSH General Haematology Task Force.** Guidelines for investigation of the alpha and beta thalassaemia traits. *Journal of Clinical Pathology*. 1994;**47**: 289–295.

58. **Coleman E, Inusa B.** Sickle cell anemia: targeting the role of fetal hemoglobin in therapy. *Clinical Pediatrics*. 2007;**46**: 386–391.

59. **Honig GR, Suarez CR, Vida LN, Lu SJ, Liu ET.** Juvenile myelomonocytic leukemia (JMML) with the hematologic phenotype of severe beta thalassemia. *American Journal of Hematology*. 1998; **58**:67–71.

60. **Passmore SJ, Hann IM, Stiller CA,** *et al.* Pediatric myelodysplasia: a study of 68 children and a new prognostic scoring system. *Blood*. 1995;**85**:1742–1750.

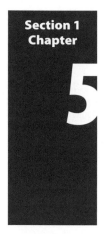

5

Hemolytic anemias

Immune- and non-immune-mediated hemolytic anemias, RBC membrane defects, and hereditary disorders due to RBC enzyme defects

Suresh G. Shelat

Introduction

Hemolysis, the destruction of red blood cells, can be categorized based on the site of hemolysis (*intravascular vs. extravascular*), the relation to the red cell (*intrinsic vs. extrinsic*), or the pattern of onset (*inherited vs. acquired*) (Fig. 5.1). The severity of the clinical findings in hemolysis depends on many factors, which are discussed below (Table 5.1). It is important to determine the underlying cause of hemolysis since the medical management may be different.

Immune-mediated hemolytic anemias

Immune-mediated hemolytic anemias result from intravascular or extravascular hemolysis triggered by various intrinsic and extrinsic factors. While the *intravascular* hemolysis occurs predominantly in the blood vessels, the *extravascular* hemolysis, which accounts for most cases of hemolytic anemia, is due to elimination of red cells by phagocytes in the spleen, liver, and bone marrow. Activation of the classic complement cascade is the main pathogenetic mechanism leading to immune-mediated hemolysis. Certain classes of antibodies are more effective than others at activating complement (IgM > IgG3 > IgG1 > IgG2). More commonly, the red cell is coated with complement C3b and C3d, and, less frequently, the activation of the complement cascade leads to the formation of membrane attack complex and red cell lysis [1, 2]. Since the liver macrophages do not harbor a C3d receptor, the red cells are not prematurely destroyed. Different antibody classes mediate the hemolytic process differently. In *IgG-mediated hemolysis*, the antibody that binds to the red cell membrane is recognized by the Fc receptors on splenic macrophages, leading to the formation of spherocytes that are eventually removed by the splenic macrophages [2]. On the other hand, in *IgM-mediated hemolysis*, the antibody binds the red cell membrane, leading to complete or incomplete activation of the complement cascade. These sensitized red cells are not removed by macrophages, which do not harbor an Fc receptor specific for the IgM molecule [2]. The immune-mediated hemolytic anemias can be categorized as autoimmune, alloimmune, and drug-induced.

Laboratory findings in immune-mediated hemolytic anemia

Findings are summarized in Table 5.2. Evidence of *in vivo* increased red cell destruction includes hemoglobinemia, hemoglobinuria, decreased serum haptoglobin, and an elevated level of serum unconjugated bilirubin or lactate dehydrogenase, especially LD1. The peripheral blood changes can reflect the underlying pathogenic mechanism of hemolysis. For example, an increased number of red cell fragments (schistocytes, helmet cells) is more frequently seen in intravascular hemolysis and thrombotic microangiopathies, whereas spherocytosis is characteristic of extravascular hemolysis [3]. Reticulocytosis and polychromasia, indicating effective erythropoiesis, are present regardless of the cause of hemolysis.

The direct destruction of the red cells results in release of free hemoglobin that is scavenged by haptoglobin [4]. The hemoglobin–haptoglobin complex is transported to the liver, where the heme group is metabolized to bilirubin, resulting in elevated levels of unconjugated bilirubin. When haptoglobin is depleted, heme groups are bound by *hemopexin* or, alternatively, they can be oxidized to *methemoglobin*, which then dissociates into oxidized heme (*hemin*) and globin chains. Hemoglobinemia, an accumulation of free hemoglobin in the plasma, occurs in brisk hemolysis when the level of free hemoglobin exceeds the capacity of haptoglobin or hemopexin. As a result, hemoglobinuria, free hemoglobin in the urine, can occur. The heme iron can accumulate in the renal tubular cells as hemosiderin. These cells slough off in the urine (*hemosiderinuria*) and are detectable using iron stains of urine sediment. In chronic hemolysis, hemosiderinuria may occur without hemoglobinuria [5].

Diagnostic Pediatric Hematopathology, ed. Maria A. Proytcheva. Published by Cambridge University Press.
© Cambridge University Press 2011.

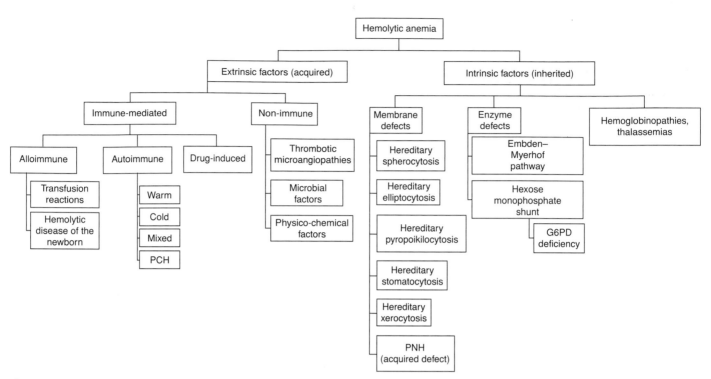

Fig. 5.1. Categories of hemolytic anemias. Abbreviations: PCH, paroxysmal cold hemoglobinuria; PNH, paroxysmal nocturnal hemoglobinuria; G6PD, glucose 6-phosphate dehydrogenase.

Table 5.1. Clinical findings in hemolytic anemias[a].

Pallor, fatigue, tachycardia
Jaundice and scleral icterus
Gallstones (chronic hemolysis)
Dark-colored or pink-colored urine

Evidence of extramedullary hematopoiesis (seen in chronic hemolytic conditions)
   Expansion of bone marrow and thinning of cortical bone
   Skeletal abnormalities

Splenomegaly
Hepatomegaly

[a] The presence and severity of clinical findings will depend on the pathophysiology of hemolysis.

Table 5.2. Laboratory findings in hemolytic anemias[a].

Reticulocytosis
Spherocytes and/or schistocytes
Bone marrow erythroid hyperplasia
Hyperbilirubinemia
Hemoglobinemia
↑ Serum lactate dehydrogenase (LDH)
↓ Haptoglobin
↓ Hemopexin
Hemoglobinuria
Hemosiderinuria
↑ Urine and fecal urobilinogen

[a] The presence of laboratory findings will depend on the pathophysiology of hemolysis.

In extravascular hemolysis, hemoglobinemia, hemoglobinuria, or hemosiderinuria is often absent, since the heme group and globin chains do not enter the plasma, but are catabolized in the phagocyte. The heme group is degraded to release iron and biliverdin (the latter of which binds to albumin), and is hepatically excreted.

Diagnostic workup of immune hemolytic anemias

The *direct antiglobulin test (DAT)* ("direct Coombs test") detects antibody or complement bound to the red cell surface *in vivo*, and is an essential part of the workup of immune hemolytic anemias. Polyspecific and anti-IgG reagents detect as few as 100–500 molecules of IgG per red cell and 400–1100 molecules of

Cd3 per red cell [6]. Monospecific AHG (antihuman globulin) reagents (anti-IgG and anti-complement) are needed to determine whether the positive reaction is due to presence of IgG, complement, or both. The most frequent causes for positive DAT are summarized in Table 5.3 [6].

A negative DAT does not necessarily mean that the red cells have no attached globulins. For example, the DAT may appear negative if the antibody-bound red cells are cleared from the circulation or if the IgG autoantibodies have low affinity or low density [7]. Alternatively, a positive DAT may be present but the red cell lifespan may not be reduced. This may occur if

Table 5.3. Causes of a positive direct antiglobulin test (DAT) with or without shortened red cell survival.

Autoantibodies to intrinsic red cell antigens
Alloantibodies in a recipient's circulation reacting with antigens on recently transfused donor red cells
Alloantibodies in donor plasma, plasma derivatives, or blood fractions which react with antigens on the red cells of a transfusion recipient
Alloantibodies in maternal circulation that passed the placenta
Antibodies directed against certain drugs, which bind to red cell membrane (e.g., penicillin)
Absorbed proteins, including immunoglobulins, which attach to the abnormal RBC membrane modified by certain drugs
Patients with hypergammaglobulinemia or recipients of high-dose intravenous gamma globulin
Antibodies produced by passenger lymphocytes in solid organ or hematopoietic stem cell recipients

Table 5.4. Warm versus cold autoimmune hemolytic anemia (AIHA).

	Cold AIHA	Warm AIHA
Optimal temperature for reactivity	<30 °C	37 °C
Autoantibody	IgM	IgG
Autoantibody specificity	Ii antigen system (anti-P in PCH)	Complex Rh-like
Eluate	Non-reactive	Pan-reactive
Complement activation	Yes	Little/none
Peripheral blood smear	Red cell agglutinates	Spherocytes
Primary site of hemolysis	Intravascular	Extravascular

the phagocytes cannot respond to a low titer of bound IgG or complement; if the thermal amplitude of the antibody is below 37 °C; or as a result of non-specific binding of immune globulins after intravenous immune globulin administration, hypergammaglobulinemia, or secondary to drugs such as α-methyldopa.

The *indirect antiglobulin test (IAT)* detects alloantibodies (from previous transfusion or pregnancy) or autoantibodies in patient's serum or plasma. Most unexpected alloantibodies are IgG, which alone do not cause agglutination, but incubation with polyspecific AHG results in agglutination in the presence of IgG [6].

Autoimmune hemolytic anemia (AIHA)

AIHA occurs when an immune response is mounted to "self" red cell antigens, resulting in premature destruction and anemia. The incidence of AIHA is 1–3 per 100 000 population [8]. AIHA is classified as "cold" or "warm" depending on the temperature at which the autoantibody demonstrates optimal reactivity (Table 5.4). In children, the highest incidence of AIHA is seen in the first four years of life [9]. Since antibody production is minimal in the first few months of life, AIHA is extremely rare in infants younger than six months of age.

Cold-reacting antibodies exhibit reactivity at low temperatures and can be either pathologic or benign (Table 5.4). Most children have cold autoantibodies that are not clinically significant. These include antibodies to P_1, Lewis A and B, and autoanti-I and IH [10]. However, pathologic cold agglutinins, either polyclonal or monoclonal, that have a broader thermal range (up to 31 °C), and which can be present in higher titer (>1 : 1000), can also be seen in children, and it is important that they are identified properly. Such antibodies should be suspected if the titer exceeds 1 : 256 and the DAT reaction to complement is positive. Cold-reacting antibodies are important to the pathogenesis of hemolytic anemia in the cold hemagglutinin disease and paroxysmal cold hemoglobinuria.

Cold hemagglutinin disease (CHD)

CHD, also known as idiopathic cold AIHA or cold agglutinin syndrome, accounts for approximately 16–32% of AIHA [11, 12]. It can occur as a chronic, idiopathic condition, or it can be associated with other diseases such as *Mycoplasma pneumoniae*, infectious mononucleosis, acute and chronic leukemia, and non-Hodgkin lymphoma. The cold antibody is usually reactive to the I antigen and less commonly to i antigen or the Pr antigens [9]. Cold agglutinins can cause agglutination of the red cells seen on the peripheral blood smear and can interfere with the automated hematology analyzer, as shown in Figure 5.2. Warming of the blood sample results in amelioration of these findings.

Paroxysmal cold hemoglobinuria (PCH)

PCH is rare and accounts for approximately 2% of AIHA cases [11, 12]. It can be idiopathic or develop secondary to childhood viral infections (measles, mumps, varicella, and influenza) and non-Hodgkin lymphoma [9]. PCH is mediated by the Donath–Landsteiner (D–L) "biphasic" antibody (Table 5.5). At the lower temperatures (<20 °C), the D–L antibody binds the red cell and early complement cascade proteins. As the red cell returns to the warmer body core temperature (37 °C), the D–L antibody dissociates and activates the complement cascade to proceed to completion, which results in red cell lysis. The autoantibody classically has specificity for the red cell P-antigen. Other reported reactivities include anti-I and anti-Pr-like [6]. PCH predominantly occurs in children and young adults. The episodes of intravascular hemolysis can be *paroxysmal*, triggered by *cold*, and cause moderate–severe anemia and *hemoglobinuria*. Management of PCH includes avoidance of cold temperatures, and treatment of the underlying disease. Transfusion is usually not necessary unless the hemolysis is significant.

Warm autoantibodies occur in children and adults and account for approximately 70% of AIHA cases [11, 12]. Sixty percent of warm autoimmune hemolytic anemia (WAIHA) cases are idiopathic [1, 9, 11]. However, a warm autoantibody may be present in Hodgkin or non-Hodgkin lymphoma, ulcerative colitis, and autoimmune disease such as scleroderma, systemic lupus erythematosus, and rheumatoid arthritis [12].

Table 5.5. Characteristics of cold-reacting antibodies.

	Benign cold agglutinins	Pathologic cold agglutinins	Paroxysmal cold hemoglobinuria (PCH)
DAT reactivity	Complement C3 – negative/ weak positive IgG – negative	Complement C3 – positive IgG – negative	Complement C3 – positive IgG – negative
Antibody type (specificity)	IgM (anti-I)	IgM monophasic (anti-I or anti-i)	Donath–Landsteiner (D–L) "biphasic" IgG (anti-P)
Antibody characteristic	Polyclonal	Monoclonal (idiopathic) Polyclonal (e.g., *Mycoplasma pneumoniae*)	Polyclonal
Titer	Low–Moderate (<1 : 64)	High (>1 : 256–1 : 1000)	Moderate (<1 : 64)
Thermal amplitude	0–4 °C optimal Rarely up to 20–24 °C	Broad range, up to 31 °C	Up to 20 °C
Donath–Landsteiner test	Negative	Negative	Positive
Hemolysis	No	Chronic, intravascular or extravascular hemolysis	Acute, intravascular
Clinical features	Benign	Acrocyanosis	Acute hemolytic episodes triggered by cold
Patient population	Children and adults	Adults mostly	Children; young adults
Etiology	Naturally occurring	Idiopathic Associated with *Mycoplasma pneumoniae*, infectious mononucleosis, lymphoproliferative diseases	Idiopathic Associated with viral infections
Treatment	Not required	Avoid cold	Treat underlying disease

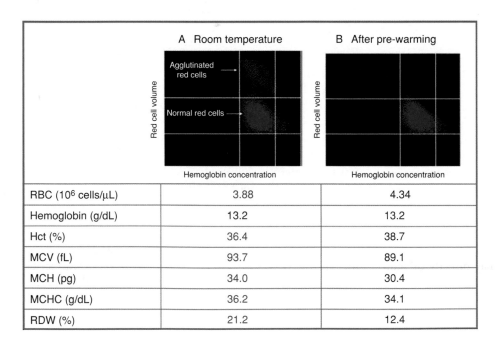

	A Room temperature	B After pre-warming
RBC (10^6 cells/μL)	3.88	4.34
Hemoglobin (g/dL)	13.2	13.2
Hct (%)	36.4	38.7
MCV (fL)	93.7	89.1
MCH (pg)	34.0	30.4
MCHC (g/dL)	36.2	34.1
RDW (%)	21.2	12.4

Fig. 5.2. Advia 2120 Hematology System (Siemens) scatter plots demonstrating the effect of cold agglutinins on the red cell parameters. (A) Prior to warming the sample (i.e., at room temperature), the hematology analyzer reported a falsely low red cell (RBC) count and a falsely elevated red cell distribution width (RDW). Consequently, other parameters such as mean corpuscular hemoglobin (MCH) and mean corpuscular hemoglobin concentration (MCHC) that are mathematically derived from the red cell count are falsely elevated. Likewise, the hematocrit (Hct) may be inaccurate. However, the hemoglobin value is not affected since it is based on direct measurement of lysed red blood cells, regardless of the agglutination. (B) After pre-warming of the sample and diluents to 37 °C, these aberrant results are corrected.

Autoantibodies often exhibit reactivity to high-incidence antigens and have a broad specificity to Rh or to Rh system antigens, although other specificities (Kell, U, Vel, Gerbich) have been described [1, 13]. In contrast to patients with alloantibodies alone, patients with AIHA demonstrate incompatibility with their own cells and all donor red cell units, and require a careful pre-RBC-transfusion workup since the presence of auto-antibodies may mask an underlying alloantibody. If an allo-antibody is detected, its specificity should be determined. In addition, phenotyping of the patient's red cells to identify the presence of clinically significant antigens such as Rh, Kidd, Kell, Duffy, and MNS is performed in order to select red cell units for transfusion that lack any identified alloantibody specificity [14]. Adjunct treatment to reduce the level of autoantibodies

Table 5.6. Pathogenic mechanisms of drug-induced hemolytic anemias[a].

	Hapten type	Immune complex mediated	Autoantibody induced
DAT reactivity	IgG mediates hemolysis IgM – no hemolysis	C3d – positive	IgG – positive
IAT reactivity [1]	Non-reactive; reactive if reagent RBC coated with drug	Reactive in drug presence	Reactive in drug absence
Mechanism of hemolysis	Extravascular	Intravascular or extravascular	Extravascular
Inciting drug	Penicillin (large intravenous doses)	Quinidine, quinine Some intravenous third generation cephalosporins (e.g., cefotetan) Some non-steroidal anti-inflammatory drugs	α-methyldopa Fludarabine Procainamide Mefenamic acid
Presence of drug necessary for hemolysis to occur	Yes	Yes	No

[a] A fourth type, *membrane modification*, can occur when certain first-generation cephalosporins alter the red cell membrane so that other plasma proteins, complement components, or immunoglobulins can adhere to the membrane in a non-immunologic and non-specific manner. Such proteins on the red cell surface may be detectable by reagent specific antibodies (anti-IgG, anti-complement, anti-albumin, anti-fibrinogen, etc.).

includes immunosuppression, intravenous immune globulin, or plasma exchange. Refractory warm AIHA may benefit from splenectomy.

Mixed autoimmune hemolytic anemia (AIHA)

The mixed AIHA exhibits characteristics of warm-reacting IgG and cold-reacting IgM antibodies. It accounts for approximately 7% of AIHA cases and is either idiopathic or occurs in association with other conditions (e.g., collagen vascular disease, systemic lupus erythematosus, chronic lymphocytic leukemia (CLL), or non-Hodgkin lymphoma) [9, 11, 12]. The red cell is sensitized with warm-reacting IgG (complex specificity) and cold-reacting IgM (autoanti-I specificity or not specified). These patients have DAT positive for C3d and IgG, and with a cold antibody of high thermal amplitude (30 °C), but low titer (<1 : 64). Most patients with mixed AIHA present with severe acute anemia. Chronic disease with sporadic episodes can also be seen. Management of such patients includes immunosuppression, though transfusion is usually not necessary.

Drug-related hemolytic anemia

Exposure to a drug or drug metabolite may directly or indirectly cause lysis or premature removal of blood cells. Drug-induced hemolytic anemia should be considered in cases of unexplained hemolysis, and should be differentiated from the (non-immune) hemolysis that occurs in red cells with inherited defects (e.g., G6PD deficiency or unstable hemoglobins) that render them susceptible to hemolysis by certain drugs. The patient may be on multiple medications, and identifying the inciting drug may be challenging and requires a special workup in a few specialized laboratories [15]. In general, drug-induced hemolytic anemias are less common in children than adults, since the inciting drugs are less commonly prescribed [9]. Three mechanisms of drug-related hemolytic anemia are described in Table 5.6.

Polyagglutination

Polyagglutination is a type of AIHA in which normally hidden cryptic antigens on red cells are exposed and then bound by naturally occurring antibodies found in virtually all patients ("*polyagglutinate*"). It can occur following a viral or bacterial infection (e.g., necrotizing enterocolitis). For example, bacterial neuraminidase from *Clostridium perfringens* cleaves red cell surface antigen *N*-acetyl-neuraminic acid to create a T-neoantigen [16]. An "acquired-B" phenotype, in which bacterial enzymes cleave the group A antigen to form the group B antigen, is another example that may result in discrepancy of the forward and reverse blood typing. Pollyagglutinins can be identified by specific lectin reagents. Children are not routinely tested for polyagglutination, since T-activation does not necessarily result in hemolysis. If the child demonstrates a clinically significant anemia or hemolysis due to T-activation, then donor platelets and red cells must be washed to remove accompanying anti-T antibodies.

Alloimmune hemolytic anemias

This anemia results from the destruction of red cells by alloantibodies. Alloimmunization in children is uncommon (approximately 1.2%) [17], but may be higher in patients with sickle cell anemia and thalassemia major that require multiple transfusions. In alloimmune hemolytic anemia the hemolysis is usually extravascular, though intravascular hemolysis can occur if there is an activation of the complement cascade.

Hemolytic transfusion reactions result when a patient with alloantibodies is transfused with RBCs containing the corresponding antigen (Table 5.7). Based on the time of hemolysis and clinical presentation, they can be divided into acute hemolytic transfusion reactions (AHTRs) and delayed hemolytic transfusion reactions (DHTRs).

Most AHTRs occur after transfusing red cells harboring major blood group antigens to a recipient who has preexisting complement-activating IgM and IgG antibodies (usually

Table 5.7. Acute versus delayed hemolytic transfusion reactions.

	Acute	Delayed
Onset of signs/symptoms	Within minutes to a few hours of transfusion	7–28 days (initial exposure) <2–3 days (anamnestic response)
Incompatible antigen	A or B	Previous foreign red cell antigens
Antibody	Naturally occurring iso-hemagglutinins: IgM and IgG	IgG
Agglutinates red cells	Yes	No
Site of hemolysis	Intravascular	Usually extravascular Can be intravascular

Table 5.8. Management of hemolytic transfusion reactions.

Action	Rationale
Stop transfusion immediately!	Severity of transfusion reaction is proportional to the amount of incompatible red cells transfused
Maintain venous access	Rapid administration of medications and resuscitative fluids to maintain organ (e.g., kidney) perfusion
Clerical check	To ensure correct identification of patient, specimens, and red cell unit
Return remaining blood products and tubing to the blood bank.	Blood bank transfusion reaction workup: Repeat the required testing to ensure pre-transfusion specimens were correctly identified and tested DAT on post-transfusion specimens
Visual inspection of plasma	Check for free hemoglobin in plasma (pink)
Analysis of urine	Hemoglobinuria indicates intravascular hemolysis Microscopy of urine sediment to distinguish hemoglobinuria due to hematuria Hemosiderinuria – indicative of chronic hemolysis

anti-A or anti-B) in his or her plasma. This results in rapid intravascular hemolysis, causing hemoglobinemia and hemoglobinuria, leading to acute renal failure and activation of the coagulation cascade, cytokine release, and disseminated intravascular coagulation (DIC). The AHTR can occur minutes after an incompatible transfusion of <20 mL of red cells. The signs and symptoms vary widely from none to various degrees of fever, rigors, shortness of breath, tachycardia, pallor, fatigue, and jaundice, hypotension or hypertension, profound cardiac failure, and respiratory failure. Death occurs in 10–50% of patients with AHTR [18].

The DHTR occurs from an immune response to antigens on donor red cells to which the patient was previously exposed. The DHTR may occur a few days to weeks following *initial* exposure to red cell antigens (e.g., Rh, Kell, Duffy, Kidd) [4]. Normally, these alloantibodies are detected by the pre-transfusion testing, but they may be missed if the titer is very low. Consequently, re-exposure to the foreign red cell antigens leads to an anamnestic response within hours to days of the exposure [6]. The hemolysis is usually extravascular, but can be intravascular with certain alloantibodies (e.g., anti-Kidd). The DHTR is rarely fatal and can show few signs or symptoms several days after transfusion, except for an unexplained fever or decline in hemoglobin (comparable to that of the transfused units). The DHTR can also be incidentally discovered when an antibody screen reveals a new antibody.

The management of a suspected transfusion reaction is summarized in Table 5.8. After the transfusion is stopped, the diagnostic workup includes repeat testing of the pre- and post-transfusion ABO/Rh type, antibody screen, DAT, cross-matches, alloantibody identification, and retyping of the donor units. The urine is analyzed for hemoglobinuria and hemosiderinuria.

Transfusion practices in neonates and children

Transfusion in pediatric patients poses special challenges and is more fully discussed elsewhere [19]. A thorough transfusion history (of mother and child) will aid in the pre-transfusion testing and may help to explain unexpected serologic results. For example, a positive DAT (for IgG) in infants less than four months of age is most likely due to passively transferred antibodies; for instance, antenatally administered Rh immune globulin, or intravenous immune globulin (IVIG) in the treatment of idiopathic thrombocytopenic purpura (ITP). In children, "minor" incompatible hemolytic transfusion reactions can occur if a child is transfused with blood products, for example platelets, with sufficient volume of plasma that contains a high titer of incompatible antibodies [20, 21].

Hemolytic disease of the fetus/newborn (HDF/HDN)

While the transport of maternal IgG antibodies across the placenta during pregnancy is usually protective for the developing fetus, maternal antibodies against a fetal red cell antigen can cause red cell hemolysis. During pregnancy, a small number of fetal red cells cross the placenta, and if they express paternal antigens that are recognized by the maternal immune system as foreign, an alloimmunization of the mother can occur. The risk of alloimmunization increases during the course of pregnancy from 3% during the first trimester to 12% in the second trimester, 45% at the third trimester, and 64% at delivery [22].

The types of HDN and their characteristic features are summarized in Table 5.9.

HDN is more frequently due to ABO incompatibility and is more common but less clinically severe. It occurs in newborns of group O mothers who harbor a naturally occurring anti-A, anti-B, or anti-A,B IgG. While ABO incompatibility occurs in 15% of pregnancies of group O mothers, less than

Table 5.9. ABO versus Rh hemolytic disease of the newborn.

	ABO	Rh
Affects first pregnancy [23]	Common (~45%)	Uncommon (<5%)
Affecting subsequent pregnancies	Common, but unpredictable	Common
Maternal red cell type	Group O	Rh negative
Fetal red cells	Group A, B, or AB	Rh positive
DAT	Negative/weak positive	Positive
Maternal antibody screen	Negative	Positive
IgG antibody specificity	Anti-A,B; anti-A; anti-B	Anti-Rh
Prenatal monitoring	Not necessary	Serial titers (anti-Rh); amniocentesis
Clinical severity	Mild–moderate	Moderate–severe; more severe with subsequent antigen-positive pregnancy
Peripheral blood findings in neonate	Occasional nucleated RBCs Reticulocytosis Spherocytes	Early erythropoietic progenitors, nucleated RBCs – "erythroblastosis fetalis" Reticulocytosis; infrequent spherocytes
Treatment	Phototherapy Exchange transfusion (rare)	Intrauterine transfusions Phototherapy Exchange transfusion

10% of infants with detectable maternal ABO antibodies are symptomatic, and only a small fraction of these (< 10%) exhibit severe disease [24]. Since the maternal antibodies are naturally occurring, HDN can be seen with first pregnancy, and the risk of hemolytic disease in subsequent pregnancies is the same.

The more severe from of HDN is due to Rh incompatibility and requires alloimmunization of the mother during pregnancy or after transfusion with Rh-positive blood. Rh(D) is a highly immunogenic antigen leading to alloimmunization of the mother and generation of IgG anti-D. These antibodies can cross the placenta and lead to hemolytic disease in the fetus. Exposure to D$^+$ red cells in subsequent pregnancies can lead to more robust IgG production and more severe HDF/HDN. The severe anemia leads to increased erythropoietin levels resulting in an increase in the extramedullary hematopoiesis in the fetal liver and spleen, with subsequent portal hypertension, compromised hepatic albumin production, and generalized edema (anasarca). If the fetus cannot compensate for the sequelae of hemolysis, either by endogenous red cell production or via intrauterine transfusions, heart failure and hydrops fetalis can occur. The severity of Rh-HDN is proportional to the degree of anemia at birth. The peripheral blood demonstrates marked reticulocytosis, increased nucleated red cell count (50-fold increased), and elevated white cell count [2]. Hyperbilirubinemia can accompany the hemolysis. In the first day of life, unconjugated bilirubin levels rise (peaking on third

to fourth day of life), due to the immaturity of hepatic enzymes that conjugate and clear it from the body. In the most serious case, bilirubin accumulates in the cerebellum and basal ganglia, leading to kernicterus (at bilirubin >20–25 mg/dL), and possibly death. Premature infants are more prone to bilirubin encephalopathy at lower bilirubin levels [23].

In addition to ABO and Rh(D) incompatibilities, HDN can result from other alloantibodies to antigens in the Rhesus (E, c, C) or other systems (Kell, Kidd, Duffy, and MNS) [25]. Severe fetal anemia due to anti-Kell is less common (only ~10% of individuals are Kell positive), but may be severe, since, in addition to antibody-mediated hemolysis, anti-Kell antibodies suppress fetal erythropoiesis [26].

Rh immune globulin (RhIg) is a preparation of high-titer anti-D antibodies that has significantly reduced the incidence of HDF/HDN [27]. RhIg should be administered to D$^-$ pregnant mothers at approximately 28 weeks of gestation and within 72 hours after potentially sensitizing events (e.g., amniocentesis, cordocentesis, abortion, placenta previa, abruption), and delivery of D$^+$ infants. The RhIg is thought to bind to D$^+$ fetal red cells that enter the maternal circulation, targeting them for removal by the spleen, and thus preventing a maternal immune response. The dose of RhIg to administer can be calculated by determining the number of fetal cells in the maternal circulation using flow cytometry or the traditional Kleihauer–Betke method.

Laboratory workup of HDN

The post-partum diagnostic workup includes ABO/Rh typing of the neonate, maternal IAT, neonatal DAT, and eluate to determine the antigen specificity of the maternal antibody. In ABO-HDN, the maternal antibody screen is usually negative (does not routinely evaluate maternal serum for ABO IgG antibodies), but positive in alloimmune HDN. The DAT usually identifies maternal antibodies on the infant's red cells in both ABO- and alloimmune HDN. The results of blood typing should be interpreted cautiously since neonatal red cells heavily sensitized with maternal IgG may interfere with Rh typing reagents and thus appear Rh negative. In Rh-HDN, the DAT usually indicates the presence of IgG, whereas in ABO-HDN, the DAT is due to anti-A,B antibodies (but not complement). If HDN is clinically suspected but the DAT and maternal antibody screen are negative, the maternal serum or an antibody-containing eluate prepared from the infant's red cells may be tested against the biological father's red cells. Although asymptomatic infants who are incompatible with their mother's ABO type may have negative DATs, almost all infants with ABO-HDN and clear evidence of a hemolytic anemia have a positive DAT. Consequently, significant jaundice and anemia in an infant with a negative DAT should not be attributed to ABO incompatibility without appropriate investigation for other causes of hemolysis [28].

Prenatal monitoring includes spectrophotometric analysis of amniotic fluid (Liley nomograms) for bilirubin levels, fetal lung maturity profiles, biophysical profiles, and middle cerebral artery peak systolic velocity [29]. Women who are

D-negative may also have a repeat antibody screen at 28 weeks of pregnancy, prior to RhIg administration, to check that the mother has not produced any active anti-D. Note that low titers (<1 : 4) of anti-D can occur following administration of RhIg. However, these titers should not be used to distinguish passive versus active anti-D antibody, nor assumed to solely account for reactivity in an antibody screen.

Non-immune hemolytic anemias

Hemolytic anemias can occur as a result of thrombotic microangiopathies, microbial toxins, and physico-chemical agents.

Thrombotic thrombocytopenic purpura (TTP)

TTP is a thrombotic microangiopathy which occurs idiopathically or in association with infections, pregnancy, malignancy, medications (clopidogrel, ticlopidine), rheumatologic conditions, and bone marrow transplant. It has been described with a classical pentad of qualifying symptoms, including microangiopathic hemolytic anemia (MAHA), thrombocytopenia, renal dysfunction, neurologic symptoms, and fever. Some patients may present with MAHA and thrombocytopenia and may not meet all criteria. With prompt treatment (plasma exchange), the mortality from TTP has been reduced from 80% to less than 20%.

It is currently believed that TTP results from the effects of unusually large von Willebrand factor (VWF) multimers in the circulation due to the absence of, or an autoantibody to, the VWF-cleaving protease known as ADAMTS13 (**13**th member of the metalloprotease family, **a d**isintegrin **a**nd **m**etalloproteinase with **t**hrombospondin type 1 repeats) [30]. Defects or absence of ADAMTS13 result in formation of platelet-rich microthrombi that occlude the microcirculation in multiple organs. The moderate–severe anemia results from red cells shearing as they traverse the microthrombi. There is a rare congenital form of TTP (Upshaw–Schulman syndrome), wherein ADAMTS13 gene mutations result in abnormal production or function of the protein [31]. Despite this evidence, it is controversial as to whether ADAMTS13 is a specific marker for TTP [32].

Hemolytic uremic syndrome (HUS)

HUS is another form of microangiopathic anemia seen affecting infants and young children. HUS shares many of the findings of TTP, including a moderate–severe anemia with schistocytes, reticulocytosis, thrombocytopenia, and elevated lactate dehydrogenase (Fig. 5.3). There is debate as to whether these two conditions represent a clinical continuum with a similar underlying pathophysiology [33].

HUS affects previously healthy infants and young children, who develop bloody diarrhea, moderate to severe MAHA, hematuria, acute renal failure, and anuria. In addition, patients can develop hypertension, abdominal pain, petechiae, jaun-

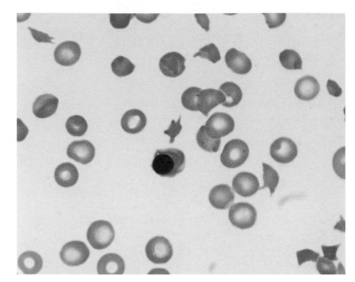

Fig. 5.3. Thrombotic thrombocytopenic purpura (TTP). Photograph kindly provided by Marybeth Helfrich MT(ASCP).

dice, and fever. Microthrombi in several organs can compromise the function of kidneys, brain, and pancreas [34]. There are several forms of HUS with different clinical presentation and underlying pathophysiology. Based on the presence or absence of preceding bloody diarrhea, HUS has been categorized into D$^+$ and D$^-$ HUS. The D$^+$ HUS is more common in children less than two years old and usually results from *Shigella dysenteriae* serotype I or enterohemorrhagic *Escherichia coli* O157:H7. The D$^-$ HUS ("atypical HUS") occurs in adults and in some children, and has been associated with infections, pregnancy, bone marrow transplant, and certain immunosuppressive and chemotherapeutic medications. A third form of HUS, a rare congenital deficiency of Factor H, a protein involved in regulating the alternative complement pathway, has also been described.

Disseminated intravascular coagulation (DIC)

DIC is characterized by aberrations in coagulation, resulting in activation of thrombin (thrombosis) and plasmin (fibrinolysis and bleeding), resulting in fibrin deposition and a consumptive coagulopathy. DIC can cause (or result from) damage to the microvasculature in multiple organ systems [35]. Etiologies include bacterial infections (Gram-negative bacteremia, streptococcus, meningococcus), viral infections (cytomegalovirus, varicella, hepatitis), fungal infections, rickettsial infections, cancer (acute promyelocytic leukemia, Kasabach–Merritt syndrome), intravascular red cell hemolysis, shock, burns, certain venoms, and connective tissue diseases [36]. Unlike TTP, DIC exhibits a prolonged prothrombin time, activated partial thromboplastin time, and thrombin time, hypofibrinogenemia, positive D-dimers, and increased fibrin degradation products [37]. The peripheral blood shows thrombocytopenia and schistocytes. The treatment of DIC requires management of the underlying disorder and transfusion of platelets, plasma, and cryoprecipitate if needed.

Table 5.10. Microorganisms causing hemolytic anemias.

Etiology	Description	Clinical–pathologic features
Plasmodium falciparum	(See text)	(See text)
Babesia [38] (*B. microti*; *B. gibsoni*; *B. divergens*)	Zoonotic hemoparasite transmitted by *Ixodes* tick Can be transmitted to human via infected RBC unit from (asymptomatic) blood donor	Fever, hemolysis (extravascular) and anemia Clinical course usually self-limited More severe in asplenic or immunocompromised patients – intravascular and extravascular hemolysis, higher parasitemia, DIC, renal failure
Clostridium [2] (*C. perfringens*; *C. septicum*)	Produces toxin that lyses the red cell membrane lipids	Brisk hemolysis, hemoglobinuria, and renal damage Spherocytes, schistocytes, helmet cells
Bartonella bacilliformis [39]	Coccobacillus transmitted by sandfly vector in Peru and Ecuador Infection causes invagination of red cell membranes and formation of intracellular vacuoles	Fever, hemolysis
Venoms (brown recluse spider; snake venom)	Venom cleaves glycoporins from red cell membrane	Intravascular hemolysis Snake bite: hemolysis, either directly or secondary to DIC

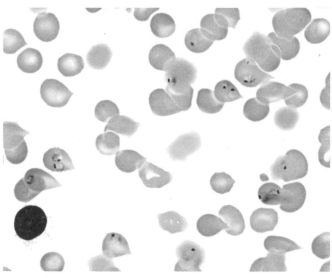

Fig. 5.4. *Plasmodium falciparum* malaria. Photograph kindly provided by Marybeth Helfrich MT(ASCP).

Table 5.11. Physical and chemical agents causing hemolytic anemias.

Etiology	Description
Prosthetic devices (e.g., heart valves)	Turbulent blood flow around valves increases shear stress → red cell fragments
Malignant hypertension	Etiology not defined (possibly related to fibrin deposition or fibrinoid necrosis in vasculature) Thrombocytopenia and red cell fragmentation Condition resolves with normalization of blood pressure
Thermal damage	Burn injury → red cell membrane proteins damage → intravascular hemolysis occurs within 48 hours May result from transfusion of packed red cells through uncalibrated blood warmers Peripheral blood smear shows schistocytes, spherocytes, RBC budding, fragments
March hemoglobinuria due to vigorous exercise on hard surface	Transient intravascular hemolysis but anemia is uncommon Red cell fragments absent
Freezing red cell units without appropriate preservation agents	Red cell hemolysis upon thawing
Inappropriate dilution or mixing of red cells with intravenous solutions	Mixing red cell units with other solutions (diluted albumin, dextrose) may cause osmotic lysis or clotting (lactated Ringer solution)

Hemolytic anemias due to microbial and physico-chemical causes

Several microorganisms can cause hemolytic anemia (Table 5.10). Perhaps the most significant of them is malaria. The *Plasmodium* parasite causes >300 million cases of malaria annually and >1 million deaths [40]. It occurs mainly in Africa, Asia, and Latin America. Though four species of *Plasmodium* infect humans (*P. vivax*, *P. ovale*, *P. malariae*, and *P. falciparum*), most deaths result from *P. falciparum* (Fig. 5.4). Diagnosis continues to be via microscopy, although immunochromatographic methods also detect and differentiate *P. falciparum* from other malarial species. Hemolytic anemia can also be caused by physical and chemical forces on the red cell (Table 5.11) [2].

Hemolytic anemia due to membrane defects

Hemolytic anemia can result from defects in the lipid and/or protein components of the red cell membrane, most of which are inherited. The resulting abnormalities in the shape, permeability, flexibility, and deformability of the red cell can compromise its integrity as it traverses the vasculature, thus rendering it susceptible to removal by the reticuloendothelial system.

Hereditary spherocytosis (HS)

HS is a common hereditary cause of hemolytic anemia among northern Europeans, occurring in approximately 1 in 5000 individuals [41]. It is inherited in an autosomal dominant manner (70%) with variable penetrance, or can occur, less frequently, as a result of a spontaneous mutation. HS is most

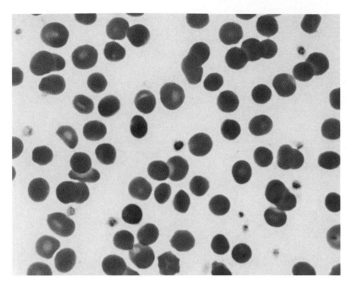

Fig. 5.5. Hereditary spherocytosis (HS). Photograph kindly provided by Marybeth Helfrich MT(ASCP).

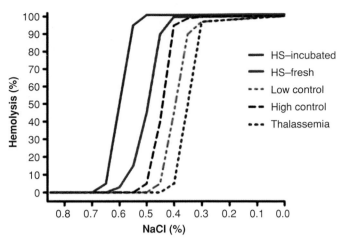

Fig. 5.6. Osmotic fragility test. Freshly drawn anticoagulated blood is incubated at room temperature for one hour with a series of buffered salt solutions of decreasing osmolarity. After centrifugation, the percentage of hemolysis is measured by spectrophotometry ($A_{540\,nm}$). Normal red cell hemolysis is shown in the area between the "low" and "high" controls. Freshly prepared red cells from patients with hereditary spherocytosis ("HS – fresh") show slightly increased osmotic fragility. Incubating red cells at 37 °C for 24 hours ("HS – incubated") prior to saline incubations increases the assay's sensitivity. Thalassemia and other conditions exhibit decreased osmotic fragility. Note, osmotic fragility should not be used in neonates as a screening test without age-matched controls.

commonly associated with a primary or secondary deficiency of red cell spectrin β-chain or another structural protein (ankyrin, AE1/band 3, protein 4.1, protein 4.2), leading to uncoupling of the cytoskeleton from the lipid bilayer at certain sites. This leads to formation of unsupported membrane microvesicles that are removed by the spleen, leading to loss of membrane (Fig. 5.5). In addition, HS red cells have lower total lipid levels and are abnormally permeable to sodium ions [42]. HS is characterized by chronic hemolysis, ranging from mild to severe. In approximately 30% of the patients the hemolysis is compensated, and severe anemia is seen in approximately 10%. Most affected infants and >75% of older children and adults exhibit jaundice and splenomegaly and can develop cholelithiasis.

Laboratory diagnosis of HS

The peripheral blood analysis shows spherocytes and an elevated mean corpuscular hemoglobin concentration (MCHC), due to loss of membrane without proportionate loss of hemoglobin. The anemia is variable, depending on the degree of hemolysis and the compensatory marrow response. Reticulocytosis (5–15%) is characteristic and may exceed that of other hemolytic anemias with comparable hemoglobin levels.

The diagnosis of HS can be confirmed by the presence of increased osmotic fragility (Fig. 5.6) [43]. Spherocytes have increased osmotic fragility, whereas in conditions with target cells (increased surface-area-to-volume ratio), such as thalassemia and certain hemoglobinopathies or in iron deficiency, the red cells exhibit decreased osmotic fragility. HS also can be diagnosed by measuring of red cell cytoskeletal protein AE1 using fluorescent dye eosin-5-maleimide (EMA) by flow cytometry [44]. AE1 is decreased in patients with HS as compared to normal individuals.

The differential diagnosis of HS includes immune-mediated hemolytic anemias, microangiopathic hemolytic anemia (MAHA), and anemia due to burn injuries. A positive direct

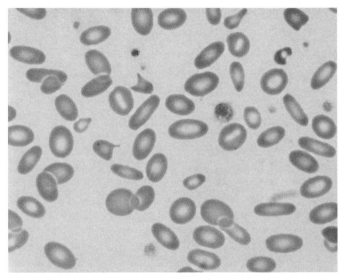

Fig. 5.7. Hereditary elliptocytosis (HE). Photograph kindly provided by Marybeth Helfrich MT(ASCP).

antiglobulin test (DAT) distinguishes immune-mediated hemolytic anemias from HS. Mild HS does not usually require treatment. Red cell transfusions may be necessary in more severe hemolytic episodes and following aplastic episodes. Splenectomy is curative and should restore the normal red cell lifespan.

Hereditary elliptocytosis (HE)

HE comprises a heterogeneous group of red cell membrane disorders characterized by an abundance of elliptocytes (Fig. 5.7).

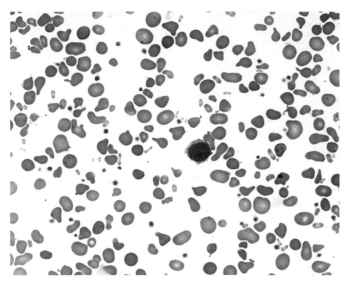

Fig. 5.8. Hereditary pyropoikilocytosis (HPP). Photograph kindly provided by Marybeth Helfrich MT(ASCP).

HE is usually transmitted in an autosomal dominant manner with variable penetrance. Abnormalities in membrane interactions between α-spectrin, band 4.1, glycoporin C, and anion transport protein (band 3) can prevent the red cell from re-establishing its normal biconcave shape after traversing the microvasculature. HE rarely presents in the neonate, and <10% of HE patients exhibit clinically significant hemolysis. However, severe HE demonstrates numerous elliptocytes, poikilocytosis, and spherocytes, and may need transfusion support or splenectomy.

Hereditary pyropoikilocytosis (HPP)

HPP is a severe form of hereditary elliptocytosis that presents in infancy with hemolytic anemia. It is commonly seen in individuals of African descent. It is due to an α-spectrin deficiency in addition to an abnormality in spectrin tetramer assembly. The red cell fragmentation and poikilocytes in HPP (Fig. 5.8) share morphologic similarities to thermally damaged red cells. In the laboratory, HPP red cells undergo fragmentation at lower temperatures (45 °C, or following incubation at 37 °C for >6 hours) than normal red cells (50 °C). The MCV is reduced (<50 fL) due to the presence of red cell fragments and microspherocytes. The HPP red blood cells have increased osmotic fragility (in the 24-hour incubated test) [45]. The neonate with HPP can exhibit hyperbilirubinemia at birth, requiring exchange transfusion and phototherapy [45].

Rare forms of membrane defects

Hereditary stomatocytosis is a rare autosomal dominant disorder with variable degrees of hemolysis, anemia, hyperbilirubinemia, and splenomegaly. Laboratory findings include stomatocytosis (up to 50% of red cells), decreased MCHC, and increased osmotic fragility [45]. The differential diagnosis of stomatocytosis includes Rh null disease, Tangier disease, alcoholic cirrhosis, and cardiovascular disease. Treatment includes transfusion support or splenectomy in severe cases.

Hereditary xerocytosis is another rare red cell membrane defect in which the net decrease in intracellular cation content results in intracellular loss of water and cellular dehydration (xerocyte). The peripheral blood smear includes spiculated red cells with condensed hemoglobin, and an increased MCHC. Clinically, it can present with moderate hemolytic anemia.

Paroxysmal nocturnal hemoglobinuria (PNH)

PNH is a rare acquired membrane disorder (approximately 0.1–1 per 10^5 persons) affecting mostly adults, but can also been seen in the pediatric population. A somatic mutation in the X-linked *PIG-A* (phosphatidyl inositol glycan, class A) gene in a hematopoietic stem cell results in neutrophils, platelets, and red cells that are more susceptible to lysis by complement. Different *PIG-A* mutations result in impaired glycosylphosphatidyl-inositol (GPI) linkage of several proteins, including decay accelerating factor (DAF/CD55), membrane inhibitor of reactive lysis (MIRL/CD59), and C8 binding protein (C8bp or homologous restriction factor) [46]. PNH is a clonal disease, as hematopoietic progenitor cells with certain *PIG-A* mutations also demonstrate a growth advantage. The abnormal clone in PNH may arise idiopathically or secondary to marrow damage seen with aplastic anemia.

Clinically, PNH is characterized by intermittent episodes of intravascular hemolysis, hemoglobinuria, and venous thrombosis, which may occur idiopathically or associated with infection, surgery, and so on. PNH can be characterized by hemolysis, infections (due to leukopenia), and marrow hypoplasia. Despite the somatic mutation causing thrombocytopenia, patients can develop venous thrombosis (cerebral, mesenteric, or hepatic vein thrombosis) contributing to morbidity and mortality.

PNH patients may show different clinical severity because their hematopoietic cells express varying levels of GPI-linked proteins. PNH cells are categorized by the level of cell-surface expression of GPI-linked proteins: type "I" PNH cells (normal/mildly reduced), type "II" PNH cells (moderately reduced), and type "III" PNH cells (no expression). Similarly, type I, II, and III PNH cells demonstrate little, moderate, or significant sensitivity to complement lysis, respectively. The relative percentages of type I, II, and III PNH cells in any one patient (mosaicism) can vary with time and correlates with disease severity. A subset of PNH patients can develop acute myeloid leukemia or myelodysplasia. Treatment includes transfusions, antimicrobials, thrombolytic therapy, and allogeneic bone marrow transplant (curative).

The intravascular hemolysis in PNH can result in moderate–severe anemia. The bone marrow can demonstrate erythroid hyperplasia or hypocellularity, depending on whether there is concurrent aplastic anemia. Neutrophils express reduced leukocyte alkaline phosphatase (LAP), a GPI-linked protein. The

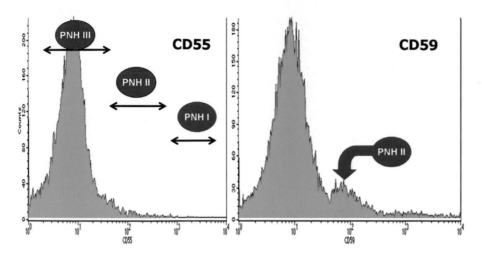

Fig. 5.9. Flow cytometry of a patient with PNH showing decreased cell-surface expression of GPI-linked proteins CD55 and CD59: shown are the relative populations of type I PNH cells (normal/mildly reduced), type II PNH cells (moderately reduced), and type III PNH cells (no expression). Figure courtesy of A. Bagg, University of Pennsylvania.

DAT is negative for IgG but may be positive for complement binding.

Diagnostic tests for PNH include the sucrose-hemolysis (screening) and Ham acidified serum test (confirmatory). The latter is also positive in congenital dyserythropoietic anemia type II (HEMPAS). With the advance of technology, more sensitive tests detecting the reduced expression of GPI-linked proteins on the surface of cells by flow cytometry have been developed. This includes CD55 (expressed on neutrophils) and CD59 (expressed on neutrophils and red cells) since they are physiologically involved in complement-mediated lysis (Fig. 5.9).

Hemolytic anemia due to red cell enzyme defects

Hemolysis can occur from defects in the red cell enzymes involved in the Embden–Meyerhof (EM) glycolytic pathway or hexose monophosphate (HMP) shunt. These pathways are essential for energy production via the anaerobic metabolism of glucose. Since red cells lack a nucleus and mitochondria, they cannot synthesize new enzymes or undergo oxidative phosphorylation to produce the adenosine triphosphate (ATP) needed to maintain membrane stability and deformability, ionic equilibrium, and so on. As such, an enzyme defect can shorten the lifespan of a red cell [3]. Deficiencies in the glycolytic enzymes are uncommon (e.g., pyruvate kinase) or rare (e.g., hexokinase, glucose 6-phosphate isomerase, phosphofructokinase, aldolase, phosphoglycerate kinase, triphosphate isomerase, and diphosphoglycerate kinase) (Table 5.12) [47]. Most are inherited in an autosomal recessive manner, except for phosphoglycerate kinase (X-linked). The deficiencies of glycolysis can impair red cell metabolism and produce a congenital non-spherocytic hemolytic anemia (CNSHA) with normal osmotic fragility. Other causes of CNSHA include defects in the hexose monophosphate (HMP) shunt, glutathione pathways, and certain hemoglobinopathies and unstable hemoglobins. Clinically, infants or children with glycolytic enzyme defects demonstrate varying degrees of hemolytic anemia, jaundice, gallstones, and splenomegaly, and can have systemic complications and other

Table 5.12. Red cell glycolytic enzyme deficiencies exhibiting hemolysis and congenital non-spherocytic hemolytic anemia (CNSHA).

Deficient enzyme	Description
Pyruvate kinase	Responsible for 90% of the cases of glycolytic enzyme deficiency which cause hemolysis Severe hemolysis *in utero* can cause hydrops fetalis
Glucose 6-phosphate isomerase	Second most common disorder of glycolytic pathway Associated with myopathy, neuropathy Severe hemolysis *in utero* can cause hydrops fetalis Partial response to splenectomy
Hexokinase	First enzyme in Embden–Meyerhof (EM) pathway Hemolytic type: responds to splenectomy Non-hemolytic type: multiple other abnormalities (decreased 2,3 diphosphoglycerate) with poorly tolerated anemia
Aldolase	May show defective hepatic glycogen storage
Phosphofructokinase	May demonstrate myoglobinuria May affect glycogen storage and myofiber function
Phosphoglycerate kinase	X-linked inheritance Mental retardation in males (milder disease in females)
Triphosphate isomerase	Abnormalities in striated muscle and central nervous system Can result in death during infancy
Diphosphoglycerate kinase	May show polycythemia

factors (e.g., suppression of marrow erythropoiesis by parvovirus B19). Treatment depends on the severity of disease and may include transfusions and splenectomy.

Laboratory diagnosis

A red cell enzyme defect causes a chronic hemolytic anemia (of variable severity) without spherocytes or Heinz bodies. With a

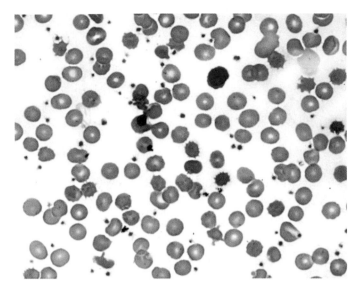

Fig. 5.10. Pyruvate kinase (PK) deficiency. Photograph kindly provided by Marybeth Helfrich MT(ASCP).

Table 5.13. G6PD deficiency: clinical classification of common variants.

Class	Isoenzyme (population commonly affected)	Percentage of normal G6PD level	Clinical effect
I		<10	Severe, chronic hemolytic anemia and with congenital non-spherocytic hemolytic anemia in infancy
II	G6PD-Mediterranean	<20	Acute, episodic hemolytic anemia associated with drugs, infection
III	G6PD-Canton (Asians) G6PD-Mahidol (Asians) G6PD-A$^-$ (10% of African-Americans): unstable enzyme	10–60	Moderate–severe, acute episodic hemolytic anemia associated with oxidant stress
IV	G6PD-B G6PD-A$^+$ (20% of African-American males)	60–150	None
V		100	None

normal marrow response, the peripheral blood shows reticulocytosis and polychromasia. Red cell enzyme assays measure an increase in spectrophotometric absorbance, reflecting production of NADPH or NADH. These assays are useful to detect severe enzyme deficiencies, since mild deficiencies are not likely to be clinically significant. Other testing can help differentiate an enzyme defect versus other conditions, including PNH, autoimmune hemolytic anemia (positive DAT), and hereditary spherocytosis (abnormal osmotic fragility). Other causes of CNSHA can be ruled out, including hemoglobinopathies, or unstable hemoglobins. Family studies may be useful in some cases, although fewer family members may be symptomatic with an autosomal recessive inheritance pattern.

Deficiency of pyruvate kinase (PK)

PK deficiency is the most common enzyme defect of the EM pathway. The peripheral blood contains echinocytes, which are removed by the spleen (Fig. 5.10). The PK activity is determined using a fluorescence screening test that measures production of pyruvate and the subsequent conversion of NADH (fluorescent) to NAD+ (non-fluorescent). Other testing includes a spectrophotometric assay for PK activity, or molecular analysis of the PK isoforms.

Glucose 6-phosphate dehydrogenase (G6PD)

G6PD deficiency is the most common red cell enzyme defect. It is an X-linked disorder more prevalent in certain ethnic groups (African, Middle Eastern, Mediterranean, Southeast Asian, Latin American). In the red cell, the hexose monophosphate (HMP) shunt provides reducing potential in the form of reduced nicotinamide adenine dinucleotide phosphate (NADPH), which is necessary to prevent oxidative damage in red cells. Deficiencies in G6PD lead to a decrease in reduced glutathione (GSH), which normally counteracts the damage to cellular enzymes due to oxygen radical formation, in

addition to the formation of methemoglobin, which denatures and precipitates (Heinz bodies), thus damaging the membrane. The two main G6PD isoforms, "A" and "B" have normal activity but are distinguishable by electrophoretic mobility. The A-isoform is found in 20% of blacks, while the B-isoform is found in all populations. Numerous mutations (usually amino acid substitutions) in the G6PD gene differentially affect enzyme activity and electrophoretic mobility, and account for the heterogeneity of the clinical and laboratory features (Table 5.13) [48]. The hemolysis in G6PD deficiency is usually sporadic and self-limited (e.g., G6PD-A$^-$), reflecting the greater susceptibility of older red cells (they express less G6PD activity) to oxidant stress initially. However, patients with G6PD-Mediterranean (class II) have very low (<1%) G6PD activity of all red cells including the reticulocytes, and can develop severe, not self-limited, hemolysis [3]. Heterozygote females possess two populations of red cells – normal enzyme and deficient – due to lyonization in the stem cell. Thus, the severity of disease varies (asymptomatic vs. clinically severe) depending on the proportion of red cells with deficient versus normal G6PD activity.

During hemolytic episodes, anisopoikilocytosis, bite cells, eccentrocytes, reticulocytosis, and Heinz bodies are seen. The latter are visualized by supravital staining. Testing is aimed at measuring the production of NADPH from glucose 6-phosphate and NADP. Testing should occur after active hemolysis has resolved, since G6PD-deficient red cells have been removed from the circulation and the younger red cells and reticulocytes have normal activity. Alternatively, reticulocyte-poor samples can be used. This is relevant to G6PD-A$^-$ enzymes and less so with G6PD-Mediterranean, wherein young red cells are also affected.

Most G6PD-deficient persons are neither symptomatic nor anemic unless exposed to an oxidant stress from foods (fava beans), infection, medications (acetanilide, sulfonamides, sulfones, nitrofurantoin, para-aminosalicylic acid, nalidixic acid), certain antimalarials (primaquine, quinacrine, etc.), and other agents (naphthalene, phenylhydrazine, methylene blue, toluidine blue). Treatment for hemolytic episodes may include simple or exchange transfusion (e.g., in severe neonatal jaundice).

References

1. **Jefferies LC, Eder AF**. Transfusion therapy in autoimmune hemolytic anemia. In Mintz PD, ed. *Transfusion Therapy: Clinical Principles and Practice*. Bethesda, MD: AABB Press; 1999, 43–64.

2. **Smith LA**. Hemolytic anemias: nonimmune defects. In McKenzie SB, ed. *Clinical Laboratory Hematology*. Upper Saddle River, NJ: Prentice Hall; 2004, 369–382.

3. **Bessmer D**. Hemolytic anemias: enzyme deficiencies. In McKenzie SB, ed. *Clinical Laboratory Hematology*. Upper Saddle River, NJ: Prentice Hall; 2004, 332–344.

4. **Blaylock RC**. Autoimmune hemolytic anemia. In Kjeldsberg CR, ed. *Practical Diagnosis of Hematologic Disorders* (4th edn.). Chicago, IL: ASCP Press; 2006, 177–188.

5. **Cines DB, Kaywin P, Bina M, Tomaski A, Schreiber AD**. Heparin-associated thrombocytopenia. *New England Journal of Medicine*. 1980;**303**:788–795.

6. Brecher M (ed.). *AABB Technical Manual* (15th edn.). Bethesda, MD: AABB Press; 2005.

7. **Freedman AM**. Unusual forms of malaria transmission. A report of 2 cases. *South African Medical Journal*. 1987;**71**:183–184.

8. **Gehrs BC, Friedberg RC**. Autoimmune hemolytic anemia. *American Journal of Hematology*. 2002;**69**:258–271.

9. **Vaglio S, Arista MC, Perrone MP**, *et al.* Autoimmune hemolytic anemia in childhood: serologic features in 100 cases. *Transfusion*. 2007;**47**: 50–54.

10. **Johnson ST, Pugh TM**. Serologic investigation of unexpected antibodies. In Hillyer CD, Strauss RG, Luban NL, eds. *Handbook of Pediatric Transfusion Medicine*. San Diego, CA: Elsevier; 2004, 73–84.

11. **Petz L, Garratty G**. *Acquired Immune Hemolytic Anemias*. New York: Churchill Livingstone; 1980, 28–37.

12. **Sokol RJ, Hewitt S, Stamps BK**. Autoimmune haemolysis: an 18-year study of 865 cases referred to a regional transfusion centre. *British Medical Journal (Clinical Research Ed.)*. 1981; **282**:2023–2027.

13. **Garratty G**. Target antigens for red cell bound autoantibodies. In Nance SJ, ed. *Clinical and Basic Science Aspects of Immunohematology*. Arlington, VA: AABB Press; 1991, 33–72.

14. **Ness PM**. How do I encourage clinicians to transfuse mismatched blood to patients with autoimmune hemolytic anemia in urgent situations? *Transfusion*. 2006;**46**:1859–1862.

15. **Blaylock RC**. Extrinsic hemolytic anemia: general concepts and transfusion reactions. In Kjeldsberg CR, ed. *Practical Diagnosis of Hematologic Disorders* (4th edn.). Chicago, IL: ASCP Press; 2006, 149–157.

16. **Judd WJ**. Review: polyagglutination. *Immunohematology*. 1992;**8**:58–69.

17. **Johnson ST, Pugh TM**. Pretransfusion compatibility testing. In Hillyer CD, Strauss RG, Luban NL, eds. *Handbook of Pediatric Transfusion Medicine*. San Diego, CA: Elsevier; 2004, 63–72.

18. **Schwartz RS, Berkman EM, Silberstein LE**. The autoimmune hemolytic anemias. In Hoffman R, Benz E, Shattil SJ, Furie B, Cohen HJ, eds. *Hematology: Basic Principles and Practice*. New York: Churchill Livingstone; 1991, 710–725.

19. **Goodstein M**. Neonatal red cell transfusion. In Herman JH, Manno CS, eds. *Pediatric Transfusion Therapy* (1st edn.). Bethesda, MD: AABB Press; 2002, xiv, 422.

20. **Angiolillo A, Luban NL**. Hemolysis following an out-of-group platelet transfusion in an 8-month-old with Langerhans cell histiocytosis. *Journal of Pediatric Hematology/Oncology*. 2004; **26**:267–269.

21. **Lozano M, Cid J**. The clinical implications of platelet transfusions associated with ABO or Rh(D) incompatibility. *Transfusion Medicine Reviews*. 2003;**17**:57–68.

22. **Bowman JM, Pollock JM, Penston LE**. Fetomaternal transplacental hemorrhage during pregnancy and after delivery. *Vox Sanguinis*. 1986;**51**: 117–121.

23. **Ramasethu J**. Hemolytic disease of the newborn. In Hillyer CD, Strauss RG, Luban NL, eds. *Handbook of Pediatric Transfusion Medicine*. San Diego, CA: Elsevier; 2004, 191–208.

24. **Vengelen-Tyler V** (ed.). The serologic investigation of hemolytic disease of the newborn caused by antibodies other than anti-D. In Garratty G, ed. *Hemolytic Disease of the Newborn*. Arlington, VA: AABB Press; 1984, 145.

25. **Geifman-Holtzman O, Wojtowycz M, Kosmas E, Artal R**. Female alloimmunization with antibodies known to cause hemolytic disease. *Obstetrics and Gynecology*. 1997;**89**: 272–275.

26. **Vaughan JI, Manning M, Warwick RM**, *et al.* Inhibition of erythroid progenitor cells by anti-Kell antibodies in fetal alloimmune anemia. *New England Journal of Medicine*. 1998;**338**: 798–803.

27. **Chavez GF, Mulinare J, Edmonds LD**. Epidemiology of Rh hemolytic disease of the newborn in the United States. *JAMA*. 1991;**265**:3270–3274.

28. **Herschel M, Karrison T, Wen M, Caldarelli L, Baron B**. Isoimmunization is unlikely to be the cause of hemolysis in ABO-incompatible but direct antiglobulin test-negative neonates. *Pediatrics*. 2002;**110**:127–130.

29. **Bullock R, Martin WL, Coomarasamy A, Kilby MD**. Prediction of fetal anemia in pregnancies with red-cell alloimmunization: comparison of middle cerebral artery peak systolic velocity and amniotic fluid OD450. *Ultrasound in Obstetrics & Gynecology*. 2005;**25**:331–334.

30. **Levy GG, Motto DG, Ginsburg D**. ADAMTS13 Turns 3. *Blood*. 2005;**106**: 11–17.

31. **Shelat SG, Ai J**, *et al.* Molecular biology of ADAMTS13 and diagnostic utility of

ADAMTS13 proteolytic activity and inhibitor assays. *Seminars in Thrombosis and Hemostasis.* 2005;**31**:659–672.

32. **Remuzzi G**. Is ADAMTS-13 deficiency specific for thrombotic thrombocytopenic purpura? No. *Journal of Thrombosis and Haemostasis.* 2003;**1**:632–634.

33. **Remuzzi G**. HUS and TTP: variable expression of a single entity. *Kidney International.* 1987;**32**:292–308.

34. **Baker KR, Moake JL**. Thrombotic thrombocytopenic purpura and the hemolytic-uremic syndrome. *Current Opinion in Pediatrics.* 2000;**12**:23–28.

35. **Reilly MP, Taylor SM, Hartman NK,** *et al.* Heparin-induced thrombocytopenia/thrombosis in a transgenic mouse model requires human platelet factor 4 activation through FcgRIIA. *Blood.* 2001;**98**: 2442–2447.

36. **Franchini M**. Pathophysiology, diagnosis and treatment of disseminated intravascular coagulation: an update. *Clinical Laboratory.* 2005;**51**: 633–639.

37. **Levi M, Ten Cate H**. Disseminated intravascular coagulation. *New England Journal of Medicine.* 1999;**341**:586–592.

38. **Homer MJ, Aguilar-Delfin I, Telford SR 3rd, Krause PJ, Persing DH**. Babesiosis. *Clinical Microbiology Reviews.* 2000;**13**:451–469.

39. **Hendrix LR**. Contact-dependent hemolytic activity distinct from deforming activity of *Bartonella bacilliformis*. *FEMS Microbiology Letters.* 2000;**182**:119–124.

40. **Kain KC, Keystone JS**. Malaria in travelers. Epidemiology, disease, and prevention. *Infectious Disease Clinics of North America.* 1998;**12**:267–284.

41. **Iolascon A, Miraglia del Giudice E, Camaschella C**. Molecular pathology of inherited erythrocyte membrane disorders: hereditary spherocytosis and elliptocytosis. *Haematologica.* 1992;**77**: 60–72.

42. **De Franceschi L, Olivieri O, Miraglia del Giudice E,** *et al.* Membrane cation and anion transport activities in erythrocytes of hereditary spherocytosis: effects of different membrane protein defects. *American Journal of Hematology.* 1997;**55**:121–128.

43. Perkins S (ed.). Disorders of hematopoiesis. In Collins RD, Swerdlow SH, eds. *Pediatric Hematopathology* (1st edn.). New York: Churchill Livingstone; 2002, 105–140.

44. **Perkins S**. Hereditary erythrocyte membrane defects. In Kjeldsberg CR, ed. *Practical Diagnosis of Hematologic Disorders* (4th edn.). Chicago, IL: ASCP Press; 2006, 93–103.

45. **Cochran-Black D**. Hemolytic anemias: membrane defects. In McKenzie SB, ed. *Clinical Laboratory Hematology.* Upper Saddle River, NJ: Prentice Hall; 2004, 313–331.

46. **Nakakuma H, Kawaguchi T**. Paroxysmal nocturnal hemoglobinuria (PNH): mechanism of intravascular hemolysis. *Critical Reviews in Oncology/ Hematology.* 1996;**24**:213–229.

47. **Brugnara C, Platt OS**. The neonatal erythrocyte and its disorders. In Nathan DG, Oski FA, eds. *Nathan and Oski's Hematology of Infancy and Childhood* (6th edn.). Philadelphia, PA: Saunders; 2003, 19–55.

48. **Beutler E, Yoshida A**. Genetic variation of glucose-6-phosphate dehydrogenase: a catalog and future prospects. *Medicine.* 1988;**67**:311–334.

6

Inherited and acquired bone marrow failure syndromes associated with multiple cytopenias

Sa A. Wang and Victor Zota

Overview

Bone marrow failure syndrome consists of a group of rare diseases with the defining features of ineffective/defective hematopoiesis by the bone marrow and resultant peripheral cytopenia [1, 2]. Bone marrow failure can be attributed to a variety of mechanisms, such as loss of pluripotent hematopoietic stem cells; bone marrow replacement by metastatic carcinoma, lymphoma, leukemia or fibrosis; nutritional/metabolic disorder leading to maturation arrest or clonal hematopoietic stem neoplasm such as myelodysplastic syndromes. Aplastic anemia is the paradigm of the human bone marrow failure syndrome, characterized by peripheral cytopenia and a hypocellular marrow [1, 3, 4]. Injury to or loss of pluripotent hematopoietic stem cells, in the absence of an infiltrative disease of the bone marrow, is the major pathophysiologic characteristic of the disease [3, 4]. Aplastic anemia can result from either inherited or acquired causes. This chapter will discuss the bone marrow failure syndromes, both inherited and acquired, that are associated with multiple cytopenias.

Inherited bone marrow failure syndromes

The inherited bone marrow failure syndromes in children comprise a group of rare congenital disorders in which the bone marrow is unable to produce blood cells effectively resulting in unilineage or multilineage cytopenia (Table 6.1). These syndromes may present with or without physical anomalies [5]. Patients with inherited bone marrow failure syndromes are at risk for severe cytopenia, development of marrow cytogenetic abnormalities, myelodysplastic syndromes (MDS), and other malignancies [6]. Over the last decade, the genetic basis and molecular pathogenesis are identified in many of the inherited marrow failure syndromes [7, 8] (Table 6.1). These advances are facilitating better diagnosis of patients with these disorders. The bone marrow failure (which may involve all or a single lineage) may present at birth or any time thereafter including adulthood in some cases. The diagnosis of inherited bone marrow failure syndromes is established by bone marrow examination in

conjunction with clinical history review, physical examination, laboratory data, molecular genetic testing.

Bone marrow failure associated with congenital disorders, such as Fanconi anemia (FA), Dyskeratosis congenita (DC), Shwachman-Diamond syndrome (SDS), and Pearson's syndrome (Table 6.1) often manifests as more than one lineage cytopenia, often pancytopenia. It has been known that FA and DC can have late presentation in individuals in their 5th and 6th decades of life, therefore, they must be considered even in adults, particularly in any young adults with characteristic physical anomalies, pancytopenia, unexplained macrocytosis, myelodysplastic syndromes (MDS), or squamous cell carcinoma even in the absence of a positive family history [9, 10].

Fanconi anemia

Fanconi anemia (FA), while rare, is the most common form of inherited bone marrow failure syndrome. It is characterized by cytopenia, congenital anomalies (e.g., radial ray anomalies, poor growth, genitourinary problems), short stature, abnormal skin pigmentation (café-au-lait and hypo- or hyperpigmented spots), and predisposition to malignancy [5]. It is an autosomal recessive disorder without racial or ethnic predisposition. The carrier frequency is estimated to be approximately 1 per 300 people. Among Ashkenazi Jews, the carrier frequency is approximately 1 per 90 people. Multiple genes appear to be responsible for FA. FA is caused by mutation in any of the thirteen complementation group genes (*FANC-A* to *FANC-N*). These genes are widely dispersed throughout the genome. The function of most of the FA proteins is to protect the genome by forming a single large multi-protein nuclear complex. Eight of the known FA proteins (FANCA, B, C, E, F, G, L, and M) bind together in a complex and monoubiquitinate FANCD2 and FANCI [11]. The ubiquitin-tagged FANCD2–FANCI complex moves to chromatin, where it assembles into nuclear DNA-repair foci. In these foci, the protein complex interacts with other downstream FA proteins (FANCD1, FANCN, and FANCJ) and additional DNA-repair proteins including BRCA1, BRCA2, and RAD51, which are known to protect cells from cross-linking agent and oxidation-induced genotoxicity

Diagnostic Pediatric Hematopathology, ed. Maria A. Proytcheva. Published by Cambridge University Press.
© Cambridge University Press 2011.

Table 6.1. Inherited bone marrow failure syndromes presenting with multiple cytopenias.

	Pattern of inheritance	Gene/locus	Physical anomalies	Hematologic findings	Other biomarkers
Fanconi anemia (FA)	Autosomal recessive	Biallelic inactivation of any of 11 FA genes	Café-au-lait spots, skeletal anomalies, short stature, microcephaly	Macrocytic anemia, mild to moderate thrombocytopenia, neutropenia	↑Hb FCγ
Dyskeratosis congenita (DC)	Autosomal dominant/X-linked/autosomal recessive	Missense mutation of *DKC1* gene on Xq28	Nail dystrophy, macular or reticular hypopigmentation, mucosal leukoplakia	Thrombocytopenia or anemia followed by pancytopenia	↑von Willebrand factor antigen
Shwachman–Diamond syndrome (SDS)	Autosomal dominant	*SBDS* (7p10–7q11) gene mutation	Pancreatic insufficiency, metaphyseal dysostosis, short stature, hepatic dysfunction	Neutropenia (>95%), anemia (40–50%), thrombocytopenia (30–40%), pancytopenia (20%)	↓pancreatic enzymes
Pearson marrow–pancreas syndrome	Sporadic	Deletion of mitochondrial DNA	Failure to thrive, exocrine pancreatic dysfunction, malabsorption, acidosis	Sideroblastic anemia, neutropenia, vacuolated marrow precursors	3-Methylglutaconic aciduria
Dubowitz syndrome	Unknown	Increased chromosomal breakage	Microcephaly, growth and mental retardation, facial anomaly, eczema	10% of patients with aplastic anemia, recurrent neutropenia	↓IgA and IgG with an increased level of IgM
Seckel syndrome	Autosomal recessive	Mutations in *ATA* and RAD3-related protein	Microcephaly, severe growth and mental retardation	25% of patients with aplastic anemia	
Nijmegen breakage syndrome (NBS)	Autosomal recessive	Mutation in *NBS1* gene on 8q21	Microcephaly, growth retardation	Approximately 3% with cytopenia	↓immunoglobulin, immunodeficiency

[12–19]. As a result, FA proteins can normalize cellular growth and restore cell sensitivity to chromosomal breakage induced by DNA-crosslinking agents such as mitomycin C.

FA patients have a wide range of phenotypic abnormalities. In the past it was thought that the type of mutations – whether null or ones leading to a partially functional gene product – was more critical than the specific gene involved. Recent studies have shown that the variability is due, at least in part, to the specific FA subtype, which has important implications for patients' clinical management [20]. For example, FA-A patients tend to experience milder disease and may develop BM failure later in life. By contrast, FA-C patients may experience more severe disease and an early onset of bone marrow failure and hematologic malignancy [21]. Furthermore, FA-D1 patients have higher propensity to develop brain tumors, Wilms' tumors, and acute leukemia early in childhood.

Clinical and hematologic features

Most children with FA are diagnosed between 6 and 9 years of age; the median age for boys is 6.5 years and for girls 8 years [5]. However, increasingly patients are being diagnosed in adulthood [10]. Affected individuals may have one or more somatic abnormalities involving skin, skeletal, genitourinary, gastrointestinal, cardiovascular, and nervous systems. Approximately one third of FA patients have no somatic abnormalities. In 25% of patients with FA who have developed malignancy, the diagnosis of leukemia or a solid tumor may precede

the diagnosis of FA [21, 22]. The first sign of a hematologic manifestation of the disease is usually petechiae and bruises, with later onset of pallor, fatigue, and infections. Macrocytosis usually precedes thrombocytopenia and leukopenia may precede pancytopenia. Reticulocytopenia is common. Serum alpha-fetoprotein levels are markedly increased, distinguishing FA from other acquired or inherited bone marrow failure syndromes [23]. Hemoglobin electrophoresis usually shows increased concentrations of hemoglobin F [24]. Elevation of hemoglobin F is a result of stress hematopoiesis in the bone marrow.

Bone marrow examination

Approximately 70% of children with FA will show evidence of bone marrow failure by the age of 10 years. Bone marrow aspirate and biopsy performed for evaluation of a hematologic abnormality often shows a hypocellular marrow (Fig. 6.1A), with loss of myeloid and erythroid precursors and megakaryocytes, or full-blown aplasia with a fatty marrow. On aspirate smears, small lymphocytes, plasma cells, mast cells, and macrophages are usually the predominant cellular components (Fig. 6.1B). The biopsy may show residual islands of hematopoietic elements on a background of hypocellularity. Erythroid precursors often show megaloblastoid maturation (Fig. 1C). Other dysplastic morphologic features, such as nuclear fragmentation, ring sideroblasts, are not common but can be occasionally seen (Fig. 6.1C and 6.1D). In the absence of increased blasts or

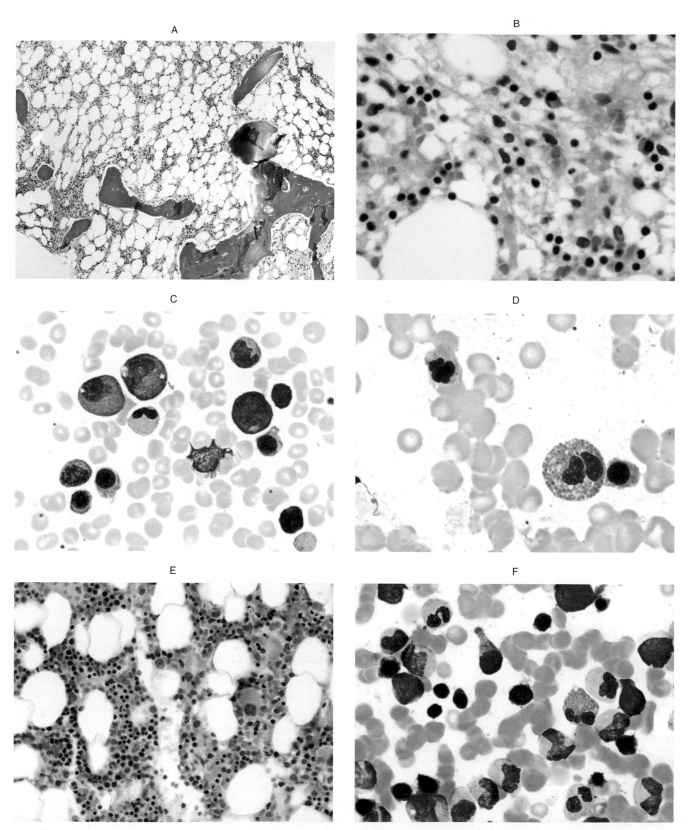

Fig. 6.1. Fanconi anemia. (A) Bone marrow biopsy showing a hypocellular marrow with approximately 20% cellularity. (B) The marrow elements are mainly comprised of lymphocytes, plasma cells, and stromal cells. (C) The marrow aspirate revealing megaloblastoid changes in erythroid precursors and occasional hypogranulated neutrophils. (D) Occasional erythroid dysplasia (nuclear budding) also can be seen in Fanconi anemia. These changes should not be interpreted as myelodysplastic syndrome. (E) Myelodysplastic syndrome arising in Fanconi anemia. The marrow often shows an increased cellularity. (F) Myelodysplastic syndrome arising in Fanconi anemia. Mild increase in myeloblasts (5–6%) is seen, and granulocytes are hypogranulated.

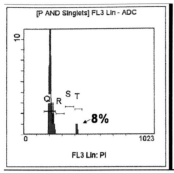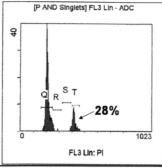

Fig. 6.2. Cell cycle analysis. Peripheral blood mononuclear cells are incubated with phytohemagglutinin and stained with propidium iodide fluorescence, and measured by a flow cytometer. A normal control shows 8% G2 cells, while a Fanconi anemia patient shows 28% G2 cells.

evolved cytogenetic abnormalities, these changes should not be interpreted as myelodysplastic syndromes.

It is noteworthy that some patients presented with hematologic abnormalities may show a normal or hypercellular marrow [21, 22]. Approximately one third of FA patients will develop hematologic neoplasm, and a small number of them may have developed MDS or acute leukemia even on the first bone marrow examination [21, 22]. Signs of MDS including dyserythropoiesis, dysmyelopoiesis, and dysplastic megakaryocytes (please see Chapter 14, myelodysplastic syndromes), and have to be evaluated carefully. However, in many cases, mild dysplasia can be seen in FA, especially in patients who have received treatment. MDS evolution should only be diagnosed if bone marrow shows new emerging clonal chromosomal abnormalities (not transient): hypercellularity (Fig. 6.1E) but persistent peripheral cytopenia, or increase in blasts (Fig. 6.1F).

Immunophenotype

There are no characteristic immunophenotypic changes identified in FA. Flow cytometric study in analyzing myelomonocytic maturation patterns may help in differentiating MDS from aplastic anemia [25]. The common immunophenotypic changes identified in MDS are discussed in Chapter 14. Cell cycle analysis by flow cytometry of FA cells cultured with nitrogen mustard and other clastogens demonstrates a cell cycle disturbance with a G2 block (Fig. 6.2). It has been shown that cell cycle analysis by flow cytometry can be a simple and rapid test, which is specific and probably more sensitive than the diepoxybutane (DEB) test [26, 27].

Diagnostic molecular genetics

Chromosome breakage is usually examined in short-term cultures of peripheral blood lymphocytes in the presence of DNA cross-linkers, such as diepoxybutane or mitomycin C. These agents lead to increased numbers of breaks, gaps, rearrangements, and quadric radii in FA homozygote cells [28]. When the FA gene mutations are known for a family, genetic sequence analysis may detect mothers who are carriers of FA genes. Care must be taken to distinguish FA from other chromosomal breakage syndromes, such as Nijmegen breakage syndrome [29], which also manifests some increase in chromosomal breakage in response to mitomycin C.

Clonal cytogenetic abnormalities are detected in approximately 30–35% bone marrows at the time of bone marrow failure, with or without morphologic dysplasia. Loss of chromosome 7, rearrangement or loss of 7q, rearrangements of lp36 and 1q24–34 are the common aberrations while rearrangements of 11q22–25 are more frequent in patients who developed MDS or AML [22, 30]. Gain of chromosome 3q is associated with shorter patient survival and increased risk for development of MDS and AML [31]. The presence of clonal chromosomal abnormalities is a risk factor for developing MDS or AML within 3 years from time of bone marrow failure development [21, 22, 30]. Cytogenetic clones identified in the bone marrow should be interpreted in the context of bone marrow morphology.

Management and prognosis

Patients with FA are at increased risk for malignancies [21, 32, 33], approximately 60% of which are of hematologic origin (e.g., acute myeloid/or lymphoblastic leukemia, MDS). Treatment of aplastic anemia with supportive use of blood products, and stem cell transplantation increases the life expectancy beyond the projected median of approximately 30 years. Hematopoietic stem cell transplantation is the only current curative treatment for bone marrow failure [34].

Dyskeratosis congenita

Dyskeratosis congenita (DC) is a rare inherited disorder characterized by hematological abnormalities and a triad of mucocutaneous anomalies: reticulated hyperpigmentation of the skin, nail dystrophy, and oral leukoplakia [35–37]. Additional abnormalities involving central nervons system, lungs, bone and teeth, gastrointestinal and genitourinary systems can be present [38–41]. Characteristic skin anomalies, e.g. nail changes and abnormal skin pigmentation, are often not present at birth but occur in the first decade of life. Other clinical findings in DC include eye abnormalities, hyperhidrosis, premature hair graying, and tooth loss [42].

There are three patterns of inheritance in DC: (1) X-linked recessive; (2) autosomal recessive; (3) autosomal dominant. X-linked recessive DC is the most common form of inheritance which results in a male to female ratio of 4.5 to 1.0 of patients affected by DC [42]. The disease is caused by missense mutations in the *DKC1* gene located on chromosome Xq28. Dyskerin, the product of the *DKC1* gene, is a nuclear protein that is a component of telomerase and involved in rRNA modification [43–46]. Telomerase is present in germ cells, stem cells, and in proliferating somatic cells of renewal tissues such as bone marrow, epidermis, endometrium, and gastrointestinal tract [47]. Its function is to maintain the telomeric ends of chromosomes in allowing cells to replicate indefinitely. Decrease in telomerase activity results in shortening of telomeres with each cell division leading to replicative senescence [48, 49]. In patients with X-linked DC, the cells have a lower level of telomerase RNA component (TERC), which produce lower levels of telomerase activity, and have shorter telomeres [50]. The disease severity directly correlates with the telomere length [51]. Defects in telomerase in DC patients result in a reduced proliferation potential of the hematopoietic stem cells, explaining bone marrow failure in DC.

In patients with autosomal dominant inheritance, heterozygous mutations in the TERC gene were identified [51, 52]. The disease can manifest itself over several generations due to progressive telomere shortening (disease anticipation) [53, 54].

DC with autosomal recessive inheritance has a wide range of clinical manifestations, of which the specific genetic defect is not identified. In some cases of DC the pattern of disease inheritance is not apparent. In these cryptic DC cases mucocutaneous features are absent and only the hematopoietic system is affected.

Clinical and hematologic features

Approximately 50% of patients develop severe aplastic anemia and more than 90% of patents develop at least a single cytopenia by age of 40 [55]. In most patients with DC, bone marrow failure begins with thrombocytopenia or anemia followed by pancytopenia, which often develops in the third decade of life and is the major cause of death. Bone marrow failure more commonly affects patients with the X-linked variant of DC and less frequently in the other forms [41, 42, 56]. Ten percent of patients with DC have predisposition to develop malignancies, particularly patients with the X-linked trait. Malignant neoplasms occur usually in the third and fourth decades of life and include MDS, AML, squamous cell carcinoma of the skin, tongue and oropharynx, and adenocarcinomas of gastrointestinal tract [41, 56]. Pulmonary fibrosis occurs in 20% of patents, and it has been linked to short dysfunctional telomeres leading to alveolar cell death [55]. Clinical manifestations of the DC vary from moderate nail dystrophy and mild blood abnormalities to a very severe variant of the X-linked syndrome, known as the Hoyeraal–Hreidarsson (HH) syndrome. HH syndrome represents early onset of bone marrow failure, intrauterine growth retardation, microcephaly, cerebellar hypoplasia, mental retardation, immune deficiency and is associated with very poor prognosis [57]. A subgroup of DC patients with or without BM hypoplasia may have significant immunologic abnormalities with lymphopenia, abnormal immunoglobulin level, and abnormal T-cell responses to phytohaemagglutinin (PHA) [58].

Bone marrow examination

BM failure occurs in a very high proportion of DC cases, either in the first or second decade of life [7], and it is the principal cause of early mortality. Patients with DC have reduced numbers of all progenitors (erythroid, myeloid, and megakaryocytic) with decline over time. The hypocellularity is a result of cell apoptosis and senescence. Like FA, although hypoplasia is the main abnormality seen in the BM, there is a predisposition to both MDS and AML in patients with DC. In patients with

DC, surveillance bone marrow studies should be performed annually.

DC is not associated with a specific diagnostic immunophenotype and DC patients do not develop paroxysmal nocturnal hemoglobinuria (PNH) clones.

Diagnostic molecular genetics

For patients with X-linked and autosomal dominant forms of DC, sequencing of genomic DNA is available. The coding region for TERC is in exon 1 and mutations in DC include large and small deletions, single base changes, and missense mutations. Testing for DKC1 mutations (missense, splice site mutations, a large deletion, and a promoter mutation) involves sequencing of 15 exons. Large deletions of DKC1 may be missed by using sequence analysis in carrier females and may also be missed in the TERC gene [59].

Chromosomal abnormalities, such as unbalanced translocation, can be detected in cultured bone marrows obtained from DC patients, and the abnormalities are often present both in bone marrow stromal cells and hematopoietic stem cells [60, 61]. Therefore, the presence of chromosomal abnormalities is not necessarily indicative of a clonal evolution, such as evolving to MDS. MDS will be suspected if there is a new clonal cytogenetic abnormality detected on serial bone marrow examination.

Prognosis and management

BM failure and complications of its treatment are the main causes of death. The second most common cause of death is pulmonary complications either as a result of pulmonary fibrosis or pulmonary complications in the context of a bone marrow transplant setting. Therapeutic strategies in DC are focused on management of patients bone marrow failure symptoms. Transfusion support and stimulation of bone marrow with androgens, granulocyte colony-stimulating factor, and granulocyte–macrophage colony-stimulating factor have been used with some temporary successes. Hematopoietic stem cell transplantation remains the only option to cure bone marrow failure.

Shwachman–Diamond syndrome

Shwachman–Diamond syndrome or Shwachman-Diamond-Oski syndrome (SDS) is an autosomal recessive disorder characterized by a triad of symptoms: exocrine pancreatic insufficiency, bone marrow failure, and skeletal changes [62]. In addition, patients with SDS can also have hepatic abnormalities, dental dysplasia, and lower IQ scores [63–66]. Immunodeficiency is a prominent component of the syndrome. Defects in B-cell and T-cell lymphocytic function with low immunoglobulin G (IgG) levels, lymphopenia, and a lack of specific antibody production have been described [66]. Patients suffer from multiple infections that may progress to sepsis particularly early in life [67–70].

After cystic fibrosis, SDS is the second most common cause of exocrine pancreatic insufficiency in childhood. The insufficiency is due to failure of pancreatic acini to develop with

Table 6.2. Major causes of acquired aplastic anemia.

Idiopathic (70% of aplastic anemia)
Cytotoxic drugs and radiation
- Chemotherapy and radiation
- Antibiotics: chloramphenicol, sulfonamides
- Non-steroidal anti-inflammatory drugs (NSAIDs): phenylbutazone, indometacin
- Anticonvulsants: felbamate, carbamazepine, phenytoin
- Toxic chemicals: gold, arsenicals, benzene, lindane, glue vapors

Viral infections
- Parvovirus B19
- Hepatitis A, B, G
- Human immunodeficiency virus infection (HIV)
- Epstein–Barr virus (EBV), cytomegalovirus (CMV)

Immune disorders
- Eosinophilic fasciitis
- Systemic lupus erythematosus
- Graft versus host disease (GvHD), including transfusion-related GvHD

Miscellaneous
- Paroxysmal nocturnal hemoglobinuria (PNH)
- Thymoma, thymic carcinoma
- Pregnancy

subsequent replacement of the hypoplastic acini with adipose tissue (congenital lipomatosis of the pancreas). Paradoxically pancreatic function improves with age, abolishing the need for pancreatic enzyme replacement therapy [64]. The estimated incidence of SDS is 1 in 75 000 [71]. The ratio of males to females diagnosed with SDS is 1.7 : 1. There is no racial predilection identified in this syndrome [72].

The SDS locus has been mapped to the centromeric region of chromosome 7 (7p10–7q11) [73] and is termed Shwachman-Bodian–Diamond Syndrome gene (*SBDS*) [74, 75]. The *SBDS* gene is highly conserved throughout evolution and ubiquitously expressed in human tissues at both the mRNA and protein levels [76]. It has nuclear and cytoplasimic localization, shuttles in and out of the nucleolus in a cell cycle–dependent manner and possibly is involved in RNA metabolism in the nucleolus [75–77]. *SBDS* mutations include missense, nonsense, frameshift, splice site mutation, as well complex rearrangements comprising of deletion/insertion, 40% of which lead to production of a truncated protein [74, 75]. There is no correlation between *SBDS* genotype and disease severity [78].

Hematological abnormalities in patients with SDS are attributed to abnormally high levels of Fas antigen expression by the hematopoietic stem cells. Signaling through the Fas mediated pathway results in high rate of apoptosis in SDS bone marrow [16]. As a result, CD34$^+$ stem cells are decreased in numbers, and their ability to generate hematopoietic colonies is impaired [79]. Neutrophil progenitors undergo apoptosis before they become fully mature [73]. Erythroid progenitor apoptosis results in ineffective erythropoiesis with shift in hemoglobin production from adult to fetal type.

Clinical and hematologic features

Patents with SDS present with varying degrees of cytopenia (Table 6.1). Neutropenia is the most common hematologic abnormality and can be present at birth. In most cases the neutropenia is intermittent with fluctuating granulocytes counts from severely low to normal levels [79]. Mild normochromic–normocytic anemia with low reticulocytes can be seen in up to 80% of cases. Thrombocytopenia is usually mild and present in 24%–88% of patents. Severe thrombocytopenia is rare and often seen in cases with MDS or AML evolution [78]. 10%–65% cases exhibit pancytopenia with severe neutropenia and milder degrees of anemia and thrombocytopenia. Pancytopenia reflects a poor prognosis and carries a higher risk of developing MDS and transformation to AML [64].

Bone marrow examination

All patients with SDS demonstrate varying degrees of bone marrow failure presenting early in life. A bone marrow biopsy is often performed in order to exclude other causes of cytopenia. There are no specific findings on bone marrow examination. The cellularity of the bone marrow can range from hypoplastic with fat infiltration to normal or hypercellular, particularly in young patients. The bone marrow cellularity has a poor correlation with degree of peripheral cytopenias [63, 65, 79, 80]. Shift to immaturity or hypoplasia of myeloid lineage is present in 15–50% of patients [63–65].

Myelodysplastic syndromes and leukemia

The risk of MDS evolution or leukemic transformation in patients with SDS is between 15% and 69% [81, 82]. Some reports have linked the occurrence of MDS/AML in SDS patients receiving growth factor such as G-CSF therapy for severe neutropenia [83, 84]. Mild dysplastic changes in the erythroid, myeloid, and megakaryocytic lineages in SDS are common and may fluctuate over time, and they should not prompt a diagnosis of MDS. To establish a MDS diagnosis in the context of SDS, the minimal diagnostic criteria recommended by the pediatric WHO classification scheme [85] should be followed: the marrow should show prominent dysplasia of more than one lineage or clonal marrow cytogenetic abnormalities or increase in leukemic blasts ($\geq$5%). MDS secondary to SDS encompasses all the pediatric MDS categories, including refractory cytopenia, refractory anemia with excess blasts, and refractory anemia with excess blasts in transformation [82].

Secondary acute leukemias described in SDS patients include AML-M2, AML-M4, AML-M5, AML-M6, AML-non-specific, acute lymphoblastic leukemia (ALL), and juvenile myelomonocytic leukemia (JMML). Acute erythroid leukemia (AML-M6) is particularly common, occurring in about 30% of cases [82, 86]. SDS-related leukemia carries a poor prognosis.

Immunophenotype

Unlike in cases of acquired bone marrow failure, PNH clones are not detectable, indicating that bone marrow failure in SDS does not select for PNH progenitor cells [87].

Diagnostic molecular genetics

The diagnosis of SDS is based upon characteristic clinical features and laboratory findings. The diagnosis requires evidence of both exocrine pancreatic dysfunction and characteristic hematologic abnormalities [65]. Short stature, skeletal abnormalities, hepatomegaly or biochemical abnormalities of the liver are supportive findings of the diagnosis. At the present time, there is no single disease characteristic or laboratory test that definitely establishes the diagnosis. Clinical genotyping may be used for diagnostic confirmation and screening family members of an affected patient with a known SBDS gene mutation. However, a negative test for SBDS gene mutations does not exclude the diagnosis because 10% of patients clinically diagnosed with SDS lack SBDS mutations.

Isochromosome 7 is the most frequent cytogenetic abnormality present in patients with SDS. However no progression to RAEB/AML has been reported in the presence of i(7q), rasing the question if this abnormality is a true clonal phenomenon. It is an extremely uncommon cytogenetic abnormality rarely described in MDS, AML, or acute lymphoblastic leukemia patients without SDS [88]. It may be an acquired breakage of chromosome 7 secondary to recombination between *SBDS* and its pseuodogene *SBDSP*. The prognostic significance of these cytogenetic findings in the absence of morphologic evidence for MDS is unclear. Interestingly acquired marrow cytogenetic abnormalities in SDS can fluctuate and become undetectable at a later stage [89, 90].

Other inherited bone marrow failure syndromes with pancytopenia

Pearson marrow–pancreas syndrome is a rare congenital multisystemic mitochondrial cytopathy, which is associated with severe anemia, neutropenia, thrombocytopenia, exocrine pancreatic insufficiency, and variable hepatic, renal, and endocrine failure [91]. Pearson syndrome is caused by defects in oxidative phosphorylation due to deletions of certain components of the electron transport chain, encoded by mitochondrial DNA. These deletions impair the biosynthesis of various components of the mitochondrial respiratory chain critical to mitochondrial function [92]. The bone marrow often shows erythroid hyperplasia; the hematopoietic precursors show cytoplasmic vacuolization and numerous ring sideroblasts. The vacuoles are probably the manifestations of cellular degeneration and death. Pancreatic deficiency in Pearson syndrome is due to pancreatic fibrosis rather than lipomatosis seen in SDS [91].

Dubowitz syndrome is an autosomal recessive disorder with the main features of intrauterine and postnatal growth retardation, eczema, microcephaly, mild to moderate mental retardation, hyperactivity, and short attention span [93]. Neither the gene location nor the pathogenesis is yet known. Some patients with manifestation of bone marrow failure have been reported [94, 95].

Nijmegen breakage syndrome (NBS) shares overlapping clinical features with FA, principally developmental delay, microcephaly, and cancer predisposition. The diagnosis has relied on chromosomal instability following exposure to ionizing radiation. Bone marrow failure has been rarely reported [96].

Seckel's syndrome is a rare form of primordial dwarfism [97] and in some patients, bone marrow failure has been reported [98].

Acquired aplastic anemia

Acquired aplastic anemia (AA), characterized by pancytopenia and hypocellular bone marrow in the absence of abnormal infiltrates or increased reticulum, accounts for most cases of AA in children and young adults. It is a disease that preferentially affects young adults and individuals over the age of 60 years. The incidence of AA is estimated at two per million annually, and at higher rates in countries with increased rates of viral hepatitis [99]. There are small peaks at two to five years (due to inherited causes) and 20 to 25 years, with the majority of patients presenting beyond 55 to 60 years of age [100]. Historically, acquired AA has been strongly associated with exposure to chemicals and drugs in the environment [101]. However, no clear cause can be determined in more than 70 percent of children with acquired AA. Studies showed that in children with severe or very severe AA who underwent hematopoietic stem cell transplantation or immunosuppressive therapy, 80% are idiopathic, 9% post-hepatitis, 7% postviral infection, and 4% due to drugs or other toxins [102]. Table 6.2 lists the possible causes of acquired AA in childhood.

Pathophysiology of AA

Despite numerous, diverse possible causes, from chemicals and drugs to viruses, pregnancy, and collagen vascular disease, a plausible, unified model of the pathophysiology of aplastic anemia has been drawn from clinical observations of therapeutic efficacy and systematic laboratory experimentation.

Most cases of acquired AA can be pathophysiologically characterized as T-cell mediated, with specific destruction of bone marrow hematopoietic cells [3]. Sometimes, the aberrant immune response can be linked to a viral infection or to drug or chemical exposure. Autoreactive T-lymphocytes from the bone marrow of patients with AA can inhibit hematopoiesis when co-cultured with normal marrows [1, 103]. This inhibition may be mediated by the release of marrow-suppressing cytokines, such as interferon gamma (IFN-gamma), tumor necrosis factor (TNF), and interleukin-2. IFN-gamma gene expression is specifically prevalent in the bone marrow of patients with acquired AA, and disappears with response to immunosuppression. Altered immunity results in destruction, specifically Fas-mediated CD34 cell death, and in activation of intracellular pathways leading to cell-cycle arrest. Telomeric attrition results in critically shortened telomeres, prompting cellular senescence or crisis. Inherited heterozygous mutations in the genes

Table 6.3. Aplastic anemia grading: moderate, severe, and very severe.

	Moderate aplastic anemia	Severe aplastic anemia	Very severe aplastic anemia
Anemia	Variable	Severe	Severe
Absolute neutrophil count ($\times 10^9$/L)	<1200	<500	<200
Platelets ($\times 10^9$/L)	<80–100	<20	
Reticulocytes ($\times 10^9$/L)	<40–60	<40	
Bone marrow cellularity (%)	<50	<25 or <50 but hematopoietic cells <30%	
Median survival and outcome	60–70 months, spontaneous recovery may occur	Most patients <12 months if untreated Spontaneous recovery is unlikely	
Treatment	Recommendation unclear	Hematopoietic cell transplantation Immunosuppressive therapy if no matched sibling	

that repair or protect telomeres may limit marrow stem cell self-renewal and predispose some patients to marrow failure [104, 105]. There is much less evidence for other mechanisms, such as direct toxicity for stem cells or a deficiency of stromal-cell or hematopoietic growth factor function.

Clinical presentation and laboratory findings

The clinical presentation of acquired AA is variable. The onset is often insidious, and the initial symptom is related to anemia or bleeding, though fever or infections are also often noted at presentation. Serologic testing for hepatitis and other viral entities, such as Epstein–Barr virus (EBV), cytomegalovirus (CMV), and human immunodeficiency virus (HIV), and an autoimmune-disease evaluation for evidence of collagen-vascular disease may be helpful. The association between onset of AA and exposure to the offending agent varies greatly, and only rarely an environmental etiology is identified. Anemia is usually normocytic but occasionally may be macrocytic, with absolute reticulocytopenia. Patients usually do not have splenomegaly or lymphadenopathy. Magnetic resonance imaging (MRI) of the vertebrae shows uniform replacement of marrow with fat.

The clinical outcome and management decision for acquired AA is dependent in part upon the severity of AA. AA can be graded as moderate, severe, and very severe. The management and clinical outcome is illustrated in Table 6.3.

Bone marrow examination

Bone marrow biopsy is performed in addition to aspiration to assess cellularity both qualitatively and quantitatively. Aspiration samples alone can be inaccurate for cellularity assessment: they may appear hypocellular because of technical reasons (e.g., dilution with peripheral blood), or they may appear cellular because of areas of focal residual hematopoiesis. By comparison, core biopsy can much better evaluate the actual cellularity. Bone marrow cellularity is included in the grading of AA severity, upon which the clinical outcome and management decision is dependent at least in part (Fig. 6.3A and B). In addition, on bone marrow biopsy, a relative or absolute increase in mast cells

may be observed around the hypoplastic spicules. Increased lymphocytes and plasma cells are common (Fig. 6.3C).

There is extensive overlapping between AA and hypocellular MDS, and in some cases, it is virtually impossible to separate them apart clinically and morphologically. In addition, the aspirate specimen obtained from a hypocellular marrow is often suboptimal, and to recognize dyspoiesis can be difficult. In AA, the residual hematopoietic cells are often morphologically normal, but some mild dyserythropoiesis with megaloblastoid maturation may be observed (Fig. 6.3D). Thus, the presence of mild dyserythropoiesis does not exclude a diagnosis of AA and warrant a diagnosis of hypocellular MDS. Megakaryocytes in AA are within the normal limits morphologically, however the low number of megakaryocytes present in the marrow may make the evaluation of megakaryocytic dysplasia difficult. Morphologic assessment on myeloid series can be performed on a peripheral smear in addition to aspirate. A CD34 stain by immunohistochemistry often reveals decreased hematopoietic stem cells [106] (Fig. 6.3E) while they are normal or increased in hypocellular MDS.

After MDS evolution, the marrow morphology is characterized by a diffuse or patchy increase in cellularity, while continued hypocellularity is found in one third of the patients. Morphological evidence of dyspoiesis can be seen in a majority of the patients. However, in a minority of the cases, there are no morphologic changes suggestive of MDS, in the settings of a clonal cytogenetic evolution [107]. In some cases, an increase in blasts is readily seen.

Immunophenotyping

Flow cytometric studies show that the bone marrow of AA patients has a decreased CD34+ cell count. The myelomonocytic maturation analyzed by flow cytometry is often normal in AA but may show non-specific changes [25]. Blood cells deficient in glycosyl phosphatidylinositol anchored membrane proteins (GPI proteins) – paroxysmal nocturnal hemoglobinuria (PNH) cells-have been detected in 30–60% of AA patients [100, 108]. The PNH clones are often below 1%; less than 10% of total cells (Fig. 6.4). Since most of these clones are small, they do not lead to clinical manifestations of hemolysis or thrombosis.

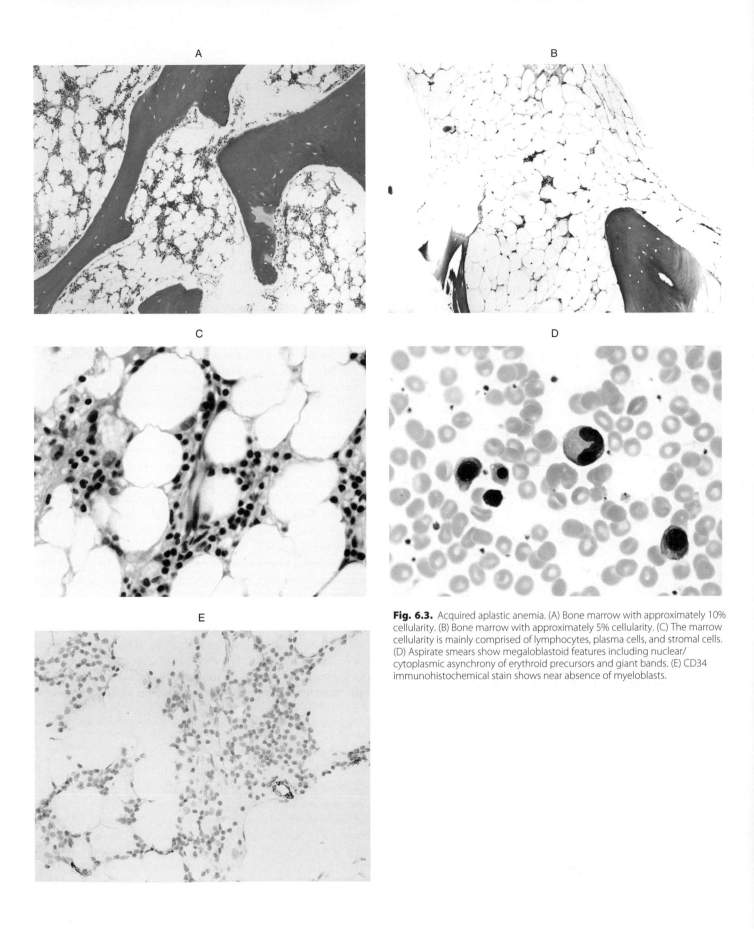

Fig. 6.3. Acquired aplastic anemia. (A) Bone marrow with approximately 10% cellularity. (B) Bone marrow with approximately 5% cellularity. (C) The marrow cellularity is mainly comprised of lymphocytes, plasma cells, and stromal cells. (D) Aspirate smears show megaloblastoid features including nuclear/cytoplasmic asynchrony of erythroid precursors and giant bands. (E) CD34 immunohistochemical stain shows near absence of myeloblasts.

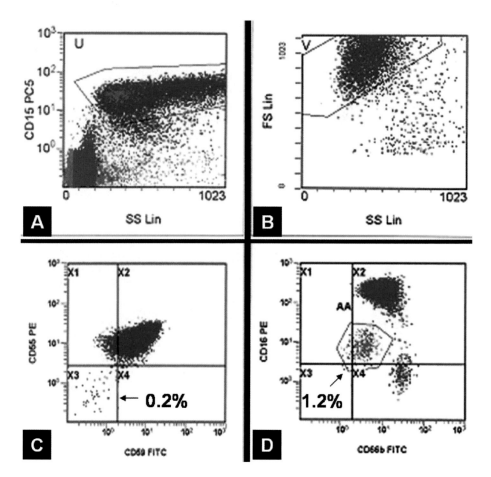

Fig. 6.4. Flow cytometric analysis in detection of a small paroxysmal nocturnal hemoglobinuria (PNH) clone in acquired aplastic anemia patients. (A) Use of CD15 to define granulocytes. (B) Further define a CD15-positive granulocyte population by forward vs. side scatter. (C) 0.2% CD55-negative and CD59-negative PNH cells were detected. (D) In another patient with acquired aplastic anemia, 1.2% CD16-negative and CD66b-negative PNH cells were detected.

Association of an expanded PNH clone in acquired aplastic anemia suggests that PNH cells escape the immune attack, a pathophysiology proposed for acquired AA [4]. The presence of a minor population of PNH-type cells in AA represents a reliable marker of a positive immunosuppressive therapy response and a favorable prognosis among patients with AA [109]. The detection of a small PNH clone relies on a high sensitivity flow cytometric analytic method which requires:

1. To analyze 100 000 granulocytes and/or red blood cells;
2. To analyze multiple GPI-proteins, such as CD55, CD59, CD14, CD16, CD66b, CD24, or FLARE assay (fluorescent aerolysin);
3. To use cell population-specific markers, such as CD15, CD11b to define granulocytes, and glycophorin for red blood cells;
4. To eliminate the damaged and dead cells by forward scatter/side scatter.

It is noteworthy that classic PNH can be dominated by marrow failure – the "aplastic anemia/PNH syndrome" – and all PNH patients show evidence of hematopoietic deficiency [110]. It has been suggested that an immune mechanism, in a human leukocyte antigen-restricted manner, plays an important role in the occurrence or selection of a PNH clone and GPI may be a target for cytotoxic-T lymphocytes [111].

Disease evolution and clonal chromosomal abnormalities

With the introduction of immunosuppressive therapy and hematopoietic growth factor treatment for AA, the survival of patients has improved significantly [1]. With long-term observation, evolution of AA to other hematologic diseases has been recognized as a serious late complication of this disease. The development of PNH is considered the most common clonal complication of AA. MDS are the second most common clonal stem cell disease occurring in the context of AA. The estimation of the evolution rate is 10% in all patients, which has been associated with immunosuppressive therapy and hematopoietic growth factor treatment [112–115].

Cytogenetic abnormalities have been infrequently reported at the time of AA diagnosis with an incidence of approximately 4–5% [116–119]. The common abnormalities include del(6), del(5), del(13), del(20), −7 or +6. Except for +6 which often shows no response to immunosuppressive therapy [118, 119], AA with other clonal chromosomal abnormalities shows a similar responsiveness to immunosuppressive treatment or a comparable risk to develop MDS or AML to AA with a normal karyotype. Cytogenetic abnormalities detected after MDS evolution included −7, 11q23 abnormalities and chromosomal 9 abnormalities [112, 120]. The occurrence of a new karyotypic abnormality objectively heralds the progression of disease to MDS.

Management and prognosis

The outcome of patients with AA has substantially improved because of improved supportive care. The natural history of AA suggests that as many as one fifth of the patients may spontaneously recover with supportive care; however, observational and/or supportive care therapy alone is rarely indicated. Immunosuppression with antithymocyte globulins (ATG) and cyclosporine is effective at restoring blood-cell production in the majority of patients. The estimated 5-year survival rate for patients receiving immunosuppression is typically 75% [121]. However, relapse and especially evolution of clonal hematologic diseases remain problematic [122, 123]. Allogeneic stem-cell transplant from histocompatible sibling donors is curative in the great majority of young patients with severe AA.

References

1. **Young, N.S.**, Acquired aplastic anemia. *Annals of Internal Medicine*, 2002. **136**(7): 534–546.

2. **Brodsky, R.A.** and **R.J. Jones**, *Aplastic anaemia*. Lancet, 2005. **365**(9471): p. 1647–56.

3. **Young, N.S.** and **J. Maciejewski**, *The pathophysiology of acquired aplastic anemia*. The New England journal of medicine, 1997. **336**(19): p. 1365–72.

4. **Young, N.S., R.T. Calado**, and **P. Scheinberg**, *Current concepts in the pathophysiology and treatment of aplastic anemia*. Blood, 2006. **108**(8): p. 2509–19.

5. **Alter, B.**, *Inherited bone marrow failure syndromes. In Nathan DG, Orkin SH, Look AT, Ginsburg D* Nathan and Oski's Hematology of Infancy and Childhood 6th edn., ed. O.S. Nathan DG, Look AT, **Ginsburg D.** 2003, Philadelphia, PA: WB Saunders. 280–365.

6. **Steele, J.M.**, *et al.*, *Disease progression in recently diagnosed patients with inherited marrow failure syndromes: a Canadian Inherited Marrow Failure Registry (CIMFR) report*. Pediatric blood & cancer, 2006. **47**(7): p. 918–25.

7. **Bagby, G.L.**, JM Sloand, EM Schiffer, CA *Marrow failure.*, in *Hematology* 2004, Am Soc Hematol Educ Program. p. 318–36.

8. **Lieberman, L.** and **Y. Dror**, *Advances in understanding the genetic basis for bone-marrow failure*. Current opinion in pediatrics, 2006. **18**(1): p. 15–21.

9. **Huck, K.**, *et al.*, *Delayed diagnosis and complications of Fanconi anaemia at advanced age – a paradigm*. British journal of haematology, 2006. **133**(2): p. 188–97.

10. **Alter, B.**, *Bone marrow failure: a child is not just a small adult (but an adult can have a childhood disease)*. 2005, Am Soc Hematol Educ Program: Hematology. p. 96–103.

11. **D'Andrea, A.D.**, *Susceptibility pathways in Fanconi's anemia and breast cancer*. N Engl J Med. **362**(20): 2010. p. 1909–19.

12. **Davies, A.A.**, *et al.*, *Role of BRCA2 in control of the RAD51 recombination and DNA repair protein*. Molecular cell, 2001. **7**(2): p. 273–82.

13. **Godthelp, B.C.**, *et al.*, *Impaired DNA damage-induced nuclear Rad51 foci formation uniquely characterizes Fanconi anemia group D1*. Oncogene, 2002. **21**(32): p. 5002–5.

14. **Faivre, L.**, *et al.*, *Association of complementation group and mutation type with clinical outcome in Fanconi anemia. European Fanconi Anemia Research Group*. Blood, 2000. **96**(13): p. 4064–70.

15. **Meetei, A.R.**, *et al.*, *A human ortholog of archaeal DNA repair protein Hef is defective in Fanconi anemia complementation group M*. Nature genetics, 2005. **37**(9): p. 958–63.

16. **Taniguchi, T.** and **A.D. D'Andrea**, *Molecular pathogenesis of Fanconi anemia: recent progress*. Blood, 2006. **107**(11): p. 4223–33.

17. **Tamary, H.** and **B.P. Alter**, *Current diagnosis of inherited bone marrow failure syndromes*. Pediatric hematology and oncology, 2007. **24**(2): p. 87–99.

18. **Xia, F.**, *et al.*, *Deficiency of human BRCA2 leads to impaired homologous recombination but maintains normal nonhomologous end joining*. Proceedings of the National Academy of Sciences of the United States of America, 2001. **98**(15): p. 8644–9.

19. **Gowen, L.C.**, *et al.*, *BRCA1 required for transcription-coupled repair of oxidative DNA damage*. Science 1998. **281**(5379): p. 1009–12.

20. **Shimamura, A.** and **A.D. D'Andrea**, *Subtyping of Fanconi anemia patients: implications for clinical management*. Blood, 2003. **102**(9): p. 3459.

21. **Kutler, D.I.**, *et al.*, *A 20-year perspective on the International Fanconi Anemia Registry (IFAR)*. Blood, 2003. **101**(4): p. 1249–56.

22. **Butturini, A.**, *et al.*, *Hematologic abnormalities in Fanconi anemia: an International Fanconi Anemia Registry study*. Blood, 1994. **84**(5): p. 1650–5.

23. **Cassinat, B.**, *et al.*, *Constitutive elevation of serum alpha-fetoprotein in Fanconi anemia*. Blood, 2000. **96**(3): p. 859–63.

24. **Giampietro, P.F.**, *et al.*, *The need for more accurate and timely diagnosis in Fanconi anemia: a report from the International Fanconi Anemia Registry*. Pediatrics, 1993. **91**(6): p. 1116–20.

25. **Stetler-Stevenson, M.**, *et al.*, *Diagnostic utility of flow cytometric immunophenotyping in myelodysplastic syndrome*. Blood, 2001. **98**(4): p. 979–87.

26. **Fabio, T.**, *et al.*, *Cell cycle analysis in the diagnosis of Fanconi's anemia*. Haematologica, 2000. **85**(4): p. 431–2.

27. **Bechtold, A.**, *et al.*, *Prenatal exclusion/confirmation of Fanconi anemia via flow cytometry: a pilot study*. Fetal diagnosis and therapy, 2006. **21**(1): p. 118–24.

28. **Auerbach, A.D.**, *Fanconi anemia diagnosis and the diepoxybutane (DEB) test*. Experimental hematology, 1993. **21**(6): p. 731–3.

29. **Digweed, M.** and **K. Sperling**, *Nijmegen breakage syndrome: clinical manifestation of defective response to DNA double-strand breaks*. DNA repair, 2004. **3**(8–9): p. 1207–17.

30. **Maarek, O.**, *et al.*, *Faconi anemia and bone marrow clonal chromosome abnormalities*. Leukemia, 1996. **10**(11): p. 1700–4.

31. **Tonnies, H.**, *et al.*, *Clonal chromosomal aberrations in bone marrow cells of Fanconi anemia patients: gains of the chromosomal segment 3q26q29 as an adverse risk factor*. Blood, 2003. **101**(10): p. 3872–4.

32. **Alter, B.P.**, *Leukemia and preleukemia in Fanconi's anemia*. Cancer genetics

and cytogenetics, 1992. **58**(2): p. 206–8; discussion 209.

33. **Alter, B.P.**, *Fanconi's anemia and malignancies.* American journal of hematology, 1996. **53**(2): p. 99–110.

34. **Guardiola, P.**, *et al.*, *Outcome of 69 allogeneic stem cell transplantations for Fanconi anemia using HLA-matched unrelated donors: a study on behalf of the European Group for Blood and Marrow Transplantation.* Blood, 2000. **95**(2): p. 422–9.

35. **Zinsser, F.**, *Atropha cutis reticularis cum pigmentatione, dystrophia ungiumet leukoplakia oris.* Ikonogr Dermatol 1906. **5** p. 219–223.

36. **Engman, M.F.**, *A unique case of reticular pigmentation of the skin with atrophy.* Archives of Dermatology and Syphiligraphie., 1926. **13** p. 685–687.

37. **Cole, H.N.**, **Rauschkolb, J.C.**, **Toomey, J**, *Dyskeratosis congenita with pigmentation, dystrophia unguis and leukokeratosis oris.* Archives of Dermatology and Syphiligraphie., 1930. **21** p. 71–95.

38. **Dokal, I.**, *Dyskeratosis congenita: an inherited bone marrow failure syndrome.* British journal of haematology, 1996. **92**(4): p. 775–9.

39. **Sirinavin, C.** and **A.A. Trowbridge**, *Dyskeratosis congenita: clinical features and genetic aspects. Report of a family and review of the literature.* Journal of medical genetics, 1975. **12**(4): p. 339–54.

40. **Drachtman, R.A.** and **B.P. Alter**, *Dyskeratosis congenita.* Dermatologic clinics, 1995. **13**(1): p. 33–9.

41. **Knight, S.**, *et al.*, *Dyskeratosis Congenita (DC) Registry: identification of new features of DC.* British journal of haematology, 1998. **103**(4): p. 990–6.

42. **Alter, B.**, *Inherited Bone Marrow Failure Syndromes.* Nathan and Oski's Hematology of Infancy and Childhood, ed. D. Nathan, Orkin, SH, Ginsburg, D, Look, AT. 2003, **Philadelphia W.**B. Saunders. 280.

43. **Heiss, N.S.**, *et al.*, *X-linked dyskeratosis congenita is caused by mutations in a highly conserved gene with putative nucleolar functions.* Nature genetics, 1998. **19**(1): p. 32–8.

44. **Knight, S.W.**, *et al.*, *X-linked dyskeratosis congenita is predominantly caused by missense mutations in the DKC1 gene.* American journal of human genetics, 1999. **65**(1): p. 50–8.

45. **Heiss, N.S.**, *et al.*, *Dyskerin localizes to the nucleolus and its mislocalization is unlikely to play a role in the pathogenesis of dyskeratosis congenita.* Human molecular genetics, 1999. **8**(13): p. 2515–24.

46. **Youssoufian, H.**, V. Gharibyan, and M. Qatanani, *Analysis of epitope-tagged forms of the dyskeratosis congenital protein (dyskerin): identification of a nuclear localization signal.* Blood cells, molecules & diseases, 1999. **25**(5–6): p. 305–9.

47. **Aisner, D.L.**, W.E. Wright, and J.W. Shay, *Telomerase regulation: not just flipping the switch.* Current opinion in genetics & development, 2002. **12**(1): p. 80–5.

48. **Blackburn, E.H.**, *Telomeres and telomerase: their mechanisms of action and the effects of altering their functions.* FEBS letters, 2005. **579**(4): p. 859–62.

49. **Shay, J.W.** and **W.E. Wright**, *Senescence and immortalization: role of telomeres and telomerase.* Carcinogenesis, 2005. **26**(5): p. 867–74.

50. **Mitchell, J.R.**, E. Wood, and K. Collins, *A telomerase component is defective in the human disease dyskeratosis congenita.* Nature, 1999. **402**(6761): p. 551–5.

51. **Vulliamy, T.J.**, *et al.*, *Mutations in dyskeratosis congenita: their impact on telomere length and the diversity of clinical presentation.* Blood, 2006. **107**(7): p. 2680–5.

52. **Vulliamy, T.**, *et al.*, *The RNA component of telomerase is mutated in autosomal dominant dyskeratosis congenita.* Nature, 2001. **413**(6854): p. 432–5.

53. **Armanios, M.**, *et al.*, *Haploinsufficiency of telomerase reverse transcriptase leads to anticipation in autosomal dominant dyskeratosis congenita.* Proceedings of the National Academy of Sciences of the United States of America, 2005. **102**(44): p. 15960–4.

54. **Vulliamy, T.**, *et al.*, *Disease anticipation is associated with progressive telomere shortening in families with dyskeratosis congenita due to mutations in TERC.* Nature genetics, 2004. **36**(5): p. 447–9.

55. **Dokal, I.**, *Dyskeratosis congenita in all its forms.* British journal of haematology, 2000. **110**(4): p. 768–79.

56. **Dokal, I.**, *Dyskeratosis congenita: recent advances and future directions.* Journal of pediatric hematology/oncology, 1999. **21**(5): p. 344–50.

57. **Aalfs, C.M.**, *et al.*, *The Hoyeraal-Hreidarsson syndrome: the fourth case of a separate entity with prenatal growth retardation, progressive pancytopenia and cerebellar hypoplasia.* European journal of pediatrics, 1995. **154**(4): p. 304–8.

58. **Knudson, M.**, *et al.*, *Association of immune abnormalities with telomere shortening in autosomal-dominant dyskeratosis congenita.* Blood, 2005. **105**(2): p. 682–8.

59. **Bagby, G.C.**, *et al.*, *Marrow failure.* Hematology / the Education Program of the American Society of Hematology. American Society of Hematology, 2004: p. 318–36.

60. **Friedland, M.**, *et al.*, *Dyskeratosis congenita with hypoplastic anemia: a stem cell defect.* American journal of hematology, 1985. **20**(1): p. 85–7.

61. **Marsh, J.C.**, *et al.*, *"Stem cell" origin of the hematopoietic defect in dyskeratosis congenita.* Blood, 1992. **79**(12): p. 3138–44.

62. **Shwachman, H.**, *et al.*, *The Syndrome of Pancreatic Insufficiency and Bone Marrow Dysfunction.* The Journal of pediatrics, 1964. **65**: p. 645–63.

63. **Aggett, P.J.**, *et al.*, *Shwachman's syndrome. A review of 21 cases.* Archives of disease in childhood, 1980. **55**(5): p. 331–47.

64. **Mack, D.R.**, *et al.*, *Shwachman syndrome: exocrine pancreatic dysfunction and variable phenotypic expression.* Gastroenterology, 1996. **111**(6): p. 1593–602.

65. **Ginzberg, H.**, *et al.*, *Shwachman syndrome: phenotypic manifestations of sibling sets and isolated cases in a large patient cohort are similar.* The Journal of pediatrics, 1999. **135**(1): p. 81–8.

66. **Dror, Y.**, *et al.*, *Immune function in patients with Shwachman-Diamond syndrome.* British journal of haematology, 2001. **114**(3): p. 712–7.

67. **Hudson, E.** and **T. Aldor**, *Pancreatic insufficiency and neutropenia with*

associated immunoglobulin deficit. Archives of internal medicine, 1970. **125**(2): p. 314–6.

68. **Maki, M.**, *et al.*, *Hepatic dysfunction and dysgammaglobulinaemia in Shwachman-Diamond syndrome.* Archives of disease in childhood, 1978. **53**(8): p. 693–4.

69. **Kornfeld, S.J.**, *et al.*, *Shwachman-Diamond syndrome associated with hypogammaglobulinemia and growth hormone deficiency.* The Journal of allergy and clinical immunology, 1995. **96**(2): p. 247–50.

70. **Aggett, P.J.**, *et al.*, *An inherited defect of neutrophil mobility in Shwachman syndrome.* The Journal of pediatrics, 1979. **94**(3): p. 391–4.

71. **Goobie, S.**, *et al.*, *Shwachman-Diamond syndrome with exocrine pancreatic dysfunction and bone marrow failure maps to the centromeric region of chromosome 7.* American journal of human genetics, 2001. **68**(4): p. 1048–54.

72. **Alter, B.**, *Inherited Bone Marrow Failure Syndromes.* Nathan and Oski's Hematology of Infancy and Childhood, ed. D. Nathan, Orkin, SH, Ginsburg, D, Look, AT. 2003, Philadelphia: W.B. Saunders. p. 280.

73. **Rothbaum, R.J.**, D.A. Williams, and C.C. Daugherty, *Unusual surface distribution of concanavalin A reflects a cytoskeletal defect in neutrophils in Shwachman's syndrome.* Lancet, 1982. **2**(8302): p. 800–1.

74. **Woloszynek, J.R.**, *et al.*, *Mutations of the SBDS gene are present in most patients with Shwachman-Diamond syndrome.* Blood, 2004. **104**(12): p. 3588–90.

75. **Boocock, G.R.**, *et al.*, *Mutations in SBDS are associated with Shwachman-Diamond syndrome.* Nature genetics, 2003. **33**(1): p. 97–101.

76. **Austin, K.M.**, R.J. Leary, and A. Shimamura, *The Shwachman-Diamond SBDS protein localizes to the nucleolus.* Blood, 2005. **106**(4): p. 1253–8.

77. **Boocock, G.R.**, M.R. Marit, and J.M. Rommens, *Phylogeny, sequence conservation, and functional complementation of the SBDS protein family.* Genomics, 2006. **87**(6): p. 758–71.

78. **Hall, G.W.**, P. Dale, and J.A. Dodge, *Shwachman-Diamond syndrome: UK*

perspective. Archives of disease in childhood, 2006. **91**(6): p. 521–4.

79. **Dror, Y.** and M.H. Freedman, *Shwachman-Diamond syndrome: An inherited preleukemic bone marrow failure disorder with aberrant hematopoietic progenitors and faulty marrow microenvironment.* Blood, 1999. **94**(9): p. 3048–54.

80. **Smith, O.P.**, *et al.*, *Haematological abnormalities in Shwachman-Diamond syndrome.* British journal of haematology, 1996. **94**(2): p. 279–84.

81. **Woods, W.G.**, *et al.*, *The occurrence of leukemia in patients with the Shwachman syndrome.* The Journal of pediatrics, 1981. **99**(3): p. 425–8.

82. **Dror, Y.**, *Shwachman-Diamond syndrome.* Pediatric blood & cancer, 2005. **45**(7): p. 892–901.

83. **Davies, S.M.**, *et al.*, *Unrelated donor bone marrow transplantation for children and adolescents with aplastic anaemia or myelodysplasia.* British journal of haematology, 1997. **96**(4): p. 749–56.

84. **Freedman, M.H.**, *et al.*, *Myelodysplasia syndrome and acute myeloid leukemia in patients with congenital neutropenia receiving G-CSF therapy.* Blood, 2000. **96**(2): p. 429–36.

85. **Hasle, H.**, *et al.*, *A pediatric approach to the WHO classification of myelodysplastic and myeloproliferative diseases.* Leukemia, 2003. **17**(2): p. 277–82.

86. **Dokal, I.**, *et al.*, *Adult onset of acute myeloid leukaemia (M6) in patients with Shwachman-Diamond syndrome.* British journal of haematology, 1997. **99**(1): p. 171–3.

87. **Keller, P.**, *et al.*, *Bone marrow failure in Shwachman-Diamond syndrome does not select for clonal haematopoiesis of the paroxysmal nocturnal haemoglobinuria phenotype.* British journal of haematology, 2002. **119**(3): p. 830–2.

88. **Mertens, F.**, B. Johansson, and F. Mitelman, *Isochromosomes in neoplasia.* Genes, chromosomes & cancer, 1994. **10**(4): p. 221–30.

89. **Dror, Y.**, *et al.*, *Clonal evolution in marrows of patients with Shwachman-Diamond syndrome: a prospective 5-year follow-up study.* Experimental hematology, 2002. **30**(7): p. 659–69.

90. **Smith, A.**, *et al.*, *Intermittent 20q- and consistent i(7q) in a patient with Shwachman-Diamond syndrome.* Pediatric hematology and oncology, 2002. **19**(7): p. 525–8.

91. **Pearson, H.A.**, *et al.*, *A new syndrome of refractory sideroblastic anemia with vacuolization of marrow precursors and exocrine pancreatic dysfunction.* The Journal of pediatrics, 1979. **95**(6): p. 976–84.

92. **Fleming, M.D.**, *The genetics of inherited sideroblastic anemias.* Seminars in hematology, 2002. **39**(4): p. 270–81.

93. **Dubowitz, V.**, *Familial Low Birthweight Dwarfism with an Unusual Facies and a Skin Eruption.* Journal of medical genetics, 1965. **42**: p. 12–7.

94. **Berthold, F.**, W. Fuhrmann, and F. Lampert, *Fatal aplastic anaemia in a child with features of Dubowitz syndrome.* European journal of pediatrics, 1987. **146**(6): p. 605–7.

95. **Walters, T.R.** and F. Desposito, *Aplastic anemia in Dubowitz syndrome.* The Journal of pediatrics, 1985. **106**(4): p. 622–3.

96. **Resnick, I.B.**, *et al.*, *Nijmegen breakage syndrome: clinical characteristics and mutation analysis in eight unrelated Russian families.* The Journal of pediatrics, 2002. **140**(3): p. 355–61.

97. **Harper, R.G.**, E. Orti, and R.K. Baker, *Bird-beaded dwarfs (Seckel's syndrome). A familial pattern of developmental, dental, skeletal, genital, and central nervous system anomalies.* J Pediatr, 1967. **70**(5): p. 799–804.

98. **Dohlsten, M.**, *et al.*, *Immunological abnormalities in a child with constitutional aplastic anemia.* Pediatric hematology and oncology, 1986. **3**(1): p. 89–96.

99. **Nathan DG**, *Hematology of Infancy and Childhood.* 2009, Philadelphia, PA: WB Saunders, Inc.

100. **Young, N.S.**, *et al.*, *The relationship of aplastic anemia and PNH.* International journal of hematology, 2002. **76** Suppl 2: p. 168–72.

101. **Young, N.**, *Drugs and chemicals.*, in *Aplastic Anemia: Acquired and Inherited.*, A.B. **Young NS**, Editor. 1994, WB Saunders: Philadelphia. p. 100–32.

102. **Fuhrer, M.**, *et al.*, *Immunosuppressive therapy for aplastic anemia in children: a more severe disease predicts better survival.* Blood, 2005. **106**(6): p. 2102–4.

103. **Shimamura, A.**, Guinan, EA., *Acquired aplastic anemia.*, in *Hematology of Infancy and Childhood*, D. Nathan, Orkin, SH Editor. 2003, WB Saunders: Philadelphia. p. 256.

104. **Ly, H.**, *et al.*, *Functional characterization of telomerase RNA variants found in patients with hematologic disorders.* Blood, 2005. **105**(6): p. 2332–9.

105. **Yamaguchi, H.**, *et al.*, *Mutations in TERT, the gene for telomerase reverse transcriptase, in aplastic anemia.* The New England journal of medicine, 2005. **352**(14): p. 1413–24.

106. **Orazi, A.**, *et al.*, *Hypoplastic myelodysplastic syndromes can be distinguished from acquired aplastic anemia by CD34 and PCNA immunostaining of bone marrow biopsy specimens.* American journal of clinical pathology, 1997. **107**(3): p. 268–74.

107. **Maciejewski, J.P.**, *et al.*, *Distinct clinical outcomes for cytogenetic abnormalities evolving from aplastic anemia.* Blood, 2002. **99**(9): p. 3129–35.

108. **Nakao, S.**, C. Sugimori, and H. Yamazaki, *Clinical significance of a small population of paroxysmal nocturnal hemoglobinuria-type cells in the management of bone marrow failure.* International journal of hematology, 2006. **84**(2): p. 118–22.

109. **Sugimori, C.**, *et al.*, *Minor population of CD55-CD59- blood cells predicts response to immunosuppressive therapy and prognosis in patients with aplastic anemia.* Blood, 2006. **107**(4): p. 1308–14.

110. **Shichishima, T.** and H. Noji, *A new aspect of the molecular pathogenesis of paroxysmal nocturnal hemoglobinuria.* Hematology (Amsterdam, Netherlands), 2002. **7**(4): p. 211–27.

111. **Young, N.S.**, *Paroxysmal nocturnal hemoglobinuria: current issues in pathophysiology and treatment.* Current hematology reports, 2005. **4**(2): p. 103–9.

112. **Fuhrer, M.**, *et al.*, *Relapse and clonal disease in children with aplastic anemia (AA) after immunosuppressive therapy (IST): the SAA 94 experience. German/Austrian Pediatric Aplastic Anemia Working Group.* Klinische Padiatrie, 1998. **210**(4): p. 173–9.

113. **Yamazaki, E.**, *et al.*, *The evidence of clonal evolution with monosomy 7 in aplastic anemia following granulocyte colony-stimulating factor using the polymerase chain reaction.* Blood cells, molecules & diseases, 1997. **23**(2): p. 213–8.

114. **Doney, K.**, *et al.*, *Primary treatment of acquired aplastic anemia: outcomes with bone marrow transplantation and immunosuppressive therapy. Seattle Bone Marrow Transplant Team.* Annals of internal medicine, 1997. **126**(2): p. 107–15.

115. **Socie, G.**, *et al.*, *Malignant tumors occurring after treatment of aplastic anemia. European Bone Marrow Transplantation-Severe Aplastic Anaemia Working Party.* The New England journal of medicine, 1993. **329**(16): p. 1152–7.

116. **Ohga, S.**, *et al.*, *Treatment responses of childhood aplastic anaemia with chromosomal aberrations at diagnosis.* British journal of haematology, 2002. **118**(1): p. 313–9.

117. **Mikhailova, N.**, *et al.*, *Cytogenetic abnormalities in patients with severe aplastic anemia.* Haematologica, 1996. **81**(5): p. 418–22.

118. **Appelbaum, F.R.**, *et al.*, *Clonal cytogenetic abnormalities in patients with otherwise typical aplastic anemia.* Experimental hematology, 1987. **15**(11): p. 1134–9.

119. **Moormeier, J.A.**, *et al.*, *Trisomy 6: a recurring cytogenetic abnormality associated with marrow hypoplasia.* Blood, 1991. **77**(6): p. 1397–8.

120. **Kojima, S.**, *et al.*, *Risk factors for evolution of acquired aplastic anemia into myelodysplastic syndrome and acute myeloid leukemia after immunosuppressive therapy in children.* Blood, 2002. **100**(3): p. 786–90.

121. **Bacigalupo, A.**, *et al.*, *Treatment of acquired severe aplastic anemia: bone marrow transplantation compared with immunosuppressive therapy – The European Group for Blood and Marrow Transplantation experience.* Seminars in hematology, 2000. **37**(1): p. 69–80.

122. **Socie, G.**, *et al.*, *Late clonal diseases of treated aplastic anemia.* Seminars in hematology, 2000. **37**(1): p. 91–101.

123. **Piaggio, G.**, *et al.*, *Coexistence of normal and clonal haemopoiesis in aplastic anaemia patients treated with immunosuppressive therapy.* British journal of haematology, 1999. **107**(3): p. 505–11.

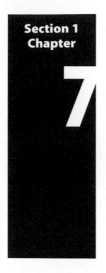

Inherited bone marrow failure syndromes and acquired disorders associated with single peripheral blood cytopenia
Pure red cell aplasia, agranulocytosis, and thrombocytopenias

Maria A. Proytcheva

Congenital anemias due to impaired red cell production

Congenital anemias are a heterogeneous group of rare disorders due to impaired red cell production, resulting from either pure red cell aplasias and lack of erythroid progenitors in the marrow, or from ineffective erythropoiesis, dyserythropoiesis, and an increased cell death (Table 7.1). Either pathogenic mechanism leads to a variable degree of anemia with a low reticulocyte count. The peripheral blood findings are non-specific, and the diagnosis requires a bone marrow evaluation and ancillary studies. Anemias due to hemoglobinopathy, nutritional deficiency, increased red cell destruction, or bone marrow metastases are discussed in other chapters.

Diamond–Blackfan anemia [Online Mendelian Inheritance in Man (OMIM) 105650]

Epidemiology and clinical presentation

Diamond–Blackfan anemia (DBA), also known as congenital hypoplastic anemia, is a clinically and genetically heterogeneous group of disorders manifested in early infancy with anemia and reticulocytopenia due to absolute erythroid hypoplasia in otherwise normocellular bone marrow (BM). DBA is the first and, so far, the only known disease of abnormal ribosome biogenesis. It is characterized by mutations at structural ribosomal proteins, which result in intrinsic disorders of erythropoiesis, congenital anomalies, and an increased predisposition to malignancies [1, 2].

One large American study and the European DBA Registry reported an estimated incidence of DBA of 4–10 per million live births [3–5]. The majority of cases are sporadic, and only approximately 10–25% of DBA cases are familial. More than 90% of individuals with DBA are diagnosed in the first year of life, and the median age at presentation is 8 weeks (range, birth–26 years).

Major clinical signs of DBA include pallor, failure to thrive, persistent diarrhea, and, less frequently, refusal to eat [6]. Congenital anomalies are present in 37–45% of individuals with DBA. They include thumb malformations (subluxation, supernumary, bifid, triphalangeal, flat thenar eminence with or without absent radial pulse); craniofacial anomalies (cleft or high arched palate, hypertelorism with flat nasal bridge, strabismus, ptosis, cataracts), giving a characteristic facial appearance of some patients; urogenital anomalies; or multiple anomalies [3, 6, 7]. Low birth weight has been reported in about a fifth of the babies with DBA.

Patients with DBA have a higher predisposition to develop hematologic and non-hematologic malignancies [6, 8]. Whether this predisposition is due to the primary genetic defects in DBA, or is instead a consequence of corticosteroid therapy or chronic iron overload is yet to be determined. However, patients with thalassemia and nephrotic syndrome, treated with similar regimens and/or having iron overload, do not have an increased risk of such malignancy. This suggests that the increased risk of hematologic and non-hematologic malignancies is associated with the primary genetic defects leading to DBA.

Laboratory findings

A consistent finding at diagnosis of DBA is normochromic, usually macrocytic anemia with reticulocytopenia, that develops early in childhood (Table 7.2; Fig. 7.1). The mean hemoglobin level is 6.1 g/dL (range from 1.5 to 12.4 g/dL), the mean hematocrit is 19.3%, and the reticulocyte count ranges from 0 to 4.5% [5, 6]. Macrocytosis, although considered characteristic for DBA, may not be present in the first year of life due to residual fetal hematopoiesis, iron deficiency, or beta-thalassemia minor.

Table 7.1. Causes of pure red cell aplasia in children.

Primary pure red cell aplasia
  Inherited
    Diamond–Blackfan anemia
    Anemia in the setting of Pearson syndrome
    Congenital dyserythropoietic anemias (CDAs)
      CDA type I
      CDA type II, hereditary erythroblastic multinuclearity with a
        positive acidified serum test (HEMPAS)
      CDA type III
  Acquired
    Transient erythroblastopenia of childhood (TEC)
    Pure red cell aplasia due to infection
      Human parvovirus B19
    Idiopathic

Secondary red cell aplasia associated with:
  Hematologic malignancies
    Hodgkin lymphoma
    Non-Hodgkin lymphoma
    Acute lymphoblastic leukemia
    Chronic myeloid leukemia
  Thymoma
  Solid tumors
    Small blue cell tumors of childhood
  Infections
    HIV
    Epstein–Barr virus
    Viral hepatitis
    Mumps
    Cytomegalovirus
    T-cell leukemia lymphoma virus (HTLV-1)
    Meningococcemia
    Staphylococcemia
    Chronic hemolytic anemia (usually associated with parvovirus B19)
  Medical diseases
    Collagen vascular diseases
    Severe renal failure
    Post-ABO incompatible hematopoietic stem cell transplantation

Table 7.2. Laboratory findings in patients with Diamond–Blackfan anemia.

Laboratory abnormality	Comment
Normochromic macrocytic anemia Reticulocytopenia	Macrocytosis may be absent during the first year of life or in patients with iron deficiency or thalassemia
Elevated erythrocyte adenosine deaminase (eADA) activity (>3 SD[a])	Weak independent predictor of DBA – also elevated in immune deficiencies, hemolytic anemias, chronic myeloproliferative disorders, dyskeratosis, or megaloblastic anemia
Elevated fetal hemoglobin (Hb F)	Non-specific – also elevated during early infancy, stress erythropoiesis, and in hereditary persistence of hemoglobin F
Strong expression of i antigen	Non-specific – also elevated during early infancy and stress erythropoiesis
Other abnormalities ↑ serum erythropoietin level ↓ red blood cell survival ↓ haptoglobin ↓ plasma iron clearance ↓ red cell iron utilization	Non-specific

[a] SD = standard deviation.

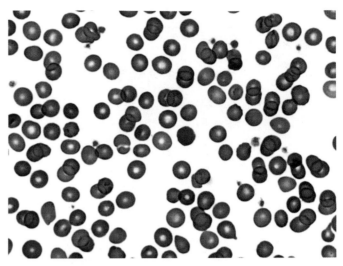

Fig. 7.1. A peripheral blood smear from a two-month-old girl with Diamond–Blackfan anemia. Notice the macrocytic red blood cells, mild anisopoikilocytosis, and the absence of polychromasia (Wright–Giemsa stain).

While the anemia may improve with age, the macrocytosis persists and, in some patients, may be the only peripheral blood abnormality. Up to one-quarter of the patients are neutropenic. While the platelet counts are usually normal, thrombocytopenia or thrombocytosis may be present as well.

Eighty to eighty-five percent of individuals classified as having DBA have elevated erythrocyte adenosine deaminase (eADA) activity [9, 10]. In such patients, eADA levels are more than three standard deviations higher than normal. However, while elevated eADA is a helpful supporting criterion of DBA in the workup of children having macrocytic anemia with reticulocytopenia, this parameter is not a strong independent predictor for the presence of disease. Elevated eADA can also be seen in immune deficiencies, hemolytic anemias, chronic myeloproliferative disorders, dyskeratosis, and megaloblastic anemias. Lastly, elevated eADA levels can be seen in normal relatives of patients with DBA, and can be used for screening of potential donors for hematopoietic stem cells for transplant.

Patients with DBA also have elevated Hb F levels for their age, and a strong expression of i antigen on their erythrocytes. However, these parameters may have a limited utility since most of the DBA workup is on infants, for whom an increased Hb F level and a strong expression of i antigen are expected. Furthermore, similar findings are associated with stress erythropoiesis or other types of anemia. Other laboratory abnormalities in DBA include an increased serum erythropoietin level; decreased red cell survival; decreased haptoglobin level, indicating mild intravascular hemolysis; delay in plasma iron clearance; and low red cell iron utilization [11].

In DBA, the bone marrow is normocellular for age. It shows reduced erythropoiesis, with preserved myelopoiesis and megakaryopoiesis (Fig. 7.2). The erythroid hypoplasia is profound, and while some immature forms such as proerythroblasts are seen, orthochromic erythroblasts are virtually absent. Dyserythropoiesis, including ring sideroblasts, may be present

A

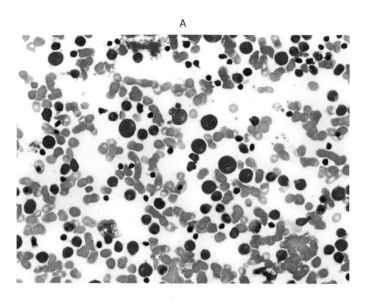

B

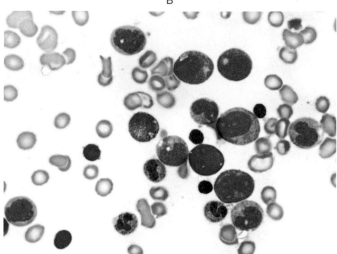

C

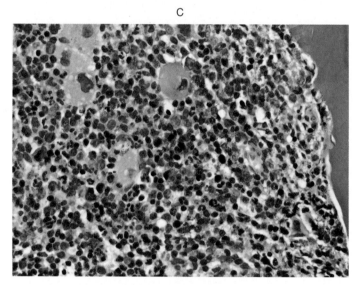

Fig. 7.2. Bone marrow from a five-month-old girl with Diamond–Blackfan anemia, transfusion dependent since birth. (A) Bone marrow aspirate shows virtually absent erythropoiesis and preserved myelopoiesis (Wright–Giemsa stain). (B) Rare proerythroblasts among myeloid progenitors are seen. The more mature orthochromic erythroblasts are markedly reduced (Wright–Giemsa stain). (C) Bone marrow biopsy showing slightly hypercellular marrow for age with myeloid hyperplasia and absolute erythroid hypoplasia. Notice the increased number of small lymphocytes. Flow cytometric studies show an increased number of normal B-cell progenitors (not shown). Megakaryocytes are present in adequate numbers. Notice the presence of several large hemosiderin granules as a result of the increased iron load after several red cell transfusions. At this age, the bone marrow shows no stainable iron.

but is not characteristic. The storage iron is increased in patients receiving multiple transfusions. The myeloid progenitors show complete maturation and the megakaryocytes are adequate in number and have unremarkable morphology. The number of normal B-cell progenitors, hematogones, may be elevated.

Genetics

Approximately 75% of cases of DBA are sporadic and the rest are familial [6]. The autosomal dominant form of inheritance is most frequently reported in DBA. Furthermore, a careful genetic analysis of DBA-affected pedigrees for the presence of macrocytosis, increased Hb F, increased eADA, and congenital anomalies in other family members strongly suggests a greater number of autosomal dominant cases than previously thought. This observation is supported by a mutation analysis suggesting an autosomal dominant type of inheritance in from 10% to 45% of individuals with DBA [2].

Different molecular defects can result in the DBA phenotype. At present, mutations at six such genes have been identified in more than half of the patients with DBA. The mutations seen in the largest number of cases (25%) are at the *RPS19* gene, followed by mutations at *RPL5* (10%), *RPL11* (6.5%), *RPL35a* (3%), *RPS24* (2%), and *RPS17* (1%) [2, 12, 13]. These genes encode for proteins that are required for the maturation of their respective ribosomal subunits. Three of the genes – *RPS17*, *RPS19*, and *RPS24* – encode proteins for the 40S ribosomal subunit, and the rest – *RPL5*, *RPL11*, and *RPL35a* – encode proteins for the 60S ribosomal subunit. Most of the mutations – deletions, nonsense, or frameshifts – result in a loss of function. The mutant proteins have varying degrees of decreased stability and compromised nucleolar localization [14]. As a result of this faulty maturation, there is increased cell death through apoptosis of the erythroid progenitors, and the development of anemia.

How mutations at ribosomal structural proteins result in a selective erythropoietic proapoptotic phenotype has not yet

Table 7.3. Diagnostic criteria for Diamond–Blackfan anemia.

Diagnostic criteria for DBA[a]
    Age less than one year
    Macrocytic anemia with no other significant cytopenias
    Reticulocytopenia
    Normal bone marrow cellularity with lack of erythroid progenitors

Major supporting criteria
    Gene mutation consistent with classical DBA
    Positive family history

Minor supporting criteria
    Elevated erythrocyte adenosine deaminase (eADA) activity
    Congenital anomalies consistent with classical DBA
    Elevated Hb F
    No evidence of another inherited bone marrow failure syndrome

[a] *Classical DBA*: diagnosis requires all diagnostic criteria; *Non-classical DBA*: not all diagnostic criteria are met, but there is positive family history and confirmed mutation; *Probable DBA* if: three diagnostic criteria are met and there is a positive family history; two diagnostic criteria and three minor supporting criteria are met; or positive family history and three minor supporting criteria are met, even in the absence of diagnostic criteria.
Adapted from Vlachos *et al.* [13].

been determined. Recent animal models of knockout rps19 in zebra fish recapitulate the phenotype of DBA and show that disruption of ribosomal assembly results in the diversion of the ribosomal proteins from their normal fates [2]. Since the 60S ribosomal subunit proteins RPL5, RPL11, and RPL35a are important signaling molecules, they can interact with and activate MDM2 (murine double minute), a potent regulator of p53 levels and activity. Thus, the abnormal activation of p53 may explain the high apoptotic rate. However, it is still unclear as to why the erythropoiesis is affected almost exclusively and why mutations at ribosomal structural proteins can lead to an increased susceptibility to malignancy in patients with DBA. Of the 150 reported cases of DBA, at least 30 cases of malignancies including acute myeloid leukemia, Hodgkin and non-Hodgkin lymphomas, acute lymphoblastic leukemia, osteogenic sarcoma, breast cancer, hepatocellular carcinoma, colon carcinoma, and gastric carcinoma have been reported in the literature [2].

Diagnostic criteria of Diamond–Blackfan anemia

The diagnostic criteria for DBA are summarized in Table 7.3. The presence of marked anemia with reticulocytopenia before the first birthday, normal neutrophil and platelet counts, and normal bone marrow cellularity with a paucity of erythroid progenitors defines the DBA [13]. If all of the criteria are met, the diagnosis of classical DBA is made. However, some affected individuals may present with anemia after the first birthday, or have only mild hematologic abnormalities, that is, macrocytosis without anemia. Such individuals are considered to have non-classical DBA. The diagnosis of non-classical DBA is therefore more challenging and requires more careful weighing of clinical findings, even more so in the light of the increased risk of malignancies in such individuals or in the event that the individual is considered a potential donor for a hematopoietic stem cell transplant. The diagnosis of DBA is probable, with a

decreased degree of certainty, if three diagnostic criteria are met along with a positive family history; or two diagnostic criteria and three minor supporting criteria; or a positive family history and three minor supporting criteria, even in the absence of any diagnostic criteria [13].

Currently, molecular diagnosis is not routinely performed to confirm the diagnosis of DBA since it is expensive and provides a diagnosis in only about 50% of patients. Molecular diagnosis is reserved for patients with a family history of DBA, prenatal diagnosis, or screening of family members who may be potential hematopoietic stem cell donors. For donors, the presence of macrocytosis and elevated eADA is suggestive of a carrier state with a low penetrance of the disease.

Differential diagnosis

In an infant with straightforward red cell failure with macrocytosis and reticulocytopenia, DBA should be suspected after other acquired disorders – for example, parvovirus B19 infection, transient erythroblastopenia of childhood (TEC), infections such as HIV, drug or toxic suppression of the marrow – are excluded (Table 7.4). Shwachman–Diamond and Fanconi anemia may be considered as well, since these disorders also present with macrocytosis and reticulocytopenia. While DBA is most frequently diagnosed in infancy, it may present later in life.

Red cell aplasia due to human parvovirus B19 infection

Parvovirus B19 is the only virus of the parvovirus family known to cause transient aplastic crisis and anemia in humans with impaired red cell production. The clinical manifestation of the infection is variable, from asymptomatic to serious diseases depending on the immunologic status of the host [15].

Parvovirus B19 is endemic throughout the world, and more than 50% of children by age 15 and 90% of elderly individuals are seropositive. Most infections are asymptomatic. In children, the virus causes erythema infectiosum, also known as fifth disease, and in adults polyarthropathy syndrome. Infection during pregnancy results in hydrops fetalis. During early infection, the virus is present in the blood but viremia is rare. After infection, immunocompetent individuals develop virus-specific IgM and IgG antibodies.

Parvovirus B19 has high tropism to early erythroid progenitors and enters the red cells via a cellular receptor, globoside, also known as blood group P. An infection results in red cell aplasia that lasts 5–10 days and does not produce significant anemia in individuals with a normal, 120 day red blood cell lifespan. However, in individuals with impaired red cell production and a shorter erythrocyte lifespan due to underlying hemoglobinopathy – such as thalassemia, sickle cell disease, SC disease, hereditary spherocytosis, elliptocytosis, immune-mediated hemolytic anemia, or iron deficient anemia – Parvovirus B19 infection can result in a transient aplastic crisis leading to serious anemia [16].

Table 7.4. Acquired pure red cell aplasia in children.

Disorder	Pathogenesis	Characteristic features
Parvovirus B19 infection	Direct infection of early progenitors Acute transient aplastic crisis in individuals with impaired red cell production Chronic anemia in immunosuppressed individuals Congenital infection	Almost complete absence of erythroid progenitors, particularly orthochromic erythroblasts Rare proerythroblasts, occasional giant forms with inclusion Characteristic intranuclear inclusions in formalin-fixed tissue
Immune mediated Transient erythroblastopenia of childhood (TEC)	Acquired anemia in previously healthy children Most children have autoantibodies against red cell progenitors after infection with unknown virus different from parvovirus B19 Rare genetic form	Temporal reticulocytopenia; rarely leukopenia or platelet abnormalities Normal eADA levels Bone marrow – erythroblastopenia Increased number of hematogones Spontaneous recovery is a rule During recovery phase – marked reticulocytosis with high MCV Excellent prognosis
Associated with autoimmune diseases (rare in children)	Rheumatoid arthritis Systemic lupus erythematosus As part of a paraneoplastic syndrome Thymoma, Hodgkin lymphoma	Anemia, reticulocytopenia
After hematopoietic stem cell transplant	ABO incompatibility between donor and recipient Major – the recipient has antibodies directed against the donor red cells Minor – the donor has antibodies directed to the recipient red blood cells	Delay in red cell engraftment and reticulocyte recovery
Acquired somatic mutation Initial manifestation of pre-leukemia syndromes 5q–	Haploinsufficiency of *RPS14* leading to a loss of function of a structural ribosomal protein	Phenotype strikingly similar to Diamond–Blackfan anemia
Drug induced Phenytoin, azathioprine, isoniazid	Pathogenesis largely unknown – Direct toxicity? – Immune mediated?	More frequently macrocytosis, rarely cause anemia Effect reversible after discontinuation of the offending drug

In parvovirus B19 infection, the peripheral blood shows anemia with reticulocytopenia and, rarely, neutropenia or thrombocytopenia. In the *bone marrow aspirate* smears one finds rare early proerythroblasts but almost no mature erythroid progenitors, such as orthochromic erythroblasts. A characteristic feature of Parvovirus B19 infection in the marrow is the presence of giant proerythroblasts with granular chromatin, large prominent nucleoli, and abundant blue cytoplasm with irregular cytoplasmic borders (Fig. 7.3). Though characteristic, such cells are rare, and examination of the BM aspirate smears at low magnification is particularly helpful in identifying them. The *bone marrow biopsy* confirms the presence of marked erythroid hypoplasia. Furthermore, relatively small cells with characteristic intranuclear inclusions have been identified in formalin-fixed material [17]. Such inclusions are not apparent in bone marrows fixed with other fixatives or in air-dried Wright–Giemsa-stained aspirate smears. Giant proerythroblasts and intracytoplasmic inclusions are seen in the fetal liver and bone marrow of a congenital parvovirus infection (Fig. 7.4). Immunohistochemical stain with antibodies against parvovirus B19 is positive and highlights the small proerythroblasts, whereas the gigantic forms are characteristically negative.

With the resolution of the anemia, the characteristic proerythroblasts disappear and marrow becomes hypercellular due to erythroid hyperplasia. Non-specific BM changes due to parvovirus B19 infection include a mild increase in the number of megakaryocytes, many of which have oddly shaped nuclei. Rarely, parvovirus infection can manifest with bone marrow necrosis.

The infection can be confirmed by immunohistochemistry or *in situ* hybridization [18, 19]. Positive PCR confirms the diagnosis. Immunocompetent individuals develop protective virus-specific IgM and later, with resolution of the infection, IgG antibodies appear as a result of Parvovirus B19 infection. A positive IgM and a negative IgG titer confirm recent infection. However, negative IgM and a high titer of IgG is indicative of a previous infection.

Individuals with immune deficiency, either congenital or acquired due to human immunodeficiency virus infection, or hematopoietic or solid organ transplant recipients, have an impaired immune response to Parvovirus B19 and may develop a persistent infection [20]. Such individuals present with pancytopenia rather than anemia, and the antibody studies are often negative. Thus, in the settings of immune deficiency, serologic studies have a limited use and the presence of Parvovirus B19 should be confirmed by immunohistochemical and/or *in situ* hybridization studies, or by a molecular detection of the virus by polymerase chain reaction (PCR).

Transient erythroblastopenia of childhood

Transient erythroblastopenia of childhood (TEC) is a rare disorder characterized by a sudden decrease in red cell production,

A

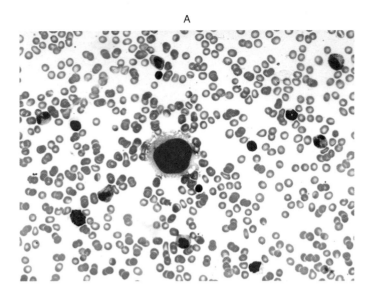

B

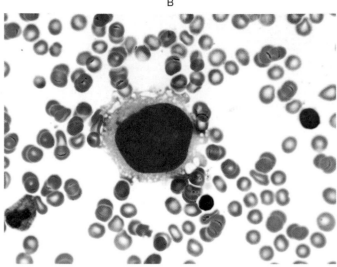

C

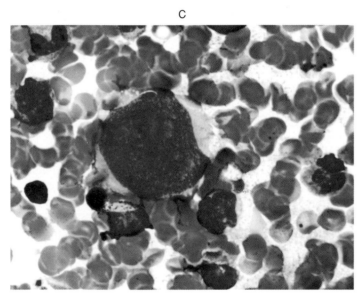

Fig. 7.3. Bone marrow from a 16-year-old girl with human parvovirus B19 infection leading to marked anemia with reticulocytopenia, leukopenia, and thrombocytopenia. The parvovirus infection was confirmed serologically by the presence of elevated IgM and negative IgG at the time of diagnosis. This was followed by a seroconversion several months later and a resolution of the peripheral blood cytopenias. (A) Bone marrow aspirate shows a paucity of erythroid progenitors and rare giant proerythroblasts. (B, C) Examples of giant proerythroblasts with intranuclear inclusions and a moderate amount of basophilic cytoplasm with irregular cytoplasmic borders. Cytoplasmic vacuolization may be present (Wright–Giemsa stain).

manifested by anemia with reticulocytopenia, followed by a spontaneous recovery within one to two months [21]. TEC is most frequent in children between four months and four years of age, and it is usually associated with pure red cell aplasia. However, accompanying white blood cell and platelet abnormalities may also be present [22, 23].

The etiology of TEC is still unknown. Immune-mediated mechanisms and viral infection, such as *human herpesvirus 6* (HHV-6) or parvovirus B19, although reported have not been proven [24–27]. A growing body of evidence suggests that TEC occurs as a result of environmental exposure to an unknown agent in genetically predisposed individuals. Rarely, siblings with TEC, or a family history of anemia suggesting an underlying genetic susceptibility transmitted in an autosomal dominant pattern, have been reported [28].

During the recovery phase, the peripheral blood shows an improvement of the anemia, marked reticulocytosis, and high MCV. At that time, the red blood cells have some characteristics of fetal erythrocytes, such as high MCV, increased Hb F production, and the presence of i antigen. As a result, distinguishing TEC from other forms of congenital pure red cell aplasia, such as DBA, may be difficult. Unlike DBA, the erythrocytes in TEC have normal eADA levels.

The prognosis of TEC is excellent. The disease is self-limited and rarely requires transfusion or bone marrow examination. TEC should be suspected in otherwise healthy children with anemia and reticulocytopenia and no other abnormalities suggestive of leukemia or other specific disease.

Other causes of acquired pure red cell aplasia in children

Drug-induced red cell aplasia is by far the most frequent cause of pure red cell aplasia in children. Treatment with azathioprine

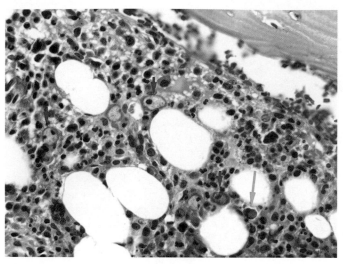

Fig. 7.4. Bone marrow biopsy from a child with human Parvovirus B19 infection. Normocellular bone marrow with absolute erythroid hypoplasia and the presence of giant erythroblasts with large intranuclear inclusions (short blue arrows). Rare cells with a central lucent area and condensation of the periphery of the nucleus (lantern cell) are also seen in a formalin-fixed biopsy (long green arrow) (H&E stain).

for renal transplant rejection is one of the most common offending agents. It generally causes megaloblastic anemia; it can result in pure red cell aplasia, but more rarely. Thymoma or B-cell lymphoproliferative disorders may present with pure red cell aplasia. However, chronic lymphocytic leukemia/lymphoma, the most common lymphoproliferative disorder associated with pure red cell aplasia, is almost never seen in the first 25 years of life and, thus, it is not a diagnostic consideration in the workup of a child with pure red cell aplasia.

Proper diagnosis and distinction between a congenital and acquired pure red cell aplasia is required for further management. In infants and young children, the main distinction is between DBA and TEC. For older children, a drug history, functional activity, physical examination, serology for autoimmune diseases, and bone marrow morphology are required for proper diagnosis. Serial measurements of Parvovirus B19 IgM and IgG, and bone marrow examination for giant erythroblasts should be performed as well. However, until a firm diagnosis is established, the management of these two disorders is very similar, which allows the flexibility to complete the investigation and observe spontaneous remission of the anemia due to TEC or other self-limiting conditions.

Congenital dyserythropoietic anemias

Congenital dyserythropoietic anemias (CDAs) are a heterogeneous group of disorders manifested by congenital or hereditary anemia/jaundice, ineffective erythropoiesis, and a typical morphologic appearance of bone marrow erythroblasts [29–31]. Based on the morphologic and ultrastructural abnormalities and the results of the acidified serum test, CDA has been divided in to three major and several minor types. The

characteristic features of the three major types of CDA are presented in Table 7.5.

Congenital dyserythropoietic anemia type I (OMIM 224120)

More than 150 individuals – mostly from Western Europe but also from the Middle East (Israeli Bedouins, Lebanese, Kuwaitis, and South Arabians), India, Japan, and China – have been reported to have CDA type I [29, 32]. This rare disorder is diagnosed from birth to late adulthood, with the majority of cases presenting during early childhood and adolescence [33, 34].

The major clinical symptoms of CDA type I include mild to moderate anemia, mild jaundice, high bilirubin levels, and a tendency to develop gallstones. In addition, individuals with CDA type I exhibit an increased iron absorption which, along with the ineffective erythropoiesis, results in increases of serum ferritin levels, in the range of 600–1500 µg/L [31]. The iron overload is a genuine feature of the disease and is present even in non-transfused patients or those that have been transfused only rarely.

A palpable spleen is present in 80–90% of cases. Congenital anomalies such as brown skin pigmentation, syndactyly in the feet, absence of phalanges and nails in the fingers and toes, additional phalanx, short stature, and others are present in a proportion of patients with CDA type I [31, 35]. While rare, skeletal deformities such as parietal and frontal bossing can be present in patients with marked erythroid hyperplasia.

The hemoglobin baseline levels vary between 6.6 g/dL and 11.6 g/dL (mean, 9.2 g/dL), and there is consistent reticulocytopenia [36]. The MCV is increased in the majority of cases and there is moderate to marked anisopoikilocytosis of the red blood cells, including the presence of macroovalocytes, normocytes, microspherocytes, and teardrop-shaped erythrocytes (Fig. 7.5). Macrocytes are present even in cases with normal MCV. Basophilic stippling, both fine and coarse, is frequently present.

The bone marrow shows erythroid hyperplasia with megaloblastoid erythroid maturation and characteristic morphologic changes seen predominantly in the polychromatophilic erythroblasts [30]. These include the presence of internuclear chromatin bridges and bi- or multinucleate forms, some of which have nuclei of unequal size, others nuclei that are overlapping or stuck together, or nuclei at different stages of maturation (Fig. 7.6). While these dyserythropoietic changes of CDA type I are characteristic, they are present in a minority of erythroblasts and thus require an assessment of a large number of cells. For instance, the prevalence of binucleated forms in the bone marrow of the first 12 patients with CDA type I in the United Kingdom is 4.87% (range 3.5–7.02%) as compared to only 0.31% (range 0–0.57%) in 10 normal subjects [36]. In the same study, internuclear chromatin bridges were found in 1.59% (range 0.60–2.83%) of patients with CDA type I, but in none of the normal controls.

Electron microscopy shows a characteristic "spongy" appearance of the heterochromatin, enlargement of the nuclear

Table 7.5. Characteristic features of the major subtypes of congenital dyserythropoietic anemias.

	Type I	Type II (HAMPAS)	Type III (familial)
Peripheral blood	Moderate anemia Elevated MCV (70%) Macrocytes present even if MCV is normal Marked anisopoikilocytosis Basophilic stippling Cabot ring (rare) Rare nucleated RBC	Mild to moderate anemia MCV – normal or minimally elevated Moderate anisopoikilocytosis Basophilic stippling Rare nucleated RBC	Mild macrocytic anemia due to ineffective erythropoiesis and intravascular hemolysis Moderate anisopoikilocytosis Basophilic stippling
Bone marrow findings	Megaloblastoid erythroid maturation Polychromatic erythroblasts – binucleated forms <10% Multiple nuclei have different sizes Intranuclear chromatin bridges (rare)	Normoblastic maturation Binucleated forms 10–45%, orthochromic erythroblasts Multiple nuclei have similar size	Giant multinucleated erythroblasts[a] with up to 12 nuclei per cell and DNA content up to 14 C[b] The individual nuclei of some multinucleated cells vary in size and DNA content
Ultrastructural studies	Spongy, "Swiss cheese" chromatin Typical binucleated forms Intranuclear chromatin bridges Peripheral condensation of the nuclear chromatin due to apoptosis Iron-loaded mitochondria	Peripheral double membrane due to excess of rough endoplasmic reticulum	Non-specific – intranuclear clefts and karyorrhexis
Laboratory abnormalities	Ham test negative High bilirubin Increased ferritin Decreased glycosylation	Ham test positive (characteristic) High bilirubin Increased ferritin Impaired globin chain synthesis Defective glycosylation	Ham test negative Slightly increased bilirubin Normal iron, ferritin, and transferrin Evidence of intravascular hemolysis: Decreased or absent haptoglobin Markedly elevated LDH Hemosiderinuria
Other abnormalities	Iron overload Gallstones 80–90% splenomegaly Congenital anomalies	Iron overload ~20% develop liver cirrhosis Gallstones Splenomegaly Congenital anomalies (infrequent)	No iron overload High incidence of lymphoproliferative disorders
Inheritance	Autosomal recessive	Autosomal recessive South Italy, founder effect	Autosomal dominant Several families in northern Sweden, North America, and Argentina Autosomal recessive in sporadic forms
Locus/gene	15q15.1 (CDAN1)	Linkage to 20q11.2	Linkage to 15q22 in multiplex families

[a] A non-specific finding that can be seen in myelodysplastic syndromes.
[b] C = haploid DNA content.

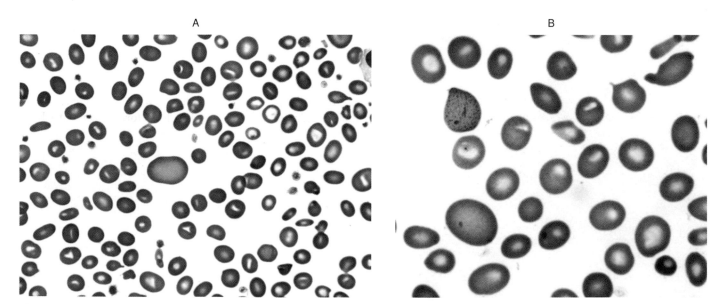

Fig. 7.5. A peripheral blood smear from a five-year-old boy with congenital dyserythropoietic anemia, type I (Wright–Giemsa stain). (A) Notice the presence of macroovalocytes, normocytes, microspherocytes, and teardrop-shaped erythrocytes. (B) Coarse basophilic stippling.

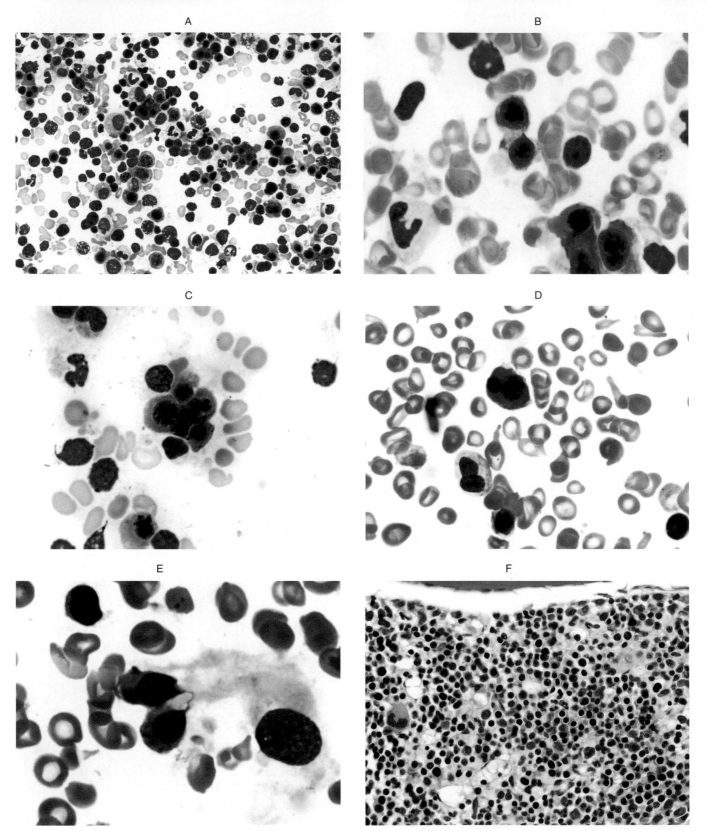

Fig. 7.6. Bone marrow from the same child as Fig. 7.5. (A) Notice the marked erythroid hyperplasia and dyserythropoiesis (Wright–Giemsa stain). (B–E) Examples of dyserythropoiesis, intranuclear bridges, karyorrhexis, and the uneven size of the dysplastic nuclear lobes (Wright–Giemsa stain). (F) A bone marrow biopsy shows hypercellular bone marrow with marked erythroid hyperplasia and myeloid hypoplasia (H&E stain).

A   B

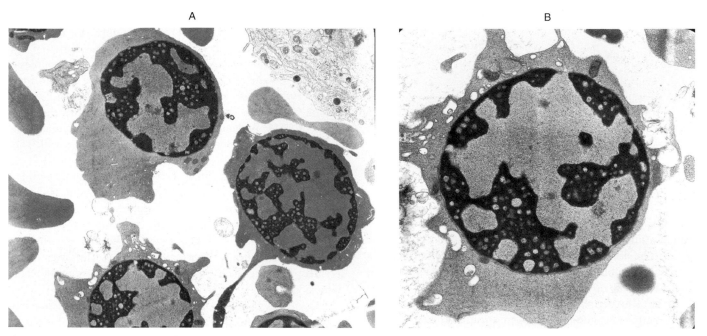

Fig. 7.7. Electron microscopy of the bone marrow of the same child as Fig. 7.5 shows erythroblasts with the characteristics of congenital dyserythropoietic anemia, type I "Swiss cheese" (spongy) appearance of the heterochromatin.

pores, and marked invagination of the nuclear membrane, carrying cytoplasm and cytoplasmic organelles into the nuclear territory. These changes result in a "Swiss cheese" appearance of the erythroblasts (Fig. 7.7). Typical binucleated forms with nuclear bridges can also be seen. Peripheral condensation of heterochromatin and disruption of nuclear pores, features characteristic of apoptosis, indicating an increased cell death, are present as well. Iron-loaded mitochondria can also be seen.

CDA type I is inherited as an autosomal recessive disorder. The disease gene has been identified and designated as *CDAN1*, and mutations were identified in affected Israeli Bedouin and European individuals [37, 38]. The *CDAN1* gene encodes codanin-1, a protein of still-unknown function. The majority of the mutations at the *CDAN1* gene are missense mutations resulting in a single amino acid substitution. Nonsense mutations, splice site mutations, and nucleotide insertions and deletions are uncommon. No cases of homozygosity for null-type mutation have been reported, thus indicating that the function of codanin-1 is essential during fetal development [32]. There is no correlation between the level of codanin-1 expression, or the nature of the mutation, and the severity of the disease. While mutations at *CDAN1* have been reported in both familial and sporadic cases of CDA type I, other gene(s) may be involved in the pathogenesis of the disease, since no mutations in the coding region of this gene have been detected in some sporadic cases of confirmed CDA type I [39].

Congenital dyserythropoietic anemia type II (OMIM 224100)

CDA type II, also known as hereditary erythroblastic multinuclearity with a positive acidified serum test (HEMPAS), is the most common type of CDA. It occurs in approximately 1 in 100 000 births per year [31]. The disease is inherited in autosomal recessive fashion. A high proportion of reported families are from south Italy, suggesting a founder effect. Cases from northwest Europe, North Africa, and India have also been reported [29, 31].

CDA type II presents with anemia and/or jaundice in childhood or young adults, somewhat later in life than is so for the CDA type I. In a large collection of patients, the mean age of diagnosis was 18.2 years (with a range from 0.1 to 78 years), and most of the individuals were diagnosed in the first three decades of life [40]. A majority of individuals with CDA type II develop progressive splenomegaly, gallstones, and iron overload as a consequence of the ineffective erythropoiesis and increased red cell destruction. In about 20% of the patients, iron overload leads to liver cirrhosis or cardiac failure [31, 40]. Dysmorphic features are less frequent in CDA type II as compared to CDA type I.

The anemia in CDA type II is mild to moderate, and most cases have baseline hemoglobin levels between 8 and 11 g/dL [31]. MCV is normal in most of the cases, but rare cases have been reported with elevated MCV. There is moderate-to-marked anisocytosis, anisochromasia, and poikilocytosis of the red blood cells, including tear-drop shaped forms, microcytes, spherocytes, and macroovalocytes. Basophilic stippling is present. There is no significant polychromasia, and the reticulocyte count is inappropriately low for the degree of anemia.

The bone marrow shows marked hypercellularity due to erythroid hyperplasia and pronounced dyserythropoiesis. Ten to forty-five percent (median, 20%) of the late polychromatophilic erythroblasts are binucleated, and a small number are multinucleated. The multiple nuclei have similar size. A proportion of the orthochromic erythroblasts show basophilic stippling.

Table 7.6. Diagnostic criteria for CDA type II: presence of all A criteria and at least one B criterion is required.

A criteria
  A1 : Evidence of congenital or hereditary anemia/jaundice
  A2 : Evidence of ineffective erythropoiesis
  A3 : Typical morphology of bone marrow erythroblasts, with at least 10% binucleated precursors

B criteria
  B1 : Positive acid lysis test with at least 20% of normal serum
  B2 : Typical abnormalities of bands 3 and 4.5 in SDS-PAGE
  B3 : Double membrane running internally from the cell membrane of late erythroblasts seen on electron microscopy

Reprinted with permission from Heimpel et al. [40].

A small number of lipid-laden macrophages, pseudo-Gaucher cells, can be seen in some cases. Electron microscopy shows stretches of double membrane (peripheral cisternae) running parallel to, 40–60 nm away from, the membrane of the erythroblasts [31]. The peripheral cisternae represent excess of rough endoplasmic reticulum. It has been speculated that a functional/maturation abnormality of endoplasmic reticulum may account for the defective glycosylation of the red cell membrane seen in CDA type II [31].

The acidified serum test is characteristically positive in CDA type II, but a sucrose hemolysis test is negative. This helps in distinguishing CDA type II from paroxysmal nocturnal hemoglobinuria (PNH). CDA type II erythrocytes have decreased glycosylation and, as a result, they have an abnormal band 3 (the anion transport protein) and band 4.5 (glucose transporter 1) migration on sodium dodecyl sulfate polyacrylamide gel electrophoresis (SDS-PAGE) [31]. These abnormalities are due to abnormal processing of N-glycans [41].

For over 30 years, biochemical studies have failed to clearly reveal a CDA type II gene, and genetic analysis has not found causative mutation in the genes coding for the proposed enzymes. In 1997, a genome-wide linkage analysis localized the CDA type II locus to a 5 cM region on chromosome 20q11.2 [42]. Nevertheless, more than 10 years later, the CDA type II gene still has not been found in this region. Several genes have been sequenced but have failed to confirm the presence of mutation [43].

The diagnostic criteria of CDA type II are summarized in Table 7.6. They include evidence of congenital or hereditary anemia/jaundice, ineffective erythropoiesis, and typical morphology of bone marrow erythroblasts, with at least 10% binucleated precursors, along with at least one of the following: a positive acid lysis test with at least 20% of normal serum, or typical abnormalities of bands 3 and 4.5 on sodium dodecyl sulfate polyacrylamide gel electrophoresis (SDS-PAGE), or characteristic electron microscopy findings [40].

Congenital dyserythropoietic anemia type III (OMIM 1056000)

CDA type III is the least common form of congenital dyserythropoietic anemia. Both familial and sporadic cases have been reported. The majority of the known patients belong to several families living in a northern Swedish county (Västerbotten), North America, and Argentina [44]. As with types I and II, CDA type III patients present with anemia and dyserythropoiesis. However, the anemia is never severe and is due to both ineffective erythropoiesis and mild intravascular hemolysis [29]. As a result, there is no significant iron overload. Unlike the other forms of CDA, patients with type III also have a higher incidence of lymphoproliferative disorders, the causes of which are poorly understood [44].

Mild to moderate anemia, with normal or slightly elevated MCV and a normal or slightly low reticulocyte count, is characteristic. The blood film shows moderate-to-marked anisopoikilocytosis, characteristic large macrocytes, and basophilic stippling. The bilirubin is slightly increased in most patients but there are no significant abnormalities in the serum iron, transferrin, or ferritin. The haptoglobin is low or absent and there is hemosiderinuria.

Despite its rarity, CDA type III should be considered in neonates, children, and adults with anemia with normal or slightly elevated MCV having marked anisopoikilocytosis and evidence of hemolysis, particularly if there is a family history of anemia. A bone marrow examination is usually diagnostic and should be performed early. It shows characteristic giant erythroblasts with either a single nucleus or with up to 12 nuclei per cell. Other dysplastic features are often seen, such as basophilic stippling, nuclear lobulation, and karyorrhexis.

Unlike the other types of CDA, the familial cases of type III follow autosomal dominant inheritance with full penetrance. Linkage analysis of a large multiplex family localized the disease gene (CDAN3) to a locus on chromosome 15q22, distal to the CDAN1 gene.

Other types of congenital dyserythropoietic anemia

Some of the reported cases of CDA cannot be classified as type I–III, and these patients have been tentatively classified based on their phenotypic characteristics into CDA groups IV, V, VI, and VII [36, 45, 46]. The characteristic features of these types are summarized in Table 7.7.

Differential diagnosis of CDA

The differential diagnosis of CDA includes other congenital and acquired disorders associated with dyserythropoiesis, such as thalassemia; certain hemoglobinopathies, for example hemoglobin C and hemoglobin E diseases; anemia due to unstable hemoglobins; hereditary sideroblastic anemia; nutritional deficiencies such as B_{12} and folic acid deficiencies; heavy metal poisoning; liver disease; or myelodysplastic syndrome (MDS).

Disorders of granulopoiesis

Neutrophils, produced in the bone marrow under the direction of cytokines – the most important of which is the granulocyte colony stimulating factor (G-CSF) – are an essential part

Table 7.7. Characteristic features of congenital dyserythropoietic anemia groups IV to VI.

	CDA group IV	CDA group V	CDA group VI
Anemia	Severe transfusion-dependent anemia present at birth	Normal or near normal hemoglobin	Normal to near normal hemoglobin
MCV	Normal or slightly elevated	Normal or slightly elevated	Marked macrocytosis (MCV 120–130 fL)
Erythropoiesis	Normoblastic or slightly megaloblastic	Usually normoblastic	Megaloblastoid
Bone marrow	Non-specific dyserythropoiesis Absence of changes characteristic of CDA types I–III	Marked erythroid hyperplasia with minimal or mild dyserythropoiesis	Erythroid hyperplasia with marked megaloblastoid maturation
Laboratory abnormalities	Negative Ham test	Negative Ham test Unconjugated hyperbilirubinemia	Negative Ham test

Data from Wickramasinghe *et al.* [36, 45], and Renella *et al.* [46].

of the immune system. Neutropenia or abnormal neutrophil function results in an inadequate innate immune host response to bacterial and fungal infections. The total white blood cell count and the absolute neutrophil count (ANC) depend upon age and, as has recently been discovered, are genetically determined [47, 48]. At birth, newborns have a relatively high ANC that decreases gradually to reach a nadir at 72 hours of life and then increases to reach a stable level by five days of life [49]. The low limit of ANC in term Caucasian infants, aged two weeks to one year of life, is lower than that of adults (1×10^9/L vs. 1.5×10^9/L), and this difference is even more dramatic in African-American infants. Their ANC low limits are 0.2–0.6×10^9/L lower, as compared to Caucasian children [50]. The absolute neutrophil count of premature newborns is even lower than this. Thus, the cut off for ANC-defining neutropenia in children will vary depending upon both the age and race of the child.

The degree of neutropenia determines its clinical significance. When mild (ANC $< 1.5 \times 10^9$/L) or moderate (ANC $< 1 \times 10^9$/L), neutropenias are clinically asymptomatic. Severe neutropenia (ANC $< 0.5 \times 10^9$/L) and "agranulocytosis," a term reserved for ANC below 0.2×10^9/L, lead to serious bacterial and fungal infections such as cellulitis, furunculosis, superficial and deep abscesses, pneumonia, and septicemia. Since the neutrophils are not an essential part of the host defense against viruses and parasites, neutropenic patients are not at an increased risk of developing such infections.

Neutrophils have a half life of about four hours. A constant production by the bone marrow and proper distribution in the periphery are necessary to keep the neutrophil count in the peripheral blood steady. Neutropenia occurs when either the bone marrow production is impaired, the distribution is altered and neutrophils shift from the marginated to tissue pool, or when there is an increased peripheral utilization or destruction. Depending upon the factors leading to ineffective granulocytopoiesis, the neutropenias can be divided into *intrinsic* – arising as a single abnormality or as a part of a broader bone marrow failure syndrome – or *acquired* due to increased clearance or destruction by antineutrophil antibodies, drugs, infection,

or other causes (Tables 7.8 and 7.9). Based on the molecular pathogenesis and underlying genetic defect, the neutropenias can be classified into disorders of granulocytopoiesis, disorders due to ribosomal dysfunction, vesicular transport, metabolism, and abnormal immune function.

Severe congenital neutropenia (OMIM 202700)

Severe congenital neutropenia (SCN) is genetically and phenotypically a heterogeneous group of bone marrow failure disorders characterized by maturation arrest of the granulopoiesis at the promyelocyte–myelocyte stage, which results in isolated low neutrophil counts and frequent bacterial infectious during early infancy and an increased risk of developing leukemia. The disorder was first described as an autosomal recessive infantile congenital agranulocytosis in several consanguineous Swedish families more than 50 years ago [54]. Following Kostmann's report, multiple cases with the same phenotype but with other types of inheritance, such as autosomal dominant, as well as sporadic forms have been reported. Currently, the term *severe congenital neutropenia* (OMIM 202700) is used to define the entire disorder regardless of the mode of inheritance or genotype. *Kostmann disease* (OMIM 610738) is reserved for the autosomal recessive form of severe congenital neutropenia only.

The diagnosis of SCN requires repeat differential counts indicating persistent neutropenia with an ANC range from 0 to 0.5×10^9/L [52]. Clinically, SCN presents with frequent episodes of fever, skin infections, stomatitis, pneumonia, or perirectal abscesses in the first three months of life. Stomatitis, gingivitis, and periodontitis may be the initial presentation of the disease.

In SCN, the peripheral blood ANC is usually below 0.2×10^9/L. Relative monocytosis and eosinophilia are usually present, but anemia and thrombocytopenia are infrequent. The levels of serum immunoglobulins are often elevated. Antineutrophil antibodies are usually absent, although not always. The bone marrow of such patients shows a maturation arrest of the granulopoiesis at the promyelocyte–myelocyte stage (Fig. 7.8).

Table 7.8. Selected neutropenias due to intrinsic defects in granulocytes or their precursors.

	Genes/locus	Clinical features
Neutropenia associated with disorders of granulopoiesis		
Severe congenital neutropenia (AD, AR)	ELA2 (19p13.3) GFI1 (1p21) G-CSFR (1p35–p34.3)	Neutropenia, MDS, AML
Kostmann disease (AR)	HAX1 (1q21.3)	
Cyclic neutropenia (AD)	ELA2 (19p13.3)	Alternate 21 day cycles of neutrophils and monocytes
Neutropenia associated with disorders of ribosomal dysfunction (covered in Chapter 6)		
Shwachman–Diamond syndrome (AR)	SBDS (7q11)	Pancreatic insufficiency; moderate to severe neutropenia; normochromic, normocytic anemia (~50%); thrombocytopenia (~50%); pancytopenia (10–40%)
Dyskeratosis congenita (XLR, AD, AR)	DKC (Xq28) TERC (3q21–q28) TERT (5p15.33)	Abnormal skin pigmentation, nail dystrophy, oral leukoplakia, pancytopenia
Congenital neutropenias as a component of immune deficiency syndromes		
Reticular dysgenesis	AK2 on 1p34	Severe agranulocytosis and lymphopenia, defective humoral immunity, absence of secondary lymphoid organs
Hyper IgM syndrome (XLR)	CD40L (Xp26)	Neutropenia, pancytopenia
Cartilage hair hypoplasia (AR)	RMRP (9p21–p12)	Neutropenia, lymphopenia, macrocytic anemia
Common variable immunodeficiency (probably AR)	TNFRSF13B (17p11.2)	Neutropenia, decreased IgG and IgM
Disorders of vesicular transport (albinism/neutropenia syndromes)		
Chédiak–Higashi syndrome (AR)	LYST/CHS1 (1q42.1–q42.2)	Partial oculocutaneous albinism, mild bleeding diathesis, predisposition to life-threatening hemophagocytic syndrome following EBV infection, moderate neutropenia
Cohen syndrome (AR)	COH1 (8q22–q23)	Mental retardation, pigmentary retinopathy, facial dysmorphism, neutropenia
Griscelli syndrome, type II (AR)	RAB27A (15q15–q21.1)	Varying degree of neutropenia, hypogammaglobulinemia, partial albinism, predisposition to terminal lymphohistiocytic proliferation with hemophagocytic syndrome
Hermanski–Pudlak syndrome, type 2	AP3B1 (5q14.1)	Oculocutaneous albinism, platelet defects, neutropenia
Neutropenia associated with disorders of metabolism		
Barth syndrome (XLR)	TAZ1 (Xq28)	Dilated cardiomyopathy, 3-methylglutaconic aciduria, growth retardation, neutropenia, may be cycling
Glycogen storage disease type 1B (AR)	G6PT1 (11q23)	Severe neutropenia, neutrophil functional abnormality
Pearson syndrome	Mitochondrial DNA deletion	Macrocytic anemia, neutropenia and or thrombocytopenia; striking vacuolations of the erythroid and myeloid precursors

Abbreviations: AD, autosomal dominant; AR, autosomal recessive; XLR, X-linked recessive.
Data from Boxer *et al.* [51], Berliner *et al.* [52], Dinauer *et al.* [53], and Online Mendelian Inheritance in Man, OMIM.

While the number of promyelocytes is increased, no mature forms beyond a myelocyte stage are present. Dysgranulopoiesis manifested by large atypical nuclei and cytoplasmic vacuoles is frequently seen. The overall bone marrow cellularity is appropriate or mildly decreased for age. The erythropoiesis and megakaryopoiesis are not usually affected. Since most of the patients are diagnosed early in life, a large number of normal B-cell progenitors are also present (Fig. 7.9). These morphologic characteristics, independently of the underlying genetic defect, are consistently present in all patients with SCN.

Another clinical phenotype of SCN manifested in infancy or early childhood is *cyclic neutropenia (CN)*. With CN, the numbers of neutrophils and monocytes undulate in opposite directions in approximately 21-day cycles [55]. During the period of neutropenia, patients present with fever and infections that resolve when the neutrophil counts improve. Even so, peak neutrophil counts may or may not reach normal levels. The neutropenia is usually associated with monocytosis as well as some anemia and thrombocytopenia. Consequentially,

cyclic hematopoiesis has been proposed as a term to define this disorder.

In CN, the bone marrow findings vary depending on the peripheral blood counts. During the time of neutropenia, the bone marrow shows an absence of granulocyte precursors or maturation arrest. This is followed by restoration of the granulopoiesis and improvement of the ANC in the peripheral blood. The differential diagnosis includes other disorders, such as cyclic fever with neutropenia and hyper IgM syndrome, where neutropenia is a part of the syndrome. However, the neutropenia in these disorders follows a different pattern. To establish the diagnosis of CN, the neutrophil count should be monitored at least once and preferentially twice per week for six to eight weeks.

Current data suggest that SCN is a multigene disorder. Mutational analysis of 122 patients with SCN, followed up by the European Branch of the Severe Congenital Neutropenia International Registry, is shown in Fig. 7.10 [56]. A quarter of the patients with SCN have no identifiable mutations so far.

Table 7.9. Causes of acquired neutropenia in children.

Disorders	Characteristic features
Neonatal alloimmune neutropenia	Neutrophil-specific maternal IgG due to maternal alloimmunization Affected infants may be asymptomatic
Autoimmune neutropenia	Primary, most frequent in infants and young children Secondary, as a part of autoimmune disorder (hemolytic anemia, immune-mediated thrombocytopenia, Evans syndrome) Antineutrophil antibodies, presumed peripheral destruction of antibody-coated neutrophils

Drug-induced neutropenia	Most common classes
	Antimicrobials:
	    Trimethoprim/sulfamethoxazole[a]
	    Penicillins
	    Chloramphenicol
	Anticonvulsant – valproic acid
	Anti-thyroid – *propylthiouracil*
	Anti-psychotics – *clozapine*
	Idiosyncratic reactions, immune-mediated destruction, or direct toxicity

Infection	Most frequently viral infection (EBV, hepatitis A and B, HIV, influenza A and B, measles, RSV, parvovirus B19, rubella, varicella) Sepsis, neonatal bacterial sepsis
Nutritional deficiencies	B_{12} or folic acid deficiency Bone marrow – megaloblastoid maturation
Reticuloendothelial sequestration	Hypersplenism due to portal hypertension, moderate neutropenia
Bone marrow infiltration	Bone marrow involvement by leukemia, lymphoma, or solid tumors Granulomatous infections, lysosomal storage diseases, osteopetrosis
Chronic idiopathic neutropenia	Poorly understood disorders with variable clinical features, bone marrow findings, and clinical history

[a] Italicized are the drugs with highest relative risk of causing neutropenia.
RSV = respiratory syncytial virus.

The most common genetic abnormality is a heterozygous mutation at the *ELA2* (19p13.3) gene, encoding neutrophil elastase (NE) [56–58]. *ELA2* is specifically transcribed in promyelocytes and promonocytes of the marrow, but its protein, NE, persists in the cell through terminal differentiation to a mature neutrophil or monocyte [59]. NE is a potent serine protease localized primarily to the azurophilic neutrophil granules and to the cell surface and intracellular membranes.

Heterozygous mutations at *ELA2* are found in approximately 50–60% of patients with SCN, suggesting a dominant mechanism of inheritance. These mutations, however, are also found in sporadic cases. Furthermore, mutations at *ELA2* are found in patients with SCN and CN (both inherited in autosomal dominant fashion); they are not present in patients with autosomal recessive SCN or Kostmann syndrome. Genetic analysis show mutations at the same site of the *ELA2* gene in both

SCN and CN, thus suggesting a lack of genotype–phenotype correlation [60].

The mechanism by which a heterozygous mutation at *ELA2* results in neutropenia is still not well understood. While various mutations at the gene have been identified, the lack of genotype–phenotype correlation suggests that structural rather than enzymatic activity of the NE is responsible for development of neutropenia. Recent studies have hypothesized that mutations at *ELA2* lead to production of misfolded NE protein in the endoplasmic reticulum, which induces unfolded protein response (UPR) and subsequent UPR-dependent apoptosis [61, 62]. However, the pathogenic mechanism responsible for the development of different phenotypes, congenital or cyclic neutropenia, is still unknown.

Homozygous mutations at another gene, *HAX1*, are identified in about one-third of patients with SCN, including some of the original families reported by Kostmann, thus supporting at molecular level the autosomal recessive type of inheritance [63]. *HAX1* encodes a mitochondrial protein that has a distant structural similarity with the anti-apoptotic members of the *BCL2* family. HAX1 protein is a critical regulator of the mitochondrial membrane potential and cellular viability, so that a homozygous mutation at *HAX1* results in a loss of function and increased apoptosis [60]. However, how mutations at *HAX1* lead specifically to premature neutrophil death and neutropenia in humans is uncertain and still under active investigation.

Rare mutations at other genes, such as *G6PC3*, *GFI1*, *WASP*, *p14*, and *TAZ*, have also been shown to result in severe congenital neutropenia (for in-depth review see [56, 64]). In addition, inherited mutations in the G-CSF receptor gene (*G-CSFR*) have been reported in SCN [52, 65]. However, such mutations rarely cause SCN.

Genetic testing is commercially available and clinically useful in discriminating between acquired and hereditary neutropenia, and in identifying patients who are candidates for hematopoietic stem cell transplant.

G-CSF is a standard treatment for *SCN* that has greatly improved the survival of these patients. More than 90% of patients respond to the therapy with an increase in the ANC of more than 1×10^9/L and clinical resolution of infections [66]. For those who do not respond to such therapy, the only currently available option is hematopoietic stem cell transplantation.

It is well established that a significant portion of patients with SCN develop leukemia, but the underlying mechanisms are yet to be discovered [67, 68]. Myelodysplastic syndrome/acute myeloid leukemias are the most frequent type of leukemia, and abnormalities of chromosome 7 are the most frequent cytogenetic abnormality [69].

The risk of malignant transformation seams to correlate with the length of G-CSF therapy, and is further increased in less-responsive patients that require higher doses [56]. In addition, more than 80% of the patients with SCN who develop acute leukemia have acquired *G-CSFR* mutations (*CSF3R*), suggesting that such mutations play a role in the leukemogenesis [60, 70].

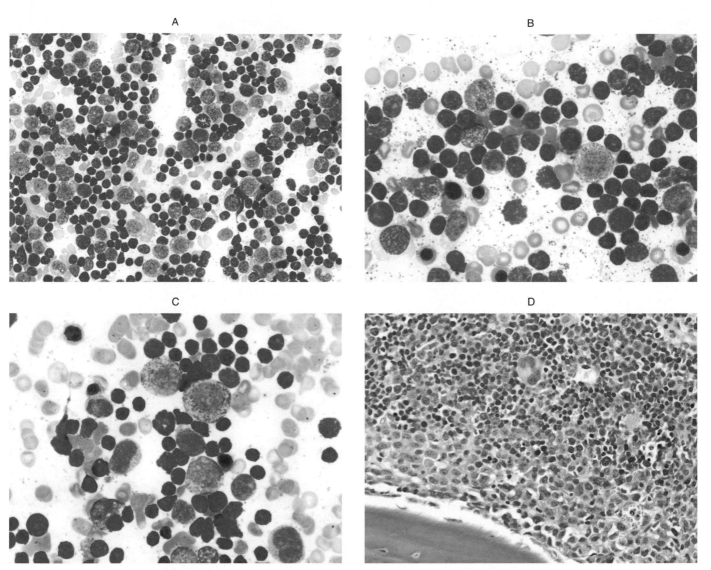

Fig. 7.8. Bone marrow from a child with severe congenital neutropenia due to a heterozygous *ELA2* mutation. (A) Bone marrow aspirate at diagnosis at five months of age shows a striking paucity of mature granulocytes. Small numbers of promyelocytes and an occasional myelocyte are present. Notice the unremarkable eosinophils (Wright–Giemsa stain). (B) There is an increased number of hematogones (Wright–Giemsa stain). (C) Bone marrow aspirate after treatment with high doses of G-CSF for three years shows an increased number of granulocytes with a marked shift to immaturity (Wright–Giemsa stain). (D) The bone marrow is hypercellular and shows a marked granulocytic shift to immaturity (H&E stain).

This risk of leukemia is present in sporadic, autosomal recessive, and autosomal dominant forms of SCN, and is unrelated to the mutational status of *ELA2* or *HAX1* [71]. However, patients with CN, who have a mutation at *ELA2*, are not at increased risk of developing leukemia.

Congenital neutropenia as a component of immune deficiency syndromes

Congenital neutropenia may be a component of many congenital immune deficiency syndromes, such as reticular dysgenesis, hyper IgM syndrome, X-linked agammaglobulinemia, cartilage syndrome, and Wiscott–Aldrich syndrome (WAS).

Reticular dysgenesis (RD) is an extremely rare autosomal recessive form of congenital neutropenia associated with severe combined immune deficiency [72, 73]. Such patients have a defective cellular and humoral immunity due to lymphoid tissue depletion, including thymic dysplasia, and thus can develop overwhelming infections and die shortly after birth.

While the peripheral blood shows consistent leukopenia from birth, the number of lymphocytes varies from none to normal. When present, B-cells, particularly CD5+ naïve B-cells, are the predominant lymphocyte population, and the T-cells are virtually absent (Fig. 7.11) [73]. The bone marrow in RD is hypocellular and shows maturation arrest at the promyelocyte–myelocyte stage. There is a conspicuous absence of mature

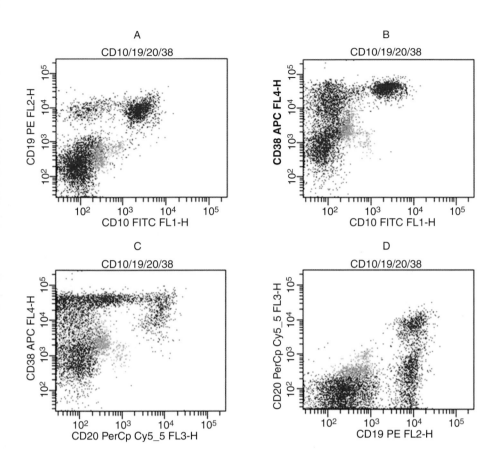

Fig. 7.9. Multiparameter flow cytometry of bone marrow from the same child as Fig. 7.8 shows an increased number of CD10+/CD19+ normal B-cell progenitors (A) with bright CD38 expression (B and C) and a heterogeneous expression of CD20 (C and D) consistent with B-cell maturation characteristic for hematogones. Recognizing the maturation pattern is particularly important in such cases, in order to avoid misdiagnosis of acute lymphoblastic leukemia.

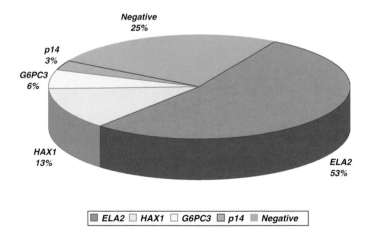

Fig. 7.10. Genetic distribution of 122 patients with SCN from the European Branch of the Severe Chronic Neutropenia International Registry tested for *ELA2, HAX1, G6PC3,* or *p14.* (Redrawn with permission from Welte, Zeidler [56].)

neutrophils, while the number of the normal B-cell progenitors, hematogones, is markedly increased. The erythropoiesis and megakaryopoiesis are unaffected.

With respect to RD, recent studies show mutations at the *adenylate kinase 2 (AK2)* gene, encoding a protein involved in mitochondrial energy metabolism [74]. Unlike the other congenital neutropenias, patients with RD do not respond to growth factor therapy (G-CSF or GM-CSF). Bone marrow transplantation is the only form of successful therapy [73].

Disorders of vesicular transport (albinism/neutropenia syndromes)

This is a group of rare autosomal recessive disorders caused by defects in the formation or trafficking of lysosome-related organelles, which clinically manifest with a constellation of neutropenia, and partial albinism.

Chédiak–Higashi syndrome (CHS), the prototype of the disorder, is characterized by severe immune deficiency, recurrent pyogenic infections, abnormal NK function, bleeding diathesis, variable forms of albinism, and neuropathies [75]. The hematologic abnormalities of CHS, summarized in Table 7.10, extend beyond the granulocytic lineage. The syndrome is lethal. The patients either succumb from bacterial infection or develop a poorly understood lymphohistiocytic proliferative syndrome and macrophage activation termed "accelerated phase" [76]. The only therapeutic option for CHS is a bone marrow transplantation.

The morphologic hallmark of CHS is the presence of giant, abnormally enlarged granules or lysosome-related organelles such as lysosomes, melanosomes, platelet-dense granules, and cytoplasmic granules in the cells, which in the peripheral blood are manifested as giant granules of the mature granulocytes (Fig. 7.12). The number of granules varies. Some patients may have only a few granules. The presence of giant peroxidase-positive lysosomal granules in the peripheral blood

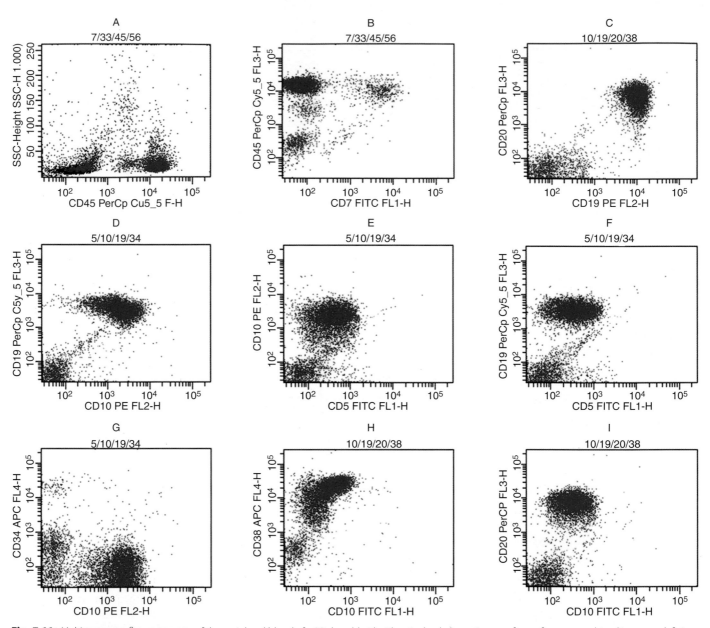

Fig. 7.11. Multiparameter flow cytometry of the peripheral blood of a 39-day-old girl with reticular dysgenesis, a rare form of severe combined immune deficiency. (A) A CD45 side scatter histogram shows a paucity of granulocytes and a large lymphocytic population (CD45 bright). (B) Only a small number of them are CD7+ T-cells. (C–F) Instead, the majority are CD19+/CD20+ B-cells with moderate expression of CD10 and dim expression of CD5. (G) These cells are CD34 negative. (H–I) While the CD10/CD38 expression pattern suggests some degree of maturation, these cells have a uniform CD20 expression, suggesting that they are mature B-cells. Hematopoietic stem cell transplant and successful engraftment resulted in normalization of the peripheral blood lymphocyte subsets.

neutrophils and bone marrow myeloid progenitors in patients with hypopigmentation of the hair, recurrent infections, bleeding diathesis, and unexplained hepatosplenomegaly is diagnostic of CHS.

CHS is caused by mutations in the lysosomal trafficking regulator gene *LYST* [77, 78]. Such mutations affect the morphology and function of lysosome-related organelles. The nature of the mutation can predict the severity of the disease

Other disorders of vesicular transport are extremely rare causes of clinically significant congenital neutropenia.

Inherited disorders associated with abnormal white blood cell morphology

Pelger–Huët anomaly (PHA) is an autosomal dominant disorder characterized by functionally normal, but abnormally segmented neutrophils and eosinophils [79]. The clinical significance of this anomaly lies in the need to distinguish Pelger–Huët (PH) forms from immature granulocytes such as bands or pseudo-PH forms that are seen in primary or secondary dysgranulopoiesis.

Table 7.10. Hematologic manifestation of Chédiak–Higashi syndrome.

Peripheral blood
  Neutropenia, mild to moderate
    Abnormal neutrophils with giant azurophilic-specific granules
    Abnormal neutrophil function
    Decreased bactericidal activity due to decreased hemotaxis *in vivo*
      and *in vitro*
    Delayed and incomplete degradation
  Monocytes/macrophages
    Ring-shaped lysosomes
    Decreased chemotaxis
  Lymphocytes/NK-cells
    Giant cytoplasmic granules
    Decreased natural killer function
    Decreased antibody-dependent cell-mediated cytolysis
  Platelets
    Giant cytoplasmic granules
    Abnormal aggregation as a result of storage pool deficiency of ADP
      and serotonin

Bone marrow abnormalities
  Ineffective granulopoiesis
    Vacuolization of marrow neutrophils
    Increased intramedullary destruction of granulocytes

Accelerated phase (lymphoproliferative disorder)
  Worsening multiple cytopenias (neutropenia, thrombocytopenia,
    anemia)
    Hepatosplenomegaly
    Bone marrow lymphocytosis
    Hemophagocytosis

In the peripheral blood, almost all neutrophils and eosinophils have only two lobes. They either overlap or are connected by a thin thread giving the characteristic "pince-nez" appearance (Fig. 7.13). Mononuclear variants are also present. The PH forms have condensed, mature chromatin and normal granules in the cytoplasm, features helping to distinguish them from immature/band forms. Regardless of the number of lobes, these cells are mature neutrophils and need to be reported as such.

PHA is due to mutations at the lamin B receptor (*LBR*) gene, a protein essential for the nuclear segmentation of granulocytes [80]. A single dominant mutation at the *LBR* gene results in a lack of segmentation and bilobed PH neutrophils and eosinophils. Individuals with homozygous mutations completely lack segmentation and, as a result, most of their neutrophils have a single oval nucleus (Fig. 7.14). While LBR protein is required for the nuclear segmentation of the neutrophils, it is not essential for neutrophil functions such as chemotaxis or microbicidal activity, including respiratory burst [81, 82].

The differential diagnosis of PHA includes a variety of acquired conditions manifested by hyposegmented neutrophils, or pseudo-Pelger–Huët (p-PH) forms, summarized in Table 7.11. In such conditions, p-PH forms are a minority and rarely exceed 25–30% of the neutrophils. By contrast, in PHA, almost all neutrophils and eosinophils are hyposegmented [79]. In primary myelodysplasia, in addition to hyposegmentation, the neutrophils have abnormal granularity and other features of dysgranulopoiesis. Such changes are present in a small subset of neutrophils, and normally segmented forms are also present. In addition, dyserythropoiesis and abnormal platelets, as well as peripheral cytopenias, are usually present.

The distinction of PH forms from immature neutrophils/ bands is particularly important in neonates and infants, in order to avoid an erroneous diagnosis of a severe bacterial infection and unnecessary treatment [83]. The exclusive presence of mononuclear or bilobed neutrophils and absence of toxic granulations, vacuolations, or Döhle bodies, is supportive of PHA. On the other hand, leukocytosis, neutrophilia with shift to immaturity including myelocytes and metamyelocytes, and toxic changes support the presence of infection. Some drugs such as valproic acid, mycophenolate mofetil, and ganciclovir, alone or in combination, have been shown to induce secondary p-PH changes [84–86]. Proper recognition of these changes is of paramount importance since these individuals are at high risk of infections.

The simplest way to confirm the inherited nature of PHA in a child is to demonstrate the same anomaly in the peripheral blood of the biologic parents, since the anomaly is inherited in autosomal dominant fashion.

Congenital thrombocytopenias

The congenital thrombocytopenias are a heterogeneous group of disorders with various modes of inheritance that are characterized by thrombocytopenia and variable bleeding tendency, as well as an array of physical stigmata. While some of these disorders are associated with mutations at specific genes, for most the cause is still unknown. A complete characterization of all congenital thrombocytopenias is beyond the scope of a single chapter. Here, we will focus on the more frequent and diagnostically challenging of these ordinarily rare disorders. More comprehensive reviews on the topic can be found elsewhere [87–89].

The degree of thrombocytopenia and platelet function will determine the clinical presentation and need for further workup. While mild congenital thrombocytopenia with adequate platelet function is asymptomatic and may be discovered accidentally, moderate and marked thrombocytopenias leading to increased bleeding will require a workup early in life. The thrombocytopenia or abnormal platelet function leads to petechiae, easy bruising, and mucous membrane bleeding such as epistaxis, gastrointestinal hemorrhage, hematuria, and menorrhagia.

The workup of patients with suspected thrombocytopenia or abnormal platelet function begins with CBC and a careful examination of a well-stained peripheral blood film. The size of the platelets defined by the mean platelet volume (MPV) is genetically determined and can be used to subclassify the thrombocytopenias into those associated with large platelets (macrothrombocytopenias), normal size platelets, or small platelets (microthrombocytopenias) (Table 7.12).

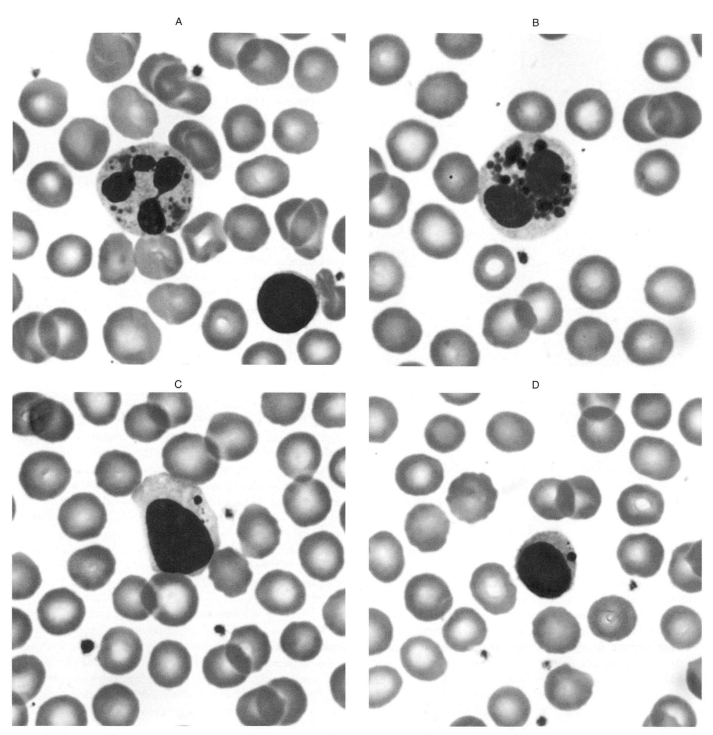

Fig. 7.12. Peripheral blood from a child with Chédiak–Higashi syndrome (Wright–Giemsa stain). (A) A granulocyte with abnormally large lilac cytoplasmic granules. (B) An eosinophil with giant granules. Smaller eosinophilic granules are also present. (C) A monocyte with a single large granule. (D) A lymphocyte with a large granule.

Thrombocytopenias associated with large platelets (macrothrombocytopenia)

The macrothrombocytopenias include clinically and genetically heterogeneous disorders presenting with variable degrees of thrombocytopenia along with consistently large platelets (MPV greater than 11 fL). These disorders are extremely rare. They result from mutations at various unrelated genes that encode proteins with completely different functions. Included among them are the cytoskeleton proteins (*MYH9*-related disorders), glycoprotein GPIb/IX/V complex (Bernard–Soulier syndrome, Mediterranean macrothrombocytopenia/Bernard–Soulier syndrome carrier, and DiGeorge/velocardiofacial syndrome), transcription factors (Paris–Trousseau thrombocytopenia/Jacobsen

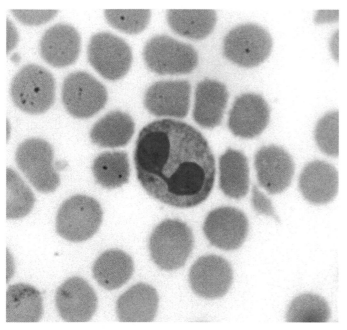

Fig. 7.13. Peripheral blood from a child with Pelger–Huët anomaly shows an abnormally segmented neutrophil with the characteristic "pince-nez" appearance (Wright–Giemsa stain).

syndrome and X-linked macrothrombocytopenia with dyserythropoiesis), or mutations at still undiscovered genes (Gray platelet syndrome).

Macrothrombocytopenia with leukocyte inclusions/ *MYH9*-related disorders

This group of rare disorders, characterized by a triad of thrombocytopenia, giant platelets, and Döhle body-like cytoplasmic inclusions, are caused by various mutations at the *MYH9* gene encoding the heavy chain of the non-muscle myosin IIA (NMMHC-IIA) [90]. The disorders present with a spectrum of clinically overlapping features that were initially described as May–Hegglin, Fechtner, Sebastian, and Epstein syndromes [90–94]. Currently, these are not considered to be separate entities but rather to represent a single disease with a heterogeneous spectrum varying from a mild form of macrothrombocytopenia with leukocyte inclusions to a severe form complicated by hearing loss, cataracts, and/or microscopic hematuria that can develop into severe renal failure [89]. The estimated prevalence of *MYH9*-related disorders in Japan and Italy was found to be approximately 1 in 100 000. Most of the cases are inherited in an autosomal dominant pattern; a minority (about 20%) are due to sporadic germline mutations [87].

Almost all affected subjects have mild to moderate thrombocytopenia as well as leukocyte inclusions, and the patients rarely present with bleeding diathesis. While the platelets are large, they have normal granularity. Examination of a Wright–Giemsa or May–Grünwald–Giemsa-stained peripheral blood film shows bluish opacities or Döhle body-like structures in the cytoplasm of the neutrophils that are otherwise unremarkable. These inclusions consist of mutant NMMHC-IIA protein

(Fig. 7.15). The Döhle-like bodies are best seen on Giemsa-based stained blood films, and may not be present on smears stained with water-based stains. Furthermore, the intensity of the inclusions fades with time, particularly when the blood is stored in ethylenediaminetetraacetic acid (EDTA). Thus, if congenital macrothrombocytopenia is a clinical consideration, direct blood film or immediate preparation of blood films of blood anticoagulated with EDTA would be preferred. The cytoplasmic inclusions vary in size and shape as well as in their ultrastructural characteristics. While in May–Hegglin anomaly the Döhle-like bodies are most prominent, in Epstein syndrome they are not visible on routine Wright–Giemsa staining. Ultrastructural studies show two patterns of Döhle-like bodies – clusters of ribosomes aligned along parallel filaments, as seen in May–Hegglin anomaly, and randomly distributed filaments typical for Sebastian and Fechtner syndromes [89].

All of these disorders result from mutations at the *MYH9* gene encoding NMMHC-IIA, an important cytoskeletal contractile protein in hematopoietic cells. Genotype–phenotype analysis of *MYH9* shows no clear relationship between the site of mutations and clinical presentation and whether the patient will develop Alport syndrome or not [87, 88]. Although the molecular mechanism for macrothrombocytopenia in these patients is not known, it most likely results from defective cytoplasmic blebbing of mature megakaryocytes.

The diagnosis of *MYH9*-related macrothrombocytopenias is based on the examination of peripheral blood smears, the presence of macrothrombocytopenia, and presence of cytoplasmic inclusions (Fig. 7.16). Detection of an abnormal pattern of NMMHC-A by immunofluorescence or molecular studies is confirmatory [95].

Abnormalities in the GPIb/IX/V complex

The disorders are shown in Table 7.13. *Bernard–Soulier syndrome (BSS)*, also known as giant platelet syndrome and platelet glycoprotein Ib deficiency, is a rare bleeding disorder of large platelets with quantitative or qualitative abnormalities of the platelet membrane von Willebrand receptor complex glycoprotein (GP) Ib-IX-V. Clinically, BSS is manifested by severe, mostly mucocutaneous bleeding early in infancy.

BSS is inherited as an autosomal recessive disorder. Parental consanguinity is frequent. While the disease is rare, and the estimated frequency based on the literature is less than 1 in a million, the heterozygosity, or carrier state, is estimated to be 1 in 500. That makes this disorder the most common congenital macrothrombocytopenia [96]. Heterozygote family members are usually asymptomatic or have mild bleeding and have half of the normal levels of GPIb/IX/V complex.

The GPIb/IX/V complex comprises four transmembrane polypeptide subunits – GPIbα, GPIbβ, GPIX, and GPV – which are products of four distinct genes [96]. The expression of GPIb/IX/V is mostly limited to megakaryocytes and platelets. The GPIb/IX/V complex has two important roles: it mediates platelet adhesion to the vessel walls at the site of injury by binding to von Willebrand factor (VWF), and also facilitates the

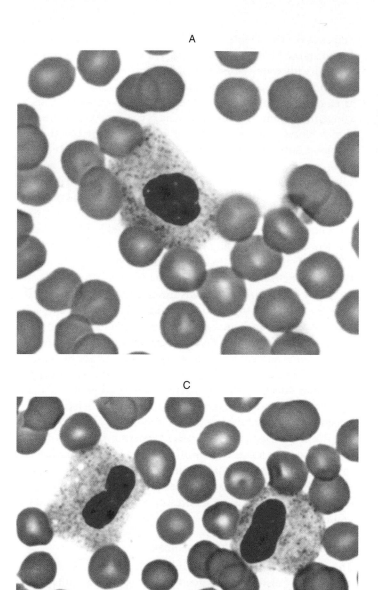

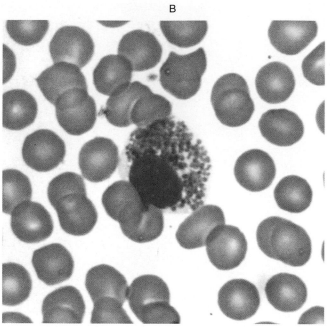

Fig. 7.14. Peripheral blood smear from a child with familial Pelger–Huët anomaly (Wright–Giemsa stain). (A) Neutrophils are mostly monolobated, as is the one shown here. (B) A monolobated eosinophil is also present. (C) Two monolobated neutrophils with band-shaped nuclei reminiscent of band neutrophils. Notice the condensed nuclear chromatin and cytoplasm which indicates that these cells are mature neutrophils.

ability of thrombin to activate platelets at low concentrations. A lack of GPIb/IX/V complex results in abnormal platelet aggregation in response to ristocetin, a feature characteristic of BSS. However, this abnormality may be difficult to demonstrate in the setting of thrombocytopenia, since some of the techniques determining platelet function require a normal platelet count. Furthermore, because a large amount of blood is required to obtain a sufficient amount of platelet-rich plasma for platelet aggregation studies, the limited blood availability in small children may make such testing impossible. In small children, an alternative solution is to perform platelet aggregation studies on whole blood.

The abnormal platelet aggregation studies can be confirmed by assessment of the expression of GPIb through flow cytometry or other techniques such as surface labeling of washed platelets by sodium dodecyl sulfate polyacrylamide gel electrophoresis (SDS-PAGE) and autoradiography, or Western blot of platelet lysates, and/or demonstration of abnormal genotype by molecular studies.

BSS is frequently misdiagnosed as idiopathic thrombocytopenic purpura (ITP) based on the prolonged bleeding time and presence of macrothrombocytopenia [97, 98]. However, unlike BSS, ITP platelets have normal function.

BSS carriers are *heterozygotes for GPIb/IX* mutations. They are asymptomatic and their platelet count ranges from very low to normal. Furthermore, the platelets are functionally normal and sufficient to support platelet–VWF interactions, since the residual amount of normal GPIb/IX/C complex is adequate.

Table 7.11. Differential diagnosis of Pelger–Huët anomaly.

Congenital (Pelger–Huët anomaly)
  Autosomal dominant – mutation at lamin B receptor (1q41–43)

Acquired (pseudo-Pelger–Huët forms)
  Neoplastic
    Myelodysplastic syndrome
    AML with abnormalities at chromosome 17
    Myeloproliferative syndromes (CML)
  Drugs
    Mycophenolate mofetil (CellCept)
    Valproate
    Ganciclovir
    Ibuprofen
    Colony stimulating factors
      G-CSF and GM-CSF
  Infections
    Severe bacterial infections
    HIV
    Mycoplasma pneumoniae
    Tuberculosis

While BSS carriers have varying numbers of large platelets, this is not an absolute rule, and the platelet size of some carriers can be normal.

A form of autosomal dominant macrothrombocytopenia, also known as *Mediterranean macrothrombocytopenia*, shares clinical and molecular features with the heterozygous BSS phenotype. Genetic analysis of Italian families with this disorder showed a founder mutation at the *GP1BA* (Ala156Val) gene [99]. However, this disorder is somewhat enigmatic since not all of the families included in this study have mutations at *GP1BA*, and BSS carriers with the same level of GP1BA expression are asymptomatic. It is possible that other factors play a role in the Mediterranean macrothrombocytopenia phenotype. The diagnostic criteria for this disorder include moderate thrombocy-topenia (70–150×10^9/L), increased mean platelet volume, and mild bleeding.

Macrothrombocytopenia without bleeding tendency is also a feature of DiGeorge/velocardiofacial syndrome, which is due to a microdeletion of 22q11.2 with resultant heterozygocity for the *GP1BB* gene.

Type 2B von Willebrand disease (VWD 2B) is another disorder manifesting with spontaneous bleeding due to abnormal binding of GP1b/IX/V complex to the von Willebrand factor (VWF). Unlike the previously described disorders, however, here the mutation is at the VWF GP1b/IX/V complex binding site. This mutation results in an unusual gain of function and increased aggregation with ristocetin.

Other congenital macrothrombocytopenias

X-linked macrothrombocytopenia with *GATA1* mutation

This is a relatively recently described entity of macrothrombocytopenia with mild to moderate dyserythropoiesis transmitted as an X-linked disorder [100–102]. The cause of the disorder is an inherited mutation at the *GATA1* gene, a critical transcription factor involved in megakaryopoiesis and erythropoiesis. As a result of the mutation, GATA1 is unable to bind its essential cofactor, FOG1.

Peripheral blood shows mild anemia and severe thrombocytopenia with platelet count between 10×10^9/L and 40×10^9/L. Using flow cytometry, the platelets show abnormal distribution and reduction of GPIb complex. Very immature platelets may have a complete lack of expression of GPIb. Platelet aggregation shows weak ristocetin-induced aggregation. Ultrastructural studies reveal giant platelets with cytoplasmic clusters consisting of smooth endoplasmic reticulum and abnormal membrane complex [102]. The bone marrow in patients with

Table 7.12. Inherited thrombocytopenias classified by platelet size.

Large platelets (>11 fL)	Normal platelets (7–11 fL)	Small platelets (<7 fL)

Abnormalities in platelet cytoskeleton (*MYH9*-related disorders)
  May–Hegglin anomaly
  Fechtner syndrome
  Epstein syndrome
  Sebastian syndrome
	Familial platelet disorder with associated myeloid malignancy
	  RUNX1
	  Haploinsufficiency
		Wiscott–Aldrich syndrome
		  WAS

Abnormalities in GP1b/IX/V
  Bernard–Soulier syndrome
  Mediterranean thrombocytopenia/Bernard–
    Soulier syndrome carrier
  DiGeorge/velocardiofacial syndrome
	Thrombocytopenia 2; THC2
	  MASTL gene encoding microtubule-associated serine/threonine kinase
		X-linked thrombocytopenia, disorder allelic to Wiskott–Aldrich syndrome resulting from mutation in *WAS*

Abnormalities in transcription factors
  Paris–Trousseau thrombocytopenia/Jacobsen syndrome
    FLI1
  X-linked macrothrombocytopenia with dyserythropoiesis
    GATA1
	Congenital amegakaryocytic thrombocytopenia (CAMT)
	  MPL gene encoding thrombopoietin receptor	

Unknown cause Gray platelet syndrome, platelet alpha granules deficiency	Thrombocytopenia with absent radii Chromosome 1q21.1 deletion syndrome	

Data from Online Mendelian Inheritance in Man, OMIM.

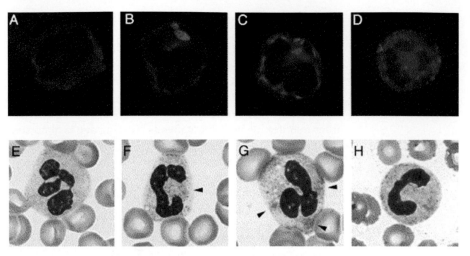

Fig. 7.15. Immunofluorescence patterns of anti-platelet non-muscle myosin heavy chain A (NMMHC-A) antibodies in a normal control and individuals with *MYH9*-related disorders (A–D) compared to various types of inclusion bodies in neutrophils stained with May–Grünwald–Giemsa (E–H). The abnormal patterns can be classified into three groups (types I to III) according to the number, size, and shape of fluorescence-labeled NMMHC-A granules. (A) In normal neutrophils NMMHC-A is homogeneously distributed in the cytoplasm and the neutrophils lack inclusion bodies (E). (B) Type I localization shows one or two intensely stained cytoplasmic foci and a prominent leukocyte inclusion (F). (C) Type II localization shows several cytoplasmic spots with circular-to-oval shape and several inclusion bodies (G). (D) Type III or speckled staining consists of a diffuse, speckled staining of the neutrophil cytoplasm and no inclusion bodies (H). Type III staining pattern is seen in patients with Epstein syndrome in which Wright or May–Grünwald–Giemsa-stained inclusion bodies have never been identified. (Reprinted with permission from Kunishima, Saito [87].)

GATA1 mutation, which may be hypercellular, shows dyserythropoiesis and dysmegakaryopoiesis.

GATA1 mutation should be suspected in male children with mild anemia, severe thrombocytopenia with normal to large platelets, and dyspoiesis involving the erythroid and megakaryocytic progenitors. Sequencing of *GATA1* and identification of mutation is the only confirmatory test and is available through specialized laboratories [88].

Gray platelet syndrome (GPS)

This is a very rare form of macrothrombocytopenia for which the etiology and genetics are yet to be discovered. GPS platelets are giant and lack platelet α granules, which results in a variable bleeding tendency. Many cases are transmitted in an autosomal dominant pattern, yet some recessive forms are also present, suggesting heterogeneity of the disorder. The most characteristic feature of GPS is agranular platelets whose lack of α granules can be demonstrated by ultrastructural studies. Furthermore, secretion-dependent platelet aggregation studies are abnormal.

Approach to patients with macrothrombocytopenia

The proper diagnosis of macrothrombocytopenias requires a systematic approach in order to avoid unnecessary expensive testing and lengthy workups. Fig. 7.17 depicts a helpful algorithm in the workup of a child with bleeding and macrothrombocytopenia. The initial steps in the workup of any thrombocytopenia include detailed clinical history and CBC with a careful examination of a well-stained peripheral blood film prepared either directly or very shortly after the blood was drawn. The acquired thrombocytopenias, such as idiopathic thrombocytopenia (ITP), should be excluded first. The presence of gran-

ulocyte inclusions is suggestive of *MYH9*-related thrombocytopenias and further workup with mutational analysis of *MYH9* will be helpful. A history of severe bleeding and macrothrombocytopenia is suggestive of GPIb/IX/V abnormalities with the result that platelet aggregation studies should be performed. The lack of aggregation with ristocetin and the absence of GPIb/IX/V complex by flow cytometry is diagnostic of BSS. If the aggregation with ristocetin is increased, VWD 2B should be considered. The morphologic appearance and lack of granules would suggest gray platelet syndrome. If the patient is male and there is dyserythropoiesis, *GATA1* mutations should be considered.

Inherited thrombocytopenias associated with normal platelet size

Congenital amegakaryocytic thrombocytopenia (CAMT) (OMIM 139090)

This is an autosomal recessive thrombocytopenia due to a virtual absence of megakaryocytes as a result of mutations at the thrombopoietin receptor (*MPL*). The type of the mutation at *MPL* predicts the clinical presentation and course of the disease [103–105]. For example, patients with *MPL* nonsense mutations have a lower platelet count at birth (18×10^9/L), worsening of the thrombocytopenia resulting in easy bruising and bleeding diathesis, and develop bone marrow failure and aplastic anemia by age 22 months (range 6–53 months). By contrast, patients with missense mutations have a slightly higher platelet count at birth (21×10^9/L), a spontaneous increase in the platelet count to over 50×10^9/L during early infancy, and ultimately a slower

A

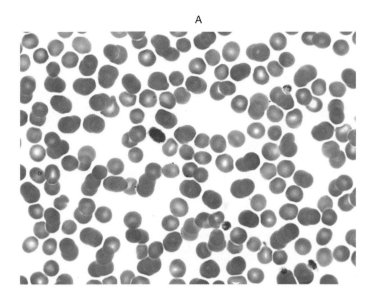

B

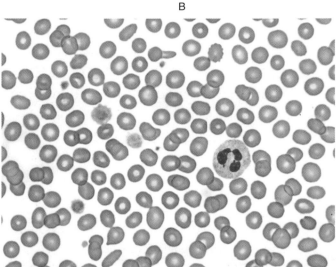

C

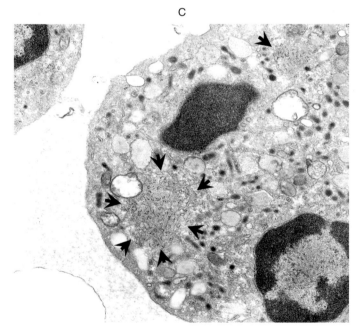

Fig. 7.16. Peripheral blood and bone marrow from a 10-month-old boy with *MYH9*-related disorder (May–Hegglin anomaly) (Wright–Giemsa stain). (A) A peripheral blood smear shows large platelets. (B) A neutrophil with faint Döhle-like bodies. (C) Electron microscopy shows a neutrophil with clusters of dispersed filaments and randomly distributed ribosomes in an area free of specific granules (arrows).

progression to aplastic anemia by age 48 months (range 36–82 months) [104].

In patients with CAMT, peripheral blood smear review shows moderate to severe thrombocytopenia with normal platelet size and granulation. In a cohort of 20 patients, King *et al.* found a median platelet count at birth to be 21×10^9/L (range 7–87×10^9/L), the median hemoglobin level to be 13.3 g/dL (range 7.6–18.4 g/dL), and a median WBC 10.7×10^9/L (range 4.9 to 32×10^9/L) [105].

The bone marrow is normocellular and the megakaryocytes are virtually absent or markedly reduced in number. While the cytogenetic studies are normal in most patients, at least two cases with clonal cytogenetic abnormalities have been reported [105]. These include t(2;11) in one case and the presence of

a marker chromosome in 94% of the metaphases in another case.

MPL signaling is important in the production of mature megakaryocytes and the maintenance of the hematopoietic stem cell population [106]. Thus, mutation at this gene results in marked thrombocytopenia. Some of the mutations result in a complete absence of a receptor or function and lead to severe thrombocytopenia and lack of megakaryopoiesis; others result in a residual function of MPL and present as milder forms. For definitive diagnosis, homozygous mutation at *MPL* should be demonstrated.

About 40% of patients with CAMT develop bone marrow failure. Even though CAMT has been referred to as a pre-leukemic syndrome, AML and MDS are rare.

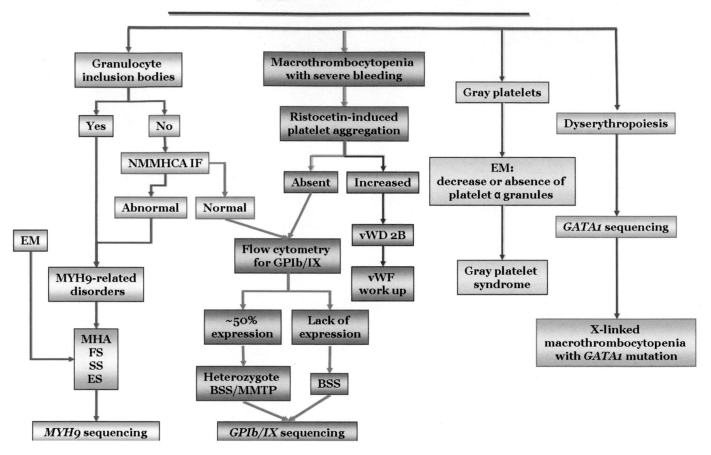

Fig. 7.17. A flowchart for a diagnostic workup of non-syndromic congenital macrothrombocytopenias. Abbreviations: EM, electron microscopy; NMMHC-A IF, anti-non-muscle myosin heavy chain A immunofluorescence; MHA, May–Hegglin anomaly; FS, Fechtner syndrome; SS, Sebastian syndrome; ES, Epstein syndrome; BSS Bernard–Soulier syndrome; MMTP Mediterranean macrothrombocytopenia; GPIb/IX, glycoprotein Ib/IX; VWF, von Willebrand factor; VWD, von Willebrand disease.

Table 7.13. Disorders associated with mutations in glycoprotein Ib-IX-V complex.

Disorder	Platelet function abnormalities	Gene
Bernard–Soulier syndrome, type A (AR)	No ristocetin-induced platelet aggregation; loss of function	GPIa GPIb GP9
Mediterranean macrothrombocytopenia/ Bernard–Soulier syndrome, carrier (AD)	Mild thrombocytopenia with normal ristocetin-induced platelet aggregation	GPIa GPIb GP9
von Willebrand disease, platelet type (AD)	Quantitative abnormality of plasma VWF multimers and platelets; increased ristocetin aggregation due to gain of function	GPIb

Abbreviations: AD, autosomal dominant; AR, autosomal recessive.

Familial platelet disorder with associated myeloid malignancy (FPD/AML) (OMIM 601399)

The familial platelet disorder associated with myeloid malignancy (FPD/AML) is an autosomal dominant disorder characterized by quantitative and qualitative platelet abnormalities and a propensity to develop MDS/AML. The disorder is due to heterozygous mutations at *CBFA*, also known as the *RUNX1* gene, resulting in abrogation of DNA binding of the runt domain [107]. *RUNX1* is a transcription factor and a key regulator of hematopoietic cell proliferation, cytoskeleton stability, and genomic stability so that its deregulation can result in hematologic malignancies [108].

Haploinsufficiency for *RUNX1* leads to decreased megakaryocyte colony formation as well as smaller megakaryocytic colonies in these individuals, presumably as a result of abnormal regulation of downstream genes, that regulate platelet production. The platelets of affected individuals demonstrate

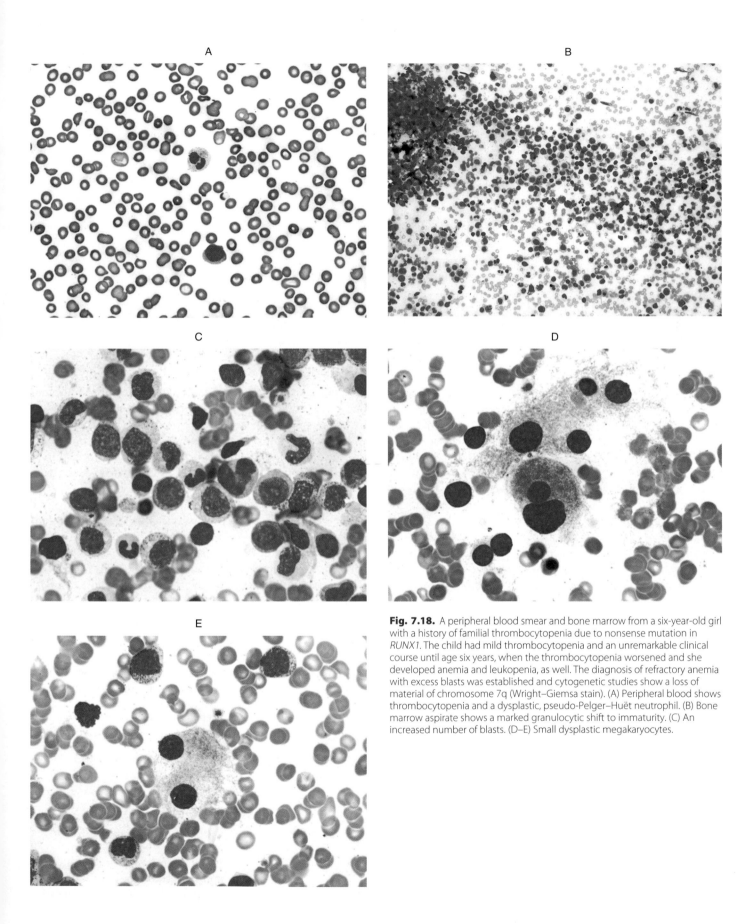

Fig. 7.18. A peripheral blood smear and bone marrow from a six-year-old girl with a history of familial thrombocytopenia due to nonsense mutation in *RUNX1*. The child had mild thrombocytopenia and an unremarkable clinical course until age six years, when the thrombocytopenia worsened and she developed anemia and leukopenia, as well. The diagnosis of refractory anemia with excess blasts was established and cytogenetic studies show a loss of material of chromosome 7q (Wright–Giemsa stain). (A) Peripheral blood shows thrombocytopenia and a dysplastic, pseudo-Pelger–Huët neutrophil. (B) Bone marrow aspirate shows a marked granulocytic shift to immaturity. (C) An increased number of blasts. (D–E) Small dysplastic megakaryocytes.

functional abnormalities causing prolonged bleeding times and abnormal response to platelet agonists. A mild microtubule defect might partially explain the platelet defect in individuals with FPD/AML, since microtubules are necessary at several stages of megakaryopoiesis, including endomitosis, production of platelets from polyploid megakaryocytes, and release of platelet granule content. Furthermore, haploinsufficiency for *RUNX1* predisposes to the development of myelodysplastic syndrome or acute myeloid leukemia in FPD/AML kindreds (Fig. 7.18). The disruption of largely unknown biologic pathways controlled by *RUNX1* is likely to be responsible for the development of acute leukemia [108]. Even so, how the haploinsufficiency contributes to the development of acute leukemia is not well understood. It is known that translocations involving *RUNX1* are a recurrent cytogenetic abnormality in acute myeloid [t(8;21)(q22;q22)] and B-lymphoblastic leukemia/lymphoma [t(12;21)(p13;q22)]. Both types are associated with a relatively good response to therapy.

Thrombocytopenia with small platelets (microthrombocytopenias)

Wiskott–Aldrich syndrome (WAS) (OMIM 301000)

This is a rare, X-linked disorder generally characterized by eczema, microthrombocytopenia, and immune deficiency, due to mutation at the WAS protein *(WASP)* gene [109]. A minor form of X-linked thrombocytopenia (XLT) exists in which eczema and immune deficiency are not clinically significant [110].

In WAS, the platelet count varies from as low as 5×10^9/L to as high as 50×10^9/L, with a mean platelet volume of 3.8–5.0 fL (normal 7–11 fL) [110]. Also, iron deficient anemia is a frequent finding because of chronic blood loss. Diagnosis should be suspected in any male child presenting with thrombocytopenia or immune deficiency.

WASP has no enzymatic activity but contains numerous protein-interacting domains and plays an important role in actin polymerization, the development of hematopoietic cells, cell signaling, and lymphocyte apoptosis [110]. Thus, mutations at *WASP* result in a complex phenotype with abnormalities involving multiple lineages and cell types. Mutations producing a single amino acid substitution lead to a milder phenotype, XLT; whereas, a lack of expression of WASP or expression of truncated protein results in a severe phenotype [109, 110]. Rarely, there are reports of girls having microthrombocytopenia with or without other components of WAS. Spontaneous mutations at *WASP* with skewed X-inactivation of the hematopoietic cells have been reported [111].

To establish the diagnosis of WAS, an absence or reduced quantity of WASP in lymphocytes identified by flow cytometry or Western blot is the best confirmatory test. Lymphopenia is a consistent finding in young children with WAS. Of note, some of the mutations at *WASP* may result in proteins with abnormal function that may be detected by flow cytometry. Ultimately, mutation at *WASP* is essential for diagnosis.

Summary

In conclusion, the inherited bone marrow failure syndromes that manifest with a single cytopenia, once considered a rarity, are recognized to occur more frequently and to include a wider spectrum of clinical presentations ranging from severe diseases in neonates to mild conditions usually identified incidentally later in life. Our understanding of the underlying pathogeneses of these disorders has increased as a result of determining specific molecular defects in many of them. Some of these genetic alterations are associated with a higher risk of developing myeloid malignancies along with the complications of the specific cytopenia. Thus, specific diagnosis followed by adequate management is critical for such patients. In making specific diagnoses, one approach is to develop and use diagnostic algorithms. They can greatly facilitate the process and overcome some of the challenges, thereby reducing unnecessary and costly testing.

References

1. **Gazda HT, Sieff CA.** Recent insights into the pathogenesis of Diamond-Blackfan anaemia. *British Journal of Haematology.* 2006;**135**:149–157.

2. **Lipton JM, Ellis SR.** Diamond-Blackfan anemia: diagnosis, treatment, and molecular pathogenesis. *Hematology/Oncology Clinics of North America.* 2009;**23**:261–282.

3. **Ball SE, McGuckin CP, Jenkins G, Gordon-Smith EC.** Diamond-Blackfan anaemia in the U.K.: analysis of 80 cases from a 20-year birth cohort. *British Journal of Haematology.* 1996;**94**:645–653.

4. **Young NS.** *Bone Marrow Failure Syndromes.* Philadelphia, PA: WB Saunders; 2000.

5. **Janov AJ, Leong T, Nathan DG, Guinan EC.** Diamond-Blackfan anemia: natural history and sequelae of treatment. *Medicine.* 1996;**75**:77–87.

6. **Willig T-NMD, Gazda HMD, Sieff CAMBB.** Diamond-Blackfan anemia. *Current Opinion in Hematology.* 2000;7:85–94.

7. **Halperin DS, Freedman MH.** Diamond-Blackfan anemia: etiology, pathophysiology, and treatment. *American Journal of Pediatric Hematology/Oncology.* 1989;**11**:380–394.

8. **Lipton JMM, Federman NBA, Khabbaze YMD,** *et al.* Osteogenic sarcoma associated with Diamond-Blackfan anemia: a report from the Diamond-Blackfan Anemia Registry. *Journal of Pediatric Hematology/Oncology.* 2001;**23**:39–44.

9. **Glader BE, Backer K, Diamond LK.** Elevated erythrocyte adenosine deaminase activity in congenital hypoplastic anemia. *New England Journal of Medicine.* 1983;**309**:1486–1490.

10. **Willig TN, Perignon JL, Gustavsson P,** *et al.* High adenosine deaminase level among healthy probands of Diamond Blackfan anemia (DBA) cosegregates

with the DBA gene region on chromosome 19q13. *Blood*. 1998;**92**: 4422–4427.

11. **Bessler M, Mason PJ, Link DC, Wilson DB**. Inherited bone marrow failure syndromes. In Orkin SH, Nathan DG, Ginsburg D, *et al.*, eds. *Nathan and Oski's Hematology of Infancy and Childhood* (7th edn.). Philadelphia: Saunders/Elsevier; 2009, 307–395.

12. **Dianzani I, Loreni F**. Diamond-Blackfan anemia: a ribosomal puzzle. *Haematologica*. 2008;**93**:1601–1604.

13. **Vlachos A, Ball S, Dahl N**, *et al.* Diagnosing and treating Diamond Blackfan anaemia: results of an international clinical consensus conference. *British Journal of Haematology*. 2008;**142**:859–876.

14. **Dianzani I, Loreni F**. Diamond-Blackfan anemia: a ribosomal puzzle. *Haematologica*. 2008;**93**:1601–1604.

15. **Brown MKE, Young MNS**. Parvovirus B19 in human disease. *Annual Review of Medicine*. 1997;**48**:59–67.

16. **Kudoh T, Yoto Y, Suzuki N**, *et al.* Human Parvovirus B19-induced aplastic crisis in iron deficiency anemia. *Acta Paediatrica Japonica*. 1994;**36**: 448–449.

17. **Krause JR, Penchansky L, Knisely AS**. Morphological diagnosis of Parvovirus B19 infection. A cytopathic effect easily recognized in air-dried, formalin-fixed bone marrow smears stained with hematoxylin-eosin or Wright-Giemsa. *Archives of Pathology and Laboratory Medicine*. 1992;**116**:178–180.

18. **Morey AL, O'Neill HJ, Coyle PV, Fleming KA**. Immunohistological detection of human Parvovirus B19 in formalin-fixed, paraffin-embedded tissues. *Journal of Pathology*. 1992;**166**: 105–108.

19. **Liu W, Ittmann M, Liu J**, *et al.* Human Parvovirus B19 in bone marrows from adults with acquired immunodeficiency syndrome: a comparative study using in situ hybridization and immunohistochemistry. *Human Pathology*. 1997;**28**:760–766.

20. **Frickhofen N, Chen ZJ, Young NS**, *et al.* Parvovirus B19 as a cause of acquired chronic pure red cell aplasia. *British Journal of Haematology*. 1994;**87**: 818–824.

21. **Gerrits GP, van Oostrom CG, de Vaan GA, Bakkeren JA**. Transient erythroblastopenia of childhood. A review of 22 cases. *European Journal of Pediatrics*. 1984 **142**:266–270.

22. **Rogers ZR, Bergstrom SK, Amylon MD, Buchanan GR, Glader BE**. Reduced neutrophil counts in children with transient erythroblastopenia of childhood. *Journal of Pediatrics*. 1989;**115**:746–748.

23. **Cherrick IMD, Karayalcin GMD, Lanzkowsky PMD**. Transient erythroblastopenia of childhood: prospective study of fifty patients. *American Journal of Pediatric Hematology/Oncology*. 1994;**16**: 320–324.

24. **Freedman MH**. Pure red cell aplasia in childhood and adolescence: pathogenesis and approaches to diagnosis. *British Journal of Haematology*. 1993;**85**:246–253.

25. **Penchansky L, Jordan JA**. Transient erythroblastopenia of childhood associated with human herpesvirus type 6, variant B. *American Journal of Clinical Pathology*. 1997;**108**:127–132.

26. **Skeppner G, Kreuger A, Elinder G**. Transient erythroblastopenia of childhood: prospective study of 10 patients with special reference to viral infections. *Journal of Pediatric Hematology/Oncology*. 2002;**24**: 294–298.

27. **Rogers BB, Rogers ZR, Timmons CF**. Polymerase chain reaction amplification of archival material for Parvovirus B19 in children with transient erythroblastopenia of childhood. *Pediatric Pathology & Laboratory Medicine*. 1996;**16**:471–478.

28. **Shaw J, Meeder R**. Transient erythroblastopenia of childhood in siblings: case report and review of the literature. *Journal of Pediatric Hematology/Oncology*. 2007;**29**:659–660.

29. **Heimpel H**. Congenital dyserythropoietic anemias: epidemiology, clinical significance, and progress in understanding their pathogenesis. *Annals of Hematology*. 2004;**83**:613–621.

30. **Heimpel H, Wendt F**. Congenital dyserythropoietic anemia with karyorrhexis and multinuclearity of erythroblasts. *Helvetica Medica Acta*. 1968;**34**:103–115.

31. **Wickramasinghe SN, Wood WG**. Advances in the understanding of the congenital dyserythropoietic anaemias. *British Journal of Haematology*. 2005; **131**:431–446.

32. **Tamary H, Dgany O, Proust A**, *et al.* Clinical and molecular variability in congenital dyserythropoietic anaemia type I. *British Journal of Haematology*. 2005;**130**:628–634.

33. **Parez N, Dommergues M, Zupan V**, *et al.* Severe congenital dyserythropoietic anaemia type I: prenatal management, transfusion support and alpha-interferon therapy. *British Journal of Haematology*. 2000;**110**:420–423.

34. **Shalev HMD, Kapelushnik JMD, Moser AMD**, *et al.* A comprehensive study of the neonatal manifestations of congenital dyserythropoietic anemia type I. *Journal of Pediatric Hematology/ Oncology*. 2004;**26**:746–748.

35. **Wickramasinghe SN**. Congenital dyserythropoietic anemias. *Current Opinion in Hematology*. 2000;**7**:71–78.

36. **Wickramasinghe SN**. Dyserythropoiesis and congenital dyserythropoietic anaemias. *British Journal of Haematology*. 1997;**98**:785–797.

37. **Dgany O, Avidan N, Delaunay J**, *et al.* Congenital dyserythropoietic anemia type I is caused by mutations in codanin-1. *The American Journal of Human Genetics*. 2002;**71**:1467–1474.

38. **Tamary H, Shalmon L, Shalev H**, *et al.* Localization of the gene for congenital dyserythropoietic anemia type I to a <1-cM interval on chromosome 15q15.1–15.3. *American Journal of Human Genetics*. 1998;**62**:1062–1069.

39. **Ahmed MR, Chehal A, Zahed L**, *et al.* Linkage and mutational analysis of the *CDAN1* gene reveals genetic heterogeneity in congenital dyserythropoietic anemia type I. *Blood*. 2006;**107**:4968–4969.

40. **Heimpel H, Anselstetter V, Chrobak L**, *et al.* Congenital dyserythropoietic anemia type II: epidemiology, clinical appearance, and prognosis based on long-term observation. *Blood*. 2003; **102**:4576–4581.

41. **Fukuda MN, Papayannopoulou T, Gordon-Smith EC, Rochant H, Testa U**. Defect in glycosylation of erythrocyte membrane proteins in congenital dyserythropoietic anaemia

type II (HEMPAS). *British Journal of Haematology.* 1984;**56**:55–68.

42. **Gasparini P, Miraglia del Giudice E, Delaunay J**, et al. Localization of the congenital dyserythropoietic anemia II locus to chromosome 20q11.2 by genomewide search. *American Journal of Human Genetics.* 1997;**61**:1112–1116.

43. **Denecke J, Marquardt T**. Congenital dyserythropoietic anemia type II (CDAII/HEMPAS): Where are we now? *Biochimica et Biophysica Acta (BBA) – Molecular Basis of Disease.* 2009;**1792**: 915–920.

44. **Sandstrom H, Wahlin A**. Congenital dyserythropoietic anemia type III. *Haematologica.* 2000;**85**:753–757.

45. **Wickramasinghe SN**. Congenital dyserythropoietic anaemias: clinical features, haematological morphology and new biochemical data. *Blood Reviews.* 1998;**12**:178–200.

46. **Renella R, Wood WG**. The congenital dyserythropoietic anemias. *Hematology/ Oncology Clinics of North America.* 2009;**23**:283–306.

47. **Reich D, Nalls MA, Kao WHL**, et al. Reduced neutrophil count in people of African descent is due to a regulatory variant in the Duffy antigen receptor for chemokines gene. *PLoS Genetics.* 2009;**5**:e1000360.

48. **Nalls MA, Wilson JG, Patterson NJ**, et al. Admixture mapping of white cell count: genetic locus responsible for lower white blood cell count in the Health ABC and Jackson Heart studies. *American Journal of Human Genetics.* 2008;**82**:81–87. Erratum appears in *American Journal of Human Genetics.* 2008;**82**:532.

49. **Schmutz N, Henry E, Jopling J, Christensen RD**. Expected ranges for blood neutrophil concentrations of neonates: the Manroe and Mouzinho charts revisited. *Journal of Perinatology.* 2008;**28**:275–281.

50. **Hsieh MM, Everhart JE, Byrd-Holt DD, Tisdale JF, Rodgers GP**. Prevalence of neutropenia in the U.S. population: age, sex, smoking status, and ethnic differences. *Annals of Internal Medicine.* 2007;**146**:486–492.

51. **Boxer LA, Newburger PE**. A molecular classification of congenital neutropenia syndromes. *Pediatric Blood & Cancer.* 2007;**49**:609–614.

52. **Berliner N, Horwitz M, Loughran TP Jr**. Congenital and acquired neutropenia. *Hematology/the Education Program of the American Society of Hematology.* 2004: 63–79.

53. **Dinauer MC, Newberger PE**. The phagocyte system and disorders of granulopoiesis and granulocyte function. In Orkin SH, Nathan DG, Ginsburg D, et al., eds. *Nathan and Oski's Hematology of Infancy and Childhood* (7th edn.). Philadelphia, PA: Saunders/Elsevier; 2009, 1109–1217.

54. **Kostmann R**. Infantile genetic agranulocytosis; agranulocytosis infantilis hereditaria. *Acta Paediatrica.* 1956: 1–78.

55. **Dale DC, Hammond WP**. Cyclic neutropenia: a clinical review. *Blood Reviews.* 1988;**2**:178–185.

56. **Welte K, Zeidler C**. Severe congenital neutropenia. *Hematology – Oncology Clinics of North America.* 2009;**23**:307–320.

57. **Bellanne-Chantelot C, Clauin S, Leblanc T**, et al. Mutations in the ELA2 gene correlate with more severe expression of neutropenia: a study of 81 patients from the French Neutropenia Register. *Blood.* 2004;**103**:4119–4125.

58. **Ancliff PJ, Gale RE, Liesner R, Hann IM, Linch DC**. Mutations in the ELA2 gene encoding neutrophil elastase are present in most patients with sporadic severe congenital neutropenia but only in some patients with the familial form of the disease. *Blood.* 2001;**98**:2645–2650.

59. **Horwitz MS, Duan Z, Korkmaz B, Lee H-H, Mealiffe ME, Salipante SJ**. Neutrophil elastase in cyclic and severe congenital neutropenia. *Blood.* 2007; **109**:1817–1824.

60. **Zeidler C, Germeshausen M, Klein C, Welte K**. Clinical implications of ELA2-, HAX1-, and G-CSF-receptor (CSF3R) mutations in severe congenital neutropenia. *British Journal of Haematology.* 2009;**144**:459–467.

61. **Berliner N**. Lessons from congenital neutropenia: 50 years of progress in understanding myelopoiesis. *Blood.* 2008;**111**:5427–5432.

62. **Xia J, Link DC**. Severe congenital neutropenia and the unfolded protein response. *Current Opinion in Hematology.* 2008;**15**:1–7.

63. **Klein C, Grudzien M, Appaswamy G**, et al. HAX1 deficiency causes autosomal recessive severe congenital neutropenia (Kostmann disease). *Nature Genetics.* 2007;**39**:86–92.

64. **Schaffer AAa, Klein Cb**. Genetic heterogeneity in severe congenital neutropenia: how many aberrant pathways can kill a neutrophil? *Current Opinion in Allergy & Clinical Immunology.* 2007;**7**:481–494.

65. **Ward AC, van Aesch YM, Gits J**, et al. Novel point mutation in the extracellular domain of the granulocyte colony-stimulating factor (G-CSF) receptor in a case of severe congenital neutropenia hyporesponsive to G-CSF treatment. *The Journal of Experimental Medicine.* 1999;**190**:497–508.

66. **Dale DC, Cottle TE, Fier CJ**, et al. Severe chronic neutropenia: treatment and follow-up of patients in the Severe Chronic Neutropenia International Registry. *American Journal of Hematology.* 2003;**72**:82–93.

67. **Freedman MH, Bonilla MA, Fier C**, et al. Myelodysplasia syndrome and acute myeloid leukemia in patients with congenital neutropenia receiving G-CSF therapy. *Blood.* 2000;**96**:429–436.

68. **Rosenberg PS, Alter BP, Bolyard AA**, et al. The incidence of leukemia and mortality from sepsis in patients with severe congenital neutropenia receiving long-term G-CSF therapy. *Blood.* 2006; **107**:4628–4635.

69. **Kalra R, Dale D, Freedman M**, et al. Monosomy 7 and activating RAS mutations accompany malignant transformation in patients with congenital neutropenia. *Blood.* 1995;**86**: 4579–4586.

70. **Aprikyan AAG, Kutyavin T, Stein S**, et al. Cellular and molecular abnormalities in severe congenital neutropenia predisposing to leukemia. *Experimental Hematology.* 2003;**31**: 372–381.

71. **Rosenberg PS, Alter BP, Link DC**, et al. Neutrophil elastase mutations and risk of leukaemia in severe congenital neutropenia. *British Journal of Haematology.* 2008;**140**:210–213.

72. **Roper M, Parmley RT, Crist WM, Kelly DR, Cooper MD**. Severe congenital leukopenia (reticular dysgenesis). Immunologic and morphologic characterizations of leukocytes. *American Journal of Diseases of Children.* 1985;**139**:832–835.

73. **De La Calle-Martin O, Badell I, Garcia A**, *et al.* B cells and monocytes are not developmentally affected in a case of reticular dysgenesis. *Clinical & Experimental Immunology.* 1997;**110**: 392–396.

74. **Pannicke U, Honig M, Hess I**, *et al.* Reticular dysgenesis (aleukocytosis) is caused by mutations in the gene encoding mitochondrial adenylate kinase 2. *Nature Genetics.* 2009;**41**:101–105.

75. **Kaplan J, De Domenico I, Ward DM.** Chediak-Higashi syndrome. *Current Opinion in Hematology.* 2008;**15**:22–29.

76. **Spritz RA.** Chediak-Higashi syndrome. In Ochs HD, Smith CIE, Puck JM, eds. *Primary Immunodeficiency Diseases: A Molecular and Genetic Approach.* New York: Oxford University Press; 1999, 389–396.

77. **Nagle DL, Karim MA, Woolf EA**, *et al.* Identification and mutation analysis of the complete gene for Chediak-Higashi syndrome. *Nature Genetics.* 1996;**14**: 307–311.

78. **Faigle W, Raposo G, Tenza D**, *et al.* Deficient peptide loading and MHC class II endosomal sorting in a human genetic immunodeficiency disease: the Chediak-Higashi syndrome. *The Journal of Cell Biology.* 1998;**141**:1121–1134.

79. **Cunningham JM, Patnaik MM, Hammerschmidt DE, Vercellotti GM.** Historical perspective and clinical implications of the Pelger-Huet cell. *American Journal of Hematology.* 2009; **84**:116–119.

80. **Hoffmann K, Dreger CK, Olins AL**, *et al.* Mutations in the gene encoding the lamin B receptor produce an altered nuclear morphology in granulocytes (Pelger-Huet anomaly). *Nature Genetics.* 2002;**31**:410–414.

81. **Johnson CA, Bass DA, Trillo AA, Snyder MS, DeChatelet LR.** Functional and metabolic studies of polymorphonuclear leukocytes in the congenital Pelger-Huet anomaly. *Blood.* 1980;**55**:466–469.

82. **Cohen TV, Klarmann KD, Sakchaisri K**, *et al.* The lamin B receptor under transcriptional control of C/EBPepsilon is required for morphological but not functional maturation of neutrophils. *Human Molecular Genetics.* 2008;**17**: 2921–2933.

83. **Mohamed ISI, Wynn RJ, Cominsky K**, *et al.* White blood cell left shift in a neonate: a case of mistaken identity. *Journal of Perinatology.* 2006;**26**:378–380.

84. **Ganick DJ, Sunder T, Finley JL.** Severe hematologic toxicity of valproic acid. A report of four patients. *American Journal of Pediatric Hematology/Oncology.* 1990;**12**:80–85.

85. **Kennedy GA, Kay TD, Johnson DW**, *et al.* Neutrophil dysplasia characterised by a pseudo-Pelger-Huet anomaly occurring with the use of mycophenolate mofetil and ganciclovir following renal transplantation: a report of five cases. *Pathology.* 2002;**34**: 263–266.

86. **Banerjee R, Halil O, Bain BJ, Cummins D, Banner NR.** Neutrophil dysplasia caused by mycophenolate mofetil. *Transplantation.* 2000;**70**:1608–1610.

87. **Kunishima S, Saito H.** Congenital macrothrombocytopenias. *Blood Reviews.* 2006;**20**:111–121.

88. **Drachman JG.** Inherited thrombocytopenia: when a low platelet count does not mean ITP. *Blood.* 2004; **103**:390–398.

89. **Balduini CL, Iolascon A, Savoia A.** Inherited thrombocytopenias: from genes to therapy. *Haematologica.* 2002;**87**:860–880.

90. **Kunishima S, Kojima T, Matsushita T**, *et al.* Mutations in the NMMHC-A gene cause autosomal dominant macrothrombocytopenia with leukocyte inclusions (May-Hegglin anomaly/Sebastian syndrome). *Blood.* 2001;**97**:1147–1149.

91. **Peterson LC, Rao KV, Crosson JT, White JG.** Fechtner syndrome – a variant of Alport's syndrome with leukocyte inclusions and macrothrombocytopenia. *Blood.* 1985;**65**:397–406.

92. **Greinacher A, Nieuwenhuis HK, White JG.** Sebastian platelet syndrome: a new variant of hereditary macrothrombocytopenia with leukocyte inclusions. *Blut.* 1990;**61**: 282–288.

93. **Kelley MJ, Jawien W, Ortel TL, Korczak JF.** Mutation of MYH9, encoding non-muscle myosin heavy chain A, in May-Hegglin anomaly. *Nature Genetics.* 2000;**26**:106–108.

94. **Epstein CJ, Sahud MA, Piel CF**, *et al.* Hereditary macrothrombocytopathia, nephritis and deafness. *American Journal of Medicine.* 1972;**52**:299–310.

95. **Kunishima S, Matsushita T, Kojima T**, *et al.* Immunofluorescence analysis of neutrophil non-muscle myosin heavy chain-A in MYH9 disorders: association of subcellular localization with MYH9 mutations. *Laboratory Investigation.* 2003;**83**:115–122.

96. **Lopez JA, Andrews RK, Afshar-Kharghan V, Berndt MC.** Bernard-Soulier Syndrome. *Blood.* 1998;**91**:4397–4418.

97. **Bader-Meunier BMD, Proulle VMD, Trichet CMD**, *et al.* Misdiagnosis of chronic thrombocytopenia in childhood. *Journal of Pediatric Hematology/Oncology.* 2003;**25**: 548–552.

98. **Biner B, Devecioglu O, Demir M.** Pitfalls in the diagnosis of immune thrombocytopenic purpura in children: 4 case reports. *Clinical and Applied Thrombosis/Hemostasis.* 2007;**13**:329–333.

99. **Savoia A, Balduini CL, Savino M**, *et al.* Autosomal dominant macrothrombocytopenia in Italy is most frequently a type of heterozygous Bernard-Soulier syndrome. *Blood.* 2001;**97**:1330–1335.

100. **Nichols KE, Crispino JD, Poncz M**, *et al.* Familial dyserythropoietic anaemia and thrombocytopenia due to an inherited mutation in GATA1. *Nature Genetics.* 2000;**24**:266–270.

101. **Yu C, Niakan KK, Matsushita M, Stamatoyannopoulos G, Orkin SH, Raskind WH.** X-linked thrombocytopenia with thalassemia from a mutation in the amino finger of GATA-1 affecting DNA binding rather than FOG-1 interaction. *Blood.* 2002; **100**:2040–2045.

102. **Freson K, Devriendt K, Matthijs G**, *et al.* Platelet characteristics in patients with X-linked macrothrombocytopenia because of a novel GATA1 mutation. *Blood.* 2001;**98**:85–92.

103. **Germeshausen M, Ballmaier M, Welte K.** MPL mutations in 23 patients suffering from congenital amegakaryocytic thrombocytopenia: the type of mutation predicts the course of the disease. *Human Mutation.* 2006; **27**:296.

104. **Ballmaier M, Germeshausen M, Schulze H**, *et al.* c-mpl mutations are the cause of congenital amegakaryocytic thrombocytopenia. *Blood.* 2001;**97**:139–146.

105. **King S, Germeshausen M, Strauss G, Welte K, Ballmaier M.** Congenital amegakaryocytic thrombocytopenia: a retrospective clinical analysis of 20 patients. *British Journal of Haematology.* 2005;**131**:636–644.

106. **Kaushansky K**. Thrombopoietin and hematopoietic stem cell development. *Annals of the New York Academy of Sciences.* 1999;**872**:314–319.

107. **Song W-J, Sullivan MG, Legare RD**, *et al.* Haploinsufficiency of CBFA2 causes familial thrombocytopenia with propensity to develop acute myelogenous leukaemia. *Nature Genetics.* 1999;**23**:166–175.

108. **Michaud J, Simpson K, Escher R**, *et al.* Integrative analysis of RUNX1 downstream pathways and target genes. *BMC Genomics.* 2008;**9**:363.

109. **Lemahieu V, Gastier U, Francke JM**. Novel mutations in the Wiskott-Aldrich syndrome protein gene and their effects on transcriptional, translational, and clinical phenotypes. *Human Mutation.* 1999;**14**:54–66.

110. **Ochs HD, Thrasher AJ**. The Wiskott-Aldrich syndrome. *Journal of Allergy and Clinical Immunology.* 2006;**117**:725–738.

111. **Parolini O, Ressmann G, Haas OA**, *et al.* X-linked Wiskott-Aldrich syndrome in a girl. *New England Journal of Medicine.* 1998;**338**:291–295.

Peripheral blood and bone marrow manifestations of metabolic storage diseases

Andrea M. Sheehan

Introduction and general considerations

Metabolic storage diseases are rare disorders that have a wide spectrum of clinical and pathologic findings, depending on the genetic mutation inherited and the biochemical pathway disrupted. Most involve deficiency of a lysosomal enzyme, cofactor, or transport protein, resulting in accumulation of glycolipid or glycoprotein substances in the lysosome. As the presenting signs and symptoms can be variable, the peripheral blood smear or bone marrow findings may be the first clue that the patient has one of these disorders. Although the morphologic features for many of these are quite characteristic, none are entirely specific, and the diagnosis is best made utilizing a combination of clinical features, blood and marrow morphology, and biochemical testing of peripheral blood leukocytes or cultured skin fibroblasts. Targeted molecular diagnostic studies for specific mutations may be helpful to confirm the diagnosis for certain disorders, especially if there is an already characterized mutation within a family. Accurate diagnosis is important, as enzyme replacement therapy or other treatment has become available for several of these disorders.

Although the sites of accumulation of excess glycoprotein or glycolipid may vary, nearly all of these disorders involve the reticuloendothelial system to some extent, and many present with splenomegaly or hepatosplenomegaly. Splenomegaly may be quite pronounced, and cytopenias, specifically thrombocytopenia and anemia, are commonly seen at some stage at least in part due to hypersplenism. Lymph node and thymic involvement are also commonly seen, although prominent lymphadenopathy is unusual.

General features of the peripheral blood and bone marrow in storage diseases

Although early papers highlighted the presence of cytoplasmic vacuoles or prominent inclusions within granulocytes or mononuclear cells as common in some of these disorders, in reality the presence of vacuolated lymphocytes or the Alder–Reilly anomaly on peripheral smear is seen in only a subset of cases and only in certain stages of the disease for an individual patient. By contrast, most of these disorders will show some degree of marrow involvement, whether focal or extensive. The degree of marrow involvement depends on the specific

Table 8.1 Differential diagnosis of storage disease-type cells.

Cell type	Differential diagnosis
Gaucher cell or pseudo-Gaucher cell	Gaucher disease Chronic myelogenous leukemia Acute leukemias Myelodysplastic syndrome Hodgkin lymphoma Congenital dyserythropoietic anemias Hemoglobinopathies/thalassemias Mycobacterial infection
Foamy histiocyte	Niemann–Pick type A or B Hereditary hypercholesterolemias Farber disease (disseminated lipogranulomatosis) Tangier disease Polyvinylpyrrolidone storage disease Hydroxyethyl starch
Sea blue histiocyte	Niemann–Pick type C Fabry disease Sandhoff disease Wolman disease Hyperlipoproteinemia Total parenteral nutrition (TPN) Myelodysplastic syndromes Myeloproliferative neoplasms Idiopathic thrombocytopenia purpura
Peripheral blood vacuolated lymphocyte	Tay–Sachs disease Batten–Spielmeyer–Vogt disease Pompe disease (type II glycogen storage disease) (PAS positive) Niemann–Pick disease Mucopolysaccharidoses (types I–VI) Galactosialidosis Acute lymphoblastic leukemia

References: [1–14].

Table 8.2 Clinical features of metabolic storage diseases.

Disease	Deficient enzyme	Mode of inheritance	Clinical features
Gaucher disease	Glucocerebrosidase	Autosomal recessive	*Type I:* Hepatosplenomegaly Bone disease Bleeding Bruising May have growth retardation Anemia Pancytopenia *Type II and III:* Central nervous system involvement Hepatosplenomegaly Bone disease Bleeding Bruising Anemia Pancytopenia
Niemann–Pick	Type A & B: sphingomyelinase Type C: unknown	Autosomal recessive	*Type A and B:* Hepatosplenomegaly Macula with cherry red spot Pulmonary infiltrates Central nervous system involvement (type B) Anemia Pancytopenia Failure to thrive (type A) Type C: Hepatosplenomegaly Pulmonary disease Neonatal jaundice Central nervous system involvement
Fabry disease	α-galactosidase A	X-linked recessive	Angiokeratomas Renal failure Cardiomyopathy Vascular disease Corneal deposits Painful neuropathy Anemia

Mucopolysaccharidoses (MPS I–IX)	MPS I (Hurler, Scheie): Iduronidase
	MPS II (Hunter): Iduronate-2-sulfatase
	MPS III (Sanfilippo):
	   IIIA – heparin-*N*-sulfatase
	   IIIB – *N*-acetyl-glucosaminidase
	   IIIC – acetyl CoA glucosamine *N*-acetyl transferase
	   IIID – *N*-acetyl-glucosamine 6-sulfatase
	MPS IV (Morquio):
	   IVA – galactose-6-sulfatase
	   IVB – β-galactosidase
	MPS VI (Maroteaux–Lamy):
	Galactosamine-4-sulfatase
	MPS VII (Sly): β-glucuronidase
	MPS IX: Hyaluronidase
		Autosomal recessive: MPS I, III–IX
		
		X-linked: MPS type II
			Central nervous system involvement
			Hepatosplenomegaly
			Dysmorphic facies
			Skeletal abnormalities
			(Variable depending on disorder)

References: [15, 16].

disorder and its severity. It may be patchy or diffuse. Certain cytologic characteristics may be best appreciated on Wright–Giemsa-stained smear, although trephine core biopsy will give a better assessment of the degree of involvement.

There are essentially three types of storage disease histiocytes: Gaucher cells, highly vacuolated foamy histiocytes, and sea blue histiocytes. Although Gaucher cells are relatively the most specific, pseudo-Gaucher cells can certainly be seen in a variety of disorders that are not storage diseases. Some storage disorders will have more than one type of storage disease histiocyte. For example, foamy histiocytes and sea blue histiocytes may be seen together along with cells demonstrating intermediate features. Some cases show more foamy histiocytes, and others more sea blue histiocytes. Like pseudo-Gaucher cells, these cells may also be seen in a variety of disorders that are not storage diseases (Table 8.1).

Table 8.3 Pathologic findings in metabolic storage disorders.

Disease	Peripheral blood	Bone marrow smears	Special characteristics and special stains
Gaucher disease	Rarely, circulating Gaucher cells may be seen following splenectomy	*Gaucher cells* 20–100 μm in size Small, bland nucleus (few may be multinucleated) Fibrillar, striated, "crinkled" or "rumpled tissue paper" cytoplasm Occasional phagocytosis of platelets or erythrocytes May have hemosiderin pigment	Positive birefringence with polarized light PAS positive (with and without diastase), Prussian blue variably positive Masson trichrome may highlight striations in paraffin sections CD68 positive (KP1 and PGM1) S100 negative Fite negative Ziehl–Neelsen negative *Cytochemical stains* Sudan black B positive Acid phosphatase positive (tartarate resistant) Non-specific esterase positive (alpha naphthyl butyrate esterase stain)
Niemann–Pick	Foam cells or vacuolated lymphocytes may be seen	Type A and B: *Foamy histiocytes/ foam cells* 20–90 um in size Small, bland nucleus "bubbly," "foamy," vacuolated histiocytes Rarely erythrophagocytosis Type C: *Sea blue histiocytes* Small, bland nucleus Globular blue-gray to blue-green pigment Note: few foamy histiocytes and intermediate forms also seen	Luxol fast blue positive Oil red O positive PAS positive (with and without diastase) *Cytochemical stains* Sudan black B positive *Type A and B:* Positive birefringence on fresh unstained smears *Type C:* Cells may be faint yellow to brown on H&E stain
Fabry disease		*Sea blue histiocytes* Small, bland nucleus Globular blue-gray to blue–green pigment Note: cells appear foamy in paraffin tissue sections	PAS positive (with and without diastase) Luxol fast blue weakly positive Acid fast (Ziehl–Neelsen) *Cytochemistry* Sudan black B positive Acid phosphatase positive
Mucopolysaccharidoses (types I–VI)	Deep-lilac inclusions in lymphocytes and monocytes Vacuolated lymphocytes Alder–Reilly anomaly Single or small clusters of deep-lilac inclusions in neutrophils	Histiocytes with dark-lilac or dark-purple inclusions ("Gasser cells") Plasma cells with dark-lilac or dark-purple inclusions ("Buhot cells")	Deep-lilac inclusions metachromatic with toluidine blue (not all cases) PAS negative Sudan black B negative
Pompe disease (type II glycogen storage disease)	Vacuolated lymphocytes	Osteoblasts with cytoplasmic vacuoles (PAS positive)	

Abbreviations: PAS, periodic acid–Schiff; H&E, hematoxylin and eosin.
References: [1–4, 17, 18, 19].

Specific metabolic storage disorders

Detailed discussion of the clinical, genetic, and biochemical features of the lysosomal storage disorders is beyond the scope of this chapter, but a brief clinical summary of the following disorders is provided in Table 8.2. The pathologic features are summarized in Table 8.3.

Gaucher disease

Gaucher disease is the most common of the lysosomal storage disorders. It stems from a deficiency of glucocerebrosidase (also called acid beta-glucosidase or GBA) that results in the accumu-lation of glucosylceramide (also called glucocerebroside) within the lysosomes of the reticuloendothelial system and the central nervous system (in neuronopathic forms). There are three clinical types, broadly divided into the neuronopathic (types II and III) and non-neuronopathic (type I) forms. The most common form is the non-neuronopathic type, or type I [20].

The characteristic finding in the bone marrow is the Gaucher cell (Fig. 8.1). On a Giemsa- or Wright-stained bone marrow aspirate smear, Gaucher cells are large histiocytic cells (20–100 μm in size) with striated, fibrillar pale-blue to gray cytoplasm that has been likened to "crinkled" or "rumpled tissue paper," "wrinkled silk," or "paint brush strokes." They usually have a single, bland nucleus, although multinucleated cells

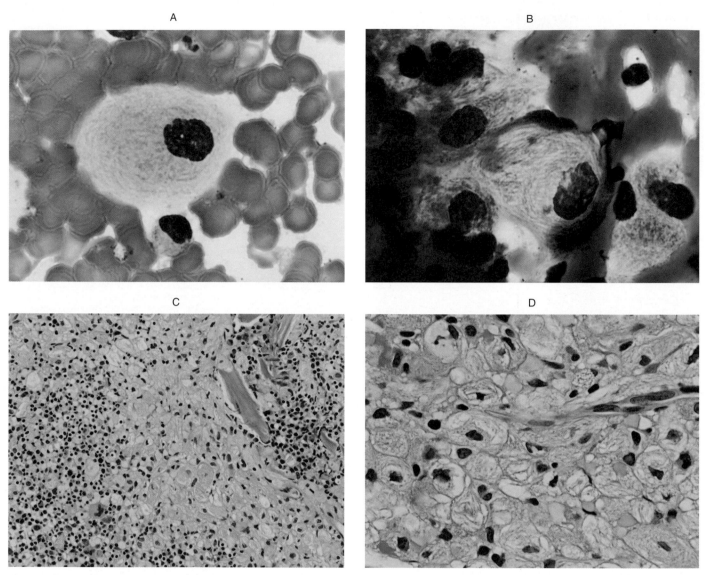

Fig. 8.1. Gaucher disease. (A, B) Bone marrow aspirate smear (Wright–Giemsa stain). Gaucher cells with pale-gray, striated cytoplasm. (C) Bone marrow core biopsy (H&E stain). Patchy infiltrate of Gaucher cells with abundant eosinophilic cytoplasm. (D) Bone marrow core biopsy (H&E stain). Gaucher cells with striated eosinophilic cytoplasm.

can be seen. Occasional hemosiderin pigment, erythrophagocytosis, or ingested platelets may be within the cytoplasm. Special stains for PAS (with and without diastase) and iron will be positive. Although Sudan black B is positive, other lipid stains will be negative [3]. Immunohistochemistry for CD68 is positive, but S100 is negative [19].

Niemann–Pick disease

Niemann–Pick encompasses two groups of diseases. Types A and B are both due to deficiency of acid sphingomyelinase, while type C is due to deficiency of a protein involved in intracellular processing and transport of low-density lipoprotein (LDL)-derived cholesterol (defective *NPC1* or *NPC2* gene) [21, 22]. All types result in hepatosplenomegaly, and many have

pulmonary involvement [23]. Peripheral blood foam cells or vacuolated lymphocytes have been described, but are not reliably present. Bone marrow involvement is invariably present in all types in most cases. The characteristic "Niemann–Pick cell," "foam cell," or foamy histiocyte is seen in types A and B, while sea blue histiocytes are more prevalent in type C. There is, however, overlap with some foam cells as well as intermediate forms being present in type C, and sea blue histiocytes can be seen in types A or B.

On a Giemsa- or Wright-stained bone marrow aspirate smear, foam cells or "Niemann–Pick cells" are large histiocytic cells 20–90 μm in size with small, bland, centrally located or eccentric nuclei (see Fig. 8.2). The cytoplasm is clear to pale blue and diffusely, finely vacuolated. Rare cells may show erythrophagocytosis. PAS is positive (with and without diastase),

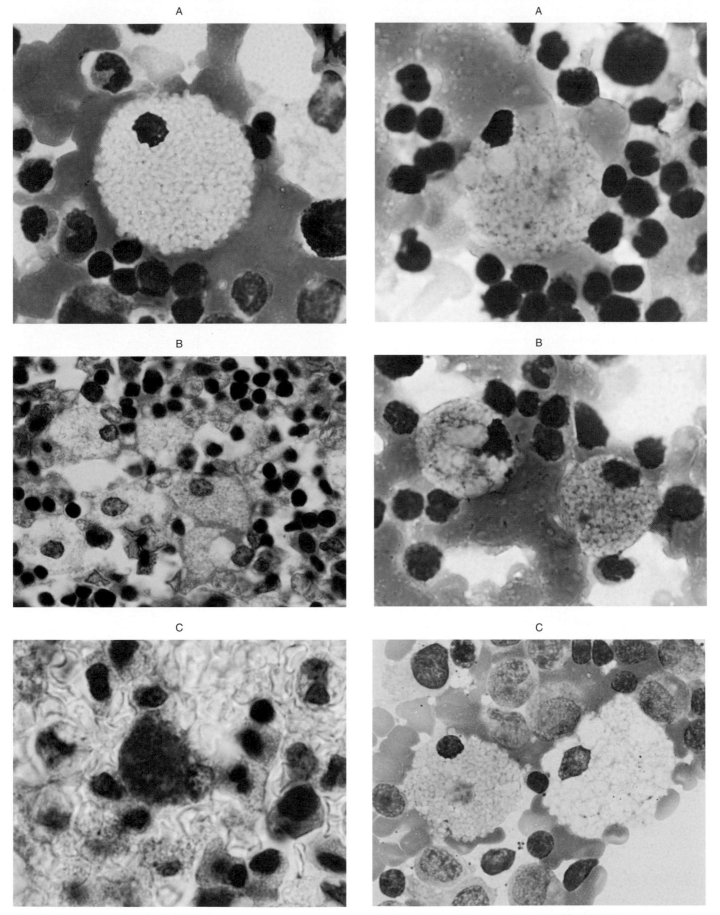

Fig. 8.2. Foam cells in Niemann–Pick. (A) Bone marrow aspirate smear (Wright–Giemsa stain). Large foamy histiocyte with abundant cytoplasm filled with uniform cytoplasmic vacuoles. (B) Bone marrow biopsy (H&E stain). Histiocytes with abundant foamy to finely granular cytoplasm. (C) Bone marrow biopsy (PAS stain). Strong PAS positivity in a storage foamy histiocyte.

Fig. 8.3. Sea blue histiocytes in Niemann–Pick type C. Bone marrow aspirate smear (Wright–Giemsa stain). (A, B) Sea blue histiocytes with abundant cytoplasm filled with variably sized blue–green to sea blue granules. (C) Sea blue histiocyte and foam cell in the same case. Focal erythrophagocytosis is noted.

as is Sudan black B and Oil red O (Fig. 8.2C) [3]. Sea blue histiocytes are slightly smaller than the foam cells and have coarse granules of variable size that stain blue–green or sea blue (Fig. 8.3). Similar to the foam cells, sea blue histiocytes stain with Oil red O and Sudan black B [24].

Fabry disease (also called Anderson–Fabry disease)

Fabry disease is an X-linked storage disorder resulting from a deficiency of α-galactosidase A (GALA). Patients present with relatively non-specific multisystem symptoms, and the diagnosis is often delayed years after the onset of symptoms. The most prominent findings are those of progressive renal failure, cardiac dysfunction, neuropathic pain, and vascular involvement with an increased risk for stroke [25]. Unlike many of the lysosomal storage disorders, prominent reticuloendothelial involvement with splenomegaly or markedly increased marrow histiocytes is uncommon. If performed, bone marrow aspirate examination usually will show the presence of sea blue histiocytes [26].

Mucopolysaccharidoses

The mucopolysaccharidoses are a group of 11 disorders resulting from deficiency of enzymes that break down glycosaminoglycans. The clinical spectrum is broad and variable in severity, depending on the specific deficiency and level of residual enzyme. Peripheral blood and bone marrow findings, although very characteristic, are not commonly seen. The morphologic findings, when present, are more prominent in the peripheral blood than the bone marrow. Vacuolated lymphocytes, lymphocytes containing cytoplasmic dark purple to lilac granules, the Alder–Reilly anomaly, and smaller numbers of dark-purple to lilac granules within neutrophils constitute the main peripheral blood findings (Fig. 8.4) [3]. The dark granules seen in lymphocytes, monocytes, and neutrophils are often surrounded by a clear halo, and may exhibit metachromatic staining with toluidine blue. Similar granules may be seen within histiocytes in the bone marrow. The Alder–Reilly anomaly consists of numerous, dark-lilac granules present within granulocytes that resemble toxic granulation or G-CSF effect, but the granules are somewhat bigger and increased in number. Similar granules are seen in basophils and eosinophils, which may make them difficult to distinguish from one another, although in some cases eosinophils show abnormal green-gray granules. Unlike the deep-lilac colored granules seen in the lymphocytes and monocytes, the granules of Alder–Reilly anomaly are not metachromatic with toluidine blue [3].

Differential diagnosis

Histiocytic infiltrates may be seen in the bone marrow associated with a variety of other conditions and may be distinguished from storage disease histiocytes by the clinical and morphologic features. The differential diagnosis would include, but is

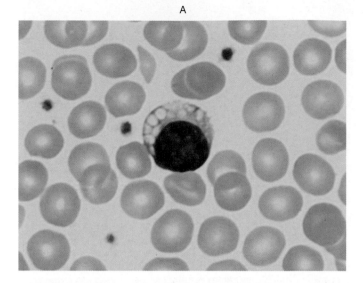

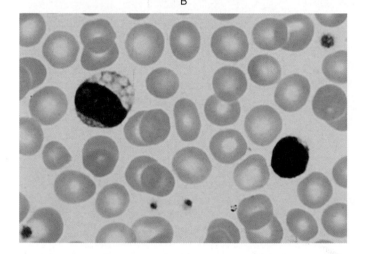

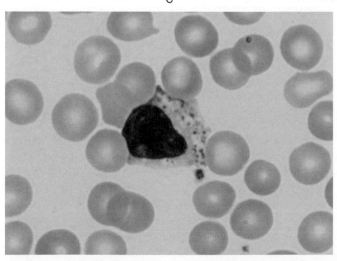

Fig. 8.4. Vacuolated lymphocytes and lymphocyte inclusions in a case of galactosialidosis. Peripheral blood smear (Wright stain). (A, B) Mature lymphocytes with multiple, large, prominent cytoplasmic vacuoles. (C) Mature lymphocytes with abundant cytoplasm containing prominent, pale eosinophilic granules surrounded by halos.

not limited to, granulomatous inflammation, lipogranulomas, hemophagocytic lymphohistiocytosis, Langerhans cell histiocytosis, Hodgkin lymphoma, and T-cell/histiocyte-rich diffuse large B-cell lymphoma, which may all have variable histiocytic infiltrates within the bone marrow.

Pseudo-Gaucher cells, sea blue histiocytes, and foamy macrophages, although very characteristic of the storage diseases, are not specific for them and can be seen associated with a variety of neoplastic and non-neoplastic conditions (see Table 8.1). However, when such cells are seen in a setting other than a storage disease, they are usually less prominent and not as numerous, although exceptions do occur. Pseudo-Gaucher cells, in particular, are seen associated with situa-tions of increased cell turnover or ineffective hematopoiesis, particularly leukemias and myelodysplastic syndromes [9] as well as some thalassemias and hemoglobinopathies [27, 28]. The striated inclusions seen in pseudo-Gaucher cells represent cell membranes and other cellular material from ingested cells. Some have proposed that the mechanism for the pseudo-Gaucher appearance lies in the supply of cell membranes overwhelming the capacity of the enzyme to break them down, leading to a localized enzyme deficiency within the cell. However, this has yet to be proven. Although pseudo-Gaucher cells are histologically and immunophenotypically identical to Gaucher cells [18], their ultrastructural features are distinct [4].

References

1. **Ziyeh S**, **Harzer K**. Bone marrow cytological storage phenomena in lipidoses. *European Journal of Pediatrics*. 1994;**153**:224–233.

2. **Takahashi K**, **Naito M**. Lipid storage disease: Part II Ultrastructural pathology of lipid storage cells in sphingolipidoses. *Acta Pathologica Japonica*. 1985;**35**:385–408.

3. **Brunning RD**. Morphologic alterations in nucleated blood and marrow cells in genetic disorders. *Human Pathology*. 1970;**1**:99–124.

4. **Lee RE**. Histiocytic diseases of bone marrow. *Hematology/Oncology Clinics of North America*. 1988;**2**:657–667.

5. **Bigorgne C**, **Le Tourneau A**, **Vahedi K**, *et al*. Sea-blue histiocyte syndrome in bone marrow secondary to total parenteral nutrition. *Leukemia and Lymphoma*. 1998;**28**:523–529.

6. **Van Dorpe A**, **Broeckaert-van Orshoven A**, **Desmet V**, **Verwilghen RL**. Gaucher-like cells and congenital dyserythropoietic anemia, type II (HEMPAS). *British Journal of Haematology*. 1973;**25**:165–170.

7. **Sharma P**, **Khurana N**, **Singh T**. Pseudo-Gaucher cells in Hb E and thalassemia intermedia. *Hematology*. 2007;**12**:457–459.

8. **Howard MR**, **Kesteven PJ**. Sea blue histiocytosis: a common abnormality of the bone marrow in myelodysplastic syndromes. *Journal of Clinical Pathology*. 1993;**46**:1030–1032.

9. **Kelsey PR**, **Geary CG**. Sea-blue histiocytes and Gaucher cells in bone marrow of patients with chronic myeloid leukemia. *Journal of Clinical Pathology*. 1988;**41**:960–962.

10. **Zidar BL**, **Hartsock RJ**, **Lee RE**, *et al*. Pseudo-Gaucher cells in the bone marrow of a patient with Hodgkin's disease. *American Journal of Clinical Pathology*. 1987;**87**:533–536.

11. **Kuo TT**, **Hu S**, **Huang CL**, *et al*. Cutaneous involvement in polyvinylpyrrolidone storage disease: a clinicopathologic study of five patients, including two patients with severe anemia. *American Journal of Surgical Pathology*. 1997;**21**:1361–1367.

12. **Stewart AJ**, **Jones RD**. Pseudo-Gaucher cells in myelodysplasia. *Journal of Clinical Pathology*. 1999;**52**:917–918.

13. **Dunn P**, **Kuo M-C**, **Sun C-F**. Pseudo-Gaucher cells in mycobacterial infection: a report of two cases. *Journal of Clinical Pathology*. 2005;**58**:1113–1114.

14. **Auwerda JJA**, **Leebeek FWG**, **Wilson JHP**, *et al*. Acquired lysosomal storage caused by frequent plasmapheresis procedures with hydroxyethyl starch. *Transfusion*. 2006;**46**:1705–1711.

15. **Wraith JE**. Lysosomal disorders. *Seminars in Neonatology*. 2002;**7**:75–83.

16. **Weibel TD**, **Brady RO**. Systematic approach to the diagnosis of lysosomal storage disorders. *Mental Retardation and Developmental Disabilities Research Reviews*. 2001;**7**:190–199.

17. **Volk BW**, **Adachi M**, **Schneck L**. The pathology of sphingolipidoses. *Seminars in Hematology*. 1972;**9**:317–348.

18. **Florena AM**, **Franco V**, **Campesi G**. Immunophenotypical comparison of Gaucher's and pseudo-Gaucher cells. *Pathology International*. 1996;**46**:155–160.

19. **Ortiz J**, **Abad M**, **Muriel M**, *et al*. Gaucher's disease: morphological findings in a case studied with fine needle aspiration. *Cytopathology*. 2002;**13**:371–374.

20. **Chen M**, **Wang J**. Gaucher disease. Review of the literature. *Archives of Pathology and Laboratory Medicine*. 2008;**132**:851–853.

21. **Kolodny EH**. Niemann-Pick disease. *Current Opinion in Hematology*. 2000;**7**:48–52.

22. **Ikonen E**, **Holtta-Vuori M**. Cellular pathology of Niemann-Pick type C disease. *Seminars in Cell and Developmental Biology*. 2004;**15**:445–454.

23. **Schuchman EH**. The pathogenesis and treatment of acid sphingomyelinase-deficient Niemann-Pick disease. *Journal of Inherited Metabolic Diseases*. epub 2007;**30**:654–663.

24. **Chang KL**, **Gaal KK**, **Huang Q**, **Weiss LM**. Histiocytic lesions involving the bone marrow. *Seminars in Diagnostic Pathology*. 2003;**20**:226–236.

25. **Ries M**, **Gupta S**, **Moore DF**, *et al*. Pediatric Fabry disease. *Pediatrics*. epub 2005;**115**:e344–e355.

26. **Oliveira JP**, **Valbuena C**, **Moreira AB**, *et al*. Splenomegaly, hypersplenism, and peripheral blood cytopenias in patients with classical Anderson-Fabry disease. *Virchows Archiv*. epub 2008;**453**:291–300.

27. **Zaino EC**, **Rossi MB**, **Pham TD**, **Azar HA**. Gaucher's cells in thalassemia. *Blood*. 1971;**38**:457–462.

28. **Carrington PA**, **Stevens RF**, **Lendon M**. Pseudo-Gaucher cells. *Journal of Clinical Pathology*. 1992;**45**:360.

9

Reactive lymphadenopathies

Maria A. Proytcheva

Introduction

Lymphadenopathies occur frequently during childhood, and their incidence varies with age. In a majority of children, lymph node enlargement is transient, self-limited, and resolves without sequel, and lymph node biopsies are rarely performed. When a lymph node biopsy is performed, the primary goal of histologic examination is to determine the nature of the process: whether it is a malignant or benign, lymphoid or non-lymphoid proliferation.

This chapter focuses on reactive lymphoid proliferations in children. The chapter will first summarize key points in the development and functional anatomy of lymph nodes, then will discuss the epidemiology of pediatric lymphadenopathies and finally will describe the most frequent types of reactive lymphoid proliferations in children. Since characterization of all lymphadenopathies is beyond the scope of a single chapter, here we will focus on those entities that present major diagnostic challenges in distinguishing benign from malignant disorders, as well as those pediatric lymphadenopathies that are seen in conjunction with specific syndromes.

Embryonal development of lymph nodes

Lymph nodes, similarly to the other secondary lymphoid organs, have a specialized architecture and microenvironment promoting controlled interactions of immune cells in order to elicit a rapid and appropriate immune response to infectious agents. Knowledge of the development and functional anatomy of lymph nodes is important since many of the morphologic changes observed in reactive conditions reflect lymph node function and its role in the normal immune response.

Lymph nodes develop independently of antigen or pathogen recognition during the embryonal period and shortly after birth. While our understanding of the programmed development of lymph nodes has expanded significantly in the last decade, some elements of the developmental scheme are still to be discovered. According to the latest model based on transgenic animal studies as well as on the study of patients with primary immune deficiencies, lymph nodes develop as a result of a highly coordinated series of interactions between various hematopoietic, mesenchymal, and endothelial cells [1–4].

The lymph node development occurs concurrently with the process of lymphatic vascularization. Initially, the lymphatic endothelial cells evolve out of venous endothelial cells at predetermined sites, to form loose, confluent connections of capillary plexuses or lymphatic spaces that will later develop into lymph nodes [5]. In mice, this process is controlled by transcription factor Prox1 which is expressed exclusively on the lymphatic endothelial cells [6]. In the early stages of lymph node development, homeostatic cytokines, including CXCL13, CCL19, and CCL21 recruit IL-R7R+CD3−CD4+CD45+ hematopoietic cells, known as "lymphoid tissue inducers" (LTis) to the lymph sacs. LTis are derived from interleukin-7 receptor α (IL-7Rα)-positive multipotent hematopoietic cells from the fetal liver that have been shown to be the precursors of all lymphocyte subsets (B, T, and NK) and dendritic cells (DCs). The LTis aggregate near the endothelium of the future lymph nodes and trigger the differentiation of VCAM1+ICAM1+immature mesenchymal cells, also known as "lymphoid tissue organizers" (LTos) that form the stromal matrix of the developing lymph nodes. The unstructured collection of LTi and LTo cells formed at the sites of the secondary lymphoid organs is called primitive lymph node anlagen. In mice, this process occurs around embryonic day (E) 12.5 [3].

The interactions between the LTi and LTo cells are orchestrated by several key signaling pathways, such as transcription factor Ikaros, IL-7, tumor necrosis factor-related activation-induced cytokine (TRANCE), and lymphotoxin signaling. Failure of proper differentiation of IL-7Rα-positive cells due to alterations in these signaling pathways results in global defects in the immune system and impaired development of lymph nodes and Peyer patches in the gastrointestinal tract. For example, transcription factor Ikaros-deficient transgenic mice lack B-, T-, NK-, and dendritic cells, and do not develop lymph nodes or Peyer patches, and lymphotoxin-deficient, Lta −/− mice lack Peyer patches and most lymph nodes [3].

Once sufficient cell clustering occurs, interactions between the LTi and LTo cells allow a further differentiation of these cells as well as of the surrounding cells. This stimulating microenvironment promotes the development of high endothelial venules (HEVs), which regulate lymphocyte trafficking into the lymph node. The HEVs are specialized venules found in lymphoid tissue that are the site of entry for lymphocytes from the bloodstream into the lymph nodes. The lymphotoxin pathway is essential for the formation of HEVs by promoting the expression of LTαβ on the endothelial cells, in addition to its role in the formation and maturation of stromal cells and dendritic cells, and in maintaining the number of dendritic cells [1].

The next step in lymph node development is *lymphocyte-independent initiation of follicle formation*. The initial follicle formation also requires proper lymphotoxin pathway activation, and while it occurs independently of B- and T-cells, it is cytokine dependent [7]. CXCL13, CCL19, and CCL21 direct the migration of CXCR5-expressing B-cells, and CCR7 attracts the T-cells [2]. The last step in the *development of fully mature secondary lymphoid organs* involves the recruitment of lymphocytes, the segregation of B- and T-cell areas, and the formation of mature B-cell follicles, and is antigen dependent.

During *B-cell ontogeny*, the generation of B-cells secreting specific antibodies proceeds in two stages. The first stage is antigen independent and occurs in the bone marrow, where B-lymphoblasts undergo immunoglobulin (Ig) VDJ gene rearrangement and mature to surface-immunoglobulin-positive naïve B-cells [8]. These naïve B-cells, often CD5+, are small, resting lymphocytes that circulate in the peripheral blood. The second stage is antigen dependent and occurs in the secondary lymphoid organs. There, the naïve B-cells encounter antigen that fits their surface Ig receptors and transform, proliferate, and ultimately become memory B-cells and antibody-secreting plasma cells.

The *T-cells* also arise in the bone marrow, but their maturation occurs in the thymus via a series of well-defined independent stages [8]. There, through the processes of beta selection, positive selection, and negative selection, T-cells mature and become effector T-cells, able to respond to foreign antigens and develop self-tolerance. The least mature cortical thymocytes express CD1a, cytoplasmic CD3, CD5, CD7, and TdT, and are CD4 and CD8 double negative. During that stage, the TCR gene rearrangement is completed; the cells express surface CD3. The T-cells that have not properly rearranged their TCRs die by apoptosis (beta selection). The cells that survive the beta selection express surface TCRs, but not all of the receptors are functional. Only T-cells whose TCRs are capable of binding major histocompatibility complex (MHC) molecules survive. During this process, called positive selection, CD4 and CD8 are upregulated and co-expressed (double positive). The double-positive thymocytes undergo lineage commitment, maturing into CD8+ T-cells capable of binding MHC class I, and CD4+ cells capable of binding MHC class II molecules. These T-cells leave the thymus and circulate through the blood and lymphoid tissue looking for matching antigen.

The developmental pathways for peripheral lymph nodes, mesenteric lymph nodes, and Peyer patches differ in their requirements for chemokines, cytokines, and growth factors. The development is also confined to a temporal window in embryogenesis that varies depending on the type and location of these lymphoid organs. For example, in mice, mesenteric lymph nodes develop first, followed by brachial, axillary, and popliteal lymph nodes [1]. Once a specific temporal window has passed, the particular lymph node group associated with that time period cannot develop, regardless of whether key signaling pathways, such as the lymphotoxin pathway, are activated or not.

Structure and function of lymph nodes

Lymph nodes are located throughout the body. Usually they are less than 1 cm in diameter, except in early childhood, specifically ages 2 to 10 years, when they may be larger. Lymph nodes are solitary structures surrounded by a dense fibrous capsule with inner trabecular structures of similar composition branching off to cross the interior of the node. The capsule is pierced by several afferent lymphatics that drain lymph containing lymphocytes and antigen-presenting cells. The lymph flows slowly and unceasingly from the draining area through the afferent lymphatics to the subcapsular, intermediate, and medullary sinuses; it exits as efferent lymph through the lymph node hilum. The lymph node sinuses are lined by sinus endothelial cells that have flat endothelium forming a discontinuous layer allowing free trafficking of small molecules.

Lymph nodes are highly specialized organs, and their schematic structure is shown in Fig. 9.1. The lymph node has defined B- and T-cell-dependent compartments and distinct cortical, paracortical, and medullary regions. The outer region of the node, the *cortex*, contains multiple follicles that are very dense accumulations of B-lymphocytes associated with follicular dendritic cells (FDCs). Prior to antigenic stimulation, these collections are composed predominately of naïve B-cells, and are known as "primary" follicles. After stimulation by an antigen which fits their surface receptor, the naïve B-cells undergo transformation and proliferate to form a germinal center (GC), thereby transforming the primary follicle into a "secondary" follicle. Some of these antigen-stimulated B-cells ultimately mature into antibody-secreting plasma cells and memory B-cells. B-cells that do not gain access to the antigen die by apoptosis. The follicles are unstable structures that undergo changes in size, composition, and dimension in accordance with the degree of antigenic stimulation, state of health, and age.

The *paracortex*, the area between the cortex and medulla, is composed of a less-dense accumulation of T-cells and dendritic cells (DCs). The tissue in the central part of the lymph node, the *medulla*, is loose and contains lymphoid cells and plasma cells that are arranged in the form of irregular strands called medullary cords. The *sinuses* are composed of small and broader, continuous and interconnected ducts and spaces crowded by cells. According to their location, the sinuses are divided into subcapsular (marginal), trabecular, and medullary sinuses.

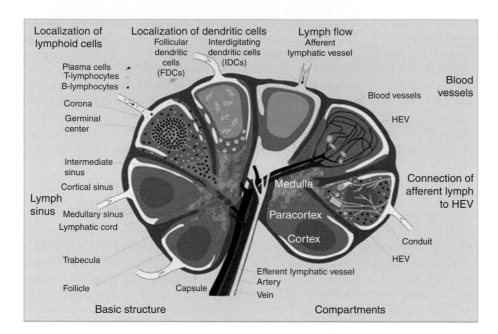

Fig. 9.1. Schematic representation of a lymph node. The cortex contains predominantly B-cells organized in primary or secondary follicles. The paracortex contains a less-dense accumulation of T-cells and dendritic cells. The medulla contains mostly plasma cells and B-lymphocytes. The lymphocytes enter the lymph node via afferent lymphatic vessels or through transmigration of the high endothelial venules (HEVs). The lymphatic vasculature and blood vasculature are connected via a conduit system, and both ultimately drain into the medullary sinus and then to an efferent lymphatic vessel. (Reprinted from Blum, Pabst [2], with permission.)

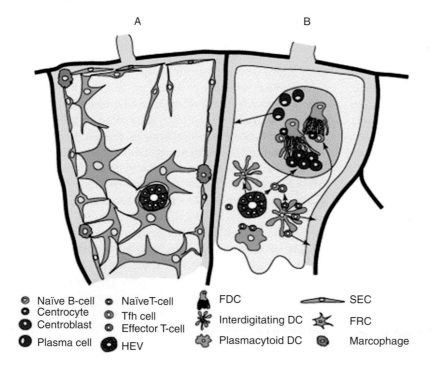

Fig. 9.2. Schematic representation of the lymph node conduit system. (A) The left panel shows the three-dimensional network of fibroblastic reticular cells (FRCs) that provide cellular bases for the conduit system which connects the subcapsular and intermediate sinuses to the high endothelial venules (HEVs) and allows efficient trafficking and rapid transfer of antigens, cytokines, and immune complexes from the subcapsular sinuses to the deep cortex. (B) In the right panel, naïve B- and T-cells enter the lymph node through the HEV in response to a specific chemoattractant, and are directed to designated areas of the lymph node. The naïve B-cells are attracted to the B-cell follicles in the cortex in response to CXCL13 cytokine secreted by the follicular dendritic cells (FDCs). The FDCs form the meshwork of the secondary follicles. The T-cell differentiation occurs in the paracortex and is driven by dendritic cells (DCs). Plasma cells and effector T-cells leave the lymph node via medullary sinuses. Abbreviations: SEC, sinus endothelial cell; Tfh, follicular B-helper T-cell. (Reprinted from Crivellato et al. [9], with permission.)

The lymph nodes are composed of two components: stroma, consisting of a meshwork of collagenous and reticular fibrils and stromal cells; and parenchyma comprised of migrating cells (lymphocytes and antigen-presenting cells). The function of the stroma is to support lymphocyte trafficking and promote the production of homing cytokines for T-cells, B-cells, and DCs. To achieve this function, the major stromal cell population, the fibroblast reticular cells (FRCs), along with the collagenous and reticular fibrils, forms an internal three-dimensional framework of interconnected channels, called the FRC conduit system, that "directs" the traffic of lymphocytes and facilitates their movement along preformed "corridors." Schematic representation of the conduit system of the lymph node is shown in Fig. 9.2. This system connects the subcapsular and intermediate sinuses to HEVs and allows for efficient and rapid transfer of antigens, chemokines, and immune complexes from the subcapsular sinus into the deep cortex. The FRCs are also deeply involved in matrix reorganization and remodeling of the lymph node architecture during an immune response [9]. The B- and T-lymphocytes enter the lymph node by extravasation across the HEVs, while soluble antigens and DCs enter the lymph node via the afferent lymphatics at multiple sites along the capsule [10].

Functional organization of the cortex, B-cell compartment

The functional organization of the lymph node follicles is highly dependent on the presence of follicular dendritic cells (FDCs). These cells occupy the outer layers of the primary and secondary follicles and express CXCL13, which is essential for follicular clustering of B-cells and for attracting a unique CD4+ T-cell subset known as follicular B-helper T (Tfh) cells, which promote the terminal differentiation of B-cells [9]. The FDCs, with the adjacent FRC, form a three-dimensional sponge-like meshwork that plays an essential role in antigen presentation and in promoting B-cell proliferation and differentiation into the GC.

The naïve B-cells enter the lymph node via the HEVs in the T-cell zone, where they are directed to the follicles in response to CXCL13. Upon antigenic stimulation, B-cells migrate to the border of the primary follicles to meet antigen-specific CD4+ Tfh cells, and initiate the formation of the GC. In the GCs, the B-cells undergo clonal expansion, somatic hypermutation in the B-cell Ig variable region genes, selection of B-cells on their ability to receive antigen-specific signals, and subsequent differentiation to memory B-cells and plasma cells [11].

The GCs contain at least two morphologically distinct cell types: large centroblasts with scant cytoplasm; and small centrocytes with a dense, cleaved nucleus and abundant, pale cytoplasm, as shown in Fig. 9.3. The centroblasts are actively prolif-

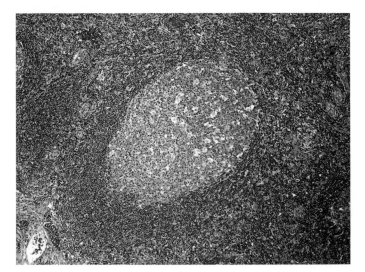

Fig. 9.3. A secondary follicle with well-defined germinal center (GC) and mantle zone. The dark zone (top right) of the GC contains actively proliferating centroblasts that undergo clonal expansion and diversification of their immunoglobulin B-cell receptors. The resulting B-cells migrate to the light zone (lower left) of the GC and become centrocytes. The B-cells expressing low affinity immunoglobulin B-cell receptors undergo apoptosis and are eliminated by tingible body macrophages seen in the dark zone. The mantle zone is well defined and thicker in the area covering the light zone, a feature called polarization that is frequently present in reactive but absent in neoplastic follicles (H&E stain).

erating cells that undergo clonal expansion and diversification of their B-cell receptor repertoire through somatic hypermutation of *IG* genes. The resulting B-cells move to the light zone of the GC and become centrocytes. Both centroblasts and centrocytes are BCL2 negative, and as a result are programmed to die unless they are rescued by high-affinity interactions between their antigen receptor and a given antigen. The GC B-cells express CD10 and BCL6, a nuclear transcription factor which plays a critical regulatory role in the proliferation and differentiation of the B-cells in the GC. The *BCL6* gene also undergoes somatic mutations but with lower frequency compared to *IG variable* genes.

Centrocytes expressing Ig with high affinity to antigen are rescued from apoptosis by re-expression of BCL2. They switch off BCL6 protein expression after interactions with FDCs (via CD23) and T-cells (via CD40 ligand), and differentiate into memory and antibody-producing B-cells. The late centrocytes express IRF4/MUM1. The antibody-producing cells migrate to the medullary cords where they become plasma cells that eventually will leave the lymph node through the medullary sinuses and home to the bone marrow. They lack surface Ig but contain cytoplasmic IgG or IgA and express IRF4/MUM1, CD79a, CD38, and CD138. The plasma cells are CD20 negative.

Functional organization of the T-cell compartment (paracortex)

The adaptive immune response begins in the paracortex after the interaction between naïve T-cells and DCs that have migrated from the inflamed areas to the lymph node. The naïve T-cells constantly circulate through the blood and lymphoid tissue looking for their cognate antigens and, similarly to the B-cells, they enter the lymph node via the HEVs as a result of homing cytokines secreted by HEVs, stromal cells, and DCs. The DCs present antigens and provide co-stimulatory signals to the naïve CD4+ and/or CD8+ T-cells to become specialized effector T-cells that either leave the lymph node, or stay within the lymph node proper as memory T-cells or CD4+ Tfh cells.

The DCs are potent antigen-presenting cells. Using real-time two-proton microscopy it has been shown that one DC can contact approximately 500 T-cells [9]. DCs are a heterogeneous group of bone marrow-derived antigen-presenting cells. In humans, there are two primary types of DC – conventional and plasmacytoid. Conventional DCs (cDCs) are HLA-DR+ cells that express high levels of CD11c [8]. Human HLA-DR+ plasmacytoid DCs (pDCs), also known in the past as plasmacytoid monocytes/plasmacytoid T-cells, are defined by lack of expression of CD11c and high expression of CD123. The pDCs are typically found in cell clusters in the T-cell-dependent paracortical and interfollicular areas and around HEVs.

The pDCs have recently drawn more attention, since prominent clusters of such cells called plasmacytoid monocytes have been recognized as features of Kikuchi–Fujimoto disease [12] and the hyaline vascular type of Castleman disease [13]. These cells secrete large amounts of type I interferon (interferon-α),

Table 9.1. Common microorganisms causing lymphadenitis in children.

Bacteria
Staphylococcus aureus
Streptococcus (group A)
Bartonella henselae (cat scratch disease)
Brucella abortus (brucellosis)
Francisella tularensis (tularemia)
Yersinia pseudotuberculosis (yersiniosis)
Salmonella species (typhoid fever)
Gram-negative rods
Treponema pallidum (syphilis)
Chlamydia trachomatis (lymphogranuloma venereum)

Mycobacterium
Mycobacterium tuberculosis complex

Viruses
Epstein–Barr virus (EBV) [human herpesvirus 4 (HHV-4)]
Cytomegalovirus (CMV)
Herpes simplex virus (HSV)
Human immunodeficiency virus (HIV)
Measles virus
Rubella virus

Fungi
Histoplasma capsulatum
Coccidioides immitis
Cryptococcus neoformans
Aspergillus spp.

Protozoa
Toxoplasma gondii (toxoplasmosis)
Plasmodium spp. (malaria)

Table 9.2. Pattern approach in classification of lymphadenopathy in children.

Predominantly follicular pattern
Follicular hyperplasia
Giant follicular hyperplasia
Juvenile rheumatoid arthritis
Progressive transformation of germinal centers
Castleman disease
Kimura disease

Predominantly paracortical pattern
Nodular paracortical hyperplasia
   Dermatopathic and non-dermatopathic lymphadenopathy
Diffuse paracortical expansion
   Infectious mononucleosis
   Infectious mononucleosis-like lymphadenopathy
   Atypical lymphoproliferative disorders in children

Predominantly sinus pattern
Sinus histiocytosis
Sinus histiocytosis with massive lymphadenopathy (Rosai–Dorfman disease)
Benign lymph node lesions mimicking metastatic pediatric renal tumors

Stromo-vascular lesions
Inflammatory pseudotumor of lymph nodes
Vascular transformation of sinuses

Necrotizing lymphadenitis
Histiocytic necrotizing lymphadenitis (Kikuchi–Fujimoto disease)
Systemic lupus lymphadenopathy
Cat scratch disease
Kawasaki disease

accounting for their extensive rough endoplasmic reticulum and plasmacytoid cytoplasm. Normal and neoplastic pDCs in human tissue express the adaptor protein CD2AP, which is essentially restricted to this cell population [14]. The pDCs can arise from both lymphoid and myeloid progenitors, and they show features associated with several lineages – T-cells, B-cells, and myeloid cells. As a consequence, the cellular origin of pDCs has been a subject of controversy in the past.

Lymph node plasticity

Once established, the lymph nodes cannot be ablated. However, they are not stationary structures and they undergo substantial remodeling after an inflammatory insult. Following antigenic stimulation, lymph nodes increase in size, cellularity, efferent lymph flow, and number and dimension of HEVs, and once the antigenic stimulation is resolved, the lymph node gradually returns to normal [4]. The intensity and pattern of reaction depends on the age, type, and duration of antigenic stimulation, and immune competency of the patient. For these reasons, marked lymphoid hyperplasia is common in children and young adults, and is a result of the normal antigenic stimulation that occurs early in life.

Classification for reactive lymphadenopathies

There is no standard classification of reactive lymphadenopathies in either children or adults. The etiology of lymph-

adenopathy can be broadly divided into infectious, autoimmune, iatrogenic, or unknown. Table 9.1 lists the common microorganisms causing various types of lymphadenitis in children. Based on this approach, the lymphadenitis can be divided into bacterial, viral, mycobacterial, and so on. While such classification is very important from a therapy prospective, establishing it may be problematic, since genetically related microorganisms may demonstrate different morphologic patterns. For example, lymphadenitis due to closely related viruses, that is, cytomegalovirus (CMV), Epstein–Barr virus (EBV), or herpes simplex virus (HSV), has morphologically distinctive features. Furthermore, most of the infectious diseases show a spectrum of morphologic changes depending upon the host response. Therefore, the morphologic findings will depend on when the tissue is sampled in respect of the immune response as well as the immune competence of the individual.

Discussion of benign enlargement of lymph nodes has traditionally followed architectural patterns in the context of normal anatomy and physiology of the lymph node [15]. Thus, the cellular composition and morphology of the cortex, paracortex, and/or sinuses of the lymph node allows classification of the lymphadenopathies into mostly follicular, diffuse, sinusoidal, or mixed (Table 9.2).

A challenging step in evaluation of lymph nodes is the identification of the various lymph node compartments, particularly when they are obscured by the pathologic process. A small panel of *immunohistochemical stains* can facilitate this process. CD20 highlights the B-cells in the follicles as well as scattered B-cells in the interfollicular areas. CD21 or CD35, follicular dendritic cell markers, highlight the follicular dendritic cell meshwork. The paracortex can be identified by T-cell antibodies such as CD3 or CD5. The interdigitating reticulum cells are S100 positive, and HECA-452 is helpful to demonstrate the endothelial cells of the HEVs. CD68 confirms the presence of macrophages and other cells of monocytic origin. CD123 is very helpful in detection of plasmacytoid dendritic cells.

Epidemiology of lymphadenopathies in children

Lymphadenopathies are frequent during childhood. Palpable lymph nodes are found in 34% of neonates and 57% of children aged 1 to 12 months [16]. Forty-four percent of children younger than five years seen during well-child visits had lymphadenopathy. In children seen during a "sick visit," this percentage has been reported to be as high as 64% [17]. The most frequent sites of involvement are the head and neck regions.

While lymphadenopathy is common during childhood, lymph node biopsy is infrequent. Indications for a lymph node biopsy in a child include lymph nodes larger than 2.5 cm; a node that increases in size despite appropriate therapy; rapid increase in the size of hard, matted lymph nodes in the pre-auricular or supraclavicular regions, or in the posterior triangle of the neck; the presence of massive generalized lymphadenopathy; or when the lymphadenopathy is associated with systemic symptoms such as fever or persistent night sweats and/or with worrisome clinical and laboratory findings [18, 19].

Despite worrisome symptoms, most of the lymph node biopsies in children are non-neoplastic. In a series of 239 children, 55% had reactive hyperplasia with undetermined etiology, 32% granulomatous diseases including cat scratch disease, atypical mycobacterial infection, tuberculosis, toxoplasmosis, and fungal infection, and only 13% of the lymphadenopathies were neoplastic [18]. Similarly, Moore and colleagues, in a series of 1877 surgical specimens from children with cervical lymphadenopathy, found a malignant process in approximately one of every eight lymph node biopsies [19].

The location and number of enlarged lymph nodes may suggest the nature of the process. While submandibular and upper cervical lymph nodes are more frequently involved by a reactive process, lower cervical, supraclavicular, axillary, and inguinal lymphadenopathy are more frequently malignant. However, no site of lymph node enlargement is completely immune from serious disease. In children, generalized lymphadenopathy with systemic symptoms is more frequently reactive in nature, and lymphadenopathy due to neoplasm is more frequently localized.

The specific cause of the lymphadenopathy in a child should be sought. Reactive hyperplasia occurs most frequently in the upper cervical lymph nodes. The age of the child is not particularly useful in helping to determine the cause of lymph node enlargement. Exceptions to this general rule include histiocytosis X, which occurs primarily in children less than three years of age; atypical mycobacterial infection, which is seen most fre-

Table 9.3. Pediatric malignancies involving lymph nodes.

Hematopoietic malignancies
Precursor lymphoid neoplasms
   T-lymphoblastic lymphoma
   B-lymphoblastic lymphoma
Mature B- or T-cell neoplasms
   Burkitt lymphoma
   Diffuse large B-cell lymphoma
   Anaplastic large cell lymphoma, ALK positive
   Peripheral T cell lymphoma
Hodgkin lymphoma

Non-hematopoietic malignancies
Neuroblastoma
Rhabdomyosarcoma
Wilms tumor
Thyroid carcinoma
Nasopharyngeal carcinoma
Malignant melanoma

quently in children between one and six years; and Hodgkin lymphoma, which has a high incidence in the teenage years [18].

Lymphoma (lymphoblastic, Hodgkin, or non-Hodgkin lymphoma) is the most common malignancy, and it is seen in about two-thirds of the malignant cases. Metastatic neuroblastoma, rhabdomyosarcoma, or local spread of thyroid tumors, nasopharyngeal carcinoma, Wilms tumor, melanoma, and ovarian tumors account for the remaining cases (Table 9.3).

The clinical history, physical examination, and the results of other laboratory tests are helpful in determining the cause of lymphadenopathy. Knowledge of previous surgery/biopsy, vaccination, exposure to pets, and duration of the lymphadenopathy is helpful in the diagnostic workup of a child with enlarged lymph nodes. Duration of symptoms, fever and weight loss, sore throat, presence of toothache or lesion in the region drained by the enlarged lymph node may be helpful in determining the underlying cause. In the presence of peripheral lymphadenopathy, a mediastinal mass, abdominal lymphadenopathy, and/or hepatosplenomegaly are more often seen in neoplastic than reactive conditions.

Diagnostic approach

The workup of a child with lymphadenopathy should include a thorough clinical history and physical examination as well as laboratory tests, if clinically indicated. Some of the most frequently ordered laboratory studies include a complete blood cell count, erythrocyte sedimentation rate, serologic studies for infectious agents and immune disorders, and flow cytometry, not all of which may be helpful.

Complete blood cell count (CBC), including an evaluation of the peripheral blood smear, while non-specific, can contribute to determining the cause of reactive lymphadenopathies in children. If anemia is present, it is usually mild, normochromic, normocytic. However, severe immune-mediated hemolytic anemia with or without thrombocytopenia may be present in patients with lymphadenopathies due to underlying immune deficiency, either congenital or acquired.

The *white blood cell (WBC) count* and white blood cell differential count may also be helpful in the investigation of the cause of lymph node enlargement. Bacterial infection can be suspected if there is leukocytosis with neutrophilia, particularly if the neutrophils show toxic changes such as toxic granulation, vacuolation, and Döhle bodies, and/or a shift to immaturity in the granulocytes. Patients with viral infections, particularly due to EBV and CMV, often have lymphocytosis including circulating transformed, atypical, reactive lymphocytes. In other acute and chronic viral infections, transformed lymphocytes and plasma cells are frequently found. Chronic infections, particularly *Mycobacterium tuberculosis*, are associated with peripheral blood monocytosis. The presence of blasts on the peripheral blood smear from a child is not always indicative of leukemia/lymphoma. However, in the setting of normochromic, normocytic anemia with or without thrombocytopenia, generalized lymphadenopathy, and/or hepatosplenomegaly, the identification of blasts in the peripheral blood is worrisome and requires further investigation to rule out acute leukemia.

The *erythrocyte sedimentation rate (ESR)* is often requested, but is rarely helpful in distinguishing between benign and neoplastic lymphadenopathy. This test is non-specific and can be elevated in either clinical setting.

Serologic studies for infectious agents and autoimmune disorders can be particularly helpful. The presence of IgM and absence of IgG antibodies specific for EBV, CMV, *Bartonella henselae*, or *Toxoplasma gondii*, points to an acute infection with one of these organisms rather than history of past infection and anamnestic immune response. While positive monospot test demonstrating heterophile antibodies confirms the diagnosis of infectious mononucleosis, a negative test does not exclude an acute EBV infection. This test, while very specific, is not sensitive, and is negative in 10–15% of patients, particularly children under 10 years of age. *Tuberculin skin* tests or an *in vitro* gamma interferon test for tuberculosis may be considered in the proper clinical settings.

Fine needle aspiration (FNA), a minimally invasive procedure for obtaining material for cytologic examination and flow cytometry, is used widely in adults. In children, however, its use has been limited to the workup of metastatic solid tumors, obtaining specimens for microbiologic studies in suppurative lymphadenitis, and, to lesser degree, in some hematologic malignancies such as lymphoblastic lymphoma. Several reasons contribute to the limited utility of FNA in children. In this age group, most of the lymphadenopathies are due to reactive causes and an increased number of transformed lymphocytes is frequent. Thus, limited sampling and lack of examination of all lymph node compartments may result in erroneous diagnosis of lymphoma in the settings of florid lymphoid hyperplasia. As a result, FNA in children is often inconclusive and requires a subsequent lymph node biopsy. Low viability due to crush artifact limits the use of material obtained by FNA for cytogenetic studies and flow cytometry. Lastly, the main advantage of FNA in adults, lack of sedation, is not applicable for most children.

Attempts have been made to utilize FNA in the diagnosis of reactive lymphadenitis with characteristic histologic features such as Kikuchi–Fujimoto disease (KFD). However, the studies are small and the results are mixed. In one such study of 27 cases in adolescents and adults, FNA was successful in making the diagnosis of KFD by identifying plasmacytoid monocytes and karyorrhectic debris intermixed with "crescentic" histiocytes with abundant cytoplasm containing karyorrhectic debris and/or eosinophilic material [20]. In another study, a retrospective review of 44 cases of KFD, the overall accuracy of FNA was only 56.2%, with a false-negative rate of 50%, and a false-positive rate of 37.5% [21]. Lastly, in a study of 10 Taiwanese children with lymphadenopathy, FNA was unsuccessful and a subsequent excisional biopsy was required for the establishment of the diagnosis of KFD in all patients [22]. Thus, FNA has not been established as a useful tool in the diagnosis of reactive lymphadenopathies in children.

Ancillary studies such as *flow cytometry* and *gene rearrangement* studies can contribute and establish the presence of heterogeneous B- and/or T-cell populations, and will be discussed as a part of the lymphoma workup. However, these studies by themselves are insufficient in concluding that the lesion is a reactive or neoplastic process.

Lymphoma workup

A lymph node biopsy in a child is performed when there is high suspicion of lymphoma or metastatic tumor and, less frequently, for microbiologic studies. In either situation, the tissue should be delivered fresh to the laboratory and processed without delay. It is mandatory that it is handled properly to allow optimal preservation of the tissue for histologic examination and ancillary studies [23]. In general, a lymphoma workup in a child does not differ significantly from that in adults. Both include gross examination of the lymph node, evaluation of Diff-Quik-stained touch imprints, proper fixation, and banking frozen material for future studies. If, based on the touch imprint examination, there is high suspicion of lymphoma, then flow cytometry and cytogenetic studies should be performed. However, these and other ancillary studies should be used judiciously since they are time consuming, expensive, and contribute little in most cases of reactive lymphadenopathy. If enough tissue is available, a piece should be frozen in liquid nitrogen, since it is an excellent source of DNA and RNA that may be needed for further characterization of the pathologic process.

Special efforts need to be made to prevent the tissue from drying, to maximize cell viability and antigen preservation, since some of the studies, such as flow cytometry and cytogenetics, require viable cells. For best results, the entire lymph node should be submitted in either culture medium (RPMI-1640) or sterile normal saline. Receiving the tissue in a saline-soaked gauze is an acceptable, but less preferable, alternative. Gross examination of the tissue and careful documentation of size, shape, cut surface, and presence of hemorrhage or necrosis is important and helpful in formulating an initial impression.

A   B

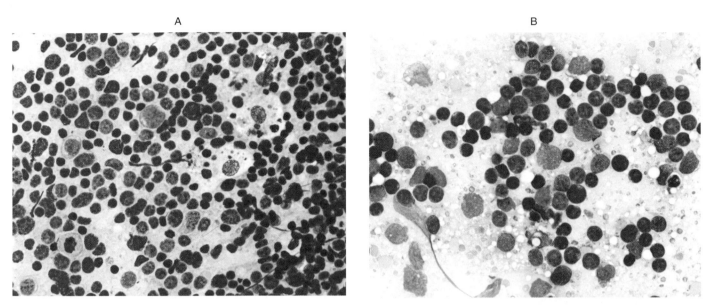

Fig. 9.4. Diff-Quik-stained touch imprints of lymph nodes. (A) Reactive lymphoid proliferation showing a mixture of small, medium, and large lymphocytes, immunoblasts, and tingible body macrophages. (B) Neoplastic proliferation showing a monotonous population of variable-size blasts with finely speckled chromatin, inconspicuous nucleoli, and scant basophilic cytoplasm on a background of cytoplasmic fragments. Flow cytometric and cytogenetic studies would be appropriate.

The highest priority of the lymphoma workup is proper fixation of the tissue for histologic examination, with ancillary studies such as flow cytometry and/or cytogenetics secondary, particularly since many of the more important studies can be performed on routinely processed tissues. Specifically, a wide variety of paraffin-reactive antibodies have been developed to detect lymphoid and myeloid antigens in paraffin-embedded tissues. Furthermore, some specific cytogenetic abnormalities can also be identified in routinely processed tissues by fluorescent *in situ* hybridization (FISH), although, for cytogenetics, fresh cells are preferable. However, the development of ancillary tests for routinely processed material allows for more extensive analysis of even limited tissue specimens.

Examination of well-stained touch imprints provides invaluable information for further triaging of the tissue. The presence of a mixed cellular infiltrate composed of small, medium, and large lymphocytes, immunoblasts, a few plasma cells as well as neutrophils, eosinophils, and histiocytes in a lymph node biopsy of a child suggests a reactive process (Fig. 9.4). By contrast, the presence of a monotonous population of cells (Fig. 9.4B) is more likely to be a neoplastic proliferation, thereby requiring cytogenetic studies and flow cytometry. If the tissue is limited and one must choose between the two, the cytogenetic studies should be chosen over the flow cytometry.

Flow cytometry and/or gene rearrangement studies of pediatric lymph nodes should be interpreted carefully and only in conjunction with the morphologic features of the routinely processed specimen (either an H&E section or FNA smear). While clonal B- or T-cell populations are present in lymphomas, they can also be seen in reactive processes such as follicular hyperplasia, particularly in children. For instance, light chain restricted, follicle center-type B-cells have been demonstrated by four color flow in histologically reactive lymph nodes in

young patients with no known immunologic abnormalities [24, 25]. Similarly, clonal immunoglobulin heavy chain or T-cell receptor gene rearrangements have also been detected by PCR analysis or the Southern blot hybridization technique [25]. Thus, one should bear in mind that identification of a monotypic B-cell proliferation by flow cytometry, even if confirmed by the presence of a clonal population in gene rearrangement studies, does not always equate to lymphoma.

In the remaining sections of this chapter, the most frequent lymphadenopathies diagnosed in children, as well as those lymphoid proliferations that require distinction from lymphoma will be discussed. These entities are organized based on the morphologic changes seen in one or more lymph node compartments.

Predominantly follicular lesions

Follicular hyperplasia

Follicular hyperplasia (FH) is a non-specific manifestation of a B-cell response to antigenic stimulation in the presence of intact T-cell help. FH is a common finding in lymph nodes of children and adolescents, and may be quite extensive. In adults, extensive follicular hyperplasia is uncommon and is more frequently seen in the settings of autoimmune disorders, such as rheumatoid arthritis, or acquired immune deficiency.

The hallmark of the *histologic examination* in FH is the marked increase in the number and size of follicles that occupy the cortex, paracortex, and even the medulla (Fig. 9.5). The follicles vary in size and shape and may show polarization, a feature attributed to reactive cause of the proliferation. The follicles are composed of well-defined germinal centers and preserved mantle zones. The germinal centers contain a mixture of centrocytes,

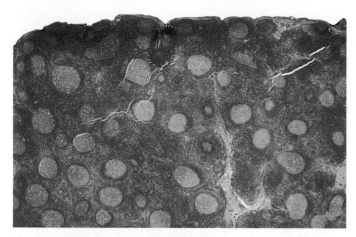

Fig. 9.5. Reactive follicular hyperplasia. Numerous follicles in the cortex, paracortex, and medulla of a lymph node. The follicles vary in size and have well-defined GC and mantle zone (H&E stain).

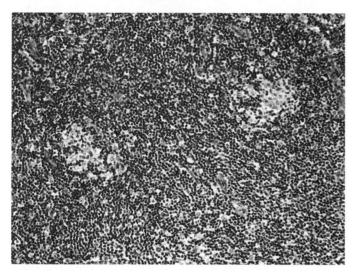

Fig. 9.6. Follicle lysis: GC infiltrated by small lymphocytes, a mixture of T-lymphocytes, and a smaller number of mantle B-lymphocytes (H&E stain).

centroblasts, plasma cells, and histiocytes. Numerous tingible body macrophages containing karyorrhectic debris and apoptotic bodies, as well as scattered mitotic figures, are frequently, but not always, present. The follicles are composed predominantly of B-lymphocytes, and only a small number of CD4+ T-lymphocytes are seen in the germinal centers.

As was presented earlier, the lymph nodes are dynamic structures, and after antigenic stimulation different follicles are at various stages of activation. While some of the follicles have small emerging germinal centers with a prominent mantle zone, others are large, composed mostly of a germinal center, and with only a thin, attenuated mantle zone. The ultimate fate of the follicles at the end of immune reaction is follicle dissolution, a process known as *follicle lysis* (Fig. 9.6). Morphologically, in follicle lysis the germinal centers are infiltrated by "tongues" of small lymphoid cells with clumped nuclear chromatin and scant cytoplasm, which by immunostaining have been shown to be primarily CD3+ BCL2+ T-cells admixed with a smaller number of BCL2+ mantle B-cells [26].

The germinal centers can undergo regressive changes in which they are burned out or *regressively transformed*. This is due to the progressive disappearance of the lymphoid component of the germinal centers with sclerosis and crowding of vessels, and an increased number of follicular dendritic cells, either by concentration as a result of the collapse of the germinal center, or due to proliferation of the FDCs as documented by expression of Ki-67. These cells are positive for follicular dendritic cell markers (CD21 and CD23), and are negative for macrophage markers such as CD14, CD15, and lysozyme.

Epithelioid germinal centers are found in some cases of angioimmunoblastic lymphadenopathy and sometimes in lymph nodes from young children who have succumbed as a result of a fulminant infection [27, 28]. In children dying from a variety of causes, marked follicular hyperplasia with prominent nuclear fragmentation can also be seen along with epithelioid germinal centers (Fig. 9.7). Such changes are particularly prevalent in young children between the ages of one and three years. While the cause of death does not correlate with the changes, evidence of shock is present in the majority of cases [28]. Nuclear fragmentation and epithelioid change in germinal centers have also been described with the sudden infant death syndrome. While infections, glucocorticoids, shock, and acute breakdown of immune defenses have been speculated to play a role, the etiology of these changes is still unclear.

The interfollicular area may be expanded in parallel, or compressed by the hyperplastic follicles. It is composed of a mixture of small- and medium-sized lymphocytes, immunoblasts, plasma cells, and a small number of histiocytes, as well as eosinophils. Prominent vascular proliferation and HEVs with plump endothelium are characteristic and are in accord with the reactive nature of the process. Numerous plasma cells can be seen in the medullary sinuses.

Giant follicular hyperplasia

In children, follicular hyperplasia can be exuberant and manifested by very large follicles composed of two or more fused adjacent germinal centers, forming oddly shaped geographic outlines (Fig. 9.8). The mantle zone is attenuated or completely replaced by the germinal center, and the interfollicular area is compressed. In rare cases, particularly in young males, coalescence of large serpentine germinal centers may result in the formation of one giant follicle occupying the entire lymph node. The nature of such giant follicular hyperplasia, however, is unclear. While some consider this phenomenon a distinct clinicopathologic entity [29], others view it as an extreme manifestation of reactive follicular hyperplasia [30].

Juvenile rheumatoid arthritis (JRA)

Follicular hyperplasia with interfollicular plasmacytosis is characteristic of lymphadenopathy in patients with autoimmune diseases and particularly *rheumatoid arthritis* (RA) [31]. Similarly to adults, children with systemic *juvenile rheumatoid arthritis* (JRA) may present with FH with plasmacytosis. In such

A

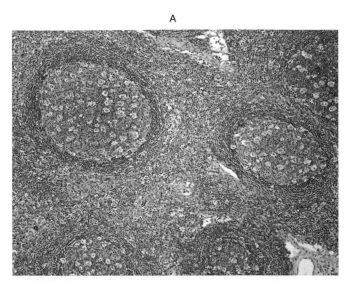

B

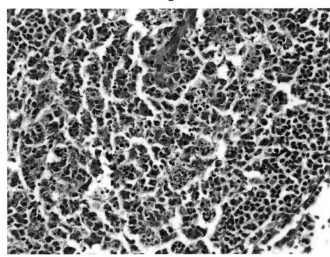

C

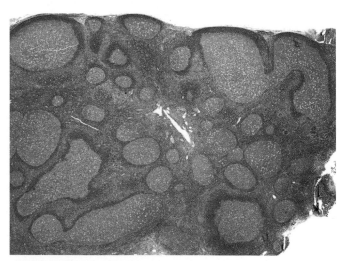

Fig. 9.7. (A, B) Post-mortem lymph node demonstrating follicular hyperplasia with striking nuclear fragmentation. (C) Epithelioid change of germinal centers (H&E stain).

Fig. 9.8. Exuberant follicular hyperplasia in a seven-year-old boy with recurrent lymphadenopathy. Extensive immune deficiency workup was negative. Note the oddly shaped expanded follicles and attenuated mantle zones. Similar changes can be seen in the lymph nodes of patients with congenital or acquired immune deficiency (H&E stain).

lymph nodes, the follicles vary in size and shape as shown in Fig. 9.9A. The germinal centers can be very prominent with numerous tingible body macrophages and mitotic figures. The mantle zone, when present, can be attenuated. Cracking artifact surrounding large follicles has been reported, but is not always seen. The interfollicular areas are infiltrated by variable numbers of polytypic plasma cells, as shown in Fig. 9.9B–C. Some follicles may contain an increased number of plasma cells as well. Collections of neutrophils and focal microabscesses in patients with severe disease may be present. There is moderate proliferation of HEVs that demonstrate hyperplastic plump endothelium. The sinuses are patent, but may be dilated and contain histiocytes and neutrophils.

The etiology of JRA is still unclear, and multiple factors, both genetic and environmental, play a role in this disease. While some mechanisms are shared between children and adults, there are unique factors playing a role in this disease in children. At least 10% of children with systemic JRA develop macrophage activation syndrome, a complication that contributes

A

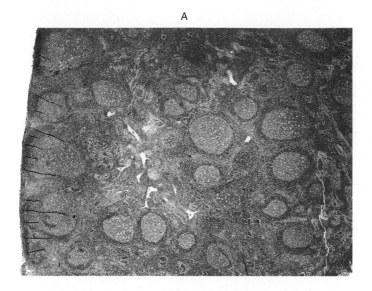

B

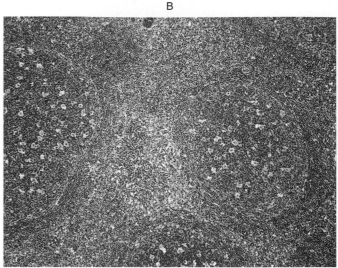

C

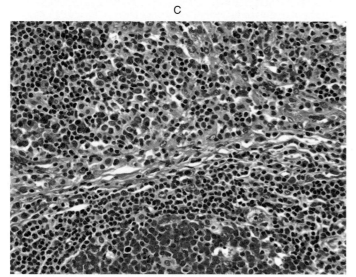

Fig. 9.9. Juvenile rheumatoid arthritis lymphadenopathy. (A) Low-power view showing marked follicular hyperplasia with expanded paracortex. Note the variable size and shape of follicles. (B) Well-defined germinal centers with numerous tingible body macrophages and interfollicular plasma cells. (C) High-power view showing sheets of plasma cells (H&E stain).

significantly to the morbidity and mortality of the disease [32]. In such patients, abnormal NK function and characteristic polymorphism at the *MUNC13–4* have been reported. In lymph nodes of such patients, bland-appearing histiocytes containing phagocytized erythrocytes, platelets, or other cellular elements may be present.

Progressive transformation of germinal centers

Progressive transformation of germinal centers (PTGC) is a benign, poorly understood condition that is present in 3–15% of lymph nodes with reactive follicular hyperplasia [26, 33–36]. It is usually seen in young adults, and the diagnosis is established solely on morphologic criteria.

While there are many similarities between the clinical presentation of PTGC in children and adults, some age-specific differences exist. The condition is more frequent in children, and the median age at diagnosis is 11 years [34]. Similarly to adults, PTGC is more frequent in males than in females and usually

presents as a single, asymptomatic, enlarged lymph node in the cervical, inguinal, or, less frequently, axillary region. However, in children PTGC can also present as generalized lymphadenopathy and there is a higher recurrence rate compared to adults (50% vs. 23%). Two or more recurrences, usually in the same lymph node region, have been reported in about 20% of the children with PTGC [34].

Lymph nodes vary in size from 1 to 5 cm, and the cut surface of the lymph node is nodular to lobulated in appearance, as shown in Fig. 9.10A. The progressively transformed GCs are at least three- to four-times larger than normal GCs, and are present in the context of reactive follicular hyperplasia. Therefore, they are best recognized on low magnification (Fig. 9.10B–C). The number of transformed GCs varies, with most affected lymph nodes having from one to three abnormal follicles. Less frequently there are between 4 and 11 transformed GCs per lymph node [36]. In a small number of cases (<5%), mostly adolescent boys and young men, lymphoid hyperplasia with florid PTGC has been reported [33]. In such cases, the number

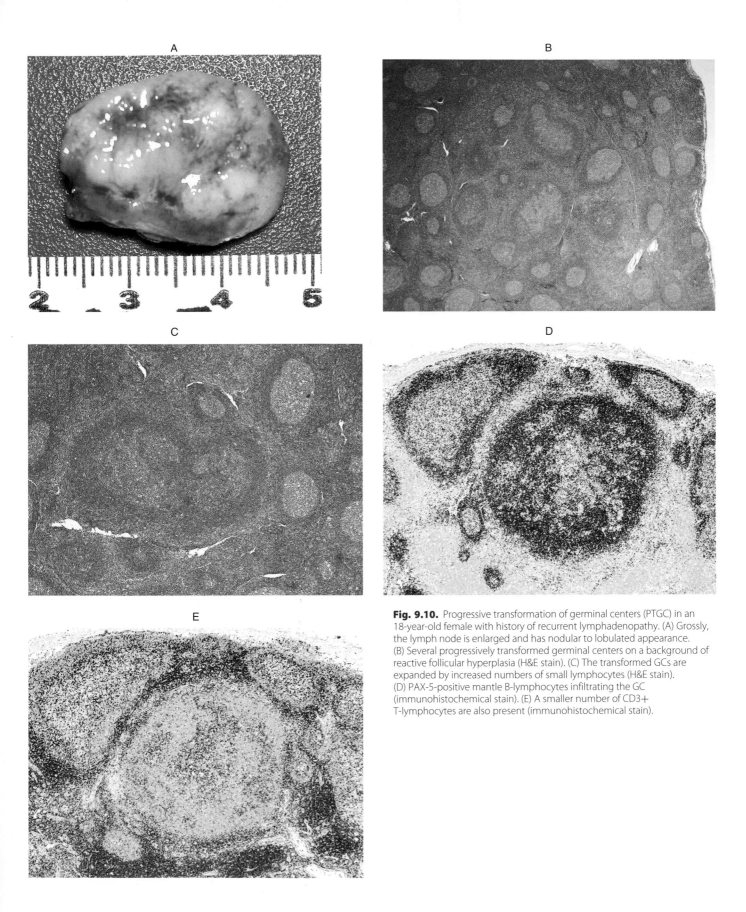

Fig. 9.10. Progressive transformation of germinal centers (PTGC) in an 18-year-old female with history of recurrent lymphadenopathy. (A) Grossly, the lymph node is enlarged and has nodular to lobulated appearance. (B) Several progressively transformed germinal centers on a background of reactive follicular hyperplasia (H&E stain). (C) The transformed GCs are expanded by increased numbers of small lymphocytes (H&E stain). (D) PAX-5-positive mantle B-lymphocytes infiltrating the GC (immunohistochemical stain). (E) A smaller number of CD3+ T-lymphocytes are also present (immunohistochemical stain).

F

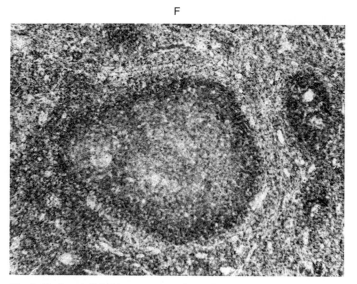

G

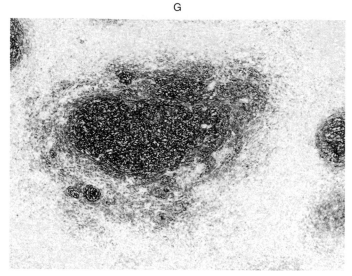

Fig. 9.10. (*cont.*) (F) BCL2-positive mantle B-cells and T-cells infiltrating the progressively transformed GC (immunohistochemical stain). (G) CD21 highlights the disrupted follicular dendritic cell meshwork of PTGC (immunohistochemical stain).

of progressively transformed GCs has ranged from 10 to 123 per specimen. In nearly half of the pediatric PTGC, clusters of epithelioid histiocytes rim the progressively transformed GCs [34, 36]. This feature appears to be unique to children.

PTGC is a part of the spectrum of reactive follicular hyperplasia and possibly the ultimate fate of a follicular center in response to antigen stimulation [37]. Progressively transformed GCs are enlarged as a result of increased numbers of predominantly BCL2+ small mantle B-lymphocytes, and to a lesser degree of CD3+ T-lymphocytes, which results in breaking-up of the germinal centers into ill-defined clusters (Fig. 9.10D–G). Similar to the reactive GCs, most of the cells in these clusters of progressively transformed GCs are B-cells, which have undergone somatic hypermutation, clonal expansion, and selection, but are clonally unrelated [38]. It is still unclear whether progressively transformed GCs are descendants of classical GCs or develop independently as a distinct type of immune reaction.

The majority of cases of PTGC resolve without sequelae. However, PTGC has consistently been associated with the nodular lymphocyte-predominant type of Hodgkin lymphoma (NLPHL), which is one of the reasons for the great interest in this disorder in the past [33, 34, 36, 39]. Currently, based on single cell molecular analysis, PTGC shows no evidence of clonal expansion beyond the limits of individual progressively transformed GCs, and is not considered to be a premalignant lesion [38].

The association between PTGC and NLPHL is based on the morphologic and immunohistochemical similarities between the two disorders. The distinction between the two lesions occasionally can be difficult. The most important difference is the presence of popcorn (lymphocytic and histiocytic; L&H) cells in NLPHL and their absence in PTGC. With the combination of pan-B- and pan-T-cell markers, most cases of NLPHL can

be distinguished from PTGC by the irregular distribution of B-cells and the presence of numerous aggregates of CD3+, CD4+, CD57+ T-cells, often forming rosettes around the L&H cells. While T-cell rosettes may be present in PTGC, they are notably fewer than those in NLPHL. In addition, the T-cells are frequently in clusters in NLPHL, and in PTGC the CD57+ cells are usually scattered throughout the node.

Castleman disease

Castleman disease (CD), known also as angiofollicular hyperplasia, is a lymphoproliferative disorder associated with characteristic, but not diagnostic, histopathologic findings and clinical symptoms (as they can be seen in other clinical settings). While the disease affects all ages, there are differences in CD between children and adults. Although this discussion will focus on children, some general comments about CD, including comments about the process in adults, will also be included.

Histologic variants and clinical presentation

The diagnosis of CD is based on histopathologic features supported by clinical findings and follow-up. CD has two *histologic variants*: hyaline vascular (HV) and plasma cell (PC) variants; however, mixed forms showing features of both histologic variants (i.e., mixed type) can also be seen. These histologic variants can present either as *unicentric or multicentric disease*. The HV variant is by far the most common and is seen in up to 91% of the cases [40, 41]. Most HV cases show hyperplasia of lymphoid follicles with abnormalities involving both the germinal center and the mantle zone (Fig. 9.11A). The follicles are composed of expanded mantle zones and germinal centers surrounded by concentric layers of small lymphocytes ("onion skin"). One follicle may contain one or multiple well-demarcated germinal centers (Fig. 9.11B–C). All stages and

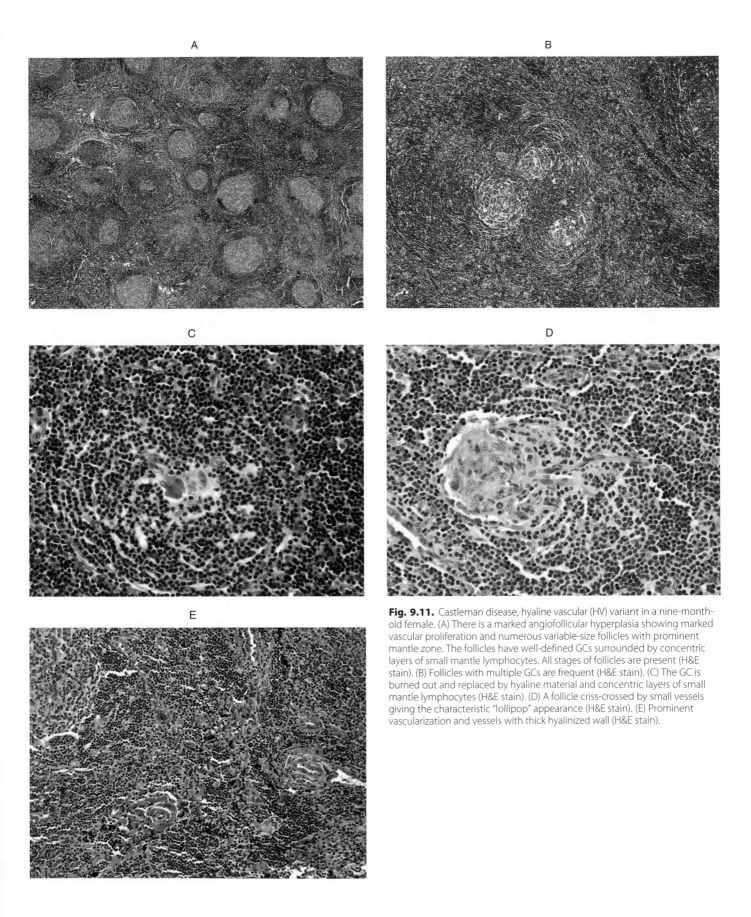

Fig. 9.11. Castleman disease, hyaline vascular (HV) variant in a nine-month-old female. (A) There is a marked angiofollicular hyperplasia showing marked vascular proliferation and numerous variable-size follicles with prominent mantle zone. The follicles have well-defined GCs surrounded by concentric layers of small mantle lymphocytes. All stages of follicles are present (H&E stain). (B) Follicles with multiple GCs are frequent (H&E stain). (C) The GC is burned out and replaced by hyaline material and concentric layers of small mantle lymphocytes (H&E stain). (D) A follicle criss-crossed by small vessels giving the characteristic "lollipop" appearance (H&E stain). (E) Prominent vascularization and vessels with thick hyalinized wall (H&E stain).

forms of follicles are present: from large follicles with well-demarcated germinal centers to small ones composed of pale eosinophilic cells with a few or no follicular dendritic cells and an expanded mantle zone. Completely burned-out follicles composed of fibrotic scars with radiating vessels, with or without hyalinized walls, are also present (Fig. 9.11D). Some of the nodules are criss-crossed by small vessels that penetrate into the follicles and form a characteristic "lollypop" appearance (Fig. 9.11E).

The interfollicular areas in the HV type show an increased vascular network. Most of these vessels have flat endothelium and thicker wall due to the hyaline deposition, but vessels with plump endothelium may also be seen (Fig. 9.11F). Areas with increased fibrosis and large sclerotic bands may also be present [40].

The diagnosis of HV type of CD is based on the presence of the combination of vascular proliferation and characteristic follicles, and not on the individual features that can be seen in other disorders. For example, occasionally, isolated germinal centers with the above described morphology or "onion skin" layering of mantle lymphocytes can be seen in otherwise nondescript reactive nodes. Small, regressively transformed germinal centers may be seen in HIV-associated lymphadenopathy [42] or in children who die of sepsis or systemic illness [28]. Increased vascularity is a common feature of reactive lymphadenopathies. Thus, neither of the above mentioned features alone is sufficient for the diagnosis of CD.

The morphologic features of the PC variant of CD are quite distinctive and differ from the morphologic features of the HV type (Fig. 9.12). The hallmark of this type of CD is the presence of sheets of mature plasma cells in the interfollicular areas in a background of reactive follicular hyperplasia [40]. In most of the cases the plasma cells are polytypic. However, cases with foci of monotypic plasma cells in a background of polytypic plasma cells have been reported [43]. In some cases, amyloid deposits are found either in the lymphoid mass, the liver, spleen, or systemically throughout the body [40].

Follicular hyperplasia and plasmacytosis are non-specific features and may be seen in lymphadenopathies in rheumatoid arthritis and other autoimmune diseases, syphilis, lymph nodes draining malignancy, and skin disorders. Therefore, the diagnosis of PC variant of CD is appropriate only after these possibilities have been excluded and the clinical presentation is consistent with that of CD.

In most cases, CD is localized or unicentric, with or without systemic symptoms, and it has an excellent prognosis. Less frequently, CD manifests as disseminated or multicentric disease involving multiple sites. Systemic symptoms and unfavorable prognosis are characteristic for the multicentric type of CD. The HV type of CD is almost always unicentric. However, the PC variant can present clinically either as unicentric or as multicentric disease.

The PC variant of CD is more frequently associated with systemic symptoms than the HV type. These include fever, night sweats, and fatigue, and laboratory abnormalities such as mild normochromic, normocytic anemia, leukocytosis, thrombocytopenia, elevated erythrocyte sedimentation rate, hyperglobulinemia, hypoalbuminemia, hypoferritinemia, hypotransferrinemia, hypergammaglobulinemia, elevated alpha-2-globulin levels, hyperfibrinogenemia, elevated IL-6 levels, and elevated levels of other cytokines [40, 44].

Pathogenesis

While the pathogenesis of HV type is poorly understood, our understanding of the pathogenesis of PC type, particularly the multicentric form of CD, has advanced greatly. The key element responsible for the clinical symptoms of CD is the deregulated overproduction of IL-6, from either endogenous or viral sources [45]. It has been shown that the serum IL-6 level correlates with the degree of lymph node hyperplasia and the clinical and laboratory abnormalities in CD. After a localized tumor is excised, complete recovery of the IL-6 level and clinical improvement follows. In contrast, in the HV variant of CD, the patients do not have increased serum levels of IL-6, which most likely accounts for the paucity of plasma cells in this histologic type, and paucity of systemic symptoms [46].

Furthermore, our understanding of the multicentric form of CD has advanced greatly with the discovery of its association with the Kaposi sarcoma-associated herpesvirus/*human herpesvirus 8* (KSHV/HHV-8) [47, 48]. HHV-8 is thought to play an etiologic role in the multicentric form of CD, as it produces a human IL-6 homolog, viral IL-6, that functions similarly to human IL-6. Furthermore, 100% of the HIV-positive patients and 40–50% of immunocompetent patients with multicentric CD are found to be infected with HHV-8, by a variety of means including immunostaining of CD lymph nodes for the latent nuclear antigen (LANA) of the virus.

Castleman disease in children

Pediatric CD is rare, and less than 100 reports occurring in children under 18 years of age are found in the literature [49–52]. As such, there is very little information on the actual incidence of the disease in children. In one retrospective study from South Africa, the proven cases of CD comprised less than 2% of all pediatric lymph node biopsies examined in that institution [52]. CD appears to be slightly more frequent in girls compared to boys. Although most of the children in the literature are older than 13 years of age, occurrences in children as young as 2 months have been reported [50, 53].

A slow-growing mass is present in a quarter of the children with CD. The most frequent sites of involvement are the mesenteric, mediastinal, retroperitoneal, and peripheral lymph nodes. General symptoms such as fever, fatigue, failure to thrive, and weight loss are the initial symptoms in almost a half of the reported cases [50, 53]. Similarly, laboratory abnormalities are more frequently present in children in comparison to adults, and are reported in 23% of patients with the HV type, 55% of the localized cases, 82% of children with the mixed cell type, and in all children with the PC variant [50]. In a fifth of the children

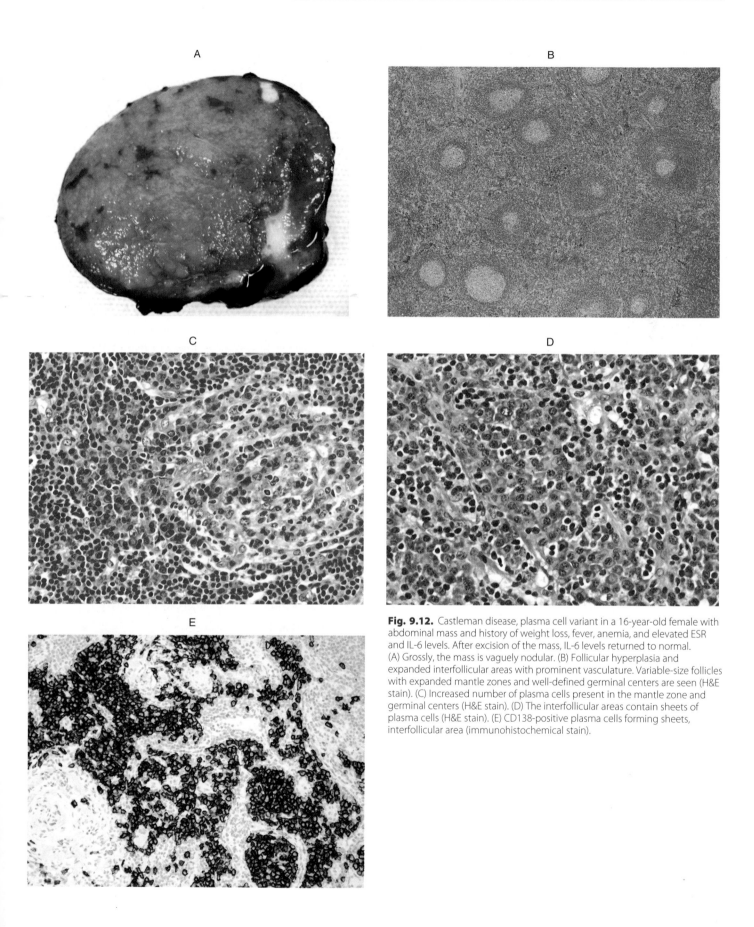

Fig. 9.12. Castleman disease, plasma cell variant in a 16-year-old female with abdominal mass and history of weight loss, fever, anemia, and elevated ESR and IL-6 levels. After excision of the mass, IL-6 levels returned to normal. (A) Grossly, the mass is vaguely nodular. (B) Follicular hyperplasia and expanded interfollicular areas with prominent vasculature. Variable-size follicles with expanded mantle zones and well-defined germinal centers are seen (H&E stain). (C) Increased number of plasma cells present in the mantle zone and germinal centers (H&E stain). (D) The interfollicular areas contain sheets of plasma cells (H&E stain). (E) CD138-positive plasma cells forming sheets, interfollicular area (immunohistochemical stain).

diagnosed with CD, there is an association between anemia, hypergammaglobulinemia, and failure to thrive. All children with multicentric CD have laboratory abnormalities, as mentioned, including neutropenia and thrombocytopenia. In some children with multicentric disease, positive *in situ* hybridization with EBV-encoded RNA or, rarely, clonal Ig heavy chain rearrangements have been reported [51]. The rare pediatric multicentric CD cases examined for the presence of HHV-8 were consistently negative. Thus, HHV-8 most likely does not play a role in the pathogenesis of pediatric multicentric CD, in contrast to adults. Furthermore, the lower frequency of multicentric CD in children supports the hypothesis that pediatric CD may represent an earlier form of the disease where other environmental factors play a role in its pathogenesis.

Most of the children with CD present with unicentric disease. Similarly to adults, HV variant is the most frequent histologic type and the PC variant comprises a minority of pediatric cases. However, the mixed cell type is more frequent in children than in adults. Unicentric CD is a benign disorder. As a result, a complete excision of the mass is usually curative. A few cases of spontaneous remission have been reported as well [50]. Rarely, symptoms due to mass compression may require radiation therapy.

Multicentric CD is extremely rare in children [51]. It is a serious disease and requires medical treatment in most cases. Even so, its prognosis in children is more favorable than in adults and the morbidity and mortality are lower. Of the 12 pediatric cases of multicentric CD reported in the literature, there is only one early death occurring shortly after excision of the mass [50, 51, 54]. Prednisone alone or in combination with methotrexate, intravenous immunoglobulin, interferon, and plasmapheresis have been used for successful therapy.

Overall, multicentric CD in children as compared to adults is more frequently present in mesenteric lymph nodes and less frequently located in the thorax. The disease is less often, if ever, associated with HIV infection or other immunodeficiency states. Unlike adults, in children CD is not associated with HHV-8 and has a good response to treatment with an overall favorable outcome [50, 51].

Patients with multicentric CD have an increased risk of developing lymphoma, whereas the unicentric form, particularly the HV type, usually has excellent prognosis. However, rarely, patients with HV type of CD complicated by lymphoma have been reported, as in the case of a 17-year-old female with unicentric CD, HV type, who developed follicular lymphoma [55].

CD is rarely reported in children from the developing countries, and the manifestation of the disease may be different in these children when compared to children from developed countries [52]. It is unclear whether the disease is underreported or overlooked in pre-pubertal children where constitutional symptoms are common and the lymphadenopathies may be under-investigated. Taylor *et al.* report six confirmed and five probable cases of CD diagnosed in a single institution in South Africa during a 10-year period [52]. All of the cases were unicentric CD, five of the six cases with overt CD were of the PC variant, and only one was HV. All of the cases in the probable category were of mixed type and had features of both histologic types. In three cases, the lymph nodes were in areas draining malignancy – two with Kaposi sarcoma and one with B-cell lymphoma. In one of the patients with Kaposi sarcoma, the CD recurred. All cases were in boys and none of the tested patients were HIV positive. While basing conclusions on a report from a single institution may be skewed, it is also possible that, similarly to Burkitt lymphoma, CD in children from developing countries has different pathogenesis and clinical course as compared to developed countries.

Kimura disease

Kimura disease is a rare, chronic inflammatory disorder seen predominately in young Asian males, which presents with the triad of painless subcutaneous nodules or unilateral cervical lymphadenopathy, tissue eosinophilia, and markedly elevated serum immunoglobulin E (IgE) [56]. While the clinical course of the disease is generally benign and self-limited, Kimura disease can be complicated by renal involvement. *Histologically*, florid germinal center hyperplasia with the presence of Warthin–Finkeldey-type polykaryocytes, eosinophils, eosinophilic deposits of IgE, increased numbers of HEVs, and sclerosis in the paracortex are characteristic of Kimura disease. However, these morphologic findings are non-specific and the diagnosis should be supported by a clinical history of a long-lasting, painless, deep soft tissue mass or lymphadenopathy, eosinophilia, and elevated IgE levels.

Differential diagnosis of a predominantly nodular pattern

The differential diagnosis of a predominantly nodular pattern in a lymph node of a child includes both reactive and malignant proliferations. While reactive follicular hyperplasia is frequent, follicular lymphomas and other lymphomas with a nodular pattern are extremely rare in children. For that reason, the diagnosis should be made based on strict morphologic criteria and the demonstration of clonality. The nodular lymphomas in children are reviewed more extensively in Chapter 21.

Follicular lymphoma (FL) comprises less than 3% of the pediatric non-Hodgkin lymphomas [57, 58]. Males are more frequently affected, with a reported male to female ratio of 4 : 1; the median age at diagnosis varies in different reports from approximately 7 to 12 years of age. Unlike adults, most of the pediatric FL cases are stage I at presentation, yet exhibit a high histologic grade (II or III).

Features helpful in making the distinction between reactive follicular hyperplasia and pediatric follicular lymphoma

Table 9.4. Comparison of reactive follicular hyperplasia and pediatric follicular lymphoma.

Reactive follicular hyperplasia	Follicular lymphoma
Architecture	
Preserved lymph node architecture with increased number of follicles	Total or partial effacement of nodal architecture Nodules with "expansile" growth pattern In a lymph node with partial involvement, the neoplastic nodules are distinctly different from the small residual follicles
Follicles	
Uneven distribution, mostly cortical	Even distribution of neoplastic nodules
Variability in size and shape	Uniformity of size and shape of follicles
Polymorphous cellular composition, frequent polarization	Monomorphic cellular composition
Frequent tingible body macrophages in the dark zone of the germinal center	Lack of tingible body macrophages
Mitosis frequent	Mitosis infrequent
Polytypic B-cells	Monotypic, light chain restricted plasma cells
BCL2-negative follicles	BCL2 usually negative in the follicles, but may be positive
Interfollicular areas	
Proliferation of immunoblasts, histiocytes, and plasma cells, to a variable degree	The neoplastic nodules bland into the interfollicular area; lack of reactive background
Lack of CD10+ and/or BCL6+ B-cells	Presence of CD10+ and/or BCL6+ B-cells
Vascularity not increased, high endothelial venules with plum endothelium	Increased vascularity, most likely due to displacement and crowding together
Sclerosis	
May be present, but not characteristic	Mild fibrosis with fine trabecular pattern Fibrosis enclosing single cells or small clusters may be present Less frequently, large collagen bands
Capsule	
Thin	Neoplastic expansion involving capsule

are summarized in Table 9.4. In reactive processes the follicles exhibit predominately cortical distribution, are varied in size and shape, and are composed of a heterogeneous cell population including tingible body macrophages. In follicular lymphoma, there is a total or an extensive replacement of the nodal architecture by follicles of neoplastic cells; even distribution of the follicles throughout the entire node; uniformity in the size and shape of the nodules; crowding of the nodules with small interfollicular areas; monomorphic cytologic composition of the nodules; and lack of tingible body macrophages in comparison to follicular hyperplasia as outlined above. In addition, in follicular lymphoma there is a striking lack of reactive lymphoid cells, immunoblasts, and plasma cells in the interfollicular areas, which are present in reactive processes [58].

Ancillary studies are less helpful in distinguishing between reactive and neoplastic nodular proliferations in children. The vast majority of the pediatric FL cases lack BCL2 expression and BCL2/immunoglobulin heavy chain translocations are most frequently negative. Thus, BCL2 is typically not helpful in establishing the diagnosis of pediatric FL. The presence of BCL6- and/or CD10-positive B-cells in the interfollicular area is more helpful and supports the diagnosis of lymphoma. Flow cytometry studies in FL usually identify a monotypic B-cell population based on light chain restriction. However, a light chain restricted B-cell population may be seen in reactive FH in children, and should be interpreted with caution and in conjunc-

tion with the morphologic features. The immunoglobulin heavy chain (IgH) gene rearrangement analysis by PCR may be not be contributory either, since not all cases of pediatric FL have IgH gene rearrangement. Thus, to make the diagnosis of follicular lymphoma in a child, one should rely more on the morphology than on ancillary studies.

Nodal marginal zone B-cell lymphoma in children is also infrequent. The median age of diagnosis is 16 years [59]. Most of the children are males (M : F = 5 : 1), with no underlying disease, that present with localized lymphadenopathy. Histologic examination shows total or partial effacement of the nodal architecture by expanded marginal zones and a polymorphous population of centrocyte-like cells, plasma cells, and scattered large cells in the interfollicular areas. The residual follicles may be expanded and show progressive-transformation-of-germinal-center-like changes. Features that favor a neoplastic process include: expansion, at least focally, of the interfollicular areas, and destruction of follicles; an increased number of interfollicular B-cells that are CD10 and BCL6 negative; and aberrant expression of CD43, a preferential T-cell marker, which is frequent. BCL2, if present, is generally weak. Immunoglobulin heavy chain gene rearrangements are present, but *BCL2* is in the germline configuration.

The differentiation of PTGC from the *florid variant of follicular lymphoma* can be a problem in adults but usually not in children, since these lymphomas rarely have been reported in individuals below 40 years of age.

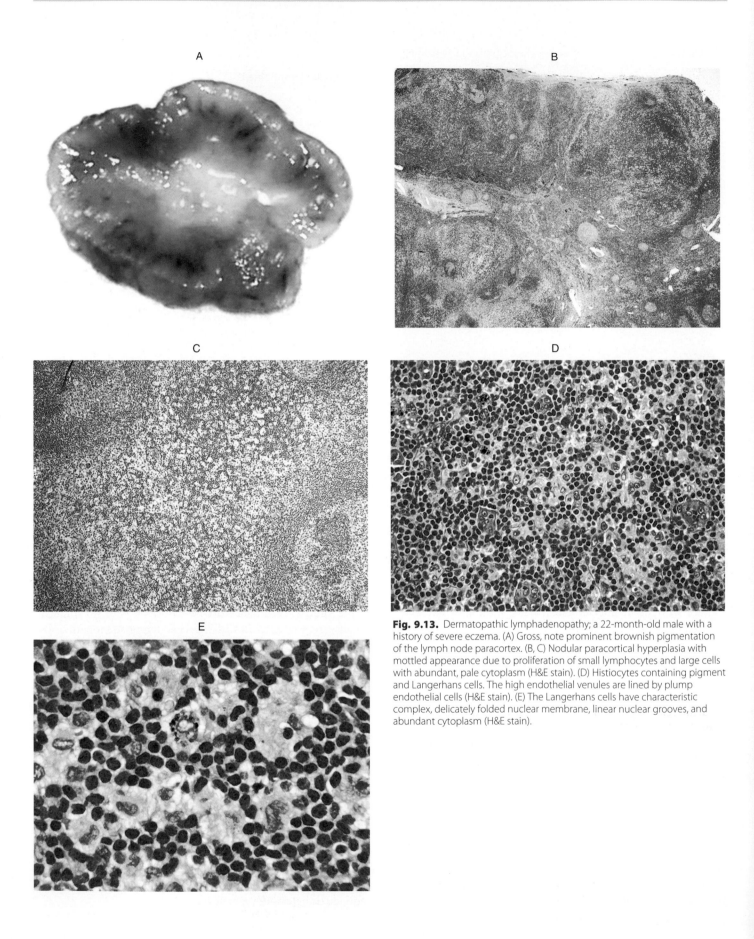

A

B

C

D

E

Fig. 9.13. Dermatopathic lymphadenopathy; a 22-month-old male with a history of severe eczema. (A) Gross, note prominent brownish pigmentation of the lymph node paracortex. (B, C) Nodular paracortical hyperplasia with mottled appearance due to proliferation of small lymphocytes and large cells with abundant, pale cytoplasm (H&E stain). (D) Histiocytes containing pigment and Langerhans cells. The high endothelial venules are lined by plump endothelial cells (H&E stain). (E) The Langerhans cells have characteristic complex, delicately folded nuclear membrane, linear nuclear grooves, and abundant cytoplasm (H&E stain).

F

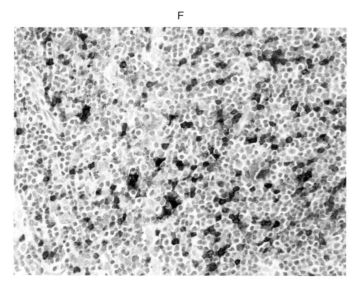

G

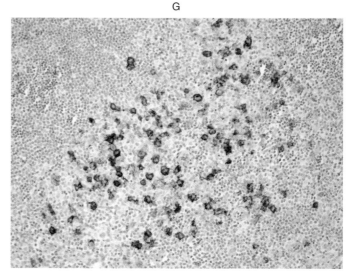

Fig. 9.13. (*cont.*) (F) S100 (immunohistochemical stain). (G) CD1a (immunohistochemical stain).

Predominantly paracortical lesions

Paracortical proliferations are frequent in pediatric lymph nodes and can be seen either in isolation or in conjunction with marked follicular hyperplasia. Depending on the extent and nature of these reactive proliferations, they may represent a serious diagnostic problem, since they may be mimicking a neoplastic process.

Nodular paracortical proliferations

Nodular paracortical expansion is seen in lymph nodes draining inflammatory skin lesions (dermatopathic) or tumors. However, in children such a pattern may be seen in reactive lymphadenopathies with no associated apparent skin lesion. The lymph nodes vary in size and gross examination may show vague nodularity and, in exuberant cases of skin lesions, pigmentation (Fig. 9.13A).

Histologically, the paracortical areas are expanded by nodules of cells, known also as *tertiary follicles or T-nodules*. These nodules consist of T-cells, predominately CD4 positive, intermixed with histiocytes, Langerhans cells, and interdigitating dendritic cells (Fig. 9.13B–C). Histiocytes contain melanin pigment (Fig. 9.13D). Variable numbers of eosinophils and plasma cells are also present. Follicular hyperplasia may be present, and when the paracortical expansion is prominent, the follicles may be compressed in the outer cortex. The HEVs are prominent and lined by plump endothelial cells. The presence of histiocytes and other large cells with abundant cytoplasm in a lymphocytic background gives mottled appearance to the lymph node at low magnification.

An increased number of Langerhans cells may be present (Fig. 9.13E). These cells have characteristic complex, delicately folded nuclear membranes, linear nuclear grooves, and express the CD1a, CD68, Langerin (CD207), HLA-DR, and S100 antigens (Fig. 9.13F–G) [60]. It has been postulated that the Langer-

hans cells migrate to the lymph node from draining inflammatory skin lesions and are part of the immune response during chronic inflammation [61].

The differential diagnosis, particularly at low magnification, includes interfollicular Hodgkin lymphoma. The presence of reactive lymphocytic background composed of small and medium lymphocytes and immunoblasts is the most reassuring feature that supports reactive rather than neoplastic proliferation. In Hodgkin lymphoma, the background lymphocytes are predominantly small and immunoblasts are not present. While Reed–Sternberg (RS)-like cells may be present, for the diagnosis of Hodgkin lymphoma, a proper background is required.

In children, Langerhans cell histiocytosis (LCH) is another diagnostic consideration. While the reactive and neoplastic Langerhans cells have the same immunophenotype and express CD1a and Langerin [60], morphologically they differ. Furthermore, in LCH, the neoplastic cells form large clusters as compared to the scattered Langerhans cells seen in a reactive condition.

Diffuse paracortical proliferations

Diffuse paracortical expansion, associated with numerous immunoblasts and prominent HEVs, is a feature of the lymph node response to antigenic stimulation, particularly in florid viral, drug-induced, or post-vaccinial lymphadenopathies. The prototype of such lesions is infectious mononucleosis.

Infectious mononucleosis

Infectious mononucleosis (IM), an acute lymphoproliferative process caused by the Epstein–Barr virus (EBV), is frequent in children. While lymphadenopathy is a characteristic feature of the disease, lymph node biopsies are performed in rare cases with unusual clinical presentation or negative serology. These latter patients are usually older and, as such, the suspicion of lymphoma is high.

Young children with IM usually have a mild viral respiratory illness that rarely requires medical attention. The classical clinical presentation of IM is usually seen in adolescents and young adults. Malaise, fever, sore throat, lymphadenopathy, hepatosplenomegaly, and skin rash are the main clinical symptoms. The most characteristic feature of IM is the presence of symmetric, moderately enlarged, slightly tender lymph nodes, particularly in the posterior cervical region. The nodes are not matted and there are no signs of inflammation such as redness, heat, or fluctuation. The axillary, epitrochlear, and inguinal lymph nodes are also frequently involved. Rarely, IM may present with mediastinal lymph node enlargement. The hallmark of IM in the peripheral blood is the presence of atypical lymphocytes composed of CD8-positive T-cells (Fig. 9.14A). Anemia is rare, as well as immune-mediated thrombocytopenia.

The most frequently seen *morphologic findings* in IM are non-uniform expansion of the interfollicular areas without obliteration of the lymph node architecture, only mild activation of the germinal centers, an abundance of HEVs, and the presence of single cell necrosis (Fig. 9.14B). The interfollicular expansion is due to the proliferation of a polymorphous lymphoid population composed of small- and medium-size lymphoid cells, immunoblasts, as well as tingible body macrophages, variable numbers of plasma cells, eosinophils, and an occasional neutrophil. Focal sheets of immunoblasts are often present (Fig. 9.14C). Single cell necrosis and frequent mitotic figures are present as well. Intermixed with the reactive transformed lymphocytes are rare, large binucleated immunoblasts that resemble Reed–Sternberg (RS) cells (Fig. 9.14D). RS-like cells can also be seen in lymph node touch imprints as shown in Figure 9.14E.

Some degree of reactive follicular hyperplasia is present. This is more frequently seen in the tonsils, and to a lesser degree in the lymph nodes where the germinal centers are ill defined and mildly reactive. The lymphoid sinuses are usually easily recognized, although they may be compressed. The sinuses are filled with small and large lymphocytes in variable numbers. The lymph node capsule may be infiltrated by small and large lymphoid cells in rare cases.

Immunohistochemical studies show that the transformed cells are a mixture of B- and T-cells. This is a reflection of the pathogenesis of IM, where primary EBV infection produces transformed B-lymphoblasts that differentiate via the germinal center to become latently infected resting memory B-cells. Expression of EBV-related antigens by the virally infected B-cells results in an aggressive cytotoxic T-cell response, as well as rapid killing of B-immunoblasts [62]. Necrosis, most frequently single cell and less frequently patchy or diffuse, is also present. In the tonsils, ulceration of the surface mucosa may occur.

In situ hybridization for EBV-encoded RNA (using an EBER probe) shows a variable number of EBV-positive cells (Fig. 9.14F). The number of these cells varies from as low as 1% in some cases, to as high as 90% in others [63]. However, the presence of EBV-positive cells is not sufficient for the diagnosis of IM, since memory B-cells with latent EBV infection may persist for a long time and may be seen in patients with a previous acute EBV infection. As a result, serologic confirmation of the acute infection is needed.

Differential diagnosis of infectious mononucleosis

The differential diagnosis of IM includes non-Hodgkin lymphoma, Hodgkin lymphoma, and a variety of reactive lymphoid proliferations. In *diffuse large B-cell lymphoma* (*DLBCL*), the neoplastic proliferation is monomorphous and shows monotypic surface Ig expression. By contrast, in IM, the transformed immunoblasts are both T- and B-cells that show no restricted surface Ig expression. Extensive necrosis, capsular infiltration, and/or complete effacement of the architecture favor a neoplastic process rather than a reactive proliferation. The presence of prominent mitotic activity and an abundance of small vessels composed of post-capillary venules in the interfollicular areas is not helpful, since it can be seen in both DLBCL and IM.

Classical Hodgkin lymphoma (HL) may present a differential diagnostic consideration when Reed–Sternberg-like cells are present. A feature helpful in distinguishing between HL and IM is the type of background lymphocytes: the presence of small lymphocytes that lack maturation is characteristic for HL, whereas numerous transformed lymphocytes and immunoblasts are seen in IM. In IM, the large, atypical cells are a mixture of CD45+ B- and T-lymphocytes. While many of these activated lymphocytes will be CD30+, an activation marker, the cells in IM are consistently CD15−. This immunophenotype, in conjunction with the morphologic features, will support IM and help exclude classical HL. Detection of EBV-positive cells does not help to distinguish between the two, since the Reed–Sternberg cells in HL may also be EBV positive. However, the EBV-positive cells are usually large and usually substantially fewer in number in HL. In IM, the number of EBV-positive cells may be large and will include both small and large lymphocytes.

Similar histologic changes can be seen in other viral infections such as cytomegalovirus (CMV) and *Herpes simplex* lymphadenitis. While *CMV infection* is usually occult, it may present as an IM-like syndrome in immunocompetent children. Single or multiple enlarged and tender lymph nodes may be present, but a lymph node biopsy is rarely performed. The histologic features include a variable degree of paracortical expansion and follicular hyperplasia (Fig. 9.15A). The paracortex is expanded by proliferation of immunoblasts focally forming sheets (Fig. 9.15B). Patches of monocytoid B-cells associated with small collections of neutrophils are also present. The most characteristic finding of CMV lymphadenitis is the presence of rare large, virally infected cells with prominent intranuclear and intracytoplasmic inclusions (Fig. 9.15C). Immunohistochemical stains with anti-CMV antibodies or *in situ* hybridization confirm that the CMV is the causative agent (Fig. 9.15D). The differential diagnosis of CMV lymphadenitis may include Hodgkin lymphoma (HL) since the infected large cells

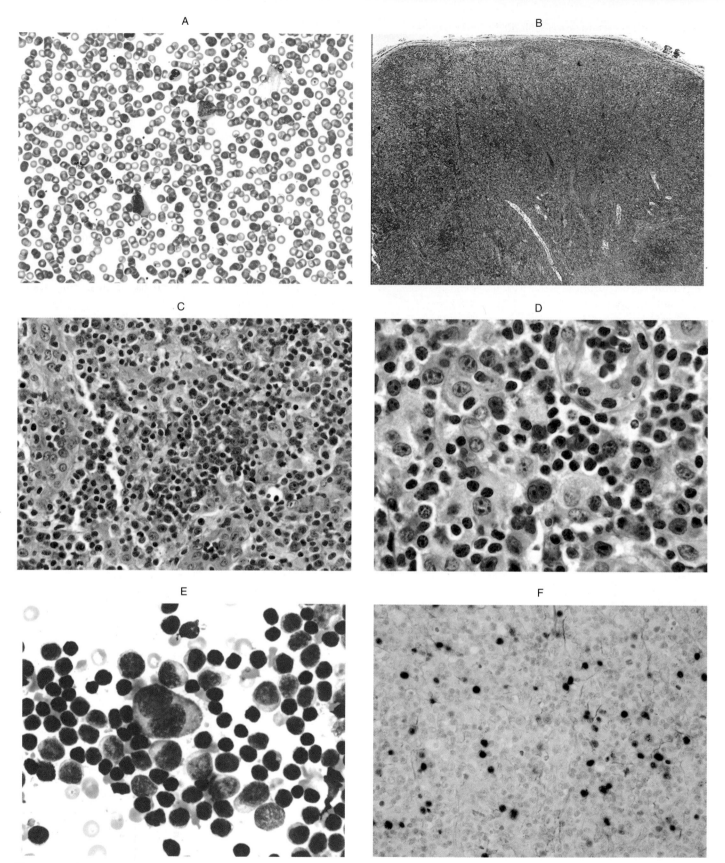

Fig. 9.14. Infectious mononucleosis. (A) Peripheral blood film showing characteristic atypical lymphocytes with abundant basophilic cytoplasm, along with unremarkable red blood cells and adequate platelet counts (Wright–Giemsa stain). (B) Lymph node with expanded interfollicular area and preserved nodal architecture, low magnification. Note residual follicles in the cortex, open sinuses, prominent vascularity, and polymorphous cell proliferation (H&E stain). (C) Numerous immunoblasts forming sheets. Note scattered single cell necrosis (H&E stain). (D) An RS-like cell present on a background of numerous immunoblasts (H&E stain). (E) An RS-like cell on touch imprints of lymph node (Diff-Quik stain). As with the histologic section, this cell is accompanied by numerous immunoblasts and activated lymphocytes, a feature supporting the benign nature of this process (Diff-Quik stain). (F) Numerous EBV-positive cells; *in situ* hybridization with EBV-encoded RNA (EBER probe).

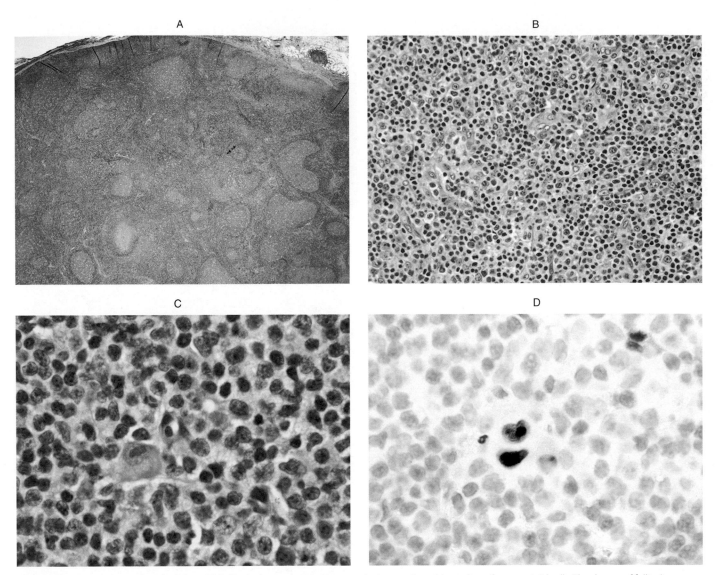

Fig. 9.15. Cytomegalovirus lymphadenitis. (A) Follicular hyperplasia and paracortical expansion with patches of monocytoid cells. The degree of follicular hyperplasia varies from minimal to more prominent as in this example (H&E stain). (B) The paracortex is expanded by proliferation of transformed cells and immunoblasts that focally form sheets. Mitotic features are frequent and the vascular endothelium prominent (H&E stain). (C) Rare large cells with prominent intranuclear inclusion and granular cytoplasm are present. These cells may resemble Reed–Sternberg cells (H&E stain). (D) CMV-positive cells are diagnostic of CMV lymphadenitis (immunohistochemical stain).

resemble the Reed–Sternberg cells morphologically and, similarly to the real RS cells, express CD15 [64]. The most helpful feature in distinguishing viral lymphadenitis from HL is the presence of numerous background immunoblasts in reactive proliferations, and the characteristic background of small lymphocytes, histiocytes, and other inflammatory cells in HL.

Herpes simplex lymphadenitis usually presents with extensive geographic necrosis and large characteristic cells with ground-glass nuclei (Fig. 9.16A–B). Immunohistochemical stains can confirm the etiologic agent in many cases.

Rare cases of IM with extensive necrosis have to be distinguished from necrotizing histiocytic lymphadenitis, such as seen in Kikuchi–Fujimoto, systemic lupus, or Kawasaki disease.

Atypical lymphoproliferative disorders in children

Rarely, children can present with diffuse effacement of the lymph node architecture at the border between reactive lymphoid proliferation and bona fide lymphomas. Such an exuberant reaction can be seen in the setting of an extreme immune response to a viral infection, drug hypersensitivity, or another undetermined cause. While such a reaction most likely is due to abnormal immune response that progresses unchecked due to an underlying immune abnormality, no specific associated immune aberration has been identified in most of the cases. Similar abnormalities can be seen in lymph nodes from patients on immunosuppressive therapy for solid organ or bone marrow

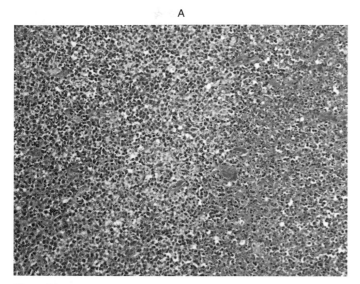

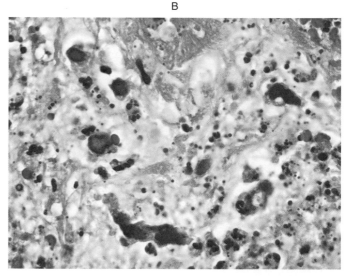

Fig. 9.16. Herpes simplex lymphadenitis. (A) Diffuse paracortical proliferation with extensive necrosis (H&E stain). (B) Along the edge of necrosis, large cells with characteristic ground-glass nuclei are present (H&E stain).

transplantation as well as in some patients on immunomodulating therapy.

Frizzera and colleagues call such pattern pseudoobliterative, and describe the key features as (1) marked expansion of the germinal centers and paracortex, resulting in compression of the sinuses and blurring of the topographic landmarks of the lymph node; (2) florid proliferation of immunoblasts and an increase in the number and prominence of HEVs, both of which encroach on the follicles; and (3) concurrent abnormal reaction of the germinal centers, such as follicle lysis, regressive transformation of germinal centers, or follicular dissolution [15]. These changes in the follicular dendritic meshwork can be demonstrated by staining with CD21 and CD23.

The combination of these features suggests an exuberant immune response rather than lymphoma. In the case of lymphoma, the topographic landmarks are completely destroyed, germinal centers are absent or, if present, show no abnormal reaction, and the lymphoid proliferation is monomorphous and is easily recognizable as atypical. In the pseudoobliterative pattern, the immunoblastic proliferation is composed of a mixture of B- and T-lymphocytes that have minimal atypia, the germinal centers are expanded, and the HEVs are numerous and are lined with prominent plump endothelial cells.

It is important to recognize the pseudoobliterative pattern in order to exclude lymphoma as well as to identify patients that may be at increased risk of developing lymphoma in the future.

Predominantly sinusoidal lesions

Sinus histiocytosis

Dilation of the sinuses containing an increased number of histiocytes (macrophages) is a common non-specific finding in pediatric lymph nodes. While it can be the single most prominent finding, it can also be seen in the setting of follicular hyper-

plasia and/or paracortical expansion. While most of the time the cause is not apparent, sinus histiocytosis can be seen in lymph nodes draining tumors, infection, or prosthesis. Histologically, the sinuses are dilated and filled with large histiocytes that are uniform in size and have abundant cytoplasm (Fig. 9.17). Depending on the underlying condition, the histiocytes may contain pigment, hemosiderin, or display erythrophagocytosis. The degree of follicular hyperplasia and/or paracortical expansion varies from non-apparent to prominent. In general, the capsule is thin and there is no fibrosis or granulomata present.

Sinus histiocytosis with massive lymphadenopathy

Sinus histiocytosis with massive lymphadenopathy (SHML), also known as Rosai–Dorfman disease, is a rare histiocytic disorder that frequently affects children. It involves both nodal and extranodal sites and shows significant clinical heterogeneity [65]. A more extensive discussion on this entity in children is presented in the chapter on histiocytic disorders (Chapter 25).

While the etiology of the Rosai–Dorfman disease is still unknown, the presence of immunologic abnormalities in some patients [66], immune dysfunction in others [67], and overlap between the clinical and morphologic features of SHML with autoimmune lymphoproliferative syndrome (ALPS) [68] suggests an underlying immune dysregulation. As a result, an abnormal proliferation of histiocytes with features intermediate between Langerhans/interdigitating cells and mononuclear phagocytes (S100+, CD14+, CD11c+, CD68+, CD1a−) is present [69], both in the lymph nodes and extranodal sites.

The histologic findings of Rosai–Dorfman disease are quite characteristic [65]. The lymph node architecture is generally preserved and the sinuses are expanded by a proliferation of histiocytes with round to oval vesicular nuclei, a single, small

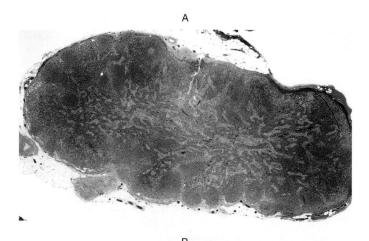

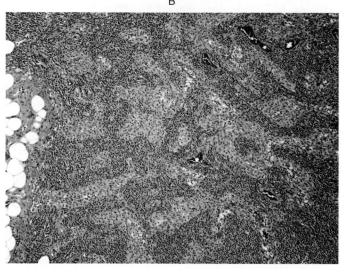

Fig. 9.17. Sinus histiocytosis. (A) Markedly dilated sinuses, paracortical expansion, and mild follicular hyperplasia, low magnification (H&E stain). (B) The sinuses are filled with large histiocytes with abundant eosinophilic cytoplasm (H&E stain).

nucleolus and abundant, pale-pink cytoplasm (Fig. 9.18). The majority of the histiocytes contain well-preserved lymphocytes and occasional neutrophils, plasma cells, and erythrocytes in their cytoplasm, a phenomenon known as emperipolesis. These cells are characteristically S100 positive and CD1a negative. The distended sinuses and medullary cords contain numerous plasma cells. Reactive germinal centers may be present. In some cases, an increased number of neutrophils throughout the lymph node and focal microabscesses may be seen. The capsule can be fibrotic and the fibrosis can extend into the surrounding soft tissue. Intranodal fibrosis, however, is usually minimal or absent.

The morphologic features and clinical presentation are quite characteristic, although SHML is sometimes difficult to separate from Langerhans cell histiocytosis based on morphology alone. In such cases, immunostaining for S100 and CD1a is helpful and demonstrates CD1a-positive neoplastic Langerhans cells. SHML has, on rare occasions, been identified in lymph nodes affected by malignant lymphoma, both non-Hodgkin and

Hodgkin lymphomas [70–73]. While foci with the characteristic features of SHML are identified within sinuses between the areas replaced by the neoplastic process, such foci usually represent only a minor portion of the lymph node (<10%) [70]. Hodgkin lymphoma may be more difficult to appreciate, particularly nodular lymphocyte-predominant type if the lymph node is only partially involved [71]. Characteristic S100+ histiocytes demonstrating emperipolesis may be present, scattered in irregular clusters or individually within lymphoid tissue adjacent to the nodules of NLPHL.

Benign lymph node lesions mimicking metastatic pediatric renal neoplasms

A variety of benign lesions mimicking metastases have been reported in regional lymph nodes of children with renal tumors [74]. The most common sources of error include: the presence of a complex of epithelial cells with Tamm–Horsfall protein (THP); mature squamous cells; and mesothelial inclusions. THP is synthesized by the kidney and is absent from other tissues [75]. In lymph nodes, the THP can accumulate and present as dense proteinaceous material containing well-differentiated, cuboidal epithelial cells arranged in small alveolar or tubular configurations that are confined to the sinuses (Fig. 9.19). While finding benign epithelia/THP inclusions in the lymph node should not be mistaken for metastatic renal tumor, their presence however does not exclude metastatic disease.

Less frequently, mesothelial inclusions consisting of small, cytologically benign glandular structures may be present within a connective tissue extension of lymph node capsules (Fig. 9.20). Unlike true metastases, these glands are confined to the capsule and do not extend to the lymph node sinuses. Similarly, benign squamous cells present in lymph nodes of patients with ulcerated metaplastic calyceal urothelium. Proper identification of all these changes is important, since misdiagnosing them as a metastatic renal tumor will result in unnecessary upstaging of the patient and intensification of chemotherapy.

Predominantly stromo-vascular lesions

Inflammatory pseudotumor of lymph nodes

Inflammatory pseudotumor of lymph nodes, a benign proliferation of spindle and inflammatory cells involving the connective tissue framework of the lymph node, is rare in children, and most information on this lesion is based on studies consisting primarily of adults and only occasionally including pediatric cases [76–81]. The youngest child reported with inflammatory pseudotumor of the lymph node was five years old [76]. The clinical presentation is variable, although most children present with isolated lymphadenopathy. A small number of patients are completely asymptomatic except for lymphadenopathy at presentation. However, more frequently, the patients present with fever, including rare reported cases of intermittent episodes of fever and night sweats, once or twice

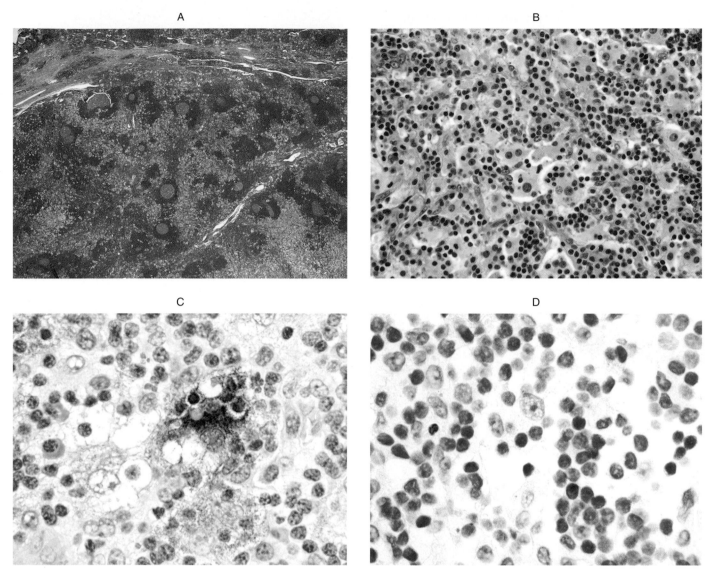

Fig. 9.18. Sinus histiocytosis with massive lymphadenopathy (Rosai–Dorfman disease) in a 12-month-old male who presented with marked lymphadenopathy. (A) Markedly distended sinuses filled with large cells with eosinophilic cytoplasm. Reactive germinal centers are also present. Focal fibrosis is present (H&E stain). (B) Characteristic large cells with pale nucleus, with prominent nucleolus and abundant cytoplasm containing intact lymphocytes, a phenomenon known as emperipolesis (H&E stain). (C) These cells express S100 (immunohistochemical stain). (D) However, they are CD1a negative (immunohistochemical stain).

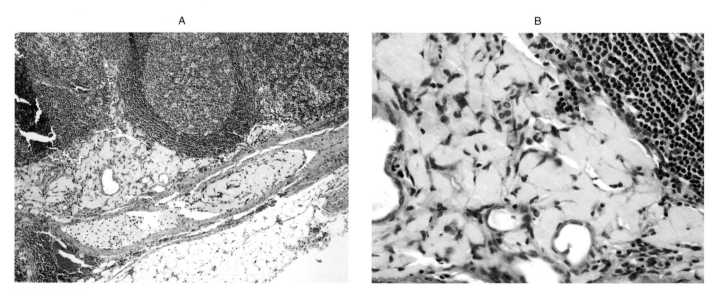

Fig. 9.19. Epithelial cells with Tamm–Horsfall protein in the lymph node of a child with Wilms tumor. These types of inclusions are benign and should not be mistaken for metastatic Wilms tumor. (A) Epithelial glands embedded in protein matrix (H&E stain). (B) Higher magnification (H&E stain). (The case is a generous contribution of Dr. Elizabeth Perlman.)

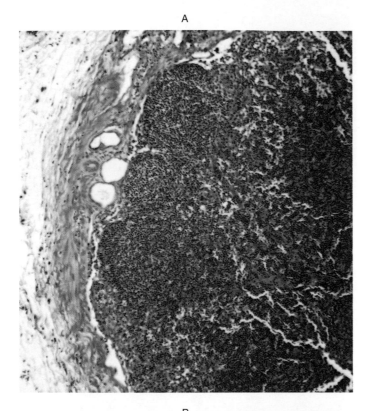

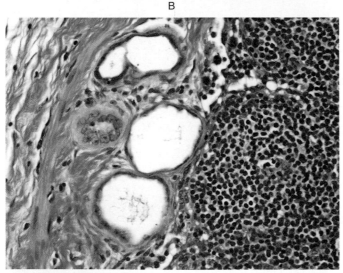

Fig. 9.20. Mesothelial inclusions in a child with Wilms tumor, another mimicker of tumor metastatic to the lymph node (H&E stains). (A) Note that the inclusions are confined to the capsule and are not present in the lymph node sinuses. (B) Higher magnification. (The case is a generous contribution of Dr. Elizabeth Perlman.)

a year for several years prior to diagnosis [77]. Abdominal pain and vomiting can be present as well. Laboratory abnormalities are present and include anemia, hypergammaglobulinemia, and elevated ESR. In such patients, a hematologic malignancy may be suspected.

The cause of the disorder is not known. *In situ* hybridization for EBV-encoded RNA has been positive in a small number of inflammatory pseudotumors of the lymph node, and the possibility of EBV as a causative agent has been entertained [81].

The hallmark of inflammatory pseudotumor of the lymph node is the presence of a spindle cell proliferation expanding the connective tissue framework of the lymph node, variable amounts of fibrosis, and the presence of a mixed inflammatory infiltrate [78]. Vasculitis with or without microthrombi may be present. The morphologic findings vary depending on the stage of the disease. During the early stage (stage I), there are sharply circumscribed discrete nodules of proliferating fibroblastic spindle cells, a fine collagenous network composed of eosinophilic acellular material, and inflammatory cells such as small lymphocytes, plasma cells, and histiocytes. These changes are seen on a background of reactive follicular hyperplasia with mild paracortical expansion [78]. In more advanced disease (stage II), there is extensive replacement of the lymph node by a prominent fibroblastic/myofibroblastic proliferation that extends along subcapsular and trabecular sinuses in a radial fashion (Fig. 9.21A). The capsule is frequently involved. At the end, stage III, the lymph node is replaced by dense sclerosis with a minimal inflammatory component (Fig. 9.21B).

Most of the spindle cells are myofibroblastic in nature and express smooth muscle actin (Fig. 9.21C–D) and vimentin. Small, round and spindle-shaped CD68-positive histiocytes are also seen throughout the lesion. The inflammatory component consists of small B- and T-lymphocytes with a predominance of T-cells. Scattered CD15-positive mononuclear cells, as well as CD138-positive plasma cells are also present. CD31 demonstrates an increased number of capillaries. The inflammatory pseudotumor of lymph nodes is consistently ALK1 negative, unlike similar lesions at extranodal sites.

The list of malignant and benign diseases that may present with a mixed inflammatory component, fibrosis, and/or vasculitis is extensive and should be considered in the differential diagnosis of inflammatory pseudotumor of the lymph node [82]. According to New *et al.*, only about a third of the inflammatory pseudotumors were correctly diagnosed initially; the remaining were usually thought to be Hodgkin and non-Hodgkin lymphomas or benign reactive conditions [82]. Since inflammatory pseudotumor of lymph node may present with worrisome clinical and laboratory findings and protracted clinical course in children, the correct diagnosis is mandatory. The overall prognosis is excellent.

Vascular transformation of sinuses

Vascular transformation of sinuses (VTS) is a rare benign change in the lymph nodes that can be seen in children as well as in adults [83]. As the name suggests, it is characterized by vascular transformation of the lymph node sinuses into vascular channels (Fig. 9.22A). Segmental or total involvement of the lymph nodes can be present and the vasoproliferative process results in variable expansion of the subcapsular, medullary, or intermediate sinuses. The intervening parenchyma shows mild to striking lymphocyte depletion. The vascular spaces may form

A

B

C

D

E

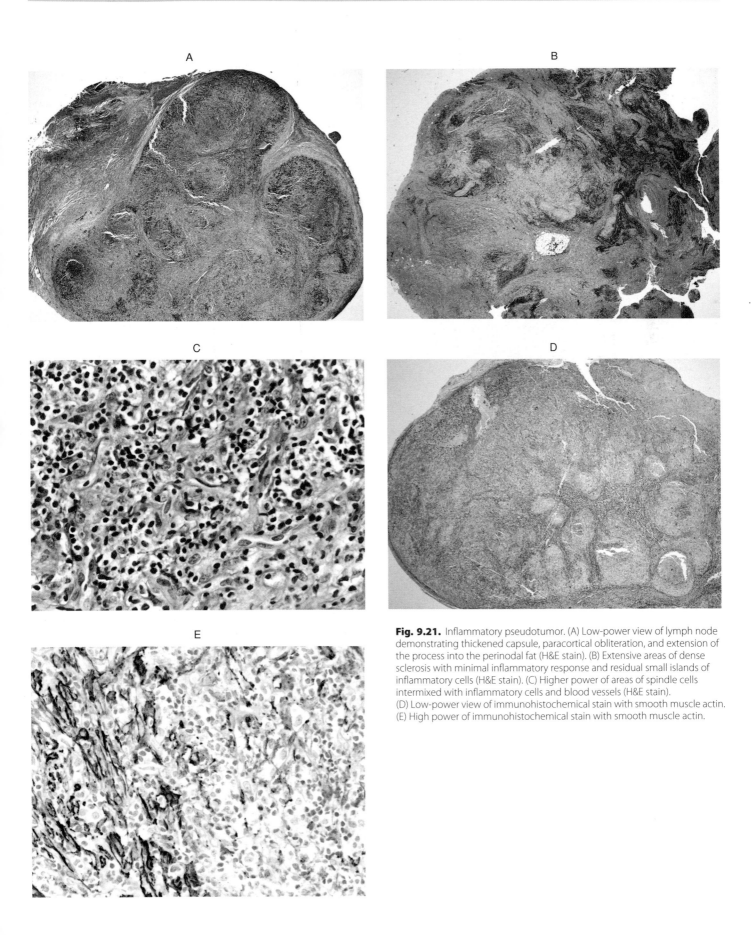

Fig. 9.21. Inflammatory pseudotumor. (A) Low-power view of lymph node demonstrating thickened capsule, paracortical obliteration, and extension of the process into the perinodal fat (H&E stain). (B) Extensive areas of dense sclerosis with minimal inflammatory response and residual small islands of inflammatory cells (H&E stain). (C) Higher power of areas of spindle cells intermixed with inflammatory cells and blood vessels (H&E stain). (D) Low-power view of immunohistochemical stain with smooth muscle actin. (E) High power of immunohistochemical stain with smooth muscle actin.

A

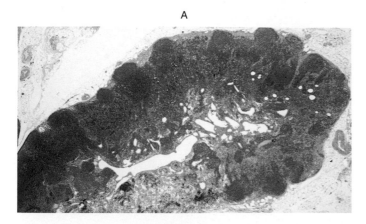

B

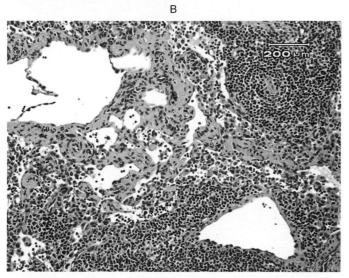

C

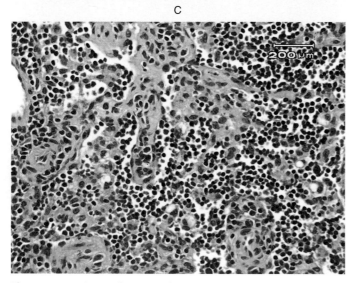

Fig. 9.22. Vascular transformation of sinuses (H&E stain). (A) Lymph node with almost complete involvement. (B) The sinuses are transformed into dilated vascular channels. (C) Cleft-like spaces filled with lymphocytes and extravasated red blood cells. (The case is a generous contribution of Dr. Elizabeth Perlman.)

cleft-like spaces, rounded spaces, a plexiform pattern, or a solid proliferation (Fig. 9.22B). The vascular spaces may be empty, filled with lymph-like fluid, congested with blood, or occasionally thrombosed (Fig. 9.22C). Extravasation of red blood cells is common. While the more cellular areas may resemble Kaposi sarcoma, in VTS there is no capsular or trabecular involvement as is commonly seen in Kaposi sarcoma. Although the cause of VTS is still unknown, it is often found associated with obstruction of veins or efferent lymphatics by lymphoma or other tumors.

Necrotizing lymphadenitis

Histiocytic necrotizing lymphadenitis (Kikuchi–Fujimoto disease)

Kikuchi–Fujimoto disease (KFD) is a benign self-limited histiocytic necrotizing lymphadenitis characterized by regional lymphadenopathy with or without fever. While the disease occurs worldwide, it is more prevalent in Asia and in individuals of Asian descent [84]. The reason for these geographic and ethnic differences is not completely understood. However, there is a high prevalence of specific HLA class II gene alleles, DPA1*01 and DPB1*0202, in Asians with KFD as compared to Caucasians, which may account for these differences [85].

KFD is rare and affects individuals of all ages. While most children with KFD are between 10 and 16 years of age [86, 87], it has been reported in a child as young as 19 months [88]. There is a male predominance, in children, which is in contrast to adults, where there is a female predominance [87, 89, 90]. However, most of the reports on pediatric KFD are small series and may not be representative for the true incidence of the disease.

Most of the children present with lymphadenopathy, typically in the head and neck area. Unilateral involvement of multiple lymph nodes is typical. The posterior cervical region is the most frequently affected area and, according to some series, is involved in 92% of the affected children [87]. The duration of the lymphadenopathy varies from several days to six months. Most of the lymph nodes do not exceed 6 cm in greatest dimension, but occasionally lymph nodes as large as 8 cm have been reported. In addition to discomfort and tenderness in the area of the lymphadenopathy, fever is common. Skin rash, headache, nausea and/or vomiting, hepatomegaly, and oral ulcers have also been reported in 20–30% of the children.

Some of the children present initially with prolonged fever of unknown origin (FUO) [89]. While most of the children have a normal white blood cell count, those with prolonged fever may have leukopenia, mild anemia, and an elevated erythrocyte sedimentation rate but a relatively low C-reactive protein. The lactate dehydrogenase may also be elevated.

The etiology of KFD is still unknown. While positive serologic test results for EBV, CMV, HHV-6, HTLV-1 (human T-cell lymphotropic virus type 1), and parvovirus B19 have suggested that these agents are etiologically related to the development of KFD, none of these viruses has been proven to cause the disease by culture or PCR. In addition, KSHV/HHV-8 has been found to be negative as well in these cases. The histologic, clinical, and laboratory overlap between KFD and systemic lupus erythematosus (SLE), however, suggest the possibility of some underlying autoimmune component in the pathogenesis of the disease [86].

Lymph node biopsy is the gold standard for the diagnosis of KFD. While fine needle aspiration (FNA) has been reported to be a reliable tool for the diagnosis of KFD in adults, its utility in children is limited. In one study from Taiwan, FNA was performed in 10 cases of children with KFD and none was diagnosed by this procedure [22].

The histologic findings in children are similar to those in adults and include the presence of discrete or confluent fibrinoid necrosis with abundant karyorrhectic debris and crescentic or "C-shaped" histiocytes (Fig. 9.23). The necrosis is patchy and, while it is present mostly in the paracortical areas, it can also affect the cortex and the follicles as well. The areas of necrosis are surrounded by immunoblasts and plasmacytoid dendritic cells (Fig. 9.23C). A characteristic feature of the disorder is a conspicuous absence of neutrophils from the necrotic areas. Plasma cells are generally rare. The lymph node capsule may be focally thickened in the areas overlying the necrosis. The necrosis occasionally may extend into the surrounding extranodal soft tissue. A variable number of reactive follicles may be present, but they are usually less conspicuous.

A spectrum of histologic phases, specifically proliferating, necrotizing, and xanthomatous, have been observed in KFD [91]. The *proliferating phase* is characterized by the presence of pale histiocytes, plasmacytoid monocytes, and lymphocytes present in variable numbers admixed with scattered cells with pyknotic nuclei and nuclear debris, but overt necrosis is absent. As the disease progresses, there is more striking karyorrhexis, and histiocytes with variable features, including the crescentic forms, are present. Nodular aggregates of cells with central coagulative necrosis and nuclear dust surrounded by histiocytes are present in the *necrotizing phase*. The *xanthomatous phase* is characterized by numerous foamy histiocytes without necrosis. Whether these phases represent stages in the natural history of KFD is not clear. One attempt to correlate the histologic findings with the duration of the disease as well as subsequent lymph node biopsies failed to confirm this hypothesis [91].

Immunohistochemical staining shows a characteristic increase in the number of CD3+ T-lymphocytes with varying proportions of CD8-positive and CD4-positive cells (Fig. 9.23D–F). The CD8-positive cells outnumber the CD4-positive T-cells and express cytotoxic molecules such as granzyme B and TIA1. B-cells are rare or absent in affected areas (Fig. 9.23G). The histiocytes in KFD express CD11b, CD11c, CD14, CD68, lysozyme, and MPO, a unique feature seen in KFD and Kikuchi-like lymphadenopathy but not in other disorders [92].

An increased number of plasmacytoid monocytes/dendritic cells (pDCs) is a characteristic feature of this disease. These cells have been the subject of interest to many pathologists, and

their origin is still controversial. The pDCs are CD43+, CD2+, CD5−, CD4+, CD8−, BCL2−, CD68+, and CD123+ (IL-3 receptor) [12, 14]. The plasmacytoid monocytes have abundant basophilic cytoplasm as a result of prominent endoplasmic reticulum, and are generally present in clusters in the T-cell-rich interfollicular areas in KFD (Fig. 9.23C, H). Identification of these cells is important since they help to exclude the presence of T-cell lymphoma and support the reactive nature of the process. The role of plasmacytoid monocytes in the pathogenesis of KFD is not completely understood, but they appear to be involved in the cell-mediated cytotoxicity and may be the first line of defense against viruses or other pathogens [14].

KFD is a self-limited disease that most frequently resolves spontaneously within several weeks to six months. Only rare fatalities from KFD have been reported [88]. The treatment is symptomatic and supportive. There is, however, a recurrence rate for KFD of 3.3% [87, 91].

KFD has been associated with SLE, and the time from the initial diagnosis of KFD to SLE in those who develop it ranges from 10 months to 3 years. KFD has also been associated with mixed connective tissue disease and, in rare cases, Still disease. In a long-term follow-up study of children with KFD, a significant percentage had new symptoms months to years following the diagnosis of KFD, most likely as a result of autoimmune phenomena [87]. Thus, the risk of evolution of KFD to an autoimmune disease in children is high, and long-term follow-up is warranted.

The difficulties of distinguishing KFD from malignant lymphoma have been the focus of several studies [93–95]. In one study, only 3 of 27 lymph node biopsies submitted for consultation were correctly diagnosed as KFD by the referring pathologists; the remaining 24 cases were initially diagnosed as non-Hodgkin lymphoma [93]. The morphologic separation of KFD from peripheral T-cell lymphoma (PTCL) may be difficult. Key features that favor KFD over PTCL include the presence of preserved architecture with paracortical expansion and partial effacement, plasmacytoid monocytes, karyorrhectic debris, abundance of histiocytes, including the crescentic forms, absence of neutrophils, numerous CD3+ CD8+ T-cells surrounding the areas of necrosis, and lack of a significant B-cell component (Table 9.5). Peripheral T-cell lymphomas generally present with total architectural effacement by proliferation of atypical T-cells; many cases lack histiocytes and plasmacytoid monocytes as well as areas of coagulative necrosis; however, some PTCLs can show some or all of these features. Most PTCLs are CD4+ positive, unlike the CD8+ proliferations seen in KFD. Loss of pan-T-cell marker, unfortunately, is not a reliable indicator of the presence of T-cell lymphoma, as it can be seen in reactive conditions including KFD. Thus, in some instances it is difficult to separate KFD from PTCL; in these cases, PCR analysis of the T-cell receptor gamma chain gene may be helpful. Luckily in children, however, the majority of T-cell neoplasms are T-cell lymphoblastic lymphoma/leukemia, which is composed of sheets of lymphoblasts, and anaplastic large cell lymphoma, which has "hallmark" cells as part of the infiltrate.

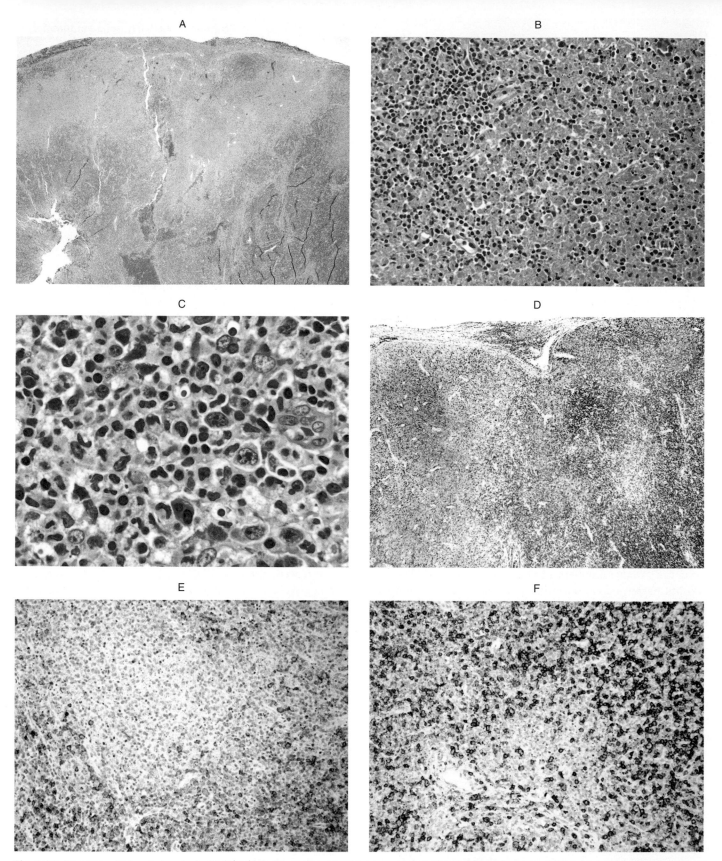

Fig. 9.23. Necrotizing histiocytic lymphadenitis (Kikuchi–Fujimoto disease). (A) Patchy necrosis in the cortex and paracortex (H&E stain). (B) Fibrinoid necrosis with abundant karyorrhectic debris and numbers of histiocytes with abundant cytoplasm filled with eosinophilic material. Note the conspicuous absence of neutrophils (H&E stain). (C) Numerous immunoblasts, plasmacytoid dendritic cells, and histiocytes surround the areas of necrosis. Many histiocytes have crescentic "C-shaped" nucleus, and cytoplasm filled with eosinophilic material (H&E stain). (D) CD3+ T-lymphocytes predominate in the areas surrounding the necrosis (immunohistochemical stain). (E) CD4+ T-cells are relatively sparse. Of note, the histiocytes also express CD4 (immunohistochemical stain). (F) CD8+ cells are the predominant T-cell subset present in the areas surrounding the necrosis (immunohistochemical stain). (G) CD20+ B-lymphocytes are present in areas unaffected by necrosis (immunohistochemical stain). (H) CD123+ plasmacytoid dendritic cells are numerous in the T-cell-rich interfollicular areas in Kikuchi–Fujimoto disease (immunohistochemical stain; the photograph is a generous contribution of Dr. Elizabeth Hyjek.)

G

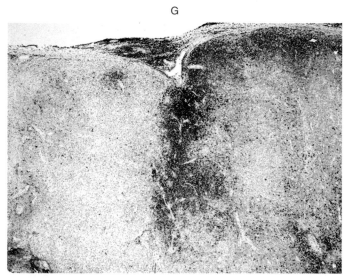

H

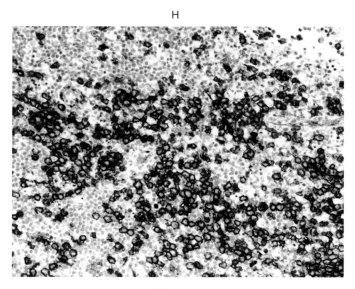

Fig. 9.23. (*cont.*)

Table 9.5. Helpful features to distinguish Kikuchi–Fujimoto lymphadenitis from peripheral T-cell lymphoma (PTCL).

Kikuchi–Fujimoto lymphadenitis	PTCL
Architecture	
Paracortical expansion with preserved architecture; partial effacement	Effaced lymph node architecture
Sinuses	
Patent in the non-pathologic areas; may be obliterated in the areas of necrosis	Obliterated
Type of necrosis	
Karyorrhectic debris; single cell necrosis; extracellular karyorrhectic material	Coagulative necrosis
Histiocytes	
Histiocytes with abundant eosinophilic cytoplasm; "C" shaped nuclei	Tingible body macrophages (intermediate- and high-grade lymphomas); epithelioid histiocytes
Major cell populations	
A mixture of immunoblasts and transformed lymphocytes with band nuclei; abundance of plasmacytoid dendritic cells (CD123+)	Monotonous population of medium to large cells with irregular nuclear contours, pleomorphic hyperchromatic or vesicular nuclei, and variable amount of cytoplasm
Immunophenotype	
Predominance of CD8+ T-cells	Usually CD4+; CD8+ rare
Inflammatory background	
Paucity of neutrophils, eosinophils, and plasma cells	Small lymphocytes, eosinophils, plasma cells, large B-cells, clusters of epithelioid histiocytes

The paucity of B-cells makes diffuse large B-cell lymphoma less frequently a diagnostic dilemma.

SLE lymphadenitis may present with very similar morphologic changes. Features that favor a diagnosis of SLE over KFD include the presence of hematoxylin bodies, plasma cells, at least some neutrophils, and vasculitis in addition to proper clinical presentation. The morphologic manifestations of lupus lymphadenitis are described later.

Herpes simplex lymphadenitis may present with extensive single cell necrosis, karyorrhectic debris, and crescentic histiocytes, but it usually presents with neutrophils and large cells with viral inclusions and ground-glass nuclei. Immunohistochemical staining with anti-HSV antibodies confirms the viral nature of the process.

Lymphadenitis due to EBV may also present with necrosis. The characteristic expansion of paracortical areas by a proliferation of immunoblasts, and *in situ* hybridization with an EBER probe to EBV-encoded RNA support the diagnosis of infectious mononucleosis as discussed previously. In necrotizing granulomatous lymphadenitis, such as cat scratch disease, tuberculosis, histoplasmosis, or leprosy, granulomata are present and the areas of necrosis are usually surrounded by palisading epithelioid histiocytes. Neutrophils are abundant.

Systemic lupus erythematosus lymphadenopathy

Localized or generalized lymphadenopathy is frequent in patients with systemic lupus erythematosus (SLE). Yet, since the diagnosis is based on clinical criteria and the presence of specific autoantibodies, lymph node biopsy is rarely performed. Lymph node biopsy is indicated in cases of unexpected lymphadenopathy or a sudden increase in the size of an existing lymph node.

In SLE, the lymphadenopathy is usually associated with more constitutional symptoms and more active disease as demonstrated by higher titers of anti-double-stranded DNA antibodies, and low complement levels [96]. Patients with SLE have three- to five-times higher risk of developing lymphoma as compared to the general population.

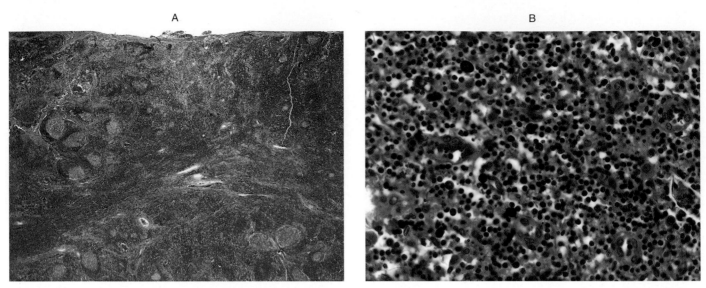

Fig. 9.24. Lymphadenopathy in systemic lupus erythematosus, necrotizing histiocytic-like (H&E stain). (A) Preserved nodal architecture with focal expansion of the paracortical areas. (B) Patchy fibrinoid necrosis with karyorrhectic debris and numerous hematoxylin bodies.

The morphologic features of SLE lymphadenitis are heterogeneous and vary depending upon the time of onset of disease as well as other factors. The most well-recognized pattern consists of paracortical coagulative necrosis, either focal or extensive, abundance of karyorrhectic debris, and numerous histiocytes, hematoxylin bodies, vasculitis, and a small number of plasma cells (Fig. 9.24). The hematoxylin bodies are composed of nuclear DNA, polysaccharides, and immunoglobulins forming extracellular clumps (5–12 μm in diameter) of amorphous material that stains heavily with hematoxylin.

Other morphologic patterns in lupus lymphadenopathy include reactive follicular hyperplasia with a Castleman disease-like pattern, follicular hyperplasia with pronounced arborizing vasculature in the expanded paracortex pattern, and non-specific follicular hyperplasia [97]. In cases of follicular hyperplasia with a Castleman disease-like pattern, the lymph nodes show a variable number of abnormal follicles with hyalinization and prominent vascular proliferation in the interfollicular areas, as shown in Figure 9.25. The interfollicular areas and medullary cords may contain numerous plasma cells. The most characteristic feature is the presence of disturbed follicular dendritic (FDC) meshworks, which can be demonstrated by immunostaining for CD21 or CD23. A similar disarray of the FDC meshworks is not specific and can be observed in individuals with profound immunologic deficits such as found in patients with HIV, Castleman disease, or who have undergone organ transplantation. Similar to those with Castleman disease, patients with SLE can present with elevated IL-6 levels; thus it and other cytokines may play a similar role in the pathogenesis of the two disorders [98]. While the causes of increased IL-6 in the two diseases may be different, it is plausible to speculate that these increased levels of IL-6 result in similar pathophysiologic changes and ultimately a similar morphology.

In some cases, the follicular hyperplasia is accompanied by pronounced paracortical arborizing vasculature. In 60% of the cases reported by Kojima *et al.*, the interfollicular areas were expanded by proliferation of CD4+ T-cells, and in the remaining cases by CD8+ T-cells [97]. Some cases of SLE lymphadenitis may present with follicular hyperplasia without other specific changes.

The differential diagnosis of SLE depends upon the morphologic changes seen in the lymph node. In cases with extensive necrosis, KFD should be considered. The presence of hematoxylin bodies and plasma cells in the proper clinical setting favors the diagnosis of SLE-related lymphadenitis. In cases with reactive follicular hyperplasia, the changes are less specific, and while SLE should be a clinical consideration, the diagnosis will ultimately depend on the clinical presentation and other laboratory abnormalities.

Cat scratch disease

Cat scratch disease (CSD) is a self-limiting infection caused by *Bartonella* (formally *Rochalimaea*) *henselae* that presents with regional lymphadenitis. The disease is caused by a cat scratch or bite, or by a flea bite, and has a worldwide distribution with a high prevalence in the fall and early winter [99]. Numerous studies show that CSD is directly linked to exposure to cats, particularly kittens, and cat fleas [100].

Children and young adults are most commonly affected. While cutaneous lesions and/or regional lymphadenitis are the most frequent presentations, visceral organ, neurologic, and/or ocular involvement can be seen in a minority of cases. In a study of 1200 patients with CSD, lymphadenopathy was present in all patients, and 11.8% of them developed suppuration [101]. Enlarged lymph nodes proximal to the inoculation site appear

A

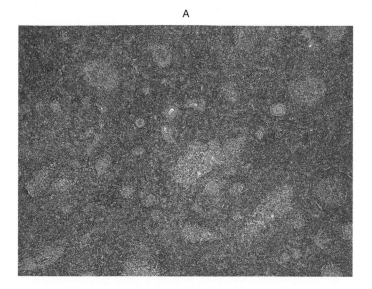

B

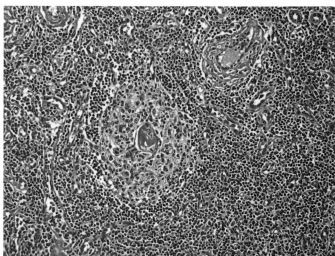

Fig. 9.25. Lymphadenopathy in systemic lupus erythematosus, Castleman disease-like (H&E stain). (A) Increased number of abnormal follicles and prominent vascular proliferation. The follicles are at different stages of maturation. (B) Many germinal centers are burned out and are composed mostly of follicular dendritic cells. Prominent vascular proliferation and hyalinization of vessels is seen. (C) Abnormal germinal centers composed of collapsed follicular dendritic cell meshwork penetrated by blood vessels.

C

several weeks after the skin has been inoculated with the organism. The nodes are almost always tender, with or without erythema of the overlying skin.

The average lymph node ranges from 1 to 5 cm in size. Lymph node biopsy is usually performed three to six weeks after the onset of the disease if antibiotic therapy does not yield an appropriate response. On sectioning, the lymph node may demonstrate multiple irregular microabscesses or more extensive necrosis. Touch preparations show a mixture of neutrophils and histiocytes. Multinucleated giant cells may be also seen.

The *morphologic findings* are quite characteristic and vary depending on the stage of the disease. Early lesions show small, focal areas of necrosis and small clusters of neutrophils surrounded by histiocytes beneath the subcapsular sinus. The necrosis may involve hyperplastic germinal centers. As the disease advances, the necrosis expands, and irregularly shaped

stellate foci with characteristic zonation are typically seen (Fig. 9.26A). There is a central area of necrosis with numerous neutrophils and karyorrhectic debris surrounded by palisading epithelioid histiocytes. Reactive lymphocytes surround the lesion. The sinuses may be distended with monocytoid B-cells. All stages of granulomatous inflammation may be seen in the same lymph node.

In the early stages of the disease, organisms can be demonstrated in the areas of necrosis or in the capillary walls using Warthin–Starry silver stain [102]. *B. henselae* is a fastidious organism and is difficult to culture. In conjunction with the morphologic features, a positive serologic or molecular (i.e., PCR) test for *B. henselae* is considered to be diagnostic.

The differential diagnosis includes tularemia, mycobacterial infection, lymphogranuloma venereum (usually affects the inguinal lymph nodes), and *Yersinia psuedotuberculosis* and *Y. enterocolitica* (usually involves mesenteric lymph nodes).

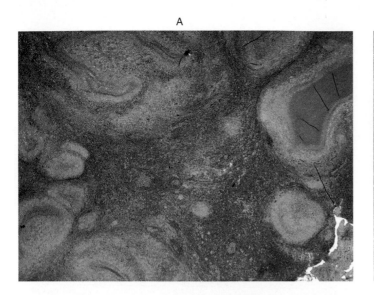

A

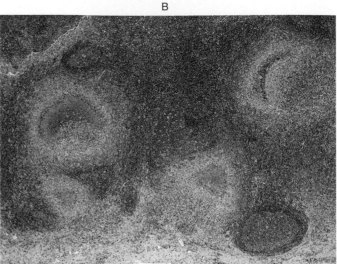

B

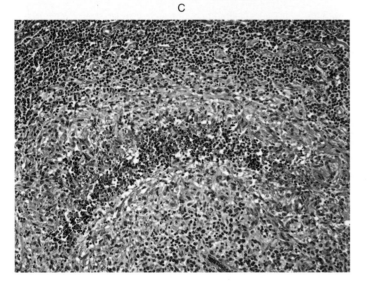

C

Fig. 9.26. Cat scratch disease (H&E stain). (A) A lymph node showing marked necrosis, with irregularly shaped stellate foci with characteristic zonation. (B) Several early granulomata with marked necrosis along with reactive germinal centers. (C) Central areas of necrosis containing karyorrhectic debris and numerous neutrophils surrounded by palisading histiocytes.

Clinical presentation, bacterial cultures, and serologic studies are helpful in separating CSD from these other entities.

Kawasaki disease (mucocutaneous lymph node syndrome)

Kawasaki disease (KD), also known as mucocutaneous lymph node syndrome, is an acute, potentially fatal vasculitis of young children that affects predominantly the coronary arteries [103]. While the disease is self-limited, about 20–25% of patients develop a serious coronary artery aneurism that, if untreated, may result in death. Treatment with IVIG in the first 10 days of the onset of fever significantly reduces the risk of coronary artery complications.

KD has a worldwide distribution. More than 85% of the patients are younger than five years; rarely are patients younger than six months or older than eight years at diagnosis. The reported annual incidence per 100 000 children younger than five years varies from 3 in South America to 134 in Japan [104]. Epidemiologically, the cases tend to occur during the winter–spring, the cases occur in clusters, and epidemics can occur. Clinically the patients with KD present with evidence of an abrupt infection which resolves in one to three weeks even without therapy. The patients often have an oligoclonal IgA immune response and recurrences are infrequent. These features suggest that the underlying cause of KD is infectious in nature. Cytoplasmic inclusion bodies have been identified in the bronchial epithelium of patients with acute illness [105], indicating that the identification of the causative infectious agent is close at hand.

The diagnosis of KD is made based on the presence of fever that lasts for at least five days, along with four of

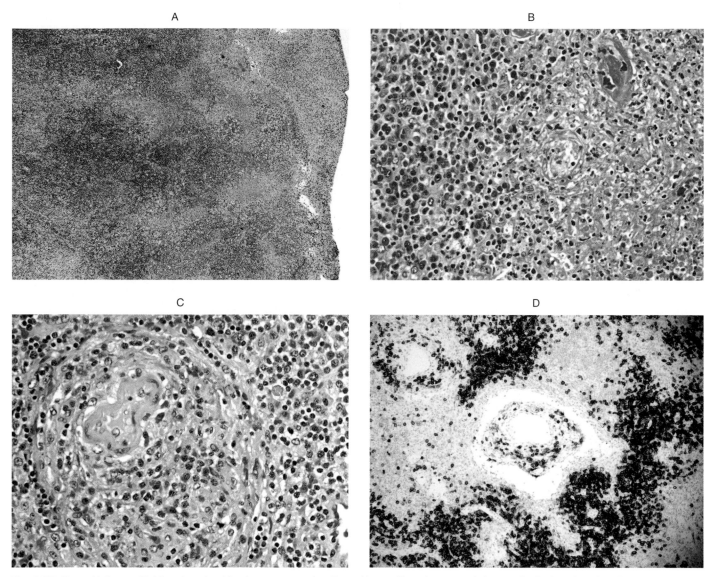

Fig. 9.27. Kawasaki disease. (A) A lymph node with edematous capsule infiltrated by small lymphocytes and plasma cells. The lymph node architecture is somewhat altered and areas of necrosis are noted (H&E stain). (B) Area of necrosis containing karyorrhectic debris surrounded by numerous lymphocytes, immunoblasts, and plasma cells (H&E stain). (C) Vasculitis; concentric layers of reactive lymphocytes and plasma cells infiltrating an intranodal arteriole (H&E stain). (D) CD138 highlights the plasma cells (immunohistochemical stain).

the following five criteria: bilateral conjunctival infection; changes in the mucus membranes of the upper respiratory tract (injected pharynx, injected, fissured lips, strawberry tongue); polymorphous rash; changes of the extremities (peripheral edema, erythema, periungual desquamation); and cervical lymphadenopathy.

The lymphadenopathy is the least consistent feature of the disease [106], and thus the name "mucocutaneous lymph node syndrome" is itself somewhat misleading. Lymph node biopsies in KD are infrequent, but sometimes performed early in the course of the disease when the other clinical features may not be apparent. The pathologic alterations in the lymph nodes of patients with KD are distinctive and possibly diag-

nostic of the disease. Thus, when a lymph node biopsy is performed, it is important that the correct diagnosis is rendered since prompt therapy is necessary to prevent the vascular complications.

The most characteristic *pathologic features* found in the cervical lymph nodes of patients with KD are the presence of edema, focal areas of necrosis consisting of karyorrhectic debris, histiocytes, immunoblasts, plasma cells, and vasculitis with fibrin microthrombi adjacent to necrotic small vessels (Fig. 9.27) [107, 108]. There may also be concentric layers of reactive lymphocytes and plasma cells surrounding and infiltrating many of the small intranodal arterioles and venules (Fig. 9.27C). Follicles can be present, and the degree of follicular hyperplasia varies. Sinus histiocytosis can also be seen. The capsule can be thickened and focally infiltrated by small lymphocytes and plasma cells. The number of plasma cells varies from a few to many, forming sheets. The plasma cells are polytypic and in some cases are predominantly IgA positive. However, IgA plasma cells are non-specific and can be seen in a variety of types of lymphadenitis.

The differential diagnosis in KD includes KFD and SLE lymphadenitis. The characteristic clinical presentation and the presence of vasculitis are suggestive of KD rather than the other diseases.

Acknowledgement: The author thanks Dr. Amy Chadburn, whose critical comments have been of extreme value for the clarity and structure of this chapter.

References

1. **Randall TD, Carragher DM, Rangel-Moreno J**. Development of secondary lymphoid organs. *Annual Review of Immunology*. 2008;**26**: 627–650.

2. **Blum KS, Pabst R**. Keystones in lymph node development. *Journal of Anatomy*. 2006;**209**:585–595.

3. **Mebius RE**. Organogenesis of lymphoid tissues. *Nature Reviews. Immunology*. 2003;**3**:292–303. Erratum in *Nature Reviews. Immunology*. 2003;3:509.

4. **Drayton DL, Liao S, Mounzer RH, Ruddle NH**. Lymphoid organ development: from ontogeny to neogenesis. *Nature Immunology*. 2006;**7**:344–353.

5. **Skandalakis JE, Skandalakis LJ, Skandalakis PN**. Anatomy of the lymphatics. *Surgical Oncology Clinics of North America*. 2007;**16**:1–16.

6. **Wilting J, Papoutsi M, Christ B**, *et al*. The transcription factor Prox1 is a marker for lymphatic endothelial cells in normal and diseased human tissues. *The FASEB Journal*. 2002;**16**:1271–1273.

7. **Yoshida H, Naito A, Inoue J-I**, *et al*. Different cytokines induce surface lymphotoxin-alphabeta on IL-7 receptor-alpha cells that differentially engender lymph nodes and Peyer's patches. *Immunity*. 2002;**17**:823–833.

8. **Blom B, Spits H**. Development of human lymphoid cells. *Annual Review of Immunology*. 2006;**24**:287–320.

9. **Crivellato E, Vacca A, Ribatti D**. Setting the stage: an anatomist's view of the immune system. *Trends in Immunology*. 2004;**25**:210–217.

10. **Randolph GJ, Ochando J, Partida-Sanchez S**. Migration of dendritic cell subsets and their precursors. *Annual Review of Immunology*. 2008;**26**:293–316.

11. **Maclennan ICM**. Germinal centers. *Annual Review of Immunology*. 1994; **12**:117–139.

12. **Facchetti F, de Wolf-Peeters C, Van Den Oord JJ, de Vos R, Desmet VJ**. Plasmacytoid monocytes (so-called plasmacytoid T-cells) in Kikuchi's lymphadenitis. An immunohistologic study. *American Journal of Clinical Pathology*. 1989;**92**:42–50.

13. **Harris NL, Bhan AK**. "Plasmacytoid T cells" in Castleman's disease. Immunohistologic phenotype. *American Journal of Surgical Pathology*. 1987;**11**:109–113.

14. **Marafioti T, Paterson JC, Ballabio E**, *et al*. Novel markers of normal and neoplastic human plasmacytoid dendritic cells. *Blood*. 2008;**111**: 3778–3792.

15. **Krishnan J, Danon AD, Frizzera G**. Reactive lymphadenopathies and atypical lymphoproliferative disorders. *American Journal of Clinical Pathology*. 1993;**99**:385–396.

16. **Nield LS, Kamat D**. Lymphadenopathy in children: when and how to evaluate. *Clinical Pediatrics*. 2004;**43**:25–33.

17. **Herzog LW**. Prevalence of lymphadenopathy of the head and neck in infants and children. *Clinical Pediatrics*. 1983;**22**:485–487.

18. **Knight PJ, Mulne AF, Vassy LE**. When is lymph node biopsy indicated in children with enlarged peripheral nodes? *Pediatrics*. 1982;**69**:391–396.

19. **Moore SW, Schneider JW, Schaaf HS**. Diagnostic aspects of cervical lymphadenopathy in children in the developing world: a study of 1,877 surgical specimens. *Pediatric Surgery International*. 2003;**19**:240–244.

20. **Tsang WY, Chan JK**. Fine-needle aspiration cytologic diagnosis of Kikuchi's lymphadenitis. A report of 27 cases. *American Journal of Clinical Pathology*. 1994;**102**:454–458.

21. **Tong TR, Chan OW, Lee KC**. Diagnosing Kikuchi disease on fine needle aspiration biopsy: a retrospective study of 44 cases diagnosed by cytology and 8 by histopathology. *Acta Cytologica*. 2001; **45**:953–957.

22. **Chiang YC, Chen RM, Chao PZ**, *et al*. Pediatric Kikuchi-Fujimoto disease masquerading as a submandibular gland tumor. *International Journal of Pediatric Otorhinolaryngology*. 2004; **68**:971–974.

23. **Perkins SL, Segal GH, Kjeldsberg CR**. Work-up of lymphadenopathy in children. *Seminars in Diagnostic Pathology*. 1995;**12**:284–287.

24. **Kussick SJ, Kalnoski M, Braziel RM, Wood BL**. Prominent clonal B-cell populations identified by flow cytometry in histologically reactive lymphoid proliferations. *American Journal of Clinical Pathology*. 2004; **121**:464–472.

25. **Orphanos V, Anagnostou D, Papadaki T**, *et al*. Detection of gene rearrangements in reactive lymphoid processes. *Leukemia and Lymphoma*. 1993;**9**:103–106.

26. **Chang CC, Osipov V, Wheaton S, Tripp S, Perkins SL**. Follicular hyperplasia, follicular lysis, and progressive transformation of germinal centers. A sequential spectrum of morphologic evolution in lymphoid hyperplasia. *American Journal of Clinical Pathology*. 2003;**120**:322–326.

27. **Howat AJ, Variend S**. Epithelioid germinal centers. *Archives of Pathology and Laboratory Medicine*. 1989;**113**:451.

28. **Howat AJ, Variend S**. Nuclear fragmentation and epithelioid change of germinal centers in the lymphoid tissue of child deaths. *Pediatric Pathology*. 1986;**5**:125–134.

29. **Osborne BM, Butler JJ, Variakojis D**, *et al*. Reactive lymph node hyperplasia with giant follicles. *American Journal of Clinical Pathology*. 1982;**78**:493–499.

30. **Kojima M, Nakamura S, Shimizu K**, *et al*. Reactive lymphoid hyperplasia of the lymph nodes with giant follicles: a clinicopathologic study of 14 Japanese cases, with special reference to

Epstein-Barr virus infection. *International Journal of Surgical Pathology*. 2005;**13**:267–272.

31. **Nosanchuk JS, Schnitzer B.** Follicular hyperplasia in lymph nodes from patients with rheumatoid arthritis. A clinicopathologic study. *Cancer*. 1969; **24**:243–254.

32. **Zhang K, Biroschak J, Glass DN,** *et al.* Macrophage activation syndrome in patients with systemic juvenile idiopathic arthritis is associated with MUNC13-4 polymorphisms. *Arthritis & Rheumatism*. 2008;**58**:2892–2896.

33. **Ferry JA, Zukerberg LR, Harris NL.** Florid progressive transformation of germinal centers. A syndrome affecting young men, without early progression to nodular lymphocyte predominance Hodgkin's disease. *American Journal of Surgical Pathology*. 1992;**16**:252–258.

34. **Osborne BM, Butler JJ, Gresik MV.** Progressive transformation of germinal centers: comparison of 23 pediatric patients to the adult population. *Modern Pathology*. 1992;**5**:135–140.

35. **Segal GH, Perkins SL, Kjeldsberg CR.** Benign lymphadenopathies in children and adolescents. *Seminars in Diagnostic Pathology*. 1995;**12**:288–302.

36. **Hicks J, Flaitz C.** Progressive transformation of germinal centers: review of histopathologic and clinical features. *International Journal of Pediatric Otorhinolaryngology*. 2002;**65**:195–202.

37. **Chang CC, Osipov V, Wheaton S, Tripp S, Perkins SL.** Follicular hyperplasia, follicular lysis, and progressive transformation of germinal centers. A sequential spectrum of morphologic evolution in lymphoid hyperplasia. *American Journal of Clinical Pathology*. 2003;**120**:322–326.

38. **Brauninger A, Yang W, Wacker HH,** *et al.* B-cell development in progressively transformed germinal centers: similarities and differences compared with classical germinal centers and lymphocyte-predominant Hodgkin disease. *Blood*. 2001;**97**:714–719.

39. **Osborne BM, Butler JJ.** Clinical implications of progressive transformation of germinal centers. *American Journal of Surgical Pathology*. 1984;**8**:725–733.

40. **Frizzera G.** Castleman's disease and related disorders. *Seminars in Diagnostic Pathology*. 1988;**5**:346–364.

41. **Keller AR, Hochholzer L, Castleman B.** Hyaline-vascular and plasma-cell types of giant lymph node hyperplasia of the mediastinum and other locations. *Cancer*. 1972;**29**:670–683.

42. **Harris NL.** Hypervascular follicular hyperplasia and Kaposi's sarcoma in patients at risk for AIDS. *New England Journal of Medicine*. 1984;**310**:462–463.

43. **Nagai K, Sato I, Shimoyama N.** Pathohistological and immunohistochemical studies on Castleman's disease of the lymph node. *Virchows Archiv – A, Pathological Anatomy & Histopathology*. 1986;**409**: 287–297.

44. **Leger-Ravet MB, Peuchmaur M, Devergne O,** *et al.* Interleukin-6 gene expression in Castleman's disease. *Blood*. 1991;**78**:2923–2930.

45. **Yoshizaki K, Matsuda T, Nishimoto N,** *et al.* Pathogenic significance of interleukin-6 (IL-6/BSF-2) in Castleman's disease. *Blood*. 1989; **74**:1360–1367.

46. **Hsu SM, Waldron JA, Xie SS, Barlogie B.** Expression of interleukin-6 in Castleman's disease. *Human Pathology*. 1993;**24**:833–839.

47. **Chadburn A, Cesarman E, Nador RG, Liu EY, Knowles DM.** Kaposi's sarcoma-associated herpesvirus sequences in benign lymphoid proliferations not associated with human immunodeficiency virus. *Cancer*. 1997;**80**:788–797.

48. **Parravicini C, Corbellino M, Paulli M,** *et al.* Expression of a virus-derived cytokine, KSHV vIL-6, in HIV-seronegative Castleman's disease. *American Journal of Pathology*. 1997; **151**:1517–1522.

49. **Palma DA, Dar AR, Millington SJ,** *et al.* Castleman's disease in children: report of 2 cases and clinicopathologic review. *Journal of Pediatric Hematology/ Oncology*. 2004;**26**:264–266.

50. **Parez N, Bader-Meunier B, Roy CC, Dommergues JP.** Paediatric Castleman disease: report of seven cases and review of the literature. *European Journal of Pediatrics*. 1999;**158**:631–637.

51. **Smir BN, Greiner TC, Weisenburger DD.** Multicentric angiofollicular lymph node hyperplasia in children: a

clinicopathologic study of eight patients. *Modern Pathology*. 1996;**9**: 1135–1142.

52. **Taylor KL, Kaschula RO.** Castleman's disease in children: the experience of a children's hospital in Africa. *Pediatric Pathology & Laboratory Medicine*. 1995;**15**:857–868.

53. **Salisbury JR.** Castleman's disease in childhood and adolescence: report of a case and review of literature. *Pediatric Pathology*. 1990;**10**:609–615.

54. **Baserga M, Rosin M, Schoen M, Young G.** Multifocal Castleman disease in pediatrics: case report. *Journal of Pediatric Hematology/Oncology*. 2005; **27**:666–669.

55. **Vasef M, Katzin WE, Mendelsohn G, Reydman M.** Report of a case of localized Castleman's disease with progression to malignant lymphoma. *American Journal of Clinical Pathology*. 1992;**98**:633–636.

56. **Shetty AK, Beaty MW, McGuirt WF Jr.,** *et al.* Kimura's disease: a diagnostic challenge. *Pediatrics*. 2002;**110**:e39.

57. **Swerdlow SH.** Pediatric follicular lymphomas, marginal zone lymphomas, and marginal zone hyperplasia. *American Journal of Clinical Pathology*. 2004; **122**(Suppl):S98–S109.

58. **Frizzera G, Murphy SB.** Follicular (nodular) lymphoma in childhood: a rare clinical-pathological entity. Report of eight cases from four cancer centers. *Cancer*. 1979;**44**:2218–2235.

59. **Taddesse-Heath L, Pittaluga S, Sorbara L,** *et al.* Marginal zone B-cell lymphoma in children and young adults. *American Journal of Surgical Pathology*. 2003;**27**:522–531.

60. **Chikwava K, Jaffe R.** Langerin (CD207) staining in normal pediatric tissues, reactive lymph nodes, and childhood histiocytic disorders. *Pediatric & Developmental Pathology*. 2004;**7**:607–614.

61. **Geissmann F, Dieu-Nosjean MC, Dezutter C,** *et al.* Accumulation of immature Langerhans cells in human lymph nodes draining chronically inflamed skin. *Journal of Experimental Medicine*. 2002;**196**:417–430.

62. **Hadinoto V, Shapiro M, Greenough TC,** *et al.* On the dynamics of acute EBV infection and the pathogenesis of infectious mononucleosis. *Blood*. 2008; **111**:1420–1427.

63. **Strickler JG, Fedeli F, Horwitz CA, Copenhaver CM, Frizzera G.** Infectious mononucleosis in lymphoid tissue. Histopathology, in situ hybridization, and differential diagnosis. *Archives of Pathology & Laboratory Medicine.* 1993;**117**:269–278.

64. **Rushin JM, Riordan GP, Heaton RB,** *et al.* Cytomegalovirus-infected cells express Leu-M1 antigen. A potential source of diagnostic error. *American Journal of Pathology.* 1990;**136**:989–995.

65. **Foucar E, Rosai J, Dorfman R.** Sinus histiocytosis with massive lymphadenopathy (Rosai-Dorfman disease): review of the entity. *Seminars in Diagnostic Pathology.* 1990;**7**:19–73.

66. **Foucar E, Rosai J, Dorfman RF, Eyman JM.** Immunologic abnormalities and their significance in sinus histiocytosis with massive lymphadenopathy. *American Journal of Clinical Pathology.* 1984;**82**:515–525.

67. **Maennle DL, Grierson HL, Gnarra DG, Weisenburger DD.** Sinus histiocytosis with massive lymphadenopathy: a spectrum of disease associated with immune dysfunction. *Pediatric Pathology.* 1991;**11**:399–412.

68. **Maric I, Pittaluga S, Dale JK,** *et al.* Histologic features of sinus histiocytosis with massive lymphadenopathy in patients with autoimmune lymphoproliferative syndrome. *American Journal of Surgical Pathology.* 2005;**29**:903–911.

69. **Eisen RN, Buckley PJ, Rosai J.** Immunophenotypic characterization of sinus histiocytosis with massive lymphadenopathy (Rosai-Dorfman disease). *Seminars in Diagnostic Pathology.* 1990;**7**:74–82.

70. **Lu D, Estalilla OC, Manning JT Jr., Medeiros LJ.** Sinus histiocytosis with massive lymphadenopathy and malignant lymphoma involving the same lymph node: a report of four cases and review of the literature. *Modern Pathology.* 2000;**13**:414–419.

71. **Maia DM, Dorfman RF.** Focal changes of sinus histiocytosis with massive lymphadenopathy (Rosai-Dorfman disease) associated with nodular lymphocyte predominant Hodgkin's disease. *Human Pathology.* 1995;**26**:1378–1382.

72. **Falk S, Stutte HJ, Frizzera G.** Hodgkin's disease and sinus histiocytosis with massive lymphadenopathy-like changes. *Histopathology.* 1991;**19**:221–224.

73. **Krzemieniecki K, Pawlicki M, Marganska K, Parczewska J.** The Rosai-Dorfman syndrome in a 17-year-old woman with transformation into high-grade lymphoma. A rare disease presentation. *Annals of Oncology.* 1996;**7**:977.

74. **Weeks DA, Beckwith JB, Mierau GW.** Benign nodal lesions mimicking metastases from pediatric renal neoplasms: a report of the National Wilms' Tumor Study Pathology Center. *Human Pathology.* 1990;**21**:1239–1244.

75. **Yunis EJ, Jaffe R.** Tamm-Horsfall protein in lymph nodes. *Human Pathology.* 1981;**12**:179–183.

76. **Kojima M, Nakamura S, Shimizu K,** *et al.* Inflammatory pseudotumor of lymph nodes: clinicopathologic and immunohistological study of 11 Japanese cases. *International Journal of Surgical Pathology.* 2001;**9**:207–214.

77. **Perrone T, De Wolf-Peeters C, Frizzera G.** Inflammatory pseudotumor of lymph nodes. A distinctive pattern of nodal reaction. *American Journal of Surgical Pathology.* 1988;**12**:351–361.

78. **Moran CA, Suster S, Abbondanzo SL.** Inflammatory pseudotumor of lymph nodes: a study of 25 cases with emphasis on morphological heterogeneity. *Human Pathology.* 1997;**28**:332–338.

79. **Kutok JL, Pinkus GS, Dorfman DM, Fletcher CDM.** Inflammatory pseudotumor of lymph node and spleen: an entity biologically distinct from inflammatory myofibroblastic tumor. *Human Pathology.* 2001;**32**:1382–1387.

80. **Chan JK, Cheuk W, Shimizu M.** Anaplastic lymphoma kinase expression in inflammatory pseudotumors. *American Journal of Surgical Pathology.* 2001;**25**:761–768.

81. **Arber DA, Kamel OW, van de Rijn M,** *et al.* Frequent presence of the Epstein-Barr virus in inflammatory pseudotumor. *Human Pathology.* 1995;**26**:1093–1098.

82. **New NE, Bishop PW, Stewart M, Banerjee SS, Harris M.** Inflammatory pseudotumour of lymph nodes. *Journal of Clinical Pathology.* 1995;**48**:37–40.

83. **Chan JK, Warnke RA, Dorfman R.** Vascular transformation of sinuses in lymph nodes. A study of its morphological spectrum and distinction from Kaposi's sarcoma. *American Journal of Surgical Pathology.* 1991;**15**:732–743.

84. **Bosch X, Guilabert A, Miquel R, Campo E.** Enigmatic Kikuchi-Fujimoto disease: a comprehensive review. *American Journal of Clinical Pathology.* 2004;**122**:141–152.

85. **Tanaka T, Ohmori M, Yasunaga S,** *et al.* DNA typing of HLA class II genes (HLA-DR, -DQ and -DP) in Japanese patients with histiocytic necrotizing lymphadenitis (Kikuchi's disease). *Tissue Antigens.* 1999;**54**:246–253.

86. **Lin HC, Su CY, Huang SC.** Kikuchi's disease in Asian children. *Pediatrics.* 2005;**115**:e92–e96.

87. **Wang TJ, Yang YH, Lin YT,** *et al.* Kikuchi-Fujimoto disease in children: clinical features and disease course. *Journal of Microbiology, Immunology & Infection.* 2004;**37**:219–224.

88. **O'Neill D, O'Grady J, Variend S.** Child fatality associated with pathological features of histiocytic necrotizing lymphadenitis (Kikuchi-Fujimoto disease). *Pediatric Pathology & Laboratory Medicine.* 1998;**18**:79–88.

89. **Lee KY, Yeon YH, Lee BC.** Kikuchi-Fujimoto disease with prolonged fever in children. *Pediatrics.* 2004;**114**:e752–e756.

90. **Scagni P, Peisino MG, Bianchi M,** *et al.* Kikuchi-Fujimoto disease is a rare cause of lymphadenopathy and fever of unknown origin in children: report of two cases and review of the literature. *Journal of Pediatric Hematology/Oncology.* 2005;**27**:337–340.

91. **Kuo TT.** Kikuchi's disease (histiocytic necrotizing lymphadenitis). A clinicopathologic study of 79 cases with an analysis of histologic subtypes, immunohistology, and DNA ploidy. *American Journal of Surgical Pathology.* 1995;**19**:798–809.

92. **Pileri SA, Facchetti F, Ascani S,** *et al.* Myeloperoxidase expression by histiocytes in Kikuchi's and Kikuchi-like lymphadenopathy. *The American Journal of Pathology.* 2001;**159**:915–924.

93. **Menasce LP, Banerjee SS, Edmondson D, Harris M.** Histiocytic necrotizing lymphadenitis (Kikuchi-Fujimoto

disease): continuing diagnostic difficulties. *Histopathology*. 1998;**33**: 248–254.

94. **Chamulak GA, Brynes RK, Nathwani BN**. Kikuchi-Fujimoto disease mimicking malignant lymphoma. *American Journal of Surgical Pathology*. 1990;**14**:514–523.

95. **Emir S, Gogus S, Guler E, Buyukpamukcu M**. Kikuchi-Fujimoto disease (histiocytic necrotizing lymphadenitis) confused with lymphoma in a child. *Medical & Pediatric Oncology*. 2001;**37**:546–548.

96. **Shapira Y, Weinberger A, Wysenbeek AJ**. Lymphadenopathy in systemic lupus erythematosus. Prevalence and relation to disease manifestations. *Clinical Rheumatology*. 1996;**15**:335–338.

97. **Kojima M, Nakamura S, Morishita Y**, *et al*. Reactive follicular hyperplasia in the lymph node lesions from systemic lupus erythematosus patients: a clinicopathological and immunohistological study of 21 cases. *Pathology International*. 2000;**50**: 304–312.

98. **Cross JT, Benton HP**. The roles of interleukin-6 and interleukin-10 in B cell hyperactivity in systemic lupus erythematosus. *Inflammation Research*. 1999;**48**:255–261.

99. **Windsor JJ**. Cat-scratch disease: epidemiology, aetiology and treatment. *British Journal of Biomedical Science*. 2001;**58**:101–110.

100. **Bass JW, Vincent JM, Person DA**. The expanding spectrum of *Bartonella* infections: II. Cat-scratch disease. *Pediatric Infectious Disease Journal*. 1997;**16**:163–179.

101. **Carithers HA**. Cat-scratch disease. An overview based on a study of 1,200 patients. *American Journal of Diseases of Children*. 1985;**139**:1124–1133.

102. **Miller-Catchpole R, Variakojis D, Vardiman JW, Loew JM, Carter J**. Cat scratch disease. Identification of bacteria in seven cases of lymphadenitis. *American Journal of Surgical Pathology*. 1986;**10**:276–281.

103. **Burns JC, Glodé MP**. Kawasaki syndrome. *Lancet*. 2004;**364**:533–544.

104. **Newburger JW, Taubert KA, Shulman ST**, *et al*. Summary and abstracts of the Seventh International Kawasaki Disease Symposium: December 4–7, 2001, Hakone, Japan. *Pediatric Research*. 2003;**53**:153–157.

105. **Rowley AH, Baker SC, Orenstein JM, Shulman ST**. Searching for the cause of Kawasaki disease – cytoplasmic inclusion bodies provide new insight. *Nature Reviews. Microbiology*. 2008;**6**:394–401.

106. **Sung RY, Ng YM, Choi KC**, *et al*. Lack of association of cervical lymphadenopathy and coronary artery complications in Kawasaki disease. *Pediatric Infectious Disease Journal*. 2006;**25**:521–525.

107. **Giesker DW, Pastuszak WT, Forouhar FA**, *et al*. Lymph node biopsy for early diagnosis in Kawasaki disease. *American Journal of Surgical Pathology*. 1982;**6**:493–501.

108. **Amano S, Hazama F, Kubagawa H**, *et al*. General pathology of Kawasaki disease. On the morphological alterations corresponding to the clinical manifestations. *Acta Pathologica Japonica*. 1980;**30**:681–694.

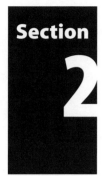

Section 2

Neoplastic hematopathology

10 Chromosome abnormalities of hematologic malignancies
A practical guide to cytogenetic analysis

Katrin Carlson Leuer

Introduction

Chromosomes have attracted many microscopists not only because these sausage-like bodies represent vehicles of genetic material (and hence, are biologically important) but also because they are hypnotically beautiful objects [1].

Chromosomes have captured the interest of scientists for well over 150 years. Initial studies of chromosomes were conducted in plants as early as the mid 1850s. At this time, technical limitations in microscopy and cytogenetic methodology precluded much advancement in the field. The first positive association between a chromosome aberration and a human disorder was made in 1959 when Lejeune and colleagues described trisomy 21 in nine cases of Down syndrome [2]. The first time that a characteristic chromosome change was associated with a specific neoplasm came in 1960 when Nowell and Hungerford identified an abnormally small G-group chromosome [the Philadelphia chromosome number 1 (Ph^1)] in cells from patients with chronic myelogenous leukemia [3]. Prior to 1971, identification of each individual chromosome was limited to segregation into seven groups, A through G, using chromosome size and centromere placement as the identifiers. Individual identification of each chromosome was made possible in 1971 by methods developed by Caspersson and colleagues [4]. Using chemical treatment and nuclear dyes, patterns of dark and light areas or "bands" could be visualized along the length of each chromosome. These patterns were both reproducible and recognizable and served as an indispensable tool in the advancement of cytogenetic studies in both the research and the clinical setting. With the aid of the newly described banding method, in 1973, Rowley determined that the Philadelphia chromosome was the product of a reciprocal translocation between chromosome 9 and chromosome 22 [5]. Shortly thereafter she identified the first recurring translocation in human acute leukemia t(8;21) and thus ushered in an exciting era in the study of hematologic disease [6].

Today, it is well known that specific numerical and structural chromosomal abnormalities are associated with distinct subtypes of leukemia and lymphoma, and that these abnormalities correlate with clinical outcome. In 2001, the World Health Organization recognized the significance of chromosome aberrations in hematologic disorders by incorporating cytogenetic data as a primary classification tool [7, 8]. This classification scheme included the subtypes: AML with t(8;21), AML with inv(16) or t(16;16), AML with t(15;17), and AML with 11q23 abnormalities. More recently, the fourth edition of *WHO Classification of Tumours of Haematopoietic and Lymphoid Tissues* includes genetic information in not only the 4 subtypes mentioned above, but in 15 other subtypes of hematopoietic malignancies [8]. This clearly illustrates the significance of cytogenetic and molecular genetic studies in the diagnosis and treatment of patients with hematopoietic disorders.

This chapter will present the basic principles, applications and limitations of both chromosome analysis and fluorescence *in situ* hybridization (FISH) testing, in order to aid the clinical pathologist in ordering practices as well as to facilitate interpretation of the cytogenetic report.

Conventional cytogenetic analysis
Background and theory

Detailed methods for the cytogenetic analysis of specimens submitted for the study of hematologic disease have been described previously [9]. Briefly, short-term cultures (24–72 h) are initiated with actively dividing cells from affected tissue. Dividing cells are arrested in the metaphase stage of mitosis through addition of a spindle fiber inhibitor (typically Colcemid). Once cell cycle arrest has occurred, a low-salt solution is added to the cell suspension; this increases cell volume and aids in chromosome spreading. The cell suspension is fixed with acetic acid and methanol to preserve the integrity of the cell membranes. A few drops of the fixed cell suspension are deposited on a microscope slide and allowed to dry. The drying process causes the cell membranes to rupture and the chromosomes to spread apart on the microscope slide (metaphase spread). The slides are treated with a protease to induce banding patterns and then stained,

Diagnostic Pediatric Hematopathology, ed. Maria A. Proytcheva. Published by Cambridge University Press.

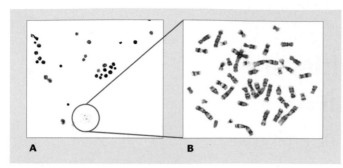

Fig. 10.1. (A) A low-power view of prepared microscope slides showing a number of interphase nuclei (round dark cells) and a metaphase spread. (B) A high-power view of the metaphase spread corresponding to the low-power image shown in A.

traditionally with Giemsa and/or Wright stain. The chromosomes are visualized using bright-field microscopy (Fig. 10.1).

Specimen collection

As summarized above, chromosome analysis depends on the analysis of actively dividing cells; therefore, the tissue received for study must be viable. Formalin-fixed tissue, frozen tissue, paraffin-embedded tissue, or necrotic tissue will result in a failed analysis. Bone marrow is the tissue of choice for leukemia studies, although peripheral blood, pleural effusions, or cerebrospinal fluid can be used in the case of circulating leukemia cells. It is important to mention that chromosome studies can be performed on bone marrow biopsy or bone core specimens. In the case of an inaspirable marrow (dry tap), a bone marrow biopsy can contain adequate numbers of viable cells for chromosome studies. However, if there is extensive bone marrow necrosis or if significant fibrosis is present, adequate numbers of viable cells may not be present. For lymphoma studies the most appropriate specimen is a biopsy of the involved tissue such as the lymph node, spleen or tonsil. Fine needle aspirates rarely result in successful chromosome studies. The analysis of bone marrow samples from patients with lymphoma rarely proves to be informative unless the lymphoma is of an aggressive nature.

For best results, tissue submitted for cytogenetic studies should be collected in a sterile manner, as bacterial and fungal contamination introduced during the processing of the specimen will also grow in culture and will preclude the successful culture and analysis of neoplastic cells. This is of particular concern in the surgical pathology setting, where sterile surfaces, forceps and scissors, or sterile cell culture media may not be readily available. In such cases surgical specimens should be placed in either sterile media or sterile saline. Surgical specimens should not be allowed to dry out as this will result in dead cells. Peripheral blood and bone marrow specimens should be placed in either cell culture media supplemented with heparin to prevent clotting and antibiotics to prevent bacterial contamination, or in standard sodium heparin collection tubes if media is not available. Specimens should not be collected in tubes containing agents such as EDTA or sodium citrate as these affect

cell viability. Specimens should be kept at room temperature and transported to the laboratory as quickly as possible to prevent undue cell death. If transport to the laboratory is delayed and there is a concern for bacterial or fungal contamination, the specimen can be stored at 4 °C. Extreme variability in temperature >37 °C or <4 °C, as well as extended transport times, will result in cell death and preclude cytogenetic analysis.

Analytical methodology

A routine chromosome analysis typically includes evaluation of 20 metaphase spreads. For each of 20 metaphase spreads, each chromosome is assessed for abnormalities in size, number, and banding. A structural abnormality or gain of a chromosome is considered clonal if it is observed in two or more cells, and a loss of a chromosome is considered a clonal abnormality only when it occurs in three or more cells. In some instances, such as inadequate sample volume, low mitotic index, or poor sample quality, the number of metaphase spreads available for analysis may be fewer than 20. In such cases, the analysis can still be informative if a clonal abnormality is detected.

Routine chromosome analysis is performed manually by microscopic evaluation at 100× magnification, using standard bright-field microscopy, by a trained technologist. In this way cytogenetics is much like anatomic pathology which requires assessment of a specimen under the microscope by a trained analyst. Because the analysis is done manually, the assessment of a particular abnormality is subjective and is dependent upon the experience of the microscopist. The time required to perform the evaluation of 20 metaphase spreads varies with mitotic index, morphology, and complexity, and can range from a few hours to days for highly complex cases.

While cytogenetic analysis can be used to monitor serial specimens from a single patient for continued presence/absence of disease, the absolute number or percentage of abnormal cells should not be used as a quantitative tool. As mentioned previously, cytogenetic evaluations are subjective, and if the technologist notices an abnormal cell with poor morphology he/she will then search for more abnormal cells until a number are found with adequate morphology to completely describe all aberrations noted. This is a biased assessment of the bone marrow; normal cells are passed over so as to find enough abnormal cells to most accurately identify the aberrations. Therefore, if 15 of 20 cells are shown to be abnormal, this number does not mean that 75% of the marrow is abnormal. Nor does it mean that more or less disease is present if, in follow-up specimens, 18 abnormal versus 13 abnormal cells are detected.

Nomenclature

The International System for Human Cytogenetic Nomenclature (ISCN) is the gold standard for the identification of chromosomes and their banding patterns. It provides a universal method of describing chromosomes and chromosomal aberrations. Now in its seventh edition, the ISCN contains

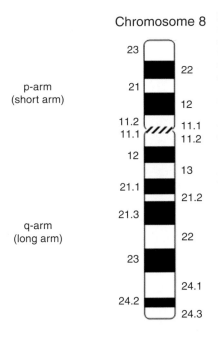

Chromosome 8

p-arm
(short arm)

q-arm
(long arm)

Fig. 10.2. Shown is a representative ideogram of chromosome 8 at a 400 band-level resolution. Band designations are as determined by the ISCN. Regions, bands, and sub-bands are numbered with lowest numbers near the centromeres and increase distally. Additional bands will be present at higher resolution. The numbering convention can be found in the ISCN.

Table 10.1. Standard cytogenetic abbreviations and interpretation [ISCN (2009)].

Abbreviation	Interpretation
add	Additional material of unknown origin
Brackets, square ([])	Surround number of cells
c	Constitutional anomaly
Comma (,)	Separates chromosome numbers, sex chromosomes, and chromosome abnormalities
cp	Composite karyotype
del	Deletion
der	Derivative chromosome
dup	Duplication
i	Isochromosome
idem	Denotes stemline karyotype in subclones
idic	iso-dicentric chromosome
ins	Insertion
inv	Inversion
mar	Marker chromosome (unidentifiable chromosome)
Minus sign (−)	Loss
Multiplication sign (×)	multiple copies of rearranged chromosome
p	Short arm of chromosome
Parentheses ()	Surround structurally altered chromosomes and breakpoints
Plus sign (+)	Gain
q	Long arm of chromosome
Question mark (?)	Questionable identification of a chromosome or chromosome structure
r	Ring chromosome
rob	Robertsonian translocation
sdl	Sideline
Semicolon (;)	Separates altered chromosomes and breakpoints in structural rearrangement involving more than one chromosome
sl	Stemline
Slant line (/)	Separates clones
t	Translocation

maps or ideograms of all the chromosomes, and outlines the numerical region, band and sub-band designations [10]. In addition to chromosome banding ideograms, the ISCN also outlines a detailed system for the naming and documentation of chromosome abnormalities. Interpretation of chromosome nomenclature, with all the numbers, punctuation, and abbreviations, can appear daunting to the untrained. It is worthwhile to become familiar with a few basic principles of the nomenclature and to refer to a trained cytogeneticist when more complex karyotypes are encountered. Briefly, each arm of a chromosome is designated "p" or "q". The p-arm (petite arm) is the shorter of the two arms, considering centromere placement. The longer arm is labeled the q-arm. By convention, the short arm or p-arm is always oriented up. Each band of a chromosome has been given a numerical designation (banding ideograms can be found in the ISCN and in other genetic resources). Numerical designations refer to regions, bands, and sub-bands. For example, 8q24.3 refers to chromosome 8, the q-arm (long arm), region 2, band 4, sub-band 3 (Fig. 10.2). Using the banding ideograms and the nomenclature as outlined in the ISCN, almost any chromosome abnormality can be uniquely and completely described. When describing the chromosome content of a cell (karyotype), the total chromosome number is always listed first. This is followed by the sex chromosome complement and a description of any abnormality noted in the cell. Abnormalities within each cell are listed in numerical chromosomal order and are described using abbreviated terms for the rearrangement. Lastly, the number of cells analyzed appears in square brackets "[. . .]" at the end of the karyotype. The most commonly used abbreviations and their definitions are listed in Table 10.1. Examples and explanations of abnormal karyotypes are shown in Figure 10.3A–D.

One source of misinterpretation that warrants clarification is the "add" terminology. "add" refers to the presence of addi-

tional material of unknown origin; it does not mean an additional copy of a particular region. For example, add(5)(q22) should be interpreted as a chromosome 5 that appears normal in the p-arm through to the centromere and then from the centromere along the q-arm until band q22. At band 5q22 material that can not be identified is present (Fig. 10.3C). The implication is that genetic material from 5q23 to the end of the chromosome, 5q35, is unaccounted for. Therefore, add(5)(q22) can be roughly equated to a deletion of the long arm of chromosome 5 from band q23 to q35.

Another source of confusion is the use of a composite karyotype (Fig. 10.3D). A composite system of nomenclature is used

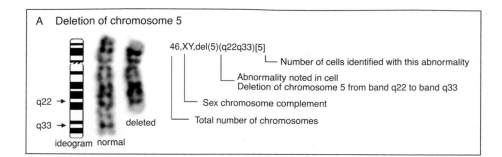

A   Deletion of chromosome 5

46,XY,del(5)(q22q33)[5]

— Number of cells identified with this abnormality

— Abnormality noted in cell
Deletion of chromosome 5 from band q22 to band q33

— Sex chromosome complement

— Total number of chromosomes

q22 →

q33 →   deleted

ideogram normal

Fig. 10.3. Examples and explanations of abnormal karyotypes.

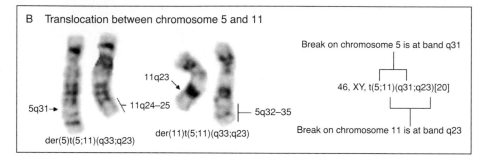

B   Translocation between chromosome 5 and 11

Break on chromosome 5 is at band q31

46, XY, t(5;11)(q31;q23)[20]

Break on chromosome 11 is at band q23

11q23

5q31→   11q24–25   5q32–35

der(5)t(5;11)(q33;q23)   der(11)t(5;11)(q33;q23)

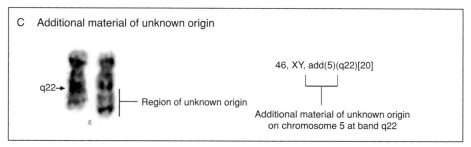

C   Additional material of unknown origin

46, XY, add(5)(q22)[20]

q22→

— Region of unknown origin

Additional material of unknown origin
on chromosome 5 at band q22

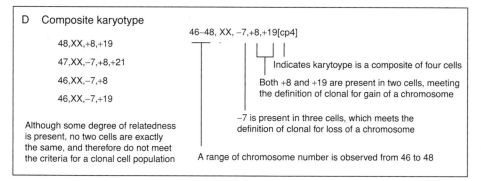

D   Composite karyotype

48,XX,+8,+19

47,XX,–7,+8,+21

46,XX,–7,+8

46,XX,–7,+19

Although some degree of relatedness
is present, no two cells are exactly
the same, and therefore do not meet
the criteria for a clonal cell population

46–48, XX, –7,+8,+19[cp4]

Indicates karytoype is a composite of four cells

Both +8 and +19 are present in two cells, meeting
the definition of clonal for gain of a chromosome

–7 is present in three cells, which meets the
definition of clonal for loss of a chromosome

A range of chromosome number is observed from 46 to 48

when there are a number of seemingly related abnormal cells, but no two are exactly the same and therefore do not meet the definition of a clonal cell population. In order to express that there are abnormal cells with some degree of relatedness, a composite karyotype is written. It is important to recognize that no cell necessarily has all the abnormalities listed in the composite karyotype, and that this is a compilation of abnormalities noted in a number of different cells.

Another important factor to keep is mind is that, due to the subjectivity of the cytogenetic methodology, breakpoint desig-

nations are somewhat dependent upon the observer. For College of American Pathologists (CAP) proficiency testing cases, ~250 different laboratories are given the same images to interpret. A certain degree of variation in the breakpoints used to describe the abnormality is always observed. CAP has determined that breakpoint designations plus or minus two bands is reasonable variation. It is helpful for the clinician and the pathologist to fully understand that breakpoint designations are not an exact science, and to consider the "two band rule" when investigating particular abnormalities.

Table 10.2. Application of cytogenetic testing (chromosome analysis).

	At diagnosis	In remission	With residual disease	At relapse
Acute leukemia	Yes	Only if a chromosome abnormality was noted in the diagnostic specimen	Only if a chromosome abnormality was noted in the diagnostic specimen	Yes
Myelodysplastic/ myeloproliferative disorders	Yes	Only if a chromosome abnormality was noted in the diagnostic specimen	Yes	Yes
Non-Hodgkin lymphoma	Yes Most appropriate on the affected tissue: lymph node, spleen, tonsil, etc. Not bone marrow	Only if a chromosome abnormality was noted in the diagnostic specimen Result is only informative if positive, a negative result must be interpreted with caution (see text)	No	Yes Most appropriate on the affected tissue: lymph node, spleen, tonsil, etc. Not bone marrow
Hodgkin lymphoma	No	No	No	No

Applications

Given the incorporation of chromosome abnormalities into the classification of hematopoietic tumors by the WHO, chromosome analysis should be performed on any specimen obtained for the purpose of the diagnosis of a hematologic neoplasm (Table 10.2). For leukemia studies, in those cases in which a chromosome abnormality has been identified in a pretreatment specimen, chromosome analysis is warranted for all follow-up specimens. Any abnormality noted at the time of diagnosis can be used as a biologic marker to monitor response to therapy. The presence or absence of this chromosome abnormality in a post-treatment specimen can be indicative of remission, residual disease, or relapsed disease. Alternatively, in those cases in which a chromosome abnormality has not been identified in a pretreatment specimen, chromosome analysis is warranted only in cases of suspected relapse. In these cases, repeating the chromosome analysis when remission or residual disease is suspected will be uninformative.

Cytogenetic studies are warranted for all possible diagnoses of non-Hodgkin lymphoma. However, the utility of the study depends upon the tissue type received by the laboratory. The study will be most informative if the diagnostic tissue, the lymph node, mass, tonsil, spleen, and so on, is submitted for evaluation. The analysis of bone marrow samples from patients with lymphoma is not optimal, even when bone marrow involvement has been confirmed by morphologic analysis. The reason for this is unclear, but may be because the normal bone marrow cells are dividing at a faster rate than the lymphoma cells and will therefore outcompete them in short-term cultures. Following this theory, the more aggressive the lymphoma, the more likely abnormal cells will be detected in short-term bone marrow cultures. If an abnormality is detected in the primary tissue and/or involved bone marrow, this can be of great utility for the classification of a lymphoid neoplasm. However, a normal karyotype must be interpreted with caution. When studying the bone marrow from a patient with lymphoma, in the face of a negative result (normal karyotype), a distinction cannot be made between the absence of lymphoma and the failure to detect the lymphoma.

Benefits and limitations

As with all tests, there are benefits and limitations to the utility of chromosome analysis. The greatest benefit of chromosome analysis is that the entire genome is surveyed in a single test. Unlike FISH, PCR, or flow cytometry, which survey specific/limited genes, loci, or markers, classic chromosome analysis surveys every chromosome for every patient. However, this global survey of the genome has some limitations. One limitation is the relatively few cells that are analyzed. Chromosome analysis is limited to the observation of 20 cells, therefore, the "sensitivity" of detecting an abnormal cell is 1 out of 20, or 5%. The second limitation of this global, whole-genome survey is the resolution of chromosome analysis. Each band can represent 1–10 Mb of DNA and can include many genes. Deletions, duplications, or other abnormalities which do not significantly alter the size of the chromosome or affect the banding pattern will not be detected using standard chromosome analysis. Lastly, chromosome analysis is subjective and, therefore, depends upon the experience and competence of the microscopist performing the study.

Fluorescence *in situ* hybridization

Background and theory

Fluorescent *in situ* hybridization (FISH) is a method which can be used in conjunction with standard chromosome analysis to provide additional information about a specific gene or locus. FISH analysis utilizes a fluorescently tagged DNA probe sequence (typically a gene of interest) and single-stranded DNA target sequences. Target sequences are most often metaphase spreads or interphase nuclei (Fig. 10.4). A variety of probe types can be used to detect chromosomal abnormalities by FISH.

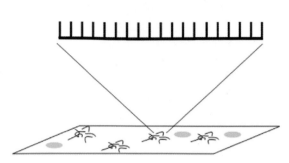

Fig. 10.4. Principle of fluorescent *in situ* hybridization (FISH) technique.

Fluorescently labeled probe in excess

Metaphase spread or interphase cells on slide

Single-strand probe sequence and single-strand target sequence anneal

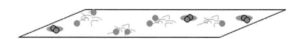

Visualize with counterstain and fluorescent microscopy

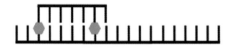

Most FISH probes used for clinical purposes are purchased from commercial vendors. Although many labs can label target sequences (BAC clones) "in house," this often is not cost effective or efficient. It is important to recognize that FISH probes are available for the common recurring abnormalities, but they will not be available for unique chromosome aberrations.

Specimen collection

The specimen used for FISH analysis is typically the same specimen collected for standard chromosome analysis. FISH can be performed on metaphase spreads or, unlike standard chromosome analysis, can also be performed on non-dividing cells. Thus, non-viable cells with preserved architecture, such as touch preparations or paraffin-embedded tissue sections, can also be used for the analysis.

Analytical methodology

Although FISH can be performed on many types of test samples, by far the most ordinary use for FISH with respect to hematologic disease is on interphase cells. The benefit of using interphase cells is that a large number of cells can be analyzed fairly quickly. Although there is no regulation for the number of cells to be analyzed, typically 200 cells are scored for each probe (range from 50 to 500). A variety of FISH probe strategies are available, each with its own limitations and benefits which are described below. For each probe and for each use of a probe, false-positive rates are calculated. False-positive rates refer to

the observation of an "abnormal" signal pattern in a normal individual, and are often calculated by using the mean number of abnormal signal patterns noted in a certain number of normal samples and adding two to three standard deviations. Each laboratory calculates their own false-positive rate, but in general the values adhere to some theoretical guidelines. Understanding the false-positive rates and the applications of different probe configurations is critical for proper interpretation of test results.

Probe types

Centromere probes

The centromeres of chromosomes are flanked by repeat DNA, termed α- and β-satellite DNA. In most cases, each chromosome contains unique sequences within these satellite regions, allowing for DNA probes which will identify each centromere specifically. Hybridization of chromosome-specific repetitive sequence probes is particularly suitable for the detection of monosomy, trisomy, and other aneuploidies.

Locus-specific probes

In contrast to centromere probes, which hybridize to repetitive segments of DNA, locus-specific probes have one target site. These probes can be used to detect the presence or absence of a specific sequence such as p53, or they can be used for detecting structural rearrangements such as a translocation of BCR and ABL.

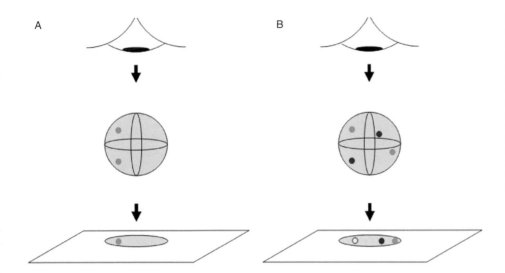

Fig. 10.5. False-positive signal patterns. (A) Schematic of a hybridization with a single-color enumeration probe. In the three-dimensional cell it is clear that there are two signals; however, in two-dimensional viewing, owing to spatial orientation of the signals, the two signals appear as one. This is a false-positive score for a deletion of this locus. (B) Schematic of a two-color single-fusion probe set. In the three-dimensional cell it is clear that there are two red signals and two green signals (normal); however, in two-dimensional viewing, due to spatial orientation of the signals, one green and one red signal appear fused (yellow). This is a false-positive score for a fusion of these two loci.

FISH strategies

Chromosome enumeration probes

Single color

Both centromere probes and locus-specific probes can be used to determine copy number. This can be useful for something straightforward such as detection of a gain of a chromosome (e.g., +8) or the loss of a chromosome (e.g., −5). The false-positive rate for the detection of a *gain of a chromosome* using a single-color probe is ∼2–5%. False-positive scoring for extra signals can be due to the false appearance of three signals in a cell due to the DNA being expanded or stretched out in interphase cells. It can also be due to technical artifacts such as nonspecific hybridization to another locus or to the presence of fluorescing debris on the cell. Using single-color probe strategy for the detection of a *loss of a chromosome or locus*, as opposed to the gain of a chromosome, has a much higher false-positive rate of ∼5–20%. The exact rate depends on the specific probe or locus being queried. The higher false-positive rate is the result of a number of factors. False-positive patterns consistent with loss of a particular locus can be the result of close proximity or random juxtaposition of target sequences in interphase nuclei. For example, if the two centromeres of chromosome 8 are near one another in an interphase cell, the hybridization signal pattern may appear as one signal, and a false-positive reading for monosomy. Some loci tend to associate in interphase more frequently than others; hence the variable false-positive rate.

False-positive scores can also be due to the technical constraints of signal visualization. For example, interphase cells are three dimensional; however, since they are affixed to microscope slides they are viewed through the microscope in two dimensions. Therefore, in a normal cell suspension, due to spatial configurations, a certain number of cells will always have a monosomic signal pattern (Fig. 10.5).

Dual color

Using two probes in two colors greatly increases the sensitivity when looking for loss or gain of a whole chromosome. For example, if a centromere probe for chromosome 8 labeled in red is used in combination with a locus-specific probe on chromosome 8 labeled in green, only those cells with three red signals *and* three green signals would be considered true positives for trisomy. The false-positive rate for this signal pattern is less than 0.5%. Similarly, a positive score for monosomy would be those cells with only one green signal *and* one red signal. This type of strategy has a false-positive rate of ∼3%; a significant improvement over the single-color strategy.

Fusion probe sets

Fusion probe sets are ideal for detection of structural chromosome abnormalities in interphase cells. These probe sets require two genes or two loci to be known; typically one is labeled in red and one in green. In the case of the fusion of BCR and ABL, t(9;22)(q34;q11.2), a normal cell will show a two-red and two-green signal pattern, corresponding to the two normal copies of ABL and the two normal copies of BCR (Fig. 10.6). In the case of a translocation, the genes are juxtaposed, moving the red and green signals near enough to appear "fused" or yellow. Fusion probes are only useful for translocations that have been cloned, meaning the specific DNA sequences on either side of the breakpoint/fusion site are known. Therefore, they cannot be used on orphan translocations, those that are non-recurring, or those for which the genes or sequences involved have not been identified. Similar to enumeration probes, fusion probes are available in different configurations.

Dual color, single fusion

The original fusion probe sets resulted in a single fusion product. In this design, the probe sequences are outside the breakpoint region, resulting in the entire probe hybridization area

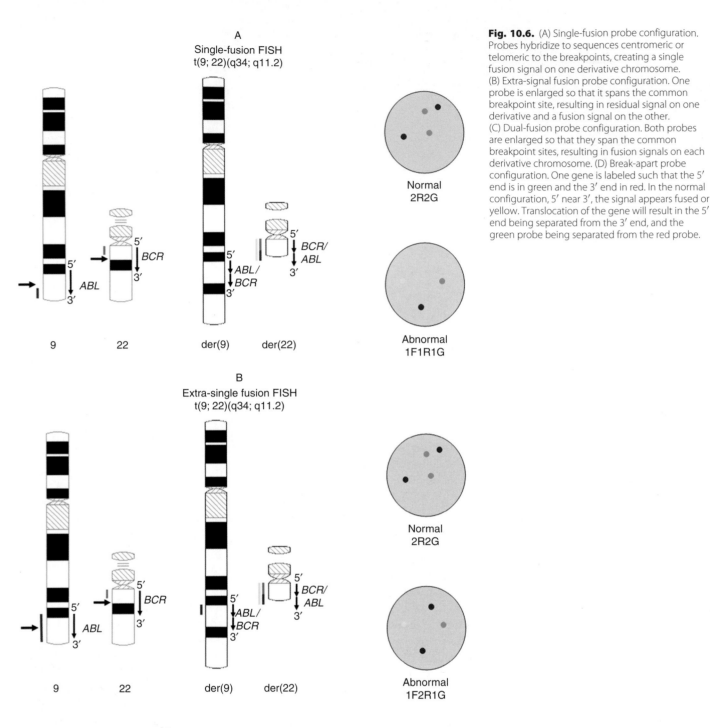

A
Single-fusion FISH
t(9; 22)(q34; q11.2)

9   22   der(9)   der(22)

Normal
2R2G

Abnormal
1F1R1G

B
Extra-single fusion FISH
t(9; 22)(q34; q11.2)

9   22   der(9)   der(22)

Normal
2R2G

Abnormal
1F2R1G

Fig. 10.6. (A) Single-fusion probe configuration. Probes hybridize to sequences centromeric or telomeric to the breakpoints, creating a single fusion signal on one derivative chromosome. (B) Extra-signal fusion probe configuration. One probe is enlarged so that it spans the common breakpoint site, resulting in residual signal on one derivative and a fusion signal on the other. (C) Dual-fusion probe configuration. Both probes are enlarged so that they span the common breakpoint sites, resulting in fusion signals on each derivative chromosome. (D) Break-apart probe configuration. One gene is labeled such that the 5' end is in green and the 3' end in red. In the normal configuration, 5' near 3', the signal appears fused or yellow. Translocation of the gene will result in the 5' end being separated from the 3' end, and the green probe being separated from the red probe.

being translocated when the rearrangement occurs (Fig. 10.6A). The result is a fusion signal on one of the abnormal chromosomes and no signal on the other abnormal chromosome. In interphase, the "positive" signal pattern is one fusion, one red, one green (1F1R1G). This type of configuration has a very high false-positive rate. This again can be due to either close proximity or random juxtaposition of the target sites in interphase nuclei or to the technical constraints of signal visualization. The false-positive rate with single-fusion probes can be greater than 15% (Fig. 10.5). Although this type of probe design is useful when a high percentage of abnormal cells are present, it is not useful for monitoring disease in patients who have been treated and may have minimal residual disease.

Dual color, extra signal

The second generation of probe design is the extra-signal probe set. This design extends the size or placement of one of the two probes to span the breakpoint. In this way, when a translocation occurs, part of the probe hybridization site will be translocated and part of the hybridization site will remain behind, giving rise to an extra signal in a single color (Fig. 10.6B). False-positive signals can be distinguished from genuine fusion

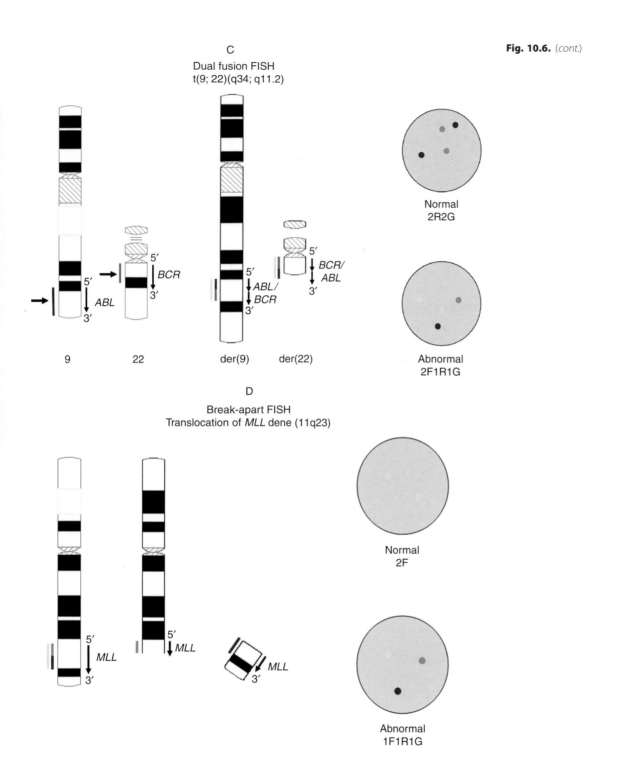

C
Dual fusion FISH
t(9; 22)(q34; q11.2)

9   22   der(9)   der(22)

Normal
2R2G

Abnormal
2F1R1G

D
Break-apart FISH
Translocation of *MLL* dene (11q23)

Normal
2F

Abnormal
1F1R1G

Fig. 10.6. (*cont.*)

signals by virtue of the absence of the extra signal. The false-positive rate of this type of probe configuration is much lower than the single-fusion probe configuration. The drawback to this probe design is that some patients have microdeletions at the site of translocation, so that the "extra signal" portion of the probe is deleted. The rate of deletion was shown to be quite frequent in CML (10–19%) [11–13]. For these patients, the probe set would then have no greater sensitivity than the single-fusion probe set.

Dual color, dual fusion

The third generation of probe expanded on the idea of the extra-signal probe configuration by extending the hybridization site of both probes. In the dual-fusion configuration, both probe hybridization sites span the breakpoint regions, resulting in the formation of two fusion signals when a translocation occurs (Fig. 10.6C). This probe configuration has a very good detection rate. Small deletions at the hybridization site would still result in abnormal patterns 2F1R1G, 1F2R1G, or 1F1R2G. The

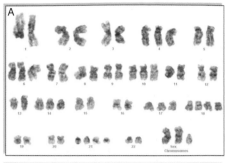

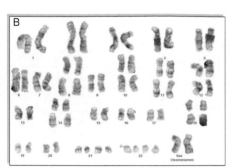

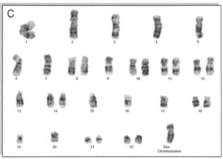

Fig. 10.7. (A) Typical pattern of "hyperdiploid" ALL. Notice extra chromosomes are usually present in three copies (sometimes four). (B) Karyotype suspicious for a doubled near-haploid. Notice that all extra chromosomes are present in four copies. (C) Near-haploid karyotype that doubled to form cell in B.

false-positive rate of dual-fusion probes can be as low as 0%, making this the most sensitive fusion probe strategy, and the most useful for monitoring residual disease.

Break-apart probes

A third type of probe strategy is the break-apart strategy. Break-apart probes are most useful when one gene needs to be queried and the specific partner is either unknown or not relevant. Unlike fusion probes, only one gene or locus is queried. For example, the *MYC* gene on chromosome 8q24 is frequently rearranged in Burkitt lymphoma. The rearrangement typically occurs with chromosome 14q32 (*IGH*) t(8:14)(q24;q32), but can also rearrange with chromosome 2 or chromosome 22: t(2;8)(p12;q24), t(8;22)(q24;q11). Instead of performing three FISH assays using three different fusion probe sets (*MYC/IGH*, *MYC/IGκ* and *MYC/IGλ*) to detect each translocation separately, it is useful in this case to employ the break-apart probe strategy. With a break-apart probe, one gene, in this case *MYC*, is labeled such that the 5′ region of the gene is labeled in one color (e.g., green), and the 3′ region in another (e.g., red). When the gene is intact the red and green colors are juxtaposed and appear as two, close red–green spots, or as a fused yellow spot. In a normal cell, it will appear as two fused spots, one for each of the two normal *MYC* genes on chromosome 8. If a translocation has occurred within the gene, separating the 5′ region from the 3′ region, the signals will appear as one red dot and one green dot in different areas of the cell (Fig. 10.6D). The break-apart probe strategy is particularly useful for those genes which have multiple translocation partners, such as *MLL* (11q23), *IGH* (14q32), *RUNX1* (*AML1*, 21q22).

Applications/limitations

FISH is a very useful and sensitive tool. It is important to note the type of probe strategy that was employed and to understand the general sensitivity of the test performed. If the application is appropriate, FISH can successfully identify abnormalities which are beyond the resolution of standard banding techniques. FISH is most useful when the analysis targets abnormalities that are known to be associated with a particular disease or are known to occur in a particular patient's tumor. Once an abnormality has been confirmed to be present in a diagnostic specimen (usually by standard chromosome analysis), FISH can be used to monitor response to therapy, detect residual disease, and in some cases detect early relapse. Another advantage of FISH is that it may be applied to both metaphase cells and interphase cells, allowing for the accurate and informative analysis of specimens for which no metaphase spreads are available. A major limitation of FISH is that the information gained from each hybridization is limited by the probe(s) used. Unlike chromosome analysis, which surveys the whole genome (albeit at a very global level), FISH analysis only queries one, or a few specific loci, the exact sequences/location of which are determined by the probe used. For example, a relatively common request is FISH analysis for loss of the long arm of chromosome 7, del(7q). Only one FISH probe is typically used to determine whether 7q is present or absent. If the probe maps to a small region on band 7q31, a normal result only means that that specific locus is present; it does not mean that other regions of 7q, even other regions within 7q31, are not deleted. It is imperative that this is clearly understood by ordering clinicians/pathologists. Lastly, as detailed above, FISH is also limited by the false-positive rates that can range from 0 to 20%.

Recurring abnormalities

There are many resources which thoroughly review recurring cytogenetic abnormalities in hematologic malignancies. One of the most useful is the web resource *Atlas of Genetics and Cytogenetics in Oncology and Haematology* at http://atlasgeneticsoncology.org/. Other useful resources include the *WHO Classification of Tumours of Haematopoietic and Lymphoid Tissues* [8], and Heim and Mitelman *Cancer Cytogenetics* [14]. In addition, in-depth discussion of cytogenetic abnormalities associated with specific clinical entities is present in the respective chapters of this book. This section will provide only a brief summary of recurring abnormalities and will highlight aspects which are of particular interest with respect to cytogenetic studies.

Myeloproliferative neoplasms

Chronic myeloid leukemia (CML)

The BCR-ABL1 transcript is required, by WHO definition, for a diagnosis of CML [8]. Nearly 95% of cases show the classic t(9;22) by standard banding methods. A small percentage of cases have a cytogenetically visible variant translocation that also results in the fusion of *BCR* and *ABL1*. Only a very few cases have a cryptic rearrangement of *BCR* and *ABL1* which requires the use of molecular methods [either reverse transcription polymerase chain reaction (RT-PCR) or FISH] to detect the transcript.

Characteristic patterns of chromosome abnormalities are associated with disease progression in CML [15], the most frequent of which is a gain of a second Ph chromosome [+der(22)], +8, −7, +19, and i(17q). These abnormalities can precede morphologic evidence of accelerated phase, warranting routine, repeat complete chromosome analysis on all patients with CML. FISH analysis, although accurate in detecting the fusion of *BCR* and *ABL1*, and invaluable in the detection of cryptic translocations, should not replace complete chromosome analysis. FISH analysis alone will not provide any information as to secondary abnormalities that may signal disease progression. FISH should also not be used to monitor minimal residual disease if methods to detect the transcript by PCR are available. FISH is not as sensitive as RT-PCR detection of fusion transcripts.

Abnormalities in other myeloproliferative neoplasms

Other than CML, MPDs as classified by the WHO are rare in children. In adults, although many patients have a normal karyotype, abnormalities such as +8, +9, or del(20q) are not uncommon. Despite the lack of knowledge regarding recurring abnormalities in pediatric myeloproliferative disorders, chromosome analysis of bone marrow from these patients is warranted in order to rule out the presence of t(9;22) and to identify those patients with 4q12 or 5q33 abnormalities involving platelet-derived growth factor receptor α (PDGFRα) and PDGFRβ (see below).

Myeloid neoplasms associated with eosinophilia with abnormalities of *PDGFRA, PDGFRB,* or *FGFR1*

Relatively recently, a cryptic fusion resulting from a submicroscopic deletion within chromosome band 4q12 was identified in a patient with hypereosinophilic syndrome [16]. This deletion, which was approximately 800 kb and included the gene *CHIC2*, resulted in the fusion of the tyrosine kinase *PDGFRA* to *FIP1L1*. The incidence of the *FIP1L1/PDGFRA* fusion in patients with hypereosinophilic syndrome/chronic eosinophilic leukemia (HES/CEL) is not clear. Study reports range from 3 to 56%, depending on study criteria. The frequency seems to be lower in children, with only one case of the *FIP1L1/PDGFRA* fusion having been identified in a pediatric patient [17]. Importantly, these patients have been shown to have response to treatment with the tyrosine kinase inhibitor imatinib. Since this deletion is beyond the resolution of standard chromosome analysis, when eosinophilia is noted and a myeloproliferative neoplasm is suspected, FISH analysis for the *FIP1L1/PDGFRA* fusion and/or *CHIC2* deletion should be requested.

Abnormalities of another imatinib-responsive tyrosine kinase, *PDGFRB*, at 5q31–33, have also been described in patients with myeloproliferative neoplasms, including at least one pediatric patient [18–20]. Unlike abnormalities of *PDGFRA* which are cryptic, to date, all reported rearrangements of *PDGFRB* have been cytogenetically visible, making standard chromosome analysis an appropriate test for the detection of these rearrangements [18]. When an abnormal karyotype involving band 5q31–33 is identified by standard chromosome analysis, FISH with a *PDGFRB* break-apart probe is warranted to confirm involvement of this gene.

Myelodysplastic/myeloproliferative neoplasms

Juvenile myelomonocytic leukemia (JMML)

As reviewed in Chapter 13, a large percentage of children with JMML have abnormalities of chromosome 7, either loss of the entire chromosome (−7), or abnormalities that result in loss of the long arm [del(7q)]. A smaller percentage, yet still a significant number, of children with JMML will have abnormalities of chromosomes other than chromosome 7 [21]. Although abnormalities of chromosome 7 are seen in a high percentage of patients with JMML, they are not unique to JMML and can be seen in all types of hematologic disorders. It is important to recognize that, although a valuable tool for monitoring disease status in these patients, with the exception of CML, cytogenetics analysis can not differentiate between a diagnosis of JMML and other myeloproliferative or myelodysplastic disorders.

Myelodysplastic syndromes

Myelodysplastic syndromes in children

The International Prognostic Scoring System (IPSS) is a useful system for the clinical management of adult patients with myelodysplastic syndrome (MDS). However, it appears to have limited utility with respect to the classification of pediatric MDS [22, 23]. The IPSS utilizes three criteria: cytogenetic abnormalities, bone marrow blast percentage, and number of cytopenias, to predict outcome [24]. The cytogenetic subgroups of the IPSS are good [normal karyotype, del(5q) only, del(20q) only, −Y only], intermediate (+8, 1–2 miscellaneous abnormalities), and poor [complex (≥ 3 abnormalities), or chromosome 7 abnormalities]. However, because distribution of cytogenetic abnormalities differs in children and adults, the IPSS system has been shown to be of limited value in the pediatric population [25]. In order to most appropriately treat pediatric patients with MDS, other pediatric-specific classification systems have been proposed, such as the CCC system, and the IPSS for childhood MDS and JMML [23, 25]. To date, there is no universally accepted classification system [26]. Regardless, cytogenetic studies are still warranted in children with MDS. Approximately 60% will have an abnormal karyotype, with the most frequent abnormality being −7 or deletions of 7q [27, 28]. If a recurring leukemia-associated abnormality is detected (see below), chromosome studies can also differentiate between those patients with MDS, and those with AML and low blast count. Any abnormality noted can also be used to monitor disease status in future bone marrow specimens.

Acute myeloid leukemia

The prognostic significance of various specific clonal chromosomal abnormalities in AML is well established [29–31]. The recurring abnormalities incorporated into the WHO classification system are thoroughly reviewed in Chapter 15 and will not be discussed in detail here. The specific cytogenetic subgroups of AML were so designated because the cytogenetic features could be associated with specific morphologic and/or prognostic features. The t(8;21)(q22;q22), inv(16)(p13q22)/t(16;16)(p13;q22) and t(15;17)(q22;q11−12) are all associated with a favorable prognosis when appropriate therapies are employed [8, 29, 31]. As a whole, patients with abnormalities of 11q23 are thought to have an intermediate prognosis. However, as mentioned previously, the *MLL* gene at chromosome band 11q23 has numerous different partner genes. Although the t(9;11) is the most common, various other translocations are observed with significant frequency. A recent international study of pediatric patients with rearrangement of *MLL* has shown that the specific 11q23 translocation partner can be used to further stratify the patients who fall into this clinical group [32]. They conclude that the t(1;11) is a favorable risk subgroup, whereas the t(6;11) and t(10;11) are poor-risk subgroups. The data were still not clear as to the prognostic significance of the t(9;11), both within this subgroup and for AML as a whole. Additional studies are needed to clarify the significance of each specific translocation involving *MLL*. It should be noted that FISH probes are readily available for the recurring translocations highlighted above, and can easily be used to monitor disease status when

more sensitive methods (such as RT-PCR) are not available or appropriate.

With the incorporation of chromosome abnormalities into the WHO classification system for acute leukemia, cytogenetic studies are appropriate for every patient with a new diagnosis of AML. Approximately 80% of pediatric patient with AML will have a detectable chromosome abnormality, many of which (e.g., +8, −7) are not specific to a single subtype of AML [31]. It is important to understand that chromosome abnormalities in pediatric AML include, but are not limited to, those highlighted by the WHO. If a patient is found to have an abnormal karyotype that is not listed in the WHO classification as a specific subgroup, then although the prognostic significance may be unclear, this abnormality can be used to monitor disease status in future bone marrow specimens.

Myeloid proliferations related to Down syndrome

As described in Chapter 16, individuals with Down syndrome can develop transient abnormal myelopoiesis (TAM), and are at a higher risk for the development of acute myeloid leukemia [33]. Transient abnormal myelopoiesis is most often characterized by absence of acquired chromosome abnormalities; however, abnormalities are sometimes identified [34]. The identification of clonal chromosome abnormalities in TAM is correlated with significant risk of future development of acute leukemia [34]. When myeloid leukemia develops in a patient with Down syndrome, a gain of chromosome 8 is the most frequent acquired abnormality noted. The t(1;22) characteristic of acute megakaryoblastic leukemia in patients without Down syndrome is not typically seen in this patient population.

All patients with Down syndrome will have three copies of chromosome 21 (+21, trisomy 21) in all or a subset of cells (mosaicism). The +21 noted in a patient with Down syndrome is a constitutional (congenital) chromosome abnormality. This is in contrast to acquired chromosome abnormalities associated with clonal neoplastic processes. A gain of chromosome 21 can also be seen as an acquired abnormality in a patient with acute leukemia. Because TAM in a patient with Down syndrome cannot be distinguished morphologically from acute leukemia in a newborn (without Down syndrome), the diagnosis of Down syndrome is critical. In many cases, a prenatal diagnosis of trisomy 21 has been made and, in other cases, the phenotypic features of the infant are sufficient to make a clinical diagnosis of Down syndrome.

However, in a few instances, a diagnosis of Down syndrome is suspected but has not been made either genetically or clinically. If chromosome analysis shows a karyotype that does not exhibit a +21, it is unlikely that the patient has Down syndrome. However, if the karyotype is positive for +21, either in all cells or in a portion of cells, and circulating blasts are present in the peripheral blood, this does not mean that the patient has Down syndrome. As mentioned previously, +21 can also be seen as an acquired abnormality associated with acute leukemia. In the presence of circulating blasts, cytogenetic analysis cannot differentiate between a constitutional +21 and an acquired +21.

Using mitogens, as is typically done for constitutional chromosome analysis, does not alter the ambiguity of the result. If circulating blasts are present, they will be dividing regardless of added mitogens. To unequivocally determine the constitutional chromosome complement, a peripheral blood specimen should be submitted when no blasts are present. Alternatively, if treatment decisions are pending a genetic diagnosis of Down syndrome, a chromosome analysis from a skin biopsy can be performed to determine the karyotype of the fibroblast (non-hematopoietic) cells. It is important to recognize that chromosome analysis of fibroblast cells requires long-term culture, and the turnaround time can be as long as three weeks. Alternatively, FISH methods on uncultured cells obtained from buccal mucosa can, in some instances, aid in the determination of the presence of a constitutional +21.

Precursor lymphoid neoplasms

B-cell lymphoblastic leukemia/lymphoma

Cytogenetic abnormalities are noted in the majority of cases of B-cell acute lymphoblastic leukemia/lymphoma, and often the chromosome abnormalities have clear clinical and/or morphologic properties and/or have important prognostic associations. Therefore, in 2008, for the first time, the WHO included cytogenetic information in the classification system for precursor lymphoid neoplasms. The recurring abnormalities noted in B-cell lymphoblastic leukemia/lymphoma are too numerous to list, and again the reader is referred to key reference resources as well as to Chapter 17 in this volume. Only the most significant with respect to frequency and prognostic information will be reviewed here.

Hyperdiploidy

"Hyperdiploid ALL" or "high hyperdiploid ALL" refers to a group of patients with a chromosome count of over 50, typically between 51 and 65 chromosomes. The extra chromosomes are non-randomly distributed, and most frequently include X, 4, 6, 10, 14, 17, 18, and 21 [35, 36]. Typically, the extra chromosomes are gained such that there is one extra of a number of chromosomes. A representative karyotype is, as such: 56,XY,+X,+Y,+4,+5,+6,+10,+14,+18,+21,+21. A pattern can be appreciated which includes single gains (trisomy) of a subset of chromosomes. The exception is chromosome 21, which can very frequently be present in four copies. "Hyperdiploid ALL" is associated with a good prognosis, and patients with simultaneous gains of 4, 10 and 17 are thought to be in an extremely good prognostic group [37, 38].

Near-haploid ALL

Near-haploid ALL refers to a group of patients with a karyotype which is similar to a haploid karyotype (one each of each chromosome), with some chromosomes present in two copies. Chromosome number is generally around 23–39 chromosomes. Quite often, the near-haploid line is accompanied by a hyperdiploid line. This line originates through a dou-

bling of the near-haploid cell line, resulting in nearly all chromosomes in the hyperdiploid line being present in two or four copies. For example, a near-haploid 26,X,+8,+14,+21 line when doubled becomes a 52,XX,+8,+8,+14,+14,+21,+21 line. The pattern of this cell line with over 50 chromosomes is in stark contrast to the "hyperdiploid ALL" karyotype described above, where affected chromosomes are most often present in three copies (Fig. 10.8). Recognition of a near-haploid karyotype is important, as data show that these patients have a high risk of relapse and so patients are treated on high-risk protocols [38–40].

t(12;21)(p13;q22)

The t(12;21)(p13;q22) is detected only by FISH, has been found in about 25% of pediatric patients with precursor B-cell ALL, and is associated with a good prognosis [38, 41, 42]. The majority of patients with the *ETV6/RUNX1* (*TEL/AML1*) fusion detected by FISH will have some other visible chromosome abnormalities, such as +21, del(6q), or del(9p), or abnormalities of the short arm of chromosome 12 [43]. If a patient has an abnormal karyotype but does not have one of the recurring chromosome abnormalities noted in B-cell ALL [hyperdiploidy, abn(11q23), t(1;19), or t(9;22)], it is imperative that FISH be performed to determine if the fusion of *ETV6* and *RUNX1* is present.

Amplification of *RUNX1*

Incidental to the identification of the *ETV6/RUNX1* fusion and the adoption of routine FISH screening methods for this cryptic translocation, an amplification of *RUNX1* was identified in approximately 1.5% of childhood precursor B-cell ALL [44]. In these cases, the sample was negative for a fusion of *ETV6* and *RUNX1*, but multiple hybridization sites were noted for *RUNX1*, suggestive of an amplification of this locus [45]. Combining cytogenetic and FISH data, the amplification of *RUNX1* most frequently arose as a result of a complex rearrangement of chromosome 21. This abnormality was shown to be indicative of a poor prognosis [44, 46].

Abnormalities of 11q23

Abnormalities of the *MLL* gene at chromosome band 11q23 are frequently noted in precursor B-cell leukemia/lymphoma. Cases are most usually associated with lack of CD10 expression. Although abnormalities of *MLL* can be seen in all age groups, the majority of children less than one year of age will have a rearrangement of this locus [47]. The most frequent rearrangement is the t(4;11), although others such as t(9;11) and t(11;19) are not uncommon. The t(4;11) is thought to portend a poor prognosis; however, it is less clear if patients with other translocations of 11q23 are similarly classified [38].

t(9;22)(q34;q11.2)

As discussed earlier, the t(9;22) involving the fusion of *BCR* and *ABL* is a hallmark of CML. However, the same translocation is also noted quite frequently in cases of precursor B-cell ALL. The

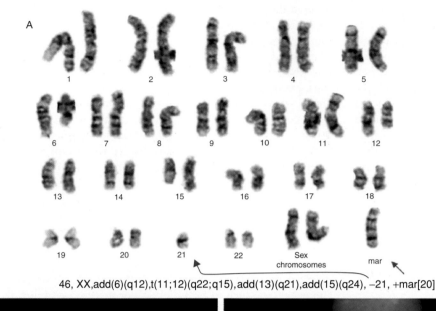

Fig. 10.8. (A) Complex karyotype with −21 and marker chromosome (mar). (B) FISH with probes to detect the cryptic t(12;21). Result shows no fusion, but instead amplification of *RUNX1* (red signal). (C) FISH to metaphase cell showing that the marker chromosome contains multiple copies of *RUNX1* (red signal).

46, XX,add(6)(q12),t(11;12)(q22;q15),add(13)(q21),add(15)(q24), −21, +mar[20]

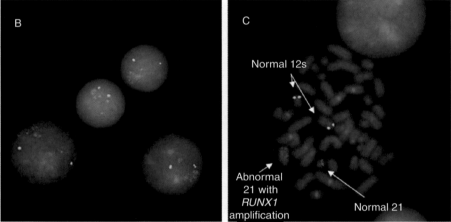

t(9;22) is present in 30% of cases of adult precursor B-cell ALL and in 3–5% of pediatric B-cell ALL. At the cytogenetic level, the translocations observed in CML and ALL are identical; however, at the molecular level the breakpoints are slightly different. In ALL the translocation typically gives rise to a 190 kDa protein product (p190), whereas in CML the protein product is most commonly 210 kDa (p210). In pediatric ALL, the t(9;22) is associated with a high white blood cell count, a high percentage of circulating blasts and a poor prognosis [38, 48]. In at least half of the cases, the t(9;22) is associated with additional chromosome abnormalities. However, except for monosomy 7, these abnormalities seem to have minimal impact on response to therapy [49]. Children with the t(9;22) are treated on high-risk protocols. Recent data show that the addition of the ABL tyrosine kinase inhibitor, imatinib, to standard treatment protocols positively impacts early event-free survival [50].

t(1;19)(q23;p13)

In early studies, the t(1;19) rearrangement and fusion of *E2A* and *PBX1* was associated with a poor prognosis. However, mod-

ern treatment regimens have moderated the prognostic significance of this abnormality. Patients with a t(1;19) are now considered to be within the standard risk group [38]. Although the prognostic significance of this abnormality has become less important, it is still considered a distinct entity by the WHO, due to the frequent association with a unique immunophenotype (CD19+, CD10+ and positive cytoplasmic μ heavy chain) [8].

T-cell lymphoblastic leukemia/lymphoma

Cytogenetic abnormalities are noted in approximately 50% of cases of T-cell acute lymphoblastic leukemia/lymphoma. A distinct pattern of non-random karyotypic abnormalities is apparent, and frequently involves the T-cell receptor genes at band 14q11.2 (*TRA@* or *TRD@*), 7q34, and 7p14 (*TRB@* and *TRG@*). The most common recurring abnormalities include t(11;14)(p13;q11.2) and t(10;14)(q24;q11.2). Other frequent abnormalities in T-cell ALL include deletions of the short arm of chromosome 9, and deletions of the long arm of chromosome 6 [51, 52]. The t(11;19)(q23;p13.3) involving the *MLL* gene at band 11q23 is noted in T-cell ALL [53]. This same translocation is also observed in B-cell ALL, acute myeloid leukemia and biphenotypic acute leukemia. Although reports indicate that the presence of the t(11;19) rearrangement confers a better prognosis, in contrast to B-cell ALL, the prognostic significance of most of the chromosomal abnormalities observed in T-cell ALL is not as clear [51, 54].

Mature lymphoid neoplasms

Very limited studies of pediatric non-Hodgkin lymphoma (NHL) have been performed, and most available data pertains to studies performed on adult disease. In adult studies, samples obtained from patients with NHL exhibit cytogenetic abnormalities in a high proportion of cases. As mentioned previously, the optimal tissue to study in the case of lymphoma is the primary affected tissue, such as lymph node, spleen, or tonsil. Many of the recurring abnormalities correlate with morphologic, histologic, and immunologic findings. For example, the t(14;18) is observed in a high proportion of follicular small cleaved cell lymphoma, whereas rearrangements of 3q27 (*BCL6*) are most frequently associated with diffuse large B-cell lymphoma. Rearrangements of *MYC* at band 8q24.1, for example t(8;14)(q24.1;q32), are most typical of Burkitt lymphoma.

The majority of recurring translocations in T-cell lymphoma involve rearrangement of the T-cell receptor genes *TRA@/TRD@*, *TRB@* and *TRG@*, located at chromosome bands 14q11.2, 7q34, and 7p14. An exception is the t(2;5)(p23;q35) noted in anaplastic large cell lymphoma, which fuses the *NPM* gene to the *ALK* tyrosine kinase, and is associated with positive expression of Ki-1 (CD30).

References

1. **Hsu TC**. *Human and Mammalian Cytogenetics: An Historical Perspective* (1st edn.). New York: Springer-Verlag; 1979.

2. **Lejeune J, Gautier M, Turpin R**. Study of somatic chromosomes from 9 mongoloid children. [Article in French.] *Comptes Rendus Hebdomadaires des Séances de l'Académie des Sciences*. 1959;**248**: 1721–1722.

3. **Nowell PC, Hungerford DA**. A minute chromosome in human chronic granulocytic leukemia. *Science*. 1960; **132**:1497–1500.

4. **Caspersson T, Lomakka G, Zech L**. The 24 fluorescence patterns of the human metaphase chromosomes – distinguishing characters and variability. *Hereditas*. 1971;**67**:89–102.

5. **Rowley JD**. A new consistent chromosomal abnormality in chronic myelogenous leukemia identified by quinacrine fluorescence and Giemsa staining. *Nature*. 1973;**243**:290–292.

6. **Rowley JD**. Identification of a translocation with quinacrine fluorescence in a patient with acute leukemia. *Annals of Genetics*. 1973: 109–112.

7. **Jaffe ES, Harris NL, Stein H, Vardiman J**. *World Health Organization Classification of Tumours: Pathology and Genetics of Tumours of Haematopoietic and Lymphoid Tissues*. Lyon: IARC Press; 2001.

8. **Swerdlow SH, Campo E, Harris NL**, *et al.* (eds.). *WHO Classification of Tumours of Haematopoietic and Lymphoid Tissues* (4th edn.). Lyon: IARC Press; 2008.

9. **Barch MJ, Knutsen T, Spurbeck JL** (eds.). *The AGT Cytogenetics Laboratory Manual* (3rd edn.). Philadelphia, PA: Lippincott-Raven; 1991.

10. **Shaffer LG, Slovak ML, Campbell LJ** (eds.). *ISCN (2009): An International System for Human Cytogenetic Nomenclature*. Basel: S. Karger; 2009.

11. **Dewald G, Wyatt W, Silver R**. Atypical BCR and ABL D-FISH patterns in chronic myeloid leukemia and their possible role in therapy. *Leukemia and Lymphoma*. 1999;**34**:481–491.

12. **Herens C, Tassin F, Lemaire V**, *et al.* Deletion of the 5′-ABL region: a recurrent anomaly detected by fluorescence *in situ* hybridization in about 10% of Philadelphia-positive chronic myeloid leukaemia patients. *British Journal of Haematology*. 2000; **110**:214–216.

13. **Sinclair PB, Nacheva EP, Leversha M**, *et al.* Large deletions at the t(9;22) breakpoint are common and may identify a poor-prognosis subgroup of patients with chronic myeloid leukemia. *Blood*. 2000;**95**:738–743.

14. **Heim S, Mitelman F** (eds.). *Cancer Cytogenetics*. New York: JohnWiley & Sons, Inc.; 1995.

15. **Johansson B, Fioretos T, Mitelman F**. Cytogenetic and molecular genetic evolution of chronic myeloid leukemia. *Acta Haematologica*. 2002;**107**:76–94.

16. **Cools J, DeAngelo DJ, Gotlib J**, *et al.* A tyrosine kinase created by fusion of the PDGFRA and FIP1L1 genes as a therapeutic target of imatinib in idiopathic hypereosinophilic syndrome. *New England Journal of Medicine*. 2003; **348**:1201–1214.

17. **Rives SMD, Alcorta IMD, Toll TMD**, *et al.* Idiopathic hypereosinophilic syndrome in children: report of a 7-year-old boy with FIP1L1-PDGFRA rearrangement. *Journal of Pediatric Hematology/Oncology*. 2005;**27**:663–665.

18. **Bain BJ, Fletcher SH**. Chronic eosinophilic leukemias and the myeloproliferative variant of the hypereosinophilic syndrome. *Immunology and Allergy Clinics of North America*. 2007;**27**:377–388.

19. **Golub TR, Barker GF, Lovett M, Gilliland DG**. Fusion of PDGF receptor beta to a novel ets-like gene, tel, in chronic myelomonocytic leukemia with t(5;12) chromosomal translocation. *Cell*. 1994;**77**:307–316.

20. **Wittman B, Horan J, Baxter J**, *et al.* A 2-year-old with atypical CML with a t(5;12)(q33;p13) treated successfully with imatinib mesylate. *Leukemia Research*. 2004;**28**:65–69.

21. **Hall G**. Cytogenetic and molecular genetic aspects of childhood myeloproliferative/myelodysplastic disorders. *Acta Haematologica*. 2002; **108**:171–179.

22. **Hasle H, Niemeyer CM, Chessells JM**, *et al.* A pediatric approach to the WHO classification of myelodysplastic and myeloproliferative diseases. *Leukemia*. 2003;**17**:277–282.

23. **Mandel K, Dror Y, Poon A, Freedman MH**. A practical, comprehensive classification for pediatric myelodysplastic syndromes: the CCC system. *Journal of Pediatric*

Hematology/Oncology. 2002;**24**: 596–605.

24. **Greenberg P, Cox C, LeBeau MM,** *et al.* International scoring system for evaluating prognosis in myelodysplastic syndromes. *Blood.* 1997;**89**:2079–2088.

25. **Hasle H, Baumann I, Bergstrasser E,** *et al.* The International Prognostic Scoring System (IPSS) for childhood myelodysplastic syndrome (MDS) and juvenile myelomonocytic leukemia (JMML). *Leukemia.* 2004;**18**:2008–2014.

26. **Elghetany M.** Myelodysplastic syndromes in children: a critical review of issues in the diagnosis and classification of 887 cases from 13 published series. *Archives of Pathology & Laboratory Medicine.* 2007;**131**:1110–1116.

27. **Martinez-Climent JA, Garcia-Conde J.** Chromosomal rearrangements in childhood acute myeloid leukemia and myelodysplastic syndromes. *Journal of Pediatric Hematology/Oncology.* 1999; **21**:91–102.

28. **Passmore SJ, Hann IM, Stiller CA,** *et al.* Pediatric myelodysplasia: a study of 68 children and a new prognostic scoring system. *Blood.* 1995;**85**:1742–1750.

29. **Grimwade D, Walker H, Oliver F,** *et al.* The importance of diagnostic cytogenetics on outcome in AML: analysis of 1,612 patients entered into the MRC AML 10 trial. *Blood.* 1998;**92**: 2322–2333.

30. **Byrd JC, Mrozek K, Dodge RK,** *et al.* Pretreatment cytogenetic abnormalities are predictive of induction success, cumulative incidence of relapse, and overall survival in adult patients with de novo acute myeloid leukemia: results from Cancer and Leukemia Group B (CALGB 8461). *Blood.* 2002;**100**:4325–4336.

31. **Ravindranath Y, Chang M, Steuber CP,** *et al.* Pediatric Oncology Group (POG) studies of acute myeloid leukemia (AML): a review of four consecutive childhood AML trials conducted between 1981 and 2000. *Leukemia.* 2005;**19**:2101–2116.

32. **Balgobind BV, Raimondi SC, Harbott J,** *et al.* Novel prognostic subgroups in childhood 11q23/MLL-rearranged acute myeloid leukemia: results of an international retrospective study. *Blood.* 2009;**114**:2489–2496.

33. **Hasle H, Clemmensen IH, Mikkelsen M.** Risks of leukaemia and solid tumours in individuals with Down's syndrome. *Lancet.* 2000;**355**:165–169.

34. **Massey GV, Zipursky A, Chang MN,** *et al.* A prospective study of the natural history of transient leukemia (TL) in neonates with Down syndrome (DS): Children's Oncology Group (COG) study POG-9481. *Blood.* 2006;**107**: 4606–4613.

35. **Heerema NA, Raimondi SC, Anderson JR,** *et al.* Specific extra chromosomes occur in a modal number dependent pattern in pediatric acute lymphoblastic leukemia. *Genes, Chromosomes and Cancer.* 2007;**46**:684–693.

36. **Mertens F, Johansson B, Mitelman F.** Dichotomy of hyperdiploid acute lymphoblastic leukemia on the basis of the distribution of gained chromosomes. *Cancer Genetics and Cytogenetics.* 1996;**92**:8–10.

37. **Sutcliffe MJ, Shuster JJ, Sather HN,** *et al.* High concordance from independent studies by the Children's Cancer Group (CCG) and Pediatric Oncology Group (POG) associating favorable prognosis with combined trisomies 4, 10, and 17 in children with NCI standard-risk B-precursor acute lymphoblastic leukemia: a Children's Oncology Group (COG) initiative. *Leukemia.* 2005;**19**:734–740.

38. **Schultz KR, Pullen DJ, Sather HN,** *et al.* Risk- and response-based classification of childhood B-precursor acute lymphoblastic leukemia: a combined analysis of prognostic markers from the Pediatric Oncology Group (POG) and Children's Cancer Group (CCG). *Blood.* 2007;**109**:926–935.

39. **Charrin C, Thomas X, Ffrench M,** *et al.* A report from the LALA-94 and LALA-SA groups on hypodiploidy with 30 to 39 chromosomes and near-triploidy: 2 possible expressions of a sole entity conferring poor prognosis in adult acute lymphoblastic leukemia (ALL). *Blood.* 2004;**104**:2444–2451.

40. **Harrison CJ, Moorman AV, Broadfield ZJ,** *et al.* Three distinct subgroups of hypodiploidy in acute lymphoblastic leukaemia. *British Journal of Haematology.* 2004;**125**: 552–559.

41. **Raimondi SP, Mauchauffe M, Le Coniat M,** *et al.* The t(12;21) of acute lymphoblastic leukemia results in a tel-AML1 gene fusion. *Blood.* 1995; **85**:3662–3670.

42. **Shurtleff S, Buijs A, Behm F,** *et al.* TEL/AML1 fusion resulting from a cryptic t(12;21) is the most common genetic lesion in pediatric ALL and defines a subgroup of patients with an excellent prognosis. *Leukemia.* 1995;**9**: 1985–1989.

43. **Attarbaschi A, Mann G, Konig M,** *et al.* Incidence and relevance of secondary chromosome abnormalities in childhood TEL/AML1+ acute lymphoblastic leukemia: an interphase FISH analysis. *Leukemia.* 2004;**18**: 1611–1616.

44. **Robinson HM, Broadfield ZJ, Cheung KL,** *et al.* Amplification of AML1 in acute lymphoblastic leukemia is associated with a poor outcome. *Leukemia.* 2003;**17**:2249–2250.

45. **Harewood L, Robinson H, Harris R,** *et al.* Amplification of AML1 on a duplicated chromosome 21 in acute lymphoblastic leukemia: a study of 20 cases. *Leukemia.* 2003;**17**:547–553.

46. **Cooley LD, Chenevert S, Shuster JJ,** *et al.* Prognostic significance of cytogenetically detected chromosome 21 anomalies in childhood acute lymphoblastic leukemia: a Pediatric Oncology Group study. *Cancer Genetics and Cytogenetics.* 2007;**175**:117–124.

47. **Biondi A, Cimino G, Pieters R, Pui C-H.** Biological and therapeutic aspects of infant leukemia. *Blood.* 2000;**96**: 24–33.

48. **Crist W, Carroll A, Shuster J,** *et al.* Philadelphia chromosome positive childhood acute lymphoblastic leukemia: clinical and cytogenetic characteristics and treatment outcome. A Pediatric Oncology Group study. *Blood.* 1990;**76**:489–494.

49. **Russo C, Carroll A, Kohler S,** *et al.* Philadelphia chromosome and monosomy 7 in childhood acute lymphoblastic leukemia: a Pediatric Oncology Group study. *Blood.* 1991; **77**:1050–1056.

50. **Schultz KR, Bowman WP, Aledo A,** *et al.* Improved early event-free survival with imatinib in Philadelphia chromosome-positive acute lymphoblastic leukemia: a Children's Oncology Group study. *Journal of Clinical Oncology.* 2009;**27**:5175–5181.

51. **Heerema NA, Sather HN, Sensel MG,** *et al.* Frequency and clinical

significance of cytogenetic abnormalities in pediatric T-lineage acute lymphoblastic leukemia: a report from the Children's Cancer Group. *Journal of Clinical Oncology*. 1998;**16**: 1270–1278.

52. **Raimondi SC, Behm FG, Roberson PK**, *et al.* Cytogenetics of childhood

T-cell leukemia. *Blood*. 1988;**72**:1560–1566.

53. **Moorman AV**, **Richards S**, **Harrison CJ**. Involvement of the MLL gene in T-lineage acute lymphoblastic leukemia. *Blood*. 2002;**100**:2273–2274.

54. **Rubnitz JE, Camitta BM, Mahmoud H**, *et al.* Childhood acute lymphoblastic leukemia with the MLL-ENL fusion and t(11;19)(q23;p13.3) translocation. *Journal of Clinical Oncology*. 1999;**17**: 191–196.

11

Expression profiling in pediatric acute leukemias

Lawrence Jennings and Chiang-Ching Huang

Introduction

DNA microarrays have proven to be a very powerful research tool. Since the term "DNA microarray" was first introduced in 1995 [1], there have been more than 12 000 publications on this new technology. The anticipated clinical utility has always been implied if not directly stated and it is notable that one of the first proof-of-principle studies to demonstrate clinical utility involved gene expression profiling of pediatric leukemias [2]. Acute leukemias have been ideal for exploring the potential of microarray technology because of the easy accessibility and purity of the neoplastic cells. This, and other early studies, investigated the differential gene expression of leukemia cells as a tool for predicting prognosis and therapy-related toxicity, and for identifying new mechanisms of pathogenesis and potential targets for therapy. Indeed, some investigators have suggested that gene expression microarray of acute leukemia will soon replace the standard diagnostic tools such as morphology, cytogenetics, and flow cytometry, in addition to establishing a molecular classification that would usher in the era of "personalized medicine." However, despite these early successes and the consequent excitement they generated, some investigators have questioned accuracy and reproducibility of microarray data, arguing that the data are at best a starting point for investigations, and translation to clinical practice will require extensive validation using more established, reproducible technologies. Nevertheless, proponents of the gene expression microarray approach continue to press on with refinements in targets, techniques, and technology, and clinical trials have begun. But is gene expression microarray ready for prime time? Will it replace or complement morphology, cytogenetics, and flow cytometry, or will it remain a research tool?

The development of the DNA microarray

DNA microarrays grew out of dot blot hybridization techniques. As far back as 1979, Kafatos *et al.* were able to demonstrate that they could determine nucleic acid sequence homol-

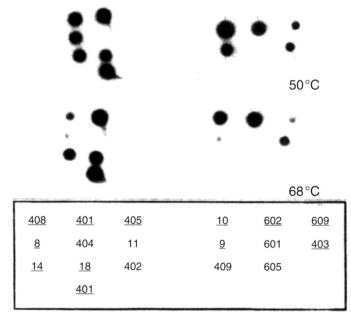

Fig. 11.1. First gene expression array. In this dot hybridization procedure, chorion cDNA clones were blotted onto nitrocellulose and intact endlabeled mRNA from mixed stages of choriogenesis was used as the probe. Ten of the 17 clones were detectable (underlined) and their intensity varied with the stringency of the wash. (Reprinted with permission [3].)

ogy and relative concentrations of mRNA in what could be called the first gene expression array [3]. They spotted multiple linearized fragments of cloned DNA onto nitrocellulose filter paper and then hybridized radioactive mRNA. In a proof of principle experiment, they spotted the nitrocellulose with equal amounts of DNA from 17 chorion complementary DNA (cDNA) clones. They were able to demonstrate variation in expression across the 17 clones, and, interestingly, autoradiography with higher stringency showed increased signal for two of the clones, which they attributed to greater sequence homology (Fig. 11.1).

Other investigators used similar "macroarray" approaches until improvements in technology and techniques allowed

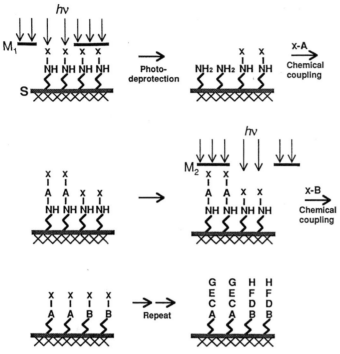

Fig. 11.2. Concept of the first synthetic oligonucleotide array. A solid support is covalently linked to a spatially addressable substrate. The substrate is chemically inert due to a photolabile protecting group. Exposure to light removes the protecting group and allows the synthetic chemical reaction to occur, but reaction only occurs at those sites that were deprotected. To deprotect some substrates but not others, "masks" are used. The pattern of masks will define the sequence of oligonucleotides that are synthesized. (Reprinted with permission [4].)

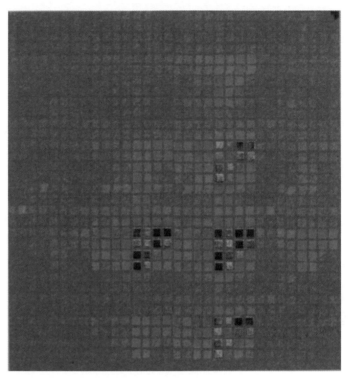

Fig. 11.3. The first "DNA Chip." One picomole of the target molecule (3′-AACCCAAACCC-fluorescein) was incubated with an array of octanucleotides. High fluorescent intensity indicates binding to the complementary probe sequence. (Reprinted with permission [5].)

greater numbers of probes to be arrayed, leading to the concept of microarrays. In 1991, Fodor *et al.* were able to demonstrate the synthesis of oligonucleotides *in situ* using technology adopted from fabrication of semiconductors (Fig. 11.2) [4]. Using such an approach, thousands of various short peptides or oligonucleotides could be synthesized *in situ* and in parallel. To the authors, the implications to clinical medicine seemed clear; they stated that such arrays would be "valuable in gene mapping, fingerprinting, diagnostics, and nucleic acid sequencing." In 1993, Fodor *et al.* went on to demonstrate that by using the "DNA chips," microarray-based sequencing was possible, although the methods and algorithms to reconstruct the target sequence from the hybridization data were still in development (Fig. 11.3) [5]. Again, the clinical implications seemed obvious as they went on to establish the first microarray company, Affymetrix (established in 1992). Affymetrix produced the first commercially available DNA microarrays (GeneChips™), and therefore the majority of early studies investigating the clinical utility of this new technology used their platform.

In 1995, Schena *et al.* produced the first spotted microarrays (and introduced the term "DNA microarray") following the dot blot hybridization techniques established years before, but they added two important improvements [1]. First, they increased the density of features per array while decreasing the area of the array by using robotic printing. Although they demonstrated

only 96 cDNA targets on their array, they argued that it was technically feasible to scale up fabrication to 20 000 cDNA targets per array using the robotic spotting technique. In addition, the smaller area allowed for far less sample volume to be hybridized to the array (2 μg of total cellular mRNA). Second, they introduced the two-color hybridization scheme. In this approach, fluorescent probes were prepared using reverse-transcriptase in the presence of fluorescent-labeled nucleotide analogs. The test mRNA would be labeled with one fluorescent molecule, while a control or reference mRNA would be labeled with another. The two probes would then be mixed in equal proportion and hybridized to a single array. The probes would compete for the same microarray cDNA, and the relative fluorescence of each probe would correspond to the relative concentration of that particular mRNA (Fig. 11.4) [6]. This approach was intended to minimize experimental variation that was inherent in the comparison of independent hybridizations. As proof of principle, these investigators demonstrated differential expression of 45 genes of the small flowering plant, *Arabidopsis thaliana* (Fig. 11.5). These investigators also noted the clinical utility of DNA microarrays, stating that they could provide "a useful link between human gene sequences and clinical medicine."

Thus, even from the inception of microarrays, expectations for clinical utility of this new technology were high. Over the last 10 years, there have been several other excellent microarray platforms developed (most notably Illumina,

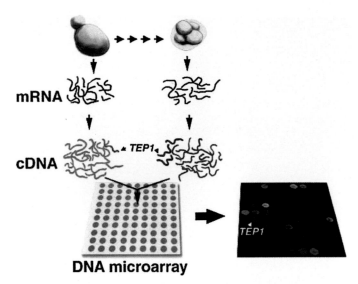

Fig. 11.4. The two-color DNA microarray approach. In this illustration, mRNA is prepared from the sample of interest and a corresponding control or reference. Each mRNA sample is labeled with a different fluor and hybridized to the microarray simultaneously. Excess abundance of one transcript relative to another would result in a corresponding increase in that fluor intensity. In this example, *TEP1* would be more abundant in the sample labeled with the red fluor. (Reprinted with permission [6].)

Agilent Technologies, and Nimblegen). However, the vast majority of studies to date that have explored gene expression profiling in pediatric leukemias have used either a version of the Affymetrix oligonucleotide arrays or the spotted arrays developed within independent laboratories or from a variety of commercial vendors.

Early studies demonstrate the potential for pediatric leukemias

One of the first demonstrations of the clinical potential for gene expression profiling by DNA microarray using acute leukemia as a test case was published in 1999 by Golub *et al.* [2]. RNA isolated from 38 diagnostic bone marrow samples (27 ALL, 11 AML) was hybridized to Affymetrix high-density oligonucleotide microarrays containing probes for more than 6800 human genes, and a quantitative expression level of each gene was determined. The first goal of this study was to determine whether the gene expression pattern could predict the type of leukemia – ALL vs. AML. The initially identified 1100 genes were narrowed down to 50 genes most closely correlating with AML–ALL. Using this approach, 36 of 38 leukemias were accurately assigned to either ALL or AML, and for the remaining 2 the score was below the defined threshold. These results indicated that microarray techniques can be used for distinction between ALL and AML in most cases. Furthermore, the 50-gene predictor was applied to an independent group of 34 leukemia samples (24 bone marrow, 10 peripheral blood), and the prediction was strong and accurate in 29 of these cases, with the remaining cases left unclassified (Fig. 11.6). The 50-gene predictor included lineage-specific genes such as *CD11c*, *CD33*,

and *MB-1*, as well as genes encoding cell cycle proteins (Cyclin D3, *Op18*, and *MCM3*), chromosome remodeling (*RbAP48* and *SNF2*), transcription factors (*TFIIEβ*), cell adhesion molecules (*CD11c*) or known oncogenes (*c-MYB*, *E2A*, and *HOXA9*) (Fig. 11.7). Thus, these findings constituted one of the first demonstrations of the feasibility of cancer classification based solely on gene expression profiles.

The gene expression patterns could be used to discover diagnostic subsets as well. Using an unsupervised statistical approach called self-organizing maps (SOMs), this initial study was able to divide the leukemias into four groups (B1–B4), primarily corresponding to AML, T-lineage ALL, B-lineage ALL, and B-lineage ALL. The gene expression profiles show that the two B-lineage ALLs (B3 and B4) are similar and can be merged together. Thus, in this early work, Golub *et al.* were able to nicely demonstrate that gene expression profiling could be used as a tool for class prediction, but could also be used for class discovery. Class prediction could be used to classify types of leukemia, but could also be used to predict outcomes, provided the eventual outcomes were known. Class discovery could be used to identify subsets that behave differently and use this separation to develop new sets of predictors.

Many other gene expression microarray studies investigating pediatric leukemias were soon to follow, and the results were very promising [7–29]. These studies have been focused on gene expression patterns in pediatric ALL, AML, and to a much lesser extent myelodysplastic syndrome (MDS). All these studies have used one of the generations of Affymetrix arrays or laboratory-developed spotted arrays, and the number of test subjects ranged from 10 to 360. The aims of these studies were primarily to classify the pediatric acute leukemias into known subsets, but also to predict response to therapy and overall prognosis, or to provide biologic insights into leukemogenesis.

The largest study came out of St. Judes. Yeoh *et al.* [28] focused on acute lymphoblastic leukemias, and went beyond classification and subtype discovery to include gene expression profiling to identify those patients that would eventually fail therapy or develop secondary AML. These investigators used Affymetrix oligonucleotide arrays including more genes (12 600) and a higher number of total samples analyzed (360) as compared to the earlier studies. In 327 diagnostic bone marrow samples, they were able to identify expression profiles using the top 40 genes per subgroup selected by a chi-squared metric, and cluster the diagnostic subgroups of ALL by hierarchical clustering: *E2A-PBX1*, *MLL*, T-ALL (T-cell acute lymphoblastic leukemia), hyperdiploid ALL (>50 chromosomes), *BCR-ABL1*, and *ETV6-RUNX1* (*TEL-AML1*), as well as a "novel" subgroup (Fig. 11.8). It should be noted that the "novel" subgroup comprised 65 samples (20% of the total). Across the subgroups, 9 genes were identified as useful in discriminating more than one subgroup, so that the total number of discriminating genes for seven subgroups was 271. To demonstrate the potential of expression profiling as a diagnostic tool, these investigators divided the 327 diagnostic samples into a

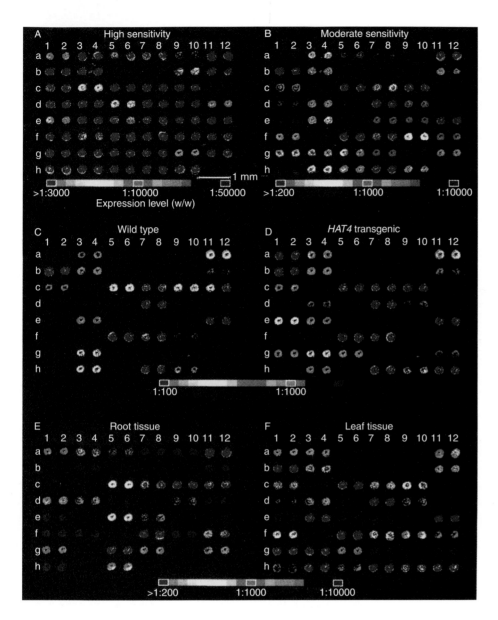

Fig. 11.5. First cDNA microarray. Fluorescent scans represented in pseudocolor correspond to hybridization intensities. Color bars were calibrated from the signal obtained with the use of known concentrations of human acetylcholine receptor (AChR) mRNA in independent experiments. Numbers and letters on the axes mark the position of each cDNA. (A) High-sensitivity fluorescein scan after hybridization with fluorescein-labeled cDNA derived from wild-type plants. (B) Same array as in A, but scanned at moderate sensitivity. (C, D) A single array was probed with a 1 : 1 mixture of fluorescein-labeled cDNA from wild-type plants and lissamine-labeled cDNA from *HAT4*-transgenic plants. The single array was then scanned successively to detect the fluorescein fluorescence corresponding to mRNA from wild-type plants (C), and the lissamine fluorescence corresponding to mRNA from *HAT4*-transgenic plants (D). (E, F) A single array was probed with a 1 : 1 mixture of fluorescein-labeled cDNA from root tissue and lissamine-labeled cDNA from leaf tissue. The single array was then scanned successively to detect the fluorescein fluorescence corresponding to mRNAs expressed in roots (E), and the lissamine fluorescence corresponding to mRNAs expressed in leaves (F). (Reprinted with permission [1].)

training set (215 cases) and a test set (112 cases) and classified these using a decision-tree format. Cases not assigned to one of these classes were excluded. For the cases that were assignable, this approach demonstrated remarkable accuracy (Table 11.1). The authors contend that the overall diagnostic accuracy of 96% exceeds that typically achieved using standard diagnostic approaches of morphology, cytogenetics, and immunophenotyping. They further suggest that gene expression profiling might even be more accurate when one considers that some of the misclassified samples actually had genetic lesions that were consistent with the gene expression profile but were missed by RT-PCR.

This study went beyond subgroup classification and discovery to use gene expression profiles to identify patients at high risk of treatment failure. For this analysis, expression profiles were compared among four groups of children with ALL: diagnostic samples of those that would eventually relapse ($n = 32$),

diagnostic samples of those that remain in complete remission ($n = 201$), diagnostic samples of those who developed therapy-related AML ($n = 16$), and leukemia samples collected at the time of relapse ($n = 25$). With some leukemia subtypes, they were able to identify distinct expression profiles that could be used to predict relapse. For both T-ALL and hyperdiploid ALL (>50 chromosomes) subgroups, these expression profiles identified those cases that went on to relapse with 97% and 100% accuracy in cross-validation, which were statistically significant when compared to results from an analysis of 1000 random permutations of the data set. In other subgroups, although the accuracies were very high, they failed to reach statistical significance, which was attributed to the low number of samples in each subgroup. The authors conclude that gene expression profiling can provide accurate diagnosis and risk stratification, but in addition could help identify patients at increased risk of drug toxicity or relapse.

Table 11.1. Acute lymphoblastic leukemia subgroup prediction accuracies using support vector machines (SVMs).

	Training set[a]		Test set[b]		
Subgroups	Apparent accuracy[c] (%)		True accuracy[d] (%)	Sensitivity[e] (%)	Specificity[f] (%)
T-ALL[g]	100		100	100	100
E2A-PBX1	100		100	100	100
ETV6-RUNX1	98		99	100	98
BCR-ABL	96		97	83	98
MLL rearrangement	100		100	100	100
Hyperdiploid ALL (>50 chromosomes)	93		96	100	93

[a] The training set consisted of 215 samples.
[b] The blinded test set consisted of 112 samples.
[c] Apparent accuracy was determined by leave-one-out cross-validation.
[d] True accuracy was determined by class prediction on the blinded test set.
[e] Sensitivity = (the number of positive samples predicted)/(the number of true positives).
[f] Specificity = (the number of negative samples predicted)/(the number of true negatives).
[g] The distribution of cases in the training and test sets is: T-ALL (28 cases, 15 cases); E2A-PBX1 (18, 9); ETV6-RUNX1 (52, 27); BCR-ABL (9, 6); MLL rearrangement (14, 6); hyperdiploid ALL (>50 chromosomes) (42, 22).
Reproduced with permission [28].

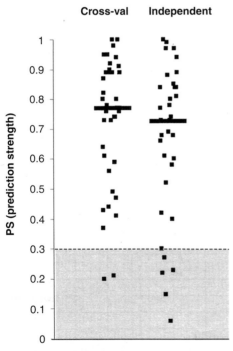

Fig. 11.6. Prediction strength (PS) in cross-validation and independent samples. The prediction of a new sample is based on "weighted votes" of a set of informative genes. Each such gene "votes" for either AML or ALL depending on whether the expression level is closer to the mean expression level of AMLs or ALLs. The votes are weighted depending on how well that given gene correlates to the class distinction, and summed up to establish "winning and losing classes." The prediction strength corresponds to the "margin of victory." As shown, the median prediction strengths for cross-validation and independent samples are quite comparable. (Reprinted with permission [2].)

The quality of microarray data is challenged

Several investigators challenged the reproducibility and data quality generated by microarrays [30–32]. Kuo *et al.* [31] compared mRNA measurements from two large-scale studies that measured gene expression in cancer cell lines. The two studies had in common data from 56 of the NCI-60 cancer cell lines, but were performed on different microarray platforms – the Stanford cDNA spotted array and Affymetrix oligonucleotide array. Overall, the inter-platform correlation was quite poor (Fig. 11.9), and led the authors to conclude that broad utilization of gene expression measurements across platforms had a "poor prognosis."

Other investigators challenged the methods of data analysis and therefore the statistical conclusions drawn from microarray data [33–37]. The risk of overfitting the data is a serious problem that is inherent in microarray analysis, yet not readily appreciated by those who wished to use microarray data in the clinical laboratory. With thousands of genes in a given microarray study, there are numerous ways to construct mathematical rules to perfectly discriminate different classes of tumors, as long as the number of genes is close to or greater than the sample size. To demonstrate how overfitting could lead to erroneous conclusions, Simon *et al.* randomly generated expression profiles comprised of 6000 genes for 20 virtual samples [37]. Ten "samples" were arbitrarily assigned to one group and the remaining 10 to another group. They then used the expression profiles of the 20 samples to create a gene signature for class prediction. Because there is no underlying difference between these two groups, class prediction should be similar to that from random guess, that is, 50% misclassification. However, when class prediction was performed back on the same 20 samples (i.e., no

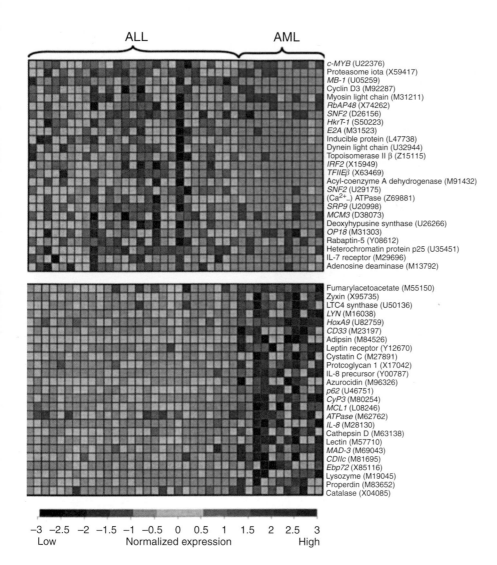

ALL AML

c-MYB (U22376)
Proteasome iota (X59417)
MB-1 (U05259)
Cyclin D3 (M92287)
Myosin light chain (M31211)
RbAP48 (X74262)
SNF2 (D26156)
HkrT-1 (S50223)
E2A (M31523)
Inducible protein (L47738)
Dynein light chain (U32944)
Topoisomerase II β (Z15115)
IRF2 (X15949)
TFIIEβ (X63469)
Acyl-coenzyme A dehydrogenase (M91432)
SNF2 (U29175)
(Ca²⁺₋) ATPase (Z69881)
SRP9 (U20998)
MCM3 (D38073)
Deoxyhypusine synthase (U26266)
OP18 (M31303)
Rabaptin-5 (Y08612)
Heterochromatin protein p25 (U35451)
IL-7 receptor (M29696)
Adenosine deaminase (M13792)

Fumarylacetoacetate (M55150)
Zyxin (X95735)
LTC4 synthase (U50136)
LYN (M16038)
HoxA9 (U82759)
CD33 (M23197)
Adipsin (M84526)
Leptin receptor (Y12670)
Cystatin C (M27891)
Protcoglycan 1 (X17042)
IL-8 precursor (Y00787)
Azurocidin (M96326)
p62 (U46751)
CyP3 (M80254)
MCL1 (L08246)
ATPase (M62762)
IL-8 (M28130)
Cathepsin D (M63138)
Lectin (M57710)
MAD-3 (M69043)
CDIIc (M81695)
Ebp72 (X85116)
Lysozyme (M19045)
Properdin (M83652)
Catalase (X04085)

-3 -2.5 -2 -1.5 -1 -0.5 0 0.5 1 1.5 2 2.5 3
Low   Normalized expression   High

Fig. 11.7. Genes distinguishing ALL from AML. The 50 genes most highly correlated with the ALL–AML class distinction are shown. Each row corresponds to a gene, with the columns corresponding to expression levels in different samples. Expression levels for each gene are normalized across the samples, such that the mean is 0 and the SD is 1. Expression levels greater than the mean are shaded in red, and those below the mean are shaded in blue. The scale indicates SDs above or below the mean. The top panel shows genes highly expressed in ALL, the bottom panel shows genes more highly expressed in AML. Although these genes, as a group, appear correlated with class, no single gene is uniformly expressed across the class, illustrating the value of a multigene prediction method. (Reprinted with permission [2].)

cross-validation), 98% of the models produced zero misclassification, demonstrating the risk of overfitting, especially when the number of test subjects remains very limited as compared to the number of genes used in the model. This result also points to the importance of validating the gene classifier on an independent data set. These two data sets are often referred to as a "training set" and a "validation set."

In 2005, Michiels et al. published an article in Lancet in which they reanalyzed data from seven of the largest published studies that had attempted to use gene expression microarray to predict prognosis of cancer patients [34]. They chose studies that included survival-related outcomes, had at least 60 patients, and had publicly available data. With this approach, they merged the published training and validation sets (N). The combined training–validation set (N) is divided into 500 training sets (n) with $n/2$ patients having each outcome (survived or died), and a corresponding validation set ($N - n$). They then identified a molecular signature for each training set, which was defined as the 50 genes for which expression was most highly

correlated with prognosis, as shown by the Pearson correlation coefficient. They used this signature to classify the validation set. Through this approach, they demonstrated that the resulting signatures were highly variable and strongly depended on the selection of patients in the training set. As can be seen in Figure 11.10, the mean and 95% confidence intervals for the proportion of misclassifications were not very impressive. Only two of the studies could be shown to have 95% confidence intervals below the 50% mark, indicating gene expression signatures that performed significantly better than chance, one of which was the St. Jude's pediatric leukemia study. These results led these investigators to conclude that the authors of these large studies were "over optimistic" in their accuracy estimates.

Standardization and technical improvements continue to evolve to address concerns

Several initiatives have been started, to standardize the approach to microarray studies and develop quality metrics

Diagnostic ALL BM samples (*n* = 327)

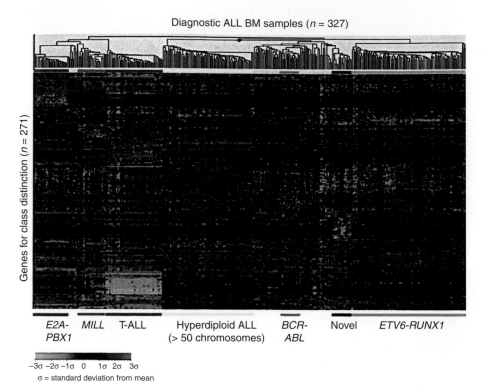

E2A-   MILL   T-ALL   Hyperdiploid ALL   BCR-   Novel   ETV6-RUNX1
PBX1   (> 50 chromosomes) ABL

−3σ −2σ −1σ 0 1σ 2σ 3σ
σ = standard deviation from mean

Fig. 11.8. Hierarchical clustering of 327 diagnostic ALL samples (columns) versus 271 genes (rows). The genes used in this analysis are the top 40 genes chosen by a chi-square statistic that are most highly correlated with the seven specific class distinctions. Nine genes were identified as useful in discriminating more than one class, but each is used only once in this analysis (thus the total is 271). The normalized expression value for each gene is indicated by a color, with red representing high expression and green representing low expression, with the scale shown at the lower left. (Reprinted with permission [28].)

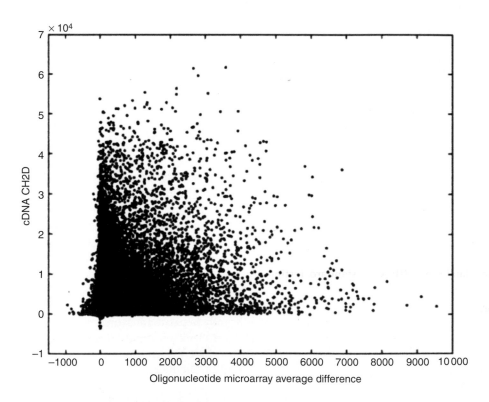

Fig. 11.9. Scatter plot of cDNA microarray and oligonucleotide microarray results for 162 120 pairs of matched measurements. As shown, the correlation was poor ($r = 0.328$). (Reprinted with permission [31].)

that will hopefully improve data quality and confidence in microarray experiments. The Microarray and Gene Expression Data (MGED) Society is an international organization of early adopters and microarray developers that was founded in 1999 to establish "standards for data quality, management, annotation and exchange" (www.mged.org, accessed December 4, 2009). In 2001, they published recommendations for standardizing the reporting of microarray experiments (called minimum information about a microarray experiment or MIAME), so that data can be easily interpreted and results can be independently

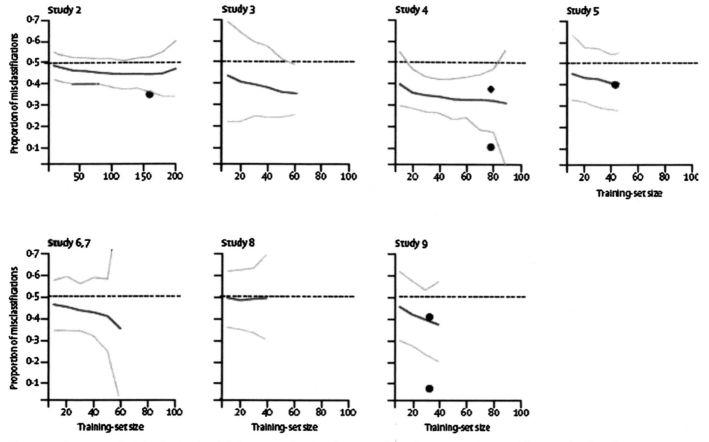

Fig. 11.10. Proportion of misclassifications in validation sets as a function of corresponding training-set sizes in seven different studies. Green lines = mean proportion of misclassifications obtained from 500 random training–validation sets as a function of the training-set size. Pale red lines = 95% confidence intervals. Dots = misclassification rates in original publications. Yeoh *et al.* correspond to study 3, and the measured outcome was relapse-free survival. (Reprinted with permission [34].)

verified [38]. MIAME is composed of six critical elements: experimental design, array design, samples, raw data, normalized data, and data processing information. Many journals now require submitting authors to meet the minimum information requirements of MIAME, and data are made publicly available at data repositories such as the European Bioinformatics Institute site, ArrayExpress (www.ebi.ac.uk/microarray-as/ae/, accessed December 4, 2009), the NCBI site GEO (www.ncbi.nlm.nih.gov/geo/, accessed December 4, 2009), and the Center for Information Biology Gene Expression Database, CIBEX (cibex.nig.ac.jp/index.jsp, accessed December 4, 2009). This initiative made the *Lancet* study, as well as others like it, possible.

In 2003, researchers involved in gene expression studies met at Stanford University to discuss the need for universal RNA standards. The attendees included more than 70 members from public, private, and academic sectors, and the meeting was sponsored by the US National Institute of Standards and Technology (NIST), Genomics Health, Inc., Affymetrix, Inc., and Agilent, Inc. They formed the External RNA Controls Consortium (ERCC), whose goal is to develop a set of external RNA control transcripts that could be spiked into gene expression assays to assess technical performance and compare

performance across platforms [39]. Since that time, the group has been actively collecting non-human and unique sequences for testing, performing preliminary testing and generating clones, and building consensus on testing protocols [40]. Towards this end, they have recently approved the Clinical and Laboratory Standards Institute (CLSI) document MM16p: *Use of External RNA Controls: Proposed Guideline*. Presently, the Test Plan has been proposed but not yet finalized, clone construction continues, and microarrays for external RNA standard testing are being designed. It should be noted that the consortium does not intend to market RNA standards but rather to develop ~100 well characterized non-mammalian sequences for which the performance criteria are established, with the expectation that the manufacturers will include these as part of the quality control of gene expression studies.

Realizing the need to increase collaboration in developing molecular signatures for cancer diagnosis and prognosis, in 2005 the National Cancer Institute (NCI) initiated a five-year program called Strategic Partnering to Evaluate Cancer Signatures (SPECS; www.cancerdiagnosis.nci.nih.gov/scientificPrograms/specs.htm, accessed June 28, 2010). This program is funding multi-institutional, multi-disciplinary teams investigating molecular signatures in breast cancer,

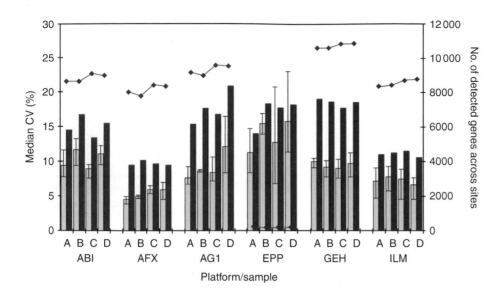

Fig. 11.11. Signal variation within and between test sites. For each of the four sample types, the replicate coefficient of variation (CV) of signal within a test site (blue bar) and the total CV of signal across and within sites (red bar) are presented. Genes detected in at least three of the replicates of a sample type at a single test site are included in the replicate CV calculation. Genes present in the intersection of these gene lists are included in the total CV calculation. The number of such genes within each platform and sample type is noted by blue dots connected by lines and is read on the secondary axis. Abbreviations: ABI, Applied Biosystems; AFX, Affymetrix; AG1, one-color microarray; EPP, Eppendorf; GEH, GE Healthcare; ILM, Illumina. (Reprinted with permission [41].)

prostate cancer, lung cancer, sarcoma, lymphoma, and leukemia. The goal of SPECS programs is to evaluate the potential clinical utility of molecular signatures correlated to recurrence, survival, and treatment response, and to develop robust, reproducible assays for the molecular signatures that can be incorporated into clinical validation trials. These teams utilize resources to obtain several hundred tumor samples from the Clinical Co-operative Groups, SPOREs (Specialized Programs of Research Excellence), Cancer Centers, NCI intramural, the National Laboratories, community hospitals, and individual academic institutions in the US and Europe. It is anticipated that refined molecular signatures may be identified by the end of the SPECS program. Of note, as genomic technology and our molecular knowledge of cancer advance, molecular signatures are not confined to the mRNA level. Indeed, the SPECS programs have used various high-throughput technologies to investigate variation in single nucleotide polymorphisms, DNA copy number, protein, and microRNA. However, large clinical trials will be needed before these molecular signatures become available in the clinical labs.

The Food and Drug Administration (FDA), recognizing the key role that microarray data would play in personalized medicine, spear-headed an ambitious project to provide quality control tools to the microarray developers and end users. This project is called the MicroArray Quality Control (MAQC) project, and involves six FDA Centers and many other private, public, and academic stakeholders, including the Environmental Protection Agency, the National Institute of Standards and Technology (NIST), major providers of microarray platforms and RNA controls, and academic laboratories (www.fda.gov/ScienceResearch/BioinformaticsTools/MicroarrayQualityControlProject/default.htm, accessed December 4, 2009).

The project has been divided into two main phases. The first phase was launched in February of 2005 and was focused on technical performance. For this phase, the objectives were to compare intra- and inter-laboratory variability across plat-

forms. The results of this phase were complete in June of 2006 and recently published [41]. For this first phase, the primary goal was to assess the imprecision of microarrays between runs, between laboratories and between platforms. A secondary goal was to assess accuracy by comparing gene call rate (i.e., proportion of genes that were detected) as well as fold change across microarray platforms and three alternative gene expression platforms (based on quantitative RT-PCR). To do this, four high-quality RNA samples were repeatedly tested on seven microarray platforms at multiple sites, and three RT-PCR platforms. The two RNA reference samples were a universal human reference RNA (UHRR) from Stratagene and a human brain reference RNA (HBRR) from Ambion. The four samples included the two reference samples and mixtures of these: Sample A, 100% UHRR; Sample B, 100% HBRR; Sample C, 75% UHRR and 25% HBRR; and Sample D, 25% UHRR and 75% HBRR. Importantly, these samples are commercially available and researchers can therefore use these as standards to assess the performance of their own experiments. Six commercially available microarray platforms were tested (Applied Biosystems, Affymetrix, Agilent Technologies, GE Healthcare, Illumina, and Eppendorf) as well as an NCI-developed spotted array using oligonucleotides obtained from Operon. The alternative gene expression platforms were TaqMan Gene Expression Assays from Applied Biosystems, StaRT-PCR from Gene Express, and QuantiGene assays from Panomics. Each RNA sample was tested five times at each of three sites (with the exception of the spotted microarray which was tested only at two sites).

As can be seen in Figure 11.11, the investigators were able to demonstrate a high intraplatform precision, both intra-site as well as intersite, for all samples. The intersite median of the coefficient of variance (CV) ranged from 10% to just over 20% across all platforms. In addition, the same genes were consistently detected (80–95% intrasite concordance and 70–85% intersite concordance, and ~74% across platforms).

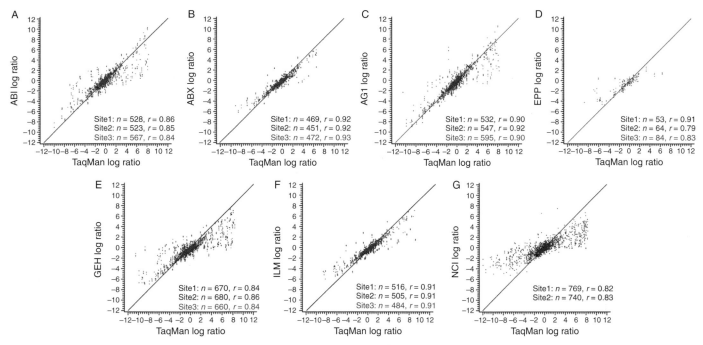

Fig. 11.12. Correlation between microarray and TaqMan data. The scatter plots compare the log ratio differential expression values (using A versus B replicates) from each microarray platform relative to values obtained by TaqMan assays. Each point represents a gene that was measured on both the microarray and TaqMan assays. The spot coloring indicates whether the data were generated in Test site 1 (black), Test site 2 (blue), or Test site 3 (red) for the microarray platform. Only genes that were generally detected in sample type A replicates and sample type B replicates were used in the comparisons. The exact number of probes analyzed for each test site and its correlation to TaqMan assays are listed in the bottom right corner of each plot. The line shown is the ideal 45° line. Abbreviations: ABI, Applied Biosystems; AFX, Affymetrix; AG1, one-color microarray; EPP, Eppendorf; GEH, GE Healthcare; ILM, Illumina; NCI, NCI Operon. (Reprinted with permission [41].)

The investigators were also able to demonstrate an impressive correlation as compared to the alternative gene expression platforms. As can be seen in Figure 11.12, when the log differential expression values of sample A versus sample B were plotted on a scatter plot of microarray versus TaqMan Gene Expression Assay, the calculated correlation coefficients (r) were quite impressive.

The MAQC investigators concluded that microarray results were repeatable within a test site and reproducible between test sites, and despite unique probes and protocols, comparable across platforms. They further suggest that discordance in detection across platforms may be partially attributable to alternative splicing and probe design, and if the biologic pathway rather than the specific gene target were considered, the concordance rate may be higher. They also emphasize that the overreliance on the statistical significance (P value) rather than the actual measured quantity of differential expression (fold change or ratio) could result in increased discordance between platforms, and suggest that this may be an important factor in previous studies that demonstrated high discordance between platforms. It should be noted that several other analyses used the MAQC-I data to generate quality control metrics. The microarray performance characteristics were compared to the alternative gene expression methods [42], the RNA titrations were used to assess the effects of normalization [43], studies using one-color and two-color gene expression microarrays were compared on the same platform [44], and spiked RNA controls were used to assess microarray performance [45]. This last analysis complements the efforts of the ERCC by providing valuable performance data from the different protocols used by Affymetrix, Agilent Technologies, and GE Healthcare. By September of 2006, Phase II of the MAQC project (MAQC-II) was launched. The aim of MAQC-II is to reach consensus on "best practices" for "real-life applications" for developing and validating predictive models based on microarray data. To achieve this aim, multiple data sets have been collected and distributed to participating organizations for independent analyses with available algorithms [46]. Thirty-six teams developed classifiers from six large training data sets, which were subsequently challenged by independent and blinded validation sets generated for MAQC-II. The performance and reproducibility of the various data analysis methods looks promising and, to date, over 10 manuscripts from the MAQC-II have been submitted to *Nature Biotechnology* for peer review (www.fda.gov/ScienceResearch/BioinformaticsTools/MicroarrayQualityControlProject/, accessed December 4, 2009).

The exploration of the potential of gene expression profiling microarray has been, and remains, a dynamic process. Seemingly small differences in samples, RNA preparation, microarray design, and data analysis can have big differences in results. This has posed a problem for those who wished to compare independent microarray studies, as the techniques, technology, and targets have continued to evolve. For this reason, the MAQC project is truly a landmark study that was

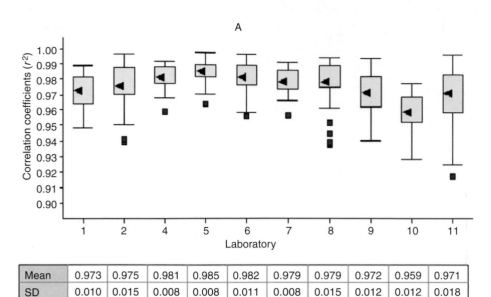

A

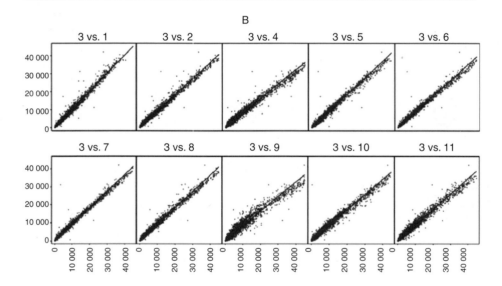

Mean	0.973	0.975	0.981	0.985	0.982	0.979	0.979	0.972	0.959	0.971
SD	0.010	0.015	0.008	0.008	0.011	0.008	0.015	0.012	0.012	0.018
Count	36	36	36	36	36	36	36	72	36	96

B

Fig. 11.13. (A) Box-and-whisker plots display the inter-laboratory squared correlation coefficients (r^2) of all probe sets represented on the HG-U133 Plus 2.0 microarray for the HepG2 cell line sample. Microarray data from Centre 3 are compared with all other laboratories. Each inter-laboratory analysis with different pairwise comparisons is represented by a single box plot (Count). Mean r^2 values (black arrow) and standard deviation (SD) values are given for each series of comparisons. Outliers are represented as red boxes. (B) Scatter plot analysis of inter-laboratory reproducibility. The graph shows 10 distinct scatter plot analyses, each displaying a comparison between Centre 3 and the other laboratories for the 5.0 μg HepG2 sample run at the stage of proficiency testing. (Reprinted with permission [47].)

critically important to demonstrate reproducibility across platforms and institutions. Only after data can be shown to be reproducible can clinical utility be assessed. The MAQC study has provided a wealth of data and information to the microarray community, and promises to bring the power of gene expression microarray from the research laboratory to the clinical laboratory. Importantly, this project has been received enthusiastically by the microarray community, in large part because it is an FDA-driven initiative. Indeed, since the FDA has identified microarrays as a core technology for the advancement of personalized medicine through its Critical Path Initiative (www.fda.gov/oc/initiatives/criticalpath/, accessed December 4, 2009), its support for the clinical utility of microarrays is evident, and this opens the door for microarray developers.

International studies demonstrating the clinical utility of microarray

Starting in 2005, the Microarray Innovations in LEukemia (MILE) study was begun, to assess the clinical utility of gene expression microarray for classifying acute and chronic leukemias as well as myelodysplastic syndromes (MDS). This study was organized around the European Leukemia Network, included 11 centers (7 in Europe, 3 in the USA, and 1 in Singapore), and was sponsored by Roche Molecular Systems, Inc. The study began with an initial 'prephase', intended to standardize process and ensure reproducibility across centers [47]. These investigators noted the importance of standardized RNA labeling protocols, with which they were able to demonstrate excellent intersite reproducibility (Fig. 11.13).

After the initial "prephase," the centers began the first of two phases for the MILE study [48]. The first phase was designed to identify gene expression profiles for acute and chronic leukemias as well as myelodysplastic syndromes. A total of 2143 adult and pediatric samples were collected, tested with the Affymetrix HG-U133 Plus 2.0 microarrays, and retrospectively compared to conventional diagnostic assays. Only 47 (2.1%) analyses failed technical quality criteria. Of the remaining 2096, the overall concordance rate was 92.1% when compared to the conventional diagnostic assays. Concordance was better with pro-B-ALL with t(11q23)/*MLL*, c-ALL (common ALL)/pre-B-ALL with t(9;22), T-ALL, ALL with t(12;21), AML with t(8;21), AML with t(15;17), AML with inv(16)/t(16;16), CLL, and CML, and worse with ALL with hyperdiploid karyotype, c-ALL/pre-B-ALL without specific genetic abnormalities, AML with complex aberrant karyotype, and MDS. The lower concordances for these subclasses were attributed to the biological heterogeneity and lack of a standardized "gold standard."

The second phase of the MILE study involved a prospective, blinded validation using a customized microarray with probe sets for 1480 genes. A total of 1156 samples were tested, and a focused classification algorithm was used to classify the acute leukemias [mature B-ALL with t(8;14), pro-B-ALL with t(11q23)/*MLL*, c-ALL/pre-B-ALL with t(9;22), T-ALL, ALL with t(12;21), ALL with t(1;19), ALL with hyperdiploid karyotype, c-ALL/pre-B-ALL without specific genetic abnormalities, AML with t(8;21), AML with t(15;17), AML with inv(16)/t(16;16), AML with t(11q23)/*MLL*, AML with normal karyotype or other abnormalities, and AML with complex aberrant karyotype]. A total of 696 acute leukemia samples were tested; the median sensitivity for this independent group was 95.5% and the median specificity was 99.5%. Once again, lower accuracy was noted for ALL with hyperdiploid karyotype, c-ALL/pre-B-ALL without specific genetic abnormalities, AML with t(11q23)/*MLL*, and AML with complex aberrant karyotype. However, it was noted that during the process of discrepancy resolution, 52 cases (7.5%) were correctly classified by microarray and were "missed" due to clerical error ($n = 12$) or initial misdiagnoses by the conventional methods ($n = 40$). It was also noted that the concordances for CLL, CML and MDS were 99.2%, 95.2%, and 81.5%, respectively. Interestingly, further analysis of discordant results led to the development of a prognostic classification model [49].

These impressive results led these investigators to conclude that gene expression profiling using standardized methods may improve the accuracy of conventional diagnostic algorithms and therefore serve to complement these methods. They also suggest that gene expression profiling may offer a reliable diagnostic/prognostic tool for many patients who do not have access to the "gold standard" conventional diagnostic methods.

The MILE study convincingly demonstrated that gene expression profiling can be used to classify acute leukemias, and even presents evidence that it may be better than the conventional diagnostic methods. Indeed, almost 6% of the total diagnostic samples were misclassified by conventional diagnostic methods and reassigned after gene expression profiling. Given these impressive results and the backing of Roche Diagnostic Systems, Inc., this method will likely be submitted to the FDA for approval and would probably get approval rather quickly. Indeed, other gene expression microarray tests have already been FDA cleared. Pathwork Diagnostics has recently obtained FDA clearance for its Tissue of Origin Test™. This test requires clinical laboratories to extract RNA, amplify and label, and hybridize to a microarray of >1500 genes. Data are then sent to the company for analysis. Agendia also has a microarray-based gene expression analysis test (MammaPrint™) that has recently been cleared by the FDA. Their 70-gene microarray panel gives a risk assessment of distant metastasis for breast cancer patients. Also, some multiplex quantitative RT-PCR assays (such as Oncotype DX™ and Allomap™) grew out of microarray gene expression studies and have been FDA cleared.

Still, if and when the MILE study assay is FDA cleared, most clinical laboratories that already have conventional diagnostic methods will not likely switch platforms for a gene expression array test that adds little more. For laboratories to adopt this technology to complement already validated diagnostic methods, or replace these methods, gene expression profiling will have to also provide additional prognostic information that is not otherwise available. This is especially important as the list of prognostically relevant recurrent genetic mutations in acute leukemias continues to increase. Recent evidence suggests that gene expression arrays will be able to provide such information and in a manner that is less labor intensive than the alternatives presently available using conventional diagnostic methods together with gene sequencing, methylation studies, and so on [50–53]. Prospective, randomized studies will hopefully validate the gene expression approach for molecular subclassification of these recurrent genetic mutations.

Gene expression microarray in the era of personalized medicine

The term "personalized medicine" is overused and misunderstood. It implies that each individual's therapy would be specific and based on genomic and proteomic data from that person as well as his or her tumor. However, unless subjects can serve as their own control, "personalized medicine" is incompatible with evidence-based laboratory medicine, and therefore the goal really is to better refine or target therapy. Although some see gene expression profiling by microarray as the bridge to targeted therapy, others may effectively argue that targeted therapy is a journey and not a destination. After all, conventional diagnostic methods classify leukemias into low-, intermediate-, and high-risk categories that will determine therapy. Gene expression profiling has the potential to further refine these classifications and therefore further refine therapy. But just as targeted therapy doesn't begin with gene expression profiling, it won't end with it either. Already there is a wealth of data supporting other targets and techniques for refining the classification of leukemias. Gene mutations in several genes, as well as promoter hypermethylation of cancer-related genes, have been shown to be independently prognostic, alone or in combination [54–57]. Indeed, recently whole genome sequencing of a cytologically normal acute myeloid leukemia was performed, and may represent the next phase of high-throughput genetic testing [58]. Using this approach, 10 tumor-specific mutations have been identified including *NPM1* and *FLT3*, but also 8 novel mutations (*CDHL4*, *PCLKC*, *GPR123*, *EBI2*, *PTPRT*, *KNDC1*, *SLC15A1*, and *GRINL1B*). Recent evidence also shows possible prognostic significance of gene copy-number variation, uniparental disomy, and single nucleotide polymorphisms [59–62]. As single nucleotide polymorphism arrays become more widely available in clinical laboratories, these targets become more attractive. Also, expression profiling of microRNA has produced some very exciting data and protocols that can readily be adapted for the clinical laboratory [63–65]. Other targets and techniques, such as proteomic analysis, promise to offer another dimension of high-throughput analyses [66]. It is likely that the interaction of transcriptomics, genomics, epigenomics, and proteomics will be highly interdependent. As the ever-increasing complexity is elucidated, the most reproducible and predictive biomarkers should emerge.

Summary

Like most new technologies, the potential of microarray technology generated tremendous excitement from the start. When applied to pediatric leukemias, early studies showed gene expression profiling in many ways to be better than the conventional methods of morphology, flow cytometry, and cytogenetics. In addition to classifying and subclassifying pediatric leukemias as well as, or better than, conventional methods, they promised to identify subgroups at risk of recurrence or secondary leukemias. However, the initial excitement has been tempered by several investigators demonstrating a lack of reproducibility and questioning the conclusions of these early studies. Nevertheless, recent efforts to demonstrate reproducibility have been quite encouraging and presently investigators are able to move to the next phase of defining and validating expression profiles. One international study has even presented prospective data that demonstrate impressive accuracy for classifying acute leukemias. However, the potential to provide additional prognostic information is yet to be proven in a prospective, randomized trial. Some may argue that gene expression profiling has therefore fallen short of expectations, but it is the expectations that historically are inappropriate. Indeed, some may remember that carcinoembryonic antigen (CEA) was initially claimed to be nearly 100% sensitive and specific for colorectal cancer screening [67]. Although subsequent studies identified sources of bias and over optimism [68, 69], CEA nevertheless became a clinically useful marker of colorectal cancer recurrence. Likewise, gene expression profiling by microarray will provide useful diagnostic and perhaps prognostic information in pediatric leukemias. However, it will likely represent only part of the high-throughput genomic and proteomic profiling contributing to the evolution of targeted therapy.

References

1. **Schena M, Shalon D, Davis RW, Brown PO**. Quantitative monitoring of gene expression patterns with a complementary DNA microarray. *Science*. 1995;**270**:467–470.

2. **Golub TR, Slonim DK, Tamayo P**, *et al*. Molecular classification of cancer: class discovery and class prediction by gene expression monitoring. *Science*. 1999;**286**:531–537.

3. **Kafatos FC, Jones CW, Efstratiadis A.** Determination of nucleic acid sequence homologies and relative concentrations by a dot hybridization procedure. *Nucleic Acids Research*. 1979;7:1541–1552.

4. **Fodor SP, Read JL, Pirrung MC**, *et al*. Light-directed, spatially addressable parallel chemical synthesis. *Science*. 1991;**251**:767–773.

5. **Fodor SP, Rava RP, Huang XC**, *et al*. Multiplexed biochemical assays with biological chips. *Nature*. 1993;**364**:555–556.

6. **Brown PO, Botstein D**. Exploring the new world of the genome with DNA microarrays. *Nature Genetics*. 1999;**21**:33–37.

7. **Andersson A, Olofsson T, Lindgren D**, *et al*. Molecular signatures in childhood acute leukemia and their correlations to expression patterns in normal hematopoietic subpopulations. *Proceedings of the National Academy of Sciences of the United States of America*. 2005;**102**:19069–19074.

8. **Andersson A, Ritz C, Lindgren D**, *et al*. Microarray-based classification of a consecutive series of 121 childhood acute leukemias: prediction of leukemic and genetic subtype as well as of minimal residual disease status. *Leukemia*. 2007;**21**:1198–1203.

9. **Armstrong SA, Staunton JE, Silverman LB**, *et al*. MLL translocations specify a distinct gene expression profile that distinguishes a unique leukemia. *Nature Genetics*. 2002;**30**:41–47.

10. **Cario G, Stanulla M, Fine BM**, *et al*. Distinct gene expression profiles determine molecular treatment response in childhood acute lymphoblastic leukemia. *Blood*. 2005;**105**:821–826.

11. **den Boer ML, Pieters R**. Microarray-based identification of new targets for specific therapies in pediatric leukemia. *Current Drug Targets*. 2007;**8**:761–764.

12. **Edick MJ, Cheng C, Yang W**, *et al*. Lymphoid gene expression as a predictor of risk of secondary brain tumors. *Genes, Chromosomes and Cancer*. 2005;**42**:107–116.

13. **Ferrando AA, Neuberg DS, Staunton J**, *et al*. Gene expression signatures define novel oncogenic pathways in T cell acute lymphoblastic leukemia. *Cancer Cell*. 2002;**1**:75–87.

14. **Flotho C, Coustan-Smith E, Pei D**, *et al*. Genes contributing to minimal residual disease in childhood acute lymphoblastic leukemia: prognostic

significance of CASP8AP2. *Blood.* 2006;**108**:1050–1057.

15. **Holleman A, Cheok MH, den Boer ML**, *et al.* Gene-expression patterns in drug-resistant acute lymphoblastic leukemia cells and response to treatment. *New England Journal of Medicine.* 2004;**351**:533–542.

16. **Lacayo NJ, Meshinchi S, Kinnunen P**, *et al.* Gene expression profiles at diagnosis in de novo childhood AML patients identify FLT3 mutations with good clinical outcomes. *Blood.* 2004; **104**:2646–2654.

17. **Lugthart S, Cheok MH, den Boer ML**, *et al.* Identification of genes associated with chemotherapy crossresistance and treatment response in childhood acute lymphoblastic leukemia. *Cancer Cell.* 2005;**7**:375–386.

18. **McElwaine S, Mulligan C, Groet J**, *et al.* Microarray transcript profiling distinguishes the transient from the acute type of megakaryoblastic leukaemia (M7) in Down's syndrome, revealing PRAME as a specific discriminating marker. *British Journal of Haematology.* 2004;**125**:729–742.

19. **Moos PJ, Raetz EA, Carlson MA**, *et al.* Identification of gene expression profiles that segregate patients with childhood leukemia. *Clinical Cancer Research.* 2002;**8**:3118–3130.

20. **Raetz EA, Perkins SL, Bhojwani D**, *et al.* Gene expression profiling reveals intrinsic differences between T-cell acute lymphoblastic leukemia and T-cell lymphoblastic lymphoma. *Pediatric Blood and Cancer.* 2006;**47**: 130–140.

21. **Roela RA, Carraro DM, Brentani HP**, *et al.* Gene stage-specific expression in the microenvironment of pediatric myelodysplastic syndromes. *Leukemia Research.* 2007;**31**:579–589.

22. **Ross ME, Zhou X, Song G**, *et al.* Classification of pediatric acute lymphoblastic leukemia by gene expression profiling. *Blood.* 2003;**102**: 2951–2959.

23. **Steinbach D, Gillet JP, Sauerbrey A**, *et al.* ABCA3 as a possible cause of drug resistance in childhood acute myeloid leukemia. *Clinical Cancer Research.* 2006;**12**:4357–4363.

24. **Stirewalt DL, Meshinchi S, Kopecky KJ**, *et al.* Identification of genes with abnormal expression changes in acute myeloid leukemia. *Genes, Chromosomes and Cancer.* 2008;**47**:8–20.

25. **Tsutsumi S, Taketani T, Nishimura K**, *et al.* Two distinct gene expression signatures in pediatric acute lymphoblastic leukemia with MLL rearrangements. *Cancer Research.* 2003;**63**:4882–4887.

26. **van Delft FW, Bellotti T, Luo Z**, *et al.* Prospective gene expression analysis accurately subtypes acute leukaemia in children and establishes a commonality between hyperdiploidy and t(12;21) in acute lymphoblastic leukaemia. *British Journal of Haematology.* 2005;**130**:26–35.

27. **Willenbrock H, Juncker AS, Schmiegelow K, Knudsen S, Ryder LP**. Prediction of immunophenotype, treatment response, and relapse in childhood acute lymphoblastic leukemia using DNA microarrays. *Leukemia.* 2004;**18**:1270–1277.

28. **Yeoh EJ, Ross ME, Shurtleff SA**, *et al.* Classification, subtype discovery, and prediction of outcome in pediatric acute lymphoblastic leukemia by gene expression profiling. *Cancer Cell.* 2002; **1**:133–143.

29. **Ross ME, Mahfouz R, Onciu M**, *et al.* Gene expression profiling of pediatric acute myelogenous leukemia. *Blood.* 2004;**104**:3679–3687.

30. **Kothapalli R, Yoder SJ, Mane S, Loughran TP Jr**. Microarray results: how accurate are they? *BMC Bioinformatics.* 2002;**3**:22.

31. **Kuo WP, Jenssen TK, Butte AJ, Ohno-Machado L, Kohane IS**. Analysis of matched mRNA measurements from two different microarray technologies. *Bioinformatics.* 2002;**18**:405–412.

32. **Tan PK, Downey TJ, Spitznagel EL Jr.**, *et al.* Evaluation of gene expression measurements from commercial microarray platforms. *Nucleic Acids Research.* 2003;**31**:5676–5684.

33. **Abdullah-Sayani A, Bueno-de-Mesquita JM, van de Vijver MJ**. Technology insight: tuning into the genetic orchestra using microarrays – limitations of DNA microarrays in clinical practice. *Nature Clinical Practice: Oncology.* 2006;**3**:501–516.

34. **Michiels S, Koscielny S, Hill C**. Prediction of cancer outcome with microarrays: a multiple random validation strategy. *Lancet.* 2005;**365**: 488–492.

35. **Ransohoff DF**. Rules of evidence for cancer molecular-marker discovery and validation. *Nature Reviews: Cancer.* 2004;**4**:309–314.

36. **Ambroise C, McLachlan GJ**. Selection bias in gene extraction on the basis of microarray gene-expression data. *Proceedings of the National Academy of Sciences of the United States of America.* 2002;**99**:6562–6566.

37. **Simon R, Radmacher MD, Dobbin K, McShane LM**. Pitfalls in the use of DNA microarray data for diagnostic and prognostic classification. *Journal of the National Cancer Institute.* 2003;**95**:14–18.

38. **Brazma A, Hingamp P, Quackenbush J**, *et al.* Minimum information about a microarray experiment (MIAME) – toward standards for microarray data. *Nature Genetics.* 2001;**29**:365–371.

39. **Cronin M, Ghosh K, Sistare F**, *et al.* Universal RNA reference materials for gene expression. *Clinical Chemistry.* 2004;**50**:1464–1471.

40. **Baker SC, Bauer SR, Beyer RP**, *et al.* The External RNA Controls Consortium: a progress report. *Nature Methods.* 2005;**2**:731–734.

41. **Shi L, Reid LH, Jones WD**, *et al.* The MicroArray Quality Control (MAQC) project shows inter- and intraplatform reproducibility of gene expression measurements. *Nature Biotechnology.* 2006;**24**:1151–1161.

42. **Canales RD, Luo Y, Willey JC**, *et al.* Evaluation of DNA microarray results with quantitative gene expression platforms. *Nature Biotechnology.* 2006;**24**:1115–1122.

43. **Shippy R, Fulmer-Smentek S, Jensen RV**, *et al.* Using RNA sample titrations to assess microarray platform performance and normalization techniques. *Nature Biotechnology.* 2006;**24**:1123–1131.

44. **Patterson TA, Lobenhofer EK, Fulmer-Smentek SB**, *et al.* Performance comparison of one-color and two-color platforms within the MicroArray Quality Control (MAQC) project. *Nature Biotechnology.* 2006;**24**: 1140–1150.

45. **Tong W, Lucas AB, Shippy R**, *et al.* Evaluation of external RNA controls for the assessment of microarray performance. *Nature Biotechnology.* 2006;**24**:1132–1139.

46. **Shi L, Perkins RG, Fang H, Tong W.** Reproducible and reliable microarray results through quality control: good laboratory proficiency and appropriate data analysis practices are essential. *Current Opinion in Biotechnology.* 2008;**19**:10–18.

47. **Kohlmann A, Kipps TJ, Rassenti LZ,** *et al.* An international standardization programme towards the application of gene expression profiling in routine leukaemia diagnostics: the Microarray Innovations in LEukemia study prephase. *British Journal of Haematology.* 2008;**142**: 802–807.

48. **Haferlach T, Kohlmann A, Basso G,** *et al.* The clinical utility of microarray-based gene expression profiling in the diagnosis and subclassification of leukemia: final report on 3252 cases from the International MILE Study Group. *Blood (ASH Annual Meeting Abstracts).* 2008;**112**:753.

49. **Mills KI, Kohlmann A, Williams PM,** *et al.* Microarray-based classifiers and prognosis models identify subgroups with distinct clinical outcomes and high risk of AML transformation of myelodysplastic syndrome. *Blood.* 2009;**114**:1063–1072.

50. **Bullinger L, Dohner K, Bair E,** *et al.* Use of gene-expression profiling to identify prognostic subclasses in adult acute myeloid leukemia. *New England Journal of Medicine.* 2004;**350**:1605–1616.

51. **Metzeler KH, Hummel M, Bloomfield CD,** *et al.* An 86-probe-set gene-expression signature predicts survival in cytogenetically normal acute myeloid leukemia. *Blood.* 2008;**112**: 4193–4201.

52. **Radmacher MD, Marcucci G, Ruppert AS,** *et al.* Independent confirmation of a prognostic gene-expression signature in adult acute myeloid leukemia with a normal karyotype: a Cancer and Leukemia Group B study. *Blood.* 2006; **108**:1677–1683.

53. **Wouters BJ, Jorda MA, Keeshan K,** *et al.* Distinct gene expression profiles of acute myeloid/T-lymphoid leukemia with silenced CEBPA and mutations in NOTCH1. *Blood.* 2007;**110**:3706–3714.

54. **Cotta CV, Tubbs RR.** Mutations in myeloid neoplasms. *Diagnostic Molecular Pathology.* 2008;**17**:191–199.

55. **Roman-Gomez J, Jimenez-Velasco A, Barrios M,** *et al.* Poor prognosis in acute lymphoblastic leukemia may relate to promoter hypermethylation of cancer-related genes. *Leukemia & Lymphoma.* 2007;**48**:1269–1282.

56. **Ferrara F, Palmieri S, Leoni F.** Clinically useful prognostic factors in acute myeloid leukemia. *Critical Reviews in Oncology/Hematology.* 2008;**66**:181–193.

57. **Gaidzik V, Dohner K.** Prognostic implications of gene mutations in acute myeloid leukemia with normal cytogenetics. *Seminars in Oncology.* 2008;**35**:346–355.

58. **Ley TJ, Mardis ER, Ding L,** *et al.* DNA sequencing of a cytogenetically normal acute myeloid leukaemia genome. *Nature.* 2008;**456**:66–72.

59. **Mullighan CG, Su X, Zhang J,** *et al.* Deletion of IKZF1 and prognosis in acute lymphoblastic leukemia. *New England Journal of Medicine.* 2009;**360**: 470–480.

60. **Serrano E, Carnicer MJ, Orantes V,** *et al.* Uniparental disomy may be associated with microsatellite instability in acute myeloid leukemia (AML) with a normal karyotype. *Leukemia & Lymphoma.* 2008;**49**:1178–1183.

61. **Pietrzyk JJ, Bik-Multanowski M, Balwierz W,** *et al.* Additional genetic risk factor for death in children with acute lymphoblastic leukemia: a common polymorphism of the MTHFR gene. *Pediatric Blood and Cancer.* 2009; **52**:364–368.

62. **Yang JJ, Cheng C, Yang W,** *et al.* Genome-wide interrogation of germline genetic variation associated with treatment response in childhood acute lymphoblastic leukemia. *JAMA.* 2009;**301**:393–403.

63. **Marcucci G, Maharry K, Radmacher MD,** *et al.* Prognostic significance of, and gene and microRNA expression signatures associated with, CEBPA mutations in cytogenetically normal acute myeloid leukemia with high-risk molecular features: a Cancer and Leukemia Group B Study. *Journal of Clinical Oncology.* 2008;**26**:5078–5087.

64. **Marcucci G, Radmacher MD, Maharry K,** *et al.* MicroRNA expression in cytogenetically normal acute myeloid leukemia. *New England Journal of Medicine.* 2008;**358**:1919–1928.

65. **Mi S, Lu J, Sun M,** *et al.* MicroRNA expression signatures accurately discriminate acute lymphoblastic leukemia from acute myeloid leukemia. *Proceedings of the National Academy of Sciences of the United States of America.* 2007;**104**:19971–19976.

66. **Kornblau SM, Tibes R, Qiu YH,** *et al.* Functional proteomic profiling of AML predicts response and survival. *Blood.* 2009;**113**:154–164.

67. **Thomson DM, Krupey J, Freedman SO, Gold P.** The radioimmunoassay of circulating carcinoembryonic antigen of the human digestive system. *Proceedings of the National Academy of Sciences of the United States of America.* 1969;**64**:161–167.

68. **Ransohoff DF, Feinstein AR.** Problems of spectrum and bias in evaluating the efficacy of diagnostic tests. *New England Journal of Medicine.* 1978;**299**: 926–930.

69. **Sackett DL.** Zlinkoff honor lecture: basic research, clinical research, clinical epidemiology, and general internal medicine. *Journal of General Internal Medicine.* 1987;**2**:40–47.

Myeloproliferative neoplasms

Robert B. Lorsbach

Introduction

Although hematologic malignancies are collectively the most common neoplasms of childhood, comprising approximately one-fourth to one-third of all cases of pediatric cancer in the USA, the myeloproliferative neoplasms, formerly termed chronic myeloproliferative disorders, are distinctly rare in the pediatric setting [1, 2]. Among the seven entities recognized by the 2008 WHO classification of myeloproliferative neoplasms (Table 12.1), chronic myelogenous leukemia and mastocytosis are the only ones encountered with any regularity in the pediatric population. Primary myelofibrosis, polycythemia vera, and essential thrombocythemia are very uncommon in children, and chronic neutrophilic leukemia and chronic eosinophilic leukemia are extraordinarily rare in this population, the description of which is limited to an occasional case report [3]. Several pediatric "myeloproliferative" disorders are not truly neoplastic, and as such they have a pathogenesis distinct from their bona fide neoplastic counterparts in adults. The application to these pediatric disorders of the same terminology employed for adult myeloproliferative neoplasms, which are by definition clonal and neoplastic, creates confusion with regard to their pathogenesis, clinical behavior, and appropriate treatment. Our discussion of pediatric myeloproliferative neoplasms will focus almost exclusively on those disorders seen in children, with emphasis on the distinctive aspects of the pediatric forms of these disorders, as well as conditions which can mimic true pediatric myeloproliferative neoplasms. Myeloproliferative neoplasms which are exceedingly rare in children (e.g., chronic neutrophilic leukemia) will not be discussed.

Chronic myelogenous leukemia

The first complete description of chronic myelogenous leukemia (CML) is generally attributed to John Hughes Bennett, who in 1845 published the autopsy findings from a patient with CML in a report evocatively entitled "Case of hypertrophy of the spleen and liver in which death took place from suppuration of the blood" [4]. Since that time, CML has been one of the most intensely studied neoplastic disorders,

the investigation of which has yielded a number of "firsts" in oncologic research. Chronic myeloid leukemia was the first human malignancy in which a specific, recurrent genetic lesion was identified. In 1960, Peter Nowell of the University of Pennsylvania and David Hungerford of the Institute for Cancer Research observed the consistent presence of an abnormally small chromosome in the leukocytes of seven patients with CML, which was subsequently designated the "Philadelphia chromosome" [5]. In 1973, Janet Rowley of the University of Chicago reported that the Philadelphia chromosome was generated through a previously unrecognized process of chromosomal translocation in which a reciprocal exchange of genetic material between chromosomes 9 and 22 had occurred [6]. This genetic event was subsequently shown to result in the juxtaposition of the BCR and ABL genes, yielding expression of the BCR–ABL fusion oncoprotein [7, 8]. BCR–ABL has tyrosine kinase activity and is now known to play a central pathogenetic role in CML. In the absence of any highly effective chemotherapeutic treatment, allogeneic hematopoietic stem cell transplantation was for many years the only curative intervention for patients with CML. However, the introduction of imatinib, an effective and specific inhibitor of BCR–ABL, has revolutionized the treatment of CML and has confirmed the feasibility and effectiveness of molecularly targeted therapy for this disease [9].

Pathogenesis

Before discussing the pathogenetic role of BCR–ABL in CML, it is helpful to review the normal biologic role of each of the partner proteins of this fusion protein. ABL is a widely expressed, 145 kDa protein with tyrosine kinase activity. ABL localizes to both the nucleus and cytoplasm, where it regulates several divergent cellular processes, including proliferation, cell survival, adhesion, and motility. In response to DNA damage, ABL translocates to the nucleus where, together with p53, it induces apoptosis. In the cytoplasm, ABL plays a key role in the transduction to the cytoskeleton of extracellular signals from certain cell-surface proteins, such as the integrins [10, 11]. Mice deficient in ABL die soon after birth and manifest runting and

Diagnostic Pediatric Hematopathology, ed. Maria A. Proytcheva. Published by Cambridge University Press.
© Cambridge University Press 2011.

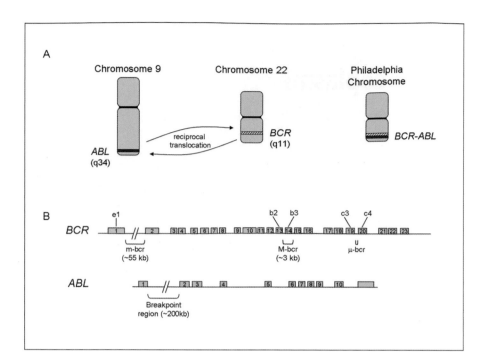

Fig. 12.1. Pathogenesis of chronic myelogenous leukemia. (A) Formation of the Philadelphia chromosome as a result of the t(9;22)(q34;q11) rearrangement is the central molecular event in CML, and results in the juxtaposition of the loci for *BCR* and *ABL*. (B) The chromosomal breakpoints in the *ABL* gene occur within the 200 kb of intronic sequence between exons 1 and 2. There is more variability in the *BCR* breakpoint. In most cases of CML, the breakpoint occurs in the so-called major breakpoint region (M-bcr), whereas it occurs in the minor breakpoint region (m-bcr) in most cases of ALLs harboring the Philadelphia chromosome.

Table 12.1. WHO classification of myeloproliferative neoplasms.

Chronic myelogenous leukemia, BCR-ABL positive
Chronic neutrophilic leukemia
Polycythemia vera
Primary myelofibrosis
Essential thrombocythemia
Chronic eosinophilic leukemia, not otherwise specified
Mastocytosis
Myeloproliferative neoplasm, unclassifiable

defective lymphoid development, particularly in B-cells [12, 13]. The latter is likely attributable to multiple mechanisms including enhanced sensitivity to proapoptotic conditions, and diminished signaling downstream of the B-cell receptor complex and other critical cell-surface molecules that regulate proliferation in B-cells [14, 15].

Surprisingly, given the intense investigation of BCR-ABL, relatively little is known about the biologic function of BCR. BCR has a GTPase activating domain, and in immune cells appears to negatively regulate the function of the Rac proteins, which have an important role in signaling to the cytoskeleton. While born at the expected frequency and phenotypically normal, BCR-deficient mice are significantly more sensitive to endotoxin challenge than their wild-type littermates, an effect that is apparently due to markedly enhanced generation of neutrophil-derived reactive oxygen intermediates secondary to defective regulation of NADPH oxidase. The relatively subtle phenotypic findings in BCR-deficient animals may be due to compensation by a related protein, ABR. Like BCR, ABR-deficient mice are phenotypically normal; however, mice defi-

cient in both proteins show inner ear defects, abnormalities in cerebellar development, and manifest severe inflammatory responses upon administration of endotoxin [16].

The pivotal pathogenetic event in CML is the occurrence of the t(9;22) within a multipotential hematopoietic stem cell (HSC) [17–19]. Mice transplanted with HSCs expressing BCR-ABL develop a myeloproliferative disorder closely resembling its counterpart in humans, indicating that expression of BCR-ABL is necessary and sufficient for development of chronic-phase CML. As alluded to above, this translocation results in the juxtaposition of the *BCR* and *ABL* genes, yielding the BCR-ABL fusion protein (Fig. 12.1) [7, 8]. The molecular details of BCR-ABL recombination have been recently reviewed [20, 21]. The chromosomal breakpoint in *ABL* occurs within a confined region of the gene, primarily within the intron preceding exon 2 (a2). There is more variability in the breakpoints within *BCR*, with most of them occurring in three regions of the gene. In nearly all cases of CML, as well as a subset of Ph-positive adult and pediatric precursor B-lymphoblastic leukemia, the breakpoint in *BCR* occurs after either exon 13 (e13 or b2) or exon 14 (e14 or b3), within the so-called *major breakpoint cluster region* or M-bcr, and results in the expression of a p210 fusion protein (Fig. 12.2). The p190 form of BCR-ABL results from utilization of breakpoints between exons 1 and 2 of *BCR*, the minor breakpoint cluster region (m-bcr), and is primarily restricted to ALL. Finally, p230 BCR-ABL is expressed in rare cases in which the BCR breakpoint occurs within intron 19, a region designated as the micro breakpoint cluster region or μ-bcr; whether those CMLs with expression of p230 BCR-ABL have atypical morphologic features is controversial [22–24].

The oncogenic activities of BCR-ABL derive largely from its dysregulated protein tyrosine kinase activity (recently

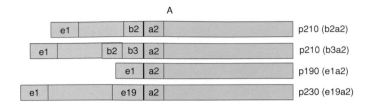

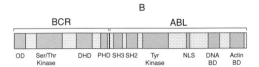

Fig. 12.2. Isoforms and domains of BCR-ABL. (A) Different isoforms of *BCR-ABL* result from the utilization of the various breakpoint cluster regions, each of which includes all of *ABL* except exon 1, and a variable amount of *BCR*. The first and last exons of *BCR* included in the various isoforms are indicated. (B) As with most fusion oncoproteins, BCR-ABL is a modular protein, containing several domains which mediate its biologic and oncogenic properties. Much of the oncogenic potential of BCR-ABL is attributable to dysregulation of the tyrosine kinase activity derived from ABL, whose activity is inhibited by imatinib mesylate. Abbreviations: OD, oligomerization domain; Ser/Thr kinase, serine/threonine-specific kinase domain; DHD, DBL homology domain; PHD, pleckstrin homology domain; SH3, Src homology domain 3; SH2, Src homology domain 2; Tyr kinase, tyrosine kinase domain; NLS, nuclear localization signal; DNA BD, DNA binding domain; Actin BD, actin binding domain.

reviewed in Goldman, Melo [21]). Motifs contributed by BCR facilitate the homodimerization of BCR-ABL, leading to the phosphorylation of critical tyrosine residues located in the activation loop of the ABL-derived tyrosine, constitutive protein tyrosine kinase activation, and ultimately dysregulated signaling through downstream signal transduction pathways. BCR-ABL exerts its oncogenic effects through several critical signaling molecules, including Ras, signal transducers and activators of transcription (STATs), phosphatidylinositol 3-kinase, mitogen-activated protein (MAP) kinases, and MYC. Details of the mechanisms by which BCR-ABL perturbs these signaling pathways is beyond the scope of our discussion, but the net result is that hematopoietic cells expressing BCR-ABL manifest enhanced growth factor-independent proliferation, reduced responsiveness to proapoptotic stimuli, and diminished cell adhesion.

In contrast to chronic phase (CP) disease, the molecular events which result in progression to accelerated phase (AP) or blast phase (BP) of CML are less well understood [25]. These latter stages of CML disease evolution are characterized by defective repair of DNA damage, increasing genomic instability, and loss of tumor suppressor function. These perturbations lead to a maturation arrest and expansion of blasts with acquisition of additional karyotypic abnormalities, features characteristic of CML disease progression.

Clinical and laboratory features

CML comprises only about 2–4% of all pediatric leukemias [1, 2, 26]. Children with CML present at a median age of

approximately 12 years; thus, CML is predominantly a disease of mid-to-late childhood [27–29]. Chronic myeloid leukemia is exceedingly rare in infants and toddlers, with only about 10% of cases in children less than five years of age, clinical features which aid in its distinction from other myeloproliferative disorders that occur predominantly in young children, such as juvenile myelomonocytic leukemia. Pediatric patients with CML commonly present with weakness, early satiety and abdominal discomfort secondary to splenomegaly, weight loss, and bleeding, including epistaxis and menorrhagia [28, 29]. On physical examination, 70–90% of affected children have palpable splenomegaly, whereas hepatomegaly and lymphadenopathy are uncommon. Of note, approximately one-quarter of children with CML are diagnosed incidentally during the clinical workup for an unrelated clinical condition.

Peripheral blood analysis in pediatric CP CML typically reveals multiple abnormalities, which are largely similar to those seen in adults (Fig. 12.3). Interestingly, affected children usually develop marked leukocytosis, with median WBC counts of $200–250 \times 10^9/L$ in most studies, a leukocyte count significantly higher than is typically encountered in adults with CML; approximately 20% of affected children have WBC counts in excess of $400 \times 10^9/L$ [28–31]. Mature, normal-appearing neutrophils usually predominate, with somewhat fewer myeloid progenitors, including metamyelocytes, myelocytes, and promyelocytes. Blasts may be seen but comprise fewer than 10% of nucleated cells in CP CML by definition (see below). Some degree of basophilia is almost always evident and provides a helpful diagnostic clue, particularly in the infrequent patient with CML who presents in blast phase. Although the platelet count is variable, most pediatric patients have mild to moderate thrombocytosis; large and giant platelets may be present. Most affected children have mild to moderate anemia, with severe anemia occurring in only about 10% of patients. Significant poikilocytosis with dacrocytes may be present when there is coexistent myelofibrosis. Patients with marked splenomegaly may have more profound anemia and thrombocytopenia, presumably secondary to splenic sequestration [29].

As alluded to above, CML is a bi- or triphasic disease, clinically and pathologically. The preponderance of pediatric patients with CML present with CP disease [28, 29]. As implied by its designation, chronic phase CML is a relatively stable state clinically. However, most patients with CP CML progress within three to five years to either AP or BP disease (Table 12.2) [32, 33]. Clinically, this progression may be manifested by progressive splenomegaly or the development of frank extramedullary disease, for example myeloid sarcoma. Laboratory studies usually show a leukocytosis with an increased frequency of blasts, and worsening anemia. The platelet count is usually normal or reduced. In contrast to myeloid BP, peripheral blood basophilia is uncommon in lymphoid BP [33, 34]. As will be discussed later, progression to AP or BP is frequently accompanied by the acquisition of cytogenetic and molecular abnormalities in addition to the Ph chromosome.

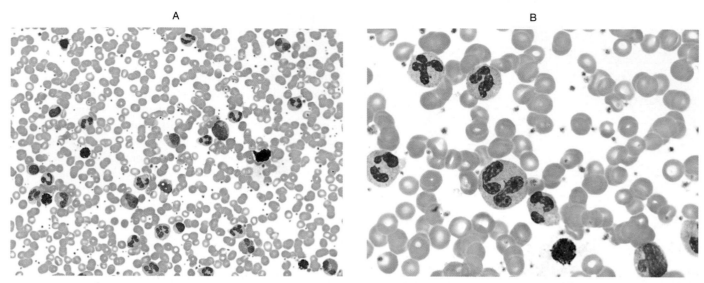

Fig. 12.3. Chronic myelogenous leukemia chronic phase, peripheral blood. (A) There is leukocytosis with the majority of cells comprised of neutrophils and fewer myeloid progenitors. Basophilia is apparent, an important diagnostic clue to CML. (B) The myeloid elements in CP CML are usually normal appearing; a basophil is present near the bottom of the field. Thrombocytosis is also present.

Table 12.2. WHO diagnostic criteria for chronic myelogenous leukemia.

Chronic phase
- Presence of BCR-ABL (detected by either cytogenetics, FISH, or molecular assay)
- Absence of diagnostic criteria for either accelerated or blast phase CML

Accelerate phase
- Presence of BCR-ABL
- Blasts comprise 10–19% of nucleated cells in blood or bone marrow
- Basophils comprising $\geq$ 20% of nucleated cells in blood
- Persistent thrombocytopenia ($<100 \times 10^9$/L) unrelated to therapy, or persistent thrombocytosis ($>1000 \times 10^9$/L) refractory to therapy
- Progressive splenomegaly and/or worsening leukocytosis ($>10 \times 10^9$/L) refractory to therapy
- Cytogenetic evidence of clonal evolution

Blast phase
- Presence of BCR-ABL
- Blasts comprising >20% of leukocytes in peripheral blood or of nucleated cells in bone marrow
- Extramedullary blast proliferation
- Large foci of blasts in the bone marrow, even if overall frequency of blasts is <20%

Pathologic features

The diagnosis of CML ultimately depends on the detection of the *BCR-ABL* fusion oncogene. Nevertheless, morphologic examination of bone marrow and other affected organs is of utility to exclude other causes of leukocytosis, to provide a rapid diagnosis, and to assess for disease progression. The bone marrow findings in pediatric CP CML are similar to those in its adult counterpart (Figs. 12.4–12.5). The bone marrow is invariably hypercellular, typically approaching 100% cellularity. Marked myeloid hyperplasia is the rule, with a commensurate decrease in erythropoiesis, resulting in an M : E ratio that is greater than 10 : 1. Myelopoiesis is complete, but usually manifests "left-shifted" maturation, that is, an increased frequency of promyelocytes, myelocytes and metamyelocytes relative to

that of mature neutrophils. In the biopsy, this perturbation of myelopoiesis in CML manifests as a prominent cuff of immature myeloid forms immediately adjacent to the bony trabeculae, up to 10 or more cells thick, which represents an exaggeration of the normal gradient of myeloid maturation that extends from the trabeculae into the intertrabecular space. A variable degree of basophilia is virtually always present in CP CML, and eosinophilia is usually present as well. The eosinophils in CML manifest complete maturation and lack significant abnormalities in either nuclear segmentation or granule content. By definition, blasts comprise fewer than 10% of cells and are not encountered in large aggregates in CP CML; in practice, blasts are only modestly increased in frequency in the majority of cases. Dysplasia in the myeloid and erythroid lineages is usually minimal in CP disease. In the pediatric setting, particularly in younger children, the presence of more pronounced dysplasia together with myelomonocytic hyperplasia raises the possibility of other disorders, such as juvenile myelomonocytic leukemia, in which dysplasia is more commonly present. Megakaryocytes are variable in frequency in CML, but there is usually a mild or moderate degree of hyperplasia, with prominent megakaryocytic clustering in the bone marrow biopsy or within aspirate spicules (Figs. 12.6–12.7). Occasional cases manifest more prominent megakaryocytic hyperplasia. The megakaryocytes in CML are frequently small and contain hypolobated nuclei, so-called "dwarf" megakaryocytes, in contrast to those of essential thrombocythemia [35, 36]. As these small and immature megakaryocytic forms can sometimes be inconspicuous in bone marrow biopsies, CD61 immunohistochemistry is helpful in some instances for their unequivocal identification (Fig. 12.7) [37]. Other forms of megakaryocytic dysplasia, for example forms with hyperchromatic or widely separated nuclei, are uncommon in chronic phase disease. It should also be mentioned that flow cytometry has little or no utility

A

B

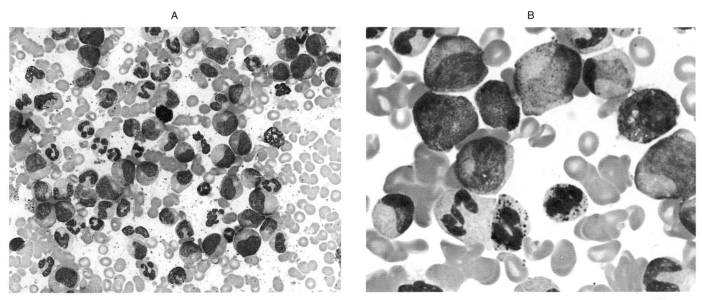

Fig. 12.4. Chronic myelogenous leukemia chronic phase, bone marrow aspirate. (A) The marrow is hypercellular with a myeloid predominance. Myelopoiesis manifests left-shifted maturation. (B) Typical features of CML are present including myeloid predominance, eosinophilia, and basophilia. The basophils may undergo partial degranulation.

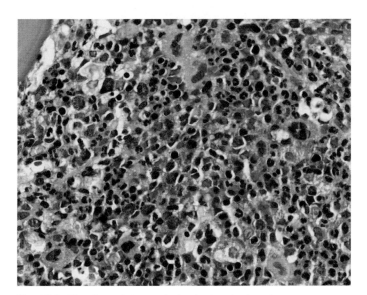

Fig. 12.5. Chronic myelogenous leukemia chronic phase, bone marrow biopsy. The marrow is hypercellular. There is myeloid hyperplasia with eosinophilia and megakaryocytic hyperplasia. Clustered megakaryocytes are a typical feature of CML.

in the evaluation of chronic phase CML, at either diagnosis or follow-up.

Pseudo-Gaucher cells are often present in the marrow in CML and may be numerous in some cases [38–40]. These histiocytes resemble the glucocerebroside-engorged cells seen in Gaucher disease, and contain abundant blue cytoplasm which is characteristically striated in appearance (Fig. 12.8). These terminally differentiated cells are derived from HSCs containing the t(9;22), and may persist in significant numbers after ther-

apy or bone marrow transplantation; however, their presence in these clinical settings is not diagnostic of persistent disease [41]. Finally, significant reticulin fibrosis is common in CML, occurring in 25–60% of cases in adults. The degree and frequency of myelofibrosis in pediatric CML has not been reported, but it is presumably comparable to that seen in adults. Myelofibrosis in the setting of CML has historically had a negative impact on prognosis, which appears to likewise hold true in the imatinib era, particularly for those patients with high grade fibrosis [42, 43].

While the determination of remission status is ultimately predicated on a negative RT-PCR or FISH result for *BCR-ABL*, the morphologic assessment of post-therapy CML bone marrows can provide a rapid assessment of response to therapy. Imatinib is the current front-line therapy for CML in adults, and will undoubtedly prove to be therapeutically important in pediatric CML as well. Several studies have examined the changes in bone marrow morphology following imatinib therapy. A robust response to imatinib is manifested by a significant reduction in the marrow cellularity and normalization of the M : E ratio [44–47]. These changes typically occur several weeks to a few months after initiation of imatinib therapy [44, 45]. Imatinib also induces the regression of reticulin fibrosis and normalization of megakaryocyte morphology and distribution [44, 46, 48]. Of note, marrow aplasia may rarely occur during imatinib therapy [49, 50].

In the past, patients with CML not infrequently underwent splenectomy for palliation or because of concern of extramedullary disease progression (Fig. 12.9). In the former instance, the spleen is massively enlarged and histologically shows infiltration of the splenic red pulp by myeloid cells. With the advent of imatinib and other tyrosine kinase inhibitors, splenectomy is now much less frequently performed.

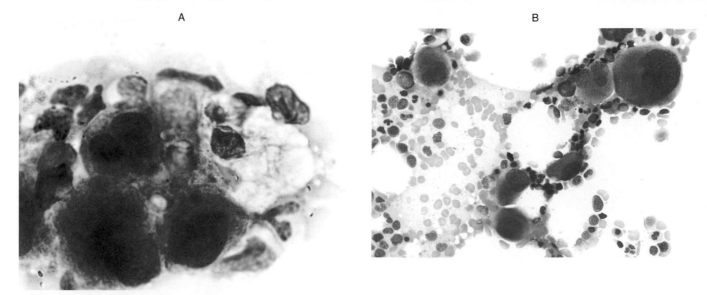

Fig. 12.6. Chronic myelogenous leukemia chronic phase, bone marrow aspirate. (A) There is usually megakaryocytic hyperplasia in CML, often with pronounced clustering, as is evident in this spicule. A pseudo-Gaucher cell is also present. (B) In addition to hyperplasia, the megakaryocytes in CML are typically smaller and contain hypolobated nuclei.

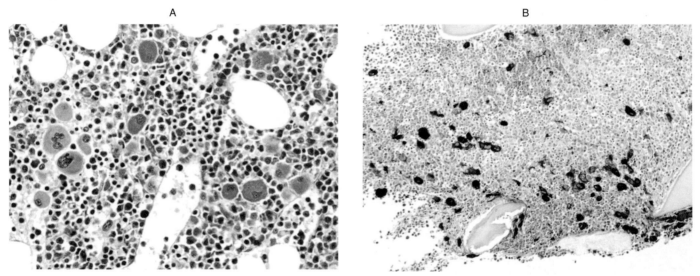

Fig. 12.7. Chronic myelogenous leukemia chronic phase, bone marrow biopsy. (A) The biopsy shows megakaryocytic hyperplasia with clustering. Most of the megakaryocytes are smaller than normal with reduced nuclear complexity. (B) These changes in megakaryocytic size and distribution in CML are highlighted by a CD61 immunohistochemical stain. Note that some megakaryocytes have an abnormal paratrabecular localization.

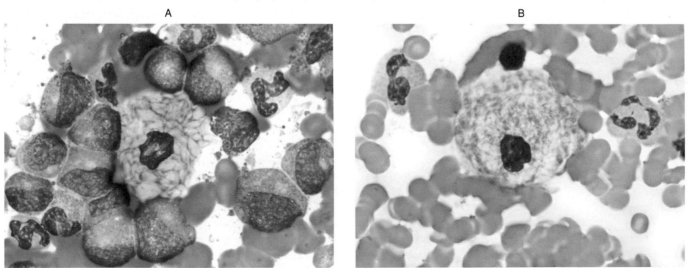

Fig. 12.8. Chronic myelogenous leukemia chronic phase, bone marrow aspirate. (A) Pseudo-Gaucher cells are frequently present in the marrow in CML. These cells contain abundant blue cytoplasm that is characteristically striated, closely resembling the glucocerebroside-engorged histiocytes seen in Gaucher disease. While common in CML, pseudo-Gaucher cells may be observed in any hematologic disorder where there is robust hematopoietic proliferation and cell death. (B) A bona fide Gaucher cell from a child with Gaucher disease is shown for comparison.

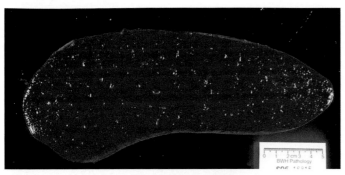

Fig. 12.9 Chronic myelogenous leukemia chronic phase, spleen. Patients with chronic phase disease typically present with splenomegaly, which can be massive in some instances. Histologically, there is red pulp infiltration by myeloid progenitors and mature neutrophils. With the advent of imatinib as an effective therapy for CML, splenectomy is now rarely performed.

Disease progression

CP CML is a labile state, and progression to either AP or BP occurs in the majority of patients within four or five years after initial diagnosis. In addition, approximately 5–10% of children with CML present with AP or BP disease [28, 29]. Several histologic, laboratory, and clinical features are recognized according to WHO criteria as being indicative of disease progression (Table 12.2). In practice, a worsening blast burden most frequently heralds CML disease progression.

In AP CML, the marrow manifests many of the features of chronic phase disease, including the hypercellularity, myeloid predominance, eosinophilia, basophilia, and megakaryocytic hyperplasia (Fig. 12.10). Blasts are increased in frequency and by definition comprise 10–19% of nucleated cells in bone marrow or peripheral blood. In some cases, progression to AP may be heralded by the development of large aggregates of blasts in the marrow, even though the overall percentage is not significantly increased. This latter finding is best appreciated in the bone marrow biopsy, although such aggregates can occasionally be observed in the aspirate smear. In some cases, there is a striking degree of megakaryocytic hyperplasia, which may be accompanied by pronounced reticulin fibrosis or even frank collagen fibrosis.

BP CML is defined as more than 20% blasts in either peripheral blood or bone marrow. In keeping with the concept that CML is a stem cell malignancy, blast crises of virtually every hematopoietic lineage have been described, including myeloid, promyelocytic, eosinophilic, basophilic, megakaryoblastic, erythroblastic, B-lymphoid, and T-lymphoid [33, 34, 51–54]. In adults, 60–70%, 20%, and 15% of blast crises have a myeloid, lymphoid, and undifferentiated (biphenotypic or bilineal) immunophenotype, respectively; the immunophenotypic frequency is presumably similar in pediatric BP CML, although there are few reported data on BP CML in children.

Morphologically, blasts are increased in frequency in the marrow by definition. Features of the antecedent chronic phase CML may persist, depending on the degree to which the blast proliferation effaces the marrow; this is more commonly encountered in myeloid BP, where the blast percentage tends to be lower than in lymphoid BP [33, 54]. In myeloid BP, the blasts have typical myeloblast or, less commonly, monoblastic morphology. Blasts may contain fine azurophilic granules in some instances; however, most cases lack Auer rods [34]. Occasional cases contain a heterogeneous blast population comprised of typical myeloblasts, including forms manifesting basophilic differentiation, erythroblasts and megakaryoblasts. While usually

A

B

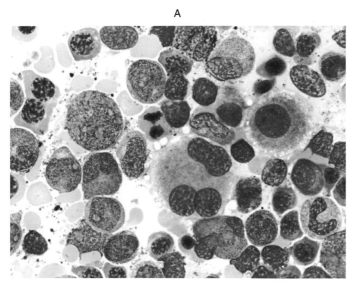

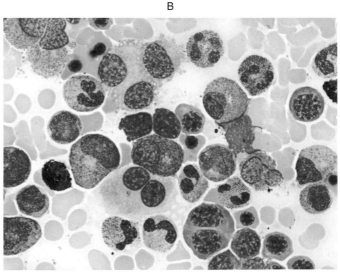

Fig. 12.10. (A, B) Chronic myelogenous leukemia accelerated phase, bone marrow aspirate. This patient presented with accelerated phase disease with 10–15% blasts in his bone marrow. In addition to the blasts, there is trilineage dysplasia, with megaloblastoid myeloid and erythroid maturation, binucleated erythroid forms, and striking megakaryocytic dysplasia. Note the presence of microcytic elements and forms containing separate nuclei, both features of megakaryocytic dysplasia. These features were initially misinterpreted at an outside institution as high-grade myelodysplasia. In addition to the t(9;22)(q34;q11), cytogenetic studies revealed monosomy 7 and a deletion of 11q in all metaphases analyzed.

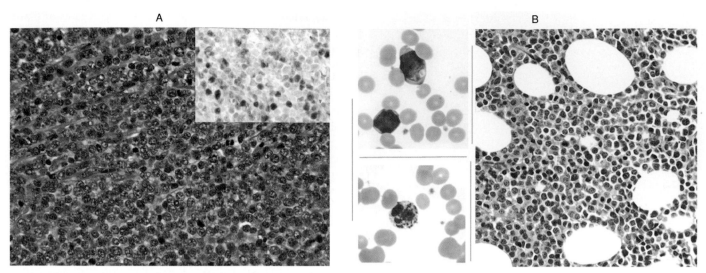

Fig. 12.11. Extramedullary manifestation of blast phase of chronic myelogenous leukemia. This previously healthy patient underwent tonsillectomy for recurrent tonsillitis. (A) The tonsil contained a diffuse infiltrate of small blasts, which expressed T-cell markers and TdT (inset), consistent with precursor T-lymphoblastic lymphoma. (B) The peripheral blood contained frequent small and intermediate-sized blasts (upper left panel); basophils comprised 3% of nucleated cells (lower left panel). Bone marrow biopsy revealed a blastic infiltrate (right panel). Flow cytometric analysis confirmed that the blasts expressed T-cell markers (cytoplasmic CD3+, CD5+, CD7+, TdT+; CD4−, CD8−) and myeloid markers (CD33+, CD13+, CD11b+), consistent with acute biphenotypic leukemia. Cytogenetic analysis of both lymph node and bone marrow cells revealed a 46,XX,r?(5)(p?15q?13),t(9;22)(q34;q11) karyotype in all metaphases analyzed.

absent or minimal in chronic phase disease, significant dysplasia can be present in accelerated and blast phase CML (Fig. 12.10), which can be misinterpreted as indicative of a myelodysplastic syndrome, particularly in patients presenting with progressive or partially treated disease in whom leukocytosis is absent. Immunophenotyping confirms the expression of progenitor and non-lineage restricted antigens (CD34, CD117, HLA-DR) and myeloid antigens (CD13, CD33, and CD11c); CD7 co-expression is frequently observed [33, 34, 55, 56]. In cases with megakaryoblastic differentiation, the blasts express megakaryocyte-specific markers, such as CD41, CD42b, and CD61. Blast phase CML can also manifest as extramedullary disease (Fig. 12.11). Finally, it should be noted that the abrupt development of BP has been described in patients receiving imatinib therapy and in whom cytogenetic and/or molecular remission had been recently documented [57–62]. Interestingly, the majority of these "sudden" BP cases have been of the lymphoid type.

Cytogenetics and molecular diagnostics

In the majority of patients presenting with chronic phase CML, the t(9;22)(q34;q11) is present as the sole cytogenetic abnormality. However, the karyotype is either apparently normal or reveals a variant translocation in 5–10% of patients with otherwise typical chronic phase disease [63–67]. In such instances, the presence of the *BCR-ABL* fusion must be confirmed using other methods, most commonly either interphase fluorescent *in situ* hybridization (FISH) or reverse transcriptase polymerase chain reaction (RT-PCR).

The advent of effective, targeted therapy for CML necessitates a more standardized approach to the initial testing and subsequent monitoring of patients for the presence of BCR-ABL. Appropriate testing is primarily determined by the clinical context and the performance characteristics of a given test. Conventional cytogenetics should be obtained at initial presentation in all cases of suspected CML. Interphase FISH permits the detection of cryptic translocations, or confirmation that an observed complex translocation targets the *BCR* and *ABL* loci; however, FISH is neither suitable for the detection of other cytogenetic lesions nor is it adequately sensitive for use in monitoring minimal residual disease. Recently, guidelines have been proposed for the cytogenetic and molecular monitoring of CML patients following initiation of tyrosine kinase inhibitor therapy [68–70].

Conventional cytogenetics also play an important role in the detection of clonal evolution in AP or BP CML. In addition to the morphologic findings described above, acquisition of additional karyotypic abnormalities often occurs during disease evolution, reflecting the progressive genomic instability characteristic of advanced phase CML. Several numerical and structural chromosomal abnormalities occur commonly in AP or BP (Fig. 12.12). In order of frequency, these include trisomy 8, an additional Ph chromosome, isochromosome 17, trisomy 19, loss of Y, trisomy 21, and monosomy 7 [32–34, 71, 72]. In addition, several cases of BP CML have been reported in which both the t(9;22) and an AML-associated translocation are present, including the inv(16), t(15;17), and t(8;21) [73–77]. The limited survival data from these reports suggest that the presence of the t(9;22) negates the relatively good

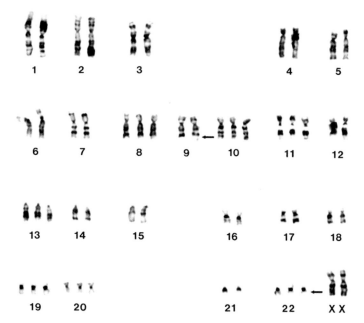

Fig. 12.12. Cytogenetic findings in accelerated phase of chronic myelogenous leukemia. Cytogenetic analysis in this case reveals typical karyotypic features of disease progression in CML, including an extra Philadelphia chromosome as well as an extra chromosome 8 and 19. (Karyotype kindly provided by Dr. Jeffrey Sawyer.)

prognosis typically associated with *de novo* AMLs harboring these translocations.

Pediatric thrombocytosis

Thrombocytosis in children is either attributable to intrinsic dysregulation of megakaryocyte proliferation or platelet production (primary thrombocytosis), or develops in the context of other disease states (secondary or reactive thrombocytosis). As in adults, reactive thrombocytosis is far more common in children than primary thrombocytosis, and is most often associated with infection, chronic inflammatory states, tissue injury, and, less often, malignancy (Table 12.3) [78–84]. In the pediatric population, the incidence of secondary thrombocytosis is highest in neonates and infants, and generally declines as a function of age [78, 80, 84].

There are two subtypes of primary pediatric thrombocytosis: familial thrombocytosis and essential thrombocythemia (ET). In a subset of familial cases, mutations are detected in either the thrombopoietin (*TPO*) gene or that of its cell-surface receptor, *MPL*, which has homology to the murine myeloproliferative leukemia retrovirus from which *MPL* derives its name. ET is rare in children, with fewer than 100 cases reported in the literature and an annual incidence approximately 65 times lower than its adult counterpart [85–87]. In a retrospective series from the Hospital for Sick Children, a major pediatric hospital in Canada, only four children were diagnosed with primary thrombocytosis over a 31-year time period [88]. Pediatric ET is somewhat heterogeneous pathogenetically, and

Table 12.3. Causes of thrombocytosis in children.

Primary thrombocytosis
Familial thrombocytosis
Essential thrombocythemia
Other myeloproliferative neoplasms (e.g., CML, polycythemia vera)
Secondary thrombocytosis
Infection
Tissue injury (trauma, surgery, burns)
Iron deficiency anemia
Inflammatory or autoimmune disorders
Low birth weight
Splenectomy
Malignancy

includes a subset of cases with mutations in the Janus kinase 2 gene (*JAK2*).

Overview of megakaryopoiesis and platelet generation

A brief overview of normal megakaryocyte development and platelet formation is helpful to provide a conceptual basis for understanding the pathogenesis of pediatric thrombocytosis. Megakaryocytes possess a number of distinct morphologic and biologic properties that enable them to fulfill their primary physiologic function, namely the production of platelets. Megakaryocytes are believed to derive from a bipotential progenitor with the capacity to subsequently undergo either megakaryocytic or erythroid differentiation (Fig. 12.13); the mechanisms governing the cell fate decision of this progenitor are poorly understood. Following commitment to the megakaryocytic lineage, progenitors undergo a unique process of endomitosis in which genomic DNA replication occurs in the absence of cell division. As a result, the mature megakaryocyte attains a ploidy of 64–128N, and accumulates a copious complement of cytoplasm which will ultimately be shed as platelets. Although incompletely understood, platelets are thought to form from long cytoplasmic extensions, or proplatelets, that protrude into vascular spaces and which contain alpha- and dense granules. The terminal segment of the proplatelet pinches off, forming a reticulated or immature platelet which contains RNA, analogous to the reticulated RBC [89–91]. These reticulated platelets subsequently mature, losing their complement of RNA. Mature platelets have a half life of four to five days [92–94].

The biology of megakaryopoiesis has been intensely investigated during the past 5–10 years. Through the analysis of genetically engineered mouse strains, it has been established that megakaryocytic lineage commitment, proliferation, maturation, and ultimately platelet production are finely coordinated through cytokine signaling, particularly that mediated by TPO-MPL, and through the regulation of downstream gene expression by a small group of transcription factors, most notably GATA1, FOG1, NF-E2, FLI-1 and RUNX1 (Fig. 12.14) [95–97]. Several rare human hematologic disorders have been

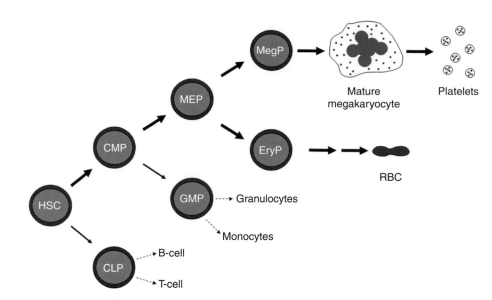

Fig. 12.13. Megakaryocytic ontogeny. Megakaryocytes derive from pluripotent hematopoietic stem cells, through a series of differentiative steps that includes a common myeloid progenitor (CMP) and a bipotential progenitor, the megakaryocytic/erythroid progenitor (MEP). The molecular events which direct commitment of the MEP to the megakaryocytic lineage are poorly understood. Abbreviations: MegP, megakaryocytic progenitor; EryP, erythroid progenitor; CLP, common lymphocytic progenitor; GMP, granulocyte/monocyte progenitor.

molecularly characterized in which there is either defective megakaryocytic development or quantitative or qualitative platelet abnormalities. In several of these disorders, mutations in the genes encoding these transcription factors and cytokine receptors have been identified. These include *MPL* mutations in congenital amegakaryocytic thrombocytopenia, *GATA1* mutations in X-linked macrothrombocytopenia, and *RUNX1* mutations in familial platelet disorder, confirming the critical role of these transcription factors and cytokines in human megakaryopoiesis and platelet generation [98–104].

Pathogenesis

Familial thrombocytosis

Given the critical role of signaling through the TPO–MPL pathway in megakaryopoiesis and platelet generation, it is not surprising that mutations in the *TPO* and *MPL* genes have been identified in several kindreds with familial thrombocytosis.

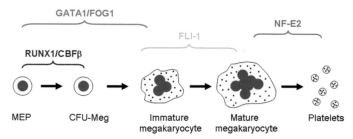

Fig. 12.14. Transcriptional regulation of megakaryopoiesis. Through the analysis of genetically engineered mouse strains, it is now established that the modulation of gene expression which dictates the differentiation and proliferative events in megakaryopoiesis results from the finely coordinated expression of several key transcription factors. Some transcription factors, such as RUNX1/CBFβ, appear to regulate early cell-fate commitment events, whereas others, for instance NF-E2, participate in later events such as the regulation of thrombogenesis. Abbreviations: CFU-Meg, megakaryocytic colony forming unit; MEP, megakaryocytic/erythroid progenitor.

These mutations are generally inherited in an autosomal dominant manner. In kindreds with mutations in *TPO*, mutations in the 5′ untranslated region of the *TPO* mRNA are the most common, and result in the generation of a transcript that is more efficiently translated, thus accounting for the markedly elevated serum TPO levels of affected family members [105–107].

Two mutations in *MPL* have been described in familial thrombocytosis. The serine 505 to asparagine 505 mutation (S505N) occurs within the transmembrane domain of MPL, and results in enhanced signaling through MPL, as evidenced by spontaneous phosphorylation of key downstream signaling molecules such as MEK protein kinases and STAT5B [108]. It is uncertain how the S505N mutation dysregulates MPL signaling, but it may be attributable in part to ligand-independent dimerization of MPL, possibly leading to aberrant activation of MPL-associated Janus kinases. Interestingly, this same mutation was shown to be oncogenic in a murine experimental system [109]; however, there is no reported predisposition to leukemia in humans harboring the S505N MPL mutation. The second MPL mutation, lysine 39 to asparagine 39 (K39N), is located in the ligand-binding domain of MPL and may result in diminished TPO binding [110]. How this mutation leads to a seemingly paradoxical thrombocytosis is unclear at present, but may be due to TPO-independent effects. Familial thrombocytosis has also been described in kindreds lacking mutations in either *TPO* or *MPL*, suggesting that perturbation of other signaling pathways may result in thrombocytosis [111]. Finally, it should be mentioned that hematopoiesis is consistently polyclonal in affected individuals with familial thrombocytosis [112, 113].

Sporadic thrombocytosis

Before addressing pediatric ET, the physiologic and pathologic aspects of JAK2 signaling will be discussed. The Janus kinase (JAK) family of protein kinases includes four members:

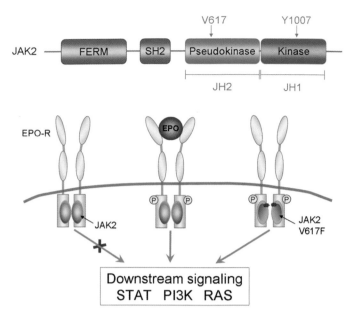

Fig. 12.15. Domain structure of JAK2 and perturbation of its signaling in myeloproliferative neoplasia. The V617F mutation is the most common in JAK2, and is detected in several types of adult myeloproliferative neoplasia and a subset of pediatric ones. This mutation disrupts the normal negative regulatory function of the pseudokinase domain of JAK2, imparting constitutive signaling to JAK2, even when the receptors with which JAK2 associates lack bound ligand. Abbreviations: FERM, band 4.1, Ezrin, radixin and moesin domain; SH2, Src homology 2 domain; JH, JAK homology domain; EPO-R, EPO receptor.

JAK1, JAK2, JAK3, and TYK2 (reviewed in Mertens, Darnell [114], and Tefferi [115]). The JAK kinases normally function to transduce cytokine-induced signals through their physical association with the cytoplasmic domains of several cell-surface cytokine receptors. These receptors lack intrinsic protein kinase activity; however, upon binding ligand, the associated JAK kinase undergoes phosphorylation and activation, inducing the recruitment and phosphorylation of STAT proteins, and ultimately resulting in the activation of downstream signaling molecules (Fig. 12.15). Each of the JAKs associates with a specific subset of cytokine receptors; for example JAK2 associates with the common β-chain (CD131) shared between the receptors for GM-CSF, EPO, TPO, IFN-γ, IL-3, and IL-5. Mice deficient in JAK2 manifest an embryonic lethal phenotype because of aborted definitive erythropoiesis [116, 117].

In a flurry of publications in 2005, a point mutation in *JAK2*, specifically the substitution of valine for phenylalanine at codon 617 of JAK2 (*JAK2V617F*), was detected at a high frequency in several types of adult myeloproliferative neoplasm [118–121]. With the reported analyses of thousands of patients with these disorders, it is now established that the *JAK2V617F* is present in approximately 95%, 50%, and 50% of adult cases of polycythemia vera, ET, and primary myelofibrosis, respectively [122]. In addition, the *JAK2V617F* is present in 5–10% of chronic myelomonocytic leukemias and less than 5% of cases of myelodysplasia and acute myeloid leukemia. This mutation occurs within the JH2 domain of JAK2, a motif that functions to inhibit the kinase activity of JAK2 (reviewed in Levine *et al.* [123]). The JAK2V617F disrupts this domain and results in

the loss of the autoinhibitory activity of JH2, endowing JAK2 with constitutive signaling activity (Fig. 12.15). As a result, signaling through receptors with which JAK2 associates is dysregulated and occurs even in the absence of ligand binding. JAK2V617F activates *in vitro* several downstream signaling pathways, including the STAT transcription factors, the Rasmitogen activated protein (MAP) kinase pathway, and phosphotidylinositol 3-kinase. Expression of JAK2V617F confers on hematopoietic cells cytokine-independent growth and cytokine hypersensitivity *in vitro*, properties characteristically observed in myeloproliferative neoplasms [118, 119].

In contrast to adults, the pathogenetic role of the *JAK2V617F* mutation in pediatric ET is less clear. In three studies to date, *JAK2V617F* has been detected in 9–38% of pediatric cases with an overall incidence of approximately 25%, significantly lower than that observed in adult ET [124–126]. Those patients with *JAK2V617F* may be more likely to have clonal hematopoiesis than those lacking it [125, 126]. Thus, ET in children is pathogenetically more heterogeneous than its adult counterpart, with dysregulation of JAK2 signaling present in only a minority of cases. The pathogenesis of pediatric ET lacking JAK2 mutations is poorly understood.

Clinical and laboratory features

In the reported cases of pediatric ET, the age at presentation ranges from 9 months to 16 years, with a median age of approximately 14 years [113, 126, 127]. Many patients are asymptomatic at presentation, and the thrombocytosis is detected during a blood analysis performed for unrelated reasons [113, 126]. The most common symptom in affected children is headache, followed by bleeding (e.g., epistaxis), and less commonly venous thrombosis. Splenomegaly is present in some patients. Laboratory studies usually reveal isolated thrombocytosis, with median platelet counts of $1100–1700 \times 10^9$/L (normal pediatric range $150–450 \times 10^9$/L). No qualitative platelet abnormalities have been described. Leukocyte and red blood cell indices are usually normal.

Pathologic features

Bone marrow examination in familial thrombocytosis typically reveals a normocellular marrow with megakaryocytic hyperplasia (Fig. 12.16). The megakaryocytes are mature, with normal nuclear morphology. Large megakaryocytes with hyperlobated nuclei are characteristic of the adult form of ET. However, while increased in frequency, the megakaryocytes in pediatric ET are often morphologically unremarkable [113, 126, 127]. It is currently unknown whether the presence of the *JAK2V617F* has any influence on megakaryocytic morphology in pediatric ET. In most cases, there is little or no reticulin fibrosis. No abnormalities in either the myeloid or erythroid lineages are usually present.

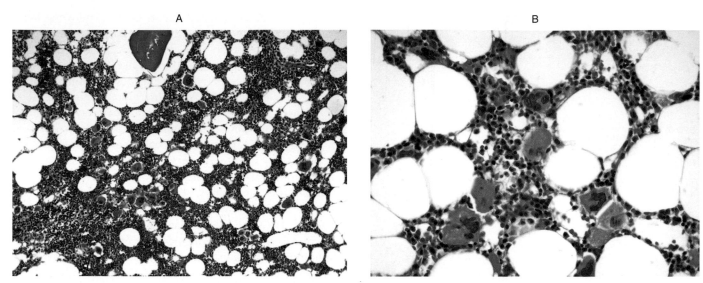

A   B

Fig. 12.16. Familial thrombocytosis, bone marrow biopsy. This 21-year-old woman has a family history significant for thrombocythemia in a sister and an aunt. Her mother has normal peripheral blood indices; however, her father died from a myocardial infarction. The patient has thrombocytosis with a platelet count of 900×10^9/L. Genetic studies identified the *MPLS505N* mutation. (A) The bone marrow is normocellular; however, megakaryocytes are increased in frequency and manifest prominent clustering. Only scattered giant forms are present. Of note, there is no significant fibrosis. (B) Higher magnification reveals that most of the megakaryocytes have normal morphology, with occasional forms containing hyperlobated nuclei. There are no morphologic abnormalities in the myeloid and erythroid lineages. (Photomicrograph kindly provided by Professor Luigi M. Larocca.)

Cytogenetics and molecular diagnostics

In virtually all cases of pediatric primary thrombocytosis, conventional cytogenetics demonstrates a normal diploid karyotype [113, 127, 128]. In patients without a family history of thrombocytosis and in whom ET is suspected, *JAK2* mutation analysis may be indicated. Several different approaches have been utilized to detect the *JAK2V617F* mutation, including DNA sequencing. However, sequencing suffers from poor sensitivity, as it cannot reliably detect a mutant allele comprising fewer than 20% of the total alleles present, and it is labor intensive and not particularly amenable to the clinical laboratory. Consequently, molecular assays with higher throughput and greater sensitivity have been developed (reviewed in Steensma [129]). These include allele-specific PCR which, with appropriately designed primers, permits preferential amplification of the mutant *JAK2* allele. Real-time PCR coupled with DNA melting curve analysis is frequently used. Melting curve analysis allows for distinction between wild-type and mutant alleles because of differences in the kinetics of melting induced by the presence of the mutation. This approach enables high-throughput analysis and, depending on the assay, can detect mutant alleles when present at levels as low as 1–10% [130].

Polycythemia vera

Erythrocytosis in the pediatric setting includes both primary disorders, in which there is intrinsically dysregulated proliferation of erythroid progenitors resulting in a significant increase in the peripheral blood red cell mass, and secondary disorders which are due to causes other than an intrinsic defect in the

Table 12.4. Classification of pediatric erythrocytoses.

Primary erythrocytosis	
Congenital	EPO receptor mutations
Acquired	Polycythemia vera

Secondary erythrocytosis	
Congenital	Hemoglobin with high oxygen affinity
	2,3-bisphosphoglycerate deficiency
	von Hippel–Lindau (VHL) gene mutations (sporadic and familial)
	Prolyl hydroxylase domain (PHD) 2 gene mutations (familial)
Acquired	Physiologically elevated EPO expression
	Paraneoplastic or ectopic expression of EPO
	Wilms tumor
	Neuroblastoma
	Hepatic tumor
	Renal cyst

regulation of erythroid proliferation (Table 12.4). The former include polycythemia vera (PV), an idiopathic neoplastic disorder characterized by erythrocytosis, which will be the subject of our discussion. Other primary erythrocytoses include the congenital erythrocytoses which are caused by mutations in proteins involved in oxygen sensing [e.g., prolyl hydroxylase domain (PHD) 2, hypoxia-inducible factor (HIF) α, von Hippel–Lindau (VHL)], or are due to dysregulated erythropoietin (EPO) signaling due to germline mutations in the EPO receptor [131–135]. These genetic disorders will only be selectively discussed here; the interested reader is referred to several recent reviews [136–138]. Secondary erythrocytoses include both congenital and acquired etiologies (Table 12.4); this group of disorders will not be discussed further.

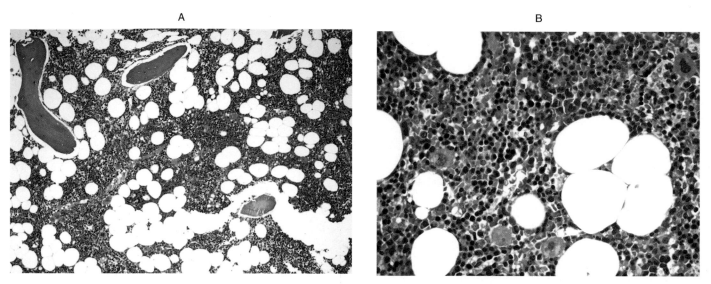

Fig. 12.17. Pediatric polycythemia vera, bone marrow biopsy. This 18-year-old male has a 6-year history of polycythemia. At the time of biopsy, he had a Hb of 17.8 g/dL, Hct 58%, and a normal serum EPO level. Genetic studies to detect the *V617F* or exon 12 JAK2 mutation were negative. The patient's father also has polycythemia. The bone marrow is normocellular (A), and there is erythroid hyperplasia with intrasinusoidal erythropoiesis (B). Megakaryocytes are present in normal numbers and are morphologically unremarkable. (Photomicrograph kindly provided by Professor Luigi M. Larocca.)

Pathogenesis

Pediatric PV is exceedingly rare, and its pathogenesis is poorly understood. Although relatively few cases have been analyzed, hematopoiesis appears to be clonal in most instances. Bone marrow cells manifest spontaneous erythroid colony forming activity in approximately one-third of cases. In contrast to its adult counterpart, where the *JAK2V617F* mutation is detected in virtually all instances, only about 30–40% of pediatric PV cases harbor this mutation [112, 139]. Little is known of the molecular pathogenesis of pediatric PV lacking the *JAK2V617F* mutation. Of note, the *JAK2V617F* mutation is not detected in the congenital erythrocytoses [140].

Clinical and laboratory features and pathologic findings

PV occurs primarily in older children. In the largest reported series, the median age at presentation was 16 years and included no children younger than 6 years of age [126]. There may be a male predominance in pediatric PV. Organomegaly is uncommon. The frequency of thrombotic events in children with PV appears to be lower than in affected adults. Laboratory studies reveal a significantly increased red cell mass, with a median Hb and Hct of 18 g/dL and 54%, respectively. The median WBC and platelet counts are usually within the normal range, although some patients may have mild leukocytosis or marked thrombocytosis, necessitating distinction of PV from other myeloproliferative neoplasms, especially CML and ET. The serum EPO level is normal in most patients. Evaluation for a positive family history is a critical part of the clinical assessment of an erythrocytotic child. A positive family history, isolated erythrocytosis, and the absence of organomegaly strongly favor

a congenital erythrocytosis and make the neoplastic condition PV much less likely. A bone marrow examination may not be indicated in this clinical setting. Finally, such patients and affected family members should undergo genetic analysis to assess for the presence of a mutation in *EPOR* or other relevant genes.

The bone marrow findings in pediatric PV are similar to those seen in adults, although there are few reported details of the bone marrow findings in pediatric cases [141]. The bone marrow is normocellular or hypercellular, usually with trilineage hyperplasia (Fig. 12.17). Erythroid hyperplasia can be pronounced, and myelopoiesis is frequently left-shifted. Significant dysplasia is not present. In addition to hyperplasia, megakaryocytes manifest clustering. A spectrum of megakaryocytic morphology, that is, small, intermediate and large, occasionally hyperlobated forms, is typical of PV. In cases with prominent megakaryocytic hyperplasia, distinction from pediatric ET on a morphologic basis alone may be difficult, as large megakaryocytes with hyperlobated nuclei characteristic of adult ET may be less frequent in pediatric cases. Prominent fibrosis has not been described. The propensity of pediatric PV to progress to spent phase or undergo blastic transformation is unknown.

Cytogenetics and molecular diagnostics

No recurrent cytogenetic abnormalities have been described in pediatric PV. As discussed above, the principal role of cytogenetics in this clinical setting is to confirm the absence of the Philadelphia chromosome and karyotypic abnormalities associated with other hematologic malignancies. With negative cytogenetic findings, the presence of the *JAK2V617F* mutation should be assessed. *JAK2* mutation analysis methods are discussed above in the section on pediatric thrombocytosis.

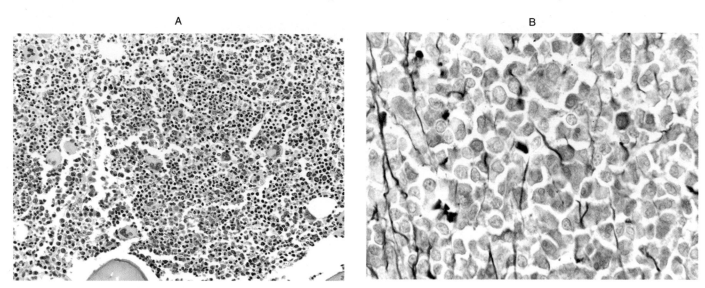

Fig. 12.18. Pediatric myelofibrosis, bone marrow biopsy. This young boy presented at 14 months of age with abdominal protuberance secondary to hepatosplenomegaly. Laboratory studies demonstrated a mildly elevated WBC count, anemia (Hb 8.3 g/dL), and thrombocytopenia (40 × 10^9/L). An initial biopsy showed myeloid and megakaryocytic hyperplasia with mild reticulin fibrosis. The current biopsy was obtained at age three years. (A) The bone marrow is hypercellular with erythroid hyperplasia and megakaryocytic clustering. (B) There is mild–moderate diffusely increased reticulin fiber deposition. At the time of this biopsy, the patient's peripheral blood indices had largely resolved. Bone marrow cytogenetics revealed a normal male karyotype. (Photomicrograph kindly provided by Dr. David Head.)

Myelofibrosis in the pediatric setting

Primary myelofibrosis (PM), also known as chronic idiopathic myelofibrosis or myeloid metaplasia with myelofibrosis, is a type of myeloproliferative neoplasia characterized by megakaryocytic and myeloid proliferation with associated, progressive marrow fibrosis. With the resultant reduction in intramedullary volume, compensatory extramedullary hematopoiesis develops, yielding the hepatosplenomegaly characteristic of the disorder. PM is predominantly a disease of older adults, with an average age at presentation of approximately 60 years. The overall incidence of PM in adults is approximately one case per 100 000 persons. In the pediatric setting, most cases of myelofibrosis appear to be secondary to metabolic, genetic, or other neoplastic disorders [142–148]. True PM is exceedingly uncommon in children, with only single cases or small series of patients described in the literature [149–154].

Pathogenesis

In contrast to its adult counterpart, virtually nothing is known regarding the pathogenesis of pediatric PM. However, several clinical observations suggest that distinct pathogenetic mechanisms for pediatric and adult PM may exist (see below). In contrast to the adult form, *JAK2* mutations have not been described in pediatric PM. No recurrent karyotypic or genetic lesions have been described in pediatric PM. However, several instances of apparently familial myelofibrosis, with presentation during infancy or childhood, have been reported [151, 155–157]. The mode of inheritance appears to be autosomal recessive in some cases; the identity of the involved gene(s) in these pedi-

grees remains unknown. Finally, while adult PM is a clonal disorder [158–160], clonality in pediatric PM has not been established.

Clinical and laboratory features

Most children with PM present in late infancy or early childhood. Signs and symptoms related to bone marrow failure are often present, including fatigue, easy bruising, and fever. Hepatosplenomegaly is common. The WBC count may be normal, increased, or occasionally decreased. Marked neutropenia has been reported frequently. Leukoerythroblastosis may be present. Anemia is usually present, frequently with pronounced anisopoikilocytosis with dacrocytes [151–153, 155, 156, 161, 162]. Thrombocytopenia, often severe, has been reported in many pediatric patients with PM [152, 161, 162]; however, the platelets are morphologically unremarkable. Rather surprisingly, many pediatric patients with PM experience spontaneous resolution of their disease after months to years of only expectant management or transfusion support [152, 153, 161]. These observations suggest that conservative management of children with PM is appropriate initially, with more aggressive therapy reserved for those individuals with evidence of disease progression.

Pathologic features

In cases with presumed idiopathic etiology, a variable degree of fibrosis may be present, ranging from moderate–marked reticulin fibrosis to overt collagen fibrosis (Figs. 12.18–12.19). In

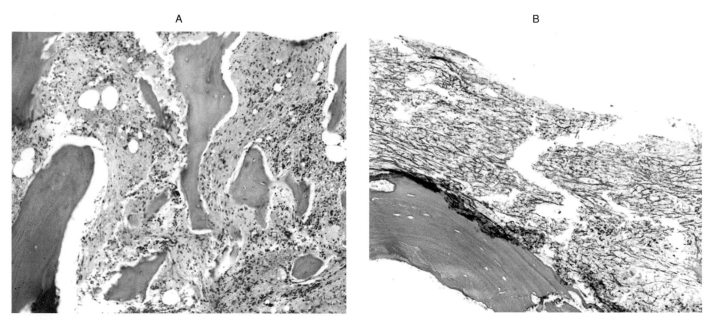

Fig. 12.19. Pediatric myelofibrosis, bone marrow biopsy. This male patient initially presented at nine months of age with splenomegaly. He was severely anemic (5.2 g/dL) and thrombocytopenic (23 × 10⁹/L). Bone marrow examination at that time revealed hypercellularity with increased and left-shifted myelopoiesis, and reticulin fibrosis. During the subsequent nine years he has intermittently required platelet and RBC transfusions secondary to mucosal bleeding. At 12 years of age, there was marked spontaneous improvement in his RBC indices. At the time of this bone marrow biopsy, he was 22 years of age and has mild anemia and severe thrombocytopenia, not requiring platelet transfusions. (A) The bone marrow is fibrotic with mild osteosclerosis. (B) Reticulin stain confirms diffuse, marked reticulin fiber deposition. (Photomicrograph kindly provided by Dr. David Head.)

the latter, the cellularity may be reduced due to obliteration of the marrow space. Due to the fibrosis, aspirate smears and biopsy touch imprints may be of limited utility for morphologic evaluation. Dyspoietic changes in the erythroid and megakaryocytic lineages can be present. Blasts are usually not significantly increased in frequency.

In the pediatric setting, the differential diagnosis of myelofibrosis is broad. When confronted with a fibrotic marrow from a child, PM should only be entertained after several much more common etiologies are excluded (Table 12.5). Clinical input may be essential in arriving at an appropriate diagnosis. In infants and toddlers, acute leukemia and metastatic solid tumor, particularly neuroblastoma, should be included in the differential diagnosis (Fig. 12.20). As described in Chapter 15, acute megakaryoblastic leukemia is frequently accompanied by myelofibrosis, which may be severe enough in some cases to obscure the blastic infiltrate. Low-grade reticulin fibrosis is not infrequent in acute lymphoblastic leukemia, particularly the precursor B-type; in rare cases of ALL, there may be marked reticulin fibrosis which can mimic PM [163, 164]. In older children, other metastatic tumors should also be considered, including Hodgkin lymphoma, which frequently has associated fibrosis. An association between vitamin D deficiency and myelofibrosis is well described, and should be considered in the differential diagnosis of a fibrotic marrow, particularly in children from resource-poor settings [146, 165, 166]. Finally, high-grade reticulin myelofibrosis may occur in association with familial or secondary hemophagocytic lymphohistiocytosis [167–169].

Table 12.5. Differential diagnosis of myelofibrosis in the pediatric setting.

Non-neoplastic etiologies
- Vitamin D-dependent rickets
- Granulomatous disease
- Osteopetrosis
- Familial hemophagocytic lymphohistiocytosis
- Primary hyperparathyroidism
- Renal osteodystrophy
- Healing fracture site or previous bone marrow biopsy site

Neoplastic etiologies
- Acute leukemia
  - acute megakaryoblastic leukemia
  - acute lymphoblastic leukemia
- Lymphoma, especially classical Hodgkin lymphoma
- Metastatic solid tumor
  - neuroblastoma
- Myeloproliferative neoplasms
  - chronic myelogenous leukemia
  - primary myelofibrosis
- Histiocytic disorders
  - Langerhans cell histiocytosis
- Systemic mastocytosis

Cytogenetics and molecular diagnostics

Recurrent numerical or structural chromosomal abnormalities have not been described in pediatric PM; however, a negative cytogenetics study is useful to exclude other etiologies of myelofibrosis. It is currently unknown whether mutations in *JAK2* play a pathogenetic role in pediatric PM, as has been observed in approximately 50% of adult cases.

A

B

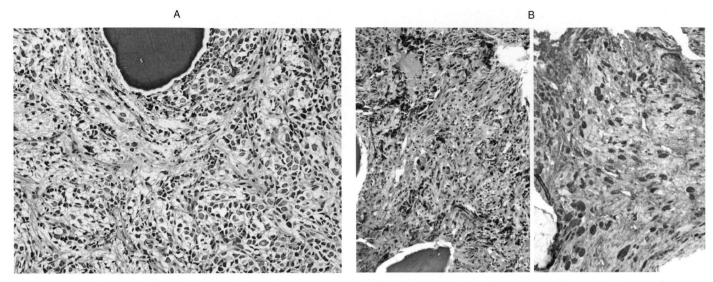

Fig. 12.20. Histologic mimics of idiopathic myelofibrosis in the pediatric setting. (A) This bone marrow biopsy shows extensive fibrosis in which nests of tumor cells are apparent (lower right-hand corner). Immunohistochemical studies confirmed a diagnosis of metastatic neuroblastoma. In some cases, the infiltrate of neoplastic cells can be masked somewhat by more pronounced fibrosis. (B) In this bone marrow biopsy from a toddler, there is marked fibrosis with significant crush artifact (left); in some areas megakaryocytes are apparent. More numerous megakaryocytic cells, including megakaryoblasts, are highlighted by a factor VII-related antigen immunohistochemical stain (right), helping to confirm the diagnosis of acute megakaryoblastic leukemia.

Table 12.6. WHO classification of mastocytosis.

Cutaneous mastocytosis
- Urticaria pigmentosa/maculopapular cutaneous mastocytosis
- Diffuse cutaneous mastocytosis
- Solitary cutaneous mastocytoma

Indolent systemic mastocytosis
Systemic mastocytosis with an associated clonal hematologic non-mast cell lineage disease (AHNMD)
Aggressive systemic mastocytosis
Mast cell leukemia
Mast cell sarcoma
Extracutaneous mastocytoma

Mastocytosis

Mast cell disease, in the form of urticaria pigmentosa, was first described clinically by Nettleship and Tay in 1869 [170]. Paul Ehrlich identified the mast cell in 1878 through his work with the aniline dyes and their application to histologic staining [171]. Ehrlich's pioneering studies facilitated the subsequent demonstration of the central pathogenetic role of the mast cell in these disorders [172–174]. Mast cell disease is clinically and pathologically heterogeneous and is relatively uncommon. Nevertheless, approximately 65% of cases develop in children. Intriguingly, there are significant differences in the clinical behavior and pathologic manifestations of mast cell disease in children and adults, which reflect differences in their underlying pathogenesis. Seven major subtypes of mast cell disease have been recognized by the WHO (Table 12.6). For practical purposes, however, only three of these entities occur with any significant frequency in children; namely, cutaneous mastocytosis, indolent systemic mastocytosis (SM), and SM with an associated clonal hematologic non-mast cell lineage disease (AHNMD). The last of these is included in Chapter 15 on acute myeloid leukemia, and will not be discussed in detail here.

Pathogenesis

Mast cells are derived from bone marrow HSCs [175–177]. KIT is expressed by HSCs and is rapidly downregulated upon lineage commitment and differentiation. However, mast cells are unique among terminally differentiated hematopoietic cells in that they express high levels of KIT (CD117), the cell-surface receptor for stem cell factor (SCF; also known as kit ligand or KITLG). KIT is a receptor tyrosine kinase comprised of an extracellular domain which participates in ligand binding and two intracellular motifs, a juxtamembrane domain with autoinhibitory function and a split tyrosine kinase domain; KIT biochemistry and signaling has been recently reviewed in Orfao *et al.* [178]. Binding of SCF induces KIT dimerization and the phosphorylation of two critical tyrosine residues in the autoinhibitory domain. This in turn leads to conformational changes in the tyrosine kinase domain, phosphorylation of key target molecules, and activation of downstream signaling pathways mediated by phosphatidylinositol 3-kinase, protein kinase C, the mitogen-activated protein kinases, and the JAK/STATs.

The importance of the SCF-KIT signaling pathway in mast cell ontogeny was confirmed by the analysis of mouse strains which harbor mutations in either the *SCF* or *KIT* gene and which have profound deficiencies of mast cells, among other abnormalities [179–184]. That perturbation of KIT signaling might likewise play a role in mast cell neoplasia was suggested by the identification of *KIT* mutations in rodent and human mast cell leukemia cell lines [185, 186]. Subsequently, *KIT* mutations were identified in urticaria pigmentosa and SM [187, 188].

KIT mutations have been detected in several human malignancies, including gastrointestinal stromal tumor, germ cell tumors, melanoma, acute myeloid leukemia and other myeloproliferative disorders [178]. *KIT* mutations in these various malignancies can be broadly categorized into two groups of mutations. The "regulatory type" mutation disrupts the function of the KIT autoinhibitory domain, resulting in dysregulated KIT signaling. The second group is the so-called "enzymatic pocket type" in which the mutation directly targets the enzymatic site of the TK2 activation loop, resulting in KIT activation and signaling in the absence of ligand binding and KIT dimerization [189]. In adults with SM, the commonest mutation is that of an A→T point mutation at nucleotide position 7176, resulting in the replacement of an aspartic acid residue by valine (D816V) [187, 188, 190, 191].

While KIT mutations are detected in nearly all cases of adult systemic mastocytosis, such mutations are generally uncommon in pediatric cutaneous mast cell disease [190, 192, 193]. Indeed, pediatric cutaneous mastocytosis harboring KIT mutations behaves clinically more like its adult counterpart, which often coexists with or progresses to systemic mastocytosis. Interestingly, *KIT* mutations (either D816V or the D816F) were detected in 83% of 14 Japanese children with seemingly indolent cutaneous disease in one study [194]. It is uncertain whether these findings reflect ethnic variations or bona fide pathogenetic differences. In summary, *KIT* mutations are generally rare in pediatric cutaneous mastocytosis and appear to represent a marker for more aggressive disease. Furthermore, the absence of *KIT* mutations suggests that perturbation of other cell signaling pathways may give rise to mast cell disease in children.

Clinical and laboratory features

Children with mast cell disease typically present at an early age, with approximately half of affected children presenting before two years of age [195, 196]. While there is no sex predilection, mast cell disease may be more common in Caucasian children. The most common clinical presentation is that of cutaneous mastocytoma, which usually develops during early infancy and may be present at birth. These manifest as single or multiple reddish-brown nodules or plaques which can be several centimeters in greatest dimension. Cutaneous mastocytomas may have associated bulla formation. Urticaria pigmentosa/maculopapular cutaneous mastocytosis (UP/MPCM) usually develops in infants, and clinically takes the form of tan-brown macules or papules distributed over the trunk and extremities (Fig. 12.21) [196]. Although the trunk is the most common site, these lesions may occur anywhere, including the mucous membranes. As with mastocytoma, there may be associated bullae. These lesions spontaneously resolve by puberty in approximately 50% of children. In UP, lesions may develop over the course of several months or years, in contrast to multiple mastocytomas which typically present as a single crop of lesions. Diffuse cutaneous mastocytosis and telangiectasia macularis eruptiva perstans are other clinical manifestations of mast cell disease which rarely occur in children.

Children with cutaneous mastocytosis most commonly present with pruritis [195, 197]. Other symptoms include flush-

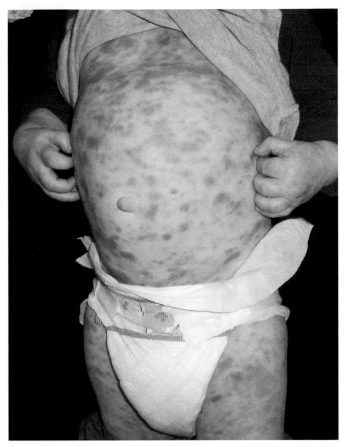

Fig. 12.21. Clinical manifestation of pediatric cutaneous mastocytosis. This 14-month-old male toddler had urticaria pigmentosa present at birth. He has had persistent involvement of over 90% of his cutaneous area with intermittent flare-ups. Numerous tan-brown macules and papules are present, which are focally confluent. His disease is generally well controlled with oral cromolyn sodium and antihistamines. (Clinical image kindly provided by Dr. Jay Kincannon.)

ing, which may be induced by physical stimuli such as stroking and temperature change (the so-called Darier sign), headache, nausea, vomiting, and irritability. Children with extracutaneous involvement may also have hepatosplenomegaly and skeletal lesions.

The criteria for the diagnosis of SM in adults and children have recently been revised as part of the 2008 WHO classification (Table 12.7); diagnosis of SM requires the fulfillment of either one major and one minor criterion, or of three minor criteria in those circumstances where the major criterion is not satisfied. As will be noted, a diagnosis of SM requires not only morphologic confirmation of an extracutaneous mast cell infiltrate but also ancillary laboratory and molecular testing, which will be discussed in this and subsequent sections.

Serum tryptase determination is of utility in the diagnosis and management of patients with mast cell disease [190, 198, 199]. Current assays measure the "total" serum tryptase, which includes precursor and mature forms of the alpha and beta isoforms; tryptase is normally present in the serum at levels less than 20 ng/mL. Because normal and neoplastic mast cells constitutively secrete precursor alpha and beta tryptase,

Table 12.7. Proposed WHO diagnostic criteria for mastocytosis.

Cutaneous
- Skin lesions with typical clinical appearance of mastocytosis
- Biopsy confirming presence of mast cell infiltrate
- No diagnostic evidence of systemic mastocytosis

Systemic[a]

Major
- Multiple, dense mast cell aggregates (≥15 cells/aggregate) in bone marrow or other extracutaneous sites

Minor
- Mast cells with atypical or spindle cell morphology comprise >25% of cells in the infiltrate at bone marrow or extracutaneous sites
- *KIT* codon 816 mutation detected in bone marrow, blood, or other extracutaneous site
- Aberrant co-expression of CD2 and/or CD25 by mast cell infiltrate in bone marrow, blood, or other extracutaneous site
- Elevated serum total tryptase (>20 ng/mL; not applicable in AHNMD)

[a] Fulfillment of the major criterion and one minor criterion, or at least three minor criteria, is required for diagnosis.

serum tryptase determination is not only useful diagnostically but also provides an accurate assessment of the overall disease burden [200]. As such, serum tryptase may be normal or only minimally elevated in patients with cutaneous mastocytosis; whereas, it is often markedly elevated in patients with disseminated disease. In typical cutaneous mastocytosis, other routine laboratory studies have limited diagnostic utility [201, 202]. Of note, hematologic abnormalities are uncommon in children with mastocytosis [203]. However, the onset of significant laboratory abnormalities, for instance, cytopenias or elevated liver enzymes, may identify patients with progression to disseminated disease involving the bone marrow and viscera. In the absence of such findings, it is uncertain as to whether bone marrow examination is warranted in a child with cutaneous mastocytosis.

Pathologic features

Morphology

As discussed above, the skin is the most common site of involvement in pediatric mast cell disease. Cutaneous involvement manifests histologically by a dermal infiltrate of mast cells of variable density. Lesions in UP are comprised of increased numbers of mast cells within the papillary dermis, often with a perivascular distribution (Fig. 12.22). In nodular lesions and in mastocytoma, a more diffuse infiltrate of mast cells is usually present which may extend into subcutaneous adipose tissue (Fig. 12.23). Cytologically, the mast cells usually have a round or spindle cell morphology. There may be associated edema of the papillary dermis. The overlying epidermis may be unremarkable, show subepidermal blister formation, or manifest hyperpigmentation of the basal cell layer.

In adults with SM, typical features of bone marrow involvement include a nodular or diffuse infiltrate of mast cells, which may have associated fibrosis, and often has associated eosinophils and lymphocytes; the mast cells themselves have polygonal or spindle cell morphology, may manifest nuclear contour irregularities, and may contain only a sparse complement of granules (Fig. 12.24) [204, 205]. Clinically significant extracutaneous disease occurs infrequently in pediatric mastocytosis. Consequently, few children undergo bone marrow examination, and as a result, the bone marrow findings in pediatric mastocytosis are poorly characterized [197, 203]. Parker and colleagues have reported that bone marrow mast cell infiltrates are present in approximately one-quarter of pediatric patients with cutaneous mastocytosis. In the biopsy, these are typically subtle lesions comprised of small perivascular mast cell aggregates containing 5–10 mast cells, often admixed with variable numbers of early myeloid cells and eosinophils; in the aspirate, mast cells may be variably increased in frequency

A

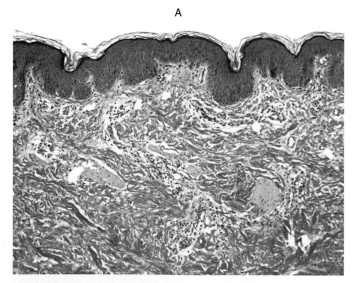

B

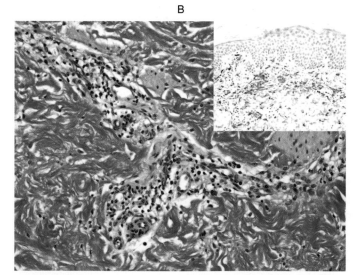

Fig. 12.22. Urticaria pigmentosa, skin biopsy. This six-year-old boy had cutaneous lesions on his upper back. (A) There is a somewhat subtle, predominantly perivascular infiltrate of mast cells present within the dermis. (B) The mast cell infiltrate and scattered admixed eosinophils are more apparent on higher magnification. Immunohistochemical staining for tryptase confirms the presence of a mast cell infiltrate (inset).

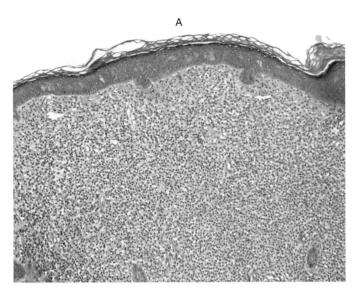
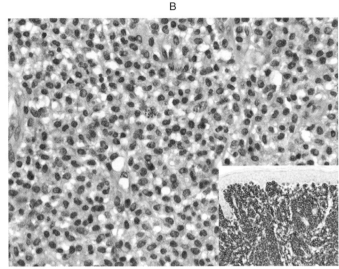

Fig. 12.23. Cutaneous mastocytoma, skin biopsy. This three-year-old female had a lesion on her right thigh. (A) There is a sheet-like infiltrate of mast cells present within the dermis extending up to the dermoepidermal junction. The overlying epidermis is unremarkable. (B) Most of the mast cells contain round or oval nuclei. Scattered admixed eosinophils are present. The mast cells strongly express KIT (CD117; inset).

[203]. The remaining marrow is usually unremarkable with the exception of eosinophilia, which occurs in about half of the cases. Under current WHO criteria, such findings would not be diagnostic of bone marrow involvement in the absence of supportive immunohistochemical and molecular data (see below). In the rare child with progressive disease, mast cell infiltrates indistinguishable to those seen in adult mastocytosis may develop, as described above (Fig. 12.24) [203].

SM with an associated clonal hematologic non-mast cell lineage disease (AHNMD) is discussed in Chapter 15 on AML. Because of the rarity of SM in children, an AHNMD should be rigorously excluded, in particular AML associated with the t(8;21), when mast cell hyperplasia or overt involvement by SM is encountered in a pediatric bone marrow. Other forms of mastocytosis recognized under current WHO criteria are rarely encountered in the pediatric setting. Mast cell sarcoma is an exceedingly rare neoplasm with only two reported cases in children [206, 207].

Immunophenotyping

In cases of suspected mastocytosis, immunophenotyping is essential for confirmation of the cell lineage of the infiltrate. While flow cytometric approaches to characterize normal and neoplastic mast cells have been described and are utilized by some laboratories [208, 209], immunohistochemistry is frequently of greater utility. This is particularly true in children, where mastocytosis is most commonly encountered in skin biopsies. Several diagnostically useful markers of normal and neoplastic mast cells have been identified. These include markers whose expression is not restricted to mast cells, such as KIT (CD117), CD33, and CD68, as well as the lineage-specific marker tryptase [209–215]. The most diagnostically useful of

these are CD117 and tryptase, which are expressed in virtually all cases of cutaneous and systemic mastocytosis. In addition, CD2 and CD25 are frequently expressed in SM, in contrast to normal mast cells [216–223]. Aberrant expression of CD25 is detected in nearly all cases of SM, whereas positivity for CD2 is more variable, which may be due to technical limitations of immunohistochemistry, since a significantly higher percentage of cases are positive for CD2 when assessed by flow cytometry [223, 224].

In pediatric and adult patients without evidence of systemic disease, CD2 and CD25 expression is detected in only about 10–15% of cutaneous mastocytosis cases [222, 224–226]. Interestingly, CD2 or CD25 co-expression in adult cases of cutaneous mastocytosis may identify patients with a propensity for systemic dissemination [222]. Whether aberrant expression of these markers will be similarly predictive of biologic behavior in pediatric cutaneous mastocytosis is currently unknown.

Cytogenetics and molecular diagnostics

No recurrent cytogenetic abnormalities have been described in pediatric mastocytosis. As discussed above, mutations in *KIT* are detected infrequently but may identify patients with a propensity to develop disseminated disease [190, 193]. Furthermore, the commonest *KIT* mutation in mastocytosis, D816V, imparts resistance to imatinib, although mast cells harboring this mutation are susceptible to second generation tyrosine kinase inhibitors [227–230]. Thus, detection of *KIT* mutations has prognostic and therapeutic importance.

Several different molecular techniques have been employed to detect *KIT* mutations, including direct sequencing, restriction fragment length polymorphism (RFLP) analysis,

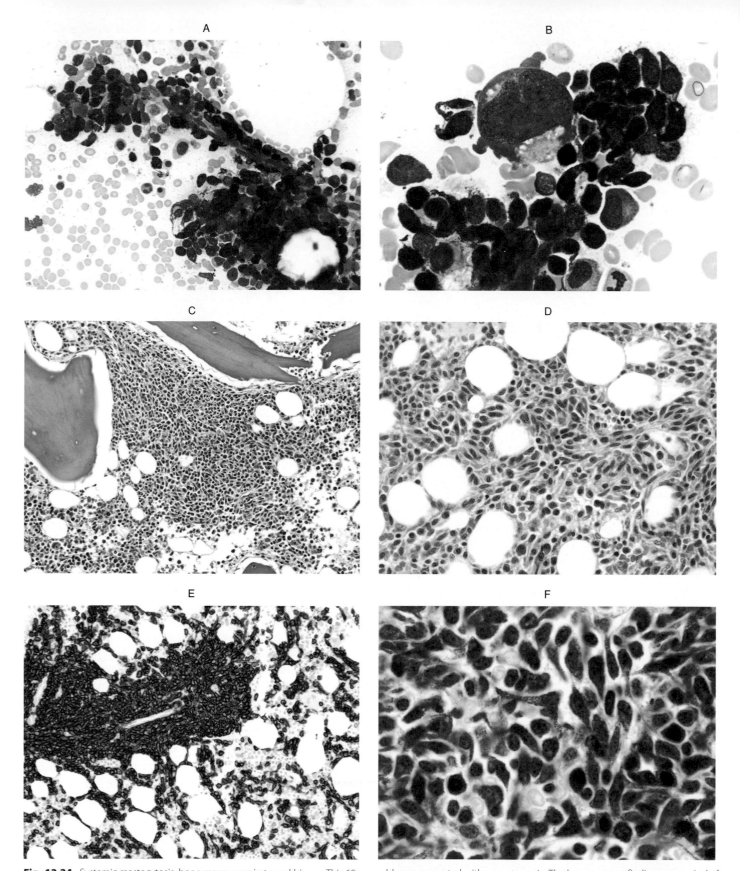

Fig. 12.24. Systemic mastocytosis, bone marrow aspirate and biopsy. This 60-year-old man presented with pancytopenia. The bone marrow findings are typical of the "adult" form of systemic mastocytosis, which also develops in a small minority of pediatric patients. (A) Low-power view of the aspirate smear showing increased numbers of mast cells within the spicules, many decorating capillaries. (B) Scattered clusters of mast cells are present focally. Large aggregates of mast cells are often not present in the aspirate, due to the difficulty in aspirating mast cell infiltrates. (C) The bone marrow biopsy revealed the presence of multiple mast cell aggregates, some of which had a paratrabecular distribution. (D) At higher power, the spindle cell morphology of many of the mast cells is apparent. In cases with pronounced spindle cell morphology or significant fibrosis, the mast cell infiltrate can be subtle. (E) The aggregates and interstitial infiltrate of mast cells are strongly positive for KIT (CD117). (F) The metachromatic granules of the mast cell infiltrate are highlighted by toluidine blue staining. Neoplastic mast cells usually contain fewer granules than do normal mast cells.

peptide–nucleic acid-mediated PCR, and allele-specific PCR [231–236]. Because of the intrinsic biologic properties of mast cell disease, limiting numbers of mast cells may be present in clinical material submitted for molecular testing. Consequently, methods used to detect *KIT* mutations in mastocytosis should have high sensitivity, and analysis of repeat biopsies may be necessary to exclude false-negative results. Because of its relatively poor sensitivity, direct sequencing has limited utility for the detection of *KIT* mutations in clinical specimens.

Acknowledgements

I thank Ms. Tina Motroni (St. Jude Children's Research Hospital, Memphis, TN) for much assistance with preparation of the photomicrographs, and Drs. David Head (Dept. of Pathology, Vanderbilt University, Nashville, TN), Jay Kincannon (Dept. of Pediatrics, Arkansas Children's Hospital, Little Rock, AR), Jeffrey Sawyer (Dept. of Pathology, University of Arkansas for Medical Sciences, Little Rock, AR) and Professor Luigi M. Larocca (Catholic University of Rome, Rome, Italy) for generously contributing images.

References

1. **Ries LAG, Smith MA, Gurney JG**, *et al.* (eds.). *Cancer Incidence and Survival Among Children and Adolescents: United States SEER Program 1975–1995*, NIH Pub. No. 99–4649. Bethesda, MD: National Cancer Institute, SEER Program; 1999.

2. **Coebergh JW, Reedijk AM, de Vries E**, *et al.* Leukaemia incidence and survival in children and adolescents in Europe during 1978–1997. Report from the Automated Childhood Cancer Information System project. *European Journal of Cancer*. 2006;**42**:2019–2036.

3. **Hasle H, Olesen G, Kerndrup G, Philip P, Jacobsen N.** Chronic neutrophil leukaemia in adolescence and young adulthood. *British Journal of Haematology*. 1996;**94**:628–630.

4. **Bennett JH.** Case of hypertrophy of the spleen and liver in which death took place from suppuration of the blood. *Edinburgh Medical and Surgical Journal*. 1845;**64**:413–423.

5. **Nowell PC, Hungerford DA.** A minute chromosome in human chronic granulocytic leukemia. *Science*. 1960;**132**:1497.

6. **Rowley JD.** A new consistent chromosomal abnormality in chronic myelogenous leukaemia identified by quinacrine fluorescence and Giemsa staining. *Nature*. 1973;**243**:290–293.

7. **Shtivelman E, Lifshitz B, Gale RP, Canaani E.** Fused transcript of abl and bcr genes in chronic myelogenous leukaemia. *Nature*. 1985;**315**:550–554.

8. **Grosveld G, Verwoerd T, van Agthoven T**, *et al.* The chronic myelocytic cell line K562 contains a breakpoint in bcr and produces a chimeric bcr/c-abl transcript. *Molecular and Cellular Biology*. 1986;**6**:607–616.

9. **Druker BJ, Talpaz M, Resta DJ**, *et al.* Efficacy and safety of a specific inhibitor of the BCR-ABL tyrosine kinase in chronic myeloid leukemia. *The New England Journal of Medicine*. 2001;**344**:1031–1037.

10. **Hervy M, Hoffman L, Beckerle MC.** From the membrane to the nucleus and back again: bifunctional focal adhesion proteins. *Current Opinion in Cell Biology*. 2006;**18**:524–532.

11. **Pendergast AM.** The Abl family kinases: mechanisms of regulation and signaling. *Advances in Cancer Research*. 2002;**85**:51–100.

12. **Schwartzberg PL, Stall AM, Hardin JD**, *et al.* Mice homozygous for the ablm1 mutation show poor viability and depletion of selected B and T cell populations. *Cell*. 1991;**65**:1165–1175.

13. **Tybulewicz VL, Crawford CE, Jackson PK, Bronson RT, Mulligan RC.** Neonatal lethality and lymphopenia in mice with a homozygous disruption of the c-abl proto-oncogene. *Cell*. 1991;**65**:1153–1163.

14. **Dorsch M, Goff SP.** Increased sensitivity to apoptotic stimuli in c-abl-deficient progenitor B-cell lines. *Proceedings of the National Academy of Sciences of the United States of America*. 1996;**93**:13131–13136.

15. **Zipfel PA, Grove M, Blackburn K**, *et al.* The c-Abl tyrosine kinase is regulated downstream of the B cell antigen receptor and interacts with CD19. *Journal of Immunology*. 2000;**165**:6872–6879.

16. **Cho YJ, Cunnick JM, Yi SJ**, *et al.* Abr and Bcr, two homologous Rac GTPase-activating proteins, control multiple cellular functions of murine macrophages. *Molecular and Cellular Biology*. 2007;**27**:899–911.

17. **Daley GQ, Van Etten RA, Baltimore D.** Induction of chronic myelogenous leukemia in mice by the P210bcr/abl gene of the Philadelphia chromosome. *Science*. 1990;**247**:824–830.

18. **Pear WS, Miller JP, Xu L**, *et al.* Efficient and rapid induction of a chronic myelogenous leukemia-like myeloproliferative disease in mice receiving P210 bcr/abl-transduced bone marrow. *Blood*. 1998;**92**:3780–3792.

19. **Zhang X, Ren R.** Bcr-Abl efficiently induces a myeloproliferative disease and production of excess interleukin-3 and granulocyte-macrophage colony-stimulating factor in mice: a novel model for chronic myelogenous leukemia. *Blood*. 1998;**92**:3829–3840.

20. **Pane F, Intrieri M, Quintarelli C**, *et al.* BCR/ABL genes and leukemic phenotype: from molecular mechanisms to clinical correlations 1. *Oncogene*. 2002;**21**:8652–8667.

21. **Goldman JM, Melo JV.** Chronic myeloid leukemia – advances in biology and new approaches to treatment. *The New England Journal of Medicine*. 2003; **349**:1451–1464.

22. **Pane F, Frigeri F, Sindona M**, *et al.* Neutrophilic-chronic myeloid leukemia: a distinct disease with a specific molecular marker (BCR/ABL with C3/A2 junction). *Blood*. 1996;**88**:2410–2414.

23. **Wilson G, Frost L, Goodeve A**, *et al.* BCR-ABL transcript with an e19a2 (c3a2) junction in classical chronic myeloid leukemia. *Blood*. 1997;**89**:3064.

24. **Mittre H, Leymarie P, Macro M, Leporrier M.** A new case of chronic myeloid leukemia with c3/a2 BCR/ABL junction. Is it really a distinct disease? *Blood*. 1997;**89**:4239–4241.

25. **Melo JV, Barnes DJ.** Chronic myeloid leukaemia as a model of disease evolution in human cancer. *Nature Reviews. Cancer*. 2007;**7**:441–453.

26. **Mejia-Arangure JM, Bonilla M, Lorenzana R**, *et al*. Incidence of leukemias in children from El Salvador and Mexico City between 1996 and 2000: population-based data. *BMC Cancer*. 2005;**5**:33.

27. **Castro-Malaspina H, Schaison G, Briere J**, *et al*. Philadelphia chromosome-positive chronic myelocytic leukemia in children. Survival and prognostic factors. *Cancer*. 1983;**52**:721–727.

28. **Chang YH, Lu MY, Jou ST**, *et al*. Forty-seven children suffering from chronic myeloid leukemia at a center over a 25-year period. *Pediatric Hematology and Oncology*. 2003;**20**: 505–515.

29. **Millot F, Traore P, Guilhot J**, *et al*. Clinical and biological features at diagnosis in 40 children with chronic myeloid leukemia. *Pediatrics* 2005;**116**: 140–143.

30. **Dow LW, Raimondi SC, Culbert SJ**, *et al*. Response to alpha-interferon in children with Philadelphia chromosome-positive chronic myelocytic leukemia. *Cancer*. 1991;**68**:1678–1684.

31. **Fioretos T, Heim S, Garwicz S, Ludvigsson J, Mitelman F**. Molecular analysis of Philadelphia-positive childhood chronic myeloid leukemia. *Leukemia*. 1992;**6**:723–725.

32. **Kantarjian HM, Keating MJ, Talpaz M**, *et al*. Chronic myelogenous leukemia in blast crisis. Analysis of 242 patients. *The American Journal of Medicine*. 1987;**83**:445–454.

33. **Cervantes F, Villamor N, Esteve J**, *et al*. 'Lymphoid' blast crisis of chronic myeloid leukaemia is associated with distinct clinicohaematological features. *British Journal of Haematology*. 1998; **100**:123–128.

34. **Khalidi HS, Brynes RK, Medeiros LJ**, *et al*. The immunophenotype of blast transformation of chronic myelogenous leukemia: a high frequency of mixed lineage phenotype in "lymphoid" blasts and a comparison of morphologic, immunophenotypic, and molecular findings. *Modern Pathology*. 1998;**11**: 1211–1221.

35. **Lorand-Metze I, Vassallo J, Souza CA**. Histological and cytological heterogeneity of bone marrow in Philadelphia-positive chronic myelogenous leukaemia at diagnosis.

British Journal of Haematology. 1987;**67**:45–49.

36. **Dickstein JI, Vardiman JW**. Hematopathologic findings in the myeloproliferative disorders. *Seminars in Oncology*. 1995;**22**:355–373.

37. **Thiele J, Kvasnicka HM, Schmitt-Graeff A**, *et al*. Bone marrow features and clinical findings in chronic myeloid leukemia – a comparative, multicenter, immunohistological and morphometric study on 614 patients. *Leukemia & Lymphoma*. 2000;**36**:295–308.

38. **Albrecht M**. "Gaucher-Zellen" bei chronisch myeloischer Leukamie. *Blut*. 1966;**13**:169–179.

39. **Dosik H, Rosner F, Sawitsky A**. Acquired lipidosis: Gaucher-like cells and "blue cells" in chronic granulocytic leukemia. *Seminars in Hematology*. 1972;**9**:309–316.

40. **Kelsey PR, Geary CG**. Sea-blue histiocytes and Gaucher cells in bone marrow of patients with chronic myeloid leukaemia. *Journal of Clinical Pathology*. 1988;**41**:960–962.

41. **Anastasi J, Musvee T, Roulston D**, *et al*. Pseudo-Gaucher histiocytes identified up to 1 year after transplantation for CML are BCR/ABL-positive. *Leukemia* 1998;**12**:233–237.

42. **Kantarjian HM, Bueso-Ramos CE, Talpaz M**, *et al*. Significance of myelofibrosis in early chronic-phase, chronic myelogenous leukemia on imatinib mesylate therapy. *Cancer*. 2005;**104**:777–780.

43. **Buesche G, Ganser A, Schlegelberger B**, *et al*. Marrow fibrosis and its relevance during imatinib treatment of chronic myeloid leukemia. *Leukemia*. 2007;**21**:2420–2427.

44. **Beham-Schmid C, Apfelbeck U, Sill H**, *et al*. Treatment of chronic myelogenous leukemia with the tyrosine kinase inhibitor STI571 results in marked regression of bone marrow fibrosis. *Blood* 2002;**99**:381–383.

45. **Braziel RM, Launder TM, Druker BJ**, *et al*. Hematopathologic and cytogenetic findings in imatinib mesylate-treated chronic myelogenous leukemia patients: 14 months' experience. *Blood* 2002;**100**:435–441.

46. **Hasserjian RP, Boecklin F, Parker S**, *et al*. STI571 (imatinib mesylate) reduces bone marrow cellularity and

normalizes morphologic features irrespective of cytogenetic response. *American Journal of Clinical Pathology*. 2002;**117**:360–367.

47. **Frater JL, Tallman MS, Variakojis D**, *et al*. Chronic myeloid leukemia following therapy with imatinib mesylate (Gleevec). Bone marrow histopathology and correlation with genetic status. *American Journal of Clinical Pathology*. 2003;**119**:833–841.

48. **Thiele J, Kvasnicka HM, Schmitt-Graeff A**, *et al*. Bone marrow changes in chronic myelogenous leukaemia after long-term treatment with the tyrosine kinase inhibitor STI571: an immunohistochemical study on 75 patients. *Histopathology*. 2005;**46**:540–550.

49. **Lokeshwar N, Kumar L, Kumari M**. Severe bone marrow aplasia following imatinib mesylate in a patient with chronic myelogenous leukemia. *Leukemia & Lymphoma*. 2005;**46**: 781–784.

50. **Srinivas U, Pillai LS, Kumar R, Pati HP, Saxena R**. Bone marrow aplasia – a rare complication of imatinib therapy in CML patients. *American Journal of Hematology*. 2007;**82**:314–316.

51. **Bain B, Catovsky D, O'Brien M, Spiers AS, Richards GH**. Megakaryoblastic transformation of chronic granulocytic leukaemia. An electron microscopy and cytochemical study. *Journal of Clinical Pathology*. 1977;**30**:235–242.

52. **Ekblom M, Borgström G, von Willebrand E**, *et al*. Erythroid blast crisis in chronic myelogenous leukemia. *Blood*. 1983;**62**:591–596.

53. **Villeval JL, Cramer P, Lemoine F**, *et al*. Phenotype of early erythroblastic leukemias. *Blood*. 1986;**68**:1167–1174.

54. **Hernandez JM, Gonzalez-Sarmiento R, Martin C**, *et al*. Immunophenotypic, genomic and clinical characteristics of blast crisis of chronic myelogenous leukaemia. *British Journal of Haematology*. 1991;**79**:408–414.

55. **Urbano-Ispizua A, Cervantes F, Matutes E**, *et al*. Immunophenotypic characteristics of blast crisis of chronic myeloid leukaemia: correlations with clinico-biological features and survival. *Leukemia*. 1993;7:1349–1354.

56. **Kosugi N, Tojo A, Shinzaki H, Nagamura-Inoue T, Asano S**. The preferential expression of CD7 and CD34 in myeloid blast crisis in chronic

myeloid leukemia. *Blood*. 2000;**95**: 2188–2189.

57. **Kantarjian H, O'Brien S, Cortes J,** *et al.* Sudden onset of the blastic phase of chronic myelogenous leukemia: patterns and implications. *Cancer*. 2003;**98**:81–85.

58. **Morimoto A, Ogami A, Chiyonobu T,** *et al.* Early blastic transformation following complete cytogenetic response in a pediatric chronic myeloid leukemia patient treated with imatinib mesylate. *Journal of Pediatric Hematology/Oncology*. 2004;**26**:320–322.

59. **Avery S, Nadal E, Marin D,** *et al.* Lymphoid transformation in a CML patient in complete cytogenetic remission following treatment with imatinib. *Leukemia Research*. 2004;**28**(Suppl 1): S75–S77.

60. **Alimena G, Breccia M, Latagliata R,** *et al.* Sudden blast crisis in patients with Philadelphia chromosome-positive chronic myeloid leukemia who achieved complete cytogenetic remission after imatinib therapy. *Cancer*. 2006;**107**:1008–1013.

61. **Jabbour E, Kantarjian H, O'Brien S,** *et al.* Sudden blastic transformation in patients with chronic myeloid leukemia treated with imatinib mesylate. *Blood*. 2006;**107**:480–482.

62. **Kim AS, Goldstein SC, Luger S, Van Deerlin VM, Bagg A.** Sudden extramedullary T-lymphoblastic blast crisis in chronic myelogenous leukemia: a nonrandom event associated with imatinib? *American Journal of Clinical Pathology*. 2008;**129**:639–648.

63. **Ganesan TS, Rassool F, Guo AP,** *et al.* Rearrangement of the bcr gene in Philadelphia chromosome-negative chronic myeloid leukemia. *Blood* 1986;**68**:957–960.

64. **Shtalrid M, Talpaz M, Blick M,** *et al.* Philadelphia-negative chronic myelogenous leukemia with breakpoint cluster region rearrangement: molecular analysis, clinical characteristics, and response to therapy. *Journal of Clinical Oncology*. 1988;**6**: 1569–1575.

65. **Morel F, Herry A,** Le Bris MJ, *et al.* Contribution of fluorescence in situ hybridization analyses to the characterization of masked and complex Philadelphia chromosome translocations in chronic myelocytic

leukemia. *Cancer Genetics and Cytogenetics*. 2003;**147**:115–120.

66. **Aoun P, Wiggins M, Pickering D,** *et al.* Interphase fluorescence in situ hybridization studies for the detection of 9q34 deletions in chronic myelogenous leukemia: a practical approach to clinical diagnosis. *Cancer Genetics and Cytogenetics*. 2004;**154**: 138–143.

67. **Costa D, Carrio A, Madrigal I,** *et al.* Studies of complex Ph translocations in cases with chronic myelogenous leukemia and one with acute lymphoblastic leukemia. *Cancer Genetics and Cytogenetics*. 2006;**166**: 89–93.

68. **Hughes T, Deininger M, Hochhaus A,** *et al.* Monitoring CML patients responding to treatment with tyrosine kinase inhibitors: review and recommendations for harmonizing current methodology for detecting BCR-ABL transcripts and kinase domain mutations and for expressing results. *Blood*. 2006;**108**:28–37.

69. **Baccarani M, Saglio G, Goldman J,** *et al.* Evolving concepts in the management of chronic myeloid leukemia: recommendations from an expert panel on behalf of the European LeukemiaNet. *Blood*. 2006;**108**:1809–1820.

70. **Kantarjian H, Schiffer C, Jones D, Cortes J.** Monitoring the response and course of chronic myeloid leukemia in the modern era of BCR-ABL tyrosine kinase inhibitors: practical advice on the use and interpretation of monitoring methods. *Blood*. 2008;**111**: 1774–1780.

71. **Derderian PM, Kantarjian HM, Talpaz M,** *et al.* Chronic myelogenous leukemia in the lymphoid blastic phase: characteristics, treatment response, and prognosis. *The American Journal of Medicine*. 1993;**94**:69–74.

72. **Johansson B, Fioretos T, Mitelman F.** Cytogenetic and molecular genetic evolution of chronic myeloid leukemia. *Acta Haematologica*. 2002;**107**:76–94.

73. **Castaigne S, Berger R, Jolly V,** *et al.* Promyelocytic blast crisis of chronic myelocytic leukemia with both t(9;22) and t(15;17) in M3 cells. *Cancer*. 1984; **54**:2409–2413.

74. **Hogge DE, Misawa S, Schiffer CA, Testa JR.** Promyelocytic blast crisis in chronic granulocytic leukemia with

15;17 translocation. *Leukemia Research*. 1984;**8**:1019–1023.

75. **Yin CC, Medeiros LJ, Glassman AB, Lin P.** t(8;21)(q22;q22) in blast phase of chronic myelogenous leukemia. *American Journal of Clinical Pathology*. 2004;**121**:836–842.

76. **Wu Y, Slovak ML, Snyder DS, Arber DA.** Coexistence of inversion 16 and the Philadelphia chromosome in acute and chronic myeloid leukemias: report of six cases and review of literature. *American Journal of Clinical Pathology*. 2006;**125**:260–266.

77. **Merzianu M, Medeiros LJ, Cortes J,** *et al.* inv(16)(p13q22) in chronic myelogenous leukemia in blast phase: a clinicopathologic, cytogenetic, and molecular study of five cases. *American Journal of Clinical Pathology*. 2005;**124**: 807–814.

78. **Chan KW, Kaikov Y, Wadsworth LD.** Thrombocytosis in childhood: a survey of 94 patients. *Pediatrics*. 1989;**84**:1064–1067.

79. **Heath HW, Pearson HA.** Thrombocytosis in pediatric outpatients. *The Journal of Pediatrics*. 1989;**114**:805–807.

80. **Vora AJ, Lilleyman JS.** Secondary thrombocytosis. *Archives of Disease in Childhood*. 1993;**68**:88–90.

81. **Yohannan MD, Higgy KE, al-Mashhadani SA, Santhosh-Kumar CR.** Thrombocytosis. Etiologic analysis of 663 patients. *Clinical Pediatrics*. 1994; **33**:340–343.

82. **Heng JT, Tan AM.** Thrombocytosis in childhood. *Singapore Medical Journal*. 1998;**39**:485–487.

83. **Chen HL, Chiou SS, Sheen JM,** *et al.* Thrombocytosis in children at one medical center of southern Taiwan. *Acta Paediatrica Taiwanica*. 1999;**40**: 309–313.

84. **Matsubara K, Fukaya T, Nigami H,** *et al.* Age-dependent changes in the incidence and etiology of childhood thrombocytosis. *Acta Haematologica*. 2004;**111**:132–137.

85. **Hasle H.** Incidence of essential thrombocythaemia in children. *British Journal of Haematology*. 2000;**110**: 751.

86. **Jensen MK, de Nully BP, Nielsen OJ, Hasselbalch HC.** Incidence, clinical features and outcome of essential thrombocythaemia in a well defined

geographical area. *European Journal of Haematology*. 2000;**65**:132–139.

87. **Dame C, Sutor AH**. Primary and secondary thrombocytosis in childhood. *British Journal of Haematology*. 2005;**129**:165–177.

88. **Gassas A, Doyle JJ, Weitzman S**, *et al*. A basic classification and a comprehensive examination of pediatric myeloproliferative syndromes. *Journal of Pediatric Hematology/Oncology*. 2005;**27**:192–196.

89. **Choi ES, Nichol JL, Hokom MM, Hornkohl AC, Hunt P**. Platelets generated in vitro from proplatelet-displaying human megakaryocytes are functional. *Blood*. 1995;**85**:402–413.

90. **Cramer EM, Norol F, Guichard J**, *et al*. Ultrastructure of platelet formation by human megakaryocytes cultured with the Mpl ligand. *Blood*. 1997;**89**:2336–2346.

91. **Junt T, Schulze H, Chen Z**, *et al*. Dynamic visualization of thrombopoiesis within bone marrow. *Science*. 2007;**317**:1767–1770.

92. **Stuart MJ, Murphy S, Oski FA**. A simple nonradioisotope technic for the determination of platelet life-span. *The New England Journal of Medicine*. 1975;**292**:1310–1313.

93. **Sinzinger H, Fitscha P, Peskar BA**. Platelet half-life, plasma thromboxane B2 and circulating endothelial cells in peripheral vascular disease. *Angiology*. 1986;**37**:112–118.

94. **Fritz E, Ludwig H, Scheithauer W, Sinzinger H**. Shortened platelet half-life in multiple myeloma. *Blood*. 1986;**68**:514–520.

95. **Shivdasani RA**. Molecular and transcriptional regulation of megakaryocyte differentiation. *Stem Cells*. 2001;**19**:397–407.

96. **Deutsch VR, Tomer A**. Megakaryocyte development and platelet production. *British Journal of Haematology*. 2006;**134**:453–466.

97. **Goldfarb AN**. Transcriptional control of megakaryocyte development. *Oncogene*. 2007;**26**:6795–6802.

98. **Ballmaier M, Germeshausen M, Schulze H**, *et al*. c-mpl mutations are the cause of congenital amegakaryocytic thrombocytopenia. *Blood* 2001;**97**:139–146.

99. **Ihara K, Ishii E, Eguchi M**, *et al*. Identification of mutations in the c-mpl gene in congenital amegakaryocytic thrombocytopenia. *Proceedings of the National Academy of Sciences of the United States of America*. 1999;**96**:3132–3136.

100. **Mehaffey MG, Newton AL, Gandhi MJ, Crossley M, Drachman JG**. X-linked thrombocytopenia caused by a novel mutation of GATA-1. *Blood*. 2001;**98**:2681–2688.

101. **Nichols KE, Crispino JD, Poncz M**, *et al*. Familial dyserythropoietic anaemia and thrombocytopenia due to an inherited mutation in GATA1. *Nature Genetics*. 2000;**24**:266–270.

102. **Song WJ, Sullivan MG, Legare RD**, *et al*. Haploinsufficiency of CBFA2 causes familial thrombocytopenia with propensity to develop acute myelogenous leukaemia. *Nature Genetics*. 1999;**23**:166–175.

103. **Tonelli R, Scardovi AL, Pession A**, *et al*. Compound heterozygosity for two different amino-acid substitution mutations in the thrombopoietin receptor (c-mpl gene) in congenital amegakaryocytic thrombocytopenia (CAMT). *Human Genetics*. 2000;**107**:225–233.

104. **van den Oudenrijn S, Bruin M, Folman CC**, *et al*. Mutations in the thrombopoietin receptor, Mpl, in children with congenital amegakaryocytic thrombocytopenia. *British Journal of Haematology*. 2000;**110**:441–448.

105. **Kondo T, Okabe M, Sanada M**, *et al*. Familial essential thrombocythemia associated with one-base deletion in the 5′-untranslated region of the thrombopoietin gene. *Blood*. 1998;**92**:1091–1096.

106. **Wiestner A, Schlemper RJ, Van Der Maas AP, Skoda RC**. An activating splice donor mutation in the thrombopoietin gene causes hereditary thrombocythaemia. *Nature Genetics*. 1998;**18**:49–52.

107. **Ghilardi N, Wiestner A, Kikuchi M, Ohsaka A, Skoda RC**. Hereditary thrombocythaemia in a Japanese family is caused by a novel point mutation in the thrombopoietin gene. *British Journal of Haematology*. 1999;**107**:310–316.

108. **Ding J, Komatsu H, Wakita A**, *et al*. Familial essential thrombocythemia associated with a dominant-positive activating mutation of the c-MPL gene, which encodes for the receptor for thrombopoietin. *Blood*. 2004;**103**:4198–4200.

109. **Onishi M, Mui AL, Morikawa Y**, *et al*. Identification of an oncogenic form of the thrombopoietin receptor MPL using retrovirus-mediated gene transfer. *Blood*. 1996;**88**:1399–1406.

110. **Moliterno AR, Williams DM, Gutierrez-Alamillo LI**, *et al*. Mpl Baltimore: a thrombopoietin receptor polymorphism associated with thrombocytosis. *Proceedings of the National Academy of Sciences of the United States of America*. 2004;**101**:11444–11447.

111. **Tecuceanu N, Dardik R, Rabizadeh E, Raanani P, Inbal A**. A family with hereditary thrombocythaemia and normal genes for thrombopoietin and c-Mpl. *British Journal of Haematology*. 2006;**135**:348–351.

112. **Teofili L, Giona F, Martini M**, *et al*. The revised WHO diagnostic criteria for Ph-negative myeloproliferative diseases are not appropriate for the diagnostic screening of childhood polycythemia vera and essential thrombocythemia. *Blood*. 2007;**110**:3384–3386.

113. **Veselovska J, Pospisilova D, Pekova S**, *et al*. Most pediatric patients with essential thrombocythemia show hypersensitivity to erythropoietin in vitro, with rare JAK2 V617F-positive erythroid colonies. *Leukemia Research*. 2008;**32**:369–377.

114. **Mertens C, Darnell JE Jr**. SnapShot: JAK-STAT signaling. *Cell*. 2007;**131**:612.

115. **Tefferi A**. JAK and MPL mutations in myeloid malignancies. *Leukemia & Lymphoma*. 2008;**49**:388–397.

116. **Neubauer H, Cumano A, Muller M**, *et al*. Jak2 deficiency defines an essential developmental checkpoint in definitive hematopoiesis. *Cell*. 1998;**93**:397–409.

117. **Parganas E, Wang D, Stravopodis D**, *et al*. Jak2 is essential for signaling through a variety of cytokine receptors. *Cell*. 1998;**93**:385–395.

118. **James C, Ugo V, Le Couedic JP**, *et al*. A unique clonal JAK2 mutation leading to constitutive signalling causes polycythaemia vera. *Nature*. 2005;**434**:1144–1148.

119. **Levine RL, Wadleigh M, Cools J**, *et al*. Activating mutation in the tyrosine

kinase JAK2 in polycythemia vera, essential thrombocythemia, and myeloid metaplasia with myelofibrosis. *Cancer Cell.* 2005;**7**:387–397.

120. **Baxter EJ, Scott LM, Campbell PJ,** *et al.* Acquired mutation of the tyrosine kinase JAK2 in human myeloproliferative disorders. *Lancet.* 2005;**365**:1054–1061.

121. **Kralovics R, Passamonti F, Buser AS,** *et al.* A gain-of-function mutation of JAK2 in myeloproliferative disorders. *The New England Journal of Medicine.* 2005;**352**:1779–1790.

122. **Khwaja A.** The role of Janus kinases in haemopoiesis and haematological malignancy. *British Journal of Haematology.* 2006;**134**:366–384.

123. **Levine RL, Pardanani A, Tefferi A, Gilliland DG.** Role of JAK2 in the pathogenesis and therapy of myeloproliferative disorders. *Nature Reviews. Cancer.* 2007;**7**:673–683.

124. **El-Moneim AA, Kratz CP, Böll S,** *et al.* Essential versus reactive thrombocythemia in children: retrospective analyses of 12 cases. *Pediatric Blood & Cancer.* 2007;**49**:52–55.

125. **Randi ML, Putti MC, Scapin M,** *et al.* Pediatric patients with essential thrombocythemia are mostly polyclonal and V617FJAK2 negative. *Blood.* 2006;**108**:3600–3602.

126. **Teofili L, Giona F, Martini M,** *et al.* Markers of myeloproliferative diseases in childhood polycythemia vera and essential thrombocythemia. *Journal of Clinical Oncology.* 2007;**25**:1048–1053.

127. **Randi ML, Putti MC, Pacquola E,** *et al.* Normal thrombopoietin and its receptor (c-mpl) genes in children with essential thrombocythemia. *Pediatric Blood & Cancer* 2005;**44**:47–50.

128. **Roy NB, Treacy M, Kench P.** Childhood essential thrombocythaemia. *British Journal of Haematology.* 2005;**129**:567.

129. **Steensma DP.** JAK2 V617F in myeloid disorders: molecular diagnostic techniques and their clinical utility: a paper from the 2005 William Beaumont Hospital Symposium on Molecular Pathology. *The Journal of Molecular Diagnostics.* 2006;**8**:397–411.

130. **Olsen RJ, Tang Z, Farkas DH, Bernard DW, Zu Y, Chang CC.** Detection of the JAK2(V617F) mutation in myeloproliferative disorders by melting

curve analysis using the LightCycler system. *Archives of Pathology & Laboratory Medicine.* 2006;**130**:997–1003.

131. **de la Chapelle A, Träskelin AL, Juvonen E.** Truncated erythropoietin receptor causes dominantly inherited benign human erythrocytosis. *Proceedings of the National Academy of Sciences of the United States of America.* 1993;**90**:4495–4499.

132. **Ang SO, Chen H, Hirota K,** *et al.* Disruption of oxygen homeostasis underlies congenital Chuvash polycythemia. *Nature Genetics.* 2002;**32**:614–621.

133. **Pastore YD, Jelinek J, Ang S,** *et al.* Mutations in the VHL gene in sporadic apparently congenital polycythemia. *Blood.* 2003;**101**:1591–1595.

134. **Percy MJ, Zhao Q, Flores A,** *et al.* A family with erythrocytosis establishes a role for prolyl hydroxylase domain protein 2 in oxygen homeostasis. *Proceedings of the National Academy of Sciences of the United States of America.* 2006;**103**:654–659.

135. **Percy MJ, Furlow PW, Beer PA,** *et al.* A novel erythrocytosis-associated PHD2 mutation suggests the location of a HIF binding groove. *Blood.* 2007;**110**:2193–2196.

136. **Gordeuk VR, Stockton DW, Prchal JT.** Congenital polycythemias/erythrocytoses. *Haematologica.* 2005;**90**:109–116.

137. **Percy MJ, Lee FS.** Familial erythrocytosis: molecular links to red blood cell control. *Haematologica.* 2008;**93**:963–967.

138. **Lee FS.** Genetic causes of erythrocytosis and the oxygen-sensing pathway. *Blood Reviews.* 2008;**22**:321–332.

139. **Park MJ, Shimada A, Asada H,** *et al.* JAK2 mutation in a boy with polycythemia vera, but not in other pediatric hematologic disorders. *Leukemia.* 2006;**20**:1453–1454.

140. **Teofili L, Foa R, Giona F, Larocca LM.** Childhood polycythemia vera and essential thrombocythemia: does their pathogenesis overlap with that of adult patients? *Haematologica.* 2008;**93**:169–172.

141. **Kvasnicka HM, Thiele J.** Classification of Ph-negative chronic myeloproliferative disorders – morphology as the yardstick of

classification. *Pathobiology* 2007;**74**:63–71.

142. **Cooperberg AA, Singer OP.** Reversible myelofibrosis due to vitamin D deficiency rickets. *Canadian Medical Association Journal.* 1966;**94**:392–395.

143. **Evans DI.** Acute myelofibrosis in children with Down's syndrome. *Archives of Disease in Childhood.* 1975;**50**:458–462.

144. **Schlackman N, Green AA, Naiman JL.** Myelofibrosis in children with chronic renal insufficiency. *The Journal of Pediatrics.* 1975;**87**:720–724.

145. **Ueda K, Kawaguchi Y, Kodama M,** *et al.* Primary myelofibrosis with myeloid metaplasia and cytogenetically abnormal clones in 2 children with Down's syndrome. *Scandinavian Journal of Haematology.* 1981;**27**:152–158.

146. **Yetgin S, Ozsoylu S.** Myeloid metaplasia in vitamin D deficiency rickets. *Scandinavian Journal of Haematology.* 1982;**28**:180–185.

147. **Pantazis CG, McKie VC, Sabio H, Davis PC, Allsbrook WC.** Down's syndrome and acute myelofibrosis. Time study of DNA content during the progression to leukemia. *Cancer.* 1988;**61**:2239–2243.

148. **Balkan C, Ersoy B, Nese N.** Myelofibrosis associated with severe vitamin D deficiency rickets. *The Journal of International Medical Research.* 2005;**33**:356–359.

149. **Mallouh AA, Sa'di AR.** Agnogenic myeloid metaplasia in children. *American Journal of Diseases of Children.* 1992;**146**:965–967.

150. **Cetingul N, Yener E, Oztop S, Nisli G, Soydan S.** Agnogenic myeloid metaplasia in childhood: a report of two cases and efficiency of intravenous high dose methylprednisolone treatment. *Acta Paediatrica Japonica.* 1994;**36**:697–700.

151. **Bonduel M, Sciuccati G, Torres AF, Pierini A, Gallo G.** Familial idiopathic myelofibrosis and multiple hemangiomas. *American Journal of Hematology.* 1998;**59**:175–177.

152. **Altura RA, Head DR, Wang WC.** Long-term survival of infants with idiopathic myelofibrosis. *British Journal of Haematology.* 2000;**109**:459–462.

153. **Sah A, Minford A, Parapia LA.** Spontaneous remission of juvenile

idiopathic myelofibrosis. *British Journal of Haematology*. 2001;**112**:1083.

154. **Walia M, Mehta R, Paul P**, *et al.* Idiopathic myelofibrosis with generalized periostitis in a 4-year-old girl. *Journal of Pediatric Hematology/Oncology*. 2005;**27**:278–282.

155. **Sekhar M, Prentice HG, Popat U**, *et al.* Idiopathic myelofibrosis in children. *British Journal of Haematology*. 1996;**93**: 394–397.

156. **Sieff CA, Malleson P**. Familial myelofibrosis. *Archives of Disease in Childhood*. 1980;**55**:888–893.

157. **Rossbach HC**. Familial infantile myelofibrosis as an autosomal recessive disorder: preponderance among children from Saudi Arabia. *Pediatric Hematology and Oncology*. 2006;**23**: 453–454.

158. **Castro-Malaspina H, Gay RE, Jhanwar SC**, *et al.* Characteristics of bone marrow fibroblast colony-forming cells (CFU-F) and their progeny in patients with myeloproliferative disorders. *Blood*. 1982;**59**:1046–1054.

159. **Jacobson RJ, Salo A, Fialkow PJ**. Agnogenic myeloid metaplasia: a clonal proliferation of hematopoietic stem cells with secondary myelofibrosis. *Blood*. 1978;**51**:189–194.

160. **Greenberg BR, Woo L, Veomett IC, Payne CM, Ahmann FR**. Cytogenetics of bone marrow fibroblastic cells in idiopathic chronic myelofibrosis. *British Journal of Haematology*. 1987;**66**: 487–490.

161. **Lau SO, Ramsay NK, Smith CM, McKenna R, Kersey JH**. Spontaneous resolution of severe childhood myelofibrosis. *The Journal of Pediatrics*. 1981;**98**:585–588.

162. **Shankar S, Choi JK, Dermody TS**, *et al.* Pulmonary hypertension complicating bone marrow transplantation for idiopathic myelofibrosis. *Journal of Pediatric Hematology/Oncology*. 2004;**26**: 393–397.

163. **Wallis JP, Reid MM**. Bone marrow fibrosis in childhood acute lymphoblastic leukaemia. *Journal of Clinical Pathology*. 1989;**42**:1253–1254.

164. **Noren-Nystrom U, Roos G, Bergh A**, *et al.* Bone marrow fibrosis in childhood acute lymphoblastic leukemia correlates to biological factors, treatment response and outcome. *Leukemia*. 2008;**22**:504–510.

165. **Stephan JL, Galambrun C, Dutour A, Freycon F**. Myelofibrosis: an unusual presentation of vitamin D-deficient rickets. *European Journal of Pediatrics*. 1999;**158**:828–829.

166. **Gruner BA, DeNapoli TS, Elshihabi S**, *et al.* Anemia and hepatosplenomegaly as presenting features in a child with rickets and secondary myelofibrosis. *Journal of Pediatric Hematology/Oncology*. 2003;**25**:813–815.

167. **Uysal Z, Ileri T, Azik F**, *et al.* Reversible myelofibrosis associated with hemophagocytic lymphohistiocytosis. *Pediatric Blood & Cancer*. 2007;**49**:108–109.

168. **Aydinok Y**. Myelofibrosis in a child with EBV-associated hemophagocytic lymphohistiocytosis. *Pediatric Blood & Cancer*. 2008;**51**:311.

169. **Friedman GK, Hammers Y, Reddy V, Pressey JG**. Myelofibrosis in a patient with familial hemophagocytic lymphohistiocytosis. *Pediatric Blood & Cancer*. 2008;**50**:1260–1262.

170. **Nettleship T, Tay W**. Rare forms of urticaria. *British Medical Journal*. 1869;**2**:323–330.

171. **Ehrlich P**. Beitrage zur Theorie und Praxis der Histologischen Farbung. Thesis. Leipzig University; 1878.

172. **Unna P**. Beitrage zur Anatomie und Pathogenese der urticaria simplex und pigmentosa. Monatschrift der praktischen. *Dermatologie*. 1887;**6**: 9–18.

173. **Touraine A, Solente G, Renault P**. Urticaire pigmentaire avec reaction splenique et myelinique. *Bulletin de la Société Française de Dermatologie et de Syphiligraphie*. 1933;**40**:1691.

174. **Ellis JM**. Urticaria pigmentosa; a report of a case with autopsy. *Archives of Pathology*. 1949;**48**:426–435.

175. **Kitamura Y, Go S, Hatanaka K**. Decrease of mast cells in W/Wv mice and their increase by bone marrow transplantation. *Blood*. 1978;**52**:447–452.

176. **Kitamura Y, Yokoyama M, Matsuda H, Ohno T, Mori KJ**. Spleen colony-forming cell as common precursor for tissue mast cells and granulocytes. *Nature*. 1981;**291**: 159–160.

177. **Kirshenbaum AS, Kessler SW, Goff JP, Metcalfe DD**. Demonstration of the origin of human mast cells from CD34+ bone marrow progenitor cells. *Journal of Immunology*. 1991;**146**:1410–1415.

178. **Orfao A, Garcia-Montero AC, Sanchez L, Escribano L**. Recent advances in the understanding of mastocytosis: the role of KIT mutations. *British Journal of Haematology*. 2007;**138**:12–30.

179. **Galli SJ, Kitamura Y**. Genetically mast-cell-deficient W/Wv and Sl/Sld mice. Their value for the analysis of the roles of mast cells in biologic responses in vivo. *The American Journal of Pathology*. 1987;**127**:191–198.

180. **Geissler EN, Ryan MA, Housman DE**. The dominant-white spotting (W) locus of the mouse encodes the c-kit proto-oncogene. *Cell*. 1988;**55**:185–192.

181. **Chabot B, Stephenson DA, Chapman VM, Besmer P, Bernstein A**. The proto-oncogene c-kit encoding a transmembrane tyrosine kinase receptor maps to the mouse W locus. *Nature*. 1988;**335**:88–89.

182. **Copeland NG, Gilbert DJ, Cho BC**, *et al.* Mast cell growth factor maps near the steel locus on mouse chromosome 10 and is deleted in a number of steel alleles. *Cell*. 1990;**63**:175–183.

183. **Huang E, Nocka K, Beier DR**, *et al.* The hematopoietic growth factor KL is encoded by the Sl locus and is the ligand of the c-kit receptor, the gene product of the W locus. *Cell*. 1990;**63**: 225–233.

184. **Zsebo KM, Williams DA, Geissler EN**, *et al.* Stem cell factor is encoded at the Sl locus of the mouse and is the ligand for the c-kit tyrosine kinase receptor. *Cell*. 1990;**63**:213–224.

185. **Furitsu T, Tsujimura T, Tono T**, *et al.* Identification of mutations in the coding sequence of the proto-oncogene c-kit in a human mast cell leukemia cell line causing ligand-independent activation of c-kit product. *The Journal of Clinical Investigation*. 1993;**92**:1736–1744.

186. **Tsujimura T, Furitsu T, Morimoto M**, *et al.* Ligand-independent activation of c-kit receptor tyrosine kinase in a murine mastocytoma cell line P-815 generated by a point mutation. *Blood*. 1994;**83**:2619–2626.

187. **Nagata H, Worobec AS, Oh CK**, *et al.* Identification of a point mutation in the catalytic domain of the protooncogene c-kit in peripheral blood mononuclear

cells of patients who have mastocytosis with an associated hematologic disorder. *Proceedings of the National Academy of Sciences of the United States of America*. 1995;**92**:10560–10564.

188. **Longley BJ, Tyrrell L, Lu SZ, et al.** Somatic c-KIT activating mutation in urticaria pigmentosa and aggressive mastocytosis: establishment of clonality in a human mast cell neoplasm. *Nature Genetics*. 1996;**12**:312–314.

189. **Longley BJ, Reguera MJ, Ma Y.** Classes of c-KIT activating mutations: proposed mechanisms of action and implications for disease classification and therapy. *Leukemia Research*. 2001;**25**:571–576.

190. **Longley BJ Jr., Metcalfe DD, Tharp M, et al.** Activating and dominant inactivating c-KIT catalytic domain mutations in distinct clinical forms of human mastocytosis. *Proceedings of the National Academy of Sciences of the United States of America*. 1999;**96**:1609–1614.

191. **Fritsche-Polanz R, Jordan JH, Feix A, et al.** Mutation analysis of C-KIT in patients with myelodysplastic syndromes without mastocytosis and cases of systemic mastocytosis. *British Journal of Haematology*. 2001;**113**:357–364.

192. **Buttner C, Henz BM, Welker P, Sepp NT, Grabbe J.** Identification of activating c-kit mutations in adult-, but not in childhood-onset indolent mastocytosis: a possible explanation for divergent clinical behavior. *The Journal of Investigative Dermatology*. 1998;**111**:1227–1231.

193. **Arceci RJ, Longley BJ, Emanuel PD.** Atypical cellular disorders. *Hematology/ the Education Program of the American Society of Hematology*. 2002;297–314.

194. **Yanagihori H, Oyama N, Nakamura K, Kaneko F.** c-kit mutations in patients with childhood-onset mastocytosis and genotype-phenotype correlation. *The Journal of Molecular Diagnostics*. 2005;**7**:252–257.

195. **Kettelhut BV, Metcalfe DD.** Pediatric mastocytosis. *The Journal of Investigative Dermatology*. 1991;**96**: 15S–18S.

196. **Wolff K, Komar M, Petzelbauer P.** Clinical and histopathological aspects of cutaneous mastocytosis. *Leukemia Research*. 2001;**25**:519–528.

197. **Kettelhut BV, Parker RI, Travis WD, Metcalfe DD.** Hematopathology of the bone marrow in pediatric cutaneous mastocytosis. A study of 17 patients. *American Journal of Clinical Pathology*. 1989;**91**:558–562.

198. **Patnaik MM, Rindos M, Kouides PA, Tefferi A, Pardanani A.** Systemic mastocytosis: a concise clinical and laboratory review. *Archives of Pathology & Laboratory Medicine*. 2007;**131**:784–791.

199. **Schwartz LB.** Clinical utility of tryptase levels in systemic mastocytosis and associated hematologic disorders. *Leukemia Research*. 2001;**25**:553–562.

200. **Schwartz LB, Min HK, Ren S, et al.** Tryptase precursors are preferentially and spontaneously released, whereas mature tryptase is retained by HMC-1 cells, Mono-Mac-6 cells, and human skin-derived mast cells. *Journal of Immunology*. 2003;**170**:5667–5673.

201. **Kanthawatana S, Carias K, Arnaout R, et al.** The potential clinical utility of serum alpha-protryptase levels. *The Journal of Allergy and Clinical Immunology*. 1999;**103**:1092–1099.

202. **Sperr WR, Jordan JH, Fiegl M, et al.** Serum tryptase levels in patients with mastocytosis: correlation with mast cell burden and implication for defining the category of disease. *International Archives of Allergy and Immunology*. 2002;**128**:136–141.

203. **Parker RI.** Hematologic aspects of mastocytosis: I: Bone marrow pathology in adult and pediatric systemic mast cell disease. *The Journal of Investigative Dermatology*. 1991;**96**: 47S–51S.

204. **Horny HP, Parwaresch MR, Lennert K.** Bone marrow findings in systemic mastocytosis. *Human Pathology*. 1985;**16**:808–814.

205. **Brunning RD, McKenna RW, Rosai J, Parkin JL, Risdall R.** Systemic mastocytosis. Extracutaneous manifestations. *The American Journal of Surgical Pathology*. 1983;**7**:425–438.

206. **Chott A, Guenther P, Huebner A, et al.** Morphologic and immunophenotypic properties of neoplastic cells in a case of mast cell sarcoma. *The American Journal of Surgical Pathology*. 2003;**27**: 1013–1019.

207. **Brcic L, Vuletic LB, Stepan J, et al.** Mast-cell sarcoma of the tibia. *Journal of Clinical Pathology*. 2007;**60**:424–425.

208. **Escribano L, Diaz-Agustin B, López A, et al.** Immunophenotypic analysis of mast cells in mastocytosis: When and how to do it. Proposals of the Spanish Network on Mastocytosis (REMA). *Cytometry. Part B, Clinical Cytometry*. 2004;**58**:1–8.

209. **Escribano L, Garcia Montero AC, Nunez R, Orfao A.** Flow cytometric analysis of normal and neoplastic mast cells: role in diagnosis and follow-up of mast cell disease. *Immunology and Allergy Clinics of North America*. 2006; **26**:535–547.

210. **Irani AM, Bradford TR, Kepley CL, Schechter NM, Schwartz LB.** Detection of MCT and MCTC types of human mast cells by immunohistochemistry using new monoclonal anti-tryptase and anti-chymase antibodies. *The Journal of Histochemistry and Cytochemistry*. 1989;**37**:1509–1515.

211. **Walls AF, Jones DB, Williams JH, Church MK, Holgate ST.** Immunohistochemical identification of mast cells in formaldehyde-fixed tissue using monoclonal antibodies specific for tryptase. *The Journal of Pathology*. 1990;**162**:119–126.

212. **Li WV, Kapadia SB, Sonmez-Alpan E, Swerdlow SH.** Immunohistochemical characterization of mast cell disease in paraffin sections using tryptase, CD68, myeloperoxidase, lysozyme, and CD20 antibodies. *Modern Pathology*. 1996;**9**: 982–988.

213. **Buckley MG, McEuen AR, Walls AF.** The detection of mast cell subpopulations in formalin-fixed human tissues using a new monoclonal antibody specific for chymase. *The Journal of Pathology*. 1999;**189**:138–143.

214. **Natkunam Y, Rouse RV.** Utility of paraffin section immunohistochemistry for C-KIT (CD117) in the differential diagnosis of systemic mast cell disease involving the bone marrow. *The American Journal of Surgical Pathology*. 2000;**24**:81–91.

215. **Hoyer JD, Grogg KL, Hanson CA, Gamez JD, Dogan A.** CD33 detection by immunohistochemistry in paraffin-embedded tissues: a new antibody shows excellent specificity and sensitivity for cells of myelomonocytic lineage. *American Journal of Clinical Pathology*. 2008;**129**:316–323.

216. **Escribano L, Orfao A, Villarrubia J, et al.** Expression of lymphoid-associated antigens in mast cells: report

of a case of systemic mast cell disease. *British Journal of Haematology*. 1995;**91**: 941–943.

217. **Escribano L, Orfao A, Diaz-Agustin B**, *et al*. Indolent systemic mast cell disease in adults: immunophenotypic characterization of bone marrow mast cells and its diagnostic implications. *Blood*. 1998;**91**:2731–2736.

218. **Jordan JH, Walchshofer S, Jurecka W**, *et al*. Immunohistochemical properties of bone marrow mast cells in systemic mastocytosis: evidence for expression of CD2, CD117/Kit, and bcl-x(L). *Human Pathology*. 2001;**32**:545–552.

219. **Sotlar K, Horny HP, Simonitsch I**, *et al*. CD25 indicates the neoplastic phenotype of mast cells: a novel immunohistochemical marker for the diagnosis of systemic mastocytosis (SM) in routinely processed bone marrow biopsy specimens. *The American Journal of Surgical Pathology*. 2004;**28**:1319–1325.

220. **Krokowski M, Sotlar K, Krauth MT**, *et al*. Delineation of patterns of bone marrow mast cell infiltration in systemic mastocytosis: value of CD25, correlation with subvariants of the disease, and separation from mast cell hyperplasia. *American Journal of Clinical Pathology*. 2005;**124**:560–568.

221. **Hahn HP, Hornick JL.** Immunoreactivity for CD25 in gastrointestinal mucosal mast cells is specific for systemic mastocytosis. *The American Journal of Surgical Pathology*. 2007;**31**:1669–1676.

222. **Hollmann TJ, Brenn T, Hornick JL.** CD25 expression on cutaneous mast cells from adult patients presenting with urticaria pigmentosa is predictive of systemic mastocytosis. *The American Journal of Surgical Pathology*. 2008;**32**: 139–145.

223. **Baumgartner C, Sonneck K, Krauth MT**, *et al*. Immunohistochemical assessment of CD25 is equally sensitive and diagnostic in mastocytosis compared to flow cytometry. *European Journal of Clinical Investigation*. 2008; **38**:326–335.

224. **Zuluaga TT, Hsieh FH, Bodo J, Dong HY, Hsi ED.** Detection of phospho-STAT5 in mast cells: a reliable phenotypic marker of systemic mast cell disease that reflects constitutive tyrosine kinase activation. *British Journal of Haematology*. 2007;**139**: 31–40.

225. **Sundram UN, Natkunam Y**. Mast cell tryptase and microphthalmia transcription factor effectively discriminate cutaneous mast cell disease from myeloid leukemia cutis. *Journal of Cutaneous Pathology*. 2007;**34**:289–295.

226. **Yang F, Tran TA, Carlson JA**, *et al*. Paraffin section immunophenotype of cutaneous and extracutaneous mast cell disease: comparison to other hematopoietic neoplasms. *The American Journal of Surgical Pathology*. 2000;**24**:703–709.

227. **Ma Y, Zeng S, Metcalfe DD**, *et al*. The c-KIT mutation causing human mastocytosis is resistant to STI571 and other KIT kinase inhibitors; kinases with enzymatic site mutations show different inhibitor sensitivity profiles than wild-type kinases and those with regulatory-type mutations. *Blood*. 2002;**99**:1741–1744.

228. **Frost MJ, Ferrao PT, Hughes TP, Ashman LK.** Juxtamembrane mutant V560GKit is more sensitive to Imatinib (STI571) compared with wild-type c-kit whereas the kinase domain mutant D816VKit is resistant. *Molecular Cancer Therapeutics*. 2002;**1**:1115–1124.

229. **Akin C, Brockow K, D'Ambrosio C**, *et al*. Effects of tyrosine kinase inhibitor STI571 on human mast cells bearing wild-type or mutated c-kit. *Experimental Hematology*. 2003;**31**: 686–692.

230. **Gleixner KV, Mayerhofer M, Sonneck K**, *et al*. Synergistic growth-inhibitory effects of two tyrosine kinase inhibitors, dasatinib and PKC412, on neoplastic mast cells expressing the D816V-mutated oncogenic variant of KIT. *Haematologica*. 2007;**92**:1451–1459.

231. **Sotlar K, Escribano L, Landt O**, *et al*. One-step detection of c-kit point mutations using peptide nucleic acid-mediated polymerase chain reaction clamping and hybridization probes. *The American Journal of Pathology*. 2003;**162**:737–746.

232. **Corless CL, Harrell P, Lacouture M**, *et al*. Allele-specific polymerase chain reaction for the imatinib-resistant KIT D816V and D816F mutations in mastocytosis and acute myelogenous leukemia. *The Journal of Molecular Diagnostics*. 2006;**8**:604–612.

233. **Tan A, Westerman D, McArthur GA**, *et al*. Sensitive detection of KIT D816V in patients with mastocytosis. *Clinical Chemistry*. 2006;**52**:2250–2257.

234. **Garcia-Montero AC, Jara-Acevedo M, Teodosio C**, *et al*. KIT mutation in mast cells and other bone marrow hematopoietic cell lineages in systemic mast cell disorders: a prospective study of the Spanish Network on Mastocytosis (REMA) in a series of 113 patients. *Blood*. 2006;**108**:2366–2372.

235. **Valent P, Akin C, Escribano L**, *et al*. Standards and standardization in mastocytosis: consensus statements on diagnostics, treatment recommendations and response criteria. *European Journal of Clinical Investigation*. 2007;**37**:435–453.

236. **Schumacher JA, Elenitoba-Johnson KS, Lim MS.** Detection of the c-kit D816V mutation in systemic mastocytosis by allele-specific PCR. *Journal of Clinical Pathology*. 2008;**61**: 109–114.

Myelodysplastic/myeloproliferative neoplasms

John Kim Choi

Introduction

Myelodysplastic/myeloproliferative neoplasms are hematopoietic diseases with features of both myelodysplastic syndrome (MDS) and myeloproliferative neoplasm (MPN). In the past, these disorders were grouped as MDS, but they are now grouped as a distinct subentity in the latest classification scheme of hematopoietic neoplasms by the World Health Organization (WHO) [1, 2]. The MDS/MPN category includes chronic myelomonocytic leukemia (CMML), atypical chronic myeloid leukemia (aCML), juvenile myelomonocytic leukemia (JMML), and myelodysplastic/myeloproliferative neoplasm, unclassifiable. This chapter will focus on JMML, which is unique to the pediatric population. CMML in children is considered a secondary or therapy-related MDS [3], and aCML does not occur in the pediatric population [4].

Juvenile myelomonocytic leukemia (JMML)

Synonyms

Juvenile chronic myelomonocytic leukemia, juvenile chronic myeloid leukemia, juvenile granulocytic leukemia, monosomy 7 syndrome, infantile monosomy 7 syndrome.

Epidemiology

JMML is a rare disorder with an incidence of 0.6 per 1 million children, and represents approximately 1.6% of childhood leukemias [5, 6]. The age of presentation ranges from 0 to 11 years, with 40%, 90%, and 98% of the cases presenting at under 1, 4, and 10 years of age, respectively [7, 8]. Boys are affected more frequently, with a male to female ratio of 2 : 1.

Clinical features

The patient with JMML often presents with hepatosplenomegaly, lymphadenopathy, macular-papular skin rash, and symptoms of infection and cytopenia (Table 13.1) [6–8]. Skin lesions also include café-au-lait spots [8], juvenile xanthogra-

nuloma [9], and JMML infiltrate [10, 11]. Approximately 16% of JMML cases are associated with various clinical abnormalities, with the most common associated syndrome being neurofibromatosis type 1, which is seen in 7–14% of all JMML. The incidence of JMML is also increased in children with Noonan syndrome [12–15].

Morphology

In JMML, myelomonocytic infiltrates involve the bone marrow, peripheral blood, liver, and spleen. The infiltrates commonly involve the skin, lymph nodes, and lung, although any organ potentially can be involved.

Peripheral blood

In all cases of JMML, the peripheral blood shows absolute monocytosis ($>1 \times 10^9$/L), with the monocyte counts ranging from 1 to 61×10^9/L (Fig. 13.1) [8]. Occasionally, the monocytes are more immature in morphology and have promonocytic features. However, these features are not very specific for JMML and can be seen in leukemoid reactions.

The WBC ranges from 5 to 260×10^9/L [8]. In 95.5% of cases, leukocytosis is present, with the WBC being $<50 \times 10^9$/L (70% of cases), 50–99 $\times 10^9$/L (22% of cases), $>100 \times 10^9$/L (8% of cases) [7, 8]. Only 4.5% of cases have WBC $<10 \times 10^9$/L. Myeloid precursors are seen in 86% of the cases, including 0–2% myeloblasts in 56% of cases and >2% myeloblasts in the remaining cases. In some cases, the neutrophils can show reactive changes (toxic granulation and Döhle bodies), or the lymphocytes can show activated forms (plasmacytoid lymphocytes and atypical, Downey II lymphocytes), consistent with a concomitant infection that can co-present with JMML.

Hemoglobin F (Hb F) is elevated in two-thirds of all JMML cases and nearly all JMML cases without the monosomy 7 karyotype [7, 8].

Other peripheral blood findings included anemia, thrombocytopenia, hypergammaglobulinemia, and increased LDH levels [7, 8]. Hemoglobin (Hb) ranges from 3.5 to 12.7 g/dL,

Diagnostic Pediatric Hematopathology, ed. Maria A. Proytcheva. Published by Cambridge University Press.
© Cambridge University Press 2011.

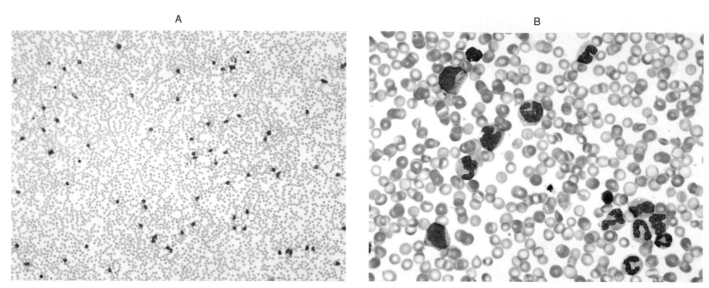

Fig. 13.1. Giemsa–Wright-stained peripheral blood smear in a patient with JMML. (A) Anemia, thrombocytopenia, and leukocytosis are present. (B) Leukocytosis consists of monocytosis, granulocytes, and myeloid precursors including occasional blasts.

Table 13.1. Clinical findings associated with JMML.

Physical signs of possible organ involvement by JMML	Frequency (percentage of cases)
Splenomegaly	87–97
Hepatomegaly	79–97
Lymphadenopathy	40–76
Skin rash	28–48
Symptoms of infection and cytopenia	
Infection	45
Cough	40
Fever	54
Pallor	64
Bleeding	46
Associated syndromes	
Neurofibromatosis type 1	7–14
Noonan syndrome	Rare
Other clinical abnormalities	**7.3**
Cyanotic heart disease	
Hypertelorism	
Hydrocephalus	
Mental retardation	
Pedal polydactyly	
Pyloric stenosis	
References: [6–8].	

children 0–1 year, 2–4 years, and 5–18 years, respectively; the variability in each group is approximately plus or minus 15% [16].

The BM usually shows myeloid hyperplasia compared to the normal M : E ratio in the pediatric population, which ranges from 5 : 1 to 2 : 1. However, a subset (10% of cases) shows erythroid hyperplasia. The megakaryocytes are usually decreased in number but can be normal or even increased in number. Hematopoiesis shows orderly maturation without significant dysplasia. In particular, the BM does not contain the hypolobated megakaryocytes that are typically seen in CML.

The BM blast percentages range from 0–9% (64% of cases), to 10–20% (26% of cases), and 21–29% (10% of cases) [7]. The last group with 21–29% blasts could be reclassified as acute myeloid leukemia with the current WHO criteria of 20% blasts for AML.

The BM monocytes range from 0 to 30% [8]. The actual percentage may be lower, since some monocytes probably represent peripheral blood contamination. In our experience, most JMML patients have <2% BM monocytes, even with the aid of non-specific esterase (NSE) cytochemical stain.

Spleen

The spleen shows red pulp expansion by a diffuse infiltrate of granulocytes, myeloid precursors, and monocytes (Fig. 13.3) [17].

While the spleen is not typically removed for diagnosis of JMML, it can be removed following chemotherapy but prior to bone marrow transplantation, in order to reduce a potential reservoir of residual JMML. A frequent clinical question for the splenectomy specimen is the level of residual JMML. Given the dismal prognosis in the absence of bone marrow transplantation, there is residual disease at some level. Histologically, the residual JMML consists of sheets of monocytes/macrophages

with nearly 80% of patients having Hb less than 12 g/dL. Most cases are normocytic, but a significant percentage of cases are microcytic (22%) or macrocytic (24%) [8]. Platelet counts range from 3 to 496 × 10⁹/L, with the count <50 × 10⁹/L in 47–57% of the cases.

Bone marrow

The bone marrow (BM) is typically hypercellular compared to the normal cellularity in the pediatric population, which varies by age (Fig. 13.2). The mean marrow cellularities in the pediatric population are approximately 80%, 70%, and 60% for

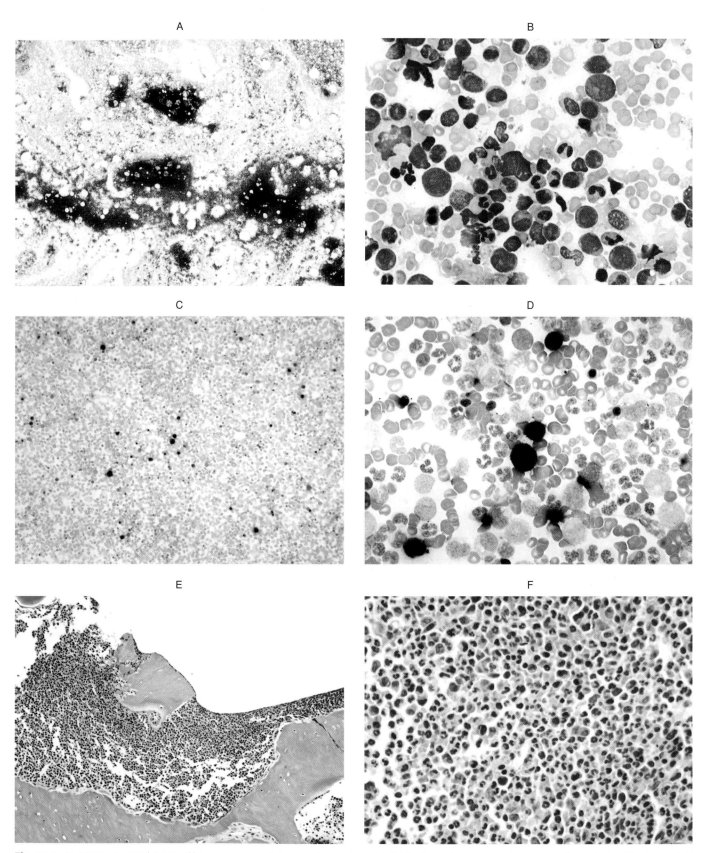

Fig. 13.2. (A–D) Giemsa–Wright-stained bone marrow aspirate smear in a patient with JMML. The aspirate smears show hypercellular spicules (A) with myeloid hyperplasia, without significant increase in blasts (B). Cytochemical stain for non-specific esterase (NSE) performed on the aspirate smear shows only occasional monocytic cells; the small, positive blobs represent artifactual stain precipitates (C, D). The accompanying PAS-stained bone marrow biopsy sections confirm the hypercellular marrow (E) with myeloid hyperplasia (F).

A

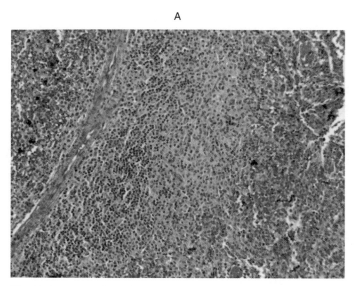

B

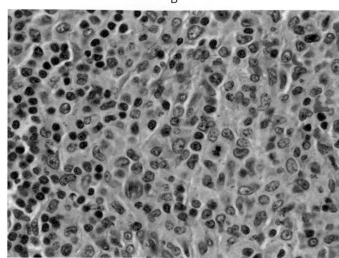

Fig. 13.3. Hematoxylin and eosin (H&E)-stained section of spleen from a patient with JMML, following chemotherapy but prior to bone marrow transplantation. (A) Mononuclear infiltrate is present at the interface between the white and red pulps. (B) The mononuclear infiltrate is composed of monocytes and macrophages consistent with residual JMML.

localized at the interface between the white and red pulps. Cytologically, the monocytes/macrophages of the residual JMML are similar to the cordal macrophages, and the distinction depends on the specific splenic localization and cell clustering.

Skin

Cutaneous involvement by JMML shows dermal perivascular, periadnexal, and interstitial infiltrates composed of monocytes/histiocytes, granulocytes, and myeloid precursors (Fig. 13.4) [10, 11]. This histology is similar to Sweet syndrome. Despite the similar histology, we favor JMML over Sweet syndrome because the composition of the infiltrate is identical to the peripheral blood manifestation of JMML.

Immunophenotype/cytochemistry

Currently, the best detection of monocytes on aspirate smears is given by the cytochemical stain for non-specific esterase, while on paraffin-embedded fixed tissue sections it is immunohistochemistry for CD163 (Fig. 13.4). The leukocyte alkaline phosphatase score is decreased in 41% of JMML cases [7]. CD1d expression is similar in JMML monocytes and normal monocytes [18]. An older report suggested that the JMML monocytes in the spleen are S100 positive [19]. Unfortunately, we have not found this finding useful because of the numerous S100-positive mononuclear cells that can be also seen in spleen without JMML. Beyond these limited findings, the immunophenotype of JMML remains poorly characterized. The possibility of an identifying abnormal immunophenotype for the JMML myelomonocytic cells similar to adult cases of MDS [20, 21] remains to be reported.

Table 13.2. WHO criteria for JMML.

(1) Peripheral monocytosis ($>1 \times 10^9$/L)
(2) Absence of t(9;22) or *BCR–ABL* (not CML)
(3) Bone marrow or peripheral blood with <20% blasts (not AML)
(4) And two of the following:
Myeloid precursors in peripheral blood
WBC $>10 \times 10^9$/L
Increased Hb F for age
GM-CSF hypersensitivity *in vitro*
Cytogenetic abnormality
References: [2, 7, 8].

Differential diagnosis and workup

The initial suspicion of JMML is based on clinical features and peripheral blood showing leukocytosis and absolute monocytosis. The major differential diagnoses for these findings are JMML, chronic myeloid leukemia (CML), acute myeloid leukemia (AML), chronic myelomonocytic leukemia (CMML), and leukemoid reaction secondary to infection (Tables 13.2, 13.3, 13.4).

Based on a large study that examined the various laboratory findings in JMML [8, 22], the WHO classification requires four laboratory diagnostic criteria in order to diagnose JMML (Table 13.2). One criterion is absolute monocytosis of 1×10^9/L, seen in all JMML. This criterion is very sensitive but not specific, since it can be seen in all other major diseases that have to be differentiated from JMML.

Two other criteria narrow the differential, since they exclude CML and AML. The exclusion of CML is relatively straightforward, because of its defining t(9;22) or *BCR-ABL* fusion transcript. However, the exclusion of AML can be controversial

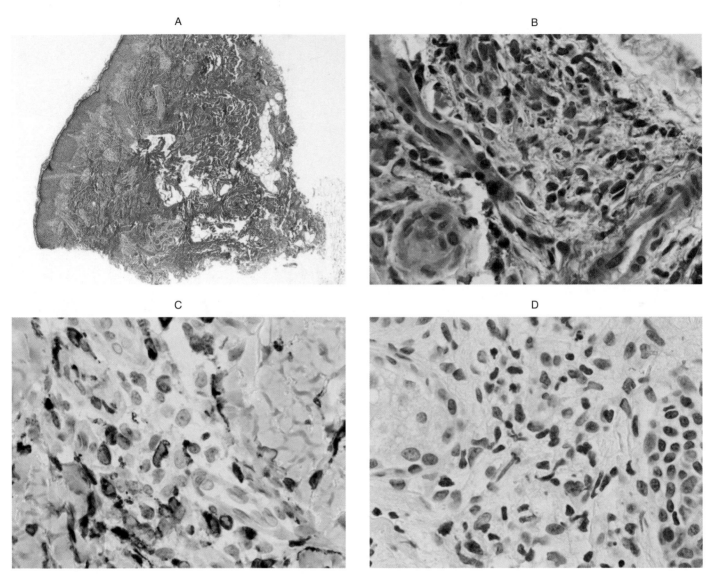

Fig. 13.4. Skin biopsy of a cutaneous rash in a patient with JMML. H&E stain shows a dermal perivascular, periadnexal, and interstitial infiltrate (A), composed of mostly mononuclear cells consistent with monocytes and histiocytes (B). Paraffin immunohistochemistry demonstrates that many of the mononuclear cells are CD163+ monocytes/histiocytes (C), with occasional MPO+ granulocytes (D).

when blasts are 20–29% of the marrow cellularity. While most JMMLs present with blast counts of <20%, occasional cases have 20% or more blasts but are otherwise typical of JMML [7]. Whether these cases represent true JMML or *de novo* AML remains unclear, and deserving of further research given their different prognosis and potentially different therapy. In fact, the exact percentage of blasts required for pediatric AML is also controversial in pediatric MDS, and the European pediatric MDS group prefers the 30% blasts of the original FAB (French–American–British) classification [3].

The last criterion requires two of five laboratory findings. Unfortunately, two of the laboratory findings are myeloid precursors in peripheral blood, and WBC count higher than $10 \times 10^9/L$, which are frequently seen in leukemoid reaction and CMML, making this last criterion unhelpful in the diagnosis of JMML. Fortunately, CMML can be excluded by clinical his-

tory and age of the patient. Pediatric CMMLs are considered to be therapy-related MDS by the European MDS group [3]. Although we have seen rare pediatric cases without prior therapy that fulfilled the WHO criteria for CMML (Table 13.4), these cases occurred in late teenagers, much older than the accepted 0–11 years of age for JMML; these rare cases remain uncharacterized, and it remains to be determined if these behave as adult CMML.

Under the current WHO criteria for JMML, leukemoid reaction secondary to infection remains the problematic differential for JMML [22]. In fact, there are case reports of infections that mimic JMML, including EBV [23, 24], CMV [25], parvovirus [26], and HHV-6 [27] infections. Given these mimics, it would be unwise to use only myeloid precursors in peripheral blood and WBC $>10 \times 10^9/L$ to meet the last criterion for JMML (Table 13.3).

Table 13.3. The frequencies of the WHO criteria for JMML in JMML [2, 7, 8] versus leukemoid reaction, probably the most problematic differential.

Criteria	Frequency in JMML (%)	Frequency in leukemoid reaction
Peripheral monocytosis ($>1 \times 10^9$/L)	100	Sometimes
Absence of t(9;22) or *BCR-ABL* (not CML)	100	Always
Bone marrow with <20% blasts (not AML)	90–100?	Always
And two of the following:		
Myeloid precursors in PBS	86–100	Always
WBC $>10 \times 10^9$/L	95.5	Always
Increased Hb F for age	66	Sometimes
GM-CSF hypersensitivity in vitro	100	Rare but possible
Cytogenetic abnormality	32–35	None

? = some cases present with 20% or more blasts but are otherwise typical of JMML.

Table 13.4. Criteria for pediatric CMML.

(1) Peripheral monocytosis ($>1 \times 10^9$/L)

(2) Absence of t(9;22) or BCR-ABL (not CML)

(3) Absence of rearrangement of PDGFRA or PDGFRB (not myeloid and lymphoid neoplasms with eosinophilia and abnormalities of PDGRA, PDGFRB, or FGFR1)

(4) Bone marrow or peripheral blood with <20% blasts (not AML)

(5) And one of the following:
Dysplasia in one or more myeloid lineages
Acquired clonal cytogenetic abnormality
Unexplained monocytosis for at least three months

(6) Prior therapy or late teen

Modified from WHO classification [1, 2] and pediatric MDS/MPS (myelodysplastic syndrome/myeloproliferative syndrome) classification [3].

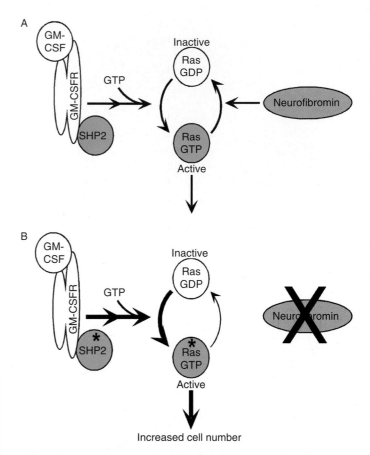

Fig. 13.5. (A) Schematic diagram of normal GM-CSF signal transduction pathway. GM-CSF binds its receptor and initiates recruitment of multiple proteins, including SHP2, to the GM-CSF receptor (GM-CSFR). These proteins convert inactive Ras (Ras-GDP) to its active form (Ras-GTP) by catalyzing the exchange of GDP for GTP. Ras-GTP activates downstream signals that result in homeostatic cell accumulation. Ras-GTP has inherent activity that hydrolyzes its GTP to GDP, leading to inactive Ras-GDP. The conversion of Ras-GTP to Ras-GDP is accelerated by neurofibromin. (B) Schematic diagram of abnormal GM-CSF signal transduction pathway in JMML. Point mutations (*) in SHP2 and Ras, as well as inactivation mutations in neurofibromin (X) lead to increased levels of active Ras-GTP, resulting in increased cell number. Modified from [7, 41].

Fortunately, the other three laboratory findings of the last criterion can distinguish JMML from leukemoid reaction (Table 13.3). Evidence of clonality excludes leukemoid reaction, and can be determined by cytogenetic abnormality, FISH for monosomy 7, or by X chromosome inactivation skewing in females by HUMURA assay. Unfortunately, JMMLs often do not have cytogenetic abnormality, and most patients are males, precluding the use of the HUMURA assay. Increased hemoglobin F (Hb F) for age is also more specific for JMML, provided that the child does not have underlying hemoglobinopathy associated with increased Hb F. Hb F, like clonality, can be normal in JMML. Unlike clonality and Hb F, the GM-CSF hypersensitivity assay is incredibly sensitive, being positive in all cases of JMML. In this assay, JMML cells (either from peripheral blood or bone marrow), cultured in methylcellulose with low concentrations of GM-CSF, form abnormally high numbers of granulocytic macrophage colonies [28]. The GM-CSF hypersensitivity is also very specific, with a false-positive result seen in some CMML [29] and rare infectious states [27]. The main disadvantages to the GM-CSF hypersensitivity assay are the long turnaround time (weeks), and its poor availability. Currently, the only laboratory officially accepting samples for GM-CSF hypersensitivity assay is the laboratory of Dr. Mignon Loh at the University of California, San Francisco.

While not part of the current criteria, some pathology laboratories are testing for specific genetic mutations that are associated with JMML (see genetics/molecular mechanisms, below).

Genetics/molecular mechanisms

Numerous cytogenetic abnormalities have been seen in 32–35% of JMML; the most frequent abnormality is monosomy 7 that is seen in 16–25% of JMML [7, 8]. Insight into the molecular mechanism for JMML has been gained from studies of congenital disorders such as neurofibromatosis type 1 (NF1) and Noonan syndrome (NS) that are associated with JMML. Neurofibromatosis type 1 is caused by loss or inactivation of the neurofibromin gene that is important for normal conversion of activated Ras to its inactive form [30, 31]. In 50% of NS, SHP2 (PTPN11) is mutated [13, 14, 32, 33]. The most common mutation in SHP2 seen in NS with JMML is Thr73Ile (9 of 19 reported cases) [12–15], which leads to increased tyrosine phosphatase activity of SHP2. Mutated SHP2 leads to increased Ras activity. In addition to the inherited mutations, somatic mutations in NF1 [34, 35], SHP2 [12, 15], and Ras [36, 37] have been identified in 30%, 33%, and 25% of JMML, respectively, indicating the importance of the Ras pathway in both sporadic and syndrome-associated JMML. Animal model systems demonstrate that NF or SHP2 mutations are sufficient to induce an MDS/MPN disorder similar to JMML [33, 38–40]. These findings indicate that JMML is induced by abnormal increase in the Ras signaling pathway (Fig. 13.5).

Postulated cell of origin

Similar to other MDSs and MPNs, the cell of origin is postulated to be the hematopoietic stem cell. The identification of chromosomal abnormalities in non-myeloid cells [42–44], blastic transformation from JMML to precursor B-lymphoblastic leukemia [45], and transformation to T-cell lymphoma [46] support this hypothesis.

Prognosis and predictive factors

In general, JMML has a poor prognosis, with the largest study showing a 10-year survival of 6% without bone marrow transplant, and 39% even with transplant [8]. Poor prognosis correlates with older age, high Hb F, low platelet counts, and increased peripheral blood or BM blasts. Chromosomal abnormality, including monosomy 7, was not predictive of outcome [8, 47]. JMML associated with NS is milder, with most patients having spontaneous remission or responding well to chemotherapy alone [13, 48, 49].

References

1. Harris NL, Jaffe ES, Diebold J, *et al.* The World Health Organization classification of neoplastic diseases of the haematopoietic and lymphoid tissues: report of the Clinical Advisory Committee Meeting, Airlie House, Virginia, November 1997. *Histopathology*. 2000;**36**(1):69–86.

2. Swerdlow SH, Campo E, Harris NL, *et al.* (eds.). *WHO Classification of Tumours of Haematopoietic and Lymphoid Tissues* (4th edn.). Lyon: IARC Press; 2008, 439.

3. Hasle H, Niemeyer CM, Chessells JM, *et al.* A pediatric approach to the WHO classification of myelodysplastic and myeloproliferative diseases. *Leukemia*. 2003;**17**(2):277–282.

4. Hernandez JM, del Canizo MC, Cuneo A, *et al.* Clinical, hematological and cytogenetic characteristics of atypical chronic myeloid leukemia. *Annals of Oncology*. 2000;**11**(4): 441–444.

5. Hasle H. Myelodysplastic syndromes in childhood – classification, epidemiology, and treatment. *Leukemia & Lymphoma*. 1994;**13**(1–2):11–26.

6. Luna-Fineman S, Shannon KM, Atwater SK, *et al.* Myelodysplastic and myeloproliferative disorders of childhood: a study of 167 patients. *Blood*. 1999;**93**(2):459–466.

7. Arico M, Biondi A, Pui CH. Juvenile myelomonocytic leukemia. *Blood*. 1997;**90**(2):479–488.

8. Niemeyer CM, Arico M, Basso G, *et al.* Chronic myelomonocytic leukemia in childhood: a retrospective analysis of 110 cases. European Working Group on Myelodysplastic Syndromes in Childhood (EWOG-MDS). *Blood*. 1997;**89**(10):3534–3543.

9. Vail JT Jr., Adler KR, Rothenberg J. Cutaneous xanthomas associated with chronic myelomonocytic leukemia. *Archives of Dermatology*. 1985;**121**(10): 1318–1320.

10. Sires UI, Mallory SB, Hess JL, *et al.* Cutaneous presentation of juvenile chronic myelogenous leukemia: a diagnostic and therapeutic dilemma. *Pediatric Dermatology*. 1995;**12**(4):364–368.

11. Matsumoto K, Miki J, Matsuzaki S, Koike K, Saida T. Skin infiltration of juvenile myelomonocytic leukemia. *The Journal of Dermatology*. 2004;**31**(9): 748–751.

12. Tartaglia M, Niemeyer CM, Fragale A, *et al.* Somatic mutations in PTPN11 in juvenile myelomonocytic leukemia, myelodysplastic syndromes and acute myeloid leukemia. *Nature Genetics*. 2003;**34**(2):148–150.

13. Jongmans M, Sistermans EA, Rikken A, *et al.* Genotypic and phenotypic characterization of Noonan syndrome: new data and review of the literature. *American Journal of Medical Genetics. Part A*. 2005;**134**(2):165–170.

14. Kratz CP, Niemeyer CM, Castleberry RP, *et al.* The mutational spectrum of PTPN11 in juvenile myelomonocytic leukemia and Noonan syndrome/myeloproliferative disease. *Blood*. 2005;**106**(6):2183–2185.

15. Loh ML, Vattikuti S, Schubbert S, *et al.* Mutations in PTPN11 implicate the SHP-2 phosphatase in leukemogenesis. *Blood*. 2004;**103**(6): 2325–2331.

16. Friebert SE, Shepardson LB, Shurin SB, Rosenthal GE, Rosenthal NS. Pediatric bone marrow cellularity: are we expecting too much? *Journal of Pediatric Hematology/Oncology*. 1998; **20**(5):439–443.

17. Hess JL, Zutter MM, Castleberry RP, Emanuel PD. Juvenile chronic myelogenous leukemia. *American Journal of Clinical Pathology*. 1996; **105**(2):238–248.

18. Metelitsa LS, Weinberg KI, Emanuel PD, Seeger RC. Expression of CD1d by myelomonocytic leukemias provides a target for cytotoxic NKT cells. *Leukemia*. 2003;**17**(6):1068–1077.

19. Ng CS, Lam TK, Chan JK, *et al.* Juvenile chronic myeloid leukemia. A malignancy of S-100 protein-positive histiocytes. *American Journal of Clinical Pathology*. 1988;**90**(5):575–582.

20. Malcovati L, Della Porta MG, Lunghi M, *et al.* Flow cytometry evaluation of erythroid and myeloid dysplasia in patients with myelodysplastic syndrome. *Leukemia*. 2005;**19**(5):776–783.

21. **Kussick SJ, Fromm JR, Rossini A**, *et al.* Four-color flow cytometry shows strong concordance with bone marrow morphology and cytogenetics in the evaluation for myelodysplasia. *American Journal of Clinical Pathology.* 2005;**124**(2):170–181.

22. **Pinkel D.** Differentiating juvenile myelomonocytic leukemia from infectious disease. *Blood.* 1998;**89**(1): 365–367.

23. **Herrod HG, Dow LW, Sullivan JL.** Persistent Epstein-Barr virus infection mimicking juvenile chronic myelogenous leukemia: immunologic and hematologic studies. *Blood.* 1983; **61**(6):1098–1104.

24. **Stollmann B, Fonatsch C, Havers W.** Persistent Epstein-Barr virus infection associated with monosomy 7 or chromosome 3 abnormality in childhood myeloproliferative disorders. *British Journal of Haematology.* 1985; **60**(1):183–196.

25. **Kirby MA, Weitzman S, Freedman MH.** Juvenile chronic myelogenous leukemia: differentiation from infantile cytomegalovirus infection. *The American Journal of Pediatric Hematology/Oncology.* 1990;**12**(3):292–296.

26. **Yetgin S, Cetin M, Yenicesu I, Ozaltin F, Uckan D.** Acute parvovirus B19 infection mimicking juvenile myelomonocytic leukemia. *European Journal of Haematology.* 2000;**65**(4): 276–278.

27. **Lorenzana A, Lyons H, Sawaf H**, *et al.* Human herpesvirus 6 infection mimicking juvenile myelomonocytic leukemia in an infant. *Journal of Pediatric Hematology/Oncology.* 2002; **24**(2):136–141.

28. **Emanuel PD, Bates LJ, Castleberry RP, Gualtieri RJ, Zuckerman KS.** Selective hypersensitivity to granulocyte-macrophage colony-stimulating factor by juvenile chronic myeloid leukemia hematopoietic progenitors. *Blood.* 1991;**77**(5):925–929.

29. **Cambier N, Baruchel A, Schlageter MH**, *et al.* Chronic myelomonocytic leukemia: from biology to therapy. *Hematology and Cell Therapy.* 1997; **39**(2):41–48.

30. **Xu GF, O'Connell P, Viskochil D**, *et al.* The neurofibromatosis type 1 gene encodes a protein related to GAP. *Cell.* 1990;**62**(3):599–608.

31. **Ballester R, Marchuk D, Boguski M**, *et al.* The NF1 locus encodes a protein functionally related to mammalian GAP and yeast IRA proteins. *Cell.* 1990;**63**(4):851–859.

32. **Niihori T, Aoki Y, Ohashi H**, *et al.* Functional analysis of PTPN11/SHP-2 mutants identified in Noonan syndrome and childhood leukemia. *Journal of Human Genetics.* 2005;**50**(4): 192–202.

33. **Mohi MG, Williams IR, Dearolf CR**, *et al.* Prognostic, therapeutic, and mechanistic implications of a mouse model of leukemia evoked by Shp2 (PTPN11) mutations. *Cancer Cell.* 2005;7(2):179–191.

34. **Side LE, Emanuel PD, Taylor B**, *et al.* Mutations of the NF1 gene in children with juvenile myelomonocytic leukemia without clinical evidence of neurofibromatosis, type 1. *Blood.* 1998; **92**(1):267–272.

35. **Miles DK, Freedman MH, Stephens K**, *et al.* Patterns of hematopoietic lineage involvement in children with neurofibromatosis type 1 and malignant myeloid disorders. *Blood.* 1996;**88**(11):4314–4320.

36. **Kalra R, Paderanga DC, Olson K, Shannon KM.** Genetic analysis is consistent with the hypothesis that NF1 limits myeloid cell growth through p21ras. *Blood.* 1994;**84**(10):3435–3439.

37. **Miyauchi J, Asada M, Sasaki M**, *et al.* Mutations of the N-ras gene in juvenile chronic myelogenous leukemia. *Blood.* 1994;**83**(8):2248–2254.

38. **Jacks T, Shih TS, Schmitt EM**, *et al.* Tumour predisposition in mice heterozygous for a targeted mutation in Nf1. *Nature Genetics.* 1994;7(3):353–361.

39. **Largaespada DA, Brannan CI, Jenkins NA, Copeland NG.** Nf1 deficiency causes Ras-mediated granulocyte/macrophage colony stimulating factor hypersensitivity and chronic myeloid leukaemia. *Nature Genetics.* 1996;**12**(2):137–143.

40. **Gitler AD, Kong Y, Choi JK**, *et al.* Tie2-Cre-induced inactivation of a conditional mutant Nf1 allele in mouse results in a myeloproliferative disorder that models juvenile myelomonocytic leukemia. *Pediatric Research.* 2004;**55**(4):581–584.

41. **Lauchle JO, Braun BS, Loh ML, Shannon K.** Inherited predispositions and hyperactive Ras in myeloid leukemogenesis. *Pediatric Blood and Cancer.* 2006;**46**(5):579–585.

42. **Amenomori T, Tomonaga M, Yoshida Y**, *et al.* Cytogenetic evidence for partially committed myeloid progenitor cell origin of chronic myelomonocytic leukaemia and juvenile chronic myeloid leukaemia: both granulocyte-macrophage precursors and erythroid precursors carry identical marker chromosome. *British Journal of Haematology.* 1986;**64**(3):539–546.

43. **Busque L, Gilliland DG, Prchal JT**, *et al.* Clonality in juvenile chronic myelogenous leukemia. *Blood.* 1995; **85**(1):21–30.

44. **Papayannopoulou T, Nakamoto B, Anagnou NP**, *et al.* Expression of embryonic globins by erythroid cells in juvenile chronic myelocytic leukemia. *Blood.* 1991;**77**(12):2569–2576.

45. **Scrideli CA, Baruffi MR, Rogatto SR**, *et al.* B lineage acute lymphoblastic leukemia transformation in a child with juvenile myelomonocytic leukemia, type 1 neurofibromatosis and monosomy of chromosome 7. Possible implications in the leukemogenesis. *Leukemia Research.* 2003;**27**(4):371–374.

46. **Cooper LJ, Shannon KM, Loken MR**, *et al.* Evidence that juvenile myelomonocytic leukemia can arise from a pluripotential stem cell. *Blood.* 2000;**96**(6):2310–2313.

47. **Hasle H, Arico M, Basso G**, *et al.* Myelodysplastic syndrome, juvenile myelomonocytic leukemia, and acute myeloid leukemia associated with complete or partial monosomy 7. European Working Group on MDS in Childhood (EWOG-MDS). *Leukemia.* 1999;**13**(3):376–385.

48. **Choong K, Freedman MH, Chitayat D**, *et al.* Juvenile myelomonocytic leukemia and Noonan syndrome. *Journal of Pediatric Hematology/Oncology.* 1999;**21**(6):523–527.

49. **Bader-Meunier B, Tchernia G, Mielot F**, *et al.* Occurrence of myeloproliferative disorder in patients with Noonan syndrome. *Journal of Pediatrics.* 1997;**130**(6):885–889.

Section 2
Chapter

Neoplastic hematopathology

14
Myelodysplastic syndromes and therapy-related myeloid neoplasms

Sa A. Wang

Myelodysplastic syndromes

Definition

Myelodysplastic syndromes (MDS) in childhood encompasses a diverse group of clonal hematopoietic stem cell disorders, characterized by ineffective hematopoiesis with morphologic dysplasia, peripheral cytopenia, and an increased propensity to evolve into acute leukemia. MDS can arise either *de novo* in a previously healthy child (primary MDS), or develop in a child with a known predisposition as secondary MDS. In adult patients, most of the secondary MDSs are therapy-related, following cytotoxic therapy for prior neoplastic or non-neoplastic conditions. Secondary MDS in childhood includes many cases associated with constitutional bone marrow failure disorders, MDS evolved from acquired aplastic anemia, and familial MDS (Table 14.1), in addition to therapy-related MDS. It is noteworthy that the distinction of primary MDS and secondary MDS may not be clear cut in pediatric patients, since some of "primary MDS" may have an underlying, yet unknown, genetic defect predisposing them to MDS at a young age.

Epidemiology

Pediatric MDS is a rare hematologic malignancy of childhood. The reported incidence of pediatric MDS comprises 1.1 to 8.7% of hematologic malignancies of childhood, with an annual incidence of 1.8 per million in children of 0–14 years of age [1]. It constitutes 4% of cases, and is the third most common hematologic malignancy in children, following acute lymphoblastic leukemia (ALL) and acute myeloid leukemia (AML). In contrast to adult MDS that shows a male predominance (1.7 : 1), MDS in children affects males and females with an equal frequency. The median age at presentation is 5–8 years, with a mean of 6.8 years [2].

Pathophysiology

MDS is defined as a clonal stem cell disorder characterized by ineffective hematopoiesis rather than a lack of hematopoiesis. A striking feature of MDS is genetic instability, which results in increased propensity to develop AML in a large proportion of cases. Three pathogenetic mechanisms in MDS have been proposed: (1) stem-cell dysfunction overlapping with AML; (2) genetic instability; and (3) deregulation of apoptosis [3]. It is noteworthy that a significant proportion of pediatric MDS is secondary to inherited bone marrow failure syndromes. Although the genetic basis for most of the inherited bone marrow failure syndromes is not well known, five major factors may govern predisposition of MDS in inherited bone marrow failure [2], including: (1) Defects in the DNA damage response. One example is Fanconi anemia with mutation in one of the 13 complementation genes, resulting in impaired DNA damage response. (2) Disturbed control of apoptosis. *HAX1*, *ELA2* mutations have been found in a subgroup of congenital neutropenia, leading to increased apoptosis. (3) Disrupted ribosome biogenesis. Mutations of the *SBDS* gene in Shwachman–Diamond syndrome and *RPS19*, *RPS24*, or *PRS17* in Diamond–Blackfan anemia are linked to ribosome biogenesis. (4) Impaired telomere maintenance. Mutations of *DKC1*, *TERC*, or *TERT* genes involved in the telomerase complex occur in dyskeratosis congenita. In addition, acquired mutations at a crucial stage in hematopoietic development predispose to additional genetic hits and facilitate leukemogenesis. The lifetime risk of developing MDS and/or AML varies from 5% in Diamond–Blackfan anemia to 30–40% in Fanconi anemia or Shwachman–Diamond syndrome [4, 5].

Pediatric MDS classification and minimal diagnostic criteria

Approximately one-third to one-half of the cases previously classified as pediatric MDS meet the diagnostic criteria of

Diagnostic Pediatric Hematopathology, ed. Maria A. Proytcheva. Published by Cambridge University Press.
© Cambridge University Press 2011.

Table 14.1. Secondary myelodysplastic syndromes in childhood.

(1)	Therapy-related myelodysplastic syndrome
	• Chemotherapy
	• Radiation therapy
	• Immunosuppressive/bone marrow transplant
(2)	MDS associated with constitutional bone marrow failure disorders
(3)	Evolution from acquired aplastic anemia
(4)	Familial myelodysplastic syndromes

juvenile myelomonocytic leukemia (JMML) that shows hybrid features of MDS and myeloproliferative neoplasm [6]. In the 2001 World Health Organization (WHO) classification scheme [3], JMML has been separated from MDS, and placed under the myelodysplastic/myeloproliferative neoplasm (MDS/MPN) category. MDS associated with Down syndrome has been reported to account for 20–25% of cases of childhood MDS in the past [7]; in the 2008 WHO classification [8], this disorder is considered as a unique biologic entity synonymous with Down syndrome related myeloid leukemia, and distinct from other cases of childhood MDS.

Although pediatric and adult MDS share many common features, they also differ in many aspects, such as clinical presentation, presence of associated morphologic abnormalities, and the spectrum of chromosomal aberrations observed [9]. The MDS subcategories defined either by the French–American–British (FAB) or WHO classification show substantial differences between pediatric and adult MDS. One example is that refractory anemia with ring sideroblasts (RARS) is exceedingly rare in children [5, 10–15]. Another example is interstitial deletion 5q; although it has occasionally been observed in children, the 5q− syndrome with BM blasts <5%, normal or elevated platelet count, an indolent course, and long survival has not been described in children [9]. Constitutional abnormalities are often observed in children with MDS but are rare in adult MDS. These differences between pediatric and adult MDS preclude pediatric MDS from being adequately categorized by the FAB or 2001 WHO classification scheme, for which the criteria are primarily based on adult MDS patients. In 2003, a pediatric approach for the WHO classification was proposed [16], where the childhood MDS is subdivided into refractory cytopenia (RC), refractory anemia with excess blasts (RAEB), and refractory anemia with excess blasts in transformation (RAEB-t). In the 2008 WHO classification [8], the differences between pediatric and adult MDS are well acknowledged. After removal of JMML and MDS associated with Down syndrome, pediatric MDS is subclassified as: refractory cytopenia of childhood (RCC) if blasts are <2% in peripheral blood, and <5% in bone marrows; and RAEB if blasts are ≥2% in peripheral blood, or ≥5% in bone marrow. RAEB is further divided into RAEB-1 and RAEB-2 based on a blast count of 2–4% versus 5–19% in peripheral blood, and 5–9% versus 10–19% in bone marrow (Table 14.1). Cases with 20–30% blasts in peripheral blood or bone marrow, theoretically AML, may have different significance in pediatric patients. This is discussed in detail

Table 14.2. Pediatric myelodysplastic syndrome subcategories defined by the 2008 WHO classification scheme, with comparison to adult myelodysplastic syndrome WHO subcategories.

	Blood findings	Bone marrow findings	Correlation with adult MDS subcategories
RCC[a]	Sustained/ unexplained cytopenia with <2% blasts	Morphologic dysplasia <5% blasts	RCUD RCMD MDS-U
RAEB RAEB-1 RAEB-2	2–19% blasts 2–4% blasts 5–19% blasts	5–19% blasts 5–9% blasts 10–19% blasts	RAEB RAEB-1 RAEB-2
20–29% blasts:[b] *De novo* AML? RAEB-t?	20–29% blasts	20–29% blasts Dysplasia No AML-related recurrent cytogenetic changes	AML

[a] Please also refer to the minimal diagnostic criteria for MDS (Table 14.3).
[b] Repeat bone marrow after a two-week interval. If blast count is stable over a period of four weeks, likely MDS; if blasts exceed 30%, likely *de novo* AML.
Abbreviations: RCC, refractory cytopenia of childhood; RCUD, refractory cytopenia of unilineage dysplasia; RCMD, refractory cytopenia with multilineage dysplasia; MDS-U, myelodysplastic syndrome-unspecified; RAEB, refractory anemia with excess blasts; RAEB-t, refractory anemia with excess blasts in transformation; AML, acute myeloid leukemia.

under Primary myelodysplastic syndrome with increased blasts, below. The correlation between pediatric and adult MDS subcategories is also shown in Table 14.2.

It is noteworthy that clinical anemia, leukopenia, and thrombocytopenia, as well as morphologic dysplasia, are not specific for MDS and may be present in reactive conditions, such as infection, exposure to drug/toxin, growth factor therapy, chronic systemic illness, or congenital bone marrow failure syndromes. In addition, features in erythroid lineage such as multinuclearity, irregular nuclear membranes, karyorrhexis, and "megaloblastoid" changes have been observed in bone marrow specimens of normal individuals or when there is brisk erythroid hyperplasia, "stress dyserythropoiesis," due to hemolysis or regeneration of the bone marrow after transplantation or chemotherapy [3]. Furthermore, the interobserver agreement among hematopathologists for recognition of dyserythropoiesis is notoriously poor [17]. In children who have a low blast cell count and no clonal cytogenetic abnormalities, to establish a diagnosis of MDS is quite challenging. To ensure diagnostic accuracy, minimal diagnostic criteria for childhood MDS have been recommended (Table 14.3) [18]. Clinically, patients should present with sustained unexplained cytopenia (neutropenia, thrombocytopenia, or anemia), and morphologically with at least bilineage dysplasia in the bone marrow and/or acquired clonal cytogenetic abnormality in hematopoietic cells, or increased blasts (≥5%). The morphologic criteria are more stringent than those for adult MDS, which define dysplasia as ≥10% dysplastic cells in a respective lineage.

Table 14.3. Minimal diagnostic criteria for myelodysplastic syndrome (MDS) in childhood.

At least two of the following:
(1) Sustained unexplained cytopenia (neutropenia, thrombocytopenia, or anemia)
(2) Acquired clonal cytogenetic abnormality in hematopoietic cells
(3) Increased blasts (≥5%)
(4) If blasts are <5%, *and* lack of clonal cytogenetic abnormalities • At least bilineage morphologic dysplasia • Or significant dysmegakaryopoiesis

Modified from Hasle *et al.* [9].

Refractory cytopenia of childhood

Refractory cytopenia of childhood (RCC) is a provisional entity in the 2008 WHO classification to describe a subtype of MDS characterized by cytopenia involving one or more lineages, dysplastic changes in the bone marrow, fewer than 2% blasts in the peripheral blood and fewer than 5% blasts in bone marrow. RCC accounts for approximately 35–65% of pediatric MDS cases [14, 19].

The presence of a clonal cytogenetic abnormality in hematopoietic cells is helpful in confirming a diagnosis of RCC. In the absence of clonal cytogenetic abnormality, a diagnosis of RCC in patients with persistent cytopenia generally requires the presence of dysplastic features in two or more lineages of the hematopoietic cells, or significant dysplasia in the megakaryocytic lineage. All other causes of cytopenia and dysplasia, such as infectious diseases and metabolic disorders, must be ruled out. The minimal diagnostic criteria recommended for pediatric MDS (Table 14.3) should be followed in establishing a diagnosis of RCC. Categories of adult MDS corresponding to pediatric RCC (Table 14.2) are MDS with blasts <5%, including refractory cytopenia with unilineage dysplasia (RCUD), refractory cytopenia with multilineage dysplasia (RCMD), and MDS-unclassifiable (MDS-U). It is noteworthy that RARS and 5q− syndrome are extremely rare in pediatric patients.

Primary myelodysplastic syndrome with increased blasts

Refractory anemia with excess blasts (RAEB) is a subcategory of MDS defined by a blast count between 5 and 19% in the bone marrow and 2–19% in the peripheral blood. RAEB is further divided into RAEB-1 and RAEB-2 by a blast count of 2–4% versus 5–19% in PB, and 5–9% versus 10–19% in BM. Unlike adult MDS, prognostic significance has not been found between RAEB-1 and -2 in children [20]. However, it is recommended to make the distinction in the current classification scheme for future investigation.

In adult patients, RAEB-t was recognized by the FAB classification as a separate entity with >5% blasts in peripheral blood and 21–29% blasts in the bone marrow. Studies comparing adult patients diagnosed as RAEB-t by the FAB criteria with patients diagnosed with MDS-related AML with 30% or more blasts have shown no significant survival differences [18, 21].

Thus in the WHO classification for adult MDS, the blasts cut off for a diagnosis of AML has been lowered from the traditional 30% to 20%, which has abolished the category of RAEB-t and reclassified most of these patients as AML with myelodysplasia related changes (AML-MRC), although the controversy regarding RAEB-t has not been completely settled [22].

In pediatric cases with 20−29% blasts in the PB or BM, if there is significant morphologic dysplasia, preexisting history of MDS, or MDS-related cytogenetic abnormalities, then these cases, although fulfilling the criteria for AML-MRC, may lack the clinical features of AML and behave more like MDS [9, 23]. The presence of organomegaly, central nervous system infiltrate, or myeloid sarcoma, is in favor of *de novo* AML over MDS. Patients with recurrent cytogenetic abnormalities typically associated with AML, such as t(15;17)(*PML/ RARA*), t(8;21)(*RUNX1/ETO*), inv(16)(*CBFB/MYH11*), t(9;11) (*MLL/AF9*), should be diagnosed and treated as AML regardless of the blast count [24].

Clinical features

Clinically, MDS manifests as isolated anemia, neutropenia, or thrombocytopenia, or as multiple cytopenias. Often, an isolated cytopenia can progress to pancytopenia over the course of the disease. Neutropenia and thrombocytopenia are found more often at the time of diagnosis, compared to adult MDS patients. Anemia is not always present, but elevated mean corpuscular volume (MCV) is observed in the majority of patients. In as many as 20% of patients, no clinical signs or symptoms are reported. Congenital abnormalities of different organ systems may be present. However, hepatosplenomegaly and lymphadenopathy are generally absent. Hb F level is frequently elevated [25].

Morphology

Bone marrow biopsy is important in evaluating a child with suspected MDS. It is performed to assess the overall cellularity and the ratio of hematopoietic series, to evaluate the marrow architecture (altered stroma) and fibrosis, as well as to detect abnormal localization of immature precursors (ALIPs). In contrast to adult MDS where the marrow is usually hypercellular or normocellular, more than 50% of pediatric MDS patients show a decreased marrow cellularity for their age, particularly patients with RCC [26]. Hypocellularity results from a proportional decrease in one or more of the hematopoietic cell lineages, and is accompanied in particular by a decrease of the myeloid, and to a lesser degree, of the megakaryocytic series [17]. Myeloid to erythroid (M : E) ratio is usually decreased but can vary from markedly decreased to markedly increased. The marrow architecture is disrupted (Fig. 14.1), and often shows increased histiocytes, lymphocytes, plasma cells, edema, or altered vasculature. Mild to moderate bone marrow fibrosis is more commonly seen at the time of initial MDS diagnosis, compared to adult MDS [27]. Marked fibrosis can be seen in

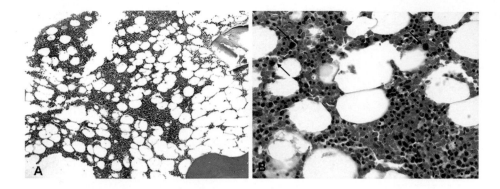

Fig. 14.1. A case of refractory cytopenia of childhood (RCC) showing (A) a hypocellular marrow under a lower power view. (B) Higher power shows dysplastic megakaryocytes (arrows). (Pictures courtesy of Dr. Victor Zota.)

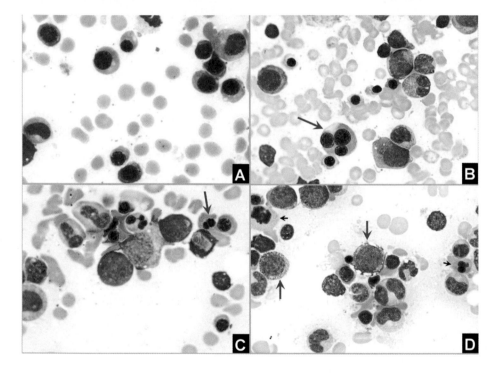

Fig. 14.2. Dyserythropoiesis. (A) Megaloblastoid maturation. (B) Trinuclear form (arrow). (C) Basophilic stippling (arrow). (D) Vacuolated erythroblasts (arrows); also, nuclear irregularity and karyorrhexis of erythroid precursors (arrow heads).

the later stage of MDS or in MDS developed from a preexisting myeloproliferative neoplasm (MPN).

Dysplastic changes can be present in one or more lineages. Dyserythropoiesis is manifested by: alterations in nuclei including budding, internuclear bridging, and karyorrhexis, multinuclearity and megaloblastoid changes; and cytoplasmic changes including vacuolization, basophilic stippling, or presence of granules (Fig. 14.2). Ring sideroblasts are very uncommon in pediatric MDS; the finding of sideroblastic anemia should prompt investigation for possible mitochondrial cytopathy or disorders of heme synthesis [28]. In myeloid series (Fig. 14.3), hypogranulation can be seen in all stages of the maturation, and is more conspicuous in the neutrophils. Abnormal granulation can also manifest as the presence of large coarse granules (pseudo-Chédiak–Higashi granules). Nuclear hypolobation often presents either as bilobed (pseudo-Pelger–Huët cells) or non-lobed nuclei in granulocytes. Nuclear hypersegmentation, abnormal segmentation, abnormal condensation of chromatin, and nuclear/cytoplasmic asynchrony are other

encountered dysplastic features. Granulocytic dysplasia may be more obvious on peripheral blood films. Megakaryocytic dysplasia is characterized by hypolobated micromegakaryocytes, non-lobated nuclei, and multiple widely separated nuclei (Fig. 14.4). The presence of dysplastic megakaryocytes is a strong indication for RCC, compared to dyserythropoiesis or dysgranulopoiesis. Hypersegmented large megakaryocytes are often seen in MPN or sometimes in megaloblastoid anemia; however, in some cases, hypersegmented megakaryocytes can be seen in MDS marrows coexisting with small hypolobated megakaryocytes. Megakaryocytes can be increased, decreased, or normal in number. In evaluating megakaryocyte dysplasia, the best approach is to make an initial evaluation based on the biopsy and then verify that impression on the BM aspirate smears. At least 30 megakaryocytes should be evaluated. It is noteworthy that regenerating, "young" megakaryocytes in patients with thrombocytopenia due to peripheral destruction can be hypolobated or monolobated and small. However, such "young" megakaryocytes often have granular and "red"

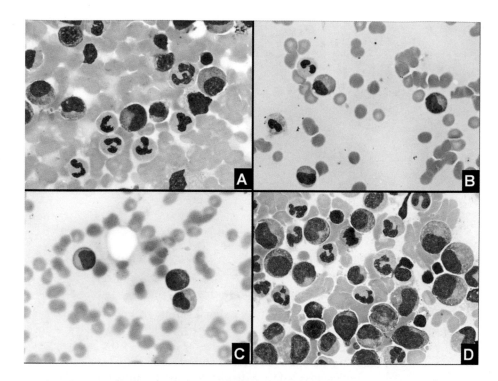

Fig. 14.3. Dysgranulopoiesis. (A) Hypogranulation. (B) Pseudo-Pelger–Huët anomaly. (C) Hypolobated forms (mononucleated neutrophils), and small myelocytes. (D) Left-shifted maturation alone should not account for dysplasia.

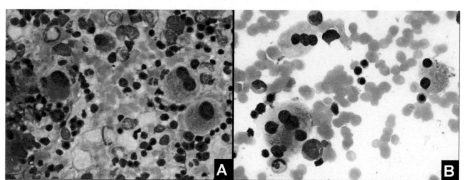

Fig. 14.4. Dysmegakaryopoiesis. (A) Small and hypolobated forms. (B) Megakaryocytes show abnormal nuclear segmentation with completely separated lobes.

cytoplasm (Fig. 14.5), and should not be interpreted as dysplastic megakaryocytes.

In MDS, cells counted as "blasts" include myeloblasts, monoblasts, and megakaryoblasts. The blasts in MDS are often variable in size, ranging from very small to large (Fig. 14.6), in contrast to a more uniform size in *de novo* AML. Myeloblasts are further defined as granular and agranular myeloblasts by the MDS international working group (IWG) [29]. Agranular blasts have high nuclear/cytoplasmic ratios, and blastic chromatin, but show conspicuous nucleoli with no granules or very scant granules in cytoplasm; while granular blasts have at least 20 azurophilic granules, and used to be called type III blasts. A minimal 500-cell count is required for an accurate blast enumeration. Abnormal localization of immature precursors (ALIPs) is defined as the presence of small clusters or aggregates of myeloblasts and promyelocytes (5–8 cells) in the marrow intertrabecular spaces, away from the vascular structures and endosteal surface of the bone trabeculae (Fig. 14.7) [9]. ALIPs can be seen frequently in pediatric MDS, especially associated

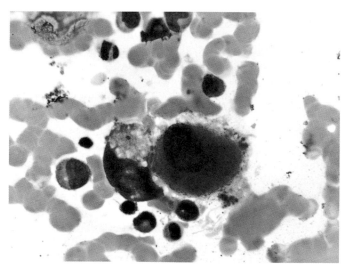

Fig. 14.5. Regenerating, "young" megakaryocytes in a patient with idiopathic thrombocytopenic purpura (ITP) can show small hypolobated nucleus but granular cytoplasm.

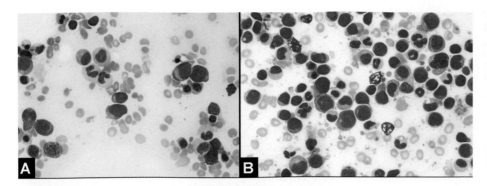

Fig. 14.6. Blasts in myelodysplastic syndrome (MDS) often show a spectrum of sizes ranging from very small to large. (A) A case of refractory anemia with excess blasts (RAEB). (B) Acute myeloid leukemia (AML) arising from preexisting myelodysplastic syndromes. Pronounced dysgranulopoiesis is present on both A and B.

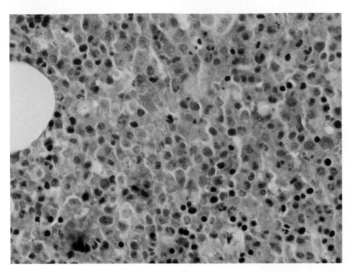

Fig. 14.7. Bone marrow biopsy shows atypical localization of immature precursors (ALIPs) in a case of refractory anemia with excess blasts (RAEB) (Wright–Giemsa stain).

with RAEB [16]. Although ALIP is not unique to MDS and can be seen in active BM regeneration or growth factor treatment, the presence of ALIPs in MDS is often associated with a poor outcome and increased risk for AML progression. The presence of Auer rods in adult MDS would classify a case as RAEB-2 regardless of blast count; however, this rule has not been clearly indicated in pediatric MDS, likely because of the rarity of such cases, and lack of significance between RAEB-1 and RAEB-2.

As described previously, in pediatric patients with blasts of 20–30%, the differential diagnosis between MDS and AML could be challenging, and the decision should be based upon clinical features, cytogenetics and serial assessments of the bone marrow. Morphologically, RAEB-t bone marrow often shows retained differentiation and maturation in the hematopoietic cells, especially in myeloid series with easily identifiable segmented neutrophils. In *de novo* AML, although megakaryocytes may be retained and erythroid series may show hyperplasia as in the FAB M6a category, there is often a lack of maturation in myeloid series with a marked decrease in segmented neutrophils. It is recommended to repeat BM examination two weeks later for patients presenting with a BM blast percentage of 20–30% and no clinical or cytogenetic changes characteristic of MDS or AML. If the blast count is stable for an arbitrary period

of four weeks, it is suggestive of RAEB-t [30]. If blasts have increased to ≥30%, the patient most likely has *de novo* AML.

Immunophenotype

Application of immunohistochemistry

Immunohistochemistry (IHC) can be very useful in assessing MDS, especially in fibrotic or hypocellular BM. CD34 is positive in the majority of blasts, regardless of MDS subtype [31]. The presence of increased and/or clustered CD34+ blasts not only helps confirm a diagnosis of MDS, but also assists in identifying ALIPs [32, 33]. CD34 also stains endothelium and sinus lining cells, so highlighting the increased angiogenesis characteristic of MDS. In rare cases, blasts in MDS are negative for CD34. In these instances, CD117/KIT can be used as an alternative blast marker; however, CD117 will also stain early erythroid precursors (pronormoblasts), some promyelocytes, and mast cells.

Paraffin section markers of megakaryocytes, including CD61, CD42b, von Willebrand factor (VWF)-associated protein, and LAT (linker of activation of T-cells), are useful in highlighting micromegakaryocytes and abnormal grouping or clustering of megakaryocytes, especially in fibrotic BM. These markers are also helpful in differentiating MDS from acute megakaryocytic leukemia where the megakaryoblasts have an abnormal phenotype, commonly CD61+ but negative for CD42 and the VWF-associated protein.

Flow cytometric immunophenotyping

Flow cytometric immunophenotyping is a highly sensitive and reproducible method for quantitative and qualitative evaluation of hematopoietic cells at different maturation stages during normal myelopoiesis. MDS patients have been found to have altered antigenic expression, as indicated by either the intensity of fluorescence or the percentage of positive cells. These abnormalities have been observed in blasts, maturing myeloid cells, and monocytes. Several groups have utilized flow cytometric immunophenotyping in diagnosing MDS, particularly in differentiating hypocellular MDS from aplastic anemia [34–37]. In MDS, the blasts can show increased fluorescence intensity of CD117, CD13, or CD33 (Fig. 14.8), decreased CD45, or aberrant lymphoid antigen (CD2, CD5, CD7, CD56 expression). The maturing myeloid cells (Fig. 14.9) can show: decreased side

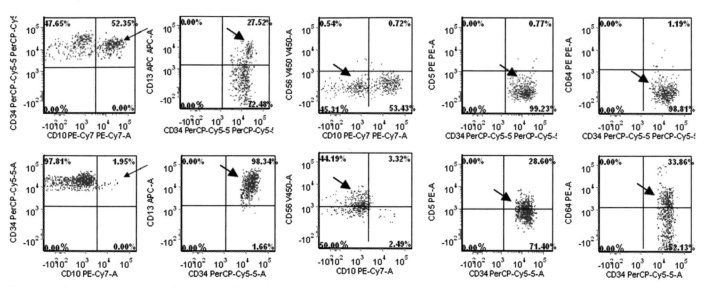

Fig. 14.8. Flow cytometric immunophenotyping of myelodysplastic syndrome – analyzing CD34+ cells. Upper panel: normal lymphoma staging bone marrow, showing many stage I hematogones (long arrow); myeloblasts (short arrow) show no aberrant antigenic expression. Lower pane: marked reduction/absence of hematogones. Compared to normal CD34+ myeloid precursors, the MDS myeloblasts (short arrows) show increased CD13, CD64 expression, aberrant CD56 and dim CD5 expression.

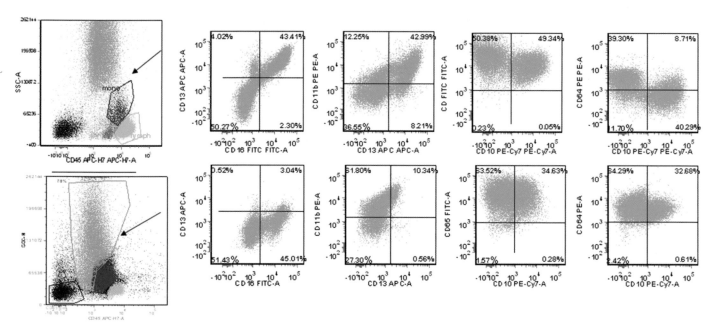

Fig. 14.9. Flow cytometric immunophenotyping of myelodysplastic syndromes – analyzing maturing myeloid cells. Upper panel: lymphoma staging normal marrow shows normal granularity, well separated myeloid and monocytic populations, and normal maturation patterns (CD13/CD16; CD11b/CD13; CD65/CD10; CD64/CD10) of maturing myeloid cells. Lower panel: bone marrow from a patient with refractory cytopenia of childhood shows: hypogranularity; merging granulocytes and monocytes; and altered CD13/CD16, CD11b/CD13, CD65/CD10, and CD64/CD10 patterns.

scatter (SS) indicative of hypogranulation; altered maturation patterns of CD13/CD16 or CD11b/CD16; or decreased fluorescence intensity of mature myeloid antigens, such as CD10, CD15, and CD33. The monocytes can be increased in numbers, show increased HLA-DR and decreased CD14, CD64, CD33, CD11b, CD13 expression, or increased CD56 expression. The normal precursor B-cells (hematogones) are usually decreased in MDS, especially the stage I hematogones (CD34+, CD10+, CD19+, CD20+/−) [38]. The utility of flow cytometric immunophenotyping as an ancillary test in diagnosing

MDS has been gradually accepted. This test is less subjective and could be particularly helpful when the morphologic evaluation is limited due to suboptimal aspirate smears, or to diagnose MDS in an early phase [39]. However, the flow cytometry analysis of immunophenotypic changes is quite complex and requires an experienced hematopathologist and extensive validation studies. Therefore, it is recommended to be utilized in experienced laboratories only. Substitution of the percentage of CD34+ cells determined by flow cytometry (FC) for a visual blast count is discouraged. Not all myeloblasts

Table 14.4. Common immunophenotypic abnormalities identified by flow cytometry in myelodysplastic syndrome bone marrows.

	Blast abnormalities	Maturing myeloid cells	Monocytes
CD45/side scatter (SS)	Increased blasts (>3%) A discrete population	Decreased SS Decreased CD45	Increased monocytes Decreased SS and/or CD45
Increased expression	CD117, CD33, CD13, CD34, CD123, CD7	HLA-DR, CD117	CD117, CD15, CD123
Decreased expression	CD45, CD38, HLA-DR	CD10, CD15, CD64, CD13, CD33, CD11b, CD16, CD38	HLA-DR, CD14, CD64, CD11b, CD13, CD33, CD123
Aberrant expression	CD2, CD5, CD7, CD10, CD56, CD15, CD65	CD2, CD5, CD7, CD56	CD2, CD5, CD7, CD56
Altered expression pattern		CD11b/CD13/CD16, CD64/CD10, CD33/CD15	CD64/CD14
Others	Decreased normal precursor B-cells (hematogones), especially stage I hematogones (CD19+, CD34+, CD10+) Decreased plasmacytoid dendritic cell precursors (CD34+, CD123+ + +, HLA-DR+)		

express CD34, and not all CD34-positive cells are myeloblasts (e.g., stage I hematogones are CD34+). Furthermore, the number of blasts enumerated by FC is affected by hemodilution, incomplete red blood cell lysis/lysis of late stage nucleated red blood cells, suboptimal cell viability due to sample aging, or cell loss due to sample processing. Recently, the European LeukemiaNet has published "Standardization of flow cytometry in myelodysplastic syndromes," and made recommendations on panel design and scoring criteria [40]. The flow cytometric immunophenotypic changes in MDS are summarized in Table 14.4.

PNH clones can be detected by flow cytometric analysis of GPI-anchored proteins, such as multiparameter fluorescent aerolysin (FLAER) analysis [41], CD55, CD59, CD24, CD16, CD66b, CD24, and CD14 [42, 43] (Fig. 14.10). Adult MDS patients with a detected PNH clone have shown overlapping features with aplastic anemia and have better responses to immunosuppressive therapy.

Cytogenetics

Chromosomal aberrations are present in 50–80% of pediatric MDS patients by conventional karyotyping [44]. This reported number may be higher than the actual frequency because of the difficulties in establishing the diagnosis of childhood RCC by morphology alone. Monosomy 7 and/or del(7q) is the most common cytogenetic abnormality in childhood MDS (>50%), and often is present as the sole abnormality. Activating *RAS* mutations or inactivation of *NF1* are found to coexist with monosomy 7/del(7q) in the bone marrows of many children with MDS, which suggests that these alterations cooperate in leukemogenesis [45]. Spontaneous disappearance of monosomy 7 and cytopenia has been reported in infants, but remains a rare event [46]. In adults, monosomy 7 is less common, and loss of chromosome 7 is frequently accompanied by multiple karyotypic rearrangements. The second most frequent chromosomal abnormality is trisomy 8. Other numeric or structural chromosomal abnormalities account for approximately 10% of karyotypic abnormalities in pediatric MDS. Karyotypic evolution is observed in some patients and is often associated

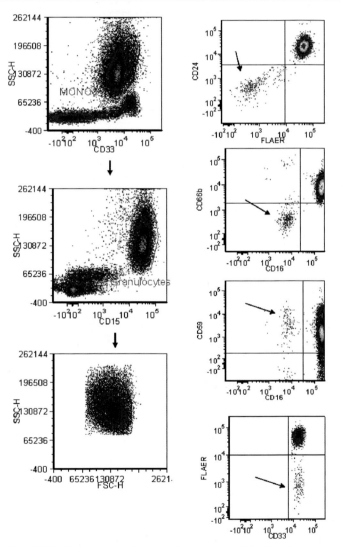

Fig. 14.10. Flow cytometry immunophenotyping in detection of paroxysmal nocturnal hemoglobinuria (PNH) cells in the peripheral blood sample obtained from a patient with aplastic anemia. Left panel: sequential gating is applied to the granulocyte population and monocytes to ensure detection accuracy (CD33/side scatter; CD15/side scatter; and forward/side scatter). Right panel: a small number (1.5%) of PNH cells are detected, both on granulocytes (FLAER negative, CD24 negative, CD16 negative, CD66b negative, CD59 negative; upper right three figures); and monocytes (loss of FLAER, lowest figure on the right).

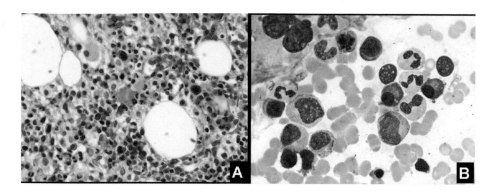

Fig. 14.11. A 14-year-old female presented with pancytopenia and later was diagnosed with systemic lupus erythematosus. (A) The bone marrow biopsy showed altered marrow stroma and some dysplastic megakaryocytes, mimicking myelodysplastic syndromes. (B) Dyserythropoiesis with karyorrhexis of erythroid precursors is also present. Plasma cells are increased. (Pictures provided courtesy of Dr. Victor Zota.)

with disease progression. Common non-random AML translocations are absent, and loss of the long arm of chromosome 5 (5q13–33) is exceedingly rare in children with MDS [3]. Cytogenetic alterations in therapy-related MDS will be discussed under therapy-related MDS/AML.

Differential diagnosis

Dysplastic features seen in cytopenic patients without a hematologic disorder

In children, morphologic dysplasia of the marrow may occur in a variety of disorders of different etiologies, such as infection [12], drug therapy [26], chronic diseases [47], nutritional deficiency, and genetic/metabolic disorders. In autoimmune disorders, such as systemic lupus erythematosus (Fig. 14.11), the bone marrow often shows altered marrow stroma with increased lymphocytes, plasma cells, stromal cells, histiocytes, and edema. Mild morphologic dysplasia, especially dyserythropoiesis, sometimes dysmegakaryopoiesis, and a left-shifted myeloid maturation are seen. Therefore, in the absence of a cytogenetic marker, the clinical course must be carefully evaluated: two bone marrow examinations with biopsies at least two weeks apart are recommended before a diagnosis of RCC can be established [2].

Dysplastic features in inherited bone marrow failure

Congenial disorders such as congenital dyserythropoietic anemia, Noonan syndrome, Dobowitz syndrome, mitochondrial disorders (Pearson syndrome) [14], reticular dysgenesis, TAR (thrombocytopenia with absent radius) syndrome, and congenital amegakaryocytic thrombocytopenia [48] can mimic MDS but are not associated with an increased risk of acute leukemia. These congenital diseases should be excluded by careful physical examination for skeletal and other organ abnormalities, past medical history, family history, and appropriate laboratory tests. It is recommended to rule out Fanconi anemia by chromosomal breakage, G2 cell cycle arrest, western blot, or mutational analysis in children with suspected primary MDS. Many inherited bone marrow failure disorders cannot be separated from RCC by morphologic criteria. It is possible that children diagnosed with hypoplastic RCC without a clonal marker may suffer from a yet undiagnosed inherited bone marrow failure disorder.

Aplastic anemia and hypoplastic myelodysplastic syndromes

Differentiating hypoplastic MDS from aplastic anemia (AA) may be very challenging. The low cellularity and often poor quality aspirates obtained from such specimens make the identification of dyspoiesis and the enumeration of blasts difficult. In some cases, it is virtually impossible to distinguish hypocellular MDS from AA [47]. In blood smears, macrocytic red blood cells are often found in both conditions, but the presence of neutrophils with pseudo-Pelger–Huët nuclei and/or hypogranular cytoplasm would favor a diagnosis of MDS. In the bone marrow, similarly, dysplastic granulopoiesis and megakaryocytopoiesis are in favor of MDS, but dyserythropoiesis has been reported in AA as well.

In hypoplastic MDS, the bone marrow biopsy shows sparsely scattered dysgranulopoietic cells, patchy islands of immature erythropoiesis, and, in most cases, decreased megakaryopoiesis with some micromegakaryocytes (Fig. 14.12) [49]. Bone marrow can be completely empty in some areas, while discernible dysplastic cellular islands are present in others. A larger and deeper biopsy may help to establish a more definitive diagnosis. Normal or increased CD34+ cells in the bone marrow are more likely seen in MDS, whereas CD34+ cells are markedly decreased in AA. Although the identification of a clonal chromosomal abnormality at the time of presentation is generally considered indicative of MDS, clonal chromosomal abnormality may occasionally be seen in AA [50], particularly in Fanconi anemia [51].

Biologically, an overlap between acquired AA and RCC has been suggested [52]. Moreover, MDS develops in 10 to 15% of those children with AA who are not treated with hematopoietic stem cell transplantation. Small populations of clones deficient in glycosyl-phosphatidyl-inositol (GPI)-anchored proteins on their cell surface may be detected in 40–50% of AA patients by flow cytometric analysis, in the absence of clinical signs of paroxysmal nocturnal hemoglobinuria (PNH) [53]. These *PIGA*-mutated cells appear to be an independent clonal expansion that arises because of a selective growth advantage under immune-mediated destruction of bone marrow hematopoietic cells. However, such small clones have been detected in approximately 20% of adult low grade MDS, such as refractory anemia (RA) [43, 54]. While it is unknown how many children with RCC harbor a PNH clone, the presence of such a PNH cell

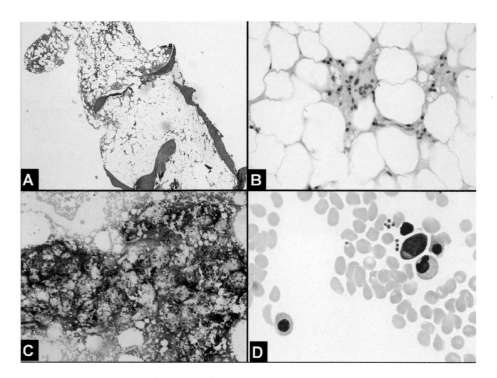

Fig. 14.12. Hypocellular myelodysplastic syndrome. (A) Bone marrow biopsy shows a hypocellularity, which could be difficult to differentiate from aplastic anemia. There are some hematopoietic islands present. (B) The cellular components are mainly of stromal cells, lymphocytes, plasma cells and a few hematopoietic cells. (C) Aspirate material comprised mainly of fat and stromal cells, reflecting the nature of hypocellularity, which should not be interpreted as "inadequate aspirate." (D) Rarely obtained hematopoietic cells showing one blast and one dysplastic neutrophil.

population is consistent and certainly does not exclude a diagnosis of MDS.

Recently, members of the French–American–British (FAB) Cooperative Leukemia Working Group met to review cases of aplastic anemia, hypocellular myelodysplastic syndrome, and hypocellular acute myeloid leukemia. Criteria were proposed and modified following the workshops [55]. The comparison of criteria of hypoplastic refractory cytopenia of childhood and aplastic anemia in childhood is listed in Table 14.5.

Diagnosis of MDS in patients with congenital bone marrow failure syndrome

MDS associated with constitutive abnormalities accounts for 29 to 45% of all pediatric MDS [56]. In patients with congenital bone marrow failure disorders, hematopoiesis can show dysplastic features, particularly dyserythropoiesis. Therefore, evolved MDS can only be diagnosed if a persistent clonal chromosomal abnormality is present, or hypercellularity in the bone marrow develops in the presence of persistent peripheral cytopenia. The incidence of secondary MDS/AML is listed in Table 14.6.

Prognosis and predictive factors

Childhood MDS with bone marrow blasts <5% and a platelet count ≥100 × 10^9/L may show a long and stable clinical course without treatment. The condition may smolder with unchanged cytopenia for months or even years, but will eventually progress in most patients [57]. Increased fetal hemoglobin (Hb F) >10%, platelet count <40 × 10^9/L, and two or more cytogenetic abnormalities are believed to be associated with an adverse outcome [57].

Pediatric patients with monosomy 7 have significantly higher risk of progression to advanced MDS. Monosomy 7 is considered to be a poor prognostic predictor irrespective of therapy [58]. The International Prognostic Scoring System (IPSS) for adult MDS weights on bone marrow blast count, cytopenia, and cytogenetics, and separates adult MDS patients into four prognostic groups: low, intermediate-1, intermediate-2, and high [59]. The IPSS has shown strong prognostic value in adults with MDS. The distribution among the IPSS groups in children is skewed towards patients in the high-risk group, due to a higher frequency of cytopenia and monosomy 7 compared to adults. IPSS can identify a small group of children with low-risk MDS and a very favorable outcome (patients with RCC, a normal karyotype, and absence of severe cytopenia); however, the scoring system has not been very informative in children [9].

In summary, pediatric MDS is a rare hematologic disease, which is not encountered often in a daily practice. The pediatric MDS diagnosis requires more stringent inclusion criteria, and the minimal diagnostic criteria recommended by the pediatric WHO classification should be followed. Pediatric MDS categorization differs from the adult MDS WHO classification, and the 2008 WHO classification for MDS in childhood is the recommended classification scheme. The comparison of adult and pediatric MDS is summarized in Table 14.7.

Therapy-related myeloid neoplasm

Definition

Therapy-related myeloid neoplasm is a late complication of cytotoxic chemotherapy and radiation therapy administered

Table 14.5. Comparison of hypoplastic refractory cytopenia of childhood and aplastic anemia in childhood.

	Aplastic anemia	Hypoplastic refractory cytopenia of childhood
Bone marrow examination		
Erythroid	Absent, or very small erythroid clusters (<10 cells/cluster), dyserythropoiesis often mild if present	Patchy distribution of erythroid clusters, left-shifted Dyserythropoiesis is often more pronounced
Megakaryocytes	Often absent, or too few to assess morphology	Reduced, but more easily identifiable, with dysplastic features
Myeloid cells	Decreased, dysgranulopoiesis is mild if present	Decreased, more pronounced dysplasia
CD34 blasts	Decreased to absent (<1%)	<5%, but more discernible than those seen in aplastic anemia
Increased mast cells, lymphocytes, and lymphoid follicles	Often present	Often present
Altered architecture	Often normal	Often altered
Reticulin fibrosis	Absent	Can present in 20% of cases
Flow cytometry immunophenotyping	Often shows normal myelomonocytic maturation. Hematogones are present. Paroxysmal nocturnal hemoglobinuria clones seen in 40–50% of cases	Often shows abnormal myelomonocytic maturation. Myeloblasts may show aberrant antigen expression. Hematogones often reduced. Paroxysmal nocturnal hemoglobinuria clones seen in 15–20% of cases
Cytogenetics	Often normal. A few can have cytogenetic abnormality	40–50% abnormal; however, markedly fatty marrows may lead to cytogenetic failures

Table 14.6. Incidence of secondary myelodysplastic syndrome/acute myeloid leukemia (t-MDS/t-AML) developed in congenital bone marrow failure syndrome.

Bone marrow failure syndrome	MDS/AML prevalence (%)
Fanconi anemia	30–40
Diamond–Blackfan anemia	5
Severe congenital neutropenia	30
Shwachman–Diamond syndrome	30–40
Congenital amegakaryocytic thrombocytopenia	10
Dyskeratosis congenita	5

for prior neoplastic or non-neoplastic disorders [60]. It includes therapy-related acute myeloid leukemia (t-AML), myelodysplastic syndrome (t-MDS) and myelodysplastic/myeloproliferative neoplasm (t-MDS/MPN).

Epidemiology

Therapy-related myeloid neoplasm accounts for 10–20% of pediatric MDS, AML, or MDS/MPN (mostly chronic myelomonocytic leukemia) [6, 15, 51]. The risk with alkylating agents or radiation therapy generally increases with age, whereas the risk for those treated with topoisomerase II inhibitors is similar across all ages [61, 62]. Therapy-related myeloid neoplasm can occur following treatment for almost any childhood cancer, it most commonly follows treatment for Hodgkin lymphoma, osteogenic sarcoma, acute lymphoblastic leukemia (ALL), non-Hodgkin lymphoma, and Ewing sarcoma

[49, 51, 59, 63–65]. It has been recognized that therapy-related myeloid neoplasm also can occur following bone marrow transplantation (both autologous and allogeneic) [66]. In children surviving at least five years following their primary cancer, the standardized incidence ratio (observed/expected) for therapy-related myeloid neoplasm is approximately 8.0 overall, with a median time to occurrence of six years [67]. Higher incidence occurs in patients treated with the regimen containing epipodophyllotoxins (topoisomerase II inhibitors). For children treated for Hodgkin lymphoma, the actuarial risk in survivors developing therapy-related myeloid neoplasm is 0.6–2.8%, and the median time to development of t-MDS/t-AML is four to five years [68]. The risk increases to 1.5–4.6% in patients who have received stem cell transplant [69–71]. The incidence of therapy-related myeloid neoplasm in patients with treated non-Hodgkin lymphoma is 0.5–5.7% in long-term survivors, with the higher incidence seen in patients treated with an epipodophyllotoxin-containing regime and/or stem cell transplantation [69, 70]. The incidence of therapy-related myeloid neoplasm in patients with treated acute lymphoblastic leukemia (ALL) ranges from 0.2 to 3% [64, 72, 73]. The improved outcome for osteogenic sarcoma and primitive neuroectodermal tumor of bone is associated with an increasing incidence of second malignancies, from 0.2 to 3.3% [74–76]. Higher incidence (7–11%) of therapy-related myeloid neoplasm in patients with Ewing sarcoma is closely associated with high-intensity chemotherapy (higher doses of doxorubicin, cyclophosphamide, and ifosfamide) received [65, 77]. t-MDS/t-AML in patients with Wilms tumor is extremely rare, and the reported incidence is 0–0.1% [49, 78, 79].

Table 14.7. Comparison between adult and pediatric myelodysplastic syndromes.

	Adult MDS	Pediatric MDS
Incidence	2 to 12 per 100 000	0.1 to <1 per 100 000
Age (median)	70 years	5–8 years
Male : female ratio	1.5–1.7 : 1	1 : 1
2008 WHO classification scheme	WHO classification scheme • RCUD • RARS • RCMD • MDS-U • RAEB-1 • RAEB-2 • 5q– syndrome	Pediatric WHO classification scheme • RCC • RAEB-1 • RAEB-2 • RAEB-t?
Morphology		
Cellularity, adjusted for age	Majority hyper- or normocellular	>50% of cases are hypocellular
Dysplasia	>10% dysplastic cells in one or more lineage	Dysplasia often pronounced and involving two or more lineages
Marrow fibrosis (%)	5–15	20–40
Clonal cytogenetic abnormalities		
Frequency of abnormalities (%)	40–50	50–70
Abnormal karyotype	del(5)(q31–33), + 8, 20q-, 3q abnormalities, 7q–, 17p–, –5, –7, 11q23– (t-MDS)	–7, (>50% of cases), +8, del(5)(q31–33), rare –5, 11q23– (t-MDS)
Prognosis scoring system	International Prognostic Scoring System (IPSS)	Category, cytology, and cytogenetics (CCC) pending further study IPSS has limited value

Abbreviations: RCC, refractory cytopenia of childhood; RCUD, refractory cytopenia of unilineage dysplasia; RCMD, refractory cytopenia with multilineage dysplasia; MDS-U, myelodysplastic syndrome-unspecified; RAEB, refractory anemia with excess blasts; RAEB-t, refractory anemia with excess blasts in transformation; AML, acute myeloid leukemia.

Over the past 30 years, the outcomes of treatment for severe acquired aplastic anemia (SAA) have been greatly improved by simultaneous administration of recombinant human granulocyte colony stimulating factor (rhG-CSF) in combination with immunosuppressive therapy. However, in the long-term follow-up of patients with aplastic anemia (AA) who had received such therapy, the development of clonal diseases, such as PNH and MDS/AML, has been observed. Clinical data to date suggest that development of MDS/AML occurs in about 5–15% of long-term survivors of aplastic anemia [80–84].

Pathophysiology

The etiology of therapy-related myeloid neoplasm in pediatric patients is probably secondary to a combination of age at the time of primary cancer diagnosis, genetic susceptibility [85], environmental exposure and prior treatment regimens [49]. Treatment with alkylating agents causes intrastrand and interstrand cross-links of DNA molecules, interfering with DNA replication, leading to cell death [30, 42, 62, 86–88]. Such agents may cause non-lethal damage to bone marrow cell precursors, thus predisposing them to malignant change. Topoisomerase II inhibitors act by binding to the topoisomerase/DNA enzyme complex at the cleavage stage induced by topoisomerase, leading to DNA strand breaks [30, 42, 62, 86–88]. Cell death is caused by unrepaired strand breaks. Chromosomal transloca-

tions may occur as a result of aberrantly repaired chromosome breakage, with subsequent predisposition to leukemia [87, 89]. Radiation-induced DNA double-strand breaks and mutagenicity may be similar to that of alkylating agents [49]. In addition, radiation may lead to t-MDS/t-AML through alteration of the *RUNX1* (*AML1*) gene [88]. The role of hematopoietic stem cell transplantation in the development of t-MDS/t-AML is complex [2, 70, 90–93]. There is evidence to suggest that the association is related to prior anticancer treatment, stem cell mobilization, and supportive measures, such as granulocyte colony stimulating growth factor (G-CSF) [92–94].

Genetic disorders may predispose children to t-MDS/t-AML secondary to poor repair of DNA. These disorders include neurofibromatosis type 1 (NF1), Fanconi anemia, Bloom syndrome, Down syndrome, Shwachman syndrome, Kostmann syndrome, Diamond–Blackfan anemia, and familial platelet disorder with predisposition to AML [95]. Genetic polymorphisms of chemotherapy drug-metabolizing enzymes are probably a more common etiology of t-MDS/t-AML [85, 96, 97]. Glutathione S-transferase (GST) has an important role in the metabolism of carcinogens and mutagens. The odds ratio of developing t-AML is increased in patients with GSTP1-Val, especially when the patients' primary tumors have been treated with a known substrate for GSTP1 (e.g., etoposide, cyclophosphamide, cisplatin, doxorubicin) [96]. In contrast to most genetic predispositions, the presence of variant cytochrome

P450 3A (CYP3A4) affords protection against topoisomerase II-related t-MDS/t-AML compared with the wild-type genotype [97, 98]. Other pharmacogenetic polymorphisms include those that decrease the function of NAD(P)H, quinone oxidoreductase 1 (NQO1), and decrease TPMT (thiopurine *S*-methyltransferase) activity [44, 85]. In t-MDS/t-AML developed in aplastic anemia patients treated with immunosuppressant and growth factors, the genetic instability in aplastic anemia patients may facilitate chromosomal loss, and the karyotypically abnormal hematopoietic clones (monosomy 7) may have a growth advantage in the presence of G-CSF [80, 82].

Clinical presentation

Patients with therapy-related myeloid neoplasm have a history of cytotoxic treatment for previous hematologic or non-hematologic malignancies, or for non-neoplastic diseases. In adults, therapy-related myeloid neoplasm secondary to alkylating agents and/or ionizing radiation most commonly occurs 5–10 years after exposure. Patients often present with t-MDS and evidence of bone marrow failure, although a minority may present with t-MDS/MPN or with overt t-AML. This category is commonly associated with unbalanced loss of genetic material, often involving chromosomes 5 and/or 7. Therapy-related myeloid neoplasm following treatment with topoisomerase II inhibitors (20–30% of cases), has a latency period of about one to five years, and most patients in this subset do not have a myelodysplastic phase but present initially with overt acute leukemia that is often associated with a balanced chromosomal translocation. In practice, many patients have received chemotherapies including both classes of drugs, and the clinicopathologic features may not be clear cut. Nevertheless, in children and adolescents, the classical distinction between alkylator-type and topoisomerase II inhibitor-type t-MDS is indistinct, clinically and cytogenetically [99, 100]. Children with t-MDS/t-AML are older, have lower white blood cell counts, and less pronounced hepatosplenomegaly than children with *de novo* MDS/AML. The t-MDS/t-AML patients usually have no central nervous system (CNS) involvement or granulocytic sarcoma (chloroma) at presentation, compared to *de novo* AML in the pediatric population [63, 65, 71, 77]. It should be noted that occasional patients assigned to the category of therapy-related myeloid neoplasms represent coincidental primary MDS, which would be expected to behave like other *de novo* disease. However, it may suggest genetic predisposition to cancer, and a confounding factor to a short overall survival in affected individuals.

Morphology

The morphologic diagnostic criteria for t-MDS/t-AML should follow the guidelines for primary MDS or *de novo* AML. With the WHO classification system, the designation is simpler [60]. Although therapy-related myeloid neoplasms can be classified as t-MDS, t-AML, or t-MDS/MPN depending on their morphology, blast counts, and peripheral monocyte counts, such subclassification may lack clinical significance [101]. Therapy-related myeloid neoplasms following alkylating agent exposure often show significant morphologic dysplasia, frequently multilineage dysplasia [18]. Compared to primary MDS, t-MDS often shows more pronounced dyspoietic and megaloblastoid erythroid changes [57]. The erythroid series is affected more often than the myeloid or megakaryocytic series, but anisopoikilocytosis and other erythrocyte abnormalities are uncommon [18]. t-AML can occasionally be the initial presentation following alkylating agent exposure, and often shows French–American–British (FAB) M0, M1, or M2 morphology. In therapy-related myeloid neoplasm secondary to topoisomerase II inhibitors, t-AML is often the initial manifestation and is associated with balanced recurrent chromosomal translocations frequently involving 11q23 (*MLL*) or 21q22 (*RUNX1*). The morphology of t-AML with recurrent chromosomal abnormalities often resembles *de novo* acute leukemia harboring the same chromosomal abnormality [89, 102–104]. Figure 14.13 illustrates the morphologic variety seen in t-AML.

To diagnose t-MDS without increased blasts or clonal cytogenetic abnormalities one has to be extremely cautious. Blood and bone marrows following chemotherapy and/or stem cell transplantation may show dysplastic features without evolution to fulfill the diagnostic criteria for t-MDS/t-AML [91, 105, 106]. Myeloid maturation arrest can occur in patients who underwent treatment for primary malignancy, and shares many clinical features with MDS (Fig. 14.14). To diagnose t-MDS/t-AML in patients with *de novo* AML that has been treated with chemotherapy with/or without bone marrow transplant may be extremely challenging. It is difficult to distinguish t-AML from "phenotypic" switch in patients with *de novo* AML that shows a different subtype of AML subsequent to initial treatment [90, 107]. The difficulty in distinguishing t-MDS/t-AML from reactive dysplasia in such a setting is further complicated by the presence of transient clonal cytogenetic abnormalities [12, 105, 108]. It has been suggested that t-MDS/t-AML should only be considered if molecular/genetic studies demonstrate an independent origin of the secondary leukemic clone [67].

Cytogenetics

Over 90% of patients with t-AML/t-MDS show an abnormal karyotype (Table 14.8). The most common cytogenetic abnormalities in t-MDS/t-AML associated with alkylating agents (approximately 70% of patients) are unbalanced chromosomal aberrations, mainly whole or partial loss of chromosomes 5 and/or 7, that are often associated with one or more additional chromosomal abnormalities [e.g., del(13q), del(20q), del(11q), del(3p), −17, −18, −21, +8] in a complex karyotype. For topoisomerase II inhibitor-associated t-MDS/t-AML (20–30% of patients), balanced chromosomal translocations that involve rearrangements of 11q23, 21q22 [including t(8;21)(q22;q22) and t(3;21)(q26.2;q22.1)], and other abnormalities such as

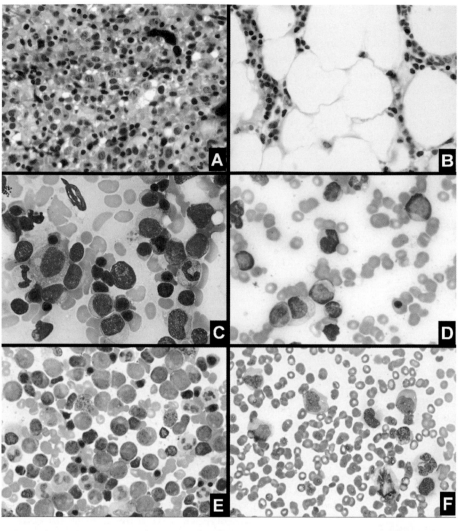

Fig. 14.13. Therapy-related/secondary acute myeloid leukemia (t-AML). (A) AML developed in a patient treated for testicular tumor. Background dysplasia is present. (B) Hypocellular AML developed in a patient with preexisting aplastic anemia. (C) a case of t-AML, FAB classification M6a. (D) A case of t-AML, FAB classification M2. (E) A case of t-AML, FAB classification M4. (F) A case of t-AML, FAB classification M5b. Background dysplasia is variably present.

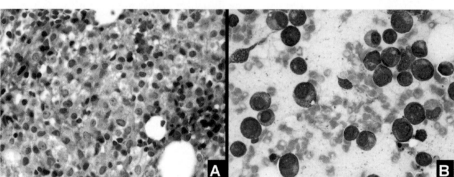

Fig. 14.14. Myeloid maturation arrest: a patient with refractory Hodgkin lymphoma who underwent bone marrow transplant and received G-CSF for supportive treatment developed neutropenia. Bone marrow showed myeloid maturation arrest with most of the cells in promyelocyte, myelocyte, and metamyelocyte stages [(A) biopsy; (B) aspirate]. Maturation arrest can share clinical and morphologic features with a myelodysplastic syndrome.

t(15;17)(q22;q12) and inv(16)(p13q22), are the common findings [87, 89, 103, 104, 109]. Of these balanced translocations, chromosomal breakage at 11q23 involving the mixed lineage leukemia (*MLL*) locus remains the most commonly associated translocation. Approximately one-third of *MLL* gene rearrangements are cryptic. The partner breakpoints of 11q23 in t-MDS/t-AML overlap with those of *de novo* MDS/AML [59, 68]. However, t(11;16)(q23;p13) appears to be found only in t-MDS/t-AML [110, 111]. Other abnormalities involving 21q22

(*RUNX1* gene) other than t(8;21) [103], or 11p15 (*NUP98* gene), chromosomes 7q, 20q, 1q, and 13q are also reported [68, 108, 112]. Reported radiation-induced cytogenetic abnormalities are generally lower than those induced by chemotherapy, and frequently include alterations of the *RUNX1* gene (21q22), del(5), or other miscellaneous cytogenetic changes [109, 112–114]. Monosomy 7 is the most frequent chromosomal abnormality seen in t-MDS/t-AML developed in patients with aplastic anemia treated with immunosuppressant and G-CSF

Table 14.8. Characteristics of therapy-related myeloid neoplasia.

	Alkylating agents	Mixed agents Stem cell transplantation	Topoisomerase II inhibitors	Radiation alone	Immunosuppressive and growth factor treatment for bone marrow failure
Latency (years)	5–7	1–4	1–4, median 2	2 to >20	Median 3–4
Presentation	MDS phase common AML with FAB M1 and M2 morphology	MDS/AML	AML with myelomonocytic differentiation; often lack an MDS phase, or present as MDS/MPN	MDS phase is common	MDS phase is common
Cytogenetics/ molecular diagnostics	−5,−7, 5q−, 7q−, 11p15 abnormalities Normal karyotype, *P53* mutation	−5,− 7, 11q23, 11p15 abnormality Normal karyotype, *FLT3* mutation	11q23 abnormalities, t(8;21), t(15;17), t(9;22), (3;21), t(8;16), inv(16)	−5, −7, 5q−, 7q−, complex, 21q22 (*RUNX1*)	−7, most common

Abbreviations: MDS, myelodysplastic syndromes; AML, acute myeloid leukemia; MDS/MPN, myelodysplastic/myeloproliferative neoplasm.

[80, 82]. The comparison of t-MDS/t-AML developed with different treatment regimens is summarized in Table 14.8.

Prognosis

Therapy-related myeloid neoplasm following the treatment of childhood cancer carries a dismal prognosis. The prognosis is not related to blast counts, regardless of whether they present as overt acute leukemia or as t-MDS [101, 115]. Neither does subclassification of t-AML/t-MDS stratify the risks. The prognosis is strongly related to the associated karyotypic abnormality as well as the comorbidity of the underlying malignancy or disease, and patient performance status. Cases associated with abnormalities of chromosome 5 and/or 7 and a complex karyotype have a particularly poor outcome. Patients with balanced translocations generally have a better prognosis, but, except for those with t(15;17)(q22;q12) and inv(16)(p13.1q22) or t(16;16)(p13.1;q22), median survival times are shorter than their *de novo* counterparts. Similar to adult t-MDs/t-AML, the treatment for childhood t-MDS/t-AML has been largely unsuccessful. The overall long-term survival rate is 10–20% [71]. Most favorable outcomes follow intensive chemotherapy and stem cell transplantation [2, 30, 63, 106]. Failure to achieve a complete remission is the most significant factor for a poor outcome [2, 30, 63, 76, 116].

References

1. **Corey SJ, Minden MD, Barber DL,** *et al.* Myelodysplastic syndromes: the complexity of stem-cell diseases. *Nature Reviews Cancer.* 2007;**7**(2):118–129.

2. **Niemeyer CM, Baumann I.** Myelodysplastic syndrome in children and adolescents. *Seminars in Hematology.* 2008;**45**(1):60–70.

3. **Jaffe ES, Harris NL, Stein H, Vardiman J.** *World Health Organization Classification of Tumours: Pathology and Genetics of Tumours of Haematopoietic and Lymphoid Tissues.* Lyon: IARC Press; 2001.

4. **Smith OP, Hann IM, Chessells JM, Reeves BR, Milla P.** Haematological abnormalities in Shwachman-Diamond syndrome. *British Journal of Haematology.* 1996;**94**(2):279–284.

5. **Hasle H, Kerndrup G, Jacobsen BB.** Childhood myelodysplastic syndrome in Denmark: incidence and predisposing conditions. *Leukemia.* 1995;**9**(9):1569–1572.

6. **Starý J, Baumann I, Creutzig U,** *et al.* Getting the numbers straight in pediatric MDS: distribution of subtypes after exclusion of Down syndrome. *Pediatric Blood and Cancer.* 2008; **50**(2):435–436.

7. **Bain BJ.** The bone marrow aspirate of healthy subjects. *British Journal of Haematology.* 1996;**94**(1):206–209.

8. **Baumann I, Niemeyer CM, Bennett JM, Shannon K.** Childhood myelodysplastic syndrome. In Swerdlow SH, Campo E, Harris NL, *et al.*, eds. *WHO Classification of Tumours of Haematopoietic and Lymphoid Tissues* (4th edn.). Lyon: IARC Press; 2008, 104–107.

9. **Hasle H, Niemeyer CM, Chessells JM,** *et al.* A pediatric approach to the WHO classification of myelodysplastic and myeloproliferative diseases. *Leukemia.* 2003;**17**(2):277–282.

10. **Chatterjee T, Mahapatra M, Dixit A,** *et al.* Primary myelodysplastic syndrome in children – clinical, hematological and histomorphological profile from a tertiary care centre in India. *Hematology.* 2005;**10**(6):495–499.

11. **Hasle H, Wadsworth LD, Massing BG, McBride M, Schultz KR.** A population-based study of childhood myelodysplastic syndrome in British Columbia, Canada. *British Journal of Haematology.* 1999;**106**(4):1027–1032.

12. **Luna-Fineman S, Shannon KM, Atwater SK,** *et al.* Myelodysplastic and myeloproliferative disorders of childhood: a study of 167 patients. *Blood.* 1999;**93**(2):459–466.

13. **Occhipinti E, Correa H, Yu L, Craver R.** Comparison of two new classifications for pediatric myelodysplastic and myeloproliferative disorders. *Pediatric Blood & Cancer.* 2005;**44**(3):240–244.

14. **Passmore SJ, Hann IM, Stiller CA,** *et al.* Pediatric myelodysplasia: a study of 68 children and a new prognostic scoring system. *Blood.* 1995;**85**(7): 1742–1750.

15. **Sasaki H, Manabe A, Kojima S,** *et al.* Myelodysplastic syndrome in childhood: a retrospective study of 189 patients in Japan. *Leukemia.* 2001;**15**(11):1713–1720.

16. **Chan GC, Wang WC, Raimondi SC,** *et al.* Myelodysplastic syndrome in children: differentiation from acute myeloid leukemia with a low blast count. *Leukemia.* 1997;**11**(2):206–211.

17. **Vardiman JW.** Hematopathological concepts and controversies in the diagnosis and classification of myelodysplastic syndromes. *Hematology/the Education Program of the American Society of Hematology.* 2006:199–204.

18. **Polychronopoulou S, Panagiotou JP, Kossiva L,** *et al.* Clinical and morphological features of paediatric myelodysplastic syndromes: a review of 34 cases. *Acta Paediatrica.* 2004;**93**(8):1015–1023.

19. **Elghetany MT.** Myelodysplastic syndromes in children: a critical review of issues in the diagnosis and classification of 887 cases from 13 published series. *Archives of Pathology & Laboratory Medicine.* 2007;**131**(7):1110–1116.

20. **Bader-Meunier B, Rötig A, Mielot F,** *et al.* Refractory anaemia and mitochondrial cytopathy in childhood. *British Journal of Haematology.* 1994;**87**(2):381–385.

21. **Mueller BU, Tannenbaum S, Pizzo PA.** Bone marrow aspirates and biopsies in children with human immunodeficiency virus infection. *Journal of Pediatric Hematology/Oncology.* 1996;**18**(3):266–271.

22. **Brichard B, Vermylen C, Scheiff JM, Ninane J, Cornu G.** Haematological disturbances during long-term valproate therapy. *European Journal of Pediatrics.* 1994;**153**(5):378–380.

23. **Yetgin S, Ozen S, Saatci U,** *et al.* Myelodysplastic features in juvenile rheumatoid arthritis. *American Journal of Hematology.* 1997;**54**(2):166–169.

24. **Tricot G, De Wolf-Peeters C, Vlietinck R, Verwilghen RL.** Bone marrow histology in myelodysplastic syndromes. II. Prognostic value of abnormal localization of immature precursors in MDS. *British Journal of Haematology.* 1984;**58**(2):217–225.

25. **Bader-Meunier B, Miélot F, Breton-Gorius J,** *et al.* Hematologic involvement in mitochondrial cytopathies in childhood: a retrospective study of bone marrow smears. *Pediatric Research.* 1999;**46**(2):158–162.

26. **Haas OA, Gadner H.** Pathogenesis, biology, and management of myelodysplastic syndromes in children. *Seminars in Hematology.* 1996;**33**(3):225–235.

27. **Baumann I.** Histopathological features of hypoplastic myelodysplastic syndrome and comparison with severe aplastic anemia in childhood. *Leukemia Research.* 1999;**23**(Suppl 1):S41.

28. **Alter BP, Scalise A, McCombs J, Najfeld V.** Clonal chromosomal abnormalities in Fanconi's anaemia: what do they really mean? *British Journal of Haematology.* 1993;**85**(3):627–630.

29. **Mufti GJ, Bennett JM, Goasguen J,** *et al.* Diagnosis and classification of myelodysplastic syndrome: International Working Group on Morphology of Myelodysplastic Syndrome (IWGM-MDS) consensus proposals for the definition and enumeration of myeloblasts and ring sideroblasts. *Haematologica.* 2008;**93**(11):1712–1717.

30. **Leone G, Voso MT, Sica S, Morosetti R, Pagano L.** Therapy related leukemias: susceptibility, prevention and treatment. *Leukemia and Lymphoma.* 2001;**41**(3-4):255–276.

31. **Ogata K, Nakamura K, Yokose N,** *et al.* Clinical significance of phenotypic features of blasts in patients with myelodysplastic syndrome. *Blood.* 2002;**100**(12):3887–3896.

32. **Oriani A, Annaloro C, Soligo D,** *et al.* Bone marrow histology and CD34 immunostaining in the prognostic evaluation of primary myelodysplastic syndromes. *British Journal of Haematology.* 1996;**92**(2):360–364.

33. **Della Porta MG, Malcovati L, Boveri E,** *et al.* Clinical relevance of bone marrow fibrosis and CD34-positive cell clusters in primary myelodysplastic syndromes. *Journal of Clinical Oncology.* 2009;**27**(5):754–762.

34. **Weiss B, Vora A, Huberty J, Hawkins RA, Matthay KK.** Secondary myelodysplastic syndrome and leukemia following 131I-metaiodobenzylguanidine therapy for relapsed neuroblastoma. *Journal of Pediatric Hematology/Oncology.* 2003;**25**(7):543–547.

35. **Kussick SJ, Fromm JR, Rossini A,** *et al.* Four-color flow cytometry shows strong concordance with bone marrow morphology and cytogenetics in the evaluation for myelodysplasia. *American Journal of Clinical Pathology.* 2005;**124**(2):170–181.

36. **Stachurski D, Smith BR, Pozdnyakova O,** *et al.* Flow cytometric analysis of myelomonocytic cells by a pattern recognition approach is sensitive and specific in diagnosing myelodysplastic syndrome and related marrow diseases: emphasis on a global evaluation and recognition of diagnostic pitfalls. *Leukemia Research.* 2008;**32**(2):215–224.

37. **Stetler-Stevenson M, Arthur DC, Jabbour N,** *et al.* Diagnostic utility of flow cytometric immunophenotyping in myelodysplastic syndrome. *Blood.* 2001;**98**(4):979–987.

38. **Clark JJ, Smith FO, Arceci RJ.** Update in childhood acute myeloid leukemia: recent developments in the molecular basis of disease and novel therapies. *Current Opinion in Hematology.* 2003;**10**(1):31–39.

39. **Truong F, Smith BR, Stachurski D,** *et al.* The utility of flow cytometric immunophenotyping in cytopenic patients with a non-diagnostic bone marrow: a prospective study. *Leukemia Research.* 2009;**33**(8):1039–1046.

40. **van de Loosdrecht AA, Alhan C, Béné MC,** *et al.* Standardization of flow cytometry in myelodysplastic syndromes: report from the first European LeukemiaNet working conference on flow cytometry in myelodysplastic syndromes. *Haematologica.* 2009;**94**(8):1124–1134.

41. **Sutherland DR, Kuek N, Azcona-Olivera J,** *et al.* Use of a FLAER-based WBC assay in the primary screening of PNH clones. *American Journal of Clinical Pathology.* 2009;**132**(4):564–572.

42. **Felix CA.** Secondary leukemias induced by topoisomerase-targeted drugs. *Biochimica et Biophysica Acta.* 1998;**1400**(1-3):233–255.

43. **Wang SA, Pozdnyakova O, Jorgensen JL,** *et al.* Detection of paroxysmal nocturnal hemoglobinuria clones in patients with myelodysplastic syndromes and related bone marrow diseases, with emphasis on diagnostic pitfalls and caveats. *Haematologica.* 2009;**94**(1):29–37.

44. **Larson RA, Wang Y, Banerjee M**, *et al.* Prevalence of the inactivating 609C–>T polymorphism in the NAD(P)H:quinone oxidoreductase (NQO1) gene in patients with primary and therapy-related myeloid leukemia. *Blood.* 1999;**94**(2):803–807.

45. **Relling MV, Yanishevski Y, Nemec J**, *et al.* Etoposide and antimetabolite pharmacology in patients who develop secondary acute myeloid leukemia. *Leukemia.* 1998;**12**(3):346–352.

46. **Mantadakis E, Shannon KM, Singer DA**, *et al.* Transient monosomy 7: a case series in children and review of the literature. *Cancer.* 1999;**85**(12):2655–2661.

47. **Hasle H, Baumann I, Bergstrasser E**, *et al.* The International Prognostic Scoring System (IPSS) for childhood myelodysplastic syndrome (MDS) and juvenile myelomonocytic leukemia (JMML). *Leukemia.* 2004;**18**(12):2008–2014.

48. **Greenberg P, Cox C, LeBeau MM**, *et al.* International scoring system for evaluating prognosis in myelodysplastic syndromes. *Blood.* 1997;**89**(6):2079–2088. Erratum appears in *Blood.* 1998; **91**(3):1100.

49. **Meadows AT, Baum E, Fossati-Bellani F**, *et al.* Second malignant neoplasms in children: an update from the Late Effects Study Group. *Journal of Clinical Oncology.* 1985;**3**(4):532–538.

50. **Bhatia S, Ramsay NK, Steinbuch M**, *et al.* Malignant neoplasms following bone marrow transplantation. *Blood.* 1996;**87**(9):3633–3639.

51. **Neglia JP, Friedman DL, Yasui Y**, *et al.* Second malignant neoplasms in five-year survivors of childhood cancer: childhood cancer survivor study. *Journal of the National Cancer Institute.* 2001;**93**(8):618–629.

52. **Barrett J, Saunthararajah Y, Molldrem J.** Myelodysplastic syndrome and aplastic anemia: distinct entities or diseases linked by a common pathophysiology? *Seminars in Hematology.* 2000;**37**(1):15–29.

53. **Maciejewski JP, Rivera C, Kook H, Dunn D, Young NS.** Relationship between bone marrow failure syndromes and the presence of glycophosphatidyl inositol-anchored protein-deficient clones. *British Journal of Haematology.* 2001;**115**(4):1015–1022.

54. **Wang H, Chuhjo T, Yasue S, Omine M, Nakao S.** Clinical significance of a minor population of paroxysmal nocturnal hemoglobinuria-type cells in bone marrow failure syndrome. *Blood.* 2002;**100**(12):3897–3902.

55. **Bennett JM, Orazi A.** Diagnostic criteria to distinguish hypocellular acute myeloid leukemia from hypocellular myelodysplastic syndromes and aplastic anemia: recommendations for a standardized approach. *Haematologica.* 2009;**94**(2):264–268.

56. **Bacigalupo A, Broccia G, Corda G,** *et al.* Antilymphocyte globulin, cyclosporin, and granulocyte colony-stimulating factor in patients with acquired severe aplastic anemia (SAA): a pilot study of the EBMT SAA Working Party. *Blood.* 1995;**85**(5):1348–1353.

57. **Barnard DR, Lange B, Alonzo TA,** *et al.* Acute myeloid leukemia and myelodysplastic syndrome in children treated for cancer: comparison with primary presentation. *Blood.* 2002;**100**(2):427–434.

58. **Brunning RD, Bennett JM, Flandrin G,** *et al.* Myelodysplastic syndromes. In Jaffe ES, Harris NL, Stein H, Vardiman J (eds.). *World Health Organization Classification of Tumours: Pathology and Genetics of Tumours of Haematopoietic and Lymphoid Tissues.* Lyon: IARC Press; 2001, 61–73.

59. **Schoch C, Schnittger S, Klaus M,** *et al.* AML with 11q23/MLL abnormalities as defined by the WHO classification: incidence, partner chromosomes, FAB subtype, age distribution, and prognostic impact in an unselected series of 1897 cytogenetically analyzed AML cases. *Blood.* 2003;**102**(7):2395–2402.

60. **Vardiman J, Arber DA, Brunning RD,** *et al.* Therapy-related myeloid neoplasms. In Swerdlow SH, Campo E, Harris NL, *et al.*, (eds.). *WHO Classification of Tumours of Haematopoietic and Lymphoid Tissues* (4th edn.). Lyon: IARC Press; 2008, 127–129.

61. **Estey E, Dohner H.** Acute myeloid leukaemia. *Lancet.* 2006;**368**(9550):1894–1907.

62. **Leone G, Mele L, Pulsoni A, Equitani F, Pagano L.** The incidence of secondary leukemias. *Haematologica.* 1999;**84**(10):937–945.

63. **Aguilera DG, Vaklavas C, Tsimberidou AM,** *et al.* Pediatric therapy-related myelodysplastic syndrome/acute myeloid leukemia: the MD Anderson Cancer Center experience. *Journal of Pediatric Hematology/Oncology.* 2009;**31**(11):803–811.

64. **Neglia JP, Meadows AT, Robison LL,** *et al.* Second neoplasms after acute lymphoblastic leukemia in childhood. *New England Journal of Medicine.* 1991;**325**(19):1330–1336.

65. **Bhatia S, Krailo MD, Chen Z,** *et al.* Therapy-related myelodysplasia and acute myeloid leukemia after Ewing sarcoma and primitive neuroectodermal tumor of bone: a report from the Children's Oncology Group. *Blood.* 2007;**109**(1):46–51.

66. **Olopade OI, Thangavelu M, Larson RA,** *et al.* Clinical, morphologic, and cytogenetic characteristics of 26 patients with acute erythroblastic leukemia. *Blood.* 1992;**80**(11):2873–2882.

67. **Andersen MK, Pedersen-Bjergaard J.** Therapy-related MDS and AML in acute promyelocytic leukemia. *Blood.* 2002;**100**(5):1928–1929.

68. **Felix CA.** Leukemias related to treatment with DNA topoisomerase II inhibitors. *Medical & Pediatric Oncology.* 2001;**36**(5):525–535.

69. **Leung W, Sandlund JT, Hudson MM,** *et al.* Second malignancy after treatment of childhood non-Hodgkin lymphoma. *Cancer.* 2001;**92**(7):1959–1966.

70. **Milligan DW, Ruiz De Elvira MC, Kolb HJ,** *et al.* Secondary leukaemia and myelodysplasia after autografting for lymphoma: results from the EBMT. EBMT Lymphoma and Late Effects Working Parties. European Group for Blood and Marrow Transplantation. *British Journal of Haematology.* 1999; **106**(4):1020–1026.

71. **Barnard DR, Woods WG.** Treatment-related myelodysplastic syndrome/acute myeloid leukemia in survivors of childhood cancer – an update. *Leukemia and Lymphoma.* 2005;**46**(5):651–663.

72. **Kimball Dalton VM, Gelber RD, Li F,** *et al.* Second malignancies in patients treated for childhood acute lymphoblastic leukemia. *Journal of*

Clinical Oncology. 1998;**16**(8):2848–2853.

73. **Löning L, Zimmermann M, Reiter A,** *et al.* Secondary neoplasms subsequent to Berlin-Frankfurt-Munster therapy of acute lymphoblastic leukemia in childhood: significantly lower risk without cranial radiotherapy. *Blood.* 2000;**95**(9):2770–2775.

74. **Pratt CB, Meyer WH, Luo X,** *et al.* Second malignant neoplasms occurring in survivors of osteosarcoma. *Cancer.* 1997;**80**(5):960–965.

75. **Aung L, Gorlick RG, Shi W,** *et al.* Second malignant neoplasms in long-term survivors of osteosarcoma: Memorial Sloan-Kettering Cancer Center Experience. *Cancer.* 2002;**95**(8):1728–1734.

76. **Leahey AM, Friedman DL, Bunin NJ.** Bone marrow transplantation in pediatric patients with therapy-related myelodysplasia and leukemia. *Bone Marrow Transplantation.* 1999;**23**(1):21–25.

77. **Rodriguez-Galindo C, Poquette CA, Marina NM,** *et al.* Hematologic abnormalities and acute myeloid leukemia in children and adolescents administered intensified chemotherapy for the Ewing sarcoma family of tumors. *Journal of Pediatric Hematology/Oncology.* 2000;**22**(4):321–329.

78. **Breslow NE, Takashima JR, Whitton JA,** *et al.* Second malignant neoplasms following treatment for Wilm's tumor: a report from the National Wilms' Tumor Study Group. *Journal of Clinical Oncology.* 1995;**13**(8):1851–1859.

79. **Pui CH, Hancock ML, Raimondi SC,** *et al.* Myeloid neoplasia in children treated for solid tumours. *Lancet.* 1990;**336**(8712):417–421.

80. **Kojima S, Ohara A, Tsuchida M,** *et al.* Risk factors for evolution of acquired aplastic anemia into myelodysplastic syndrome and acute myeloid leukemia after immunosuppressive therapy in children. *Blood.* 2002;**100**(3):786–790.

81. **Socié G, Henry-Amar M, Bacigalupo A,** *et al.* Malignant tumors occurring after treatment of aplastic anemia. European Bone Marrow Transplantation-Severe Aplastic Anaemia Working Party. *New England Journal of Medicine.* 1993;**329**(16):1152–1157.

82. **Ohara A, Kojima S, Hamajima N,** *et al.* Myelodysplastic syndrome and acute myelogenous leukemia as a late clonal complication in children with acquired aplastic anemia. *Blood.* 1997;**90**(3):1009–1013.

83. **Bacigalupo A, Bruno B, Saracco P,** *et al.* Antilymphocyte globulin, cyclosporine, prednisolone, and granulocyte colony-stimulating factor for severe aplastic anemia: an update of the GITMO/EBMT study on 100 patients. European Group for Blood and Marrow Transplantation (EBMT) Working Party on Severe Aplastic Anemia and the Gruppo Italiano Trapianti di Midolio Osseo (GITMO). *Blood.* 2000;**95**(6):1931–1934.

84. **Fuhrer M, Burdach S, Ebell W,** *et al.* Relapse and clonal disease in children with aplastic anemia (AA) after immunosuppressive therapy (IST): the SAA 94 experience. German/Austrian Pediatric Aplastic Anemia Working Group. *Klinische Padiatrie.* 1998;**210**(4):173–179.

85. **Perentesis JP.** Genetic predisposition and treatment-related leukemia. *Medical & Pediatric Oncology.* 2001;**36**(5):541–548.

86. **Pui CH, Relling MV, Behm FG,** *et al.* L-asparaginase may potentiate the leukemogenic effect of the epipodophyllotoxins. *Leukemia.* 1995;**9**(10):1680–1684.

87. **Quesnel B, Kantarjian H, Bjergaard JP,** *et al.* Therapy-related acute myeloid leukemia with t(8;21), inv(16), and t(8;16): a report on 25 cases and review of the literature. *Journal of Clinical Oncology.* 1993;**11**(12):2370–2379.

88. **Harada H, Harada Y, Tanaka H, Kimura A, Inaba T.** Implications of somatic mutations in the AML1 gene in radiation-associated and therapy-related myelodysplastic syndrome/acute myeloid leukemia. *Blood.* 2003;**101**(2):673–680.

89. **Gustafson SA, Lin P, Chen SS,** *et al.* Therapy-related acute myeloid leukemia with t(8;21)(q22;q22) shares many features with de novo acute myeloid leukemia with t(8;21)(q22;q22) but does not have a favorable outcome. *American Journal of Clinical Pathology.* 2009;**131**(5):647–655.

90. **Rege KP, Janes SL, Saso R,** *et al.* Secondary leukaemia characterised by monosomy 7 occurring post-autologous stem cell transplantation for AML. *Bone Marrow Transplantation.* 1998;**21**(8):853–855.

91. **Amigo ML, del Cañizo MC, Rios A,** *et al.* Diagnosis of secondary myelodysplastic syndromes (MDS) following autologous transplantation should not be based only on morphological criteria used for diagnosis of de novo MDS. *Bone Marrow Transplantation.* 1999;**23**(10):997–1002.

92. **Lambertenghi Deliliers G, Annaloro C, Pozzoli E,** *et al.* Cytogenetic and myelodysplastic alterations after autologous hemopoietic stem cell transplantation. *Leukemia Research.* 1999;**23**(3):291–297.

93. **Sevilla J, Rodríguez A, Hernández-Maraver D,** *et al.* Secondary acute myeloid leukemia and myelodysplasia after autologous peripheral blood progenitor cell transplantation. *Annals of Hematology.* 2002;**81**(1):11–15.

94. **Forrest DL, Nevill TJ, Naiman SC,** *et al.* Second malignancy following high-dose therapy and autologous stem cell transplantation: incidence and risk factor analysis. *Bone Marrow Transplantation.* 2003;**32**(9):915–923.

95. **Groupe Français de Cytogénétique Hématologique.** Forty-four cases of childhood myelodysplasia with cytogenetics, documented by the Groupe Français de Cytogénétique Hématologique. *Leukemia.* 1997;**11**(9):1478–1485.

96. **Bolufer P, Collado M, Barragan E,** *et al.* Profile of polymorphisms of drug-metabolising enzymes and the risk of therapy-related leukaemia. *British Journal of Haematology.* 2007;**136**(4):590–596.

97. **Rund D, Krichevsky S, Bar-Cohen S,** *et al.* Therapy-related leukemia: clinical characteristics and analysis of new molecular risk factors in 96 adult patients. *Leukemia.* 2005;**19**(11):1919–1928.

98. **Ben-Yehuda D, Krichevsky S, Caspi O,** *et al.* Microsatellite instability and p53 mutations in therapy-related leukemia suggest mutator phenotype. *Blood.* 1996;**88**(11):4296–4303.

99. **Pedersen-Bjergaard J, Andersen MK, Andersen MT, Christiansen DH.** Genetics of therapy-related myelodysplasia and acute myeloid

leukemia. *Leukemia*. 2008;**22**(2):240–248.

100. **Pedersen-Bjergaard J, Andersen MT, Andersen MK.** Genetic pathways in the pathogenesis of therapy-related myelodysplasia and acute myeloid leukemia. *Hematology/the Education Program of the American Society of Hematology.* 2007: 392–397.

101. **Singh ZN, Huo D, Anastasi J, et al.** Therapy-related myelodysplastic syndrome: morphologic subclassification may not be clinically relevant. *American Journal of Clinical Pathology.* 2007;**127**(2):197–205.

102. **Rowley JD, Olney HJ.** International workshop on the relationship of prior therapy to balanced chromosome aberrations in therapy-related myelodysplastic syndromes and acute leukemia: overview report. *Genes, Chromosomes & Cancer.* 2002;**33**(4): 331–345.

103. **Slovak ML, Bedell V, Popplewell L, et al.** 21q22 balanced chromosome aberrations in therapy-related hematopoietic disorders: report from an international workshop. *Genes, Chromosomes & Cancer.* 2002;**33**(4): 379–394.

104. **Yin CC, Glassman AB, Lin P, et al.** Morphologic, cytogenetic, and molecular abnormalities in therapy-related acute promyelocytic leukemia. *American Journal of Clinical Pathology.* 2005;**123**(6):840–848.

105. **Chu JY, Batanian JR, Gale GB, Dunphy CH, DeMello DE.** Spontaneous resolution of myelodysplastic cytogenetic abnormality developed during the treatment of leukemia. *Journal of Pediatric Hematology/Oncology.* 1998;**20**(1):88–90.

106. **Laurenti L, d'Onofrio G, Sica S, et al.** Secondary myelodysplastic syndromes following peripheral blood stem cell transplantation: morphological, cytogenetic and clonality evaluation and the limitation of FAB criteria. *Bone Marrow Transplantation.* 2000;**26**(2): 241–242.

107. **Kebelmann-Betzing C, Seeger K, Kulozik A, et al.** Secondary acute myeloid leukemia after treatment of acute monoblastic leukemia. *New England Journal of Medicine.* 2000; **343**(25):1897–1898.

108. **Seiter K, Feldman EJ, Sreekantaiah C, et al.** Secondary acute myelogenous leukemia and myelodysplasia without abnormalities of chromosome 11q23 following treatment of acute leukemia with topoisomerase II-based chemotherapy. *Leukemia.* 2001;**15**(6): 963–970.

109. **Nabhan C, Peterson LA, Kent SA, et al.** Secondary acute myelogenous leukemia with MLL gene rearrangement following radioimmunotherapy (RAIT) for non-Hodgkin's lymphoma. *Leukemia and Lymphoma.* 2002;**43**(11):2145–2149.

110. **Glassman AB, Hayes KJ.** Translocation (11;16)(q23;p13) acute myelogenous leukemia and myelodysplastic syndrome. *Annals of Clinical & Laboratory Science.* 2003;**33**(3):285–288.

111. **Rowley JD.** Rearrangements involving chromosome band 11Q23 in acute leukaemia. *Seminars in Cancer Biology.* 1993;**4**(6):377–385.

112. **Mauritzson N, Albin M, Rylander L, et al.** Pooled analysis of clinical and cytogenetic features in treatment-related and de novo adult acute myeloid leukemia and myelodysplastic syndromes based on a consecutive series of 761 patients analyzed 1976–1993 and on 5098 unselected cases reported in the literature 1974–2001. *Leukemia.* 2002;**16**(12): 2366–2378.

113. **Pedersen-Bjergaard J, Brøndum-Nielsen K, Karle H, Johansson B.** Chemotherapy-related – late occurring – Philadelphia chromosome in AML, ALL and CML. Similar events related to treatment with DNA topoisomerase II inhibitors? *Leukemia.* 1997;**11**(9):1571–1574.

114. **Harada H, Harada Y, Tanaka H, Kimura A, Inaba T.** Implications of somatic mutations in the AML1 gene in radiation-associated and therapy-related myelodysplastic syndrome/ acute myeloid leukemia. *Blood.* 2003; **101**(2):673–680.

115. **Michels SD, McKenna RW, Arthur DC, Brunning RD.** Therapy-related acute myeloid leukemia and myelodysplastic syndrome: a clinical and morphologic study of 65 cases. *Blood.* 1985;**65**(6):1364–1372.

116. **Hale GA, Heslop HE, Bowman LC, et al.** Bone marrow transplantation for therapy-induced acute myeloid leukemia in children with previous lymphoid malignancies. *Bone Marrow Transplantation.* 1999;**24**(7):735–739.

15 Acute myeloid leukemia and related precursor neoplasms

Robert B. Lorsbach

Introduction

Acute myeloid leukemia (AML) is a group of clonal malignant disorders of the bone marrow and peripheral blood that morphologically, cytochemically, and immunophenotypically manifest variable degrees of maturation resembling various stages and lineages in normal hematopoietic development. The intense research efforts of the past 30 years have led to major advances in our understanding of the pathogenesis, diagnosis, and treatment of AML. More recently, the completion of the human genome project has fueled the development of methods for the determination of global gene expression and the genome-wide assessment of DNA mutations. These techniques will enhance our knowledge of the underlying genetic lesions responsible for the development of AML, and, importantly for the pathologist, they will undoubtedly revolutionize the classification of AML. Historically, the classification of AML has had relatively little impact on patient care, since most patients with AML were treated with fairly uniform chemotherapeutic regimens and generally had a poor prognosis. However, through the research efforts alluded to above, a classification scheme for AML with clinical utility is starting to emerge. Furthermore, with the advent of chemotherapeutics for AML which specifically target the underlying genetic lesions, the paradigm being all-*trans* retinoic acid (ATRA) for the treatment of acute promyelocytic leukemia, there is now greater impetus for the precise and meaningful classification of AML.

This chapter will provide an overview of childhood AML with an emphasis on those entities which are either more common or largely restricted to the pediatric population. For each entity, a summary of our current understanding of its molecular pathogenesis will be included, as well as a description of the relevant clinical, laboratory, pathologic, and molecular diagnostic features. Because of the distinct clinical and biologic differences that exist between *de novo* AML and secondary or myelodysplasia-related AML, as well as the relative infrequency of secondary AML in the pediatric setting, discussion will be largely confined to *de novo* AMLs.

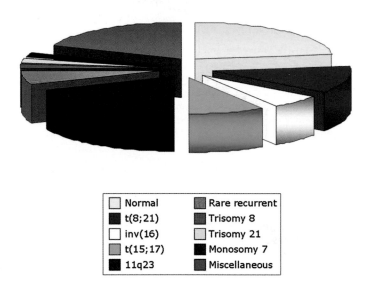

Normal	Rare recurrent
t(8;21)	Trisomy 8
inv(16)	Trisomy 21
t(15;17)	Monosomy 7
11q23	Miscellaneous

Fig. 15.1. Distribution of recurrent cytogenetic lesions in pediatric AML. Compared with adults, the overall frequency of translocation-associated AMLs is significantly higher in children, particularly those targeting the *MLL* gene at 11q23, with a commensurate decrease in the relative frequency of cytogenetically normal AMLs. The data are a compilation of the reported findings from three large pediatric AML clinical trials [5–7].

Classification of acute myeloid leukemia

For nearly 20 years, the so-called French–American–British classification was the most widely employed scheme for the categorization of AML [1–4]. The cornerstone of the FAB classification was the enumeration and morphologic and cytochemical characterization of the leukemic blasts, which was used to define eight subtypes of AML: AML M0 through M7. However, with the exception of acute promyelocytic leukemia (AML M3), classification of AMLs according to FAB criteria suffered from poor reproducibility and lacked prognostic importance. Furthermore, this reliance on morphologic features alone neglected significant advances in the cytogenetics and molecular biology of AML that have identified several common and recurrent molecular lesions, several of which have clear prognostic importance (Fig. 15.1) [5–7]. In 2001, as part of the WHO classification for hematopoietic malignancies, a new classification

Diagnostic Pediatric Hematopathology, ed. Maria A. Proytcheva. Published by Cambridge University Press.
© Cambridge University Press 2011.

Table 15.1. 2008 WHO classification of acute myeloid leukemia.

Acute myeloid leukemia with recurrent genetic abnormalities
  AML with balanced translocation/inversions[a]
    AML with t(8;21)(q22;q22) [*RUNX1/RUNX1T1*]
    AML with inv(16)(p13.1q22) or t(16;16)(p13.1;q22) [*CBFB/MYH11*]
    Acute promyelocytic leukemia, t(15;17)(q22;q12) [*PML/RARA*] or
      variant translocations
    AML with t(9;11)(p22;q23) [*MLLT3-MLL*], or other balanced
      translocations involving 11q23 (MLL)
    AML with t(6;9)(p23;q34) [*DEK-NUP214*]
    AML with inv(3)(q21q26.2) or t(3;3)(q21;q26.2) [*RPN1-EVI1*]
    AML with t(1;22)(p13;q13) [*RBM15-MKL1*]
  AML with gene mutations
    AML with mutated *NPM1*[b]
    AML with mutated *CEBPA*

Acute myeloid leukemia with myelodysplasia-related changes

Therapy-related myeloid neoplasms

Acute myeloid leukemia not otherwise specified
  AML with minimal differentiation
  AML without maturation
  AML with maturation
  Acute myelomonocytic leukemia
  Acute monoblastic and monocytic leukemia
  Acute erythroid leukemia
    Erythroleukemia (erythroid/myeloid)
    Pure erythroid leukemia
  Acute megakaryoblastic leukemia
  Acute basophilic leukemia
  Acute panmyelosis with myelofibrosis

Myeloid sarcoma

Myeloid proliferations related to Down syndrome
  Transient abnormal myelopoiesis
  Myeloid leukemia associated with Down syndrome

Blastic plasmacytoid dendritic cell neoplasm

[a] For translocation-associated AMLs, the resultant fusion transcript is indicated in brackets.
[b] Mutated NPM may be detected either by molecular studies or by immunohistochemistry to detect aberrant cytoplasmic localization of the mutated protein.

scheme was developed in which, for the first time, cytogenetic and molecular information was utilized for the classification of AMLs [8]. This WHO classification recognized as discrete entities several types of AML which are strongly associated with specific cytogenetic alterations. An updated and expanded WHO classification has recently been published and includes more recently characterized entities such as acute megakaryoblastic leukemia with t(1;22) (Table 15.1) [9].

Acute myeloid leukemia with lesions targeting the core binding factor complex genes

Intense investigation using both biochemical and genetic approaches has demonstrated that the core binding factor (CBF) complex plays a critical role in developmental hematopoiesis and lymphocyte ontogeny through its regulation of gene transcription. The CBF gene family includes four family members, *RUNX1*, *-2*, and *-3*, and *CBFB*. Each of the RUNX proteins has relatively restricted, albeit overlapping, patterns

t(8;21) RUNX1-ETO

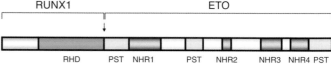

Fig. 15.2. Schematic of the RUNX1-RUNX1T1 fusion protein. This oncoprotein is expressed as a result of the t(8;21) which generates an in-frame fusion between RUNX1 and RUNX1T1. It is a modular protein containing the Runt homology domain (RHD), which mediates DNA binding, and is derived from RUNX1. Additional motifs contributed by RUNX1T1 include proline/serine/threonine-rich regions (PST) and domains, and four domains with homology to nervy (nervy homology regions, NHR). RUNX1T1-derived domains facilitate the recruitment of corepressor proteins, such as the histone deacetylases, to RUNX1/CBFβ responsive promoters, resulting in inhibition of gene expression.

of tissue-specific expression, whereas CBFβ is rather widely expressed. This complex normally exists as a heterodimer comprised of one of the RUNX proteins complexed with CBFβ. This interaction dramatically increases the DNA binding affinity of the RUNX protein and is ultimately essential for biologic function of this complex. In addition to its critical role in hematopoiesis, the genes encoding the *RUNX1/CBFB* complex, located on chromosome 21q22 and 16q22, respectively, are the most frequently targeted loci in *de novo* AML, through the t(8;21) and t(16;16)/inv(16) translocations, the latter targeting the *CBFB* gene and characteristically present in acute myelomonocytic leukemia with abnormal eosinophils (discussed below) [10–13]. Thus, these AML subtypes share a common underlying molecular pathogenesis, despite their rather disparate morphologic features.

Acute myeloid leukemia with t(8;21)(q22;q22) [t(8;21) AML]

Definition

An AML subtype containing the t(8;21)(q22;q22), which results in the in-frame fusion between the *RUNX1* gene located on chromosome 21 and the *RUNX1T1* gene (also known as *ETO*, *MTG8*, and *CBFA2T1*) on chromosome 8, yielding expression of the RUNX1-RUNX1T1 oncoprotein (Fig. 15.2). Using FAB criteria, most AMLs with the t(8;21) are classified as AML M2, and less frequently AML M4 or AML M1.

Pathogenesis

The central pathogenetic event in this AML subtype is the expression of RUNX1-RUNX1T1, which results from a balanced, reciprocal translocation between chromosomes 8q22 and 21q22 [14]. *RUNX1* is now known to be the most frequently targeted genetic locus in acute leukemia. In addition to the t(8;21) in AML, *RUNX1* is also targeted through point mutations, gene amplification events, and other translocations including the t(12;21) detected in approximately 25% of pediatric precursor B-lymphoblastic leukemia, as well as several less common chromosomal translocations associated with acute leukemia [15–19].

RUNX1 is a member of a small family of highly conserved transcription factors that also includes RUNX2 and RUNX3 [20]. In order to efficiently bind DNA, RUNX1 forms a heterodimeric complex with CBFβ. RUNX1 is required for the development of fetal hematopoiesis [21, 22]. Mice deficient in RUNX1 die at the midpoint of gestation due to anemia and hemorrhaging secondary to the complete absence of fetal liver-derived hematopoiesis [22–24], a defect that appears to be attributable to failed fetal hematopoietic stem cell formation [25]. Postnatally, RUNX1 is widely expressed within the hematopoietic system and plays a critical role in T-cell ontogeny, megakaryocytic maturation, and platelet production [26–28]. RUNX1 regulates the expression of several genes in hematopoietic cells, although the critical target genes which might account for the abrogation of hematopoiesis in the absence of RUNX1 are as yet unidentified.

RUNX1T1 was identified by virtue of its involvement in the t(8;21) [29]. RUNX1T1 is a member of a small protein family that also includes MTGX and MTG16, and is the mammalian homolog of the *Drosophila* gene *nervy*. RUNX1T1 is not physiologically expressed within the hematopoietic system, and, not surprisingly, mice deficient in RUNX1T1 have normal hematopoiesis [12, 30, 31]. The normal function of RUNX1T1 is not well defined; however, it appears to play a role in gut morphogenesis and adipocyte development [30, 32].

The RUNX1–RUNX1T1 fusion protein resulting from the t(8;21) consists of the N-terminal portion of RUNX1, including its entire DNA binding domain, fused in-frame to the C-terminal portion of RUNX1T1 (Fig. 15.2). In contrast to native RUNX1, RUNX1-RUNX1T1 does not function to activate transcription, but instead dominantly represses normal RUNX1-mediated transcriptional activation. This effect is dependent on domains contributed by both RUNX1 and RUNX1T1, and is mediated, in part, through the modification of chromatin structure at the loci of normal RUNX1 target genes [33–38].

Adult mice engineered to express RUNX1-RUNX1T1 within hematopoietic cells surprisingly manifest no significant bone marrow or peripheral blood abnormalities and fail to develop leukemia, although bone marrow cells from these animals do exhibit enhanced self-renewal properties *in vivo* [39–41]. However, the frequency of AML or granulocytic sarcoma development following mutagen administration is much greater in RUNX1-RUNX1T1 mice than in control animals. These data are consistent with the concept that the development of t(8;21) AML is a multistep process, and that while necessary, RUNX1-RUNX1T1 expression alone is insufficient for leukemogenesis, indicating the need for additional secondary mutations. Indeed, several candidate cooperating genetic lesions have been identified in t(8;21) AML, with mutations in *FLT3*, *KIT*, or *NRAS* detected in approximately 30% of cases [42]. In some instances, these mutations have been confirmed in animal models to cooperate with RUNX1-RUNX1T1 to induce AML [43]. Importantly, the presence of some of these cooperating lesions may have prognostic importance. For example,

the median survival in t(8;21) AML lacking and containing the *KIT*-D816 mutation was five years, and less than one year, respectively [44].

Clinical and laboratory features

AML with t(8;21) comprises approximately 10–15% of pediatric AML [5, 6]. Children with t(8;21) AML present at an average age of seven to nine years, with a somewhat higher frequency in males. Interestingly, this AML subtype is uncommon in infants and toddlers [45–47]. In addition to typical signs and symptoms of bone marrow failure, t(8;21) AML is more often associated with myeloid sarcoma (also known as granulocytic sarcoma, myeloblastoma or chloroma) than other AML subtypes [46, 48, 49]. Myeloid sarcoma may be present at diagnosis or recurrence, and extramedullary disease can occur in the absence of morphologically apparent bone marrow involvement. Myeloid sarcoma most frequently manifests as a skull, meningeal, or paraspinal mass, but it can develop at any anatomic site. Despite the frequent presence of extramedullary disease, hepatosplenomegaly is not common in patients with t(8;21) AML [47]. Laboratory studies usually reveal anemia and thrombocytopenia. The WBC count is typically elevated, but is usually only moderately so. Blasts are frequently present in peripheral blood, often with Auer rods.

Pathologic features

Morphology

Using FAB criteria, t(8;21) AML is classified as AML with maturation, or AML M2, in 70–80% of cases. Most of the remainder are categorized as acute myelomonocytic leukemia (AML M4), or less commonly other FAB subtypes. The t(8;21) occurs only rarely in acute monoblastic leukemia and has not been described in acute megakaryoblastic or lymphoblastic leukemia [50, 51]. A low blast percentage is observed in occasional cases, necessitating a diagnosis of refractory anemia with excess blasts when FAB criteria are invoked; however, the presence of the t(8;21) is diagnostic of this AML subtype using the WHO classification, irrespective of the blast frequency [9].

t(8;21) AML typically manifests several morphologic features which, although not diagnostic, are very characteristic of this AML subtype (Figs. 15.3 and 15.4). Blasts are variable in size, often have abundant basophilic cytoplasm, and may contain long, slender Auer rods, although the latter is not an invariant morphologic feature (Fig. 15.3) [52, 53]. Dysmyelopoiesis is present in most cases, including megaloblastoid maturation and abnormal nuclear segmentation (e.g., pseudo-Pelger–Huët cells) [54, 55]. Granulation abnormalities in myeloid intermediates may be present as well, including characteristic large, salmon-colored granules and Chédiak–Higashi-like granules (Fig. 15.5) [53]. Dyspoiesis is usually less pronounced in the erythroid and megakaryocytic lineages.

Hyperplasia of other myeloid lineages is common in t(8;21) AML. Eosinophilic hyperplasia is commonly encountered and

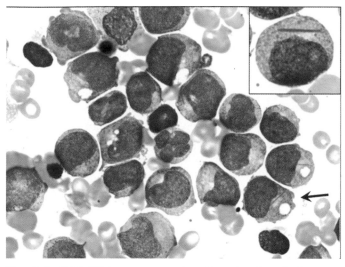

Fig. 15.3. t(8;21) AML, bone marrow aspirate. Several medium-sized myeloblasts are present, several of which contain Auer rods (arrow). The inset shows a blast at higher magnification containing a long, slender Auer rod with tapered ends, characteristic of t(8;21) AML.

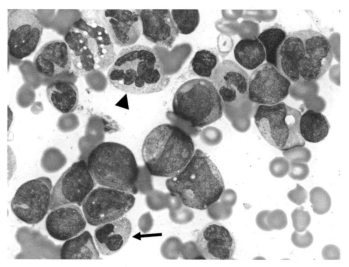

Fig. 15.4. t(8;21) AML, bone marrow aspirate. Blasts and maturing myeloid elements are present. Dysmyelopoiesis is characteristically present in this AML subtype, which includes megaloblastoid change, and neutrophils with nuclear hypersegmentation (arrowhead) and hyposegmentation (pseudo-Pelger–Huët form; arrow). Myeloid elements containing large, salmon-colored granules are also present.

may include dyspoietic forms. Mast cell hyperplasia can also occur, and in t(8;21) AMLs where this is a prominent feature, a diagnosis of systemic mastocytosis with associated clonal hematologic non-mast cell lineage disease (SM-AHNMD) is warranted (Fig. 15.6) [56]. SM-AHNMD has been described in association with several hematolymphoid malignancies; however, it appears to be more common in t(8;21) AML. In these cases, the mast cells contain the t(8;21), confirming their derivation from RUNX1-RUNX1T1-expressing leukemic stem cells [57–59]. In t(8;21) AML with SM-AHNMD, the mast cells can be cytologically atypical, with lobated or multilobated nuclei. As with isolated systemic mastocytosis, KIT gene mutations are usually present in these cases [60].

Immunophenotype

Most t(8;21) AMLs express several myeloid antigens (CD33, CD13, CD65, and CD15). While not diagnostic, nearly all t(8;21) AMLs characteristically express CD34, and most express CD117 (c-kit) [61, 62]. In addition to confirmation of myeloid lineage, flow cytometric analysis can also provide clues as to the underlying genetic lesion. CD19 and CD56 are expressed in more than 50% of t(8;21) AMLs, frequencies much higher than in other subtypes of AML [61–64]. CD56 expression may identify patients with a propensity to develop myeloid sarcoma, and it may also be a negative prognostic factor. In adults with

A

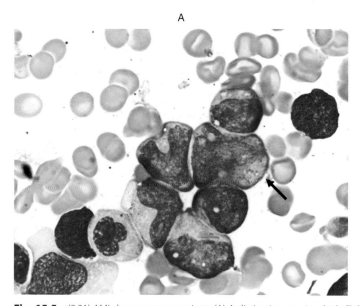

B

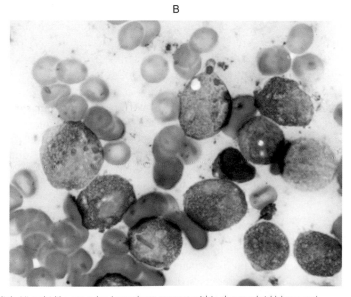

Fig. 15.5. t(8;21) AML, bone marrow aspirate. (A) A distinctive case in which Chédiak–Higashi-like granules (arrow) are present within the myeloid blasts and progenitors. (B) These granules as well as the Auer rods are intensely myeloperoxidase positive by cytochemical staining (yellow reaction product).

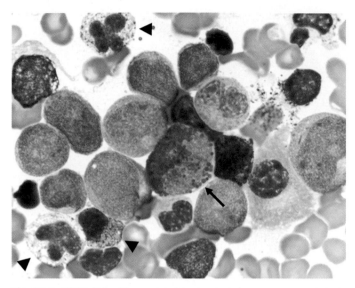

Fig. 15.6. t(8;21) AML with associated mastocytosis, bone marrow aspirate. In addition to the leukemic myeloblasts, there is pronounced mast cell proliferation in this case, consistent with systemic mastocytosis with associated clonal, hematologic non-mast cell lineage disease (SM-AHNMD). Several mast cells are depicted, some of which are partially degranulated; these mast cells manifest dyspoietic features, including nuclear lobation (arrowheads). There is also eosinophilia with dysplastic forms containing eosinophilic and basophilic granules (arrow). After chemotherapy, the mast cells persisted long after the patient's AML was in morphologic remission.

t(8;21) AML, patients with CD56-positive disease have shorter clinical remission and significantly worse overall survival than those with AML lacking CD56 expression [64, 65].

Cytogenetics and molecular diagnostics

The t(8;21) is present as the sole cytogenetic abnormality in nearly half of AMLs expressing RUNX1-RUNX1T1. Complex rearrangements targeting *RUNX1* and *RUNX1T1* are present in 10–20% of cases. Additional structural and numeric abnormalities are detected in about 50% of cases. Interestingly, the loss of either one of the sex chromosomes occurs in 35–55% of t(8;21) AMLs, a much higher frequency than is observed with other AML subtypes [47, 66, 67]. Quantitative PCR assays have been developed and are useful in confirming expression of *RUNX1-RUNX1T1*, particularly in cases harboring complex translocations, and in monitoring minimal residual disease (MRD) levels in t(8;21) AML patients [68–71]. However, the impact of MRD monitoring on the clinical management of patients with t(8;21) AML has been somewhat controversial. In some studies, MRD monitoring failed to reliably distinguish between patients in durable remission and those at risk for relapse [72]. By contrast, more recent studies have clearly demonstrated the utility of molecular monitoring for *RUNX1-RUNX1T1* transcripts in identifying those patients at risk for relapse [73–76]. The discrepant findings of these studies may reflect significant differences in the sensitivities of the assays used and in the time points at which molecular testing was undertaken following completion of therapy.

AML with inv(16)(p13q22) or t(16;16)(p13;q22) [inv(16) AML]

Definition

An AML subtype containing either the inv(16)(p13q22) or t(16;16)(p13;q22), both of which ultimately result in the expression of the CBFβ-MYH11 fusion oncoprotein. Most AMLs harboring this translocation manifest myeloid and monocytic differentiation and frequently have associated eosinophils with atypical cytologic features, and as such are designated acute myelomonocytic leukemia (AMMoL) with abnormal eosinophils, or AMMoL Eo.

Pathogenesis

The inv(16)(p13q22) and t(16;16)(p13;q22) are frequent genetic lesions in *de novo* AML. Both target the *CBFB* and *MYH11* loci, located at 16q22 and 16p13, respectively [13, 77–79]. These chromosomal rearrangements result in the expression of a chimeric transcript in which *MYH11* is fused in-frame to *CBFB*, ultimately yielding the CBFβ–MYH11 fusion oncoprotein which has a critical pathogenetic role in inv(16) AML [13, 15, 16, 19].

As discussed earlier, CBFβ is a ubiquitously expressed member of the RUNX family of transcription factors. CBFβ undergoes heterodimerization with other RUNX family members. While it lacks direct DNA binding activity, heterodimerization with CBFβ increases significantly the DNA binding affinity of the associated RUNX protein, and protects it from proteasome-mediated degradation [80–82]. Mice deficient in CBFβ manifest a spectrum of abnormalities, a subset of which is also present in each of the individual RUNX knockout mouse strains, corroborating the critical importance of heterodimerization with CBFβ for appropriate RUNX function. CBFβ is present in both the cytoplasm and nucleus, and its nuclear import is regulated by both phosphorylation and the level of RUNX1 expression [83–85].

MYH11 encodes a smooth muscle-specific myosin heavy chain, mutations of which appear to play a role in the pathogenesis of thoracic aortic aneurysm and patent ductus arteriosus [86]. MYH11 contains multiple domains, including a globular head which binds actin and has ATPase activity, and an α-helical rod domain that mediates dimerization and the formation of higher order myosin filaments [13, 87].

The chromosomal rearrangements characteristic of this AML subtype result in the formation of two reciprocal fusion genes, *CBFB-MYH11* and *MYH11-CBFB*; however, only the former is uniformly expressed in all cases, indicating that only CBFβ-MYH11 is pathogenetically relevant. The resultant fusion protein is comprised of the N-terminal portion of CBFβ fused in-frame to a variable amount of the C-terminal α-helical rod domain of MYH11 (Fig. 15.7). While the breakpoint in *CBFB* occurs consistently within either intron 4 or intron 5, the location of the *MYH11* breakpoint varies significantly; consequently, the relative amount of MYH11 included in the resultant

inv(16)/t(16;16) CBFβ-MYH11

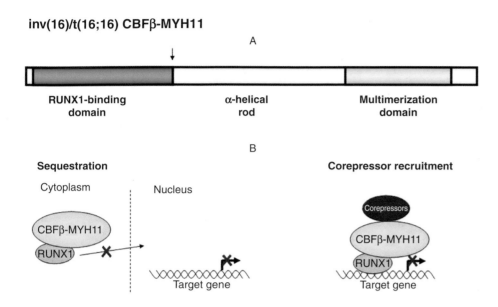

Fig. 15.7. Possible oncogenic mechanisms of CBFβ-MYH11. (A) This oncoprotein results from the in-frame fusion of CBFβ and MYH11. The former contributes the Runx1-binding domain, which is required for heterodimerization with RUNX1. CBFβ-MYH11 forms higher-order multimers, the formation of which occurs through a domain derived from MYH11. (B) CBFβ-MYH11 may contribute to leukemogenesis through two mechanisms. Because CBFβ-MYH11 can interact with cytoskeletal proteins, it may sequester RUNX1 within the cytoplasm, thereby inhibiting the expression of critical genes whose transcription is under the control of RUNX1/CBFβ. Alternatively, CBFβ-MYH11 may inhibit RUNX1/CBFβ-dependent gene transcription through the displacement of CBFβ and subsequent recruitment of transcriptional corepressors to RUNX1-responsive promoters and enhancers.

fusion protein in any given case is variable. However, the RUNX1-binding domain of CBFβ is invariably retained, enabling the CBFβ–MYH11 chimeric protein to heterodimerize with normal RUNX1 [88, 89]. In addition, the MYH11 moiety contained within the fusion protein is capable of forming homodimers and higher order multimers through intermolecular interactions of the MYH11 rod domains [13]. Experimental evidence has demonstrated the presence of high molecular weight nuclear RUNX1/CBFβ–MYH11 complexes within inv(16)-containing leukemic cells.

Biochemical and genetic data indicate that CBFβ–MYH11 induces leukemia through a dominant negative antagonism of RUNX1/CBFβ function. CBFβ–MYH11 accomplishes this indirectly by perturbing the subcellular localization and trafficking of CBFβ, resulting in the sequestration of RUNX1, and directly by inhibiting the transcriptional activation effected by RUNX1 through the recruitment of transcriptional corepressors to the promoters of RUNX1-responsive genes (Fig. 15.7) [90–93]. These effects of CBFβ–MYH11 are due, in part, to the fact that the fusion protein binds RUNX1 with higher affinity than native CBFβ [94]. That CBFβ–MYH11 functions in a dominant manner is also supported by studies of genetically engineered mice. Mice in which part of the *Myh11* cDNA is inserted into the *Cbfb* locus, yielding expression of a *CBFB-MYH11* fusion transcript identical to that seen in the human leukemia, die *in utero* at the midpoint of gestation and manifest a phenotype virtually identical to that of mice deficient in either Runx1 or Cbfβ [95]. Furthermore, while chimeric mice expressing CBFβ–MYH11 fail to spontaneously develop leukemia, mutagen administration induces AML at a high frequency in comparison to wild-type chimeras. Thus, as with RUNX1–RUNX1T1-associated AML, CBFβ–MYH11 expression alone is necessary but appears insufficient for the development of AML, implying the need for additional cooperating mutations [96, 97].

Clinical and laboratory features

AML expressing CBFβ–MYH11 comprises approximately 5–10% of pediatric AML and occurs at a median age of approximately 12 years, with no sex predilection [5, 6, 98]. This AML subtype is relatively uncommon among infants and toddlers, with fewer than 15% of cases occurring in children less than three years of age [98, 99]. Patients typically present with signs and symptoms of bone marrow failure. In contrast to t(8;21) AML, which also targets the core binding factor complex, inv(16) AML has no particular association with extramedullary disease. In peripheral blood, the leukocyte count is usually mildly or moderately elevated with myeloblasts present; Auer rods may be noted. Increased numbers of monocytes and immature monocytic forms, including monoblasts, are often present, although some cases lack significant monocytic differentiation. Eosinophilia is usually not evident in peripheral blood.

Pathologic features

Morphology

Myelomonocytic differentiation is evident morphologically in 75–90% of inv(16) AMLs, although the degree of monocytic differentiation is variable (Figs. 15.8 to 15.10) [78, 79, 88, 98, 100, 101]. In some instances, monoblasts and promonocytes predominate, and cases manifesting pure monocytic differentiation occasionally occur. In other cases, the myeloblast population is more prominent and would be classified as AML M1 or AML M2 under FAB criteria. Cases with a blast percentage of less than 20% are occasionally encountered; however, with typical morphologic findings and confirmation of *CBFB-MYH11* expression, these cases should be appropriately classified as inv(16) AML.

In the majority of cases, there is bone marrow eosinophilia, comprised of both progenitors and mature forms. Atypical

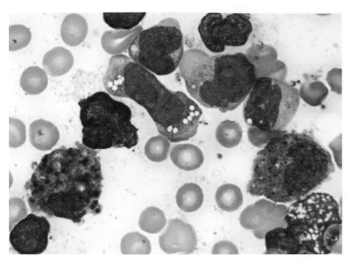

Fig. 15.8. inv(16) AML, bone marrow aspirate. In addition to myeloblasts, frequent dysplastic eosinophilic forms containing both eosinophilic and basophilic granules are present.

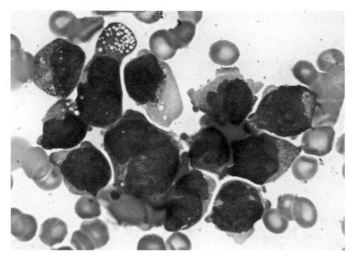

Fig. 15.9. inv(16) AML, bone marrow aspirate. Myeloid blasts, monoblasts, and monocytic forms predominate in this case, with few maturing myeloid elements.

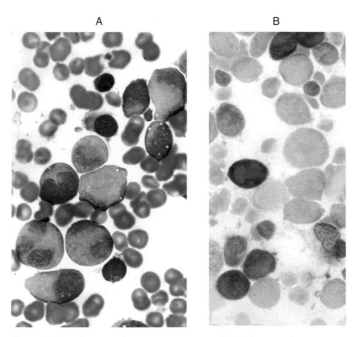

Fig. 15.10. Inv(16) AML, bone marrow aspirate. (A) Myeloperoxidase stain showing positivity in myeloid blasts as well as some monocytic cells (yellow reaction product). (B) α-naphthyl-butyrate esterase cytochemical stain highlighting intensely positive monocytic cells (red–brown reaction product).

eosinophils are usually present and characteristically contain both eosinophilic and basophilic granules and frequently other features such as nuclear lobation abnormalities (Fig. 15.8). However, the frequency of these atypical eosinophilic elements is quite variable, and in some cases, they can be very infrequent, necessitating a diligent search for them when this AML subtype is suspected [102]. Finally, it should be stressed that eosinophilia alone is insufficient for diagnosis of this AML subtype, as eosinophilia is not infrequently observed in other settings, including t(8;21) AML. The presence of abnormal

eosinophils is a much more specific morphologic clue to the presence of an underlying inv(16) or t(16;16).

Immunophenotype

Multiparameter flow cytometry in inv(16) AML often reveals discrete populations of cells that immunophenotypically mirror the relative extent of myeloid and monocytic differentiation observed morphologically. Inv(16) AMLs usually express several myeloid antigens (CD33, CD13, and CD15) and other lineage non-specific markers, such as HLA-DR. In addition, most cases express CD34 and CD117 as well. The latter marker is more frequently positive in inv(16) AMLs than in morphologically similar cases lacking this chromosomal rearrangement [103]. In cases with monocytic differentiation, expression of one or more monocyte-associated antigens, such as CD11b and CD14, is usually detected. Immunophenotyping can also provide clues as to the underlying genetic lesion. Expression of the T-cell-associated antigen CD2 is frequently detected in inv(16) AML, although the "aberrant" expression of this marker is not absolutely diagnostic of this AML subtype [104, 105]. Terminal deoxynucleotidyl transferase (TdT) is expressed in a significant minority of cases, but can likewise be detected in other AML subtypes [104]. Finally, the direct assessment of CBFβ-MYH11 expression by flow cytometry has obvious potential applications for diagnosis and minimal residual disease monitoring. Indeed, a flow cytometric assay for CBFβ-MYH11 has been reported; however, it has not been widely adopted, due mainly to the technical challenges of flow cytometric detection of this often weakly expressed fusion protein [89].

Cytogenetics and molecular diagnostics

Chromosomal recombinations targeting *CBFB* and *MYH11* include both the inv(16)(p13q22) and less commonly the t(16;16)(p13;q22) [5, 101, 106]. In approximately 70% of cases, the inv(16)/t(16;16) is the sole cytogenetic abnormality. In the remaining 30%, additional numerical and structural abnormalities are present, the most common being trisomy 22, which is present in 10–15% of cases; trisomies of chromosomes 8 and 21 occur less frequently [5, 101, 102]. Quantitative PCR assays have been developed and are useful in confirming expression of *CBFB-MYH11* in cases harboring complex or cryptic translocations [107–109]. Because of its pericentric location, the inv(16) is a relatively subtle cytogenetic change that can be difficult to detect, particularly in suboptimal chromosomal preparations. Thus, FISH or molecular assays can be of particular utility when confronted with bone marrow findings suggestive of inv(16) AML and an apparently "normal" karyotype. As with t(8;21) AML, the role of MRD monitoring in the clinical management of patients with inv(16) AML is somewhat controversial. More recent studies, however, indicate that detection of MRD in patients with this AML subtype identifies those individuals at high risk for relapse [73, 110, 111].

Acute promyelocytic leukemia (APL)

Definition

APL is characterized by the expansion of a clonal population of malignant myeloid cells blocked at the promyelocyte stage of differentiation. Genetically, APL is defined by chromosomal translocations targeting the **r**etinoic **a**cid **r**eceptor α (*RARA*) gene located on chromosome 17. In most cases, the t(15;17)(q22;q12) is identified, which results in the in-frame fusion of the **p**romyelocytic **l**eukemia (*PML*) gene on chromosome 15 with *RARA*, yielding the PML-RARα oncogene [112–115]. Variant translocations are detected in less than 5% of APL. These translocations target 11q23, 5q23, and 11q13, and fuse the *PLZF*, *NPM*, and *NUMA* genes, respectively, to *RARA*.

Pathogenesis

Perturbation of the RARα signaling cascade is the central pathogenetic event in APL [116]. With recognition of the involvement of RARα in APL and with the advent of all-*trans* retinoic acid (ATRA) as an effective therapy for this disorder, the molecular pathogenesis of APL has been the subject of intense basic and translational research. Before discussion of the pathogenesis of APL, the physiologic roles of RARα and PML will be reviewed.

RARα is a transcription factor that regulates the expression of numerous genes within hematopoietic cells, including several which play important roles in hematopoietic cell function and differentiation [117, 118]. Similar to other members of the nuclear hormone receptor superfamily of transcription factors, RARα is a modular protein containing several critical functional domains [119]. RARα normally forms heterodimers with a retinoid-X receptor (RXR) family member, thereby acquiring high-affinity DNA binding [120]. In the absence of ligand, RARα/RXR binds to response elements within the promoters of target genes and, together with corepressors, including the nuclear receptor-corepressor N-CoR/SMRT, Sin3A or Sin3B, and histone deacetylases (HDACs), induces the forma-

tion of chromatin structures that ultimately inhibit gene transcription at target loci [121–124]. The binding of retinoic acid (RA) to RARα/RXR induces the dissociation of this repressor complex and facilitates the recruitment and assembly of a multimeric complex that promotes chromatin conformational changes that ultimately enhance the transcription of target genes [124–131]. Thus, the absence or presence of RA dictates whether RARα/RXR heterodimer functions to enhance or inhibit gene expression.

PML is ubiquitously expressed and is a component of nuclear bodies, which are subnuclear organelles [132, 133]. PML is a modular protein and contains several critical domains which mediate the myriad protein–protein interactions that are central to the physiologic function of PML. PML participates in several important cellular processes, including proliferation, cellular senescence, and apoptosis [134–136]. Cells from PML-deficient mice manifest enhanced proliferation *in vitro*, and these mice develop tumors in response to mutagen treatment at a higher frequency, suggesting that PML functions as a tumor suppressor [137]. Finally, *in vitro* and *in vivo* studies with PML-deficient mice and cells indicate that PML also confers sensitivity to proapoptotic signals, such as γ-irradiation, Fas signaling and TNF, which is mediated through both p53-dependent and -independent mechanisms, the latter involving the ataxia telangiectasia-mutated (ATM) signaling pathway [138, 139].

The PML–RARα fusion oncoprotein, which results from the t(15;17), inhibits the physiologic functions of RARα and PML in a dominant negative manner (Fig. 15.11). Whereas RA binding to RARα induces the dissociation of its associated transcriptional repressors and subsequent formation of a transcriptional activation complex, the PML-RARα-associated corepressor complex fails to dissociate in response to physiologic levels of RA, resulting in the dominant negative inhibition of RARα [140–148]. Since it dimerizes with RXRs like the native protein, PML-RARα also indirectly inhibits the function of RARα, as well as other nuclear hormone receptor family members such as the vitamin D and thyroid hormone receptors, by titrating away and sequestering RXRs [149].

PML-RARα also interferes with the physiologic function of PML. PML-RARα disrupts the normal distribution of PML within nuclear bodies, which likely accounts for its inhibition of the growth regulatory properties of PML [132, 133, 150]. PML-RARα also desensitizes cells to the proapoptotic state induced by various stimuli, including growth factor deprivation or activation of the TNF and Fas signaling pathways [135, 138, 151–154]. Bcl-2 overexpression has recently been shown to accelerate the development of APL in murine models, suggesting that the anti-apoptotic effects of PML-RARα may have a significant pathogenetic role in APL [155]. In addition, PML-RARα alters gene expression through the recruitment of DNA methyltransferases which hypermethylate and silence target promoters [156]. Thus, through antagonism of both RARα and PML, PML-RARα contributes to leukemogenesis through dysregulation of gene expression critical for normal myeloid development, and enhanced cell survival through desensitization

t(15;17) PML-RARα

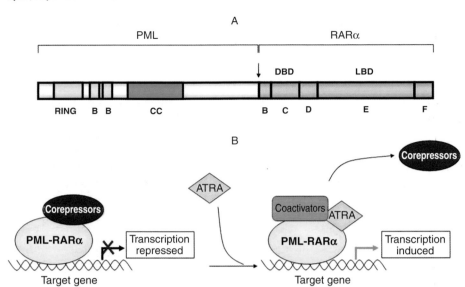

Fig. 15.11. Schematic of the PML-RARα fusion protein. (A) PML-RARα is detected in approximately 95% of all APLs and is the product of the in-frame fusion of the target genes resulting from the t(15;17). PML contributes a RING finger motif, two B-boxes, and a coiled-coil (CC) domain. The domains responsible for DNA binding (DBD) and RA binding (LBD) are derived from RARα. (B) PML-RARα contributes to oncogenesis, in part, by the inhibition of expression of RA-responsive genes. Like wild-type RARα, PML-RARα recruits corepressor molecules, such as histone deacetylases, to the promoters of target genes. In contrast to RARα, the corepressor complex associated with PML-RARα fails to dissociate in the presence of physiologic levels of RA. However, pharmacologic levels of ATRA induce its dissociation, permitting assembly of a coactivator complex and resumption of RA-induced gene expression, and ultimately permitting cells expressing PML-RARα to complete subsequent stages of myeloid maturation.

to physiologic proapoptotic stimuli, resulting in a block in myelopoiesis and expansion of malignant promyelocytes.

These pathogenetic effects of PML-RARα are overcome in the presence of superphysiologic levels of RA resulting from ATRA therapy, and are, in part, attributable to the ATRA-induced, proteasome-mediated degradation of PML-RARα [157, 158]. The resultant dissociation of the inhibitory transcriptional complex associated with PML-RARα facilitates the assembly of transcriptional coactivators and resumed expression of those RARα-responsive genes required for progression through the terminal stages of myeloid maturation [132, 133, 159]. It should be pointed out that while it potently induces terminal differentiation in APL, ATRA therapy alone does not eliminate the leukemic clone, as evidenced by the fact that patients initially treated with ATRA as a single agent achieve a high rate of remission but uniformly relapse after cessation of ATRA therapy. The development or expansion of ATRA-resistant clones, which harbor mutations abrogating RA binding to RARα-APL, may also be exacerbated by treatment with ATRA alone [160–162]. These initial observations have prompted the incorporation of ATRA into combination chemotherapeutic approaches yielding much improved clinical outcomes (discussed below).

Clinical and laboratory features

APL comprises approximately 5–10% of pediatric AML and occurs at a median age of approximately 12 years, with a higher frequency of females in some studies [5, 6, 98, 163, 164]. This AML subtype is uncommon among infants and toddlers, with fewer than 15% of cases occurring in children less than three years of age [98, 99, 165]. Although signs and symptoms of bone marrow failure are often present, the presence of a bleeding diathesis often dominates the clinical picture in most children with APL. While not uncommon in acute leukemia, coag-

ulation abnormalities occur at a higher frequency, in some 75–90% of patients, and are more severe in APL than other subtypes of pediatric AML [163, 166]. Laboratory studies usually reveal a prolonged prothrombin time (PT), decreased fibrinogen, and elevated fibrin D-dimer and fibrin degradation products (FDPs), all findings consistent with disseminated intravascular coagulation [167]. Coagulopathy is associated with both the hypergranular type and the so-called microgranular variant of APL (discussed below). Given these somewhat distinct clinical features, astute clinicians not infrequently have a strong suspicion of APL before ever receiving a confirmatory call from the pathologist. Prompt initiation of ATRA therapy ameliorates the hemorrhagic complications of APL, although it may paradoxically increase the risk of thrombosis [168–171]. Current therapy for APL includes ATRA in combination with other conventional chemotherapeutics, which yields clinical outcomes far superior to those achieved with either ATRA or chemotherapy alone and results in a cure in approximately 80–90% of patients, a remarkable achievement for a disease that 15 years ago was accompanied by high rates of morbidity and mortality [162, 172–175].

Peripheral blood analysis most often reveals pancytopenia [163–166]. Most children have moderate to severe anemia. Given the frequent coexistence of DIC in APL, severe thrombocytopenia is usually present, with median platelet counts of approximately 20×10^9/L in several reported pediatric studies [164, 165, 176]. In contrast to most other AML subtypes, the WBC count is usually decreased or within normal limits in APL, with median WBC counts in most reported pediatric series of approximately $4–5 \times 10^9$/L. A notable exception is the hyperleukocytosis characteristically present in patients with microgranular APL.

Examination of the blood smear corroborates the findings of the CBC. In cases of hypergranular APL, malignant

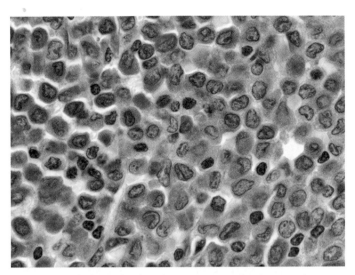

Fig. 15.12. Hypergranular APL, bone marrow biopsy. At diagnosis, the marrow is almost always hypercellular and effaced by malignant promyelocytes, and is characteristically very eosinophilic due to the heavy granulation of the promyelocytes (PAS stain).

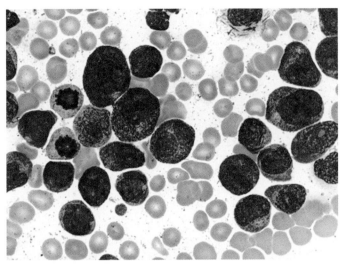

Fig. 15.13. Hypergranular APL, bone marrow aspirate. Neoplastic promyelocytes are densely granulated, obscuring cellular detail. In comparison with the microgranular variant, hypergranular APL cells are somewhat smaller in size and contain round to oval nuclei; cells with bilobed nuclei are usually infrequent.

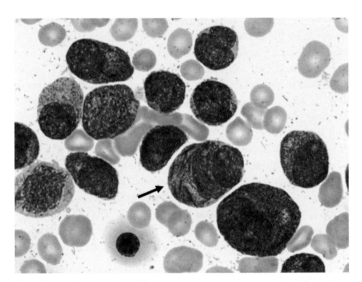

Fig. 15.14. Hypergranular APL, bone marrow aspirate. A so-called "faggot" cell is present, containing multiple Auer rods (arrow). Due to mechanical fragility, these cells are often disrupted during smear preparation and may have a degenerated appearance.

promyelocytes may be infrequent but are usually present in the peripheral blood film and readily recognized by virtue of their prominent granulation. As implied by its name, microgranular APL cells lack the heavy granulation characteristic of hypergranular APL. While the leukemic cells in this APL subtype are less subtle given their sheer number, microgranular APL is more likely to be confused with other types of acute leukemia, since microgranular promyelocytes contain a paucity of granules and have some morphologic features reminiscent of other types of acute leukemia, for instance acute monocytic leukemia (see below). The genetic basis for the morphologic differences between the hypergranular and microgranular subtypes of APL is not well understood, as both are associated with the t(15;17);

however, the frequency of FLT3 internal tandem duplication (ITD) is significantly higher in the microgranular variant and may account, in part, for its distinct morphologic and clinical features [177, 178].

Pathologic features

Morphology

The marrow in APL is almost always hypercellular and effaced by malignant promyelocytes with concomitant reduction in normal hematopoietic elements (Fig. 15.12). In hypergranular APL, the malignant promyelocytes are intermediate–large in size and contain oval or reniform nuclei; forms with bilobed nuclei are usually present as well (Figs. 15.13 and 15.14). Cytologic detail is often obscured by dense azurophilic granulation. In most cases, neoplastic cells containing multiple Auer rods, so-called "faggot" cells, are frequent. Due to the mechanical trauma of smear preparation, disrupted cells with disgorged granules or Auer rods are often present. In microgranular APL, most of the cells contain a reniform-shaped or bilobed nucleus with fine chromatin and relatively abundant, lightly basophilic cytoplasm, cytologic features which closely resemble those of monocytes (Figs. 15.15 and 15.16) [179]. Most of the malignant promyelocytes contain only sparse azurophilic granules or lack granulation altogether. However, scattered cells similar to those seen in hypergranular APL, including cells containing multiple Auer rods, are usually present in most cases of microgranular APL, providing an important clue to the diagnosis (Fig. 15.16). Analysis of myeloperoxidase expression, either by cytochemistry or flow cytometry, can be diagnostically helpful, particularly in the evaluation of a microgranular APL (Fig. 15.17). Both hypergranular and microgranular APL cells express high levels of myeloperoxidase. In cases of suspected microgranular APL, strong myeloperoxidase expression helps to exclude monocytic

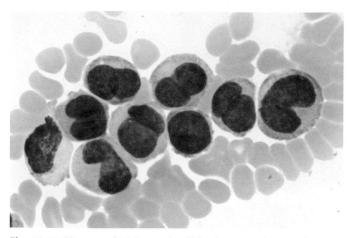

Fig. 15.15. Microgranular APL, peripheral blood smear. In this case, there was hyperleukocytosis, typical of the microgranular variant. Most of the cells have bilobed or reniform cells and contain few discernible granules. The cells of microgranular APL morphologically resemble monocytes and can lead to a mistaken diagnosis of acute monocytic leukemia.

leukemia, which is typically negative or only weakly myeloperoxidase positive.

APLs harboring variant translocations that target RARα [the t(11;17) and the t(5;17) encoding the *PLZF-RARA* and *NPM-RARA* fusion transcripts, respectively] have been reported to have distinctive morphologic features [180]. APLs with the t(11;17) have round or oval nuclei, and while nearly all are hypergranular, most cases lack Auer rods; Auer rods are similarly infrequent in cases with the t(5;17). In addition, hypolobated neutrophils are a common feature of APL expressing *PLZF-RARA*. Finally, distinction of APLs containing the t(11;17) from those with the t(15;17) is clinically important, as patients with the former do not respond to ATRA.

Immunophenotype

APL has several immunophenotypic features that facilitate its distinction from other AML subtypes. Thus, flow cytometry together with morphologic examination permits the rapid confirmation of a presumed APL diagnosis in most cases, satisfying the often urgent clinical need to initiate ATRA therapy. Because of the high granule content, hypergranular APL typically has very high side scatter in CD45 vs. side scatter plots, whereas the light scatter characteristics for microgranular APL are less distinctive. The immunophenotypic profile most often touted as "classic" for APL is positivity for myeloid antigens (primarily CD33 and CD13) and negativity for CD34 and HLA-DR. While characteristic, this immunophenotype is not uniformly present in APL and thus does not distinguish in all instances between APL and other myeloid leukemias [181–183]. Given these shortcomings, alternative immunophenotypes have been proposed that reportedly have greater diagnostic sensitivity and specificity for APL. Based on a large series of APLs, a myeloid cell population negative or only dimly positive for HLA-DR, CD11a, and CD18 has been reported to be highly specific for APL, independent of morphology and PML-RARα isoform expression [183]. The presence of a single blast population together with uniformly bright CD33 expression, heterogeneous CD13 expression, dim/negative CD15 expression, and lack of HLA-DR expression has similarly been reported to be characteristic of APL containing the t(15;17), with high specificity and sensitivity [184]. Finally, it should also be mentioned that the stem cell/progenitor antigen CD117 is expressed in most APLs, despite initial reports to the contrary.

It is now apparent that much of the immunophenotypic heterogeneity in APL reflects differences in marker expression between the hypergranular and microgranular subtypes. Whereas most hypergranular APLs are negative for CD34 and HLA-DR, a significant percentage of microgranular cases are positive for these markers. Furthermore, microgranular APLs commonly express CD2, whereas hypergranular cases are usually negative for this marker [181, 183]. This immunophenotypic heterogeneity is consistent with the results of microarray analyses of hypergranular and microgranular APL, in

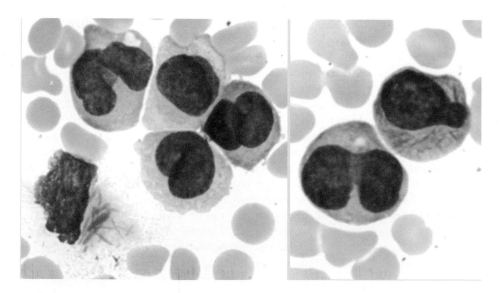

Fig. 15.16. Microgranular APL, peripheral blood smear. In this case, virtually all the promyelocytes have microgranular morphology. Although they can be quite rare, hypergranular promyelocytes are present in virtually all cases of microgranular APL; two "faggot" cells are shown.

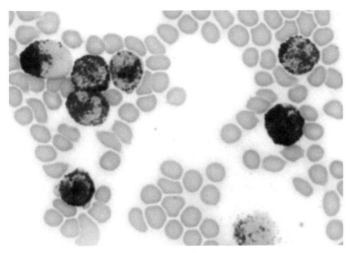

Fig. 15.17. Microgranular APL, peripheral blood smear. Microgranular promyelocytes are intensely myeloperoxidase positive by cytochemistry, a finding which can help to distinguish this APL variant from acute monocytic leukemia, which it can morphologically mimic. This seemingly paradoxical cytochemical feature is attributable to the presence of numerous granules within microgranular promyelocytes that are smaller than those of hypergranular APL and beyond the resolution of light microscopy, accounting for the apparent agranularity of this APL variant.

Cytogenetics and molecular diagnostics

The t(15;17)(q22;q12) is characteristic of APL and is detected in approximately 95% of APLs [112]. The remaining 5% contain other translocations that likewise target *RARA*, including the t(11;17)(q23;q12) [*PLZF*], t(5;17)(q35;q12) [*NPM*], t(5;17)(q13;q12) [*NUMA*], der(17) [*STAT5B*], t(3;17)(p25;q12) [uncharacterized partner gene], and cryptic events targeting *PRKAR1A* [186–191]. Of these variant translocations, only the t(11;17)(q23;q12) occurs with any significant frequency (~1% of APL cases), as descriptions of the remaining *RARA* translocations have been restricted to small series or single case reports. Despite its infrequency, detection of the t(11;17)(q23;q12) has clinical importance, because APL with this translocation is resistant to ATRA as well as newer arsenical chemotherapeutics, such as arsenic trioxide [192–194].

In the majority of cases, the t(15;17) can be readily demonstrated through conventional cytogenetics. Approximately 5% of cases contain either a complex or a cryptic rearrangement involving 15q22 and 17q12, necessitating molecular or FISH assays to confirm the expression of *PML-RARA* [195]. Secondary cytogenetic abnormalities are detected in approximately 30% of cases but appear to lack prognostic significance [196]. Given the specific and highly effective therapy available for APL, the presence of the t(15;17) can be rapidly confirmed by FISH, which can be particularly helpful in the rare case with atypical morphology or unusual immunophenotypic features. Qualitative and quantitative RT-PCR assays are available for both molecular confirmation and minimal residual disease

monitoring. Molecular monitoring has demonstrated utility in identifying APL patients at high risk of relapse [197–199]. Furthermore, such early detection may ultimately improve outcome, as survival is higher for patients in whom relapse is detected by RT-PCR versus those whose treatment is not initiated until the development of overt hematologic relapse [199].

AML with t(9;11)(p22;q23) or other balanced translocations involving 11q23 (*MLL*) [MLL-AML]
Definition
This is an AML subtype containing a balanced translocation targeting the **m**ixed **l**ineage **l**eukemia (*MLL*) gene and any one of over 50 partner genes located at other chromosomal loci, the commonest of which is the *AF9* gene located at 9p22. Irrespective of the partner gene, these translocations result in the expression of a chimeric oncoprotein in which MLL is fused in-frame to the relevant partner protein. Depending on the particular translocation, MLL-AMLs often manifest some degree of monocytic differentiation.

Pathogenesis
MLL (also referred to as HRX, ALL-1, and HTRX1) is an extraordinarily large protein, with an expansive gene located at chromosome 11q23 that is one of the most common targets of chromosomal rearrangements in AML. MLL is highly homologous to the *Drosophila* protein trithorax, which plays a critical role in embryonic development, in part through its regulation of expression of the homeobox (HOX) A genes. MLL is a modular protein containing several structural domains required for its normal biologic function, including those which mediate DNA binding, chromatin remodeling, and interactions with other proteins (Fig. 15.18). Through both intrinsic biochemical activity and that of proteins recruited by MLL, such as histone deacetylases and members of the SWI/SNF chromatin remodeling complex, MLL induces conformational changes at target loci that result in alterations in gene expression. MLL can function as either an activator or repressor of transcription, the molecular determinants of which are incompletely understood [200]. MLL undergoes proteolysis into N-terminal and C-terminal cleavage products by the endopeptidase, taspase 1, which enhances its transcriptional activating properties [201–203]. Defining the biologic role of MLL in normal hematopoiesis has been somewhat difficult, given the pleiotropic consequences of MLL deficiency and the confounding influences of hematopoietic cell-independent factors. Using techniques to circumvent these concerns, it is now established that MLL plays a critical role in the establishment of hematopoiesis during development, probably at the stage of hematopoietic stem cell formation in the aorta–gonad–mesonephros and other anatomic sites [204].

The function of AF9, whose gene is located at 9p22 and is the target of the most frequent *MLL* translocation, is poorly

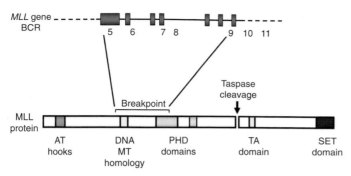

Fig. 15.18. Schematic of MLL. *MLL* is the most promiscuous of all translocation-associated genes, having been implicated as a partner gene in almost 90 different chromosomal translocations. Although MLL is encoded by a large gene, spanning over 100 kb of genomic DNA and comprised of 37 exons, these myriad translocations target a relatively small region within *MLL*, the major breakpoint region (MBR), which encompasses exons 5–11 (exons are represented as boxes in the upper figure). MLL is a large protein and comprised of multiple domains, including the AT hook domain, a region with homology to DNA methyltransferases (DNA MTs), PHD-type zinc fingers, a transactivating (TA) domain, and a SET domain. The AT hooks motif mediates DNA binding, and the TA domain mediates the transcriptional activation effected by MLL. MLL undergoes proteolysis by taspase1, resulting in the formation of an MLL heterodimer comprised of the N- and C-terminal fragments. This heterodimeric form of MLL is significantly more stable than the intact protein.

understood. AF9 contains a domain rich in serine and proline residues, as well as a nuclear localization motif, suggesting that it may function as a transcription factor [205]. Mice deficient in Af9 develop perinatal lethality and manifest multiple axial skeletal abnormalities [206]. Like MLL, AF9 similarly appears to regulate embryonic patterning through the regulation of HOX gene expression.

Nearly 90 different chromosomal translocations target *MLL*, of which more than 50 have been molecularly characterized [207]. The myriad partner genes notwithstanding, each MLL translocation generates a fusion mRNA transcript in which the 5′ portion is derived from *MLL* and is fused in-frame to a coding sequence derived from the partner gene located on the reciprocal chromosome [208–210]. Despite the size of its gene, these translocation breakpoints are confined to a relatively small 8.5 kb region of *MLL* flanked by exons 5 and 11 (Fig. 15.18). Consequently, certain MLL domains are consistently retained within the resultant fusion proteins, including the AT hooks, as well as the DNA methyltransferase homology domain, whereas other motifs are eliminated, including the zinc fingers and transactivation and SET domains. In addition to chromosomal translocations, *MLL* can also undergo partial internal duplication, which is detected mainly in AMLs with either a diploid karyotype or trisomy 11 [211].

The frequent involvement of *MLL* in leukemia-associated translocations suggests that perturbation of MLL signaling is an important mechanism of hematopoietic cell transformation. However, elucidation of the common pathways by which MLL fusion proteins induce leukemia, and determination of the biologic role, if any, of domains contributed by the partner protein is daunting given the sheer number of genes targeted by these translocations, whose products are involved in divergent

cellular processes. That certain MLL fusion proteins are consistently associated with a given type of acute leukemia, for instance MLL-AF4 and acute lymphoblastic leukemia, suggests that non-MLL derived components of these fusion proteins contribute critically to their oncogenic function. However, the exact role of the non-MLL derived component is controversial [212–217]. Finally, in addition to their intrinsic activities, the oncogenic properties of these fusion proteins may be due in part to their perturbation of the normal function of both MLL and the intact partner protein. Detailed discussion of the structural and biochemical properties of the various MLL fusion proteins is beyond the scope of this discussion; the interested reader is referred to recent comprehensive reviews [218–221].

It now appears that MLL fusion proteins may function via distinct mechanisms depending on the nature of the fusion partner [215, 222]. In fusions involving nuclear proteins, a monomeric form of the MLL fusion protein binds to DNA regulatory sequences through MLL domains, and recruits transcriptional coactivators via motifs derived from the nuclear fusion partner. MLL fusion proteins containing cytoplasmic partners similarly bind DNA through MLL motifs. However, oligomerization of the MLL chimeric protein mediated by motifs in its fusion partner leads to the recruitment of transcriptional coactivators not usually present at normal target transcriptional targets of MLL, resulting in aberrant gene expression. Internal duplication of the *MLL* gene occurs in approximately 10% of cases, leading to duplication of the MLL domains required for the enhanced cell renewal, including the CXXC domain [223–225]. In these cases, duplication of these critical domains may, in effect, mimic the dimerization which occurs in some MLL fusion proteins, ultimately leading to the aberrant recruitment of transcriptional coactivators.

Irrespective of the function of the non-MLL component, the central oncogenic role of MLL fusion proteins in this AML subtype has been confirmed experimentally. Through the use of various mouse models, enforced expression of several MLL fusion proteins within hematopoietic progenitors induces AML with a high level of penetrance [212, 213, 226–228]. With some fusion proteins, leukemia develops only after a rather protracted latency period, indicating the need for cooperating mutations for the development of frank leukemia.

The downstream signaling pathways through which the MLL fusion proteins induce leukemia remain incompletely understood. The *HOX* genes are attractive candidates, given that MLL plays an important role in their regulation in hematopoietic cells. Indeed, gene expression profiling has confirmed the overexpression of several *HOXA* genes in MLL-AMLs in comparison to other AML subtypes and normal hematopoietic cells, which normally express these genes at significantly lower levels [229–234]. Whether aberrant *HOX* gene expression plays an important pathogenetic role in MLL-AML leukemogenesis remains uncertain, however, as studies have yielded conflicting results, which could reflect differential requirements for *HOX* gene expression among the various MLL fusion proteins [234–237].

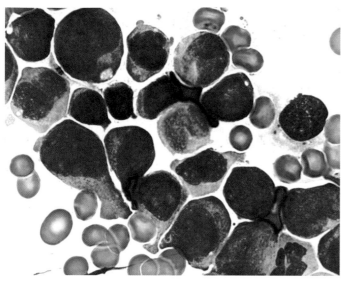

Fig. 15.19. Acute myeloid leukemia with 11q23 abnormality, bone marrow aspirate. This AML with myelomonocytic differentiation contained a rare, yet recurrent translocation involving the *TET1* gene on 10q22. The blasts contain rare Auer rods and express myelomonocytic markers by flow cytometry.

Clinical and laboratory features

As a group, MLL-AML comprises 15–20% of all pediatric AML, and as such is the most common cytogenetic AML subtype in children [5, 238, 239]. *MLL* chromosomal rearrangements are also detected in the preponderance of secondary AMLs arising after therapy containing topoisomerase II inhibitors [240–243]. Of the AML-associated translocations targeting *MLL*, the t(9;11)(p22;q23) is the most frequently encountered in the pediatric population. Other common *MLL* translocations include those targeting 10p12 (*AF10*), 19p13.1 (*ELL*), and 19p13.3 (*EEN*). For poorly understood reasons, the frequency of 11q23 translocations is particularly high in both ALL and AML arising during infancy, where they are detected in over 50% of AMLs [244–247]. Children with MLL-AML present frequently with clinical evidence of extramedullary leukemic infiltration, including hepatosplenomegaly, gingival hypertrophy, and leukemia cutis. The WBC count is often higher in MLL-AML than in morphologically similar AMLs lacking these translocations [238, 246].

Pathologic features

Morphology

Most MLL-AMLs manifest some degree of monocytic differentiation and were typically classified as either acute myelomonocytic or monocytic leukemia using FAB criteria, although *MLL* rearrangements have been detected in virtually every FAB subtype of AML (Fig. 15.19) [246, 248, 249]. Cases containing the t(9;11) are frequently classified as acute monocytic leukemia (AMoL) [238]. Infant AMLs manifesting monocytic differentiation almost invariably harbor an *MLL* translocation [246]. Other than the presence of monocytic differentiation, MLL-AMLs otherwise lack any morphologic distinctiveness.

Immunophenotype

Multiparameter flow cytometry is useful in confirming the myeloid or monocytic lineage of the leukemic blasts in MLL-AML. However, an immunophenotype diagnostic of this subtype of AML has not been described. Nearly all cases of MLL-AML express HLA-DR and the myeloid antigens CD33, CD13, and CD15, and approximately 50% of cases express CD34 and CD117 [248, 250]. In cases with monocytic differentiation, expression of CD64, CD4 (often dim), CD11b, and, less frequently, CD14 is detected. While CD56 expression is more common in AMoL and AMMoL with *MLL* translocations than in cases lacking them, CD56 expression alone is not diagnostic of the presence of an underlying MLL rearrangement.

Cytogenetics and molecular diagnostics

As with other types of AML, those associated with *MLL* chromosomal rearrangements should be characterized at diagnosis using conventional cytogenetics. This is somewhat more daunting with MLL-AMLs, given the multitude of chromosomal translocations which target the *MLL* locus, making it the most promiscuous of all leukemia-associated genes. In children, four translocations, t(9;11)(p22;q23), t(11;19)(q23;p13.1), t(11;19)(q23;p13.3), and the t(10;11)(p12;q23), account for over 60% of MLL-AMLs [5, 238]. While FISH and Southern blotting can unequivocally confirm the presence of an MLL translocation, conventional cytogenetics at diagnosis still adds important prognostic information, as pediatric AML cases with the t(9;11)(p22;q23) have a significantly better clinical outcome than those harboring other *MLL* rearrangements [238, 251, 252]. Other cytogenetic abnormalities in addition to the *MLL* translocation are detected in a significant minority of cases. By contrast, *MLL* partial tandem duplications (PTDs) are detected in AMLs which are either karyotypically normal or contain trisomy 11.

Cryptic translocations involving *MLL* occur, and they have been detected at a surprisingly high frequency in some pediatric AML series [239, 253]. In cases with complex or cryptic rearrangements, molecular testing may be essential to confirm the presence of a translocation targeting *MLL*, particularly where the pathologic or clinical features are suggestive of an MLL-AML. While Southern blotting is a useful research tool for the detection of *MLL* rearrangements, it is a time-consuming procedure and typically employs radiolabeled probes, features making it a less-than-optimal laboratory test. Alternatives to Southern blotting include RT-PCR and FISH. Reverse transcriptase PCR assays to detect several of the more common *MLL* translocations are routinely performed in many academic centers and reference laboratories [254–258]. However, a negative RT-PCR result does not exclude the possibility of a *MLL* translocation, given the plethora of potential gene partners. FISH assays to detect *MLL* rearrangements have been developed using commercially available probes, and include assays employing either a single probe that spans the *MLL* gene (so-called *break-apart probe*) or two probes that are differentially

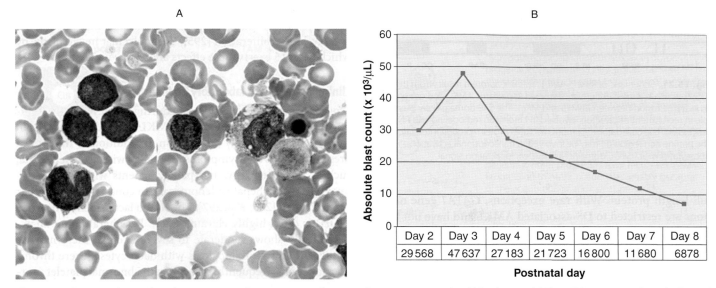

Fig. 15.22. Transient abnormal myelopoiesis in an infant constitutionally mosaic for trisomy 21, peripheral blood smear. (A) The WBC count is moderately elevated and the blood film contains a range of megakaryocytic forms, including megakaryoblasts, some of which are binucleated, and micromegakaryocytes. Nucleated RBCs and giant platelets are present as well. (B) This patient's blastemia peaked at day three of postnatal life and spontaneously resolved shortly thereafter, typical of most cases of TAM. Cytogenetics confirmed the presence of trisomy 21, as well as other numeric abnormalities. This case represents a rare, but documented occurrence of TAM in a phenotypically normal infant mosaic for trisomy 21, and it highlights the importance of including TAM in the differential diagnosis of any young infant with "acute leukemia" that manifests megakaryoblastic differentiation. (Photomicrographs and graph kindly provided by Dr. Mihaela Onciu; ©2004 American Society for Clinical Pathology.)

myelofibrosis in which only scattered nests of megakaryoblasts are present and which may closely mimic a metastatic solid tumor (Fig. 15.23) [300]. Due to the fibrosis, the bone marrow is frequently inaspirable, yielding a "dry tap"; in these instances, biopsy touch imprints may prove helpful for evaluating cytologic features of the blasts.

AMKL manifests a greater degree of heterogeneity with regard to blast morphology than most other subtypes of acute leukemia, and awareness of this morphologic spectrum is often helpful in arriving at an appropriate diagnosis. Some cases of AMKL can very closely resemble acute lymphoblastic leukemia, with small, poorly differentiated blasts. In other instances, there may be markedly increased numbers of dysplastic megakaryocytes and relatively few identifiable megakaryoblasts. Furthermore, pronounced heterogeneity in blast morphology can be present within a given case of AMKL, a finding which can serve as a subtle diagnostic feature.

Megakaryoblasts frequently manifest several characteristic cytologic features, which, although not pathognomonic, provide important diagnostic clues (Figs. 15.24 to 15.26). Megakaryoblasts tend to be somewhat cohesive, in contrast to most other types of acute leukemia. Blood films and aspirate smears may contain clumps and aggregates of blasts as a result (Fig. 15.24) [301]. The degree of cohesiveness can be sufficiently striking as to suggest metastatic solid tumor in some instances (Fig. 15.27). Although infrequent in other types of pediatric acute leukemia, binucleated blasts are frequently present in AMKL (Fig. 15.25). Megakaryoblasts often manifest cytoplasmic protrusions or blebbing, which can be broad-based extensions or more delicate projections (Fig. 15.26). These structures

reflect abortive attempts by the megakaryoblast to recapitulate proplatelet formation [302]. Finally, it should be mentioned that megakaryoblasts may contain a sparse complement of fine azurophilic granules; this finding is variable and is by no means specific to AMKL.

In children with TAM, extramedullary involvement may also occur. The most common of these extramedullary manifestations is liver involvement, which can range from isolated hepatomegaly in the absence of significant hepatic impairment, to profound hepatic dysfunction. The latter occurs in as many as 15% of affected children and is potentially fatal [303]. In these cases, liver biopsy typically reveals hepatocellular injury and fibrosis [304–306]. An intrasinusoidal infiltrate of blasts and megakaryocytic forms is usually present (Fig. 15.28). Other organs, including skin, are infrequently involved. In patients with high WBC counts, the intravascular accumulation of blasts may be readily apparent in biopsies from many anatomic sites (Fig. 15.29).

Immunophenotype and cytochemistry

Definitive diagnosis of AMKL using WHO criteria requires the demonstration of megakaryocytic differentiation. In years past, AMKLs were characterized using a combination of cytochemistry, electron microscopy-based determination of platelet peroxidase positivity, and immunofluorescence. These cumbersome assays have almost entirely been supplanted by immunophenotyping using either flow cytometry or immunohistochemistry. Utility of the latter method is limited by the availability of only a small number of antibodies appropriate for detection of megakaryocytic-specific antigens

A

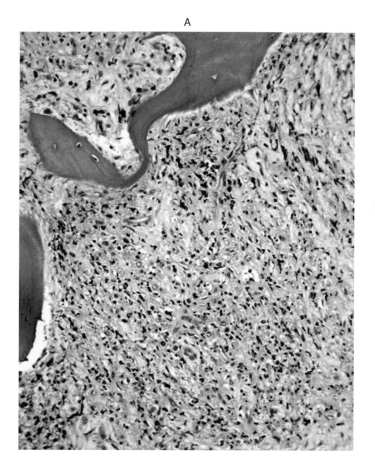

B

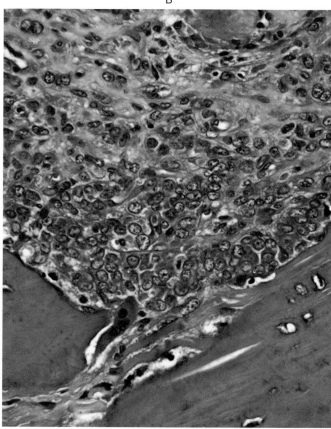

C

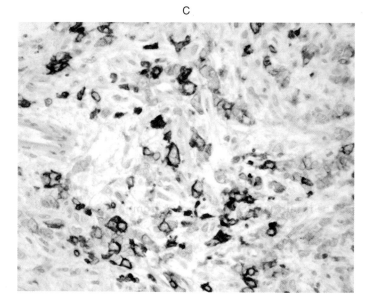

Fig. 15.23. t(1;22) AMKL, bone marrow biopsy. (A) Low-power view shows diffuse collagen fibrosis with admixed immature cells and significant crush artifact; the aspirate was a "dry tap" and contained few evaluable cells. This degree of fibrosis is characteristic of AMKLs expressing *RBM15-MKL1*. (B) Aggregates of blasts are present focally. (C) The leukemic blasts strongly express CD61, confirming their megakaryoblastic differentiation.

in paraffin-embedded bone marrow biopsies. Although not lineage specific, Factor VIII-related antigen is highly expressed in megakaryocytes and can be readily detected by immunohistochemistry. Unfortunately, most cases of pediatric AMKL are negative for factor VIII-related antigen, since this marker is expressed somewhat later in megakaryopoiesis than other megakaryocyte-specific antigens [307]. More recently, antibodies for the immunohistochemical detection of CD61, a strongly megakaryocytic-specific marker, have become available. However, the choice of fixative and decalcification method

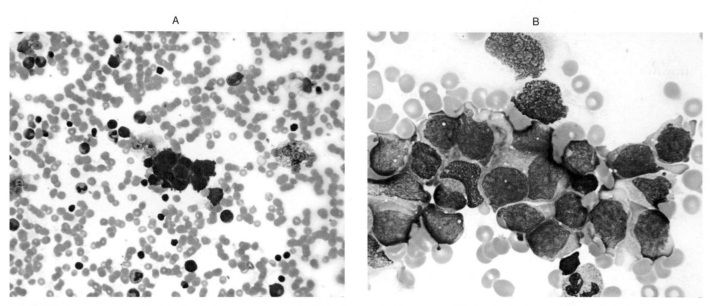

Fig. 15.24. Acute megakaryoblastic leukemia, bone marrow aspirate. (A) In this case, the blasts were strikingly cohesive both at diagnosis and relapse, a common feature in AMKL which can be confused for metastatic solid tumor. (B) High-power view of an aggregate of blasts. The blasts are large, with abundant cytoplasm; a binucleated form is present in the center of the field.

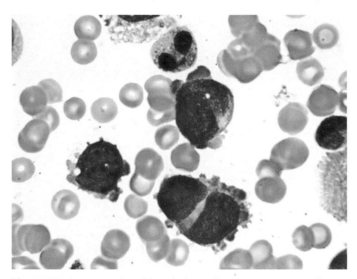

Fig. 15.25. Acute megakaryoblastic leukemia, bone marrow aspirate. The blasts in this case manifest more prominent cytoplasmic blebbing and binucleation. The latter is an uncommon cytologic feature in other types of acute leukemia.

can significantly impact on the sensitivity of CD61 immunohistochemistry. Therefore, flow cytometry is the preferred method for immunophenotyping, assuming blasts are present in peripheral blood or an adequate bone marrow aspirate is available.

Most cases of AMKL express one or more myeloid markers, including CD13, CD33 and CD11b. CD36 (thrombospondin receptor) is typically expressed at high levels in AMKL; however, this marker lacks lineage specificity since it is also expressed by monocytic and erythroid cells. Several megakaryocyte lineage-specific markers are readily detectable by flow cytometry. CD41 (platelet glycoprotein IIb/IIIa) and CD61 (glycoprotein IIIa) are early markers of the megakaryocytic lineage and are expressed in most pediatric AMKLs. CD42b (glycoprotein Ib) is expressed somewhat later in megakaryopoiesis and is less commonly positive in pediatric AMKL. The "aberrant" expression of cell-surface markers associated with other hematopoietic lineages is not infrequently observed in AMKL. For example, the T-cell markers CD7 and CD2 are frequently expressed in pediatric AMKL, and expression of CD4 and CD5 may be observed as well [263, 308, 309]. Another diagnostic pitfall is that CD45 (leukocyte common antigen) is not infrequently negative or only weakly expressed in AMKL, which could be misinterpreted by the unwary as evidence for a non-hematopoietic neoplasm. Together, these immunophenotypic properties of AMKL can be diagnostically challenging and may lead to an erroneous diagnosis, particularly when limited immunophenotyping is performed.

Our discussion of immunophenotyping is not complete without an important caveat regarding non-specific staining and its impact on the interpretation of flow cytometric studies of megakaryocyte antigen expression. All currently employed megakaryocytic markers are likewise expressed on mature platelets. As a result, adherence of platelets to the cell surfaces of an analyzed blast population can be a potential cause of spurious "positivity" for megakaryocyte markers [310]. This can be attributable to the intrinsic "stickiness" of the blasts or due to the manner in which the clinical sample is processed. In the latter instance, the analysis of other cell populations can often help to clarify whether there is a generalized problem with non-specific staining in a given specimen; inclusion of CD11b or CD14 in the same tube as the megakaryocyte marker can facilitate the identification and analysis of monocytes, which often manifest

A

B

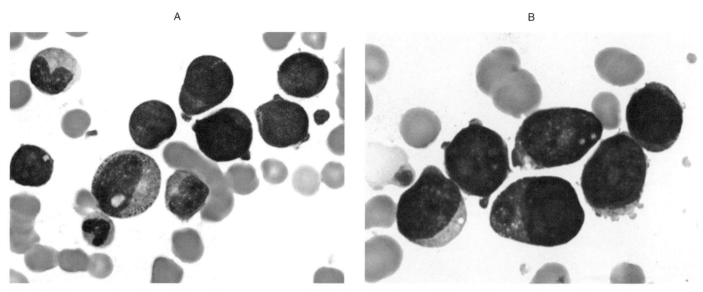

Fig. 15.26. Acute megakaryoblastic leukemia, bone marrow aspirate. (A) Small, poorly differentiated blasts predominate in this case of AMKL. (B) However, blasts with cytoplasmic blebs and projections were present as well, providing a subtle diagnostic clue.

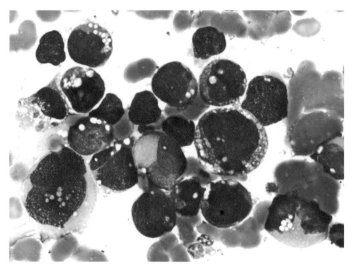

Fig. 15.27. Metastatic rhabdomyosarcoma, bone marrow aspirate. Metastatic rhabdomyosarcoma is variably cohesive and may contain cells with abundant cytoplasm and cytoplasm blebbing; these features can mimic those of AMKL or acute monocytic leukemia.

the most pronounced non-specific staining. Analysis of both the cell surface and cytoplasmic expression of a megakaryocytic marker can sometimes help to clarify matters, since bona fide megakaryocyte antigen expression should be detectable in both cytoplasmic and cell-surface analyses. When significant problems with non-specific staining are encountered, steps can be taken to assess and remedy the problem. First, platelet adhesion may be obviated in blood or bone marrow samples anticoagulated with EDTA [311]. Second, the clinical specimen can be processed so as to minimize the generation and adhesion of platelet fragments, for example, density gradient centrifugation of the specimen in lieu of whole-blood lysis.

Although not sufficient for diagnosis, cytochemical studies are of utility in some circumstances in the workup of AMKL.

Megakaryoblasts are negative for myeloperoxidase and Sudan black B. They are usually non-specific esterase positive, in contrast to ALL and AMLs lacking monocytic differentiation. When α-naphthyl-acetate is used as the esterase substrate, megakaryoblasts often manifest coarsely granular positivity in contrast to the diffuse cytoplasmic positivity characteristic of monoblasts and promonocytes (Fig. 15.30). In addition, megakaryoblasts are usually esterase negative when α-naphthyl-butyrate is used as the substrate, whereas monocytic cells are positive.

Cytogenetics and molecular diagnostics

Cytogenetic analysis is useful for confirming the presence of trisomy 21 in DS-associated megakaryoblastic disorders. In addition to trisomy 21, multiple numerical and structural chromosomal abnormalities are frequently detected in DS-AMKL [312–315]. In early small studies of TAM, constitutional trisomy 21 was identified as the sole abnormality [299]. However, it is now clear that additional numerical and structural chromosomal abnormalities may also be present in TAM [316–325]. Thus, distinction between TAM and DS-AMKL cannot be made on the basis of cytogenetic findings. Interestingly, however, the presence of additional cytogenetic changes in TAM may identify children at greater risk of progressing to AMKL [309]. Molecular monitoring of minimal residual disease in patients with DS-AMKL may not be practical given the heterogeneity of reported *GATA1* mutations, although a real-time RT-PCR assay has been described using mutation-specific primers [326]. Furthermore, in light of its excellent prognosis, the utility of minimal residual disease determination in guiding the clinical management of children with DS-AMKL is not well defined at this time.

In cases of t(1;22) AMKL, this translocation is present as the sole karyotypic abnormality finding in nearly 60% of cases [287]. Interestingly, the frequency of complex karyotypes

A

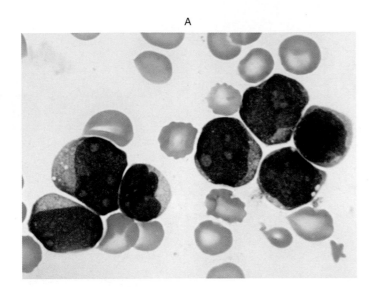

B

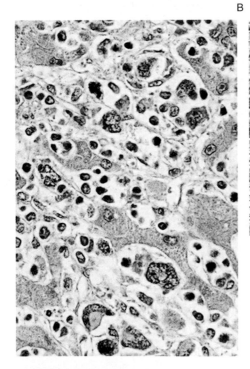
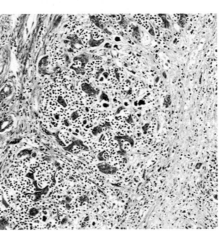

Fig. 15.28. Transient abnormal myelopoiesis of Down syndrome, peripheral blood smear and autopsy liver. This 32-week-gestation female infant was born with microcephaly, hepatosplenomegaly, and a markedly elevated WBC count comprised primarily of poorly differentiated blasts (A); however, she succumbed to hepatic failure and died at age 24 days. At autopsy, the liver contains a sinusoidal infiltrate of blasts and immature megakaryocytic elements (B, left panel) and marked fibrosis (B, right panel). (Photomicrographs kindly provided by Dr. Robert McKenna; ©2004 American Society for Clinical Pathology.)

increases with age, with approximately 80% of cases in children older than six months having complex karyotypes [287]. The *RBM15-MKL1* fusion transcript is readily detected by quantitative polymerase chain reaction (PCR) assays, and can be used to monitor minimal residual disease levels [327]. Although the t(1;22) is usually detectable by conventional cytogenetics, RT-PCR can also be useful in confirming expression of *RBM15-MKL1* in cases harboring complex or cryptic translocations targeting these loci [328, 329]. Because of the tight linkage between the t(1;22) and AMKL, *RBM15-MKL1* RT-PCR can be diagnostically useful in those instances where the availability of diagnostic clinical material is limiting. Finally, the rare occurrence in children with DS of AMKL containing the t(1;22) confirms

the importance of cytogenetic and molecular studies in all cases of AMKL [330].

AML with normal cytogenetics and mutation of nucleophosmin (NPM) [NPMc⁺ AML]

Definition

AMLs containing a normal karyotype by conventional cytogenetic analysis comprise approximately 25% of AMLs in children, and an even greater fraction of adult cases, and are typically categorized as intermediate risk in most stratification schemes employed for clinical studies. However, the lack of molecular markers to further subclassify this large

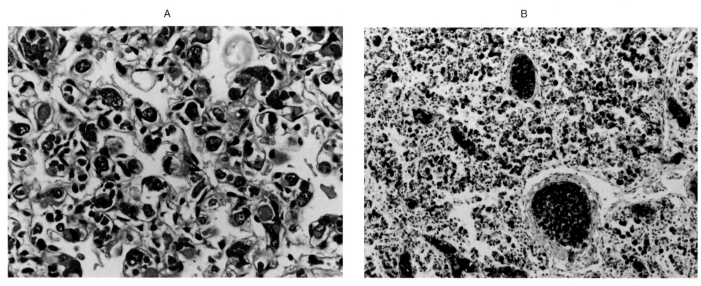

Fig. 15.29. Transient abnormal myelopoiesis of Down syndrome, fetopsy lung. This male fetus had intrauterine demise secondary to hydrops fetalis. (A) Microscopically, there is an infiltrate of immature megakaryocytic forms, including blasts, present intravascularly within the lung. (B) CD61 immunohistochemistry confirms the megakaryocytic differentiation of these cells. (Photomicrographs kindly provided by Dr. Bal Kampalath; ©2004 American Society for Clinical Pathology.)

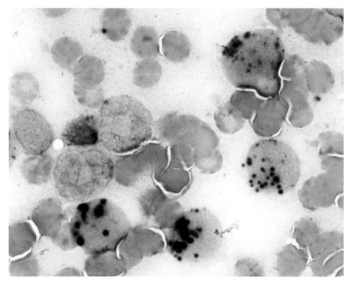

Fig. 15.30. Acute megakaryoblastic leukemia, bone marrow aspirate. Megakaryoblasts in AMKL are frequently positive cytochemically for α-naphthyl-acetate esterase. This characteristic punctate pattern of esterase positivity in megakaryoblasts aids in distinguishing them from monoblasts, which usually manifest diffuse cytoplasmic positivity.

and undoubtedly heterogeneous subset of AMLs has hindered more precise categorization and prognostication. Acute myeloid leukemia harboring mutations in *NPM1* was first identified by Falini and colleagues in 2005 [331]. These *NPM1* mutations are detected predominantly in *de novo* AMLs with normal karyotypes which lack any of the recurrent, leukemia-associated chromosomal translocations recognized elsewhere in the WHO classification.

Pathogenesis

NPM1 is located on chromosome 5q35 and is perhaps best known by virtue of its involvement in the t(2;5) translocation

characteristic of anaplastic large cell lymphoma [332]. NPM is a ubiquitously expressed, highly conserved phosphoprotein. NPM functions as a molecular chaperone and, as such, normally shuttles between the nucleus and cytoplasm; however, it is most abundant in the nucleolus. In its role as molecular chaperone, NPM prevents protein aggregation within the nucleolus and facilitates the transport of ribosomal components through the nuclear envelope. NPM also regulates centrosome duplication through cyclin E/cyclin-dependent kinase 2 phosphorylation and functions in p53-independent cell cycle regulation through its interaction with ARF (reviewed in Falini *et al.* [333]).

In adults, mutations of *NPM1* are detected in a high percentage of AML cases. Interestingly, *NPM1* mutations are almost entirely restricted to AMLs with normal karyotypes, with some 50–60% of such cases harboring mutations [331, 334]. Mutations in *NPM1* are distinctly uncommon in secondary AML [331]. Several different *NPM1* mutations have been identified. Duplication of a TCTG tetranucleotide located within exon 12, which results in a frameshift mutation, is the commonest mutation and is detected in 75% of cases. Regardless of the specific mutation, the end result is perturbation of the subcellular localization of mutant NPM due to the *de novo* formation of a nuclear export signal or ablation of the NPM nucleolar localization motif [333]. Because *NPM1* mutations are heterozygous, the mutant protein may also alter the cellular trafficking of residual wild-type NPM through the formation of mutant–wild-type NPM heterodimers. The relevant mechanism(s) by which mutant NPM contributes to leukemogenesis is currently unknown.

Clinical features and laboratory findings

NPMc⁺ AML is largely restricted to children greater than 10 years of age; this subtype of AML is distinctly uncommon in infants and toddlers [335, 336]. These observations are consistent with the reported age-related increase in *NPM1* mutations in adults. Children with NPMc⁺ AML typically present with leukocytosis, but otherwise have no distinctive peripheral blood findings [335, 336].

In comparison with adult AML, *NPM1* mutations are much less common in childhood AML, being detected in only 7% of cases, 30% of which also harbor *FLT3*-ITD mutations [335, 336]. Given the relative paucity of prognostic factors in AMLs with normal karyotype, it is significant that the presence of *NPM1* mutations has been demonstrated to have prognostic importance in at least a subset of patients. In the absence of a *FLT3*-ITD mutation, children with NPMc⁺ AML have a significantly better prognosis than those with AML lacking a *NPM1* mutation. Interestingly, the presence of *FLT3*-ITD appears to exert a dominant negative impact on prognosis, as children with AML containing the *FLT3*-ITD mutation have a poor prognosis irrespective of the presence of a *NPM1* mutation [335].

Pathologic features
Morphology
In adults, mutations in *NPM1* have been detected solely in AML and have not been demonstrated in lymphoblastic malignancies [331]. In adult AMLs, *NPM1* mutations occur in all FAB subtypes with the exception of APL; however, most NPMc⁺ cases manifest some degree of either myeloid or monocytic differentiation and, as such, are classified as either M2, M4, or M5 subtype [331, 334, 337]. Cases classified as AML M0, M6, or M7 collectively account for fewer than 5% of all NPMc⁺ AMLs. In the relatively few reported pediatric NPMc⁺ AML cases, 75% have had AML M2 or M4 morphology [336, 338]. Acute myeloid leukemias containing blasts with prominent nuclear invaginations, so-called "cuplike" nuclei, have been reported to contain *NPM1* mutations in 60% of cases [339]; however, the incidence in children of AMLs with this morphology has not been reported.

Immunophenotype
NPMc⁺ AMLs typically express myeloid antigens, including CD33, CD13, and CD15. In addition, this AML subtype is often negative or only weakly positive for several myeloid progenitor markers, including CD117, CD34, and CD133 [331, 337, 338, 340]. In adults, expression of monocytic markers is frequently detected, in concordance with the high frequency of myelomonocytic and monocytic differentiation. An immunophenotype diagnostic for NPMc⁺ AML has not been reported.

Cytogenetics and molecular diagnostics
As in adults, *NPM1* mutations are predominantly detected in pediatric AMLs with normal karyotypes; 75% of reported pediatric cases have had diploid karyotypes. In the 25% of pediatric NPMc⁺ AML cases with cytogenetic abnormalities, recurrent translocations recognized in the WHO classification [e.g., t(15;17), t(8;21), inv(16)] have not been identified. The

frequency of *FLT3*-ITD is significantly higher in AMLs containing *NPM1* mutations than in those lacking them [335, 336, 338]. By contrast, there is no significant difference in the mutation frequency of other genes, including *KIT*, *NRAS*, and *CEBPA*, in adult AMLs with and without mutated *NPM1* [337].

Robust RT-PCR assays to amplify exon 12 of *NPM1* have been described. Detection of mutations has either relied upon single-strand conformational polymorphism (SSCP) gel electrophoresis coupled with sequencing of presumptive positive samples, direct sequencing of RT-PCR products, or real-time PCR followed by melting curve analysis [331, 335, 337]. Acquisition of an *NPM1* mutation is believed to be an early oncogenic event in this AML subtype. As such, it should be a stable mutation that could serve as a potential target for minimal residual monitoring, which would be of utility in an AML subtype that lacks other "testable" molecular lesions. Indeed, recent studies have confirmed that *NPM1* mutations are stable, in contrast to mutations in *FLT3* [341]. Furthermore, detection of mutant *NPM1* using quantitative RT-PCR assays specific for the mutant allele is useful for monitoring minimal residual disease levels and appears to identify patients at increased risk for relapse [341, 342].

Acute myeloid leukemias lacking recurrent chromosomal or molecular lesions

Although the frequency of the genetic lesions discussed above is relatively high in pediatric AML, approximately one-half of cases lack the well-characterized, recurrent molecular lesions recognized in the WHO classification (Fig. 15.1). In these instances, classification depends on integration of the morphologic, immunophenotypic, and cytochemical findings. Classification is then made according to essentially the same subtypes recognized under the old FAB schema (Table 15.1). An important difference between the criteria of the WHO and FAB classifications for this group of AMLs is that the presence of 20% blasts is sufficient under the criteria of the former to render a diagnosis of AML, with the exception of acute monoblastic leukemia, where 80% or more of the cells must be either monoblasts or promonocytes. Images are included here to demonstrate the spectrum of morphology that may be encountered in acute monoblastic leukemias (Figs 15.31, 15.32 and 15.33) and also to highlight the morphology of acute erythroid leukemia, which is rarely encountered in the pediatric setting (Fig. 15.34).

Extramedullary myeloid proliferations
Definition
The extramedullary proliferation of leukemic myeloid cells can occur in association with virtually any type of AML, although it is most commonly seen in association with AMLs manifesting monocytic differentiation and certain translocation-associated AMLs. Myeloid sarcoma is defined as a mass-forming extramedullary proliferation of myeloblasts or immature

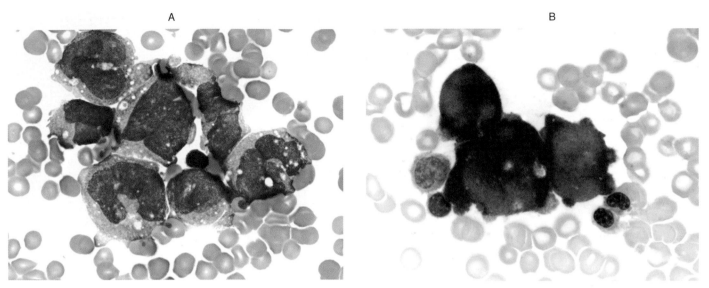

Fig. 15.31. Acute monocytic leukemia, bone marrow aspirate. (A) This distinctive case has unusually large leukemic cells, some of which are 75 μm or more in diameter. These cells are also somewhat cohesive. These cytologic features could lead to their misinterpretation as metastatic solid tumor, in particular metastatic rhabdomyosarcoma. (B) The malignant monocytes are intensely positive for α-naphthyl-butyrate esterase.

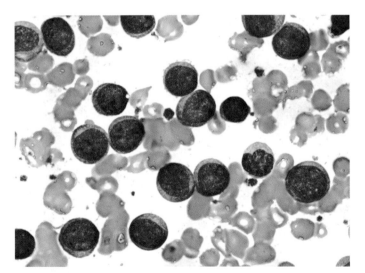

Fig. 15.32. Acute monoblastic leukemia, bone marrow aspirate. The monoblasts in this case manifest cytoplasmic blebbing, reminiscent of that seen in AMKL. Note that numerous cytoplasmic fragments are present in the background. When present in peripheral blood, automated hematologic analyzers may identify these cytoplasmic fragments as platelets, leading to a spuriously high platelet count. The serum lactate dehydrogenase level is often markedly elevated in such cases, as well.

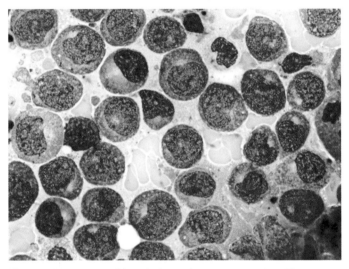

Fig. 15.33. Acute monoblastic leukemia, bone marrow aspirate. These monoblasts are relatively large with intensely basophilic cytoplasm. A rare blast with fine azurophilic granules is present (arrowhead).

myelomonocytic cells. Myeloid sarcoma may occur at any time during the disease course. It may be the presenting feature of AML or may herald its relapse, and in rare patients myeloid sarcoma develops in the absence of morphologically overt bone marrow involvement.

Clinical features and laboratory findings

Extramedullary myeloid proliferations (EMPs) occur frequently in children with AML, with a wide range of reported incidence (7–49%), which probably reflects varying definitions of EMP. Extramedullary myeloid proliferations most commonly manifest as a tumor mass (myeloid sarcoma), skin involvement (leukemia cutis), gingival infiltration, meningeal infiltration, or organ infiltration (primarily spleen or liver). Children with AML with monocytic differentiation (acute monoblastic leukemia and acute myelomonocytic leukemia) have a high incidence of gingival hypertrophy and leukemia cutis [343, 344]. Acute myeloid leukemia containing the t(8;21) is not infrequently associated with myeloid sarcoma [46, 48, 49]. When cutaneous involvement is excluded, the anatomic distribution of myeloid sarcoma in children is somewhat different

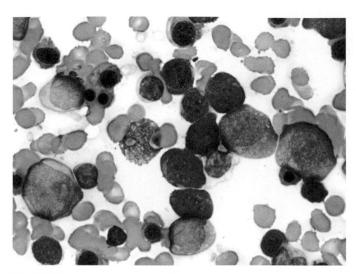

Fig. 15.34. Acute erythroid leukemia, bone marrow aspirate. Erythroid leukemia is quite rare in the pediatric setting. In this case, erythroid elements are increased in frequency and manifest megaloblastoid maturation, nuclear irregularities, and binucleation. Myeloblasts are also increased in frequency.

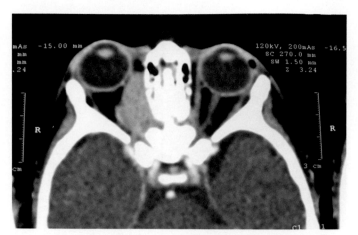

Fig. 15.35. CT scan of a child reveals a large retroorbital myeloid sarcoma. The periorbital region is a common anatomic site for myeloid sarcomas harboring the t(8;21). (Image kindly provided by Dr. Asma Quessar.)

than that seen in adults, with most cases occurring in the orbit and jaw, perhaps reflecting the proclivity of t(8;21)-associated myeloid sarcomas to develop at these anatomic sites (Fig. 15.35) [343, 345]. The prognostic significance of EMP in patients with AML is controversial; however, it is likely that the clinical outcome of children with EMP is most significantly influenced by the cytogenetics of the underlying AML, irrespective of the presence of a coexistent EMP [343].

Pathologic features

Morphology

In children, myeloid sarcomas most commonly manifest either varying degrees of myeloid maturation (designated as blastic, immature, or differentiated type), or are comprised of monoblasts and thus designated monoblastic sarcoma (Fig. 15.36). The more poorly differentiated tumors are comprised of sheets of intermediate to large blastic cells. In nodal-based myeloid sarcomas, the blasts can diffusely efface the nodal architecture or can present as a more subtle blastic infiltrate within the sinuses or paracortex. In extranodal sites of involvement, myeloid sarcoma may manifest a sheet-like growth pattern, and occasionally the blasts infiltrate surrounding tissue in a single-file fashion. Cytologically, the blasts are large with immature chromatin, usually prominent nucleoli, and variably abundant cytoplasm. Myeloid sarcoma can readily be mistaken for other types of hematolymphoid malignancy, most notably large cell lymphoma, and it is, in fact, notoriously prone to misdiagnosis, particularly when it is the initial manifestation of AML [346, 347]. In differentiating myeloid sarcomas, the presence of admixed maturing myeloid elements, such as myelocytes and metamyelocytes, provides an important clue to the

diagnosis. Other forms of myeloid sarcoma, such as those manifesting megakaryocytic or trilineage differentiation, are exceedingly rare in children.

Immunophenotype

The diagnosis of myeloid sarcoma requires immunophenotypic characterization of the neoplastic cells; this can be accomplished through either flow cytometry or immunohistochemistry, although the latter is more commonly used in this setting. Most myeloid sarcomas express the progenitor antigens CD117 and CD34, whereas monoblastic sarcomas are generally negative for these markers [346–348]. Expression of myeloperoxidase and CD68 is detected in most cases of myeloid sarcoma. Myelomonocytic or purely monoblastic sarcomas are usually positive for lysozyme as well. Negativity of myeloid sarcomas for T- and B-lineage markers helps to exclude large cell lymphoma from the differential diagnosis.

In addition to their ambiguous morphologic features, myeloid sarcomas have a few immunophenotypic properties that can lead to a misdiagnosis by the unwary pathologist. Therefore, a few caveats regarding the immunohistochemical characterization of myeloid sarcoma are in order. First, myeloid sarcomas may be negative or only weakly positive for CD45, which could lead to an erroneous diagnosis of a non-hematopoietic malignancy particularly when a limited immunohistochemical panel is performed. Second, a high proportion of myeloid sarcomas are strongly positive for CD43, a somewhat promiscuous T-cell lineage marker, which should not be misinterpreted as indicative of a T-cell malignancy in the absence of other supportive immunophenotypic findings [346, 348]. Third, myeloid sarcomas in adults, and presumably in children as well, can be positive for CD99, a marker characteristically expressed in Ewing sarcoma. Fourth, CD30 is rarely expressed in myeloid sarcomas; thus, strong CD30 expression favors other malignancies in the differential

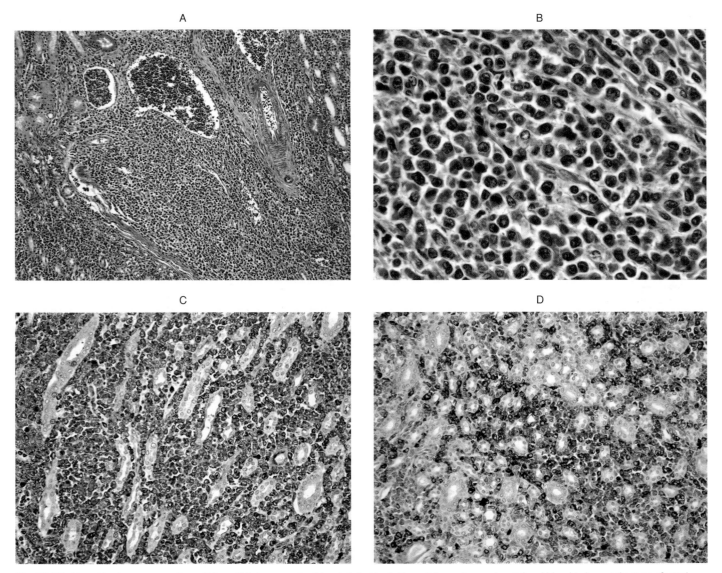

Fig. 15.36. Monoblastic sarcoma, autopsy kidney. This two-month-old male infant had skin nodules and normal peripheral blood indices at the time of initial presentation. Although the nodules spontaneously resolved three weeks later, the patient rapidly developed cytopenias, hepatosplenomegaly, and renal failure, and he died shortly thereafter. (A) Sections of kidney from post-mortem examination contain a diffuse infiltrate of large blasts obliterating the renal architecture. (B) The blasts have folded or reniform-shaped nuclei with relatively abundant cytoplasm; frequent mitotic figures are present. The blasts are diffusely, strongly positive for lysozyme (C), and a subset are positive for myeloperoxidase (D). (Photomicrographs kindly provided by Dr. Mihaela Onciu.)

diagnosis of myeloid sarcoma, such as anaplastic large cell lymphoma [346, 347]. Finally, myeloid sarcomas containing the t(8;21) can express certain B-cell markers such as PAX-5 and CD79a [349–351].

Cytogenetics and molecular diagnostics

Cytogenetics, FISH, or molecular analyses can be of great utility in confirming the diagnosis, particularly when the myeloid sarcoma harbors a recurrent leukemia-associated translocation. Although FISH can theoretically be performed on paraffin-embedded tissue, most assays are optimized for unfixed cytologic preparations; therefore, the preparation of extra touch imprints from the fresh specimen may prove

helpful in the diagnostic workup when myeloid sarcoma is suspected.

Acknowledgements

I acknowledge Ms. Tina Motroni (St. Jude Children's Research Hospital, Memphis, TN) for much assistance with preparation of the photomicrographs, and Drs. David Head (Vanderbilt University, Nashville, TN), Bal Kampalath (deceased; formerly of the Medical College of Wisconsin, Milwaukee, WI), Mihaela Onciu (St. Jude Children's Research Hospital), Asma Quessar (Hôpital du 20 Août, Casablanca, Morocco), and Robert McKenna (University of Minnesota, Minneapolis, MN) for contributing images.

References

1. **Bennett JM, Catovsky D, Daniel MT,** *et al.* Proposals for the classification of the acute leukemias. *British Journal of Haematology.* 1976;**33**:451.

2. **Bennett JM, Catovsky D, Daniel MT,** *et al.* Criteria for the diagnosis of acute leukemia of megakaryocyte lineage (M7). A report of the French-American-British Cooperative Group. *Annals of Internal Medicine.* 1985;**103**: 460–462.

3. **Bennett JM, Catovsky D, Daniel MT,** *et al.* Proposed revised criteria for the classification of acute myeloid leukemia. A report of the French-American-British Cooperative Group. *Annals of Internal Medicine.* 1985;**103**: 620.

4. **Bennett JM, Catovsky D, Daniel MT,** *et al.* Proposal for the recognition of minimally differentiated acute myeloid leukemia (AML-MO). *British Journal of Haematology.* 1991;**78**:325.

5. **Raimondi SC, Chang MN, Ravindranath Y,** *et al.* Chromosomal abnormalities in 478 children with acute myeloid leukemia: clinical characteristics and treatment outcome in a cooperative pediatric oncology group study-POG 8821. *Blood.* 1999; **94**:3707–3716.

6. **Gibson BE, Wheatley K, Hann IM,** *et al.* Treatment strategy and long-term results in paediatric patients treated in consecutive UK AML trials. *Leukemia.* 2005;**19**:2130–2138.

7. **Lange BJ, Smith FO, Feusner J,** *et al.* Outcomes in CCG-2961, a Children's Oncology Group phase 3 trial for untreated pediatric acute myeloid leukemia (AML): a report from the Children's Oncology Group. *Blood.* 2008;**111**:1044–1053.

8. **Jaffe ES, Harris RI, Stein H, Vardiman JW.** *World Health Organization Classification of Tumours: Pathology and Genetics of Tumours of Haematopoietic and Lymphoid Tissues.* Lyon: IARC Press; 2001.

9. **Swerdlow SH, Campo E, Harris NL,** *et al.* (eds.). *WHO Classification of Tumours of Haematopoietic and Lymphoid Tissues* (4th edn.). Lyon: IARC Press; 2008.

10. **Erickson P, Gao J, Chang KS,** *et al.* Identification of breakpoints in t(8;21) acute myelogenous leukemia and isolation of a fusion transcript, AML1/ETO, with similarity to *Drosophila* segmentation gene, runt. *Blood.* 1992;**80**:1825–1831.

11. **Nisson PE, Watkins PC, Sacchi N.** Transcriptionally active chimeric gene derived from the fusion of the AML1 gene and a novel gene on chromosome 8 in t(8;21) leukemic cells. *Cancer Genetics and Cytogenetics.* 1992;**63**: 81–88. Erratum in *Cancer Genetics and Cytogenetics.* 1993;**66**:81.

12. **Miyoshi H, Kozu T, Shimizu K,** *et al.* The t(8;21) translocation in acute myeloid leukemia results in production of an AML1-MTG8 fusion transcript. *The EMBO Journal.* 1993;**12**:2715–2721.

13. **Liu P, Tarle SA, Hajra A,** *et al.* Fusion between transcription factor CBF beta/PEBP2 beta and a myosin heavy chain in acute myeloid leukemia. *Science.* 1993;**261**:1041–1044.

14. **Rowley JD.** Identification of a translocation with quinacrine fluorescence in a patient with acute leukemia. *Annales de Génétique.* 1973;**16**:109–112.

15. **Osato M, Asou N, Abdalla E,** *et al.* Biallelic and heterozygous point mutations in the runt domain of the AML1/PEBP2alphaB gene associated with myeloblastic leukemias. *Blood.* 1999;**93**:1817–1824.

16. **Preudhomme C, Warot-Loze D, Roumier C,** *et al.* High incidence of biallelic point mutations in the Runt domain of the AML1/PEBP2 alpha B gene in Mo acute myeloid leukemia and in myeloid malignancies with acquired trisomy 21. *Blood.* 2000;**96**:2862–2869.

17. **Mikhail FM, Serry KA, Hatem N,** *et al.* AML1 gene over-expression in childhood acute lymphoblastic leukemia. *Leukemia.* 2002;**16**:658–668.

18. **Harewood L, Robinson H, Harris R,** *et al.* Amplification of AML1 on a duplicated chromosome 21 in acute lymphoblastic leukemia: a study of 20 cases. *Leukemia.* 2003;**17**:547–553.

19. **Zelent A, Greaves M, Enver T.** Role of the TEL-AML1 fusion gene in the molecular pathogenesis of childhood acute lymphoblastic leukaemia. *Oncogene.* 2004;**23**:4275–4283.

20. **Lorsbach RB, Downing JR.** The role of the AML1 transcription factor in leukemogenesis. *International Journal of Hematology.* 2001;**74**:258–265.

21. **Okuda T, van Deursen J, Hiebert SW, Grosveld G, Downing JR.** AML1, the target of multiple chromosomal translocations in human leukemia, is essential for normal fetal liver hematopoiesis. *Cell.* 1996;**84**:321–330.

22. **Wang Q, Stacy T, Binder M,** *et al.* Disruption of the Cbfa2 gene causes necrosis and hemorrhaging in the central nervous system and blocks definitive hematopoiesis. *Proceedings of the National Academy of Sciences of the United States of America.* 1996;**93**:3444–3449.

23. **Wang Q, Stacy T, Miller JD,** *et al.* The CBFbeta subunit is essential for CBFalpha2 (AML1) function in vivo. *Cell.* 1996;**87**:697–708.

24. **Sasaki K, Yagi H, Bronson RT,** *et al.* Absence of fetal liver hematopoiesis in mice deficient in transcriptional coactivator core binding factor beta. *Proceedings of the National Academy of Sciences of the United States of America.* 1996;**93**:12359–12363.

25. **North T, Gu TL, Stacy T,** *et al.* Cbfa2 is required for the formation of intra-aortic hematopoietic clusters. *Development.* 1999;**126**:2563–2575.

26. **Lorsbach RB, Moore J, Ang SO,** *et al.* Role of RUNX1 in adult hematopoiesis: analysis of RUNX1-IRES-GFP knock-in mice reveals differential lineage expression. *Blood.* 2004;**103**:2522–2529.

27. **Growney JD, Shigematsu H, Li Z,** *et al.* Loss of Runx1 perturbs adult hematopoiesis and is associated with a myeloproliferative phenotype. *Blood.* 2005;**106**:494–504.

28. **Taniuchi I, Osato M, Egawa T,** *et al.* Differential requirements for runx proteins in CD4 repression and epigenetic silencing during T lymphocyte development. *Cell.* 2002; **111**:621–633.

29. **Miyoshi H, Shimizu K, Kozu T,** *et al.* t(8;21) breakpoints on chromosome 21 in acute myeloid leukemia are clustered within a limited region of a single gene, AML1. *Proceedings of the National Academy of Sciences of the United States of America.* 1991;**88**:10431–10434.

30. **Calabi F, Pannell R, Pavloska G.** Gene targeting reveals a crucial role for MTG8 in the gut. *Molecular and Cellular Biology.* 2001;**21**:5658–5666.

31. **Wolford JK, Prochazka M.** Structure and expression of the human MTG8/ETO gene. *Gene.* 1998;**212**: 103–109.

32. **Rochford JJ, Semple RK, Laudes M,** *et al.* ETO/MTG8 is an inhibitor of C/EBPbeta activity and a regulator of early adipogenesis. *Molecular and Cellular Biology.* 2004;**24**:9863–9872.

33. **Frank R, Zhang J, Uchida H,** *et al.* The AML1/ETO fusion protein blocks transactivation of the GM-CSF promoter by AML1B. *Oncogene.* 1995;**11**:2667–2674.

34. **Rhoades KL, Hetherington CJ, Rowley JD,** *et al.* Synergistic up-regulation of the myeloid-specific promoter for the macrophage colony-stimulating factor receptor by AML1 and the t(8;21) fusion protein may contribute to leukemogenesis. *Proceedings of the National Academy of Sciences of the United States of America.* 1996;**93**:11895–11900.

35. **Westendorf JJ, Yamamoto CM, Lenny N,** *et al.* The t(8;21) fusion product, AML-1-ETO, associates with C/EBP-alpha, inhibits C/EBP-alpha-dependent transcription, and blocks granulocytic differentiation. *Molecular and Cellular Biology.* 1998;**18**:322–333.

36. **Lutterbach B, Sun D, Schuetz J, Hiebert SW.** The MYND motif is required for repression of basal transcription from the multidrug resistance 1 promoter by the t(8;21) fusion protein. *Molecular and Cellular Biology.* 1998;**18**:3604–3611.

37. **Lenny N, Meyers S, Hiebert SW.** Functional domains of the t(8;21) fusion protein, AML-1/ETO. *Oncogene.* 1995;**11**:1761–1769.

38. **Wang J, Hoshino T, Redner RL, Kajigaya S, Liu JM.** ETO, fusion partner in t(8;21) acute myeloid leukemia, represses transcription by interaction with the human N-CoR/mSin3/HDAC1 complex. *Proceedings of the National Academy of Sciences of the United States of America.* 1998;**95**:10860–10865.

39. **Rhoades KL, Hetherington CJ, Harakawa N,** *et al.* Analysis of the role of AML1-ETO in leukemogenesis, using an inducible transgenic mouse model. *Blood.* 2000;**96**:2108–2115.

40. **Yuan Y, Zhou L, Miyamoto T,** *et al.* AML1-ETO expression is directly involved in the development of acute myeloid leukemia in the presence of additional mutations. *Proceedings of the National Academy of Sciences of the United States of America.* 2001;**98**:10398–10403.

41. **Higuchi M, O'Brien D, Kumaravelu P,** *et al.* Expression of a conditional AML1-ETO oncogene bypasses embryonic lethality and establishes a murine model of human t(8;21) acute myeloid leukemia. *Cancer Cell.* 2002;**1**:63–74.

42. **Peterson LF, Boyapati A, Ahn EY,** *et al.* Acute myeloid leukemia with the 8q22;21q22 translocation: secondary mutational events and alternative t(8;21) transcripts. *Blood.* 2007;**110**:799–805.

43. **Schessl C, Rawat VP, Cusan M,** *et al.* The AML1-ETO fusion gene and the FLT3 length mutation collaborate in inducing acute leukemia in mice. *The Journal of Clinical Investigation.* 2005;**115**:2159–2168.

44. **Schnittger S, Kohl TM, Haferlach T,** *et al.* KIT-D816 mutations in AML1-ETO-positive AML are associated with impaired event-free and overall survival. *Blood.* 2006;**107**:1791–1799.

45. **Frenkel MA, Tupitsyn NN, Protasova AK,** *et al.* Blast cells in child and adult AML: comparative study of morphocytochemical, immunological and cytogenetic characteristics. *British Journal of Haematology.* 1994;**87**:708–714.

46. **Felice MS, Zubizarreta PA, Alfaro EM,** *et al.* Good outcome of children with acute myeloid leukemia and t(8;21)(q22;q22), even when associated with granulocytic sarcoma: a report from a single institution in Argentina. *Cancer.* 2000;**88**:1939–1944.

47. **Rubnitz JE, Raimondi SC, Halbert AR,** *et al.* Characteristics and outcome of t(8;21)-positive childhood acute myeloid leukemia: a single institution's experience. *Leukemia.* 2002;**16**:2072–2077.

48. **Wodzinski MA, Collin R, Winfield DA, Dalton A, Lawrence AC.** Epidural granulocytic sarcoma in acute myeloid leukemia with 8;21 translocation. *Cancer.* 1988;**62**:1299–1300.

49. **Tallman MS, Hakimian D, Shaw JM,** *et al.* Granulocytic sarcoma is associated with the 8;21 translocation in acute myeloid leukemia. *Journal of Clinical Oncology.* 1993;**11**:690–697.

50. **Cox-Froncillo MC, Genuardi M, Bajer J,** *et al.* First report of t(8;21)(q22;q22) in a case of de novo acute monoblastic leukemia. *Cancer Genetics and Cytogenetics.* 1995;**79**:82–85.

51. **Molero MT, Gomez Casares MT, Valencia JM,** *et al.* Detection of a t(8;21)(q22;q22) in a case of M5 acute monoblastic leukemia. *Cancer Genetics and Cytogenetics.* 1998;**100**:176–178.

52. **Berger R, Bernheim A, Daniel MT,** *et al.* Cytologic characterization and significance of normal karyotypes in t(8;21) acute myeloblastic leukemia. *Blood.* 1982;**59**:171–178.

53. **Swirsky DM, Li YS, Matthews JG,** *et al.* 8;21 translocation in acute granulocytic leukaemia: cytological, cytochemical and clinical features. *British Journal of Haematology.* 1984;**56**:199–213.

54. **Haferlach T, Bennett JM, Loffler H,** *et al.* Acute myeloid leukemia with translocation (8;21). Cytomorphology, dysplasia and prognostic factors in 41 cases. AML Cooperative Group and ECOG. *Leukemia & Lymphoma.* 1996;**23**:227–234.

55. **Nakamura H, Kuriyama K, Sadamori N,** *et al.* Morphological subtyping of acute myeloid leukemia with maturation (AML-M2): homogeneous pink-colored cytoplasm of mature neutrophils is most characteristic of AML-M2 with t(8;21). *Leukemia.* 1997;**11**:651–655.

56. **Horny HP, Sotlar K, Valent P.** Mastocytosis: state of the art. *Pathobiology.* 2007;**74**:121–132.

57. **Pullarkat VA, Bueso-Ramos C, Lai R,** *et al.* Systemic mastocytosis with associated clonal hematological non-mast-cell lineage disease: analysis of clinicopathologic features and activating c-kit mutations. *American Journal of Hematology.* 2003;**73**:12–17.

58. **Pullarkat V, Bedell V, Kim Y,** *et al.* Neoplastic mast cells in systemic mastocytosis associated with t(8;21) acute myeloid leukemia are derived from the leukemic clone. *Leukemia Research.* 2007;**31**:261–265.

59. **Nagai S, Ichikawa M, Takahashi T,** *et al.* The origin of neoplastic mast cells in systemic mastocytosis with AML1/ETO-positive acute myeloid leukemia. *Experimental Hematology.* 2007;**35**:1747–1752.

60. **Sperr WR, Escribano L, Jordan JH,** *et al.* Morphologic properties of neoplastic mast cells: delineation of stages of maturation and implication

for cytological grading of mastocytosis. *Leukemia Research*. 2001;**25**:529–536.

61. **Hurwitz CA, Raimondi SC, Head D**, *et al*. Distinctive immunophenotypic features of t(8;21)(q22;q22) acute myeloblastic leukemia in children. *Blood*. 1992;**80**:3182–3188.

62. **Kita K, Nakase K, Miwa H**, *et al*. Phenotypical characteristics of acute myelocytic leukemia associated with the t(8;21)(q22;q22) chromosomal abnormality: frequent expression of immature B-cell antigen CD19 together with stem cell antigen CD34. *Blood*. 1992;**80**:470–477.

63. **Baer MR, Stewart CC, Lawrence D**, *et al*. Expression of the neural cell adhesion molecule CD56 is associated with short remission duration and survival in acute myeloid leukemia with t(8;21)(q22;q22). *Blood*. 1997;**90**:1643–1648.

64. **Yang DH, Lee JJ, Mun YC**, *et al*. Predictable prognostic factor of CD56 expression in patients with acute myeloid leukemia with t(8;21) after high dose cytarabine or allogeneic hematopoietic stem cell transplantation. *American Journal of Hematology*. 2007;**82**:1–5.

65. **Baer R**. TAL1, TAL2 and LYL1: a family of basic helix-loop-helix proteins implicated in T cell acute leukaemia. *Seminars in Cancer Biology*. 1993;**4**:341–347.

66. **Rege K, Swansbury GJ, Atra AA**, *et al*. Disease features in acute myeloid leukemia with t(8;21)(q22;q22). Influence of age, secondary karyotype abnormalities, CD19 status, and extramedullary leukemia on survival. *Leukemia & Lymphoma*. 2000;**40**:67–77.

67. **Nishii K, Usui E, Katayama N**, *et al*. Characteristics of t(8;21) acute myeloid leukemia (AML) with additional chromosomal abnormality: concomitant trisomy 4 may constitute a distinctive subtype of t(8;21) AML. *Leukemia*. 2003;**17**:731–737.

68. **Downing JR, Margolis BL, Zilberstein A**, *et al*. Phospholipase C-gamma, a substrate for PDGF receptor kinase, is not phosphorylated on tyrosine during the mitogenic response to CSF-1. *The EMBO Journal*. 1989;**8**:3345–3350.

69. **Fujimaki S, Funato T, Harigae H**, *et al*. A quantitative reverse transcriptase polymerase chain reaction method for the detection of leukaemic cells with t(8;21) in peripheral blood. *European Journal of Haematology*. 2000;**64**:252–258.

70. **Marcucci G, Livak KJ, Bi W**, *et al*. Detection of minimal residual disease in patients with AML1/ETO-associated acute myeloid leukemia using a novel quantitative reverse transcription polymerase chain reaction assay. *Leukemia*. 1998;**12**:1482–1489.

71. **Mrozek K, Prior TW, Edwards C**, *et al*. Comparison of cytogenetic and molecular genetic detection of t(8;21) and inv(16) in a prospective series of adults with de novo acute myeloid leukemia: a Cancer and Leukemia Group B Study. *Journal of Clinical Oncology*. 2001;**19**:2482–2492.

72. **Kusec R, Laczika K, Knobl P**, *et al*. AML1/ETO fusion mRNA can be detected in remission blood samples of all patients with t(8;21) acute myeloid leukemia after chemotherapy or autologous bone marrow transplantation. *Leukemia*. 1994;**8**:735–739.

73. **Krauter J, Gorlich K, Ottmann O**, *et al*. Prognostic value of minimal residual disease quantification by real-time reverse transcriptase polymerase chain reaction in patients with core binding factor leukemias. *Journal of Clinical Oncology*. 2003;**21**:4413–4422.

74. **Leroy H, De Botton S, Grardel-Duflos N**, *et al*. Prognostic value of real-time quantitative PCR (RQ-PCR) in AML with t(8;21). *Leukemia*. 2005;**19**:367–372.

75. **Yoo SJ, Chi HS, Jang S**, *et al*. Quantification of AML1-ETO fusion transcript as a prognostic indicator in acute myeloid leukemia. *Haematologica*. 2005;**90**:1493–1501.

76. **Stentoft J, Hokland P, Ostergaard M, Hasle H, Nyvold CG**. Minimal residual core binding factor AMLs by real time quantitative PCR – initial response to chemotherapy predicts event free survival and close monitoring of peripheral blood unravels the kinetics of relapse. *Leukemia Research*. 2006;**30**:389–395.

77. **Raimondi SC, Kalwinsky DK, Hayashi Y**, *et al*. Cytogenetics of childhood acute nonlymphocytic leukemia. *Cancer Genetics and Cytogenetics*. 1989;**40**:13–27.

78. **Arthur DC, Bloomfield CD**. Partial deletion of the long arm of chromosome 16 and bone marrow eosinophilia in acute nonlymphocytic leukemia, a new association. *Blood*. 1983;**61**:994–998.

79. **Le Beau MM, Larson RA, Bitter MA**, *et al*. Association of an inversion of chromosome 16 with abnormal marrow eosinophils in acute myelomonocytic leukemia: a unique cytogenetic-clinical pathological association. *The New England Journal of Medicine*. 1983;**309**:630–636.

80. **Wang S, Wang Q, Crute BE**, *et al*. Cloning and characterization of subunits of the T-cell receptor and murine leukemia virus enhancer core-binding factor. *Molecular and Cellular Biology*. 1993;**13**:3324–3339.

81. **Ogawa E, Inuzuka M, Maruyama M**, *et al*. Molecular cloning and characterization of PEBP2 beta, the heterodimeric partner of a novel *Drosophila* runt-related DNA binding protein PEBP2 alpha. *Virology*. 1993;**194**:314–331.

82. **Huang G, Shigesada K, Ito K**, *et al*. Dimerization with PEBP2beta protects RUNX1/AML1 from ubiquitin – proteasome-mediated degradation. *The EMBO Journal*. 2001;**20**:723–733.

83. **Tanaka Y, Watanabe T, Chiba N**, *et al*. The protooncogene product, PEBP2beta/CBFbeta, is mainly located in the cytoplasm and has an affinity with cytoskeletal structures. *Oncogene*. 1997;**15**:677–683.

84. **Lu J, Maruyama M, Satake M**, *et al*. Subcellular localization of the alpha and beta subunits of the acute myeloid leukemia-linked transcription factor PEBP2/CBF. *Molecular and Cellular Biology*. 1995;**15**:1651–1661.

85. **Chiba N, Watanabe T, Nomura S**, *et al*. Differentiation dependent expression and distinct subcellular localization of the protooncogene product, PEBP2beta/CBFbeta, in muscle development. *Oncogene*. 1997;**14**:2543–2552.

86. **Zhu L, Vranckx R, Khau Van Kien P**, *et al*. Mutations in myosin heavy chain 11 cause a syndrome associating thoracic aortic aneurysm/aortic dissection and patent ductus arteriosus. *Nature Genetics*. 2006;**38**:343–349.

87. **Hajra A, Liu PP, Wang Q**, *et al*. The leukemic core binding factor b-smooth muscle myosin heavy chain (CBFb-SMMHC) chimeric protein requires

both CBFb and myosin heavy chain domains for transformation of NIH 3T3 cells. *Proceedings of the National Academy of Sciences of the United States of America*. 1995;**92**:1926–1930.

88. **Shurtleff SA, Meyers S, Hiebert SW,** *et al.* Heterogeneity in CBF beta/MYH11 fusion messages encoded by the inv(16)(p13q22) and the t(16;16)(p13;q22) in acute myelogenous leukemia. *Blood*. 1995;**85**:3695–3703.

89. **Viswanatha DS, Chen I, Liu PP,** *et al.* Characterization and use of an antibody detecting the CBFbeta-SMMHC fusion protein in inv(16)/t(16;16)-associated acute myeloid leukemias. *Blood*. 1998;**91**:1882–1890.

90. **Adya N, Stacy T, Speck NA, Liu PP.** The leukemic protein core binding factor b (CBFb)-smooth-muscle myosin heavy chain sequesters CBFa2 into cytoskeletal filaments and aggregates. *Molecular and Cellular Biology*. 1998;**18**:7432–7443.

91. **Kanno Y, Kanno T, Sakakura C, Bae SC, Ito Y.** Cytoplasmic sequestration of the polyomavirus enhancer binding protein 2 (PEBP2)/core binding factor a (CBFa) subunit by the leukemia-related PEBP2/CBFb-SMMHC fusion protein inhibits PEBP2/CBF-mediated transactivation. *Molecular and Cellular Biology*. 1998;**18**:4252–4261.

92. **Lutterbach B, Hou Y, Durst KL, Hiebert SW.** The inv(16) encodes an acute myeloid leukemia 1 transcriptional corepressor. *Proceedings of the National Academy of Sciences of the United States of America*. 1999;**96**:12822–12827.

93. **Durst KL, Lutterbach B, Kummalue T, Friedman AD, Hiebert SW.** The inv(16) fusion protein associates with corepressors via a smooth muscle myosin heavy-chain domain. *Molecular and Cellular Biology*. 2003;**23**:607–619.

94. **Lukasik SM, Zhang L, Corpora T,** *et al.* Altered affinity of CBF beta-SMMHC for Runx1 explains its role in leukemogenesis. *Nature Structural Biology*. 2002;**9**:674–679.

95. **Castilla LH, Wijmenga C, Wang Q,** *et al.* Failure of embryonic hematopoiesis and lethal hemorrhages in mouse embryos heterozygous for a knocked-in leukemia gene CBFB-MYH11. *Cell*. 1996;**87**:687–696.

96. **Castilla LH, Garrett L, Adya N,** *et al.* The fusion gene cbfb-MYH11 blocks myeloid differentiation and predisposes mice to acute myelomonocytic leukaemia. *Nature Genetics*. 1999;**23**:144–146.

97. **Kundu M, Liu PP.** Function of the inv(16) fusion gene CBFB-MYH11. *Current Opinion in Hematology*. 2001;**8**:201–205.

98. **Razzouk BI, Raimondi SC, Srivastava DK,** *et al.* Impact of treatment on the outcome of acute myeloid leukemia with inversion 16: a single institution's experience. *Leukemia*. 2001;**15**:1326–1330.

99. **Forestier E, Schmiegelow K.** The incidence peaks of the childhood acute leukemias reflect specific cytogenetic aberrations. *Journal of Pediatric Hematology/Oncology*. 2006;**28**:486–495.

100. **Costello R, Sainty D, Lecine P,** *et al.* Detection of CBFbeta/MYH11 fusion transcripts in acute myeloid leukemia: heterogeneity of cytological and molecular characteristics. *Leukemia*. 1997;**11**:644–650.

101. **Delaunay J, Vey N, Leblanc T,** *et al.* Prognosis of inv(16)/t(16;16) acute myeloid leukemia (AML): a survey of 110 cases from the French AML Intergroup. *Blood*. 2003;**102**:462–469.

102. **Larson RA, Williams SF, Le Beau MM,** *et al.* Acute myelomonocytic leukemia with abnormal eosinophils and inv(16) or t(16;16) has a favorable prognosis. *Blood*. 1986;**68**:1242–1249.

103. **Sun X, Zhang W, Ramdas L,** *et al.* Comparative analysis of genes regulated in acute myelomonocytic leukemia with and without inv(16)(p13q22) using microarray techniques, real-time PCR, immunohistochemistry, and flow cytometry immunophenotyping. *Modern Pathology*. 2007;**20**:811–820.

104. **Adriaansen HJ, te Boekhorst PA, Hagemeijer AM,** *et al.* Acute myeloid leukemia M4 with bone marrow eosinophilia (M4Eo) and inv(16)(p13q22) exhibits a specific immunophenotype with CD2 expression. *Blood*. 1993;**81**:3043–3051.

105. **Khalidi HS, Medeiros LJ, Chang KL,** *et al.* The immunophenotype of adult acute myeloid leukemia: high frequency of lymphoid antigen expression and comparison of immunophenotype, French-American-British classification,

and karyotypic abnormalities. *American Journal of Clinical Pathology*. 1998;**109**:211–220.

106. **Rowe D, Cotterill SJ, Ross FM,** *et al.* Cytogenetically cryptic AML1-ETO and CBF beta-MYH11 gene rearrangements: incidence in 412 cases of acute myeloid leukaemia. *British Journal of Haematology*. 2000;**111**:1051–1056.

107. **O'Reilly J, Chipper L, Springall F, Herrmann R.** A unique structural abnormality of chromosome 16 resulting in a CBF beta-MYH11 fusion transcript in a patient with acute myeloid leukemia, FAB M4. *Cancer Genetics and Cytogenetics*. 2000;**121**:52–55.

108. **Li S, Couzi RJ, Thomas GH, Friedman AD, Borowitz MJ.** A novel variant three-way translocation of inversion 16 in a case of AML-M4eo following low dose methotrexate therapy. *Cancer Genetics and Cytogenetics*. 2001;**125**:74–77.

109. **Merchant SH, Haines S, Hall B, Hozier J, Viswanatha DS.** Fluorescence in situ hybridization identifies cryptic t(16;16)(p13;q22) masked by del(16)(q22) in a case of AML-M4 Eo. *The Journal of Molecular Diagnostics*. 2004;**6**:271–274.

110. **Guerrasio A, Pilatrino C, De Micheli D,** *et al.* Assessment of minimal residual disease (MRD) in CBFbeta/MYH11-positive acute myeloid leukemias by qualitative and quantitative RT-PCR amplification of fusion transcripts. *Leukemia*. 2002;**16**:1176–1181.

111. **Buonamici S, Ottaviani E, Testoni N,** *et al.* Real-time quantitation of minimal residual disease in inv(16)-positive acute myeloid leukemia may indicate risk for clinical relapse and may identify patients in a curable state. *Blood*. 2002;**99**:443–449.

112. **Rowley JD, Golomb HM, Dougherty C.** 15/17 translocation, a consistent chromosomal change in acute promyelocytic leukaemia. *Lancet*. 1977;**1**:549–550.

113. **Borrow J, Goddard AD, Sheer D, Solomon E.** Molecular analysis of acute promyelocytic leukemia breakpoint cluster region on chromosome 17. *Science*. 1990;**249**:1577–1580.

114. **de Thé H, Chomienne C, Lanotte M, Degos L, Dejean A.** The t(15;17)

translocation of acute promyelocytic leukaemia fuses the retinoic acid receptor alpha gene to a novel transcribed locus. *Nature*. 1990;**347**: 558–561.

115. **Alcalay M, Zangrilli D, Pandolfi PP,** *et al.* Translocation breakpoint of acute promyelocytic leukemia lies within the retinoic acid receptor alpha locus. *Proceedings of the National Academy of Sciences of the United States of America.* 1991;**88**:1977–1981.

116. **He LZ, Bhaumik M, Tribioli C,** *et al.* Two critical hits for promyelocytic leukemia. *Molecular Cell.* 2000;**6**:1131–1141.

117. **Collins SJ.** The role of retinoids and retinoic acid receptors in normal hematopoiesis. *Leukemia.* 2002;**16**: 1896–1905.

118. **Oren T, Sher JA, Evans T.** Hematopoiesis and retinoids: development and disease. *Leukemia & Lymphoma* 2003;**44**:1881–1891.

119. **Chambon P.** A decade of molecular biology of retinoic acid receptors. *The FASEB Journal.* 1996;**10**:940–954.

120. **Leid M, Kastner P, Lyons R,** *et al.* Purification, cloning, and RXR identity of the HeLa cell factor with which RAR or TR heterodimerizes to bind target sequences efficiently. *Cell.* 1992;**68**:377–395.

121. **Horlein AJ, Naar AM, Heinzel T,** *et al.* Ligand-independent repression by the thyroid hormone receptor mediated by a nuclear receptor co-repressor. *Nature.* 1995;**377**:397–404.

122. **Kurokawa R, Soderstrom M, Horlein A,** *et al.* Polarity-specific activities of retinoic acid receptors determined by a co-repressor. *Nature.* 1995;**377**:451–454.

123. **Nagy L, Kao HY, Chakravarti D,** *et al.* Nuclear receptor repression mediated by a complex containing SMRT, mSin3A, and histone deacetylase. *Cell.* 1997;**89**:373–380.

124. **Grunstein M.** Histone acetylation in chromatin structure and transcription. *Nature.* 1997;**389**:349–352.

125. **Kamei Y, Xu L, Heinzel T,** *et al.* A CBP integrator complex mediates transcriptional activation and AP-1 inhibition by nuclear receptors. *Cell.* 1996;**85**:403–414.

126. **Shikama N, Lyon J, La Thangue N.** The p300/CBP family: integrating signals with transcription factors and chromatin. *Trends in Cell Biology.* 1997;7:230–236.

127. **Kawasaki H, Eckner R, Yao TP,** *et al.* Distinct roles of the co-activators p300 and CBP in retinoic-acid-induced F9-cell differentiation. *Nature.* 1998; **393**:284–289.

128. **Ogryzko VV, Schiltz RL, Russanova V, Howard BH, Nakatani Y.** The transcriptional coactivators p300 and CBP are histone acetyltransferases. *Cell.* 1996;**87**:953–959.

129. **Chen H, Lin RJ, Schiltz RL,** *et al.* Nuclear receptor coactivator ACTR is a novel histone acetyltransferase and forms a multimeric activation complex with P/CAF and CBP/p300. *Cell.* 1997; **90**:569–580.

130. **Pazin MJ, Kadonaga JT.** What's up and down with histone deacetylation and transcription? *Cell.* 1997;**89**:325–328.

131. **Rhodes D.** Chromatin structure. The nucleosome core all wrapped up. *Nature.* 1997;**389**:231,233.

132. **Weis K, Rambaud S, Lavau C,** *et al.* Retinoic acid regulates aberrant nuclear localization of PML-RAR alpha in acute promyelocytic leukemia cells. *Cell.* 1994;**76**:345–356.

133. **Dyck JA, Maul GG, Miller WH,** *et al.* A novel macromolecular structure is a target of the promyelocyte-retinoic acid receptor oncoprotein. *Cell.* 1994; **76**:333–343.

134. **Borden KL, Lally JM, Martin SR,** *et al.* In vivo and in vitro characterization of the B1 and B2 zinc-binding domains from the acute promyelocytic leukemia protooncoprotein PML. *Proceedings of the National Academy of Sciences of the United States of America.* 1996;**93**: 1601–1606.

135. **Borden KL, Campbell Dwyer EJ, Salvato MS.** The promyelocytic leukemia protein PML has a pro-apoptotic activity mediated through its RING domain. *FEBS Letters.* 1997;**418**:30–34.

136. **Le XF, Yang P, Chang KS.** Analysis of the growth and transformation suppressor domains of promyelocytic leukemia gene, PML. *The Journal of Biological Chemistry.* 1996;**271**:130–135.

137. **Wang ZG, Delva L, Gaboli M,** *et al.* Role of PML in cell growth and the retinoic acid pathway. *Science.* 1998; **279**:1547–1551.

138. **Wang ZG, Ruggero D, Ronchetti S,** *et al.* PML is essential for multiple apoptotic pathways. *Nature Genetics.* 1998;**20**:266–272.

139. **Yang S, Kuo C, Bisi JE, Kim MK.** PML-dependent apoptosis after DNA damage is regulated by the checkpoint kinase hCds1/Chk2. *Nature Cell Biology.* 2002;**4**:865–870.

140. **He LZ, Guidez F, Tribioli C,** *et al.* Distinct interactions of PML-RARalpha and PLZF-RARalpha with co-repressors determine differential responses to RA in APL. *Nature Genetics.* 1998;**18**:126–135.

141. **Grignani F, De Matteis S, Nervi C,** *et al.* Fusion proteins of the retinoic acid receptor-alpha recruit histone deacetylase in promyelocytic leukaemia. *Nature.* 1998;**391**:815–818.

142. **Lin RJ, Nagy L, Inoue S,** *et al.* Role of the histone deacetylase complex in acute promyelocytic leukaemia. *Nature.* 1998;**391**:811–814.

143. **Raelson JV, Nervi C, Rosenauer A,** *et al.* The PML/RAR alpha oncoprotein is a direct molecular target of retinoic acid in acute promyelocytic leukemia cells. *Blood.* 1996;**88**:2826–2832.

144. **Hong SH, David G, Wong CW, Dejean A, Privalsky ML.** SMRT corepressor interacts with PLZF and with the PML-retinoic acid receptor alpha (RARalpha) and PLZF-RARalpha oncoproteins associated with acute promyelocytic leukemia. *Proceedings of the National Academy of Sciences of the United States of America.* 1997;**94**: 9028–9033.

145. **Collins SJ.** Acute promyelocytic leukemia: relieving repression induces remission. *Blood.* 1998;**91**:2631–2633.

146. **Tobal K, Saunders MJ, Grey MR, Yin JA.** Persistence of RAR alpha-PML fusion mRNA detected by reverse transcriptase polymerase chain reaction in patients in long-term remission of acute promyelocytic leukaemia. *British Journal of Haematology.* 1995; **90**:615–618.

147. **de Thé H, Lavau C, Marchio A,** *et al.* The PML-RAR alpha fusion mRNA generated by the t(15;17) translocation in acute promyelocytic leukemia encodes a functionally altered RAR. *Cell.* 1991;**66**:675–684.

148. **Kakizuka A, Miller WHJ, Umesono K,** *et al.* Chromosomal translocation t(15;17) in human acute promyelocytic

leukemia fuses RAR alpha with a novel putative transcription factor, PML. *Cell.* 1991;**66**:663–674.

149. **Guiochon-Mantel A, Savouret JF, Quignon F**, *et al.* Effect of PML and PML-RAR on the transactivation properties and subcellular distribution of steroid hormone receptors. *Molecular Endocrinology (Baltimore, MD).* 1995;**9**:1791–1803.

150. **Koken MH, Puvion-Dutilleul F, Guillemin MC**, *et al.* The t(15;17) translocation alters a nuclear body in a retinoic acid-reversible fashion. *The EMBO Journal.* 1994;**13**:1073–1083.

151. **Fu S, Consoli U, Hanania EG**, *et al.* PML/RARalpha, a fusion protein in acute promyelocytic leukemia, prevents growth factor withdrawal-induced apoptosis in TF-1 cells. *Clinical Cancer Research.* 1995;**1**:583–590.

152. **Maeda Y, Horiuchi F, Miyatake J**, *et al.* Inhibition of growth and induction of apoptosis by all-trans retinoic acid in lymphoid cell lines transfected with the PML/RAR alpha fusion gene. *British Journal of Haematology.* 1996;**93**:973–976.

153. **Rogaia D, Grignani F, Nicoletti I, Pelicci PG**. The acute promyelocytic leukemia-specific PML/RAR alpha fusion protein reduces the frequency of commitment to apoptosis upon growth factor deprivation of GM-CSF-dependent myeloid cells. *Leukemia.* 1995;**9**:1467–1472.

154. **Rousselot P, Hardas B, Patel A**, *et al.* The PML-RAR alpha gene product of the t(15;17) translocation inhibits retinoic acid-induced granulocytic differentiation and mediated transactivation in human myeloid cells. *Oncogene.* 1994;**9**:545–551.

155. **Kogan SC, Brown DE, Shultz DB**, *et al.* BCL-2 cooperates with promyelocytic leukemia retinoic acid receptor alpha chimeric protein (PMLRARalpha) to block neutrophil differentiation and initiate acute leukemia. *The Journal of Experimental Medicine.* 2001;**193**:531–543.

156. **Di Croce L, Raker VA, Corsaro M**, *et al.* Methyltransferase recruitment and DNA hypermethylation of target promoters by an oncogenic transcription factor. *Science.* 2002;**295**:1079–1082.

157. **Nervi C, Ferrara FF, Fanelli M**, *et al.* Caspases mediate retinoic acid-induced

degradation of the acute promyelocytic leukemia PML/RARalpha fusion protein. *Blood.* 1998;**92**:2244–2251.

158. **Zhu J, Gianni M, Kopf E**, *et al.* Retinoic acid induces proteasome-dependent degradation of retinoic acid receptor alpha (RARalpha) and oncogenic RARalpha fusion proteins. *Proceedings of the National Academy of Sciences of the United States of America.* 1999;**96**:14807–14812.

159. **Jing Y, Xia L, Lu M, Waxman S.** The cleavage product deltaPML-RARalpha contributes to all-trans retinoic acid-mediated differentiation in acute promyelocytic leukemia cells. *Oncogene* 2003;**22**:4083–4091.

160. **Dermime S, Grignani F, Clerici M**, *et al.* Occurrence of resistance to retinoic acid in the acute promyelocytic leukemia cell line NB4 is associated with altered expression of the pml/RAR alpha protein. *Blood.* 1993;**82**:1573–1577.

161. **Shao W, Benedetti L, Lamph WW, Nervi C, Miller WHJ.** A retinoid-resistant acute promyelocytic leukemia subclone expresses a dominant negative PML-RAR alpha mutation. *Blood.* 1997;**89**:4282–4289.

162. **Zhou DC, Kim SH, Ding W**, *et al.* Frequent mutations in the ligand-binding domain of PML-RARalpha after multiple relapses of acute promyelocytic leukemia: analysis for functional relationship to response to all-trans retinoic acid and histone deacetylase inhibitors in vitro and in vivo. *Blood.* 2002;**99**:1356–1363.

163. **Carter M, Kalwinsky DK, Dahl GV**, *et al.* Childhood acute promyelocytic leukemia: a rare variant of nonlymphoid leukemia with distinctive clinical and biologic features. *Leukemia.* 1989;**3**:298–302.

164. **Ortega JJ, Madero L, Martin G**, *et al.* Treatment with all-trans retinoic acid and anthracycline monochemotherapy for children with acute promyelocytic leukemia: a multicenter study by the PETHEMA Group. *Journal of Clinical Oncology.* 2005;**23**:7632–7640.

165. **Mann G, Reinhardt D, Ritter J**, *et al.* Treatment with all-trans retinoic acid in acute promyelocytic leukemia reduces early deaths in children. *Annals of Hematology.* 2001;**80**:417–422.

166. **Shimizu H, Nakadate H, Taga T**, *et al.* [Clinical characteristics and treatment

results of acute promyelocytic leukemia in children (Children's Cancer and Leukemia Study Group)]. *Rinshō Ketsueki.* 1993;**34**:989–996.

167. **Falanga A, Rickles FR.** Pathogenesis and management of the bleeding diathesis in acute promyelocytic leukaemia. *Best Practice & Research. Clinical Haematology.* 2003;**16**:463–482.

168. **Kawai Y, Watanabe K, Kizaki M**, *et al.* Rapid improvement of coagulopathy by all-trans retinoic acid in acute promyelocytic leukemia. *American Journal of Hematology.* 1994;**46**:184–188.

169. **Falanga A, Iacoviello L, Evangelista V**, *et al.* Loss of blast cell procoagulant activity and improvement of hemostatic variables in patients with acute promyelocytic leukemia administered all-trans-retinoic acid. *Blood.* 1995;**86**:1072–1081.

170. **Watanabe R, Murata M, Takayama N**, *et al.* Long-term follow-up of hemostatic molecular markers during remission induction therapy with all-trans retinoic acid for acute promyelocytic leukemia. Keio Hematology-Oncology Cooperative Study Group (KHOCS). *Thrombosis and Haemostasis.* 1997;**77**:641–645.

171. **Falanga A, Rickles FR.** Management of thrombohemorrhagic syndromes (THS) in hematologic malignancies. *Hematology/the Education Program of the American Society of Hematology.* 2007;165–171.

172. **Fenaux P, Chastang C, Chevret S**, *et al.* A randomized comparison of all transretinoic acid (ATRA) followed by chemotherapy and ATRA plus chemotherapy and the role of maintenance therapy in newly diagnosed acute promyelocytic leukemia. The European APL Group. *Blood.* 1999;**94**:1192–1200.

173. **Tallman MS, Nabhan C, Feusner JH, Rowe JM.** Acute promyelocytic leukemia: evolving therapeutic strategies. *Blood.* 2002;**99**:759–767.

174. **Sanz MA.** Treatment of acute promyelocytic leukemia. *Hematology/the Education Program of the American Society of Hematology.* 2006;147–155.

175. **Adès L, Sanz MA, Chevret S**, *et al.* Treatment of newly diagnosed acute promyelocytic leukemia (APL): a

comparison of French-Belgian-Swiss and PETHEMA results. *Blood*. 2008; **111**:1078–1084.

176. **de Botton S, Coiteux V, Chevret S,** *et al.* Outcome of childhood acute promyelocytic leukemia with all-trans-retinoic acid and chemotherapy. *Journal of Clinical Oncology*. 2004;**22**:1404–1412.

177. **Gale RE, Hills R, Pizzey AR,** *et al.* Relationship between FLT3 mutation status, biologic characteristics, and response to targeted therapy in acute promyelocytic leukemia. *Blood*. 2005; **106**:3768–3776.

178. **Au WY, Fung A, Chim CS,** *et al.* FLT-3 aberrations in acute promyelocytic leukaemia: clinicopathological associations and prognostic impact. *British Journal of Haematology*. 2004; **125**:463–469.

179. **Golomb HM, Rowley JD, Vardiman JW, Testa JR, Butler A.** "Microgranular" acute promyelocytic leukemia: a distinct clinical, ultrastructural, and cytogenetic entity. *Blood*. 1980;**55**:253–259.

180. **Sainty D, Liso V, Cantù-Rajnoldi A,** *et al.* A new morphologic classification system for acute promyelocytic leukemia distinguishes cases with underlying PLZF/RARA gene rearrangements. *Blood*. 2000;**96**: 1287–1296.

181. **Guglielmi C, Martelli MP, Diverio D,** *et al.* Immunophenotype of adult and childhood acute promyelocytic leukaemia: correlation with morphology, type of PML gene breakpoint and clinical outcome. A cooperative Italian study on 196 cases. *British Journal of Haematology*. 1998; **102**:1035–1041.

182. **Foley R, Soamboonsrup P, Carter RF,** *et al.* CD34-positive acute promyelocytic leukemia is associated with leukocytosis, microgranular/ hypogranular morphology, expression of CD2 and bcr3 isoform. *American Journal of Hematology*. 2001;**67**:34–41.

183. **Paietta E, Goloubeva O, Neuberg D,** *et al.* A surrogate marker profile for PML/RAR alpha expressing acute promyelocytic leukemia and the association of immunophenotypic markers with morphologic and molecular subtypes. *Cytometry. Part B, Clinical Cytometry*. 2004;**59**: 1–9.

184. **Orfao A, Chillon MC, Bortoluci AM,** *et al.* The flow cytometric pattern of CD34, CD15 and CD13 expression in acute myeloblastic leukemia is highly characteristic of the presence of PML-RARalpha gene rearrangements. *Haematologica*. 1999;**84**:405–412.

185. **Schoch C, Kohlmann A, Schnittger S,** *et al.* Acute myeloid leukemias with reciprocal rearrangements can be distinguished by specific gene expression profiles. *Proceedings of the National Academy of Sciences of the United States of America*. 2002;**99**: 10008–10013.

186. **Chen Z, Brand NJ, Chen A,** *et al.* Fusion between a novel Kruppel-like zinc finger gene and the retinoic acid receptor-alpha locus due to a variant t(11;17) translocation associated with acute promyelocytic leukaemia. *The EMBO Journal*. 1993;**12**:1161–1167.

187. **Redner RL, Rush EA, Faas S, Rudert WA, Corey SJ.** The t(5;17) variant of acute promyelocytic leukemia expresses a nucleophosmin-retinoic acid receptor fusion. *Blood*. 1996;**87**:882–886.

188. **Wells RA, Catzavelos C, Kamel-Reid S.** Fusion of retinoic acid receptor alpha to NuMA, the nuclear mitotic apparatus protein, by a variant translocation in acute promyelocytic leukaemia. *Nature Genetics*. 1997;**17**:109–113.

189. **Arnould C, Philippe C, Bourdon V,** *et al.* The signal transducer and activator of transcription STAT5b gene is a new partner of retinoic acid receptor alpha in acute promyelocytic-like leukaemia. *Human Molecular Genetics*. 1999;**8**:1741–1749.

190. **Redner RL, Contis LC, Craig F,** *et al.* A novel t(3;17)(p25;q21) variant translocation of acute promyelocytic leukemia with rearrangement of the RARA locus. *Leukemia*. 2006;**20**:376–379.

191. **Catalano A, Dawson MA, Somana K,** *et al.* The PRKAR1A gene is fused to RARA in a new variant acute promyelocytic leukemia. *Blood*. 2007; **110**:4073–4076.

192. **Guidez F, Huang W, Tong JH,** *et al.* Poor response to all-trans retinoic acid therapy in a t(11;17) PLZF/RAR alpha patient. *Leukemia*. 1994;**8**:312–317.

193. **Licht JD, Chomienne C, Goy A,** *et al.* Clinical and molecular characterization of a rare syndrome of acute promyelocytic leukemia associated with translocation (11;17). *Blood*. 1995;**85**: 1083–1094.

194. **Koken MH, Daniel MT, Gianni M,** *et al.* Retinoic acid, but not arsenic trioxide, degrades the PLZF/RARalpha fusion protein, without inducing terminal differentiation or apoptosis, in a RA-therapy resistant t(11;17) (q23;q21) APL patient. *Oncogene*. 1999; **18**:1113–1118.

195. **Grimwade D, Biondi A, Mozziconacci MJ,** *et al.* Characterization of acute promyelocytic leukemia cases lacking the classic t(15;17): results of the European Working Party. *Blood*. 2000;**96**:1297–1308.

196. **Slack JL, Arthur DC, Lawrence D,** *et al.* Secondary cytogenetic changes in acute promyelocytic leukemia – prognostic importance in patients treated with chemotherapy alone and association with the intron 3 breakpoint of the PML gene: a Cancer and Leukemia Group B study. *Journal of Clinical Oncology*. 1997;**15**:1786–1795.

197. **Gallagher RE, Yeap BY, Bi W,** *et al.* Quantitative real-time RT-PCR analysis of PML-RAR alpha mRNA in acute promyelocytic leukemia: assessment of prognostic significance in adult patients from intergroup protocol 0129. *Blood*. 2003;**101**:2521–2528.

198. **Lee S, Kim YJ, Eom KS,** *et al.* The significance of minimal residual disease kinetics in adults with newly diagnosed PML-RARalpha-positive acute promyelocytic leukemia: results of a prospective trial. *Haematologica*. 2006;**91**:671–674.

199. **Esteve J, Escoda L, Martin G,** *et al.* Outcome of patients with acute promyelocytic leukemia failing to front-line treatment with all-trans retinoic acid and anthracycline-based chemotherapy (PETHEMA protocols LPA96 and LPA99): benefit of an early intervention. *Leukemia*. 2007;**21**:446–452.

200. **Rozenblatt-Rosen O, Rozovskaia T, Burakov D,** *et al.* The C-terminal SET domains of ALL-1 and TRITHORAX interact with the INI1 and SNR1 proteins, components of the SWI/SNF complex. *Proceedings of the National Academy of Sciences of the United States of America*. 1998;**95**:4152–4157.

201. **Hsieh JJ, Ernst P, Erdjument-Bromage H, Tempst P, Korsmeyer SJ.** Proteolytic cleavage of MLL generates a complex of N- and C-terminal

fragments that confers protein stability and subnuclear localization. *Molecular and Cellular Biology*. 2003;**23**:186–194.

202. **Yokoyama A, Kitabayashi I, Ayton PM, Cleary ML, Ohki M.** Leukemia proto-oncoprotein MLL is proteolytically processed into 2 fragments with opposite transcriptional properties. *Blood*. 2002;**100**:3710–3718.

203. **Hsieh JJ, Cheng EH, Korsmeyer SJ.** Taspase1: a threonine aspartase required for cleavage of MLL and proper HOX gene expression. *Cell*. 2003;**115**:293–303.

204. **Ernst P, Fisher JK, Avery W,** *et al*. Definitive hematopoiesis requires the mixed-lineage leukemia gene. *Developmental Cell*. 2004;**6**:437–443.

205. **Iida S, Seto M, Yamamoto K,** *et al*. MLLT3 gene on 9p22 involved in t(9;11) leukemia encodes a serine/proline rich protein homologous to MLLT1 on 19p13. *Oncogene*. 1993;**8**: 3085–3092.

206. **Collins EC, Appert A, Ariza-McNaughton L,** *et al*. Mouse Af9 is a controller of embryo patterning, like Mll, whose human homologue fuses with Af9 after chromosomal translocation in leukemia. *Molecular and Cellular Biology*. 2002;**22**:7313–7324.

207. **Meyer C, Schneider B, Jakob S,** *et al*. The MLL recombinome of acute leukemias. *Leukemia*. 2006;**20**:777–784.

208. **Downing JR, Look AT.** MLL fusion genes in the 11q23 acute leukemias. *Cancer Treatment and Research*. 1996; **84**:73–92.

209. **Waring PM, Cleary ML.** Disruption of a homolog of trithorax by 11q23 translocations: leukemogenic and transcriptional implications. *Current Topics in Microbiology and Immunology*. 1997;**220**:1–23.

210. **Rubnitz JE, Behm FG, Downing JR.** 11q23 rearrangements in acute leukemia. *Leukemia*. 1996;**10**:74–82.

211. **Schichman SA, Caligiuri MA, Strout MP,** *et al*. ALL-1 tandem duplication in acute myeloid leukemia with a normal karyotype involves homologous recombination between Alu elements. *Cancer Research*. 1994;**54**:4277–4280.

212. **Lavau C, Szilvassy SJ, Slany R, Cleary ML.** Immortalization and leukemic transformation of a myelomonocytic precursor by retrovirally transduced

HRX-ENL. *The EMBO Journal*. 1997; **16**:4226–4237.

213. **Slany RK, Lavau C, Cleary ML.** The oncogenic capacity of HRX-ENL requires the transcriptional transactivation activity of ENL and the DNA binding motifs of HRX. *Molecular and Cellular Biology*. 1998;**18**:122–129.

214. **Dobson CL, Warren AJ, Pannell R, Forster A, Rabbitts TH.** Tumorigenesis in mice with a fusion of the leukaemia oncogene Mll and the bacterial lacZ gene. *The EMBO Journal*. 2000;**19**:843–851.

215. **So CW, Lin M, Ayton PM, Chen EH, Cleary ML.** Dimerization contributes to oncogenic activation of MLL chimeras in acute leukemias. *Cancer Cell*. 2003;**4**:99–110.

216. **Martin ME, Milne TA, Bloyer S,** *et al*. Dimerization of MLL fusion proteins immortalizes hematopoietic cells. *Cancer Cell*. 2003;**4**:197–207.

217. **Eguchi M, Eguchi-Ishimae M, Greaves M.** The small oligomerization domain of gephyrin converts MLL to an oncogene. *Blood*. 2004;**103**:3876–3882.

218. **So CW, Cleary ML.** Dimerization: a versatile switch for oncogenesis. *Blood*. 2004;**104**:919–922.

219. **Hess JL.** MLL: a histone methyltransferase disrupted in leukemia. *Trends in Molecular Medicine*. 2004;**10**:500–507.

220. **Hess JL.** Mechanisms of transformation by MLL. *Critical Reviews in Eukaryotic Gene Expression*. 2004;**14**:235–254.

221. **Li ZY, Liu DP, Liang CC.** New insight into the molecular mechanisms of MLL-associated leukemia. *Leukemia*. 2005;**19**:183–190.

222. **Hsu K, Look AT.** Turning on a dimer: new insights into MLL chimeras. *Cancer Cell*. 2003;**4**:81–83.

223. **Yamamoto K, Hamaguchi H, Nagata K, Kobayashi M, Taniwaki M.** Tandem duplication of the MLL gene in myelodysplastic syndrome – derived overt leukemia with trisomy 11. *American Journal of Hematology*. 1997;**55**:41–45.

224. **Kwong YL.** Partial duplication of the MLL gene in acute myelogenous leukemia without karyotypic aberration. *Cancer Genetics and Cytogenetics*. 1997;**97**:20–24.

225. **Yu M, Honoki K, Andersen J,** *et al*. MLL tandem duplication and multiple

splicing in adult acute myeloid leukemia with normal karyotype. *Leukemia*. 1996;**10**:774–780.

226. **Corral J, Lavenir I, Impey H,** *et al*. An Mll-AF9 fusion gene made by homologous recombination causes acute leukemia in chimeric mice: a method to create fusion oncogenes. *Cell*. 1996;**85**:853–861.

227. **So CW, Karsunky H, Passegue E,** *et al*. MLL-GAS7 transforms multipotent hematopoietic progenitors and induces mixed lineage leukemias in mice. *Cancer Cell*. 2003;**3**:161–171.

228. **Zeisig BB, Garcia-Cuellar MP, Winkler TH, Slany RK.** The oncoprotein MLL-ENL disturbs hematopoietic lineage determination and transforms a biphenotypic lymphoid/myeloid cell. *Oncogene*. 2003;**22**:1629–1637.

229. **Armstrong SA, Staunton JE, Silverman LB,** *et al*. MLL translocations specify a distinct gene expression profile that distinguishes a unique leukemia. *Nature Genetics*. 2002;**30**:41–47.

230. **Ross ME, Zhou X, Song G,** *et al*. Classification of pediatric acute lymphoblastic leukemia by gene expression profiling. *Blood*. 2003; **102**:2951–2959.

231. **Park IK, He Y, Lin F,** *et al*. Differential gene expression profiling of adult murine hematopoietic stem cells. *Blood*. 2002;**99**:488–498.

232. **Pineault N, Helgason CD, Lawrence HJ, Humphries RK.** Differential expression of Hox, Meis1, and Pbx1 genes in primitive cells throughout murine hematopoietic ontogeny. *Experimental Hematology*. 2002;**30**: 49–57.

233. **Akashi K, He X, Chen J,** *et al*. Transcriptional accessibility for genes of multiple tissues and hematopoietic lineages is hierarchically controlled during early hematopoiesis. *Blood*. 2003;**101**:383–389.

234. **So CW, Karsunky H, Wong P, Weissman IL, Cleary ML.** Leukemic transformation of hematopoietic progenitors by MLL-GAS7 in the absence of Hoxa7 or Hoxa9. *Blood*. 2004;**103**:3192–3199.

235. **Ayton PM, Cleary ML.** Transformation of myeloid progenitors by MLL oncoproteins is dependent on Hoxa7

and Hoxa9. *Genes & Development.* 2003;**17**:2298–2307.

236. **Zeisig BB, Milne T, Garcia-Cuellar MP**, *et al.* Hoxa9 and Meis1 are key targets for MLL-ENL-mediated cellular immortalization. *Molecular and Cellular Biology.* 2004;**24**:617–628.

237. **Kumar AR, Hudson WA, Chen W**, *et al.* Hoxa9 influences the phenotype but not the incidence of Mll-AF9 fusion gene leukemia. *Blood.* 2004;**103**:1823–1828.

238. **Rubnitz JE, Raimondi SC, Tong X**, *et al.* Favorable impact of the t(9;11) in childhood acute myeloid leukemia. *Journal of Clinical Oncology.* 2002;**20**:2302–2309.

239. **Forestier E, Heim S, Blennow E**, *et al.* Cytogenetic abnormalities in childhood acute myeloid leukaemia: a Nordic series comprising all children enrolled in the NOPHO-93-AML trial between 1993 and 2001. *British Journal of Haematology.* 2003;**121**:566–577.

240. **Raimondi SC, Peiper SC, Kitchingman GR**, *et al.* Childhood acute lymphoblastic leukemia with chromosomal breakpoints at 11q23. *Blood.* 1989;**73**:1627–1634.

241. **Pui CH, Behm FG, Raimondi SC**, *et al.* Secondary acute myeloid leukemia in children treated for acute lymphoid leukemia. *The New England Journal of Medicine.* 1989;**321**:136–142.

242. **Pui CH, Ribeiro RC, Hancock ML**, *et al.* Acute myeloid leukemia in children treated with epipodophyllotoxins for acute lymphoblastic leukemia. *The New England Journal of Medicine.* 1991;**325**:1682–1687.

243. **Pui CH, Frankel LS, Carroll AJ**, *et al.* Clinical characteristics and treatment outcome of childhood acute lymphoblastic leukemia with the t(4;11)(q21;q23): a collaborative study of 40 cases. *Blood.* 1991;**77**:440–447.

244. **Kaneko Y, Maseki N, Takasaki N**, *et al.* Clinical and hematologic characteristics in acute leukemia with 11q23 translocations. *Blood.* 1986;**67**:484–491.

245. **Koller U, Haas OA, Ludwig WD**, *et al.* Phenotypic and genotypic heterogeneity in infant acute leukemia. II. Acute nonlymphoblastic leukemia. *Leukemia.* 1989;**3**:708–714.

246. **Sorensen PH, Chen CS, Smith FO**, *et al.* Molecular rearrangements of the MLL gene are present in most cases of infant acute myeloid leukemia and are strongly correlated with monocytic or myelomonocytic phenotypes. *The Journal of Clinical Investigation.* 1994; **93**:429–437.

247. **Martinez-Climent JA, Thirman MJ, Espinosa R, Le Beau MM, Rowley JD.** Detection of 11q23/MLL rearrangements in infant leukemias with fluorescence in situ hybridization and molecular analysis. *Leukemia.* 1995;**9**:1299–1304.

248. **Baer MR, Stewart CC, Lawrence D**, *et al.* Acute myeloid leukemia with 11q23 translocations: myelomonocytic immunophenotype by multiparameter flow cytometry. *Leukemia.* 1998;**12**:317–325.

249. **Cox MC, Panetta P, Lo-Coco F**, *et al.* Chromosomal aberration of the 11q23 locus in acute leukemia and frequency of MLL gene translocation: results in 378 adult patients. *American Journal of Clinical Pathology.* 2004;**122**:298–306.

250. **Munoz L, Nomdedeu JF, Villamor N**, *et al.* Acute myeloid leukemia with MLL rearrangements: clinicobiological features, prognostic impact and value of flow cytometry in the detection of residual leukemic cells. *Leukemia.* 2003; **17**:76–82.

251. **Martinez-Climent JA, Lane NJ, Rubin CM**, *et al.* Clinical and prognostic significance of chromosomal abnormalities in childhood acute myeloid leukemia de novo. *Leukemia.* 1995;**9**:95–101.

252. **Mrozek K, Heinonen K, Lawrence D**, *et al.* Adult patients with de novo acute myeloid leukemia and t(9; 11)(p22; q23) have a superior outcome to patients with other translocations involving band 11q23: a cancer and leukemia group B study. *Blood.* 1997; **90**:4532–4538.

253. **Watanabe N, Kobayashi H, Ichiji O**, *et al.* Cryptic insertion and translocation or nondividing leukemic cells disclosed by FISH analysis in infant acute leukemia with discrepant molecular and cytogenetic findings. *Leukemia.* 2003;**17**:876–882.

254. **Pallisgaard N, Hokland P, Riishoj DC, Pedersen B, Jorgensen P.** Multiplex reverse transcription-polymerase chain reaction for simultaneous screening of 29 translocations and chromosomal aberrations in acute leukemia. *Blood.* 1998;**92**:574–588.

255. **Strehl S, Konig M, Mann G, Haas OA.** Multiplex reverse transcriptase-polymerase chain reaction screening in childhood acute myeloblastic leukemia. *Blood.* 2001;**97**:805–808.

256. **Andersson A, Hoglund M, Johansson B**, *et al.* Paired multiplex reverse-transcriptase polymerase chain reaction (PMRT – PCR) analysis as a rapid and accurate diagnostic tool for the detection of MLL fusion genes in hematologic malignancies. *Leukemia.* 2001;**15**:1293–1300.

257. **Jansen MW, van der Velden VH, van Dongen JJ.** Efficient and easy detection of MLL-AF4, MLL-AF9 and MLL-ENL fusion gene transcripts by multiplex real-time quantitative RT-PCR in TaqMan and LightCycler. *Leukemia.* 2005;**19**:2016–2018.

258. **Olesen LH, Clausen N, Dimitrijevic A**, *et al.* Prospective application of a multiplex reverse transcription-polymerase chain reaction assay for the detection of balanced translocations in leukaemia: a single-laboratory study of 390 paediatric and adult patients. *British Journal of Haematology.* 2004; **127**:59–66.

259. **Cuthbert G, Thompson K, Breese G, McCullough S, Bown N.** Sensitivity of FISH in detection of MLL translocations. *Genes, Chromosomes & Cancer.* 2000;**29**:180–185.

260. **Arnaud B, Douet-Guilbert N, Morel F**, *et al.* Screening by fluorescence in situ hybridization for MLL status at diagnosis in 239 unselected patients with acute myeloblastic leukemia. *Cancer Genetics and Cytogenetics.* 2005;**161**:110–115.

261. **Maroc N, Morel A, Beillard E**, *et al.* A diagnostic biochip for the comprehensive analysis of MLL translocations in acute leukemia. *Leukemia.* 2004;**18**:1522–1530.

262. **Harrison CJ, Griffiths M, Moorman F**, *et al.* A multicenter evaluation of comprehensive analysis of MLL translocations and fusion gene partners in acute leukemia using the MLL FusionChip device. *Cancer Genetics and Cytogenetics.* 2007;**173**:17–22.

263. **Athale UH, Razzouk BI, Raimondi SC**, *et al.* Biology and outcome of childhood acute megakaryoblastic leukemia: a single institution's experience. *Blood.* 2001;**97**:3727–3732.

264. **Lange B**. The management of neoplastic disorders of haematopoiesis in children with Down's syndrome. *British Journal of Haematology*. 2000;**110**:512–524.

265. **Zipursky A, Poon A, Doyle J**. Leukemia in Down syndrome: a review. *Pediatric Hematology and Oncology*. 1992;**9**:139–149.

266. **Zipursky A**. Transient leukaemia – a benign form of leukaemia in newborn infants with trisomy 21. *British Journal of Haematology*. 2003;**120**:930–938.

267. **Shivdasani RA**. Molecular and transcriptional regulation of megakaryocyte differentiation. *Stem Cells*. 2001;**19**:397–407.

268. **Nichols KE, Crispino JD, Poncz M**, *et al*. Familial dyserythropoietic anaemia and thrombocytopenia due to an inherited mutation in GATA1. *Nature Genetics*. 2000;**24**:266–270.

269. **Freson K, Devriendt K, Matthijs G**, *et al*. Platelet characteristics in patients with X-linked macrothrombocytopenia because of a novel GATA1 mutation. *Blood*. 2001;**98**:85–92.

270. **Mehaffey MG, Newton AL, Gandhi MJ, Crossley M, Drachman JG**. X-linked thrombocytopenia caused by a novel mutation of GATA-1. *Blood*. 2001;**98**:2681–2688.

271. **Shivdasani RA, Fujiwara Y, McDevitt MA, Orkin SH**. A lineage-selective knockout establishes the critical role of transcription factor GATA-1 in megakaryocyte growth and platelet development. *The EMBO Journal*. 1997;**16**:3965–3973.

272. **Groet J, McElwaine S, Spinelli M**, *et al*. Acquired mutations in GATA1 in neonates with Down's syndrome with transient myeloid disorder. *Lancet*. 2003;**361**:1617–1620.

273. **Hitzler JK, Cheung J, Li Y, Scherer SW, Zipursky A**. GATA1 mutations in transient leukemia and acute megakaryoblastic leukemia of Down syndrome. *Blood*. 2003;**101**:4301–4304.

274. **Rainis L, Bercovich D, Strehl S**, *et al*. Mutations in exon 2 of GATA1 are early events in megakaryocytic malignancies associated with trisomy 21. *Blood*. 2003;**102**:981–986.

275. **Wechsler J, Greene M, McDevitt MA**, *et al*. Acquired mutations in GATA1 in the megakaryoblastic leukemia of Down syndrome. *Nature Genetics*. 2002;**32**:148–152.

276. **Xu G, Nagano M, Kanezaki R**, *et al*. Frequent mutations in the GATA-1 gene in the transient myeloproliferative disorder of Down syndrome. *Blood*. 2003;**102**:2960–2968.

277. **Ahmed M, Sternberg A, Hall G**, *et al*. Natural history of GATA1 mutations in Down syndrome. *Blood*. 2004;**103**:2480–2489.

278. **Groet J, McElwaine S, Spinelli M**, *et al*. Acquired mutations in GATA1 in neonates with Down's syndrome with transient myeloid disorder. *Lancet*. 2003;**361**:1617–1620.

279. **Hitzler JK, Cheung J, Li Y, Scherer SW, Zipursky A**. GATA1 mutations in transient leukemia and acute megakaryoblastic leukemia of Down syndrome. *Blood*. 2003;**101**:4301–4304.

280. **Rainis L, Bercovich D, Strehl S**, *et al*. Mutations in exon 2 of GATA1 are early events in megakaryocytic malignancies associated with trisomy 21. *Blood*. 2003;**102**:981–986.

281. **Wechsler J, Greene M, McDevitt MA**, *et al*. Acquired mutations in GATA1 in the megakaryoblastic leukemia of Down syndrome. *Nature Genetics*. 2002;**32**:148–152.

282. **Harigae H, Xu G, Sugawara T**, *et al*. The GATA1 mutation in an adult patient with acute megakaryoblastic leukemia not accompanying Down syndrome. *Blood*. 2004;**103**:3242–3243.

283. **Mundschau G, Gurbuxani S, Gamis AS**, *et al*. Mutagenesis of GATA1 is an initiating event in Down syndrome leukemogenesis. *Blood*. 2003;**101**:4298–4300.

284. **Xu G, Nagano M, Kanezaki R**, *et al*. Frequent mutations in the GATA-1 gene in the transient myeloproliferative disorder of Down's syndrome. *Blood*. 2003;**102**:2960–2968.

285. **Li Z, Godinho FJ, Klusmann JH**, *et al*. Developmental stage-selective effect of somatically mutated leukemogenic transcription factor GATA1. *Nature Genetics*. 2005;**37**:613–619.

286. **Carroll A, Civin C, Schneider N**, *et al*. The t(1;22) (p13;q13) is nonrandom and restricted to infants with acute megakaryoblastic leukemia: a Pediatric Oncology Group Study. *Blood*. 1991;**78**:748–752.

287. **Bernstein J, Dastugue N, Haas OA**, *et al*. Nineteen cases of the t(1;22)(p13;q13) acute megakaryblastic leukaemia of infants/children and a review of 39 cases: report from a t(1;22) study group. *Leukemia*. 2000;**14**:216–218.

288. **Mercher T, Coniat MB, Monni R**, *et al*. Involvement of a human gene related to the Drosophila spen gene in the recurrent t(1;22) translocation of acute megakaryocytic leukemia. *Proceedings of the National Academy of Sciences of the United States of America*. 2001;**98**:5776–5779.

289. **Ma Z, Morris SW, Valentine V**, *et al*. Fusion of two novel genes, RBM15 and MKL1, in the t(1;22)(p13;q13) of acute megakaryoblastic leukemia. *Nature Genetics*. 2001;**28**:220–221.

290. **Selvaraj A, Prywes R**. Megakaryoblastic leukemia-1/2, a transcriptional co-activator of serum response factor, is required for skeletal myogenic differentiation. *The Journal of Biological Chemistry*. 2003;**278**:41977–41987.

291. **Parmacek MS**. Myocardin-related transcription factors: critical coactivators regulating cardiovascular development and adaptation. *Circulation Research*. 2007;**100**:633–644.

292. **Sasazuki T, Sawada T, Sakon S**, *et al*. Identification of a novel transcriptional activator, BSAC, by a functional cloning to inhibit tumor necrosis factor-induced cell death. *The Journal of Biological Chemistry*. 2002;**277**:28853–28860.

293. **Li S, Chang S, Qi X, Richardson JA, Olson EN**. Requirement of a myocardin-related transcription factor for development of mammary myoepithelial cells. *Molecular and Cellular Biology*. 2006;**26**:5797–5808.

294. **Sun Y, Boyd K, Xu W**, *et al*. Acute myeloid leukemia-associated Mkl1 (Mrtf-a) is a key regulator of mammary gland function. *Molecular and Cellular Biology*. 2006;**26**:5809–5826.

295. **Raffel GD, Mercher T, Shigematsu H**, *et al*. Ott1(Rbm15) has pleiotropic roles in hematopoietic development. *Proceedings of the National Academy of Sciences of the United States of America*. 2007;**104**:6001–6006.

296. **Cairney AE, McKenna R, Arthur DC, Nesbit ME** Jr., **Woods WG**. Acute megakaryoblastic leukaemia in children. *British Journal of Haematology*. 1986;**63**:541–554.

297. **Ribeiro RC, Oliveira MS, Fairclough D**, et al. Acute megakaryoblastic leukemia in children and adolescents: a retrospective analysis of 24 cases. *Leukemia & Lymphoma*. 1993;**10**:299–306.

298. **Henry E, Walker D, Wiedmeier SE, Christensen RD**. Hematological abnormalities during the first week of life among neonates with Down syndrome: data from a multihospital healthcare system. *American Journal of Medical Genetics. Part A*. 2007;**143**:42–50.

299. **Hayashi Y, Eguchi M, Sugita K**, et al. Cytogenetic findings and clinical features in acute leukemia and transient myeloproliferative disorder in Down's syndrome. *Blood*. 1988;**72**:15–23.

300. **Penchansky L, Taylor SR, Krause JR**. Three infants with acute megakaryoblastic leukemia simulating metastatic tumor. *Cancer*. 1989;**64**:1366–1371.

301. **Pui CH, Rivera G, Mirro J**, et al. Acute megakaryoblastic leukemia. Blast cell aggregates simulating metastatic tumor. *Archives of Pathology & Laboratory Medicine*. 1985;**109**:1033–1035.

302. **Deutsch VR, Tomer A**. Megakaryocyte development and platelet production. *British Journal of Haematology*. 2006;**134**:453–466.

303. **Al-Kasim F, Doyle JJ, Massey GV, Weinstein HJ, Zipursky A**. Incidence and treatment of potentially lethal diseases in transient leukemia of Down syndrome: Pediatric Oncology Group Study. *Journal of Pediatric Hematology/Oncology*. 2002;**24**:9–13.

304. **Becroft DM, Zwi LJ**. Perinatal visceral fibrosis accompanying the megakaryoblastic leukemoid reaction of Down syndrome. *Paediatric Pathology*. 1990;**10**:397–406.

305. **Ruchelli ED, Uri A, Dimmick JE**, et al. Severe perinatal liver disease and Down syndrome: an apparent relationship. *Human Pathology*. 1991;**22**:1274–1280.

306. **Miyauchi J, Ito Y, Kawano T, Tsunematsu Y, Shimizu K**. Unusual diffuse liver fibrosis accompanying transient myeloproliferative disorder in Down's syndrome: a report of four autopsy cases and proposal of a hypothesis. *Blood*. 1992;**80**:1521–1527.

307. **Tomer A**. Human marrow megakaryocyte differentiation: multiparameter correlative analysis identifies von Willebrand factor as a sensitive and distinctive marker for early (2N and 4N) megakaryocytes. *Blood*. 2004;**104**:2722–2727.

308. **Carroll AJ, Crist WM, Link MP**, et al. The t(1;14)(p34;q11) is nonrandom and restricted to T-cell acute lymphoblastic leukemia: a Pediatric Oncology Group study. *Blood*. 1990;**76**:1220–1224.

309. **Massey GV, Zipursky A, Chang MN**, et al. A prospective study of the natural history of transient leukemia (TL) in neonates with Down syndrome (DS): Children's Oncology Group (COG) study POG-9481. *Blood*. 2006;**107**:4606–4613.

310. **Betz SA, Foucar K, Head DR, Chen IM, Willman CL**. False-positive flow cytometric platelet glycoprotein IIb/IIIa expression in myeloid leukemias secondary to platelet adherence to blasts. *Blood*. 1992;**79**:2399–2403.

311. **Dercksen MW, Weimar IS, Richel DJ**, et al. The value of flow cytometric analysis of platelet glycoprotein expression of CD34+ cells measured under conditions that prevent P-selectin-mediated binding of platelets. *Blood*. 1995;**86**:3771–3782.

312. **Litz CE, Davies S, Brunning RD**, et al. Acute leukemia and the transient myeloproliferative disorder associated with Down syndrome: morphologic, immunophenotypic and cytogenetic manifestations. *Leukemia*. 1995;**9**:1432–1439.

313. **Roche-Lestienne C, Dastugue N, Richebourg S**, et al. Acute megakaryoblastic leukemia with der(7)t(5;7)(q11;p11–p12) associated with Down syndrome: a fourth case report. *Cancer Genetics and Cytogenetics*. 2006;**169**:184–186.

314. **Kobayashi K, Usami I, Kubota M, Nishio T, Kakazu N**. Chromosome 7 abnormalities in acute megakaryoblastic leukemia associated with Down syndrome. *Cancer Genetics and Cytogenetics*. 2005;**158**:184–187.

315. **Ma SK, Lee AC, Wan TS, Lam CK, Chan LC**. Trisomy 8 as a secondary genetic change in acute megakaryoblastic leukemia associated with Down's syndrome. *Leukemia*. 1999;**13**:491–492.

316. **Honda F, Punnett HH, Charney E, Miller G, Thiede HA**. Serial cytogenetic and hematologic studies on a mongol with trisomy-21 and acute congenital leukemia. *The Journal of Pediatrics*. 1964;**65**:880–887.

317. **Lazarus KH, Heerema NA, Palmer CG, Baehner RL**. The myeloproliferative reaction in a child with Down syndrome: cytological and chromosomal evidence for a transient leukemia. *American Journal of Hematology*. 1981;**11**:417–423.

318. **Rogers PC, Kalousek DK, Denegri JF, Thomas JW, Baker MA**. Neonate with Down's syndrome and transient congenital leukemia. In vitro studies. *The American Journal of Pediatric Hematology/Oncology*. 1983;**5**:59–64.

319. **Coulombel L, Derycke M, Villeval JL**, et al. Characterization of the blast cell population in two neonates with Down's syndrome and transient myeloproliferative disorder. *British Journal of Haematology*. 1987;**66**:69–76.

320. **Adams RH, Lemons RS, Thangavelu M, Le Beau MM, Christensen RD**. Interstitial deletion of chromosome 5, del(5q), in a newborn with Down syndrome and an unusual hematologic disorder. *American Journal of Hematology*. 1989;**31**:273–279.

321. **Ghosh K**. Transient abnormal myelopoiesis in Down's syndrome – are some of them truly leukaemic? *Leukemia Research*. 1992;**16**:545–546.

322. **Zipursky A, Doyle J**. Leukemia in newborn infants with Down syndrome. *Leukemia Research*. 1993;**17**:195.

323. **Kounami S, Aoyagi N, Tsuno H**, et al. Additional chromosome abnormalities in transient abnormal myelopoiesis in Down's syndrome patients. *Acta Haematologica*. 1997;**98**:109–112.

324. **Shen JJ, Williams BJ, Zipursky A**, et al. Cytogenetic and molecular studies of Down syndrome individuals with leukemia. *American Journal of Human Genetics*. 1995;**56**:915–925.

325. **Groupe Français de Cytogénétique Hématologique**. Cytogenetic findings in leukemic cells of 56 patients with constitutional chromosome abnormalities. A cooperative study. *Cancer Genetics and Cytogenetics*. 1988;**35**:243–252.

326. **Pine SR, Guo Q, Yin C**, et al. GATA1 as a new target to detect minimal residual disease in both transient leukemia and megakaryoblastic leukemia of Down syndrome. *Leukemia Research*. 2005;**29**:1353–1356.

327. **Ballerini P, Blaise A, Mercher T**, *et al.* A novel real-time RT-PCR assay for quantification of OTT-MAL fusion transcript reliable for diagnosis of t(1;22) and minimal residual disease (MRD) detection. *Leukemia.* 2003; **17**:1193–1196.

328. **Dastugue N, Lafage-Pochitaloff M, Pages MP**, *et al.* Cytogenetic profile of childhood and adult megakaryoblastic leukemia (M7): a study of the Groupe Français de Cytogénétique Hématologique (GFCH). *Blood.* 2002;**100**:618–626.

329. **Duchayne E, Fenneteau O, Pages MP**, *et al.* Acute megakaryoblastic leukaemia: a national clinical and biological study of 53 adult and childhood cases by the Groupe Français d'Hématologie Cellulaire (GFHC). *Leukemia & Lymphoma.* 2003;**44**:49–58.

330. **Trejo RM, Aguilera RP, Nieto S, Kofman S**. A t(1;22)(p13;q13) in four children with acute megakaryoblastic leukemia (M7), two with Down syndrome. *Cancer Genetics and Cytogenetics.* 2000;**120**:160–162.

331. **Falini B, Mecucci C, Tiacci E**, *et al.* Cytoplasmic nucleophosmin in acute myelogenous leukemia with a normal karyotype. *The New England Journal of Medicine.* 2005;**352**:254–266.

332. **Morris SW, Kirstein MN, Valentine MB**, *et al.* Fusion of a kinase gene, ALK, to a nucleolar protein gene, NPM, in non-Hodgkin's lymphoma. *Science.* 1994;**263**:1281–1284.

333. **Falini B, Nicoletti I, Martelli MF, Mecucci C**. Acute myeloid leukemia carrying cytoplasmic/mutated nucleophosmin (NPMc+ AML): biologic and clinical features. *Blood.* 2007;**109**:874–885.

334. **Thiede C, Koch S, Creutzig E**, *et al.* Prevalence and prognostic impact of NPM1 mutations in 1485 adult patients with acute myeloid leukemia (AML). *Blood.* 2006;**107**:4011–4020.

335. **Brown P, McIntyre E, Rau R**, *et al.* The incidence and clinical significance of nucleophosmin mutations in childhood AML. *Blood.* 2007;**110**:979–985.

336. **Cazzaniga G, Dell'Oro MG, Mecucci C**, *et al.* Nucleophosmin mutations in childhood acute myelogenous leukemia with normal karyotype. *Blood.* 2005; **106**:1419–1422.

337. **Schnittger S, Schoch C, Kern W**, *et al.* Nucleophosmin gene mutations are predictors of favorable prognosis in acute myelogenous leukemia with a normal karyotype. *Blood.* 2005;**106**: 3733–3739.

338. **Mullighan CG, Kennedy A, Zhou X**, *et al.* Pediatric acute myeloid leukemia with NPM1 mutations is characterized by a gene expression profile with dysregulated HOX gene expression distinct from MLL-rearranged leukemias. *Leukemia.* 2007;**21**: 2000–2009.

339. **Chen W, Rassidakis GZ, Li J**, *et al.* High frequency of NPM1 gene mutations in acute myeloid leukemia with prominent nuclear invaginations ("cuplike" nuclei). *Blood.* 2006;**108**: 1783–1784.

340. **Mori Y, Yoshimoto G, Kumano T**, *et al.* Distinctive expression of myelomonocytic markers and down-regulation of CD34 in acute myelogenous leukaemia with FLT3 tandem duplication and nucleophosmin mutation. *European Journal of Haematology.* 2007;**79**:17–24.

341. **Chou WC, Tang JL, Wu SJ**, *et al.* Clinical implications of minimal residual disease monitoring by quantitative polymerase chain reaction in acute myeloid leukemia patients bearing nucleophosmin (NPM1) mutations. *Leukemia.* 2007;**21**:998–1004.

342. **Gorello P, Cazzaniga G, Alberti F**, *et al.* Quantitative assessment of minimal residual disease in acute myeloid leukemia carrying nucleophosmin (NPM1) gene mutations. *Leukemia.* 2006;**20**:1103–1108.

343. **Bisschop MM, Revesz T, Bierings M**, *et al.* Extramedullary infiltrates at diagnosis have no prognostic significance in children with acute myeloid leukaemia. *Leukemia.* 2001; **15**:46–49.

344. **Kobayashi R, Tawa A, Hanada R**, *et al.* Extramedullary infiltration at diagnosis and prognosis in children with acute myelogenous leukemia. *Pediatric Blood & Cancer.* 2007;**48**:393–398.

345. **Schwyzer R, Sherman GG, Cohn RJ, Poole JE, Willem P**. Granulocytic sarcoma in children with acute myeloblastic leukemia and t(8;21). *Medical and Pediatric Oncology.* 1998; **31**:144–149.

346. **Menasce LP, Banerjee SS, Beckett E, Harris M**. Extra-medullary myeloid tumour (granulocytic sarcoma) is often misdiagnosed: a study of 26 cases. *Histopathology.* 1999;**34**:391–398.

347. **Pileri SA, Ascani S, Cox MC**, *et al.* Myeloid sarcoma: clinico-pathologic, phenotypic and cytogenetic analysis of 92 adult patients. *Leukemia.* 2007;**21**: 340–350.

348. **Quintanilla-Martinez L, Zukerberg LR, Ferry JA, Harris NL**. Extramedullary tumors of lymphoid or myeloid blasts. The role of immunohistology in diagnosis and classification. *American Journal of Clinical Pathology.* 1995;**104**:431–443.

349. **Tiacci E, Pileri S, Orleth A**, *et al.* PAX5 expression in acute leukemias: higher B-lineage specificity than CD79a and selective association with t(8;21)-acute myelogenous leukemia. *Cancer Research.* 2004;**64**:7399–7404.

350. **Valbuena JR, Medeiros LJ, Rassidakis GZ**, *et al.* Expression of B cell-specific activator protein/PAX5 in acute myeloid leukemia with t(8;21)(q22;q22). *American Journal of Clinical Pathology.* 2006;**126**:235–240.

351. **Gibson SE, Dong HY, Advani AS, Hsi ED**. Expression of the B cell-associated transcription factors PAX5, Oct-2, and BOB.1 in acute myeloid leukemia: associations with B-cell antigen expression and myelomonocytic maturation. *American Journal of Clinical Pathology.* 2006;**126**:916–924.

Hematologic abnormalities in individuals with Down syndrome

John Kim Choi

Introduction

Down syndrome (DS) was first reported in 1866 [1], but likely recognized much earlier [2, 3]. DS is caused by an extra copy of chromosome 21 (whole or partial) and is the most common chromosomal abnormality in the live newborn, with a prevalence estimated at 1 in 644–733 births in the United States [4, 5]. This prevalence will likely change because of delayed maternity, which is associated with increased risk of DS [6], and because of simpler and less invasive prenatal diagnosis of DS [7, 8]. Patients with DS have numerous consistent and variable clinical presentations that include mental retardation, characteristic facies, congenital heart defects, and gastrointestinal abnormalities.

The hematologic abnormalities associated with DS and their diagnostic features are detailed in this chapter.

Hematologic abnormalities in the DS newborn

DS newborns can have transient thrombocytopenia, polycythemia, or neutrophilia. They rarely present with unexplained thrombocytosis, anemia, or neutropenia [5], which are most likely unrelated to DS.

Synonyms

Currently, no one has coined a unique term for this phenomenon and it is usually referred to descriptively as hematologic abnormalities in the newborn/neonates with DS [5, 9, 10]. This chapter will use the term *hematologic abnormalities in the newborn with DS (HANDS)*.

Epidemiology

Up to 80%, 66%, and 34% of DS newborns have neutrophilia, thrombocytopenia, and polycythemia, respectively [5, 9, 10]. These hematological abnormalities spontaneously resolve by three weeks of age [9].

Clinical features

In general, the hematologic abnormalities in newborns with DS are mild, and the clinical course is benign [5, 9, 10]. Neutrophilia rarely exceeds 30×10^9/L and is not associated with an infection. Thrombocytopenia is mild and not associated with bleeding. Only 6% of the patients have platelet counts $<50 \times 10^9$/L, while the majority have platelet counts $<150 \times 10^9$/L. Up to 34% of the DS newborns have polycythemia with hemoglobin greater than 65% (normal 40–65%) and hemoglobin greater than 22 g/dL (normal 13–22 g/dL). The polycythemia is unrelated to the cardiac defects and hypoxia that are frequently associated with DS. In some cases, DS newborns with unexplained polycythemia exhibit duskiness and cyanosis that correct with reduction/partial exchange transfusion.

Differential diagnosis

Important differentials for neutrophilia, thrombocytopenia, and polycythemia in the DS neonate include infection, platelet destructive processes, and congenital heart defects with hypoxia, respectively. Neutropenia, thrombocytosis, and anemia are rare in DS, and other causes unrelated to DS should be considered.

Uncharacterized issues

Hematologic abnormalities in DS remain poorly or not at all characterized in regards to morphology and immunophenotype. For example, what are the morphologic findings in the peripheral blood and marrow? With neutrophilia, do the myeloid cells show the characteristic morphology associated with reactive neutrophilia (toxic granulation, Döhle bodies, left-shifted maturation) or show different abnormalities as in some myeloproliferative disorders? With thrombocytopenia, are there giant platelets typical of compensatory or dysplastic thrombopoiesis? Do immunophenotypic abnormalities occur in neutrophils similar to those seen myelodysplastic syndrome [11–13] or in neonatal sepsis? The last of these is particularly

Diagnostic Pediatric Hematopathology, ed. Maria A. Proytcheva. Published by Cambridge University Press.
© Cambridge University Press 2011.

interesting because flow cytometry detection of CD64 expression in neutrophils is becoming more accepted as a biologic marker for neonatal sepsis [14–18].

The molecular mechanism for hematologic abnormalities in newborn DS is likely secondary to the extra copy of chromosome 21, and does not involve mutations to the gene *GATA1* that are seen in two other hematologic abnormalities of DS: transient abnormal myelopoiesis (TAM) and acute megakaryoblastic leukemia (AMKL) of DS. In support, *in vitro* studies of fetal liver hematopoietic precursor cells from aborted human fetuses with trisomy 21 but without *GATA1* mutations demonstrate altered hematopoiesis including increased numbers of erythro-megakryocyte progenitors [19, 20] and increased clonogenicity of CD34 [19]. The exact mechanism by which an extra copy of chromosome 21 leads to altered hematopoiesis is currently under study. Promising avenues of study are the murine models that exhibit many of the clinical features seen in patients with Down syndrome [21]. One murine model of trisomy 21, Ts65Dn, contains approximately 104 orthologs of 364 known genes of the human genes on chromosome 21, and demonstrates megakaryocytic hyperplasia and hematopoietic progenitor expansion [22], consistent with the human fetal liver studies. The Ts65Dn mouse also exhibits thrombocytosis and anemia, which is the opposite of what is usually seen in DS newborns [5, 9, 10], suggesting that some hematologic aspects of DS may not be amenable for study using this murine model.

Transient abnormal myelopoiesis (TAM)

TAM is defined as the morphologic detection of blasts in DS newborns less than three months of age. The blasts are of megakaryocytic origin in the vast majority of cases. In some cases, the megakaryoblasts are equal to or greater than 20% of the white blood cells in the peripheral blood, similar to acute megakaryoblastic leukemia (AMKL). Unlike AMKL, the megakaryoblasts in DS newborns often disappear without therapy by three months. This abnormal expansion of megakaryoblasts can initially present in the fetus [23–25], and may contribute to the 10% fetal demise associated with DS [26]. This disease entity is unique to DS newborns, and the latest WHO classification uses the designation TAM [27].

Synonyms

Other designations include transient myeloproliferative disorder (TMD) and transient leukemia (TL).

Epidemiology

TAM is usually detected in the first week of life and spontaneously resolves by three months of age. The incidence of TAM has been reported as high as 10% of all DS patients [28, 29]. However, more recent studies suggest that the percentage may be lower at 3 to 6% [5, 30, 31]. Even this percentage may not be

accurate because it does not account for cases of spontaneous fetal demise secondary to TAM [29].

Clinical features

The three largest studies to date examined the presentation of 264 patients with TAM [32–34]. The clinical presentation is variable. Some symptoms such as congenital heart disease and gastrointestinal anomalies are related to DS even in the absence of TAM. Other symptoms such as hepatosplenomegaly, effusions, and ascites are related to TAM. Although uncommon, TAM can be associated with severe diffuse lobular liver fibrosis that is associated with a high mortality rate [34–36]. TAM can also cause fetal hydrops [23–25, 34]. In contrast to all the complications, a significant portion of DS neonates (10–25%) present with only circulating blasts, with no clinical symptoms.

Morphology and cytochemistry

The percentage of blasts in TAM is usually similar or higher in the peripheral blood compared to the bone marrow, consistent with the current model that the blasts are of fetal derivation and normally reside in organs of fetal hematopoiesis such as the liver. Some cases with BM biopsies (uncommon at this age group) show few to no blasts despite the presence of numerous blasts in the peripheral blood and bone marrow aspirate smears, suggesting that blasts seen in the aspirate smears represent peripheral blood contaminants. Other bone marrow findings include megakaryocytic hyperplasia, dyspoietic megakaryocytes, and dyspoietic erythroid precursors [28, 29, 32]. Other cases show significant leukemic infiltrate of the bone marrow, skin, or liver. The histology of the liver shows increased extramedullary hematopoiesis, dysplastic megakaryocytes, and megakaryoblasts, associated with diffuse lobular fibrosis [32, 35, 36].

The blasts in TAM are medium to large sized (15 to 20 μm) with scant basophilic cytoplasm, occasional fine azurophilic granules consistent with platelet granules, and abundant cytoplasmic blebbing [29, 37] (Fig. 16.1). While TAM can have this classical megakaryoblastic morphology, including occasional binucleation and slightly round condensation of the chromatin, we have seen TAM blasts with morphologies that resemble lymphoblasts, erythroblasts, myeloblasts, and even monoblasts. Hence, the blasts in TAM are often difficult to distinguish from blasts in AML and even some ALL [38, 39].

By cytochemistry, the TAM blasts usually mark as megakaryoblasts. They are negative for Sudan black B, negative for myeloperoxidase, negative for chloroacetate esterase, occasionally granular to block positive for periodic acid–Schiff, and strongly positive for acid phosphatase (Fig. 16.2). The nonspecific esterase staining, depending on substrate used and reaction conditions, varies from negative to a multi-punctate pattern that is partially resistant to fluoride inhibition, but not the diffuse cytoplasmic pattern that is typical of monocytic differentiation [40]. In our experience, this multi-punctate staining pattern is extremely sensitive for megakaryoblasts, and

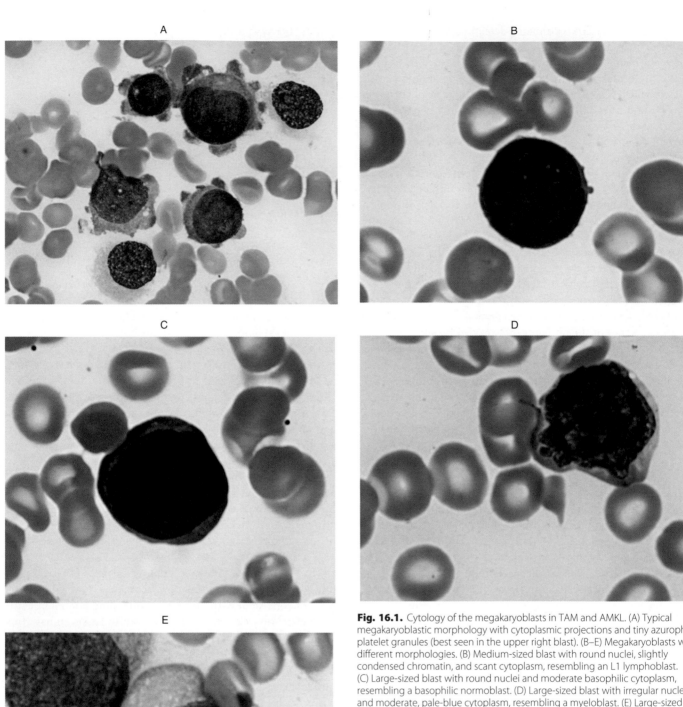

Fig. 16.1. Cytology of the megakaryoblasts in TAM and AMKL. (A) Typical megakaryoblastic morphology with cytoplasmic projections and tiny azurophilic platelet granules (best seen in the upper right blast). (B–E) Megakaryoblasts with different morphologies. (B) Medium-sized blast with round nuclei, slightly condensed chromatin, and scant cytoplasm, resembling an L1 lymphoblast. (C) Large-sized blast with round nuclei and moderate basophilic cytoplasm, resembling a basophilic normoblast. (D) Large-sized blast with irregular nuclei and moderate, pale-blue cytoplasm, resembling a myeloblast. (E) Large-sized blast with irregular nuclei, fine chromatin, and more abundant pale-blue cytoplasm, resembling a monoblast.

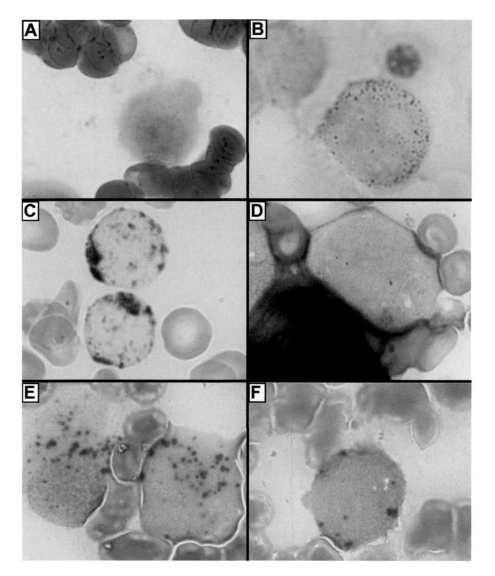

Fig. 16.2. Usual cytochemical staining patterns of megakaryoblasts in TAM and AMKL. (A) Sudan Black B. Similar negative staining is seen with myeloperoxidase and chloroacetate esterase. (B) Periodic acid–Schiff. (C) Acid phosphatase. (D) Non-specific esterase using conditions resulting in diffuse cytoplasmic staining of monocytes and macrophages. The megakaryoblast (center) is negative, while the macrophage (lower left) is strongly and diffusely positive. (E–F) Non-specific esterase using conditions resulting in multi-punctate staining of megakaryoblasts (E), which is partially resistant to sodium fluoride (F).

its absence virtually excludes AML M7. This staining pattern is relatively specific, although we have seen it on some precursor B-lymphoblastic leukemias.

On electron microscopy, most TAM blasts show cytoplasm with numerous small mitochondria, few dense granules, and few alpha granules, or demarcation membranes of megakaryocytic differentiation, while others show myeloperoxidase-positive or ferritin-containing granules [41]. By ultrastructural cytochemistry, the peroxidase activity is limited to the nuclear envelope and the endoplasmic reticulum, typical of megakaryocytic lineage; this pattern is usually referred to as the platelet peroxidase (PPO). PPO is performed in very few laboratories and has been largely replaced by flow cytometry.

Differential diagnosis

TAM with circulating blasts can be morphologically identical to acute leukemia (lymphoid or myeloid). In DS neonates less than three months of age, the diagnosis is almost always TAM.

However, the possibility that blasts are unrelated to DS cannot be completely excluded and other diagnoses such as congenital acute leukemia (myeloid or lymphoid) and myelodysplastic syndrome (MDS) need to be excluded. TAM should be considered in the differential even if DS is not suspected, because the patient may be a mosaic for trisomy 21 [42–44], and may not have the characteristic physical features. The distinction between TAM, congenital acute leukemia, and MDS can be made using immunophenotyping, cytogenetics, and molecular testing (Table 16.1).

Immunophenotype

The blasts in TAM are typically immunophenotyped by flow cytometry. TAM blasts are usually megakaryoblasts and express CD45, CD34, CD33, CD38, CD36, CD56, HLA-DR, CD7, and at least one of the megakaryocytic markers CD41, CD42a, or CD61 [32, 34, 45, 46]. Less frequently, the TAM blasts express CD13, CD11b, CD265 (glycophorin A), CD4, or CD15. In most

Table 16.1 Diagnostic approach for myeloid hematopoietic disorders in patients with suspected Down syndrome; distinctive features that aid in the diagnosis.

	HANDS	TAM	DS-MDS	DS-AML	Older DS-AML	non-DS-AML
Age[a]	0–3 wk	0–3 m	6–40 m	6 m–4 y	4–12 y	Any
Trisomy 21	Yes	Yes	Yes	Yes	Yes	9%
Increased blasts	No	Yes	Usually	Yes	Yes	Yes
FAB subtype	N/A	M7	N/A	M7 > M0–6	M0–6 > M7	M0–6 > M7
t(1;22)	?(likely no)	No	?(likely no)	No	No	2%
t(11q23)	?(likely no)	No	?(likely no)	No	No	20%
GATA1 mutation	?(likely no)	Yes	?(likely yes)	Yes	Some	Rare
JAK3 mutations	?(likely no)	Some	?(likely some)	Some	?	Some

[a] Age of the DS patient is an important distinguishing factor in the diagnosis of myeloid hematopoietic disorders. DS newborns can have either HANDS or TAM. HANDS consists of neutrophilia, thrombocytopenia, and polycythemia that usually have a benign clinical course and spontaneously resolve in three weeks. TAM consists of circulating peripheral blasts, usually has a benign clinical course and spontaneously remits before three months of age. Some TAM cases have complications leading to neonatal death; a subset of these respond to low-dose cytosine arabinoside therapy. The presence of Down syndrome/trisomy 21, megakaryocytic phenotype of the blasts, *GATA1* mutations, *JAK3* mutations, and the absence of t(1;22) and t(11q23) will favor TAM over congenital non-DS-AML. At six months or older, TAM is no longer a diagnostic possibility and DS with cytopenia or circulating blasts at this age should raise suspicions for DS-MDS or DS-AML. The same criteria used to distinguish TAM from congenital AML should be used to distinguish DS-AML from non-DS-AML. At age four or older, DS can present with AML that may lack *GATA1* mutations, unlike TAM and DS-AML.

Abbreviations: HANDS, hematologic abnormalities in the newborn with Down syndrome (DS); TAM, transient abnormal myelopoiesis; DS-MDS, DS-associated myelodysplastic syndrome; DS-AML, DS-associated acute myeloid leukemia; N/A, not applicable; wk = week, m = month, y = year; ? = no reports.

studies and in our experience, the TAM blasts do not express the more specific lymphoid markers such as CD3, CD5, CD19, and CD20. In contrast, one study suggests that TAM blasts may express specific lymphoid markers [32], but insufficient detail is presented to assess the validity of the expressions.

In general, flow cytometry detection of CD41, CD42b, or CD61 reactivity on blasts indicates megakaryocytic lineage. However, this reactivity can be seen on non-megakaryoblasts with platelet satellitosis [47], and on monoblasts. Platelet satellitosis can be excluded by examining the Wright-stained cytospin of the flow cytometry specimen, and in some laboratories by immunohistochemistry for CD61 on cytospin preparations [47]. The possibility of monoblasts can be detected by the expression of CD4, CD64, dim intracellular myeloperoxidase, and occasionally CD14, which are not expressed by megakaryoblasts; some megakaryoblasts may express isolated CD4. Lineage of the blasts can be also verified by non-specific esterase cytochemistry and platelet peroxidase electron-microscopy cytochemistry.

Genetics/molecular mechanisms

All TAM blasts contain extra copies of chromosome 21. In some patients, the TAM blasts have additional karyotypic abnormalities [32, 34]. Most abnormalities consist of complex karyotype or non-recurrent aberrations [34]. Given that TAM is seen in only a small subset of DS neonates, additional oncogenic events must collaborate with trisomy 21 to generate TAM. Recent flurrys of research have begun to identify these collaborative steps. All TAM blasts have various somatic mutations in the X-linked gene *GATA1* [48]. *GATA1* encodes a transcription factor that is critical for normal erythroid and megakaryocytic development [49]. Trisomy 21 and *GATA1* mutations are also present

in TAMs that present in neonates who are mosaic for trisomy 21 and lack the clinical feature of DS [50, 51]. A subset of TAM also has mutations in the tyrosine kinase *JAK3* [52, 53]. Additional unidentified mutations are likely present that contribute to the development of TAM.

Postulated cell of origin

The TAM blasts are thought to arise from a fetal hematopoietic progenitor cell, probably at the megakaryoblast or erythroblast–megakaryoblast progenitor stage of development. The possibility of an even earlier stage of development such as hematopoietic stem cell is currently under investigation.

Prognosis and predictive factors

In most DS neonates, TAM spontaneously resolves with the disappearance of blasts within 2 to 194 days, with a mean of 58 days [32, 54]. In 11–52% of DS neonates, TAM is associated with neonatal death secondary to liver failure, heart failure, sepsis, hemorrhage, hyperviscosity, and disseminated intravascular coagulation [32–34, 54, 55]. Death correlates with leukocytosis ($>100 \times 10^9$/L), increasing organomegaly, worsening liver function, renal failure, visceral effusions, hydrops fetalis, coagulopathy, prematurity, and low birth weight (<3 kg). Some patients with leukocytosis, ascites, preterm delivery, or bleeding responded favorably to low-dose cytosine arabinoside therapy [34].

After resolution of TAM, approximately 13 to 29% of the DS neonates develop acute megakaryocytic leukemia (AMKL) after 6 months of age, with a mean age of 20 months [32, 34, 54, 55]. In one study, additional cytogenetic abnormality beyond trisomy 21 increased the risk of developing AMKL [32], but this was not seen in another study [34]. Pleural effusion and

Table 16.2. Risk of leukemia in children without and with DS.

	Overall risk	Risk in DS	Excess risk in DS
Acute leukemia	1/2800	1/100–200	10–20×
ALL	1/3500	1/300	12×
AML	1/14 000	1/300	46×
AMKL	1/233 000	1/500	466×

Abbreviations: ALL, acute lymphoblastic leukemia; AML, acute myeloid leukemia; AMKL, acute megakaryoblastic leukemia. Modified from Lange [62].

thrombocytopenia ($<100 \times 10^9$/L) increase the risk of developing AMKL [34]; while CBC, percentage of blasts, AST (aspartate aminotransferase), ALT (alanine aminotransferase), age, and sex were not predictive [32].

Down syndrome-associated leukemias

Children with DS have increased incidence of both acute myeloid leukemia (AML) and acute lymphoid leukemia (ALL).

Epidemiology

Approximately 1 in 100–200 DS children develop acute leukemia [56–60], with roughly equal numbers of AML and ALL (Table 16.2). DS-associated AML (DS-AML) occurs at ages 6 months to 11.9 years [60, 61], with a median age of 2 years [60, 62]. Only 1–2% of DS-AML cases are diagnosed after 4 years of age [63]. The DS-associated AMKL subtype of AML occurs earlier, at ages ranging from 0 to 4.2 years [60]. In contrast, DS-associated ALL (DS-ALL) occurs throughout childhood (0 to 20.2 years), with a median age of greater than 4 years [60, 61]. Approximately 10–20% of DS-associated AMKL (DS-AMKL) cases have a preceding episode of TAM.

Clinical features

DS children with leukemia present with the same features associated with cytopenias as seen in non-DS children with leukemia. DS children with acute leukemia present with lower platelet counts than their non-DS counterparts [59, 64]. DS children with AML present with lower WBC counts and have increased preceding history of MDS [59]. DS children with ALL present with higher hemoglobin levels [64].

Morphology and cytochemistry

AML

Most DS-AMLs fulfill the FAB criteria for AMKL [58, 59, 65–68]. On aspirate smear, the morphology and cytochemical profile are similar to those seen for TAM (Figs. 16.1 and 16.2). Electron microscopic studies indicate that the megakaryoblasts in DS-AMKL have limited differentiation, with most blasts having no granules or lucent granules [41]. In contrast, TAM megakaryoblasts are of more variable differentiation, with some blasts showing alpha or dense granules [41].

On biopsy, DS-AMKL is similar to other acute myeloid leukemia, with increased numbers of mononuclear cells in a diffuse or interstitial pattern (Fig. 16.3). Often, the residual megakaryocytes are dysplastic with hypolobated or multinucleated nuclei. The megakaryoblasts can induce marrow fibrosis, resulting in a dry aspirate. Finally, AMKL can present as a nodule mimicking metastatic round blue cell tumor that may not be represented in the bone marrow aspirate smears because of minimal involvement of the specimen.

The diagnosis on biopsy alone is difficult because the current antibodies used for paraffin-fixed tissue against glycoprotein IIIa (CD61) and factor VIII related antigen (von Willebrand) may not be sufficiently sensitive to mark megakaryoblasts, although the more mature megakaryocytes are detected (Fig. 16.3). These antigens are acid labile and hence further compromised in a decalcified bone marrow biopsy. If possible, immunohistochemistry should be performed on a clot section that has not been decalcified. With only a biopsy, the diagnosis of M7 becomes a diagnosis of exclusion of other round blue cell tumors.

If an aspirate cannot be obtained, then touch imprints of the biopsy core could be used for cytochemical analysis or immunohistochemistry. Furthermore, additional biopsy cores should be submitted fresh in media, allowing the tumor cells to slowly suspend in the media with or without crushing of the core. The resulting supernatant can be analyzed as with an aspirate. In the case of a low-volume tumor, a directed biopsy and aspirate of a radiological abnormality can be tried; alternatively, time will increase the marrow and even peripheral blood involvement and a later biopsy and aspirate will provide sufficient numbers of cells.

Other DS-AMLs are classified as AML M0, M1, M2, M4, M5, or M6, but, in some cases, the blasts may still be megakaryoblasts, given the inherent shortcomings of the FAB classification, the variable morphology of megakaryoblasts, and the absence of megakaryocytic markers in the flow cytometry panel of many institutions. Non-AMKL AMLs do occur in DS children but they tend to occur in older children (>4 years old), and more resemble non-DS-AML [69]. Only one case of acute promyelocytic leukemia (APML) with the characteristic translocation has been reported in DS children, indicating that DS can both inhibit and promote the development of certain types of leukemias.

ALL

The aspirate and biopsy findings of DS-ALL are identical to those seen for other non-DS-associated ALL.

Immunophenotype

AML

Most DS-AMLs are of megakaryocytic origin and have similar immunophenotype to the TAM [45, 70, 71]. Higher frequencies of CD13 and CD11b expressions can be seen with DS-associated AMKLs compared to TAM [45].

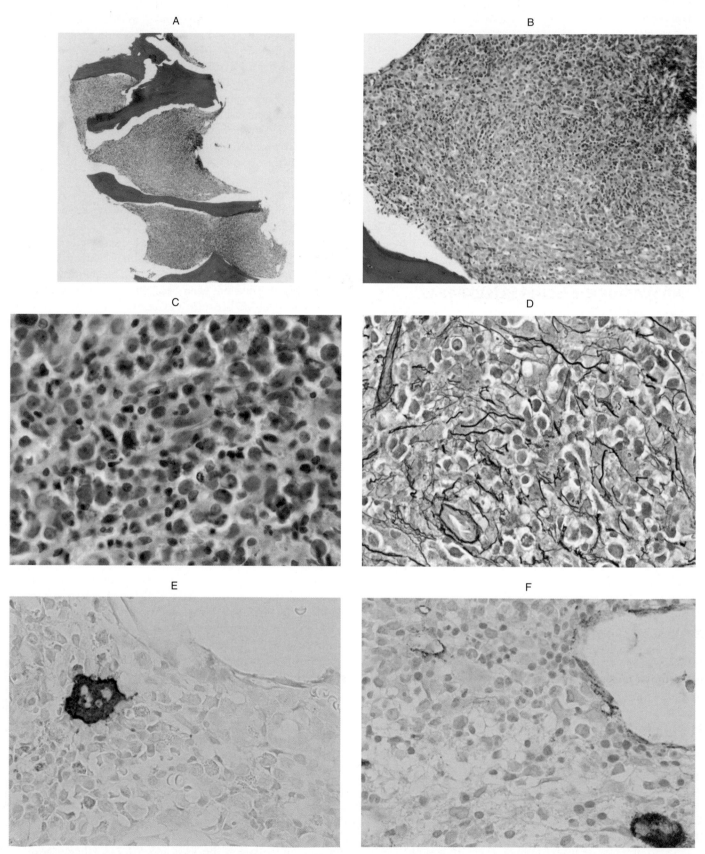

Fig. 16.3. Bone marrow biopsy findings in AMKL. (A–C) Extensive infiltration of the marrow by AMKL blasts (H&E stain). (D) Increased reticulin associated with the AMKL infiltrate (reticulin stain). (E–F) Immunohistochemistry stains for CD61 (E) and Factor VIII related antigen (F) are negative in the AMKL blasts, despite strong reactivities seen in megakaryocytes. (G–H) AMKL with an unusual nodular pattern of infiltration (H&E).

G

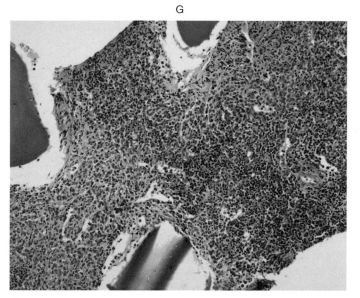

H

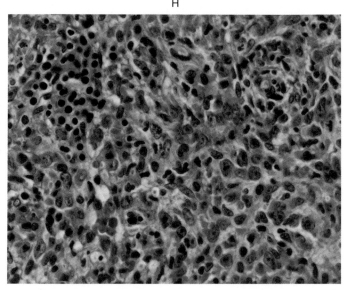

Fig. 16.3. (cont.)

ALL

Greater than 90% of the DS-ALLs are precursor B-lymphoblastic leukemia, with the remaining being precursor T-lymphoblastic leukemia [57, 60, 64, 68, 72, 73].

Genetics/molecular mechanisms

AML

Both DS- and non-DS-associated AMLs have similar frequency of normal, or constitutional, trisomy 21 karyotype (approximately 25%) [59]. In contrast, t(11q23), t(8;21), t(15;17), inv(16), and 16q22 in DS-AMLs are significantly less frequent compared to their non-DS counterparts [59, 60]. The frequencies of dup(1q), del(6q), del(7p), dup(7q), +8, +11, del(16q), +21, and −Y are increased in DS-AML compared to their non-DS counterparts [60]. The t(1;22), commonly seen in infant non-DS-associated AMKL [74, 75], is not seen in DS-AMKL or TAM [59, 60].

In addition to the similar morphology, immunophenotype, and karyotype of their blasts, TAM and most DS-AMKL also share similar molecular mechanisms. Both TAM and most DS-AMKL have trisomy 21 and *GATA1* mutations (reviewed in Vyas, Crispino [76]). Mutations in JAK3 have been identified in a small subset of the TMD and DS-AMKL [52, 53, 77, 78]. The DS-AMLs, including DS-AMKLs, that occur in patients four years or older, often lack *GATA1* mutation, suggesting that DS-AMLs in older children resemble the non-DS-AML counterparts [69].

Despite the similarities between the blasts of TAM and DS-AMKL, their clinical courses differ, suggesting fundamental molecular differences. Validating and identifying these differences would aid in the diagnosis and better understanding of these diseases. Toward these goals, transcription profiling of small numbers of TAM and DS-AMKL cases has identified mul-

Table 16.3 Partial list of transcripts with different expression levels in TAM versus DS-AMKL [79, 80] and DS-AMKL versus AMKL [81, 82].

	TAM vs. DS-AMKL	DS-AMKL vs. AMKL
MYCN	3.0 : 1.0 [80]	
CDKN2C	1.0 : 2.4 [80]	
PRAME	1.0 : > 20.0 [80]	
APOC1	1.0 : 4.2 [79]	1.0 : 5.0 [81]
TAP1	1.0 : 2.4 [79]	
SAT	1.0 : 3.0 [79]	
BACH1		2.0 : 1.0 [81]
BST2		1.0 : 7.3 [82]
BCL2		1.0 : 6.5 [82]

tiple transcripts with different expression levels [79, 80]; similar studies have identified differing transcripts in DS-AMKL versus non-DS AMKL [81, 82] (see Table 16.3 for a partial list).

Until these new markers become validated, clinical history, cytogenetics, and mutational analysis of GATA1 remain the best studies that distinguish among the megakaryoblasts of TAM, DS-AMKL, and AMKL (Table 16.1).

ALL

In half of the cases, DS-ALLs have normal constitutive karyotype [60, 83]. DS-ALL cases have decreased frequency of the common balanced translocations: t(12;21), t(1;19), t(11q23), and t(9;22), that are seen in non DS-ALL cases [60, 62, 64, 73, 84]. DS-ALL cases have increased frequencies of +21, +X, del(9p), and t(8;14)(q11;q32) [60, 85, 86]. The t(8;14), resulting in the fusion of the *CCAAT*/enhancer binding protein delta (*CEBPD*) gene with the IgH enhancer locus, is seen in 3% of DS-ALLs compared to 0.2% of non-DS-ALLs. Increased frequency of +8 was seen in one study [85], but not in another [60].

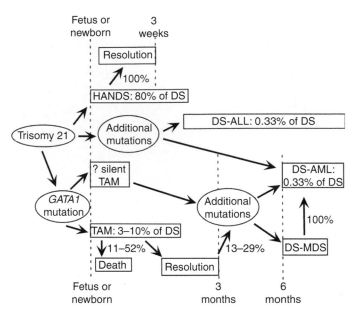

Fig. 16.4 Model of various hematopoietic abnormalities seen with DS. With trisomy 21, 80% have *hematologic abnormalities in the newborn DS* (HANDS) that spontaneously resolve within the first three weeks of life. Some DS patients acquire additional mutations and develop precursor B/T-lymphoblastic leukemia (DS-ALL) or acute myeloid leukemia (DS-AML). In DS-ALL, some cases have mutations more commonly associated with DS, such as *JAK2* mutations, +21, +X, del(9p), or t(8;14)(q11;q32), while others have mutations that are common to non-DS-ALL. In DS-AML, some cases have mutations that are common to non-DS-AML. More often, DS-AML occurs stepwise via accumulation of *GATA1* mutations followed by additional mutations. In such cases, DS with trisomy 21 is likely sufficient to lead to erythro-megakaryocytic proliferations. Acquisition of *GATA1* mutations leads to abnormal proliferation and circulation of myeloid (mostly megakaryocytic) blasts. Some of these probably escape clinical detection (? silent TAM), while others (3–10% of all DS patients) have detectible circulating blasts characteristic of transient abnormal myelopoiesis (TAM). Of the patients with TAM, 11–52% die, while the other cases spontaneously resolve within the first three months of life. After the resolution of TAM, 13–29% acquire additional mutations such as +8 or *JAK3* mutations, leading to either acute myeloid leukemia (DS-AML) or myelodysplastic syndrome (DS-MDS) that always progresses to DS-AML.

JAK2 mutations are present in 18–28% of DS-ALLs and appear to be absent in non-DS-ALLs [87–89]. The most common mutation alters the highly conserved arginine residue at position 683 (R683) that is within the pseudokinase domain. R683 mutations are distinct from the V617F mutation commonly seen in myeloproliferative disorders. Based on these findings, Malinge *et al.* proposed a model in which trisomy 21 may enhance proliferation of precursor B-progenitors and additional genetic events such as *JAK2* mutations or gain of extra chromosome X leading to precursor B-leukemogenesis [90].

Postulated cell of origin

AML

One model hypothesizes that most DS-AMKLs result from acquisition of additional genetic mutations in TAM; some TAMs are non-detectable without clinical symptoms, resulting in DS-AMKLs without an apparent preceding TAM (Fig. 16.4) [91].

ALL

DS-ALLs are of precursor B-lymphoblast derivation, similar to non-DS ALLs.

Prognosis and predictive factors

AML

DS-AMLs have a more favorable prognosis than non DS-AML (68% vs 35% four-year, event-free survival) provided that chemotherapy dosage is reduced to account for the higher toxicity in DS patients [59, 92]. Favorable prognosis is seen in patients <2 years of age (86% six-year, event-free survival compared to 64% for >2 years of age) [92]. Other variables such as rapid response to chemotherapy, cytogenetics, FAB classification (M7 vs. others), and WBC count are not significant predictors of outcome [59].

The favorable prognosis is likely due to increased sensitivity of the DS-AML blasts to cytosine arabinoside [93] because of decreased expression of cytidine deaminase (CDA), which inactivates cytosine arabinoside [94]. CDA is a potential target of GATA1 regulation, and GATA1 mutations seen in TMD and DS-AML likely decrease the expression of CDA [95].

ALL

DS-ALLs have a similar or worse prognosis compared to non-DS-ALLs [64, 73, 84]. The worse prognosis is partially secondary to decreased frequency of DS-ALLs with the favorable cytogenetics [t(12;21), hyperdiploidy, or triple trisomy of chromosomes 4, 10, and 17], because DS-ALLs have similar event-free survival to non-DS-ALLs that do not have the favorable cytogenetic findings [84]. However, the overall survival is decreased in DS-ALLs, probably because of limitations in using the more intense salvage therapy secondary to toxicity. Even the standard induction chemotherapy causes more toxicity (mucositis, hyperglycemia, and infection) in children with DS-ALLs.

DS-associated myelodysplastic syndrome (DS-MDS)

DS children can present with cytopenias, dyspoiesis, and fewer than 30% blasts in the peripheral blood or marrow, fulfilling the older FAB criteria for myelodysplastic syndrome. In some DS children, the blasts can be less than 20%, fulfilling the current WHO criteria for myelodysplastic syndrome. DS-MDSs all eventually evolve into DS-AML, and hence are usually treated the same as DS-AML.

Synonyms

The latest WHO classification and the European classification of pediatric myelodysplastic and myeloproliferative diseases do not distinguish between DS-AML and DS-MDS, grouping both as myeloid leukemia associated with DS [27, 96].

Epidemiology

Approximately 20% of the DS-AML is preceded by a history of MDS [59] that presents before 40 months of age [97].

Clinical features

Only one small study ($n = 16$) has detailed the clinical features [97]. All children with DS-MDS are clinically well at initial diagnosis and have increased blasts in the marrow (6–29% of the marrow cellularity). A subset have a history of TAM. Most present with isolated cytopenia or bicytopenia. The mean time interval for progression to AML is 6.3 months (ranging from 1 to 18 months).

Differential diagnosis

Cytopenia with unexplained increased blasts in a DS child is synonymous with DS-MDS. The only caveat is to exclude non-malignant causes of cytopenia and increased marrow blasts.

Morphology

Only one small study ($n = 11$) has detailed the marrow findings [97]. The biopsy shows increased numbers of small, monolobated megakaryocytes in most cases. The aspirate smears show occasional monolobated megakaryocytes with vacuolated cytoplasm. Myelofibrosis and dyserythropoiesis are frequently present. In our experience, we have seen focal megakaryocytic hyperplasia consisting of clusters of normal and hypolobated megakaryocytes with abnormal paratrabecular localization; findings that would be difficult to appreciate on marrow aspirate smears (Fig. 16.5).

Uncharacterized issues

Many questions remain for this poorly characterized DS-MDS. Are the clinical and morphologic findings described in one small series representative of this entity? Can DS-MDS present without increased blasts in bone marrow biopsy? We have seen cases in which a child with DS presents with unexplained cytopenia, increased dysplastic megakaryocytes, and normal blast counts, who eventually develops DS-AML

A

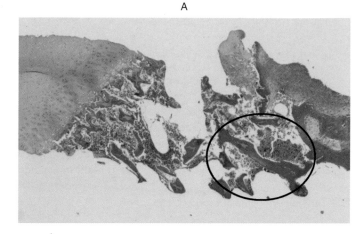

B

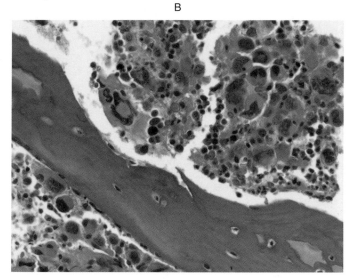

Fig. 16.5 (A, B) Focal megakaryocytic hyperplasia with megakaryocytic dysplasia (paratrabecular localization, clustering, and micromegakaryocytic forms) in a bone marrow biopsy of a six-month-old DS patient (H&E stain). The circled region in A contains the focal megakaryocytic hyperplasia represented in B. The patient had unexplained cytopenia, no increased blasts in the peripheral or bone marrow smears, and developed AMKL one month later.

(personal observations). Does the DS-MDS represent an intermediate step between TAM and DS-AML, permitting characterization of the additional genetic mutations that lead to DS-AML?

References

1. **Down J**. Observations on an ethnic classification of idiots. *London Hospital Clinical Lectures and Reports.* 1866;**3**: 259.

2. **Martinez-Frias ML**. The real earliest historical evidence of Down syndrome. *American Journal of Medical Genetics. Part A.* 2005;**132**(2):231.

3. **Levitas AS, Reid CS**. An angel with Down syndrome in a sixteenth century Flemish Nativity painting. *American Journal of Medical Genetics. Part A.* 2003;**116**(4):399–405.

4. **Centers for Disease Control and Prevention (CDC)**. Improved national prevalence estimates for 18 selected major birth defects – United States, 1999–2001. *MMWR. Morbidity and Mortality Weekly Report.* 2006;**54**(51): 1301–1305.

5. **Henry E, Walker D, Wiedmeier SE, Christensen RD**. Hematological abnormalities during the first week of life among neonates with Down syndrome: data from a multihospital healthcare system. *American Journal of Medical Genetics. Part A.* 2007; **143**(1):42–50.

6. **Hook EB, Cross PK, Schreinemachers DM**. Chromosomal abnormality rates at amniocentesis and in live-born infants. *JAMA.* 1983;**249**(15): 2034–2038.

7. **Oudejans CB, Go AT, Visser A**, *et al.* Detection of chromosome 21-encoded

mRNA of placental origin in maternal plasma. *Clinical Chemistry*. 2003;**49**(9): 1445–1449.

8. **Wataganara T, Bianchi DW.** Fetal cell-free nucleic acids in the maternal circulation: new clinical applications. *Annals of the New York Academy of Sciences*. 2004;**1022**:90–99.

9. **Miller M, Cosgriff JM.** Hematological abnormalities in newborn infants with Down syndrome. *American Journal of Medical Genetics*. 1983;**16**(2):173–177.

10. **Hord JD, Gay JC, Whitlock J.** Thrombocytopenia in neonates with trisomy 21. *Archives of Pediatrics & Adolescent Medicine*. 1995;**149**(7):824–825.

11. **Malcovati L, Della Porta MG, Lunghi M,** *et al.* Flow cytometry evaluation of erythroid and myeloid dysplasia in patients with myelodysplastic syndrome. *Leukemia*. 2005;**19**(5):776–783.

12. **Kussick SJ, Fromm JR, Rossini A,** *et al.* Four-color flow cytometry shows strong concordance with bone marrow morphology and cytogenetics in the evaluation for myelodysplasia. *American Journal of Clinical Pathology*. 2005;**124**(2):170–181.

13. **Wells DA, Benesch M, Loken MR,** *et al.* Myeloid and monocytic dyspoiesis as determined by flow cytometric scoring in myelodysplastic syndrome correlates with the IPSS and with outcome after hematopoietic stem cell transplantation. *Blood*. 2003;**102**(1): 394–403.

14. **Ng PC, Li G, Chui KM,** *et al.* Neutrophil CD64 is a sensitive diagnostic marker for early-onset neonatal infection. *Pediatric Research*. 2004;**56**(5):796–803.

15. **Fjaertoft G, Hakansson L, Ewald U, Foucard T, Venge P.** Neutrophils from term and preterm newborn infants express the high affinity Fcgamma-receptor I (CD64) during bacterial infections. *Pediatric Research*. 1999; **45**(6):871–876.

16. **Layseca-Espinosa E, Perez-Gonzalez LF, Torres-Montes A,** *et al.* Expression of CD64 as a potential marker of neonatal sepsis. *Pediatric Allergy and Immunology*. 2002;**13**(5):319–327.

17. **Skrzeczynska J, Kobylarz K, Hartwich Z, Zembala M, Pryjma J.** CD14+ CD16+ monocytes in the course of sepsis in neonates and small children:

monitoring and functional studies. *Scandinavian Journal of Immunology*. 2002;**55**(6):629–638.

18. **Ng PC, Li K, Wong RP,** *et al.* Neutrophil CD64 expression: a sensitive diagnostic marker for late-onset nosocomial infection in very low birthweight infants. *Pediatric Research*. 2002;**51**(3):296–303.

19. **Tunstall-Pedoe O, Roy A, Karadimitris A,** *et al.* Abnormalities in the myeloid progenitor compartment in Down syndrome fetal liver precede acquisition of GATA1 mutations. *Blood*. 2008;**112**(12):4507–4511.

20. **Chou ST, Opalinska JB, Yao Y,** *et al.* Trisomy 21 enhances human fetal erythro-megakaryocytic development. *Blood*. 2008;**112**(12):4503–4506.

21. **Wiseman FK, Alford KA, Tybulewicz VL, Fisher EM.** Down syndrome – recent progress and future prospects. *Human Molecular Genetics*. 2009;**18**(R1):R75–R83.

22. **Kirsammer G, Jilani S, Liu H,** *et al.* Highly penetrant myeloproliferative disease in the Ts65Dn mouse model of Down syndrome. *Blood*. 2008;**111**(2): 767–775.

23. **Robertson M, De Jong G, Mansvelt E.** Prenatal diagnosis of congenital leukemia in a fetus at 25 weeks' gestation with Down syndrome: case report and review of the literature. *Ultrasound in Obstetrics & Gynecology*. 2003;**21**(5):486–489.

24. **Smrcek JM, Baschat AA, Germer U, Gloeckner-Hofmann K, Gembruch U.** Fetal hydrops and hepatosplenomegaly in the second half of pregnancy: a sign of myeloproliferative disorder in fetuses with trisomy 21. *Ultrasound in Obstetrics & Gynecology*. 2001;**17**(5): 403–409.

25. **Zerres K, Schwanitz G, Niesen M,** *et al.* Prenatal diagnosis of acute non-lymphoblastic leukaemia in Down syndrome. *Lancet*. 1990; **335**(8681):117.

26. **Won RH, Currier RJ, Lorey F, Towner DR.** The timing of demise in fetuses with trisomy 21 and trisomy 18. *Prenatal Diagnosis*. 2005;**25**(7):608–611.

27. **Swerdlow SH, Campo E, Harris NL,** *et al.* (eds.). *WHO Classification of Tumours of Haematopoietic and Lymphoid Tissues* (4th edn.). Lyon: IARC Press; 2008, 439.

28. **Zipursky A, Brown E, Christensen H, Sutherland R, Doyle J.** Leukemia and/or myeloproliferative syndrome in neonates with Down syndrome. *Seminars in Perinatology*. 1997;**21**(1): 97–101.

29. **Zipursky A, Brown EJ, Christensen H, Doyle J.** Transient myeloproliferative disorder (transient leukemia) and hematologic manifestations of Down syndrome. *Clinics in Laboratory Medicine*. 1999;**19**(1):157–167, vii.

30. **Awasthi A, Das R, Varma N,** *et al.* Hematological disorders in Down syndrome: ten-year experience at a Tertiary Care Centre in North India. *Pediatric Hematology and Oncology*. 2005;**22**(6):507–512.

31. **Pine SR, Guo Q, Yin C,** *et al.* Incidence and clinical implications of GATA1 mutations in newborns with Down syndrome. *Blood*. 2007;**110**(6):2128–2131.

32. **Massey GV, Zipursky A, Chang MN,** *et al.* A prospective study of the natural history of transient leukemia (TL) in neonates with Down syndrome (DS): Children's Oncology Group (COG) study POG-9481. *Blood*. 2006;**107**(12): 4606–4613.

33. **Muramatsu H, Kato K, Watanabe N,** *et al.* Risk factors for early death in neonates with Down syndrome and transient leukaemia. *British Journal of Haematology*. 2008;**142**(4):610–615.

34. **Klusmann JH, Creutzig U, Zimmermann M,** *et al.* Treatment and prognostic impact of transient leukemia in neonates with Down syndrome. *Blood*. 2008;**111**(6):2991–2998.

35. **Miyauchi J, Ito Y, Kawano T, Tsunematsu Y, Shimizu K.** Unusual diffuse liver fibrosis accompanying transient myeloproliferative disorder in Down's syndrome: a report of four autopsy cases and proposal of a hypothesis. *Blood*. 1992;**80**(6):1521–1527.

36. **Ruchelli ED, Uri A, Dimmick JE,** *et al.* Severe perinatal liver disease and Down syndrome: an apparent relationship. *Human Pathology*. 1991;**22**(12):1274–8120.

37. **Jaffe ES, Harris NL, Stein H, Vardiman J.** *World Health Organization Classification of Tumours: Pathology and Genetics of Tumours of Haematopoietic and Lymphoid Tissues.* Lyon: IARC Press; 2001, 351.

38. **Weinstein HJ**. Congenital leukaemia and the neonatal myeloproliferative disorders associated with Down's syndrome. *Clinics in Haematology.* 1978;**7**(1):147–154.

39. **Ross JD, Moloney WC, Desforges JF**. Ineffective regulation of granulopoiesis masquerading as congenital leukemia in a mongoloid child. *Journal of Pediatrics.* 1963;**63**:1–10.

40. **Hayhoe FG, Quaglino D**. *Haematological Cytochemistry* (3rd edn.). New York: Churchill Livingston; 1994, 673.

41. **Eguchi M, Sakaibara H, Suda J**, *et al*. Ultrastructural and ultracytochemical differences between transient myeloproliferative disorder and megakaryoblastic leukaemia in Down's syndrome. *British Journal of Haematology.* 1989;**73**(3):315–322.

42. **Simon JH, Tebbi CK, Freeman AI**, *et al*. Acute megakaryoblastic leukemia associated with mosaic Down's syndrome. *Cancer.* 1987;**60**(10):2515–2520.

43. **Kalousek DK, Chan KW**. Transient myeloproliferative disorder in chromosomally normal newborn infant. *Medical and Pediatric Oncology.* 1987;**15**(1):38–41.

44. **Doyle JJ, Thorner P, Poon A**, *et al*. Transient leukemia followed by megakaryoblastic leukemia in a child with mosaic Down syndrome. *Leukemia & Lymphoma.* 1995;**17**(3–4):345–350.

45. **Karandikar NJ, Aquino DB, McKenna RW, Kroft SH**. Transient myeloproliferative disorder and acute myeloid leukemia in Down syndrome. An immunophenotypic analysis. *American Journal of Clinical Pathology.* 2001;**116**(2):204–210.

46. **Duchayne E, Fenneteau O, Pages MP**, *et al*. Acute megakaryoblastic leukaemia: a national clinical and biological study of 53 adult and childhood cases by the Groupe Français d'Hématologie Cellulaire (GFHC). *Leukemia & Lymphoma.* 2003;**44**(1):49–58.

47. **Betz SA, Foucar K, Head DR, Chen IM, Willman CL**. False-positive flow cytometric platelet glycoprotein IIb/IIIa expression in myeloid leukemias secondary to platelet adherence to blasts. *Blood.* 1992;**79**(9):2399–2403.

48. **Greene ME, Mundschau G, Wechsler J**, *et al*. Mutations in GATA1 in both transient myeloproliferative disorder and acute megakaryoblastic leukemia of Down syndrome. *Blood Cells, Molecules, and Diseases.* 2003;**31**(3):351–356.

49. **Orkin SH**. Hematopoiesis: how does it happen? *Current Opinion in Cell Biology.* 1995;**7**(6):870–877.

50. **Carpenter E, Valverde-Garduno V, Sternberg A**, *et al*. GATA1 mutation and trisomy 21 are required only in haematopoietic cells for development of transient myeloproliferative disorder. *British Journal of Haematology.* 2005;**128**(4):548–551.

51. **Cushing T, Clericuzio CL, Wilson CS**, *et al*. Risk for leukemia in infants without Down syndrome who have transient myeloproliferative disorder. *Journal of Pediatrics.* 2006;**148**(5):687–689.

52. **De Vita S, Mulligan C, McElwaine S**, *et al*. Loss-of-function JAK3 mutations in TMD and AMKL of Down syndrome. *British Journal of Haematology.* 2007;**137**(4):337–341.

53. **Kiyoi H, Yamaji S, Kojima S, Naoe T**. JAK3 mutations occur in acute megakaryoblastic leukemia both in Down syndrome children and non-Down syndrome adults. *Leukemia.* 2007;**21**(3):574–576.

54. **Homans AC, Verissimo AM, Vlacha V**. Transient abnormal myelopoiesis of infancy associated with trisomy 21. *The American Journal of Pediatric Hematology/Oncology.* 1993;**15**(4):392–399.

55. **Isaacs H Jr**. Fetal and neonatal leukemia. *Journal of Pediatric Hematology/Oncology.* 2003;**25**(5):348–361.

56. **Fong CT, Brodeur GM**. Down's syndrome and leukemia: epidemiology, genetics, cytogenetics and mechanisms of leukemogenesis. *Cancer Genetics and Cytogenetics.* 1987;**28**(1):55–76.

57. **Robison LL, Nesbit ME Jr., Sather HN**, *et al*. Down syndrome and acute leukemia in children: a 10-year retrospective survey from Childrens Cancer Study Group. *Journal of Pediatrics.* 1984;**105**(2):235–242.

58. **Creutzig U, Ritter J, Vormoor J**, *et al*. Myelodysplasia and acute myelogenous leukemia in Down's syndrome. A report of 40 children of the AML-BFM Study Group. *Leukemia.* 1996;**10**(11):1677–1686.

59. **Lange BJ, Kobrinsky N, Barnard DR**, *et al*. Distinctive demography, biology, and outcome of acute myeloid leukemia and myelodysplastic syndrome in children with Down syndrome: Children's Cancer Group Studies 2861 and 2891. *Blood.* 1998;**91**(2):608–615.

60. **Forestier E, Izraeli S, Beverloo B**, *et al*. Cytogenetic features of acute lymphoblastic and myeloid leukemias in pediatric patients with Down syndrome: an iBFM-SG study. *Blood.* 2008;**111**(3):1575–1583.

61. **Ross JA, Spector LG, Robison LL, Olshan AF**. Epidemiology of leukemia in children with Down syndrome. *Pediatric Blood and Cancer.* 2005;**44**(1):8–12.

62. **Lange B**. The management of neoplastic disorders of haematopoiesis in children with Down's syndrome. *British Journal of Haematology.* 2000;**110**(3):512–524.

63. **Hasle H**. Pattern of malignant disorders in individuals with Down's syndrome. *The Lancet Oncology.* 2001;**2**(7):429–436.

64. **Whitlock JA, Sather HN, Gaynon P**, *et al*. Clinical characteristics and outcome of children with Down syndrome and acute lymphoblastic leukemia: a Children's Cancer Group study. *Blood.* 2005;**106**(13):4043–4049.

65. **Ravindranath Y, Abella E, Krischer JP**, *et al*. Acute myeloid leukemia (AML) in Down's syndrome is highly responsive to chemotherapy: experience on Pediatric Oncology Group AML Study 8498. *Blood.* 1992;**80**(9):2210–2214.

66. **Kuerbitz SJ, Civin CI, Krischer JP**, *et al*. Expression of myeloid-associated and lymphoid-associated cell-surface antigens in acute myeloid leukemia of childhood: a Pediatric Oncology Group study. *Journal of Clinical Oncology.* 1992;**10**(9):1419–1429.

67. **Creutzig U, Harbott J, Sperling C**, *et al*. Clinical significance of surface antigen expression in children with acute myeloid leukemia: results of study AML-BFM-87. *Blood.* 1995;**86**(8):3097–3108.

68. **Levitt GA, Stiller CA, Chessells JM**. Prognosis of Down's syndrome with acute leukaemia. *Archives of Disease in Childhood.* 1990;**65**(2):212–216.

69. Hasle H, Abrahamsson J, Arola M, *et al.* Myeloid leukemia in children 4 years or older with Down syndrome often lacks GATA1 mutation and cytogenetics and risk of relapse are more akin to sporadic AML. *Leukemia.* 2008;**22**(7):1428–1430.

70. Yumura-Yagi K, Hara J, Kurahashi H, *et al.* Mixed phenotype of blasts in acute megakaryocytic leukaemia and transient abnormal myelopoiesis in Down's syndrome. *British Journal of Haematology.* 1992;**81**(4):520–525.

71. Litz CE, Davies S, Brunning RD, *et al.* Acute leukemia and the transient myeloproliferative disorder associated with Down syndrome: morphologic, immunophenotypic and cytogenetic manifestations. *Leukemia.* 1995;**9**(9): 1432–1439.

72. Ragab AH, Abdel-Mageed A, Shuster JJ, *et al.* Clinical characteristics and treatment outcome of children with acute lymphocytic leukemia and Down's syndrome. A Pediatric Oncology Group study. *Cancer.* 1991; **67**(4):1057–1063.

73. Dordelmann M, Schrappe M, Reiter A, *et al.* Down's syndrome in childhood acute lymphoblastic leukemia: clinical characteristics and treatment outcome in four consecutive BFM trials. Berlin-Frankfurt-Munster Group. *Leukemia.* 1998;**12**(5):645–651.

74. Ma Z, Morris SW, Valentine V, *et al.* Fusion of two novel genes, RBM15 and MKL1, in the t(1;22)(p13;q13) of acute megakaryoblastic leukemia. *Nature Genetics.* 2001;**28**(3):220–221.

75. Mercher T, Busson-Le Coniat M, Khac FN, *et al.* Recurrence of OTT-MAL fusion in t(1;22) of infant AML-M7. *Genes, Chromosomes & Cancer.* 2002;**33**(1):22–28.

76. Vyas P, Crispino JD. Molecular insights into Down syndrome-associated leukemia. *Current Opinion in Pediatrics.* 2007;**19**(1):9–14.

77. Malinge S, Ragu C, Della-Valle V, *et al.* Activating mutations in human acute megakaryoblastic leukemia. *Blood.* 2008;**112**(10):4220–4226.

78. Walters DK, Mercher T, Gu TL, *et al.* Activating alleles of JAK3 in acute megakaryoblastic leukemia. *Cancer Cell.* 2006;**10**(1):65–75.

79. Lightfoot J, Hitzler JK, Zipursky A, Albert M, Macgregor PF. Distinct gene signatures of transient and acute megakaryoblastic leukemia in Down syndrome. *Leukemia.* 2004;**18**(10): 1617–1623.

80. McElwaine S, Mulligan C, Groet J, *et al.* Microarray transcript profiling distinguishes the transient from the acute type of megakaryoblastic leukaemia (M7) in Down's syndrome, revealing PRAME as a specific discriminating marker. *British Journal of Haematology.* 2004;**125**(6):729–742.

81. Bourquin JP, Subramanian A, Langebrake C, *et al.* Identification of distinct molecular phenotypes in acute megakaryoblastic leukemia by gene expression profiling. *Proceedings of the National Academy of Sciences of the United States of America.* 2006;**103**(9): 3339–3344.

82. Ge Y, Dombkowski AA, LaFiura KM, *et al.* Differential gene expression, GATA1 target genes, and the chemotherapy sensitivity of Down syndrome megakaryocytic leukemia. *Blood.* 2006;**107**(4):1570–1581.

83. Berger R. Acute lymphoblastic leukemia and chromosome 21. *Cancer Genetics and Cytogenetics.* 1997;**94**(1):8–12.

84. Bassal M, La MK, Whitlock JA, *et al.* Lymphoblast biology and outcome among children with Down syndrome and ALL treated on CCG-1952. *Pediatric Blood and Cancer.* 2005;**44**(1): 21–28.

85. Pui CH, Raimondi SC, Borowitz MJ, *et al.* Immunophenotypes and karyotypes of leukemic cells in children with Down syndrome and acute lymphoblastic leukemia. *Journal of Clinical Oncology.* 1993;**11**(7):1361–1367.

86. Lundin C, Heldrup J, Ahlgren T, Olofsson T, Johansson B. B-cell precursor t(8;14)(q11;q32)-positive acute lymphoblastic leukemia in children is strongly associated with Down syndrome or with a concomitant Philadelphia chromosome. *European Journal of Haematology.* 2009;**82**(1): 46–53.

87. Kearney L, Gonzalez De Castro D, Yeung J, *et al.* Specific JAK2 mutation (JAK2R683) and multiple gene deletions in Down syndrome acute lymphoblastic leukemia. *Blood.* 2009; **113**(3):646–648.

88. Malinge S, Ben-Abdelali R, Settegrana C, *et al.* Novel activating JAK2 mutation in a patient with Down syndrome and B-cell precursor acute lymphoblastic leukemia. *Blood.* 2007; **109**(5):2202–2204.

89. Bercovich D, Ganmore I, Scott LM, *et al.* Mutations of JAK2 in acute lymphoblastic leukaemias associated with Down's syndrome. *Lancet.* 2008;**372**(9648):1484–1492.

90. Malinge S, Izraeli S, Crispino JD. Insights into the manifestations, outcomes, and mechanisms of leukemogenesis in Down syndrome. *Blood.* 2009;**113**(12):2619–2628.

91. Vyas P, Roberts I. Down myeloid disorders: a paradigm for childhood preleukaemia and leukaemia and insights into normal megakaryopoiesis. *Early Human Development.* 2006; **82**(12):767–773.

92. Gamis AS. Acute myeloid leukemia and Down syndrome evolution of modern therapy – state of the art review. *Pediatric Blood and Cancer.* 2005;**44**(1): 13–20.

93. Zwaan CM, Kaspers GJ, Pieters R, *et al.* Different drug sensitivity profiles of acute myeloid and lymphoblastic leukemia and normal peripheral blood mononuclear cells in children with and without Down syndrome. *Blood.* 2002; **99**(1):245–251.

94. Ge Y, Stout ML, Tatman DA, *et al.* GATA1, cytidine deaminase, and the high cure rate of Down syndrome children with acute megakaryocytic leukemia. *Journal of the National Cancer Institute.* 2005;**97**(3):226–231.

95. Taub JW, Huang X, Matherly LH, *et al.* Expression of chromosome 21-localized genes in acute myeloid leukemia: differences between Down syndrome and non-Down syndrome blast cells and relationship to in vitro sensitivity to cytosine arabinoside and daunorubicin. *Blood.* 1999;**94**(4): 1393–1400.

96. Hasle H, Niemeyer CM, Chessells JM, *et al.* A pediatric approach to the WHO classification of myelodysplastic and myeloproliferative diseases. *Leukemia.* 2003;**17**(2):277–282.

97. Zipursky A, Thorner P, De Harven E, Christensen H, Doyle J. Myelodysplasia and acute megakaryoblastic leukemia in Down's syndrome. *Leukemia Research.* 1994; **18**(3):163–171.

17

Precursor lymphoid neoplasms

Mihaela Onciu

Definition

B- and T-lymphoblastic leukemias/lymphomas comprise a family of malignant lymphoid neoplasms that morphologically and immunophenotypically recapitulate the features of early lymphoid precursors of B- or T-lineage, respectively [1]. By convention, neoplasms with predominant extramedullary involvement (defined as lacking bone marrow involvement or replacing less than 25% of the marrow cellularity) are classified as lymphoblastic lymphomas (LBLs). The remaining cases, showing bone marrow involvement of 25% or more, are staged and treated as acute lymphoblastic leukemias (ALL).

Epidemiology

Acute leukemias represent the most common type of pediatric cancer (31% of all childhood malignancies). Approximately 85% of all pediatric acute leukemias are ALLs [2]. In children, ALL shows a peak of incidence between the ages of two and five years [3]. The annual standardized rate for ALL per million population for children aged 0 to 14 years varies by geographic region, ranging from 16–18 in India and China, to 38–41 in the United States and Canada, to 46 in Costa Rica [2]. There is a slight male predominance (male : female ratio 1.2–1.5) and a striking excess incidence among white children (with the standardized rate for pediatric ALL in the United States being 20 for black children and 38 for white children) [3]. Acute lymphoblastic leukemia occurs with increased frequency in patients with certain genetic syndromes, including Down syndrome, Bloom syndrome, neurofibromatosis type 1, and ataxia telangiectasia [4]. Increased susceptibility to ALL appears to be related to certain histocompatibility groups, including HLA-DRB1*04, DQA1*0101/*0104, and DQB1*0501 (the last two in males only) [5]. Exposure *in utero* to certain environmental factors such as ionizing radiation, pesticides, and solvents has also been related to an increased risk for childhood leukemia [2]. In fact, compelling scientific evidence has demonstrated the presence of leukemia-specific fusion genes, or immunoglobulin and clonal immunoglobulin gene rearrangements in neona-tal spot (Guthrie) cards or patients who later developed ALL [6, 7].

Clinical presentation and laboratory features

The clinical onset is most often acute in children with ALL, although a small percentage of cases may develop insidiously over several months [8]. The presenting symptoms and signs typically reflect the leukemic cell burden and the degree of marrow replacement. The most common symptoms include fever (which may be caused by leukemia or secondary infections related to neutropenia), fatigue and lethargy (as a result of anemia), bone and joint pain, manifested as limping and refusal to walk, and a bleeding diathesis (due to thrombocytopenia). Patients with precursor T-cell ALL/LBL often present with a mediastinal mass that may cause respiratory distress and other signs of superior vena cava syndrome. Frequent findings on physical examination include hepatosplenomegaly, lymphadenopathy, pallor, petechiae and ecchymoses, and bone tenderness. In a minority of patients there might be ocular involvement, testicular enlargement due to leukemic infiltrates, signs of spinal cord or cranial nerve compression, enlarged tonsils and adenoids, or signs of appendicitis. Patients with extensive marrow necrosis may present with severe bone pain and tenderness, fever and very high serum lactate dehydrogenase (LDH) levels [8]. The most common laboratory abnormalities in ALL include anemia, thrombocytopenia, neutropenia, and abnormal leukocyte counts. The last of these includes leukocytosis or leukopenia, with hyperleukocytosis ($> 100 \times 10^9$/L) present in approximately 15% of the patients [8]. Of note, patients with T-cell ALL may show normal peripheral blood counts in spite of significant marrow involvement. Patients with normal or decreased leukocyte counts may show circulating leukemic blasts or may lack evidence of leukemic involvement. Other common laboratory abnormalities include elevated serum uric acid and LDH levels, correlating with the tumor burden. Imaging studies may indicate the presence of a mediastinal mass and of pleural effusions in patients with precursor T-lymphoblastic tumors.

Diagnostic Pediatric Hematopathology, ed. Maria A. Proytcheva. Published by Cambridge University Press.
© Cambridge University Press 2011.

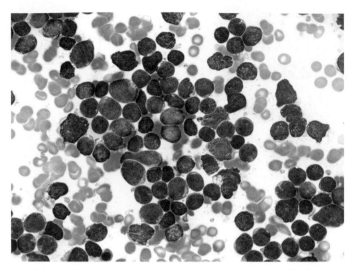

Fig. 17.1. ALL L1 (FAB classification), the most common morphologic type of pediatric ALL (Wright–Giemsa stain).

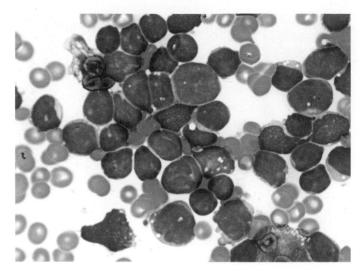

Fig. 17.2. Prominent nuclear clefts present in the blasts in a case of precursor B-cell ALL. There is no correlation between nuclear membrane irregularity and lineage of ALL (Wright–Giemsa stain).

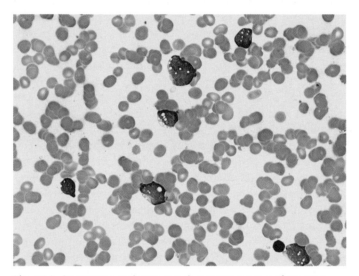

Fig. 17.3. Prominent cytoplasmic vacuoles present in a case of precursor B-cell ALL harboring the *ETV6-RUNX1* fusion gene, with ALL L1-type morphology (Wright–Giemsa stain).

Diagnostic features

Morphology

Acute lymphoblastic leukemias have a spectrum of morphologic features shared by B-lineage and T-lineage tumors. The first attempts at classifying these leukemias, made in the 1970s by the French–American–British (FAB) system [9–11], were based on the morphologic features of blood and bone marrows from untreated patients, and defined three subgroups, termed ALL L1, L2, and L3. Currently, these subgroups do not have clinical significance, as they do not correlate with the lineage or risk category, and therefore are no longer widely used. However, familiarity with their morphologic features remains important in recognizing an acute leukemia as lymphoid before immunophenotypic studies are completed, and for initiating

the appropriate differential diagnostic workup. The latter aspect is especially important in the differential diagnosis of ALL and the leukemic phase of Burkitt lymphoma, which may occasionally constitute a challenge, and has major implications for clinical management. Most pediatric ALLs (up to 85%) present with morphologic features of ALL L1 (Fig. 17.1) [9, 11, 12]. This morphologic subtype is characterized by predominantly small blast cells (up to twice the diameter of a small lymphocyte or red cell), with scanty, slightly or moderately basophilic cytoplasm, dark homogeneous nuclear chromatin, regular or cleaved and indented nuclear outlines (Fig. 17.2), and absent or small and inconspicuous nucleoli. Acute lymphoblastic leukemias that consist predominantly of large blasts but have all the other features can still be classified as ALL L1. In some cases, the blasts may contain variable numbers of cytoplasmic vacuoles (Fig. 17.3) [13, 14]. When seen in hematoxylin and eosin (H&E)-stained sections of bone marrow biopsies and other involved tissues, these leukemias consist of diffuse infiltrates of small, homogeneous lymphoid blasts with finely dispersed nuclear chromatin and small "pinpoint" nucleoli (Fig. 17.4).

The ALL L2 subtype is only present in approximately 14% of pediatric ALL (while more prevalent in adult patients) (Fig. 17.5) [11]. In this subtype, most of the blast cells are large (exceeding twice the size of a small lymphocyte), with significant heterogeneity in size and shape. Most cells show variable amounts of lightly to deeply basophilic cytoplasm, finely dispersed to coarsely condensed nuclear chromatin, often prominent nuclear clefting, indentation, and folding, and variable numbers of often prominent nucleoli. Some of the cases may show variable cytoplasmic vacuolization [13, 14]. This subtype typically raises the differential diagnosis of acute myeloid leukemia and biphenotypic leukemia. When seen in tissue sections, these leukemic blasts may resemble myeloid sarcoma infiltrates, as the blasts are larger, with vesicular nuclear chromatin and prominent eosinophilic nucleoli (Fig. 17.6).

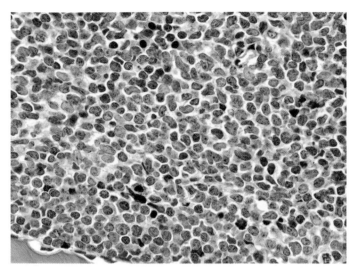

Fig. 17.4. Bone marrow biopsy sample showing ALL infiltrating and replacing the normal marrow cellularity; the blasts have characteristic lymphoid features, including small size, irregular nuclear outlines, finely dispersed nuclear chromatin and inconspicuous nucleoli. This appearance corresponds to the ALL L1 subtype seen in aspirate smears (H&E stain).

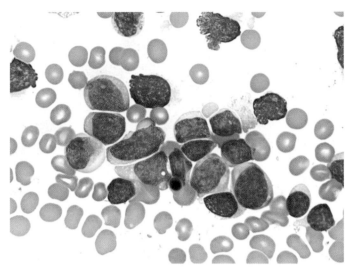

Fig. 17.5. ALL L2 (FAB classification), a less common appearance of pediatric ALL, that raises the differential diagnosis with acute myeloid leukemia (Wright–Giemsa stain).

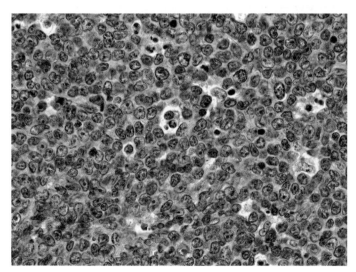

Fig. 17.6. Bone marrow biopsy sample showing ALL extensively replacing the normal marrow cellularity; the blasts are larger than those seen in Figure 17.4, with vesicular chromatin and frequent single nucleoli. This appearance corresponds to the ALL L2 subtype seen in aspirate smears, and raises the differential diagnosis with acute myeloid leukemia or myeloid sarcoma (Wright–Giemsa stain).

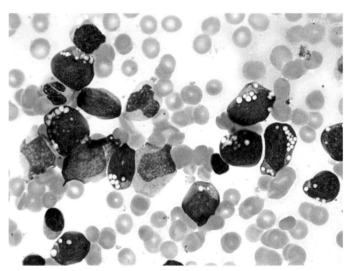

Fig. 17.7. ALL L3 (FAB classification) in a case of leukemic bone marrow involvement by Burkitt lymphoma, the most common association of this morphologic ALL subtype. Rare cases of precursor B-cell ALL with similar morphology may occur (see Figure 17.8). (Wright–Giemsa stain.)

The ALL L3 (Burkitt type) subtype is most commonly associated with leukemic bone marrow involvement by Burkitt lymphoma (so-called Burkitt leukemia; Fig. 17.7). However, occasional cases of precursor B-cell and T-cell ALL may present with similar morphologic features (Fig. 17.8). These cases are characterized by relatively homogeneous, large cells with deeply basophilic cytoplasm, which surrounds the nucleus completely and contains prominent vacuoles. They have dense and finely stippled nuclear chromatin, round or oval nuclei with regular contours, and one to several prominent nucleoli. Mitotic figures, some containing vacuoles, are frequent. Of note, in cases cor-

responding to the atypical variant of Burkitt lymphoma, the leukemic cells may be large and pleomorphic, with bi- or multi-nucleation and macronucleoli. For a detailed description of Burkitt lymphoma, the reader is referred to Chapter 20.

When bone marrow biopsy sections are examined, the marrow is typically hypercellular, with most of the normal cellularity replaced by sheets of leukemic blasts (Fig. 17.9). In cases of precursor T-cell LBL, the marrow cellularity may be largely preserved, while the leukemic blasts form non-paratrabecular aggregates of variable size. A subset of precursor B-cell ALLs may present with associated marrow fibrosis [15] that leads to hypocellular aspirate smears and may raise the differential diagnosis with acute megakaryoblastic leukemia and other non-hematopoietic neoplasms. These features are most commonly

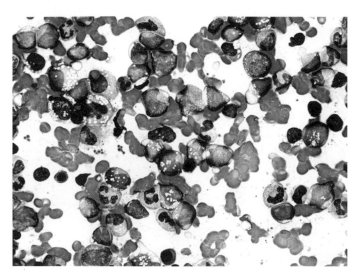

Fig. 17.8. Precursor B-cell ALL with hypodiploid (near-haploid) karyotype and morphologic features resembling those of the ALL L3 subtype. Such cases raise the differential diagnosis with Burkitt lymphoma (Wright–Giemsa stain).

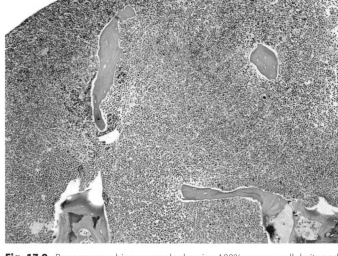

Fig. 17.9. Bone marrow biopsy sample showing 100% marrow cellularity and diffuse replacement of the normal cellularity by sheets of leukemic blasts, in a case of precursor B-cell ALL (H&E stain).

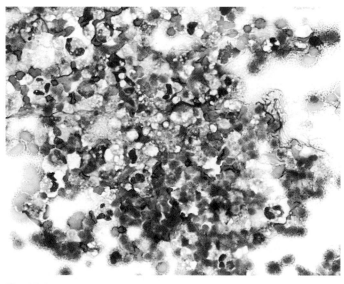

Fig. 17.10. Necrotic marrow particle in a bone marrow aspirate containing extensively necrotic ALL. Such cases may render diagnostic evaluation extremely difficult (Wright–Giemsa stain).

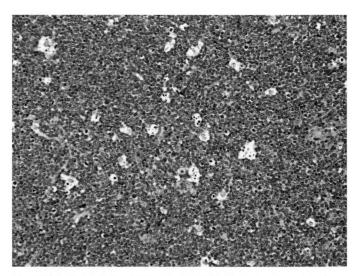

Fig. 17.11. Precursor T-cell ALL extensively infiltrating a lymph node and showing a diffuse growth pattern and a "starry sky" appearance imparted by scattered tingible body macrophages (H&E stain).

seen in hyperdiploid precursor B-cell ALL (see below). Acute lymphoblastic leukemia may also present with extensive marrow necrosis (Fig. 17.10), which may render the diagnosis difficult. Such cases may require sampling at several sites (e.g., anterior and posterior iliac crests) to obtain viable diagnostic material. Finally, rare cases of ALL may be preceded by transient bone marrow aplasia/aplastic anemia, where immunophenotypic studies may or may not uncover a population of abnormal lymphoblasts. In such cases, the bone marrow aplasia is followed by ALL within 6–15 months, typically at the time of count recovery [16, 17].

In tissues other than bone marrow, the lymphoblastic leukemic infiltrates obstruct the underlying architecture diffusely, occasionally with a partial "starry sky" appearance

(Fig. 17.11). In partially replaced lymph nodes, T-cell LBL may have an interfollicular pattern of infiltration, similar to other T-cell lymphomas. In skin lesions, lymphoblastic infiltrates diffusely infiltrate the dermis and the underlying adipose tissue, while sparing the epidermis, often with an uninvolved "Grenz zone" present in the papillary dermis (Fig. 17.12).

Several morphologic variants have been described. *Granular ALLs* are lymphoblastic leukemias with L1 or L2 morphology, that show small, azurophilic or pale-pink cytoplasmic granules in a variable proportion (typically at least 5%) of their blast cells (Fig. 17.13A) [18–22]. Granules are seen in the blasts of 5–7% of the pediatric ALL [19, 20], appear to correlate closely with a precursor B-cell immunophenotype [18, 22], although they can also be seen in T-lineage ALL, are more commonly associated with the L2 subtype, and have no prognostic

A   B

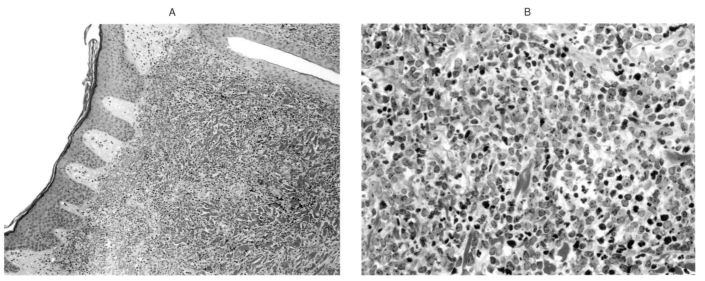

Fig. 17.12. Precursor B-cell ALL infiltrating skin, where it involves predominantly the deeper dermis, with sparing of the epidermis and papillary dermis (A), and prominent percolation of leukemic cells between collagen bundles (A and B). (H&E stain.)

A   B

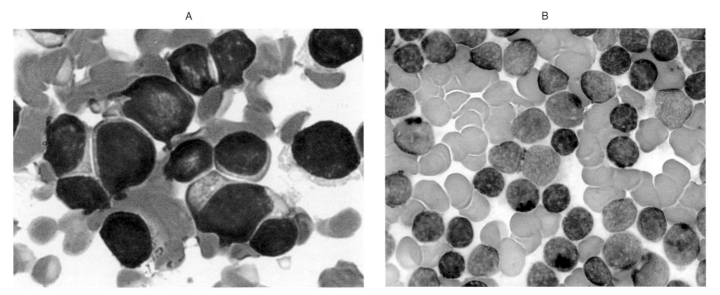

Fig. 17.13. Acute lymphoblastic leukemia with cytoplasmic granules (so-called "granular ALL"). The granules have a pale-pink color on the Wright–Giemsa stain (A) and are often positive for non-specific esterase (alpha-naphthyl butyrate esterase) (B).

significance. Rare cases of *ALL with giant cytoplasmic inclusions* have been described in children and adults (Fig. 17.14) [18, 23, 24]. These appear to represent extreme forms of granular ALL, whereby the blasts contain large (0.8–1.4 μm), rounded eosinophilic inclusions, that may be positive for periodic acid–Schiff (PAS) and non-specific esterases. Ultrastructurally, these inclusions appear to be derived from mitochondria. No prognostic significance has been associated with this morphologic variant. *Hand-mirror cell variant ALLs* are characterized by the presence of eccentric uropod-like cytoplasmic projections in at least 5–10 % of the blasts, which may have L1- or L2-type nuclear features (Fig. 17.15) [14, 25]. When defined in this manner, this variant represents 5–23% of pediatric ALL

[14, 25, 26]. It may be associated with any immunophenotypic subtype, although it is slightly more common in T-lineage ALL [14], and has no prognostic significance.

Acute lymphoblastic leukemia with eosinophilia is a subtype of precursor B-cell ALL in which the leukemic blasts are associated with numerous often dysplastic eosinophils that may obscure the acute leukemic component, occasionally leading to a misdiagnosis or hypereosinophilic syndrome [27]. In fact, this disease subtype may lead to a clinical picture similar to that associated with the hypereosinophilic syndrome [28]. In such cases, eosinophilia may also precede and announce an overt leukemia (at diagnosis or relapse). The eosinophils associated with these leukemias may show abnormal nuclear

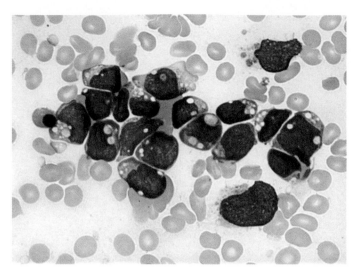

Fig. 17.14. Unusual large cytoplasmic inclusions in a case of precursor B-cell ALL (Wright–Giemsa stain).

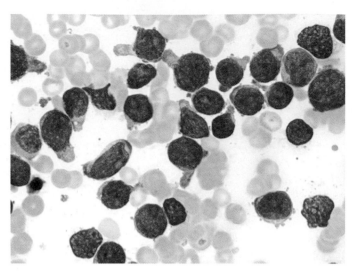

Fig. 17.15. Acute lymphoblastic leukemia with "hand mirror" morphology. Many of the leukemic cells have an eccentric uropod-like cytoplasmic extension (Wright–Giemsa stain).

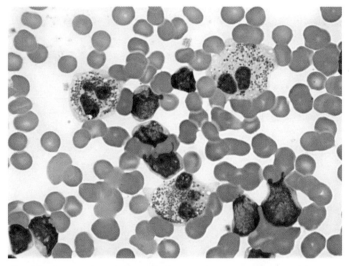

Fig. 17.16. Acute lymphoblastic leukemia with associated eosinophilia, showing lymphoid leukemic blasts and frequent dysplastic large and hypogranular eosinophils (Wright–Giemsa stain).

lobation and hypogranularity (Fig. 17.16). The blasts may have L1 or L2 morphology, and may occasionally contain granules [29]. These leukemias are typically associated with the t(5;14)(q31;q32), which leads to overexpression of the *IL3* gene located on chromosome 5q31, as a result of its rearrangement to the *IgH* gene at 14q32. This is the postulated mechanism for eosinophilia. A rare case associated with deletions of chromosomes 5 (5q) and 7 (7q) has also been reported [30]. Rare cases of T-lymphoblastic lymphoma with associated eosinophilia and the *FIP1L1-PDGFRA* fusion gene have been described [31].

Ultrastructural findings

On electron microscopy, the L1-type blasts show a high nuclear to cytoplasm ratio. Their sparse cytoplasm contains scattered organelles, including small mitochondria, a moderately sized

Golgi region, polyribosomes, rare strands of rough endoplasmic reticulum, occasional lipid inclusions, clusters of glycogen-like material, and small, electron-dense granules. These cells have peripherally condensed and clumped chromatin and typically small, but easily identified, nucleoli. The L2 blasts contain more abundant cytoplasm, but have similar cytoplasmic contents. Their nucleoli are large and may be multiple. In granular ALL cases, the granules are membrane-bound structures that contain small vesicles, glycogen-like particles, and membranous lamellae and scrolls, resembling mast cell or basophil granules. In some cases of granular ALL, the cells contain single-membrane-bound inclusions, 1.5–2.5 μm in diameter, that contain amorphous, electron-dense material [32].

Cytochemical features

While not widely used at the present time, cytochemical stains may still be informative in the diagnosis of ALL. The ALL blasts, regardless of their morphologic subtype, are typically negative for myeloperoxidase, chloroacetate esterase, Sudan black B (SBB), and non-specific esterases (NSEs). Acute lymphoblastic leukemia blasts frequently express PAS (75%) and acid phosphatase (the latter most often in T-cell ALL cases) [32]. The PAS cytoplasmic positivity seems to be associated with coarsely granular glycogen deposits [32]. In granular ALL cases, weak non-specific esterase staining may be present, localized to the granules (Fig. 17.13B) [18]; some of the latter cases may also be associated with SBB staining of the granules. These findings do not appear to have a prognostic significance. However, in rare cases of otherwise typical precursor B-cell or precursor T-cell ALL, MPO and SBB stains may highlight small numbers of leukemic blasts and even rare Auer rods. The significance of such findings is unclear at this time, since, in most of these cases, these cells cannot be identified by flow cytometry due to their low percentage, thus precluding a diagnosis of mixed-lineage leukemia. Such cases are managed clinically as ALLs, with variable degrees of success (author's unpublished observation).

Immunophenotypic features

Lymphoblastic neoplasms comprise two major immunophenotypic subgroups that correlate with distinct clinical and biologic features: B-lymphoblastic leukemia/lymphoma, and T-cell lymphoblastic leukemia/lymphoma [1]. These subgroups are identified according to their resemblance to normal lymphoid precursors, and can be further subdivided into immunophenotypic subgroups based on their resemblance to various stages of maturation encountered in the normal immune system. In addition to features similar to the normal corresponding precursors, the leukemic lymphoblasts also show immunophenotypic aberrancies that may include expression of normally encountered lymphoid antigens at abnormal intensity or by an abnormal proportion of cells, or expression of lineage-inappropriate (i.e., myeloid-associated) antigens. These aberrancies are extremely useful in the differential diagnosis with reactive expansions of benign lymphoid precursors (further detailed below).

Precursor B-cell neoplasms typically express B-lineage antigens including CD19, CD22 (surface and cytoplasmic), CD20, CD24, CD79a (cytoplasmic), and PAX-5 (the last of these evaluated by immunohistochemistry only) (Fig. 17.17). Expression of CD20, a mature B-cell antigen, in ALL may be very weak and even absent, which limits its use for B-lineage determination in paraffin-embedded tissues. In this context, antigens such as CD22, CD79a, and PAX-5 are much more useful for documenting B-lineage. Since CD79a may also be weakly expressed in T-ALL and in some acute myeloid leukemias, PAX-5 might be a better choice for this purpose. The latter is a nuclear B-lineage-specific antigen, expressed throughout B-cell ontogeny and lost only at the plasma cell stage. It appears to be highly specific for B-lineage neoplasms [33], with the notable exception of acute myeloid leukemias with the t(8;21), which may also express other B-lymphoid antigens, including CD19, CD79a, and TdT [34]. PAX-5 expression has also been reported in an exceedingly rare case of peripheral T-cell lymphoma [35], and, outside the realm of hematopoietic malignancies, in Merkel cell carcinoma, other neuroendocrine carcinomas [36–39], and a variety of other subtypes of carcinomas [37, 39, 40]. Of these neoplasms, Merkel cell carcinoma may be the most relevant in the differential diagnosis with B-lymphoblastic lymphoma, as this type of neoplasm, virtually absent in the pediatric cell population, has also been found to express TdT [41]. Precursor B-cell ALL may also show expression of immunoglobulin (Ig) molecules. According to this parameter, B-ALL can be subclassified into early pre-B- (pro-B-) ALL (absent Ig expression), pre-B-ALL (expression of cytoplasmic Igμ heavy chain only), and transitional (late) pre-B-ALL (expression of cytoplasmic and surface Igμ without Ig light chain expression or restriction). Very rare cases of otherwise classical precursor B-ALL may express complete surface IgM with light chain restriction. These cases

have to be differentiated from true mature B-cell leukemias, notably Burkitt leukemia/lymphoma. Most of the precursor B-ALLs express terminal deoxynucleotidyl transferase (TdT), a nuclear antigen specific for normal early lymphoid precursors (Fig. 17.17). Also, many pediatric ALLs express the common ALL antigen (CALLA, CD10). In addition, early precursor-associated antigens, such as CD133, CD34, HLA-DR, and CD99 are commonly present. CD45 (leukocyte common antigen) is typically expressed in B-ALL at levels lower then those seen on normal lymphocytes. Importantly, a significant percentage of pediatric precursor B-cell ALLs, especially those with hyperdiploid karyotypes (which represent 25–30% of all cases) may be CD45 negative. This becomes important in the differential diagnosis with other small blue cell tumors in tissue biopsies, where a CD45-negative, CD99-positive lymphoblastic infiltrate may be misdiagnosed as Ewing sarcoma. Including TdT in the panels used for the evaluation of such samples is typically very helpful. Myeloid antigens most commonly expressed in B-lymphoid tumors include CD11b, CD13, CD15, and CD33. These antigens have no impact on prognosis. In ALL expressing several myeloid antigens, mixed-lineage leukemia has to be considered in the differential diagnosis (see below).

Precursor T-cell neoplasms typically express T-lineage associated antigens, including CD1a, CD2, CD3 (most commonly cytoplasmic, while often weak or absent on the blast surface), CD5, CD7, and CD4 and/or CD8. Expression of CD3 is mandatory for a diagnosis of T-ALL/LBL. These CD3-positive neoplasms can be further subclassified according to their resemblance to stages of normal T-cell maturation. The EGIL (European Group for the Immunological Characterization of Leukemias) classification of T-ALL [1, 42] includes the following categories (see Table 17.1): pro-T (T-I) (CD7+, CD2−, CD5−, CD8−, CD1a−), pre-T (T-II) (CD2+ and/or CD5+, and/or CD8+, CD1a−), cortical T (T-III) (CD1a+, often CD4+ and CD8+), and mature T (post-thymic, T-IV) (CD1a−, surface CD3+, T-cell receptor αβ+ or γδ+, typically CD4+ or CD8+). It appears that T-LBLs are at late stages of late intrathymic maturation more often than T-ALLs. Many T-ALLs may express CD10, TdT, CD34, and HLA-DR. Of note, approximately 10% of T-ALLs may be negative for TdT, CD34, and HLA-DR, raising the differential diagnosis with mature (peripheral) T-cell lymphomas. In these cases, the clinical presentation (e.g., mediastinal mass), blastic morphology, and expression of CD10 may be helpful in establishing the correct diagnosis. CD45 expression in T-ALL is typically stronger than that seen in the B-ALL cases. CD45 expression, while most often weaker than seen in normal lymphocytes, occasionally may be equal in intensity, with complete overlap by flow cytometry, requiring distinct gating strategies. Myeloid antigen expression may also be seen in T-ALL. The myeloid antigens most often expressed include CD13, CD33, and CD11b. Rare cases express numerous myeloid antigens, including CD117. These cases seem to also show other recurrent immunophenotypic aberrancies (e.g., weaker CD5 expression), and appear to have a significantly less favorable prognosis than the typical T-ALL.

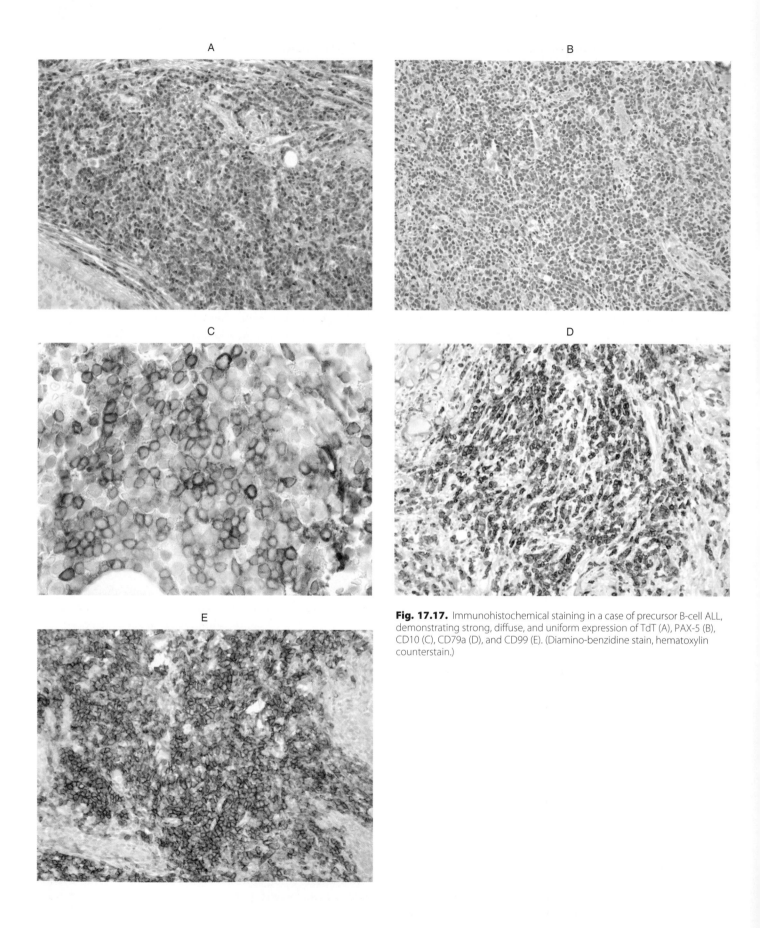

A

B

C

D

Fig. 17.17. Immunohistochemical staining in a case of precursor B-cell ALL, demonstrating strong, diffuse, and uniform expression of TdT (A), PAX-5 (B), CD10 (C), CD79a (D), and CD99 (E). (Diamino-benzidine stain, hematoxylin counterstain.)

E

Table 17.1. Subclassification of T-ALL, according to stage of maturation.

T-ALL Subtype	CD1a	CD2	cyCD3	sCD3	CD4	CD5	CD7	CD8	CD34
Pro-T (T-I)	−	−	+	−	−	−	+	−	+/−
Pre-T (T-II)	−	+/−	+	−	−	+/−	+	−	+/−
Cortical T (T-III)	+	+	+	−	+	+	+	+	−
Mature (medullary) T (T-IV)	−	+	+	+	+/−[a]	+	+	+/−[a]	−

[a] Mature T-cell and T-ALL express either CD4 or CD8.
Abbreviations: cyCD3, cytoplasmic CD3; sCD3, surface CD3.

Cytogenetic and molecular abnormalities

Immunoglobulin (*IG*) and T-cell receptor (*TCR*) gene rearrangements

Rearrangements of *IG* and/or *TCR* genes are present in the vast majority of ALL/LBL. Of note, these rearrangements may not be lineage specific, with *TCR* rearrangements present in B-ALL [43, 44], and *IG* rearrangements present in T-ALL [45]. Furthermore, 10–15% of acute myeloid leukemias may contain *IG* and/or *TCR* rearrangements[46–48]. This is likely due to continuous recombinase activity in the malignant hematopoietic cells [49]. Therefore, these gene rearrangements should not be used in isolation to determine the lineage of a leukemic process.

Precursor B-ALLs contain *IG* gene rearrangements in most cases (97%), involving the heavy chain gene (*IGH;* >95%), kappa light chain gene (*IGK;* 30%), or lambda light chain gene (*IGL;* 20%) [45]. These rearrangements may frequently be oligoclonal, rather than monoclonal (multiple *IGH* rearrangements present in 30–40%, multiple *IGK* rearrangements in 5–10%) [50]. In addition, lineage-inappropriate *TCR* rearrangements and/or deletions, involving the *TCR* –β, –γ, and/or –δ genes may be present in 35%, 55%, and 90% of the cases, respectively [44]. These may also be biclonal or oligoclonal in a small number of cases (*TCRβ* in 3%, *TCRγ* in 10%) [45]. The mechanisms for oligoclonality in these neoplasms may include continuing rearrangement processes [49] and secondary rearrangements. These mechanisms likely account for changes in the rearrangement patterns of *IG* and *TCR* genes that are often seen in B-ALL at relapse [44]. The type and pattern of *IG* and *TCR* gene rearrangements correlate with the patient's age [51].

Precursor T-ALL/LBLs frequently contain *TCR* gene rearrangements (95–100%). A lower frequency is observed in the rare pro-T-ALLs that have all *TCR* genes in a germline configuration in about 10% of the cases [45]. T-ALLs that are TCRαβ+ contain *TCRβ* (100%) and *TCRγ* (100%) gene rearrangements and have at least one deleted *TCRδ* allele (resulting from the necessary *TCRα* rearrangement), while the second allele is also deleted in 65% of the cases. T-ALLs that are TCRγδ+ have *TCRβ* and *TCRγ* rearrangements (100% of the cases for each), and most (95%) also contain *TCRβ* rearrangements. *IG* gene rearrangements are only encountered in ∼20% of T-ALLs and involve *IGH* genes, typically as incomplete (D_H–J_H) rearrangements. As opposed to B-ALL, oligoclonality is only rarely seen in diagnostic T-ALL samples [45, 52]. In relapse samples, T-ALL may show secondary rearrangements in 15 to 20% of the cases, for *TCRγ* and *TCRβ*, respectively [52].

Molecular and cytogenetic subgroups of precursor B-cell ALL

Pediatric precursor B-ALLs include several cytogenetic subgroups with distinct biologic and pharmacologic features [1] that are very important in the modern risk stratification of these patients, and therefore in the therapeutic approach to be taken (see Table 17.2). These subgroups account for ∼60–80% of cases, and can be identified by means of conventional cytogenetics, molecular diagnostics (RT-PCR), flow cytometry (cell cycle analysis/DNA index), and, currently in preclinical trials, gene expression profiling using oligonucleotide arrays. The remaining ALL cases are still characterized only on the basis of the morphologic and immunophenotypic features. Gene expression profiling studies have shown that these cytogenetic subgroups, although largely similar in morphology and immunophenotype, have vastly different gene expression signatures [53, 54]. In addition, they have distinct *in vitro* sensitivities to drugs [55–57], which correlate with different patterns of drug-metabolizing enzyme gene expression [58]. Genome-wide genetic analyses using single nucleotide polymorphism arrays and genomic DNA sequencing have found that these cytogenetic subgroups are also characterized by distinct alterations in genes encoding principal regulators of B-lymphocyte development and differentiation [59].

Hyperdiploid ALLs represent the most common cytogenetic subgroup of pediatric ALL (27–29%). These are ALLs with a modal chromosomal number of 51–65 chromosomes, corresponding to a DNA index of 1.16–1.6. Occasional cases (<1%) have near-triploid or near-tetraploid karyotypes. Approximately half of these leukemias have only numeric chromosomal changes, including, most commonly, recurring additions of chromosomes 21, 6, X, 14, 4, 18, 17, and 10. The remaining cases also have structural abnormalities that include, most

Table 17.2. Genetic subtypes important in the risk stratification of pediatric precursor B-cell acute lymphoblastic leukemia.

Cytogenetic lesion	Molecular lesion (fusion gene)	Immunophenotype	Frequency (% of pediatric ALL)	Prognostic (risk) group
Hyperdiploid (>50 chromosomes) Common trisomies: 4, 10, 18, 21	Not known	CD45− or dim+, CD10+	27–29	Low risk
t(21;21)(p13;q22)	*TEL/AML1 (ETV6/RUNX1)*	clgμ−, CD10+, CD13+, CD33+	22–25	Low risk
t(1;19)(q23;p13)	*E2A/PBX1 (TCF3/PBX1)*	clgμ+, CD20−, CD34−/dim, CD9+	3–6	Standard risk
t(9;22)(q34;q11.2) (Philadelphia chromosome)	*BCR-ABL*	No distinctive phenotype	2–3	High risk
t(4;11)(q21;q23)	*AF4/MLL*	clgμ-, CD10-, sCD22-, CD15+, CD65+, NG2+	2–3[a]	High risk
Hypodiploid (<46 chromosomes)	Not known	No distinctive phenotype	5–6	High risk

[a] This type of leukemia represents 50–80% of ALL occurring in infants (children younger than one year of age).

often, duplications of chromosome 1q and isochromosome 17q. Rare cases may show a hyperdiploid karyotype associated with the t(9;22) or the t(1;19). These cases should be assigned to the cytogenetic subgroups corresponding to these last two translocations (see below). Hyperdiploid ALLs are associated with low leukemic cell counts at diagnosis, and good response to therapy [8]. These features are possibly related to an increased propensity of the leukemic blasts to undergo apoptosis, to accumulate higher concentrations of methotrexate polyglutamates, and to a higher sensitivity to methotrexate and mercaptopurine *in vitro* [55, 60]. This feature is at least partially related to increased gene dosage of the reduced methotrexate carrier gene located on chromosome 21 (typically present as three to four copies in these cases) [61]. Genetic studies have shown that, as opposed to other cytogenetic subgroups of ALL, hyperdiploid cases only rarely harbor mutations in B-cell development genes (13%) [59].

ALL with the t(12;21)(p13;q22) TEL/AML1 (or ETV6/RUNX1) fusion transcript is the next most common cytogenetic subtype of pediatric ALL (22–25%). However, the translocation is frequently too subtle to be detected by conventional cytogenetics, and more sensitive methods such as fluorescence *in situ* hybridization (FISH) or molecular methods (RT-PCR) should be employed to search for this gene rearrangement in childhood ALL [62, 63]. Acute lymphoblastic leukemia with the *ETV6/RUNX1* fusion transcript most often occurs in patients who are 1 to 10 years of age, and is characterized by a precursor B-cell immunophenotype with frequent expression of CD10 and myeloid antigens (such as CD13 and CD33) [63–66]. In several clinical trials, this genetic feature was associated with a favorable prognosis, independent of age and leukocyte counts, and this has been attributed to the high sensitivity of the leukemic cells to asparaginase *in vitro* [56]. These tumors are characterized genetically by mono-allelic deletions in the *PAX5* gene (present in ~28% of the cases) [59].

ALL with the t(1;19)(q23;p13.3) E2A/PBX1 (or TCF3/PBX1) fusion transcript is usually associated with a pre-B (cytoplasmic Igμ-positive) immunophenotype, although cases where the blasts may lack Igμ expression are not infrequent [67, 68]. These leukemias are also frequently negative or only weakly positive for CD34, and for CD20, and show strong expression of CD9 [69]. They represent 3 to 6% of all childhood ALL cases, and 25% of all pre-B-ALL cases [8]. The adverse prognostic impact of this translocation has been largely eliminated by more effective chemotherapy treatments [55]; however, in many current clinical trials these cases are still assigned to more intensive chemotherapy regimens.

ALL with the t(9;22)(q34;q11.2) BCR–ABL1 fusion transcript (Philadelphia chromosome-positive ALL) represents 2 to 3% of all childhood ALL cases [8]. Philadelphia-positive ALL generally develops in older patients (10 years) and is associated with high initial leukocyte counts, a high incidence of CNS leukemia, L1 blast morphology, and a poor prognosis [70, 71]. In rare cases, the blasts may have abundant cytoplasm containing prominent, coarse azurophilic granules [71]. Rare Philadelphia-positive T-ALL cases have been reported [72, 73]. Allogeneic matched-related donor hematopoietic stem cell transplantation has improved the outcome of this ALL subtype [70].

ALL with 11q23 abnormalities; ALL with t(v;11q23); MLL rearranged. The translocation most commonly present in this ALL subtype is the t(4;11)(q21;q23) leading to the *AF4/MLL* fusion transcript [74–76]. This cytogenetic lesion is encountered in 2 to 3% of all pediatric ALLs, and 50 to 80% of ALL cases in infants less than one year of age [8]. These leukemias present with high leukocyte counts, bulky extramedullary disease, and frequent CNS involvement, and portend a poor prognosis [8]. They have a characteristic immunophenotype, usually CD10 negative, cytoplasmic Igμ negative, surface CD22 negative, CD15 and/or CD65 positive, and positive for the human homolog of the rat 220 kDa chondroitin sulfate proteoglycan NG2, which can be detected with the monoclonal antibody 7.1 [74, 77]. Infant ALLs with the t(4;11) appear to be preferentially sensitive to cytarabine, likely due to increased expression of cytarabine metabolizing enzymes [57, 78] and also to an increase in hENT1, which transports cytarabine across the cell membrane [79].

Hypodiploid ALLs are rare leukemias (5–6%) characterized by fewer than 46 chromosomes per cell, corresponding to a DNA index of <1.0. Occasional cases are near haploid. This cytogenetic subgroup has a distinctly poor prognosis despite contemporary therapy [80], and is considered a high-risk feature in most protocols. Genetic studies have found that most of these cases (almost 100%) carry inactivating mutations in one allele of the *PAX5* gene, while more than half of the cases also show point mutations or translocations in the other allele of this gene and deletions in up to three other B-cell development-related genes per case [59].

Molecular and cytogenetic abnormalities in T-cell ALL/LBL

Much information has accumulated in the recent years regarding the biology of pediatric T-cell lymphoblastic neoplasms. Molecular studies combined with gene expression profiling have uncovered several oncogenes that appear to play important roles in malignant transformation and correlate with disease subgroups with potential prognostic and therapeutic implications. None of the abnormalities described below has clinical applications at the current time.

Recurrent chromosomal abnormalities often include reciprocal translocations that disrupt developmentally important transcription factor genes and lead to their overexpression, as a result of rearrangements to loci for the *TCR* genes, most commonly *TCRα* (14q11.2) and *TCRβ* (7q35). For example, the *TAL1/SCL* gene (1p32) is involved in the t(1;14)(p32;q11) present in approximately 3% of T-ALLs [81]. The *HOX11* transcription factor gene (10q24) [82] is rearranged as part of the t(10;14)(q24;q11.2) [83]. Overexpression of *HOX11* in these cases appears to confer a prognostic advantage [84]. The translocation t(5;14)(q35;q32), leading to rearrangements of the related *HOX11L2* gene, appears to confer an inferior prognosis [85, 86]. The *LMO1* (11p15) and *LMO2* (11p13) oncogenes are rearranged by the t(11;14) and t(7;11), respectively [87]. Other less common translocations do not involve the *TCR* genes. The t(9;17) translocation is more commonly present in T-LBL than in T-ALL, and is associated with a more aggressive disease course. The t(10;11)(p12;q14), leading to the *AF10-CALM* fusion gene has been rarely reported in pediatric LBL cases and in T-ALL [88, 89]. It is associated with a mature or immature TCRγδ phenotype, and limited studies suggest a poor prognostic significance for the subset of patients with immature TCRγδ leukemia [90, 91].

Activating mutations of *TAL1/SCL* are found in up to 50% of all T-ALL, independent of detectable translocations, and correlate with leukemias arrested at the late cortical stage of thymocyte maturation expressing TCRαβ, and with an inferior prognosis [92, 93]. *HOX11 (TLX1)* mutations are present in ~30% of all T-ALL, are seen more commonly in adults than in children, associate with an early cortical T-ALL expressing TCRαβ, and correlate with a superior survival in limited studies [84, 92, 93]. *LYL1* is mutated in up to 22% of pediatric T-ALL, and correlates

with the double-negative early thymocyte stage of differentiation [92] and with an inferior survival. The *MLL* gene is mutated in 4–8% of T-ALL cases, associated with maturation arrest at early thymocytes stages, expression of TCRγδ, and no impact on prognosis [93]. Cryptic deletions of the *INK4/ARF* locus at 9p21, leading to alterations of the p14/p16 loci, are present in up to 75% of all T-ALL with possible defects in cell cycle control [93]. Activating mutations of the *NOTCH1* gene are present in over 50% of T-ALL [94].

Limited studies have documented a correlation between these genetic abnormalities present in T-ALL blasts and the patient age, potentially reflecting different stages of thymic development and involution [95].

Differential diagnosis of lymphoblastic leukemia/lymphoma

Lymphoblastic neoplasms must be differentiated from benign lymphoid precursors and from other neoplasms with blastic (or "small blue cell") morphology.

Benign precursor B-cell (hematogone) expansions are often important in the differential diagnosis of precursor B-ALL/LBL. Hematogones are normal precursor B-cells that reside primarily in the bone marrow, but can also be found in small numbers in extramedullary sites, including peripheral blood, lymph nodes, and tonsils [96–99]. They may increase in number (sometimes to a high percentage of the normal cells) in bone marrows from patients of any age, but are particularly common in children and young adults [100]. A variety of reactive or regenerative settings may be associated with hematogone expansions. These include viral infections and marrow recovery after infection, chemotherapy, and bone marrow transplantation [100]. Morphologically, hematogones show a range of maturation, with cells that resemble ALL L1-type lymphoblasts, and maturing or mature small lymphocytes (Fig. 17.18).

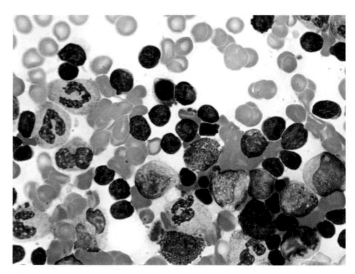

Fig. 17.18. Increased numbers of benign B-lymphoid precursors (hematogones) in the bone marrow aspirate from a child undergoing staging for retinoblastoma; the lymphoid cells demonstrate a spectrum of maturation (Wright–Giemsa stain).

Table 17.3. Stages of maturation in normal B-cell precursors ("hematogones").

Stage	CD10	CD19	CD20	CD22	CD34	CD45	TdT	clgμ	sIgM
I	Bright+	+	−	+	+	Dim+	+	−	−
II	+	+	Dim+	+	−	+	Dim+/−	+	−
III	Dim+	+	+	+	−	Bright+	−	+	+ poly
IV	−	+	Bright+	Bright+	−	Bright+	−	−	+ poly

Abbreviations: clgμ, cytoplasmic mu immunoglobulin heavy chain; sIgM, complete surface IgM; poly, polyclonal.

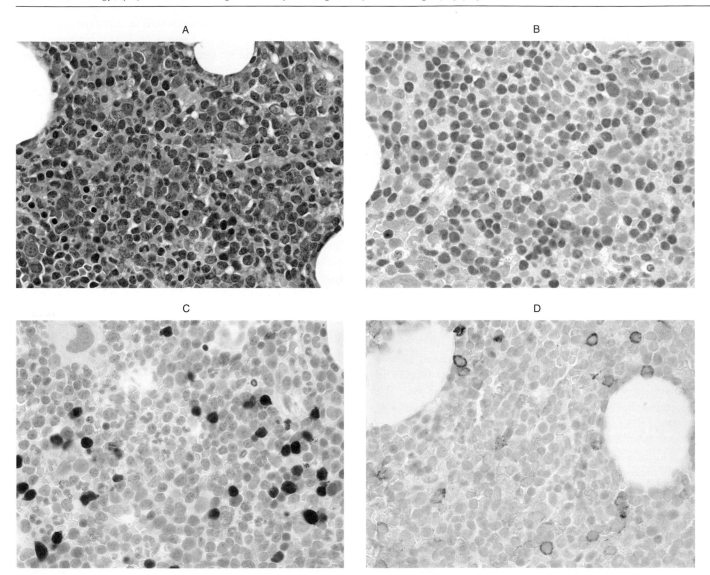

A

B

C

D

Fig. 17.19. Markedly increased numbers of benign lymphoid precursors (hematogones) in the bone marrow biopsy from a child undergoing evaluation for a benign hematologic disorder. These benign lymphoid cells have an interstitial distribution, as seen on a hematoxylin and eosin stain (A), and strongly and uniformly express PAX-5 (B), while only a small subset express TdT (C) and CD34 (D). Contrast these findings with the immunophenotypic features of ALL seen in Figure 17.17. (Images B–D, diamino-benzidine stain, hematoxylin counterstain.)

Immunophenotypically, several stages of maturation, likely corresponding to the morphologic range, have been described (see Table 17.3) [101, 102]. Cells at stage I of maturation express CD19, CD22, CD34, CD10 (bright), CD45 (dim), and TdT. Cells at stage II express CD19, CD22, variable (weak) CD20, CD10, variable (typically weak) TdT, CD45, and cytoplasmic Igμ. Cells at stage III express CD19, CD20, CD22, CD10 (dim), CD45

(bright), cytoplasmic Igμ, and surface IgM, with a polyclonal light chain pattern. Lastly, mature B-cells (stage IV) express CD19, CD22 (bright), CD20 (bright), CD45 (bright), and surface IgM (polyclonal). Typically, stage I (CD34+, TdT+ cells) represents only a very minor component of the reactive hematogone expansions (Fig. 17.19). However, in certain settings, such as recovery post-chemotherapy, this subset of immature cells

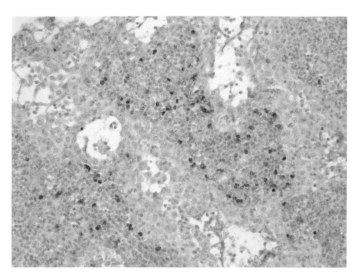

Fig. 17.20. Benign TdT+ precursor B-cells present in a reactive lymph node from a child undergoing staging for neuroblastoma. These cells are often found around sinusoidal spaces, most often in the medullary portion of the lymph node, and have an interstitial distribution. (Immunohistochemical stain for TdT, diamino-benzidine stain, hematoxylin counterstain.)

may become more prominent (or even predominant), raising the differential diagnosis with recurrent leukemia [103]. Flow cytometric analysis is typically extremely helpful in discriminating between a normal pattern of maturation and the presence of immunophenotypic aberrancies (consistent with leukemia) in a precursor B-cell population [101]. Of note, the hematogones present in tonsils and lymph nodes are typically strongly positive for TdT, and can be identified using immunohistochemistry (Fig. 17.20).

Normal cortical thymocytes are important in the differential diagnosis of precursor T-ALL/LBL, in samples obtained from mediastinal lesions, which may contain normal or hyperplastic thymic cortex, in addition to neoplastic tissue. A similar distinction should be made with thymoma (although this neoplasm is less common in children). The distinction is typically clear on morphologic examination, since normal thymocytes do not have blastic features and are set in the characteristic thymic architecture (Fig. 17.21). However, significant overlap may occur between the immunophenotype of normal thymocytes and that of precursor T-ALL/LBL at the thymic stage of differentiation (Fig. 17.22). Therefore, findings of TdT+ precursor T-cells on flow cytometry of pediatric mediastinal or cervical masses (two anatomic sites that may harbor thymic tissue in children) should always be correlated with the morphologic findings. Similar to hematogones, when examined immunophenotypically, normal thymocytes show a characteristic sequence of maturation [101]. For instance, expression of CD1a and CD4 precedes expression of surface CD3, with progression from CD1a–/CD3– cells, to CD1a+/CD3+, to CD1a–/CD3+. Thymocytes initially express CD4 only, followed by double-positive expression of CD4 and CD8, followed by expression of only CD4 or only CD8. Surface CD3 expression appears at the double-positive stage. CD10 is ini-

tially expressed dimly, and then becomes negative. And CD34 is only expressed at the CD4–/CD8–/CD1a– early thymocyte stages. T-ALL/LBLs show immunophenotypic aberrancies in all cases [101], which should be useful in the differential diagnosis.

Childhood blastic neoplasms that should be differentiated from lymphoblastic tumors include acute non-lymphoid leukemias and pediatric sarcomas, most notably Ewing sarcoma.

Acute myeloid leukemia (AML) may present as a tissue infiltrate (myeloid or monoblastic sarcoma) at virtually any anatomic location, with or without an associated leukemic process. Myeloid/monoblastic sarcoma should always be considered in the differential diagnosis of lymphoblastic leukemia/lymphoma, particularly in cases with larger blasts and prominent nucleoli (corresponding to the ALL L2 morphologic subtype). In some cases, likely corresponding to AML with inv(16), myeloid sarcoma may be associated with immature eosinophilic precursors. Flow cytometric analysis typically allows for an easy distinction between these processes. However, when only paraffin-embedded tissue samples are available, a more limited panel of immunohistochemical markers can be applied, rendering this distinction more difficult. In light of some of the immunophenotypic pitfalls likely to be encountered in childhood B-ALL/LBL, every blastic tissue infiltrate should be evaluated with a panel of hematopoietic markers, to include myeloperoxidase (MPO), lysozyme, TdT, PAX-5, and CD3. Acute myeloid leukemia with t(8;21) may be occasionally challenging in this context, as it may express CD19, CD79a, and PAX-5, in addition to MPO [34].

Acute mixed-lineage leukemias (particularly acute biphenotypic leukemias) enter the differential diagnosis of ALL aberrantly expressing several myeloid antigens. Scoring systems devised for this purpose should be applied in such cases.

Plasmacytoid dendritic cell (DC2) leukemia is a rare type of leukemia that has also been reported in children. These leukemias, thought to resemble in differentiation a subtype of antigen-presenting cells, the plasmacytoid dendritic (DC2) cells, represent <1% of all childhood leukemias [104]. Their blasts often resemble ALL L2 blasts, with occasional cases showing ample cytoplasm, with pseudopodia and peculiar cytoplasmic vacuoles lined along the cell outlines like a "string of pearls" (Fig. 17.23). These cells have a characteristic immunophenotype, expressing CD4, CD56, and HLA-DR, as well as the DC2-associated antigen CD123, and the blood dendritic cell antigens BDCA-2 and BDCA-4. In some cases, cells may express lymphoid and myeloid antigens of low specificity (such as CD2, CD22, TdT, and CD33, respectively), but are typically negative for other myeloid antigens, CD3, TCR, CD79a, and for CD34 [104, 105]. At the present time, these leukemias are treated in a fashion similar to ALL.

Ewing sarcoma is the childhood non-hematopoietic neoplasm most likely to be considered in the differential diagnosis of LBL, especially in small tissue/bone biopsies. This "small blue cell tumor" is typically composed of small blastic cells without

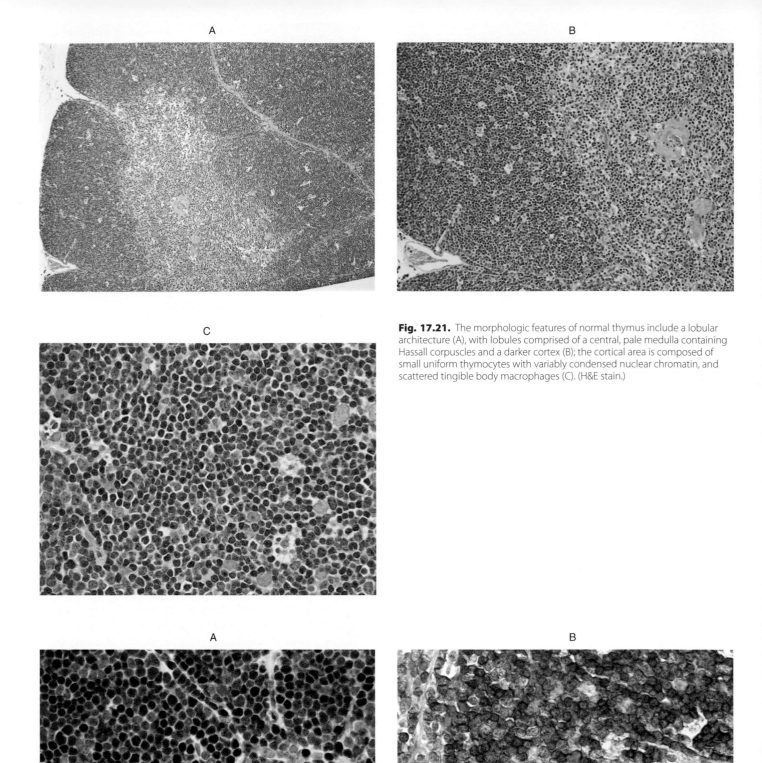

Fig. 17.21. The morphologic features of normal thymus include a lobular architecture (A), with lobules comprised of a central, pale medulla containing Hassall corpuscles and a darker cortex (B); the cortical area is composed of small uniform thymocytes with variably condensed nuclear chromatin, and scattered tingible body macrophages (C). (H&E stain.)

Fig. 17.22. The immunophenotypic features of normal cortical thymocytes include strong, uniform expression of TdT (A) and CD99 (B), and only partial weak expression of CD10 (C). Benign thymocytes should always be considered in the setting of biopsy material obtained from mediastinal masses occurring in children. (Diamino-benzidine stain, hematoxylin counterstain).

C

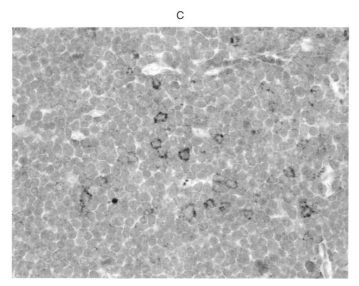

Fig. 17.22. (cont.)

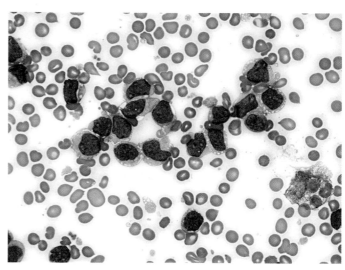

Fig. 17.23. Plasmacytoid dendritic cell (DC2) leukemia occurring in a child, and demonstrating the characteristic peripheral coalescent cytoplasmic vacuoles present in a subset of these leukemias (Wright–Giemsa stain).

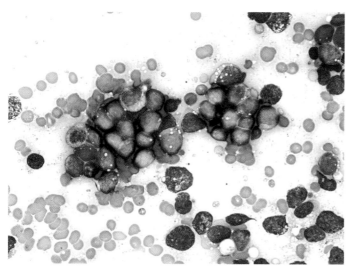

Fig. 17.24. Burkitt leukemia harboring the translocation t(8;22) and showing morphologic and immunophenotypic features intermediate between a precursor B-cell (including expression of TdT and CD34) and mature B-cell processes (including strong expression of CD20 and of surface immunoglobulin with light chain restriction), so-called "precursor B-cell Burkitt leukemia". (Wright–Giemsa stain.)

prominent nucleoli. In addition, it is CD45 negative and CD99 strongly positive, with a membrane staining pattern similar to a subset of precursor B-cell ALL. Including TdT in the immunohistochemistry panels for childhood small blue cell tumors should help in making this distinction, since TdT expression has not been reported to date in these non-hematopoietic neoplasms.

Burkitt lymphoma/leukemia. In most cases, the typical ALL L3 morphology and the dramatic clinical presentation of Burkitt tumors, with rapidly enlarging masses and high levels of serum LDH, make the distinction between precursor B-cell ALL and Burkitt lymphoma/leukemia relatively simple.

This distinction may be difficult in two situations: precursor B-cell ALL, with an otherwise typically immunophenotypic and genetic constellation of features, that has at least a subset of large deeply basophilic and vacuolated blasts with ALL L3-type morphology (Fig. 17.8); and Burkitt lymphoma with the classic Burkitt-associated chromosomal translocations, but with precursor B-immunophenotype and morphologic features (Fig. 17.24). The former seems to occur with increased frequency in hypodiploid ALL (author's unpublished observation); these cases should be treated as ALL. The latter situation, so-called precursor B-cell Burkitt lymphomas, may have clinical presentations intermediate between ALL and classical Burkitt lymphoma, and their immunophenotype includes features of precursor B-cells (e.g., expression of TdT and CD34, dim CD20 expression) and of mature B-cells (surface IgM with light chain restriction) [106]. Finding such combinations of features should prompt caution in diagnosing ALL until results of cytogenetics become available. The presence of the t(8;14) or its variants usually prompts treatment according to Burkitt lymphoma protocols [106].

Anaplastic large cell lymphoma may rarely present as a leukemic process [107] composed predominantly of small T-lymphocytes (so-called small cell variant). The lymphoma cells seen in peripheral blood and bone marrow in such cases are small, with markedly convoluted nuclei resembling those of Sézary cells (Fig. 17.25). A smaller percentage of large, atypical immunoblastic lymphoma cells, with deeply basophilic, occasionally vacuolated cytoplasm and coarsely clumped chromatin, are typically present in all of these cases. Often, these lymphoma cells are accompanied by striking neutrophilia with myeloid left shift, which may mimic an infectious process and distract from the atypical lymphoma cells. Immunophenotypic studies show a mature T-cell neoplasm (CD34−, TdT−), expressing CD30 and the anaplastic lymphoma kinase (ALK),

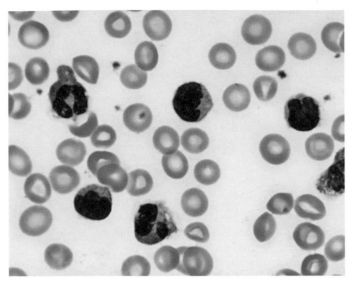

Fig. 17.25. Anaplastic large cell lymphoma, small cell variant, with leukemic involvement of the peripheral blood; the lymphoma cells are very small, with markedly convoluted, Sézary-like nuclear outlines (Wright–Giemsa stain).

and often show aberrant co-expression of myeloid antigens such as CD33 [108]. Cytogenetic studies show ALK gene rearrangements, often as a part of the t(2;5) chromosomal translocation. All of these features help in the differential diagnosis with T-ALL.

Prognosis and treatment

The prognosis of pediatric ALL has improved dramatically over the past several decades, from an overall survival of less than 10% in the 1960s to approximately 75–80% at the current time [8]. This advance has relied primarily on improving supportive care and optimizing the use of existing chemotherapy agents, accomplished by using risk-adapted strategies, and by taking into account the pharmacodynamic properties of the individual drugs. It is likely that further improvements in outcome will require the introduction of new therapeutic agents, possibly targeting specific molecular alterations found in the leukemic cells, and individualizing therapy according to various polymorphisms present in the drug-metabolizing enzyme genes (pharmacogenetics).

Risk stratification in ALL

This requires the integration of several presenting features (patient age, leukocyte counts, the presence or absence of central nervous system – CNS, or testicular involvement), leukemia features (lineage, genetic subgroup), and of early therapy response (measured, depending on the protocol, as response to prednisone, or as minimal residual disease at the end of remission induction) [8]. Patients younger than nine years of age, with leukocyte counts $<50 \times 10^9$/L, without CNS/testicular involvement, and having B-lineage leukemia with one of the

favorable genetic lesions (see Table 17.2) are typically considered low-risk for relapse and treated primarily with antimetabolite therapy. If there is persistent minimal residual disease at the end of remission induction, then they can be re-assigned to the high-risk group and receive more aggressive therapy. Patients with B-lineage ALL harboring the t(9;22) or showing induction failure or persistent minimal residual disease at the end of remission induction are classified as high-risk for relapse and are considered for allogeneic hematopoietic stem-cell transplantation. All the remaining B-ALL, and all the T-ALL, are classified as standard risk for relapse and are treated with intensive multiagent chemotherapy regimens.

Therapy of ALL

While there is not an absolute consensus regarding the risk group assignment, in most centers the treatment of ALL involves short-term intensive chemotherapy (with high-dose methotrexate, cytarabine, cyclophosphamide, dexamethasone or prednisone, vincristine, L-asparaginase, and/or an anthracycline) [8]. This is followed by intensification or consolidation therapy to eliminate residual leukemia, prevent or eradicate CNS leukemia, and ensure continuation of remission. The use of radiation for patients showing evidence of CNS or testicular leukemia is controversial, due to the significant secondary long-term effects associated with the former and the lack of a clear-cut benefit in the latter. For this reason, some treatment protocols have limited cranial radiation to CNS relapse cases, and have replaced it successfully with the use of intrathecal chemotherapy.

Pharmacogenomics of ALL

It has become evident that germline polymorphisms and mutations that affect the levels of expression and the function of drug-metabolizing genes may be related to ALL in several ways: they may increase the likelihood of leukemia in their carriers, may influence in major ways the response of ALL blasts to certain chemotherapy agents, and may also affect the probability of developing secondary (treatment-related) malignancies [109]. A few examples include the genes encoding for thiopurine S-methyltransferase (*TPMT*), glutathione S-transferase (*GST*), cytochrome P450 3A4 (*CYP3A4*), and methylene tetrahydrofolate reductase (*MTHFR*). For example, TPMT is an enzyme that converts thiopurine prodrugs (e.g., mercaptopurine) to inactive metabolites. Single nucleotide polymorphisms (SNPs) that lead to an unstable TPMT protein are present in heterozygous form in 10% of the population, and in homozygous form in 1 in 300 people. These latter patients tend to accumulate higher intracellular levels of drugs such as mercaptopurine and azathioprine, which render their leukemic cells more susceptible to therapy, but also increase the risk of toxic effects such as myelosuppression. In patients who are homozygous for these TPMT mutations, toxicities may be severe, and consequently they typically require 10–15% of the conventional doses for this drug. These latter patients are also at an increased risk for therapy-related acute myeloid leukemia. The picture is further complicated by the fact that leukemic blasts having various chromosomal abnormalities may differ from the somatic cells with respect to their production of drug metabolizing enzymes. For instance, the presence of additional chromosomes leading to additional copies of wild-type *TPMT* in the leukemic cells may increase resistance to the related drugs [61]. All these facts underscore the need for tailoring chemotherapy regimens to the patients' individual genetic background and to the specific features of their leukemia.

Minimal residual disease studies in ALL

Minimal residual disease (MRD) studies have been proven to be useful in the management of children with ALL, and encompass techniques capable of detecting amounts of residual leukemia that cannot be identified reliably using morphologic examination or conventional flow cytometry (so-called submicroscopic disease). Two technical approaches are currently used for the detection and quantification of MRD: flow cytometry and molecular analysis (polymerase chain reaction, PCR) for *IG* and *TCR* gene rearrangements, or fusion transcripts. Comparative studies indicate that, generally, there is good correlation between these methodologies for most patients, but the use of both techniques is the ideal approach for ensuring adequate MRD monitoring in all patients.

Flow cytometry

Flow cytometric detection of MRD (FC-MRD) relies on the presence of immunophenotypic aberrancies that distinguish the leukemic blasts from normal lymphoid precursors present in the bone marrow and peripheral blood. For T-ALL, since normal T-cell precursors are never encountered outside the thymus, the simple detection of cells co-expressing T-lineage antigens and TdT or CD34 in peripheral blood or marrow is sufficient to support the presence of MRD. However, as discussed above, normal precursor B-cells (hematogones) can be encountered at all sites, and more refined analyses are required to discriminate between these cells and leukemic B-lymphoblasts. Moreover, benign progenitor cells occurring in the post-chemotherapy or post-transplantation settings may have immunophenotypic features distinct from those encountered in normal individuals. This has implications in establishing panels of markers adequate for MRD analysis in this context. Aberrant leukemia-associated immunophenotypes can be identified in 95% of the pediatric ALL [110]. Markers used for this purpose in FC-MRD panels include a variety of myeloid antigens commonly co-expressed in B-cell leukemia (e.g., CD13, CD15, CD33, CD65, CD66c) as well as markers typically expressed inappropriately for stage of maturation in ALL (CD21 – normally only co-expressed on mature B-cells, CD38 – lower than normal cells, CD58 – higher than normal cells). Advantages of FC-MRD detection (when compared to PCR) include the possibility of direct quantitation and that of

excluding dying cells and cellular debris. Disadvantages include a lower sensitivity and the difficulties raised by immunophenotypic shifts in the leukemic cells, which may lead to the disappearance of some of the aberrancies used to identify MRD in a specific case [111]. The sensitivity of FC-MRD in routine clinical samples is typically 1 in 10^4 cells. Under ideal experimental conditions and in clinical situations where the leukemic cells have a very distinct immunophenotype and at least 1×10^7 cells are available, the sensitivity that can be achieved is 1 in 10^5 cells. FC-MRD detection can be applied to peripheral blood and bone marrow samples, with different results, depending on the lineage of ALL [112]. For T-ALL, the peripheral blood MRD levels always match those in the bone marrow, and are therefore acceptable substitutes for the latter samples. For B-ALL there may be bone marrow residual disease without peripheral blood MRD findings, and often the levels of MRD found in the bone marrow significantly exceed those found in the blood. These differences may stem from the distinct tissues of origin: thymus versus bone marrow for T-ALL and B-ALL, respectively. The prognostic value of FC-MRD has been demonstrated in retrospective and prospective studies. The detection of MRD of at least 0.01% at various times in therapy (but especially at the end of induction or at week 14 of continuation therapy) was found to be a strong predictor of relapse in children with uniformly treated ALL, independent of other known clinical and biologic prognostic factors. At the current time, it is expected that high-throughput methodologies for genetic analysis in ALL will lead to the discovery of new leukemia-associated markers that can be used in FC-MRD studies.

PCR for *IG* or *TCR* gene rearrangements

The detection limit of PCR (including heteroduplex and Gene-Scan strategies) is 1–5% (limited by the number of polyclonal B- or T-lymphocytes present in the sample) [45]. Since this sensitivity can be accomplished with the use of morphologic and immunophenotypic studies, alternative approaches are necessary to improve the sensitivity of this methodology and make it more suitable for MRD detection. Current strategies include using patient-specific junctional region-specific oligonucleotide probes. The generation of these probes requires sequencing of the junctional regions of the rearranged *IG* or *TCR* genes found in the leukemic cells of each patient at the time of initial diagnosis [113, 114]. Real-time quantitative PCR approaches using these probes in the follow-up samples have allowed the sensitivity of these methods to increase to 10^{-4}–10^{-6} (i.e., detection of 1–100 leukemic cells among 10^6 normal cells).

PCR for fusion transcripts

This methodology aims at detecting and quantifying fusion transcripts that result from leukemia-associated translocations such as t(9;22), t(4;11), t(1;19), or t(12;21), typically via RT-PCR assays. While the sensitivity of this methodology is as high as 10^{-4}, it remains unclear at this time to what extent this MRD

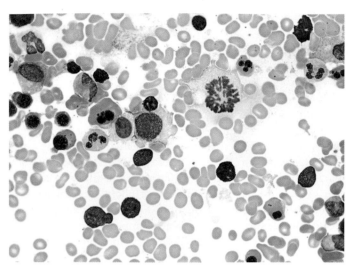

Fig. 17.26. Bone marrow aspirate from a child being treated for ALL. Erythroid precursors are increased in proportion and show megaloblastic dyserythropoiesis (Wright–Giemsa stain).

detection approach is useful in the prediction of outcome in pediatric ALL [45].

Post-chemotherapy changes in the bone marrow of ALL patients

Bone marrows of patients treated for pediatric ALL show features similar to those seen with other chemotherapy regimens (hypocellularity, variable degrees of hypoplasia and of dysplasia in one or several cell lines). In addition, they often show features associated with the administration of methotrexate, an anti-folate agent frequently used in this context. Interference with the folic acid metabolism leads to changes mimicking folate or vitamin B_{12} deficiency, which may affect the erythroid and/or myeloid cell lines. Erythroid cells are typically increased in proportion (with a myeloid : erythroid ratio of less than 1), with prominent megaloblastic dyspoiesis (Fig. 17.26). This corresponds to a peripheral blood picture that includes macroovalocytes seen on the smears, and an increased mean corpuscular volume (MCV) that becomes obvious at the time of marrow recovery (when the transfusion requirements decrease). The coexistence of these macroovalocytes with the previously transfused normal erythrocytes might impart a bimodal appearance to the red cell population. Megaloblastic changes seen in the myeloid lineage include the presence of giant metamyelocytes and bands in the bone marrow, and of large hypersegmented granulocytes seen in the peripheral blood. At the time of marrow regeneration (typically after day 21 post-chemotherapy) there may be increased numbers of hematogones, typically at stage I–II of maturation, that may mimic morphologically and immunophenotypically leukemic blasts. Correlation with the minimal residual disease studies, and, when necessary, with flow cytometry and cytogenetics might be helpful in cases where the distinction is not feasible on morphologic grounds alone.

Relapsed ALL

The overall frequency of relapse in ALL is approximately 25%, with a rate that is highly dependent on the immunophenotypic and genetic subtype of ALL [8]. These factors also determine the characteristics of the relapse, and the prognosis of these patients. For instance, relapse in patients with Philadelphia-positive ALL, representing approximately 10% of the relapsed ALL in some studies, typically occurs following a short complete remission (CR) and portends an extremely poor prognosis, as a second CR cannot be induced in many of these patients. Acute lymphoblastic leukemias with *ETV6/RUNX1* tend to relapse following a long first CR, and a second CR is relatively easy to induce and maintain, often for a long period of time.

Relapsed ALL may involve the bone marrow or extramedullary tissues (most often so-called "sanctuary sites" such as central nervous system, testis, ovary), or both. The isolated bone marrow relapses appear to correlate with a less favorable prognosis than the isolated extramedullary or combined relapses. This is, presumably, because the leukemic cells present in the microenvironment of the extramedullary sites (and possibly re-populating the marrow) have had less exposure to the chemotherapy agents and, thus, have retained their sensitivity to these drugs.

The morphologic and immunophenotypic features of relapsed ALL are often largely similar to those seen at the time of initial diagnosis. In some cases, the leukemic blasts at relapse resemble only a subset of the initial leukemic cells (e.g., a subset of blasts with vacuolated cytoplasm that becomes predominant at relapse), suggesting selection of a therapy-resistant subclone. Variable immunophenotypic shifts may also be observed by flow cytometry, whereby some antigens (most often TdT, CD10, HLA-DR, or aberrant myeloid antigens) may increase or decrease in intensity or even be lost at relapse [32]. The most extreme variations consist of lineage switch, where acquisition of myeloperoxidase expression may warrant a diagnosis of mixed lineage (biphenotypic) leukemia. In such cases, a secondary, therapy-related AML should be carefully excluded. Conventional cytogenetics and molecular analysis typically identify the translocations and fusion transcripts present at the time of initial diagnosis. In addition, cytogenetics will often (75% of cases) [32] find newly acquired chromosomal abnormalities, suggestive of clonal evolution. Very rarely, an entirely different karyotype may be identified, suggesting the possibility of a second *de novo* ALL. These observations also correlate with the data derived from PCR studies for *IG* and *TCR* rearrangements using patient-specific primers (see above) [114]. High-throughput genetic studies using SNP arrays and comparing diagnostic and relapse ALL samples have also supported all of these possibilities [115].

The therapy of relapsed ALL includes agents similar to those used for treating *de novo* disease, with 75–100% remission rates (depending on treatment protocol, time to relapse, and size of patient group reported). For patients with CNS relapse, cranial or craniospinal radiation is also frequently employed.

References

1. **Swerdlow SH, Campo E, Harris NL**, *et al.* (eds.) *WHO Classification of Tumours of Haematopoietic and Lymphoid Tissues* (4th edn.). Lyon: IARC Press; 2008.

2. **Spector LG, Ross JA, Robison LL**, *et al.* Epidemiology and etiology. In Pui C-H, ed. *Childhood Leukemias*. New York: Cambridge University Press; 2006, 48–69.

3. **Gurney JG, Severson RK, Davis S**, *et al.* Incidence of cancer in children in the United States. Sex-, race-, and 1-year age-specific rates by histologic type. *Cancer*. 1995;**75**:2186–2195.

4. **Le D, Shannon KM, Lange BJ.** Heritable predispositions to childhood hematologic malignancies. In Pui C-H, ed. *Childhood Leukemias*. New York: Cambridge University Press; 2006, 362–390.

5. **Dorak MT, Lawson T, Machulla HK**, *et al.* Unravelling an HLA-DR association in childhood acute lymphoblastic leukemia. *Blood*. 1999;**94**:694–700.

6. **Gale KB, Ford AM, Repp R**, *et al.* Backtracking leukemia to birth: identification of clonotypic gene fusion sequences in neonatal blood spots. *Proceedings of the National Academy of Sciences of the United States of America*. 1997;**94**:13950–13954.

7. **Taub JW, Konrad MA, Ge Y**, *et al.* High frequency of leukemic clones in newborn screening blood samples of children with B-precursor acute lymphoblastic leukemia. *Blood*. 2002;**99**:2992–2996.

8. **Pui CH.** Acute lymphoblastic leukemia. In Pui C-H, ed. *Childhood Leukemias*. New York: Cambridge University Press; 2006, 439–472.

9. First MIC Cooperative Study Group. Morphologic, immunologic, and cytogenetic (MIC) working classification of acute lymphoblastic leukemias. Report of the workshop held in Leuven, Belgium, April 22–23, 1985. *Cancer Genetics and Cytogenetics*. 1986;**23**:189–197.

10. **Bennett JM, Catovsky D, Daniel MT**, *et al.* Proposals for the classification of the acute leukaemias. French-American-British (FAB) co-operative group. *British Journal of Haematology*. 1976;**33**:451–458.

11. **Bennett JM, Catovsky D, Daniel MT**, *et al.* The morphological classification of acute lymphoblastic leukaemia: concordance among observers and clinical correlations. *British Journal of Haematology*. 1981;**47**: 553–561.

12. **Miller DR, Leikin S, Albo V**, *et al.* Prognostic importance of morphology (FAB classification) in childhood acute lymphoblastic leukaemia (ALL). *British Journal of Haematology*. 1981;**48**:199–206.

13. **Lilleyman JS, Hann IM, Stevens RF**, *et al.* Blast cell vacuoles in childhood lymphoblastic leukaemia. *British Journal of Haematology*. 1988;**70**:183–186.

14. **Lilleyman JS, Hann IM, Stevens RF**, *et al.* Cytomorphology of childhood lymphoblastic leukaemia: a prospective study of 2000 patients. United Kingdom Medical Research Council's Working Party on Childhood Leukaemia. *British Journal of Haematology*. 1992;**81**:52–57.

15. **Lorsbach RB, Onciu M, Behm FG.** Bone marrow reticulin fiber deposition in pediatric patients with acute lymphoblastic leukemia. *Laboratory Investigation*. 2002;**82**:252A (abstract 1048).

16. **Matloub YH, Brunning RD, Arthur DC**, *et al.* Severe aplastic anemia preceding acute lymphoblastic leukemia. *Cancer*. 1993;**71**:264–268.

17. **Wegelius R.** Bone marrow dysfunctions preceding acute leukemia in children: a clinical study. *Leukemia Research*. 1992;**16**:71–76.

18. **Cantu-Rajnoldi A, Invernizzi R, Biondi A**, *et al.* Biological and clinical features of acute lymphoblastic leukaemia with cytoplasmic granules or inclusions: description of eight cases. *British Journal of Haematology*. 1989;**73**: 309–314.

19. **Cerezo L, Shuster JJ, Pullen DJ**, *et al.* Laboratory correlates and prognostic significance of granular acute lymphoblastic leukemia in children. A Pediatric Oncology Group study. *American Journal of Clinical Pathology*. 1991;**95**:526–531.

20. **Darbyshire PJ, Lilleyman JS.** Granular acute lymphoblastic leukaemia of childhood: a morphological phenomenon. *Journal of Clinical Pathology*. 1987;**40**:251–253.

21. **Dyment PG, Savage RA, McMahon JT.** Anomalous azurophilic granules in acute lymphoblastic leukemia. *The American Journal of Pediatric Hematology/Oncology*. 1982;**4**:207–211.

22. **Stein P, Peiper S, Butler D**, *et al.* Granular acute lymphoblastic leukemia. *American Journal of Clinical Pathology*. 1983;**79**:426–430.

23. **Sharma S, Narayan S, Kaur M.** Acute lymphoblastic leukaemia with giant intracytoplasmic inclusions – a case report. *Indian Journal of Pathology & Microbiology*. 2000;**43**:485–487.

24. **Yanagihara ET, Naeim F, Gale RP**, *et al.* Acute lymphoblastic leukemia with giant intracytoplasmic inclusions. *American Journal of Clinical Pathology*. 1980;**74**:345–349.

25. **Miller DR, Steinherz PG, Feuer D**, *et al.* Unfavorable prognostic significance of hand mirror cells in childhood acute lymphoblastic leukemia. A report from the Children's Cancer Study Group. *American Journal of Diseases of Children*. 1983;**137**:346–350.

26. **Schumacher HR, Champion JE, Thomas WJ**, *et al.* Acute lymphoblastic leukemia – hand mirror variant. An analysis of a large group of patients. *American Journal of Hematology*. 1979; **7**:11–17.

27. **Hogan TF, Koss W, Murgo AJ**, *et al.* Acute lymphoblastic leukemia with chromosomal 5;14 translocation and hypereosinophilia: case report and literature review. *Journal of Clinical Oncology*. 1987;**5**:382–390.

28. **Horigome H, Sumazaki R, Iwasaki N**, *et al.* Fatal eosinophilic heart disease in a child with neurofibromatosis-1 complicated by acute lymphoblastic leukemia. *Heart Vessels*. 2005;**20**:120–122.

29. **Girodon F, Bergoin E, Favre B**, *et al.* Hypereosinophilia in acute B-lineage lymphoblastic leukaemia. *British Journal of Haematology*. 2005;**129**:568.

30. **Rezk S, Wheelock L, Fletcher JA**, *et al.* Acute lymphocytic leukemia with eosinophilia and unusual karyotype. *Leukemia & Lymphoma*. 2006;**47**:1176–1179.

31. **Metzgeroth G, Walz C, Score J**, *et al.* Recurrent finding of the FIP1L1-PDGFRA fusion gene in eosinophilia-associated acute myeloid

leukemia and lymphoblastic T-cell lymphoma. *Leukemia*. 2007;**21**:1183–1188.

32. **Brunning RD, McKenna RW.** Acute leukemias. In *Tumors of the Bone Marrow*. Washington, DC: Armed Forces Institute of Pathology; 1994, 22–142.

33. **Torlakovic E, Torlakovic G, Nguyen PL**, *et al.* The value of anti-pax-5 immunostaining in routinely fixed and paraffin-embedded sections: a novel pan pre-B and B-cell marker. *The American Journal of Surgical Pathology*. 2002;**26**:1343–1350.

34. **Tiacci E, Pileri S, Orleth A**, *et al.* PAX5 expression in acute leukemias: higher B-lineage specificity than CD79a and selective association with t(8;21)-acute myelogenous leukemia. *Cancer Research*. 2004;**64**:7399–7404.

35. **Tzankov AS, Went PT, Munst S**, *et al.* Rare expression of BSAP (PAX-5) in mature T-cell lymphomas. *Modern Pathology*. 2007;**20**:632–637.

36. **Dong HY, Liu W, Cohen P**, *et al.* B-cell specific activation protein encoded by the PAX-5 gene is commonly expressed in Merkel cell carcinoma and small cell carcinomas. *The American Journal of Surgical Pathology*. 2005;**29**:687–692.

37. **Mhawech-Fauceglia P, Saxena R, Zhang S**, *et al.* Pax-5 immunoexpression in various types of benign and malignant tumours: a high-throughput tissue microarray analysis. *Journal of Clinical Pathology*. 2007;**60**:709–714.

38. **Sica G, Vazquez MF, Altorki N**, *et al.* PAX-5 expression in pulmonary neuroendocrine neoplasms: its usefulness in surgical and fine-needle aspiration biopsy specimens. *American Journal of Clinical Pathology*. 2008;**129**:556–562.

39. **Torlakovic E, Slipicevic A, Robinson C**, *et al.* Pax-5 expression in nonhematopoietic tissues. *American Journal of Clinical Pathology*. 2006;**126**:798–804.

40. **Denzinger S, Burger M, Hammerschmied CG**, *et al.* Pax-5 protein expression in bladder cancer: a preliminary study that shows no correlation to grade, stage or clinical outcome. *Pathology*. 2008;**40**:465–469.

41. **Buresh CJ, Oliai BR, Miller RT.** Reactivity with TdT in Merkel cell carcinoma: a potential diagnostic pitfall. *American Journal of Clinical Pathology*. 2008;**129**:894–898.

42. **Bene MC, Castoldi G, Knapp W**, *et al.* Proposals for the immunological classification of acute leukemias. European Group for the Immunological Characterization of Leukemias (EGIL). *Leukemia*. 1995;**9**:1783–1786.

43. **Szczepanski T, Beishuizen A, Pongers-Willemse MJ**, *et al.* Cross-lineage T cell receptor gene rearrangements occur in more than ninety percent of childhood precursor-B acute lymphoblastic leukemias: alternative PCR targets for detection of minimal residual disease. *Leukemia*. 1999;**13**:196–205.

44. **van der Velden VH, Brüggemann M, Hoogeveen PG**, *et al.* TCRB gene rearrangements in childhood and adult precursor-B-ALL: frequency, applicability as MRD-PCR target, and stability between diagnosis and relapse. *Leukemia*. 2004;**18**:1971–1980.

45. **van Dongen JJ, Langerak AW.** Immunoglobulin and T-cell receptor gene rearrangements. In Pui C-H, ed. *Childhood Leukemias*. New York: Cambridge University Press; 2006, 210–234.

46. **Adriaansen HJ, Soeting PW, Wolvers-Tettero IL**, *et al.* Immunoglobulin and T-cell receptor gene rearrangements in acute non-lymphocytic leukemias. Analysis of 54 cases and a review of the literature. *Leukemia*. 1991;**5**:744–751.

47. **Boeckx N, Willemse MJ, Szczepanski T**, *et al.* Fusion gene transcripts and Ig/TCR gene rearrangements are complementary but infrequent targets for PCR-based detection of minimal residual disease in acute myeloid leukemia. *Leukemia*. 2002;**16**:368–375.

48. **Schmidt CA, Oettle H, Neubauer A**, *et al.* Rearrangements of T-cell receptor delta, gamma and beta genes in acute myeloid leukemia coexpressing T-lymphoid features. *Leukemia*. 1992;**6**:1263–1267.

49. **Breit TM, Verschuren MC, Wolvers-Tettero IL**, *et al.* Human T cell leukemias with continuous V(D)J recombinase activity for TCR-delta gene deletion. *Journal of Immunology*. 1997;**159**:4341–4349.

50. **Beishuizen A, Hahlen K, Hagemeijer A**, *et al.* Multiple rearranged immunoglobulin genes in childhood acute lymphoblastic leukemia of precursor B-cell origin. *Leukemia*. 1991;**5**:657–667.

51. **van der Velden VH, Szczepanski T, Wijkhuijs JM**, *et al.* Age-related patterns of immunoglobulin and T-cell receptor gene rearrangements in precursor-B-ALL: implications for detection of minimal residual disease. *Leukemia*. 2003;**17**:1834–1844.

52. **Szczepanski T, Willemse MJ, Brinkhof B**, *et al.* Comparative analysis of Ig and TCR gene rearrangements at diagnosis and at relapse of childhood precursor-B-ALL provides improved strategies for selection of stable PCR targets for monitoring of minimal residual disease. *Blood*. 2002;**99**:2315–2323.

53. **Ross ME, Zhou X, Song G**, *et al.* Classification of pediatric acute lymphoblastic leukemia by gene expression profiling. *Blood*. 2003;**102**:2951–2959.

54. **Yeoh EJ, Ross ME, Shurtleff SA**, *et al.* Classification, subtype discovery, and prediction of outcome in pediatric acute lymphoblastic leukemia by gene expression profiling. *Cancer Cell*. 2002;**1**:133–143.

55. **Pui C-H, Campana D, Evans WE.** Childhood acute lymphoblastic leukaemia – current status and future perspectives. *The Lancet Oncology*. 2001;**2**:597–607.

56. **Ramakers-van Woerden NL, Pieters R, Loonen AH**, *et al.* TEL/AML1 gene fusion is related to in vitro drug sensitivity for L-asparaginase in childhood acute lymphoblastic leukemia. *Blood*. 2000;**96**:1094–1099.

57. **Stam RW, den Boer ML, Meijerink JP**, *et al.* Differential mRNA expression of Ara-C-metabolizing enzymes explains Ara-C sensitivity in MLL gene-rearranged infant acute lymphoblastic leukemia. *Blood*. 2003;**101**:1270–1276.

58. **Kager L, Cheok M, Yang W**, *et al.* Folate pathway gene expression differs in subtypes of acute lymphoblastic leukemia and influences methotrexate pharmacodynamics. *Journal of Clinical Investigation*. 2005;**115**:110–117.

59. **Mullighan CG, Goorha S, Radtke I**, *et al.* Genome-wide analysis of genetic alterations in acute lymphoblastic leukaemia. *Nature*. 2007;**446**:758–764.

60. **Ito C, Kumagai M, Manabe A**, *et al.* Hyperdiploid acute lymphoblastic leukemia with 51 to 65 chromosomes: a distinct biological entity with a marked propensity to undergo apoptosis. *Blood.* 1999;**93**:315–320.

61. **Cheng Q, Yang W, Raimondi SC**, *et al.* Karyotypic abnormalities create discordance of germline genotype and cancer cell phenotypes. *Nature Genetics.* 2005;**37**:878–882.

62. **Romana SP, Le Coniat M, Berger R.** t(12;21): a new recurrent translocation in acute lymphoblastic leukemia. *Genes, Chromosomes & Cancer.* 1994;**9**:186–191.

63. **Shurtleff SA, Buijs A, Behm FG**, *et al.* TEL/AML1 fusion resulting from a cryptic t(12;21) is the most common genetic lesion in pediatric ALL and defines a subgroup of patients with an excellent prognosis. *Leukemia.* 1995;**9**:1985–1989.

64. **Baruchel A, Cayuela JM, Ballerini P**, *et al.* The majority of myeloid-antigen-positive (My+) childhood B-cell precursor acute lymphoblastic leukaemias express TEL-AML1 fusion transcripts. *British Journal of Haematology.* 1997;**99**:101–106.

65. **Rubnitz JE, Downing JR**, Pui C-H, *et al.* TEL gene rearrangement in acute lymphoblastic leukemia: a new genetic marker with prognostic significance. *Journal of Clinical Oncology.* 1997;**15**:1150–1157.

66. **Weir EG, Borowitz MJ.** Flow cytometry in the diagnosis of acute leukemia. *Seminars in Hematology.* 2001;**38**:124–138.

67. **Hunger SP, Galili N, Carroll AJ**, *et al.* The t(1;19)(q23;p13) results in consistent fusion of E2A and PBX1 coding sequences in acute lymphoblastic leukemias. *Blood.* 1991;**77**:687–693.

68. **Izraeli S, Henn T, Strobl H**, *et al.* Expression of identical E2A/PBX1 fusion transcripts occurs in both pre-B and early pre-B immunological subtypes of childhood acute lymphoblastic leukemia. *Leukemia.* 1993;**7**:2054–2056.

69. **Borowitz MJ, Hunger SP, Carroll AJ**, *et al.* Predictability of the t(1;19)(q23;p13) from surface antigen phenotype: implications for screening cases of childhood acute lymphoblastic leukemia for molecular analysis: a Pediatric Oncology Group study. *Blood.* 1993;**82**:1086–1091.

70. **Arico M, Valsecchi MG, Camitta B**, *et al.* Outcome of treatment in children with Philadelphia chromosome-positive acute lymphoblastic leukemia. *New England Journal of Medicine.* 2000;**342**:998–1006.

71. **Uckun FM, Nachman JB, Sather HN**, *et al.* Clinical significance of Philadelphia chromosome positive pediatric acute lymphoblastic leukemia in the context of contemporary intensive therapies: a report from the Children's Cancer Group. *Cancer.* 1998;**83**:2030–2039.

72. **Ribeiro RC, Abromowitch M, Raimondi SC**, *et al.* Clinical and biologic hallmarks of the Philadelphia chromosome in childhood acute lymphoblastic leukemia. *Blood.* 1987;**70**:948–953.

73. **Silva ML, Fernandez TS, de Souza MH**, *et al.* M-BCR rearrangement in a case of T-cell childhood acute lymphoblastic leukemia. *Medical and Pediatric Oncology.* 1999;**32**:455–456.

74. **Borkhardt A, Wuchter C, Viehmann S**, *et al.* Infant acute lymphoblastic leukemia – combined cytogenetic, immunophenotypical and molecular analysis of 77 cases. *Leukemia.* 2002;**16**:1685–1690.

75. **Chessells JM, Harrison CJ, Kempski H**, *et al.* Clinical features, cytogenetics and outcome in acute lymphoblastic and myeloid leukaemia of infancy: report from the MRC Childhood Leukaemia working party. *Leukemia.* 2002;**16**:776–784.

76. **Heerema NA, Sather HN, Ge J**, *et al.* Cytogenetic studies of infant acute lymphoblastic leukemia: poor prognosis of infants with t(4;11) – a report of the Children's Cancer Group. *Leukemia.* 1999;**13**:679–686.

77. **Hilden JM, Smith FO, Frestedt JL**, *et al.* MLL gene rearrangement, cytogenetic 11q23 abnormalities, and expression of the NG2 molecule in infant acute myeloid leukemia. *Blood.* 1997;**89**:3801–3805.

78. **Pieters R, den Boer ML, Durian M** *et al.* Relation between age, immunophenotype and in vitro drug resistance in 395 children with acute lymphoblastic leukemia – implications for treatment of infants. *Leukemia.* 1998;**12**:1344–1348.

79. **Pui C-H, Relling MV, Downing JR.** Acute lymphoblastic leukemia. *New England Journal of Medicine.* 2004;**350**:1535–1548.

80. **Nachman JB, Heerema NA, Sather H**, *et al.* Outcome of treatment in children with hypodiploid acute lymphoblastic leukemia. *Blood.* 2007;**110**:1112–1115.

81. **Bash RO, Crist WM, Shuster JJ**, *et al.* Clinical features and outcome of T-cell acute lymphoblastic leukemia in childhood with respect to alterations at the TAL1 locus: a Pediatric Oncology Group study. *Blood.* 1993;**81**:2110–2117.

82. **Kennedy MA, Gonzalez-Sarmiento R, Kees UR**, *et al.* HOX11, a homeobox-containing T-cell oncogene on human chromosome 10q24. *Proceedings of the National Academy of Sciences of the United States of America.* 1991;**88**:8900–8904.

83. **Hatano M, Roberts CW, Minden M**, *et al.* Deregulation of a homeobox gene, HOX11, by the t(10;14) in T cell leukemia. *Science.* 1991;**253**:79–82.

84. **Kees UR, Heerema NA, Kumar R**, *et al.* Expression of HOX11 in childhood T-lineage acute lymphoblastic leukaemia can occur in the absence of cytogenetic aberration at 10q24: a study from the Children's Cancer Group (CCG). *Leukemia.* 2003;**17**:887–893.

85. **Ballerini P, Blaise A, Busson-Le Coniat M**, *et al.* HOX11L2 expression defines a clinical subtype of pediatric T-ALL associated with poor prognosis. *Blood.* 2002;**100**:991–997.

86. **Bernard OA, Busson-LeConiat M, Ballerini P**, *et al.* A new recurrent and specific cryptic translocation, t(5;14)(q35;q32), is associated with expression of the Hox11L2 gene in T acute lymphoblastic leukemia. *Leukemia.* 2001;**15**:1495–1504.

87. **Valge-Archer V, Forster A, Rabbitts TH.** The LMO1 and LDB1 proteins interact in human T cell acute leukaemia with the chromosomal translocation t(11;14)(p15;q11). *Oncogene.* 1998;**17**:3199–3202.

88. **Carlson KM, Vignon C, Bohlander S**, *et al.* Identification and molecular characterization of CALM/AF10 fusion products in T cell acute lymphoblastic leukemia and acute myeloid leukemia. *Leukemia.* 2000;**14**:100–104.

89. **Narita M, Shimizu K, Hayashi Y**, *et al.* Consistent detection of CALM-AF10

chimaeric transcripts in haematological malignancies with t(10;11)(p13;q14) and identification of novel transcripts. *British Journal of Haematology*. 1999; **105**:928–937.

90. **Asnafi V, Radford-Weiss I, Dastugue N**, *et al.* CALM-AF10 is a common fusion transcript in T-ALL and is specific to the TCRgammadelta lineage. *Blood*. 2003;**102**:1000–1006.

91. **Caudell D, Aplan PD.** The role of CALM-AF10 gene fusion in acute leukemia. *Leukemia*. 2008;**22**:678–685.

92. **Ferrando AA, Neuberg DS, Staunton J**, *et al.* Gene expression signatures define novel oncogenic pathways in T cell acute lymphoblastic leukemia. *Cancer Cell*. 2002;**1**:75–87.

93. **Graux C, Cools J, Michaux L**, *et al.* Cytogenetics and molecular genetics of T-cell acute lymphoblastic leukemia: from thymocyte to lymphoblast. *Leukemia*. 2006;**20**:1496–1510.

94. **Weng AP, Ferrando AA, Lee W**, *et al.* Activating mutations of NOTCH1 in human T cell acute lymphoblastic leukemia. *Science*. 2004;**306**:269–271.

95. **Asnafi V, Beldjord K, Libura M**, *et al.* Age-related phenotypic and oncogenic differences in T-cell acute lymphoblastic leukemias may reflect thymic atrophy. *Blood*. 2004;**104**:4173–4180.

96. **Brady KA, Atwater SK, Lowell CA.** Flow cytometric detection of CD10 (cALLA) on peripheral blood B lymphocytes of neonates. *British Journal of Haematology*. 1999;**107**:712–715.

97. **Froehlich TW, Buchanan GR, Cornet JA**, *et al.* Terminal deoxynucleotidyl transferase-containing cells in peripheral blood: implications for the surveillance of patients with lymphoblastic leukemia or lymphoma in remission. *Blood*. 1981;**58**:214–220.

98. **Meru N, Jung A, Baumann I**, *et al.* Expression of the recombination-activating genes in extrafollicular lymphocytes but no apparent reinduction in germinal center reactions in human tonsils. *Blood*. 2002;**99**:531–537.

99. **Onciu M, Lorsbach RB, Henry EC**, *et al.* Terminal deoxynucleotidyl transferase-positive lymphoid cells in reactive lymph nodes from children with malignant tumors: incidence, distribution pattern, and immunophenotype in 26 patients. *American Journal of Clinical Pathology*. 2002;**118**:248–254.

100. **McKenna RW, Washington LT, Aquino DB**, *et al.* Immunophenotypic analysis of hematogones (B-lymphocyte precursors) in 662 consecutive bone marrow specimens by 4-color flow cytometry. *Blood*. 2001;**98**:2498–2507.

101. **Kroft SH.** Role of flow cytometry in pediatric hematopathology. *American Journal of Clinical Pathology*. 2004; **122**(Suppl): S19–S32.

102. **van Lochem EG, van der Velden VH, Wind HK**, *et al.* Immunophenotypic differentiation patterns of normal hematopoiesis in human bone marrow: reference patterns for age-related changes and disease-induced shifts. *Cytometry. Part B, Clinical Cytometry*. 2004;**60**:1–13.

103. **Dworzak MN, Fritsch G, Fleischer C**, *et al.* Multiparameter phenotype mapping of normal and post-chemotherapy B lymphopoiesis in pediatric bone marrow. *Leukemia*. 1997;**11**:1266–1273.

104. **Rossi JG, Felice MS, Bernasconi AR**, *et al.* Acute leukemia of dendritic cell lineage in childhood: incidence, biological characteristics and outcome. *Leukemia & Lymphoma*. 2006;**47**:715–725.

105. **Feuillard J, Jacob MC, Valensi F**, *et al.* Clinical and biologic features of CD4(+)CD56(+) malignancies. *Blood*. 2002;**99**:1556–1563.

106. **Navid F, Mosijczuk AD, Head DR**, *et al.* Acute lymphoblastic leukemia with the (8;14)(q24;q32) translocation and FAB L3 morphology associated with a B-precursor immunophenotype: the Pediatric Oncology Group experience. *Leukemia*. 1999;**13**:135–141.

107. **Onciu M, Behm FG, Raimondi SC**, *et al.* ALK-positive anaplastic large cell lymphoma with leukemic peripheral blood involvement is a clinicopathologic entity with an unfavorable prognosis. Report of three cases and review of the literature. *American Journal of Clinical Pathology*. 2003;**120**:617–625.

108. **Juco J, Holden JT, Mann KP**, *et al.* Immunophenotypic analysis of anaplastic large cell lymphoma by flow cytometry. *American Journal of Clinical Pathology*. 2003;**119**:205–212.

109. **Pui C-H, Relling MV, Evans WE.** Role of pharmacogenomics and pharmacodynamics in the treatment of acute lymphoblastic leukaemia. *Best Practice & Research. Clinical Haematology*. 2002;**15**:741–756.

110. **Campana D.** Determination of minimal residual disease in leukaemia patients. *British Journal of Haematology*. 2003;**121**:823–838.

111. **Campana D, Coustan-Smith E.** Minimal residual disease studies by flow cytometry in acute leukemia. *Acta Haematologica*. 2004;**112**:8–15.

112. **Coustan-Smith E, Sancho J, Hancock ML**, *et al.* Use of peripheral blood instead of bone marrow to monitor residual disease in children with acute lymphoblastic leukemia. *Blood*. 2002; **100**:2399–2402.

113. **Brüggemann M, van der Velden VH, Raff T**, *et al.* Rearranged T-cell receptor beta genes represent powerful targets for quantification of minimal residual disease in childhood and adult T-cell acute lymphoblastic leukemia. *Leukemia*. 2004;**18**:709–719.

114. **Szczepański T, van der Velden VH, Raff T**, *et al.* Comparative analysis of T-cell receptor gene rearrangements at diagnosis and relapse of T-cell acute lymphoblastic leukemia (T-ALL) shows high stability of clonal markers for monitoring of minimal residual disease and reveals the occurrence of second T-ALL. *Leukemia*. 2003;**17**:2149–2156.

115. **Yang JJ, Bhojwani D, Yang W**, *et al.* Genome-wide copy number profiling reveals molecular evolution from diagnosis to relapse in childhood acute lymphoblastic leukemia. *Blood*. 2008; **112**:4178–4183.

Advances in prognostication and treatment of pediatric acute leukemia

Stanley Chaleff

Leukemia is the most common cause of cancer in childhood; it accounts for approximately 40% of all cases of cancer in patients less than 18 years of age. Acute lymphoblastic leukemia (ALL) is the more prevalent in this age group, and acute myeloid leukemia (AML) is less common [1, 2].

Over the last 40 years there has been tremendous success in the treatment of leukemias in children, particularly ALL. While, in the 1950s, a child diagnosed with ALL would have had a less than 5% chance of surviving, today the survival rate for ALL is much closer to 80%; with some subgroups it is as high as 90% [3–7]. Much praise needs to be given to the pediatric oncologists who came together to perform the clinical trials and also had the vision to understand the importance of the biologic aspects of leukemia to help develop improved therapies. From this approach we have learned that ALL and AML are both heterogeneous disorders, each one including various subtypes that have different clinical progression and response to therapy. Today, leukemia therapy in children is guided by a combination of factors including age, initial white cell count, underlying cytogenetics, and response to therapy. This chapter will focus on the advances in diagnosis, prognostication, and treatment of pediatric acute leukemia from a clinician's perspective.

Acute lymphoblastic leukemia (ALL)

Epidemiology and etiology

ALL, the most common type of cancer in children, has an annual incidence of 3–4 children per 100 000, and accounts for approximately 4500 new cases per year [1]. There is a peak in occurrence of ALL between the ages of two and five years. There is also a slightly higher incidence of ALL in boys than in girls [8–13]. In the United States, ALL is more common in white than in black children, who may also have worse outcomes [8–11]. There is substantial geographic variation in the incidence of ALL. The disease is more common in industrialized countries, and the incidence is highest in the United States (among white children), Australia, and Germany. It is unclear whether the low incidence in non-industrialized countries is due to under diagnosis, or to other factors [14, 15]. Sev-

eral genetic disorders are associated with increased incidence of leukemia. Acute lymphoblastic leukemia is approximately 15 times more common in children with Down syndrome, and has also been linked to other cancer-predisposing syndromes such as Bloom syndrome, Fanconi anemia, and ataxia telangiectasia [16–18]. There are many potential agents that have been identified in the pathogenesis of ALL. Ionizing radiation has been clearly shown to incite leukemia, as seen after World War II in Japan [19, 20]. The risk of leukemia is not just related to the very high levels of exposure to radiation seen in the aftermath of the atomic bombs, but is also associated with the use of diagnostic imaging during pregnancy, with the greatest risk occurring in the first trimester [21]. Other environmental exposures have also been linked to ALL, including chemotherapy with alkylating agents, although this is more commonly associated with AML [22].

Clinical presentation

The clinical presentation of ALL varies, and while most children present with acute onset of disease, the initial signs and symptoms can be insidious and persist for months. The presenting signs depend on the degree of bone marrow involvement and the extent of the extramedullary involvement. Typically, these include anemia, thrombocytopenia, and functional neutropenia, which are clinically manifested by pallor, fatigue, petechiae, bone pain, and infections [23]. Fever is the most common finding, and is seen in 50–60% of the patients. Young infants may present with limp, bone pain, arthralgia, or refusal to walk, and initially may be evaluated for a rheumatologic disease. A small proportion of patients may present with severe bone pain and markedly elevated serum lactate dehydrogenase (LDH) due to bone marrow necrosis. Less common signs and symptoms include headache, vomiting, respiratory distress, and oligo- or anuria. Life threatening infection or bleeding can rarely occur.

Hepatosplenomegaly and lymphadenopathy are frequent and are seen in more than a half of the children at diagnosis. Mediastinal mass is frequent in T-lymphoblastic leukemia/lymphomas, which are frequently associated with high white blood cell count and central nervous system (CNS) involvement

Diagnostic Pediatric Hematopathology, ed. Maria A. Proytcheva. Published by Cambridge University Press.
© Cambridge University Press 2011.

Table 18.1. Risk stratification of acute lymphoblastic leukemia (ALL).

Variable	Low risk	High risk or very high risk
Age	1–10 years	Less than 1 and greater than 10 years
WBC count (× 10^9/L)	<50	≥50
CNS status	CNS1, CNS2	CNS3
Immunophenotype	B-lymphoblastic leukemia	T-lymphoblastic leukemia Mixed phenotype acute leukemia
Cytogenetics	t(12;21)(p13;q22); ETV6-RUNX1 Hyperdiploidy with trisomy 4, 10, 17	t(9;22)(q34;q11.2); BCR-ABL1[a] t(v;11q23); MLL rearranged Hypodiploid ALL
Response to therapy	Rapid early response	Slow early response or induction failure[a,b]
Minimal residual disease (MRD)	Negative by day 28 (<0.1%)	Positive at day 28 or beyond (>0.1%)

[a] Very high risk.
[b] Not in morphologic remission by day 28.

Table 18.2. Approximate five-year event-free survival (EFS) with current therapy for various risk groups with ALL.

Risk group	Approximate five-year EFS (%)
NCI standard risk[a]	80
NCI high risk[b]	70
ETV6-RUNX1 positive	90
Triple trisomy (+4, +10, +17)	90
Hyperdiploid (DI, DNA index >1.16)	90
Hypodiploid	60
Near haploid (24–28 chromosomes)	30
BCR-ABL positive	25
MLL positive	40
T-cell lineage	60
Infant ALL[c]	50[d]
Induction failure[e]	20

[a] Age between 1 and 10 years, WBC count <50 × 10^9/L.
[b] Age >10 years and WBC count >50 × 10^9/L.
[c] Age less than 1 year.
[d] If MLL rearranged, CD10 negative, and age <6 months, then approximate EFS of 30%.
[e] Not in morphologic remission by day 28 of induction.

[24, 25]. Less frequently, patients may present with subcutaneous nodules (leukemia cutis), salivary gland enlargement (Mikulicz syndrome), cranial nerve palsy, epidural spinal cord compression, testicular enlargement, leukemic retinopathy, or other eye abnormalities.

Laboratory abnormalities

The laboratory abnormalities will reflect the degree of bone marrow involvement. Anemia, thrombocytopenia, and abnormal leukocyte differential counts are typically present. While the white cell (WBC) count can vary from less than 0.1 to 1500 × 10^9/L, about a half of the patients present with WBC count higher than 10 × 10^9/L. Patients with markedly elevated WBC count are at risk of tumor lysis syndrome.

Not all patients present with hematologic abnormalities; in a study of 1317 white and 210 black children with newly diagnosed ALL treated at St. Jude Children's Research Hospital, a normal white blood cell count was seen in roughly half of the patients at presentation. In 20% of the patients the hemoglobin was more than 10 g/dL, and in 30% the platelet count was higher than 100 × 10^9/L. In such patients, when there is a high clinical suspicion, a bone marrow examination is necessary for the diagnosis [23–26]. Elevated serum uric acid levels and lactate dehydrogenase are common in patients with leukemia.

At diagnosis, leukemic blasts in the cerebrospinal fluid can be identified in as many as 30% of patients with ALL that lack neurologic symptoms [23]. The CNS status at diagnosis is defined as: CNS1, absence of leukemic blasts; CNS2, presence of leukemic blasts but less than 5 WBC/μL; CNS3, non-traumatic sample that contains more than 5 WBC/μL with identifiable blasts. Patients with CNS3 have a higher risk of CNS relapse and receive intense intrathecal therapy. While some studies show adverse prognosis in patients with CNS2 status, others fail to establish such an association.

Prognostic factors and risk stratification

An integral part of the modern therapy for ALL is stratification of the patients according to their risk of relapse, so that patients with high risk are treated more aggressively and those with low risk receive less aggressive chemotherapy (Table 18.1). For patients with precursor B-cell ALL, age and leukocyte count at diagnosis have been shown to be consistently important, regardless of the therapeutic regimens. Children younger than one year or older than ten years, and initial white blood cell count greater than 50 × 10^9/L are associated with adverse prognostic significance [27–29]. Race and sex also have prognostic considerations but are currently not used in the front-line protocols [8–10, 13].

Genetic abnormalities, either in the number of chromosomes or defined by specific translocations, also have important prognostic significance (Table 18.2). For example, hyperdiploidy (>50 chromosomes) or presence of ETV6/RUNX1 (TEL/AML1) fusion are associated with low risk, whereas hypodiploidy, t(9;22)(q34;q11.2) and BCR-ABL fusion, and MLL rearrangements are associated with high risk. These and other cytogenetic abnormalities are extensively covered in Chapter 10. Here, it is important to emphasize that the primary genetic features do not entirely account for treatment outcome. For example, a proportion of patients with more than 50 chromosomes or ETV6/RUNX1 fusion relapse on the current protocols, and children with t(9;22) who are one to nine years old and have low white blood cell count can be cured with chemotherapy alone. Furthermore, a subset of ALLs with *MLL* rearrangements respond well to therapy. These include children with good initial response to prednisone therapy, and patients with *MLL-ENT* fusion and T-cell phenotype. Thus, while the cytogenetic abnormalities are important for risk stratification, adjustment of chemotherapy improves the overall outcome.

Ultimately, treatment is the most important prognostic factor of ALL. The prognostic value of the initial decrease of the leukemic blasts (below 5%) has been recognized by investigators of the Children's Cancer Group and Berlin–Frankfurt–Münster (BFM) Consortium since the early 1980s. The response to therapy is measured by the disappearance of the blasts from the peripheral blood, and fewer than 5% blasts by morphologic examination in the bone marrow. With the standard protocols, the rate of remission induction is approximately 95%, and the prognosis for patients not in remission at the end of induction is very poor [30]. In addition to assessments at the end of induction (at approximately four weeks), there are more and more data from interim time points to indicate that the patients who go into remission earlier have an improved outcome.

Various ALL protocols measure the response to therapy differently. The current BFM protocols use a response in the peripheral blood after 7 days of prednisone alone to stratify patients into risk groups [31]. The Children's Oncology Group (COG) protocols use a day 14 bone marrow to risk-stratify patients into rapid early responders or slow early responders. The slow early responders are treated with additional therapy compared to the rapid responders, because they have been shown to have a worse overall prognosis [32–34].

While easily accessible, the evaluation of disease status by morphology to assess response to therapy has its limitations. For example, about 20% of patients that respond to therapy relapse, and a subset of patients with poor initial response but treated with intensified chemotherapy survive longer. Measurement of minimal residual disease (MRD) by flow cytometry or by molecular techniques proves to be more sensitive, and patients that achieve immunologic or molecular remission, defined as leukemic involvement of fewer than 10^{-4} nucleated bone marrow cells at the end of remission, have a much more favorable prognosis regardless of the underlying cytogenetic abnormalities [35]. The ability to detect MRD is changing the definition of remission. Studies have shown that patients that are considered MRD negative at different time points in induction have an improved prognosis. For that reason, MRD is currently being employed by the current COG protocols to determine therapy [36–38].

Therapy of ALL

The recognition of the heterogeneity of ALL and identification of reliable prognostic factors leads to the development of risk-directed therapy. While there are variations between different protocols, in general the therapy in ALL is directed to induction of remission, which is followed by intensification or consolidation therapy to eliminate residual leukemia, eradication

or prevention of CNS leukemia, and maintenance therapy. Each phase has a different goal which defines the degree of intensity. Patients with high risk of recurrence receive more intensive chemotherapy. The therapeutic drugs commonly used in acute lymphoblastic leukemia are shown in Table 18.3.

Remission induction is the first phase of therapy and lasts approximately four to six weeks. The goal of this phase is to induce a complete remission by elimination of more than 99% of the initial leukemic cell burden, and by restoring the normal hematopoiesis, defined by absolute neutrophil count of $>0.5 \times 10^9$/L and platelet count of $>100 \times 10^9$/L. This phase of therapy usually includes administration of dexamethasone or prednisone, vincristine, and at least a third agent (L-asparaginase or an anthracycline, or both). With the modern supportive care, 97–99% of children enter complete remission. Approximately 1% die of drug toxicity during remission induction, and another 1% of induction failure due to drug-resistant leukemia [39]. Patients with $>5\%$ blasts at the end of induction have a shorter survival, or if remission is achieved, a higher rate of relapse. These patients are often treated with very aggressive chemotherapeutic regimes or stem cell transplant [40]. The evaluation of remission has traditionally been morphologic examination of peripheral blood and/or bone marrow, which has its limitations. However, as the more sensitive techniques to detect residual disease emerge, the determination of an optimal induction may change. Current studies have shown that patients who are MRD negative at earlier time points of induction have an overall better prognosis. With improved supportive care, patients may be treated with more aggressive chemotherapy early during the course of overall therapy in order to achieve a better event-free survival (EFS) [41, 42].

The next phase of chemotherapy is *intensification (consolidation) and reinduction*. While there is a consensus on the importance of this phase of therapy, there is no uniformity in terms of which is the best regimen, or the duration of therapy. The purpose of consolidation is to continue the cytoreduction of leukemia cells and to maximize the killing of leukemia cells and reduce the likelihood of resistance by using different drugs than those used in induction. The drugs used in consolidation are very dependent on the initial risk group that the patient is in. While standard risk patients can do very well with a lower intensity consolidation, high-risk patients will need additional chemotherapy [3, 4]. The drugs that are commonly used in this phase of chemotherapy are 6 mercaptopurine (6-mp), cyclophosphamide, cytarabine (Ara-C), methotrexate (MTX), and asparaginase.

One significant breakthrough in the treatment of childhood ALL has been the incorporation of CNS therapy into the treatment protocols. Investigators at St. Jude Children's Research Hospital were first to show that with a combination of intrathecal methotrexate and 2400 cGy of radiation [43], the CNS relapse rate fell from 50% to 10% and, as a result, more than 50% of patients overall were cured. Since then, much has been learned about the significant effects of radiation on the developing brain, growth, and inciting of secondary malignancies,

Table 18.3. Therapeutic drugs commonly used in acute lymphoblastic leukemia.

Class of drug/therapy	Drugs	Mechanism of action	Phase of therapy normally used	Short- and long-term toxicity
Steroids	Dexamethasone Prednisone Hydrocortisone	Binds the steroid receptors on the nuclear membrane – leading to apoptosis of lymphocytes	Induction Consolidation Maintenance Current debate on which steroid is better	Weight gain Diabetes Avascular necrosis of the femoral heads Susceptibility to infection
Anthracyclines	Daunorubicin	Inhibition of DNA and RNA synthesis by intercalating between DNA base pairs, uncoiling of the helix, and by steric obstruction May cause free radical damage to DNA	Induction – for high-risk patients, Consolidation for all patients	Cardiovascular toxicity, short- and long-term Myelosuppression: thrombocytopenia, leukopenia, neutropenia, mild anemia Mucositis
Vinca alkaloids	Vincristine	Inhibits microtubular protein of the mitotic spindle, leading to metaphase arrest	Induction Consolidation Maintenance	Central nervous system neurotoxicity, seizures, CNS depression, cranial nerve paralysis, headache, confusion Leg and jaw pain SIADH Constipation
Alkylating agents	Cyclophoshamide	Interferes with the normal function of DNA by alkylation and cross-linking the strands of DNA, and by possible protein modification	Consolidation In the relapsed setting, multiple phases	Myelosuppression Hemorrhagic cystitis Infertility Therapy-related t-MDS/t-AML: 5–10 years after exposure, associated with unbalanced loss of genetic material, frequently chromosomes 5 and/or 7
Protein synthesis inhibitors	L-asparaginase (*Escherichia coli*) *Erwinia*-asparaginase PEG-asparaginase	Inhibits protein synthesis by deaminating asparagine and depriving tumor cells of this essential amino acid	Induction Consolidation *Erwinia* is used if there is an allergy to L-asparaginase	Pancreatitis Transient diabetes Hematologic toxicities: leukopenia, hemorrhage Coagulation abnormalities: prolonged thrombin, prothrombin, and partial thromboplastin times, hypofibrinogenemia; thrombosis
Nucleoside analogues	Cytarabine 6-Mercaptopurine 6-Tioguanine Clofarabine Nelarabine	Converted intracellularly to the active metabolite cytarabine triphosphate; inhibits DNA polymerase by competing with deoxycytidine triphosphate, resulting in inhibition of DNA synthesis; incorporated into DNA chain resulting in termination of chain elongation; cell cycle-specific for the S-phase of cell division	Consolidation Maintenance T-cell ALL For a very high-risk ALL and in the relapsed setting	Myelosuppression: leukopenia, anemia, thrombocytopenia With high doses: fevers, respiratory distress
Folic acid inhibitors	Methotrexate	An antimetabolite that binds to dihydrofolate reductase, blocking the reduction of dihydrofolate to tetrahydrofolic acid; depletion of tetrahydrofolic acid leads to depletion of DNA precursors and inhibition of DNA and purine synthesis	Consolidation Maintenance	Renal failure with high dose Hematologic toxicities: anemia, aplastic anemia, hemorrhage, leukopenia, neutropenia, myelosuppression, thrombocytopenia
Tyrosine kinase inhibitors	Imatinib Lestaurtinib Dasatinib	Blocks the signaling of BCR-ABL or other kinases	Imatinib – only in patients with BCR-ABL-positive ALL Lestaurtinib – in trials for infant ALL or patients with abnormalities at 11q23, or *FLT3* mutations	Hematologic toxicity: anemia, neutropenia, thrombocytopenia, pancytopenia May cause severe hemorrhage Joint pain
Topoisomerase II inhibitors	Etoposide	Inhibits mitotic activity; inhibits DNA type II topoisomerase producing single- and double-strand DNA breaks	Consolidation in some protocols for high-risk patients	Myelosuppression: anemia, granulocyte nadir at ~7–14 days, platelet nadir at ~9–16 days Therapy-related t-AML/t-MDS – with 11q23 (*MLL*) rearrangements Therapy-related ALL
Radiation		Generates free radicals leading to apoptosis	Consolidation in some protocols for either high-risk patients or patients with CNS-positive disease	Therapy-related secondary malignancies including t-MDS/t-AML Growth retardation Learning disabilities

Abbreviations: SIADH, syndrome of inappropriate antidiuretic hormone hypersecretion.

which has stimulated the development of new strategies for CNS therapy in order to avoid radiation-related toxicities [44]. With the advent of more aggressive systemic chemotherapy, namely high-dose methotrexate, and an increase in the number of intrathecal chemotherapies delivered, many protocols found that cranial radiation could be eliminated from the treatment of all but a selective group of patients at high risk for CNS relapse [45, 46].

Children with lymphoblastic leukemia require long-term continuous therapy of two to two-and-a-half years. Once patients get through consolidation they will continue treatment with the next phase of therapy, which is *maintenance*. This phase includes some combination of weekly methotrexate and daily mercaptopurine [47–50]. In addition, periodic steroids, vincristine, and intrathecal chemotherapy are utilized. Studies have shown that survival is improved with one or two intensive periods of chemotherapy that are similar to induction and consolidation, called delayed intensification or reinduction, but there is ongoing debate on which patients need a single or double delayed intensification [3, 4].

Hematopoietic stem cell transplantation

While it is currently accepted that stem cell transplantation is beneficial for ALL patients with a very high risk for relapse, it is still debatable which patients should be included in this category. Patients with *BCR-ABL* translocation, hypodiploidy, and induction failure are often taken towards a pathway that includes stem cell transplantation [51]. In addition, most patients who have had a relapse less than 18 months after achieving first remission undergo a stem cell transplant after remission is achieved. However, patients with a late extramedullary relapse (>18 months after achieving first remission) do well with intensive chemotherapy alone [52–54].

In summary, ALL is a heterogeneous disease that in a subset of patients has very good outcomes but in others requires intensive chemotherapy for cure. The current research is now designed to identify patients that will or will not require additional therapy, in order to minimize the long-term toxicity and improve overall outcomes. Response to therapy and presence of MRD at the end of induction chemotherapy are among the most important prognostic factors that will define the risk of relapse and guide further therapies. Stem cell transplantation is needed in some very high-risk patients, but new modalities have been investigated to make this potentially risky and toxic therapy safer, and therefore offering the potential of cure to even more patients.

Acute myeloid leukemia

In children, AML is less common as compared to ALL, although the overall incidence of the disease in adults is higher. It accounts for approximately 900 cases in children per year, or approximately 15% of all pediatric leukemias. The incidence in childhood is highest in the first year of life, where AML is as common as ALL [55, 56]. The incidence of AML in children has been growing, in large part because of an increased incidence of secondary AML as a result of previous chemotherapy [57, 58].

The distribution of AML varies among different ethnic groups. For example, there is a slightly higher incidence of AML in patients of Hispanic and black ethnicities [56]. Some subtypes, such as acute promyelocytic leukemia, are more frequent in persons from Italy, Spain, Mexico, and Central and South America. Genetic factors play a role in the leukemogenesis of AML, and some genetic disorders have a higher incidence of AML as compared to the general population. For example, AML is approximately 30 times more common in children with Down syndrome, and individuals with Bloom syndrome, Fanconi anemia, ataxia telangiectasia, Diamond–Blackfan syndrome, Shwachman–Diamond syndrome, and severe congenital neutropenia have increased risk of developing AML [59–64]. There are many different environmental factors that have been linked to AML. Radiation, prenatal exposure to cigarette smoke and marijuana, a variety of chemicals, such as benzene, pesticides, and herbicides [65–69] have been linked to the development of AML. Furthermore, previous chemotherapy, in particular administration of alkylating agents, like cyclophosphamide and busulfan, and epipodophyllotoxins, such as etoposide, increase the risk of AML [57–58].

The diagnosis and classification of AML have been evolving with time, and the advances in cytogenetics and immunophenotyping have shown that, biologically and clinically, AML is a heterogeneous group of disorders. An extensive discussion on the classification, cytogenetics, and diagnosis of AML is present in Chapter 10 and [15], as well as in other relevant chapters. Here we will focus on the clinical presentation and therapeutic approaches in AML according to the risk stratification.

Clinical presentation of AML

While the clinical presentation is very similar to that of ALL, there are some features that are more common in AML, including some that are, somewhat, AML-subtype dependant. Just as in ALL, patients with AML present with symptoms related to the bone marrow and extramedullary involvement, such as fatigue, bleeding, bone pain, fevers, weight loss, and infections [70]. One of the rarer presenting features of patients with AML is that of the myeloid sarcoma, also called granulocytic sarcomas or chloroma. A chloroma is an extramedullary tumor mass consisting of myeloid blasts with or without maturation that can manifest prior to the bone marrow involvement by several weeks. While it can present anywhere in the body, it frequently involves the orbits or the spinal canal where it can cause compression of adjacent structures [71–73]. Another unique manifestation of AML, particularly of monoblastic/monocytic leukemia, includes gingival hypertrophy, which is seen in 10% of children with the disease.

Some subtypes of AML have characteristic clinical features. For example, patients presenting with acute promyelocytic leukemia with t(15;17)(q22;q12) and acute monoblastic/acute monocytic leukemia often present in frank diffuse intravascular coagulation (DIC) due to the granules in those leukemic blasts [74–76]. Patients with acute megakaryoblastic leukemia (FAB classification: AML M7) often present with low peripheral blood counts and a marrow aspiration that is very difficult to obtain due to bone marrow fibrosis. In such patients, the diagnosis is established on a bone marrow biopsy.

AML, more frequently than ALL, presents with markedly increased white blood cell counts, leading to complications in the lung and brain, such as hyperviscosity syndrome [77, 78]. Patients with acute monoblastic/acute monocytic leukemia that present with high initial white blood cell counts are therefore at highest risk. The pathogenesis of hyperviscosity syndrome is still not completely understood. Obstruction of small vessels of the lung and brain by the viscous blood, leading to respiratory distress and seizures, as well as activation of adhesion molecules on the vascular endothelium, most likely play a role. The type of blasts is also important. For example, in AML, a WBC count greater than 100×10^9/L may lead to hyperviscosity syndrome, whereas, in ALL, counts greater than 300×10^9/L lead to symptoms. Thus, patients with AML and high counts are at increased risk of such complications.

Laboratory evaluation of children with AML is similar to those with ALL. A complete blood count, a coagulation profile, and a complete set of chemistry to assess kidney function, as well as bone marrow aspiration and a biopsy and spinal tap to assess CNS are usually done. In patients with acute promyelocytic leukemia, the mortality in induction can be as high as 10%, in large part due to the abnormalities in the coagulation system, and careful monitoring is warranted. Unlike ALL, children with AML are less likely to have a significant tumor lysis syndrome; because the AML blasts are slower growing and more stable, they are also unfortunately more resistant to chemotherapy. Still, AML patients are at risk, and require careful monitoring of renal function, calcium, phosphorus, and uric acid.

Important subgroups of AML in children

For many years, AML in adults and children was considered a similar disease. However, based on recent studies, it is becoming clear that pediatric AML differs in many ways from the disease in adults. For example, there are differences in the frequencies of different subtypes of AML in children as compared to adults. Acute myeloid leukemia with recurrent balanced translocations involving 11q23 comprises almost 80% of AML in infants and 15% of AML in older children; whereas such abnormalities are present in a small subset of adult AML. Myeloid leukemia of Down syndrome is another unique pediatric entity that has a unique clinical presentation and excellent response to chemotherapy [79].

Risk stratification of AML

Similarly to ALL, age is an important prognostic factor. Children younger than one year old, and patients who are in their late teenage years have a poorer prognosis [80]. The reasons are not completely understood. Perhaps infants do not tolerate the chemotherapy as well as other children or, perhaps, infants have disproportionately higher rates of acute megakaryoblastic leukemia, which has a poor prognosis independent of age [81, 82]. It is also unclear why teenagers do so poorly; perhaps, since they are closer to adults, their AML may have a different biology. On the other hand, patients with Down syndrome, who frequently present with acute megakaryoblastic leukemia, have a very good prognosis. Patients with Down syndrome and AML are very responsive to Ara-C, and in fact current protocols are examining if patients with Down syndrome can be treated with less chemotherapy because they have a very significant toxic death rate with current therapy for AML [83].

Cytogenetic abnormalities are found in approximately 50% of AML, and represent the biggest determinant of risk stratification at diagnosis [84]. Patients with t(8;21) and inversion 16 (FAB subclass AML M4Eo) have a very good prognosis, with approximately 70% EFS at five years with current chemotherapy [85, 86]. The third cytogenetic abnormality that confers a favorable outcome is the t(15;17), acute promyelocytic leukemia. Patients with such a translocation respond to chemotherapy in combination with all-*trans* retinoic acid (ATRA), with a five-year event-free survival of approximately 80% [87, 88].

Cytogenetic abnormalities that confer a poor prognosis include partial or complete loss of chromosomes 5 and 7. Such abnormalities are related to myelodysplasia, and patients in this group have a five-year EFS of approximately 25% with current therapy [85, 86, 89]. The presence of dysplasia or AML arising in the settings of myelodysplastic syndrome (MDS) or in syndromes that lead to bone marrow failure (for example Fanconi anemia) carries a very poor prognosis. Children with AML secondary to exposure to alkylating agents also have a very poor prognosis [77]. Secondary AML which is linked to previous exposure to epipodophyllotoxins has specific cytogenetic abnormalities, such as t(9;11)(p22;q23). This form of AML has a very poor prognosis and many patients do not even go into remission, despite aggressive chemotherapy.

In addition to balanced translocations, molecular studies have shown that mutation at specific genes such as *FLT3* can occur in AML. FLT3 is a tyrosine kinase that is linked to several intracellular pathways, and specifically the RAS signal transduction pathway, and the mutations that are described as activation lead to a poor prognosis in AML [90–92]. There are two types of mutations seen in the *FLT3* gene: point mutations, and internal tandem duplications (ITDs). While the prognostic significance of the point mutations is still unclear, patients who have the ITD mutations have a poor prognosis, and these are seen in about 15% of children with AML and 30% of adults with AML. Fortunately, potential therapeutic options for this subgroup of patients are currently under development: a new class of tyrosine kinase inhibitors may block the Ras signal transduction pathway that is activated by the FLT3 ITD mutations.

Similarly to ALL, in AML the response to therapy is the most important prognostic indicator. Patients that respond and enter remission with the first or second cycle of therapy have a much better prognosis that those who do not [85, 86, 93–96]. The detection of minimal residual disease in AML, however, is less successful as compared to ALL and, as a result, its clinical significance is still to be determined. In a study from the German BFM group, where MRD was determined by flow cytometry at different time points, they found that patients who had negative MRD results at all time points had an overall survival of 71%, as compared to 31% for those with multiple positive results. In this study, MRD was detected in only 3% of the 150 patients that were followed. On further analysis, detection of MRD at day 15 of induction, and prior to the second induction appeared to be the most important time points to predict EFS. Due to the small sample size, multivariate analysis of MRD, while very close to being significant, failed to determine the statistical significance of these findings [97]. While specific genetic translocations and fusion transcripts [t(8;21), t(15;17), and inversion [16] can be detected by PCR, only a small subset of AML patients have such alterations. For example, t(8;21) is seen in approximately 10% of patients with AML [98, 99]. In a study by Leroy et al., of 21 adult patients, 5 of 6 patients who had a positive MRD (at a level of 0.001%) at the start of consolidation relapsed, compared to only 1 of 15 patients who were negative. This study also demonstrated that quantitative PCR can be used to predict the relapse [98]. In another study by Perea et al., patients with either t(8;21) or inversion 16 MRD greater than 0.1% had a relapse rate of 67%, compared to 21 % for patients who had levels lower than 0.1%. Patients were also followed, and the later in treatment that a PCR product could be found, the higher the relapse rate [99].

Therapy

The therapy for AML, with or without hematopoietic stem cell transplant, while shorter – approximately six months – is much more intensive as compared to ALL (Table 18.4). As a result, patients develop severe neutropenia for prolonged periods of time and are at risk for fungal and bacterial infections [100, 101]. Even with the advances in supportive care, approximately 5% of patients will die in induction due to infection or complications with the therapy. The development of newer antifungals that can be given orally and are well tolerated will broaden the ability to both treat fungal infections and provide effective prophylaxis. The chemotherapy is given over prolonged periods of time, and often patients need significant nutritional support as they deal with nausea and not wanting to eat.

The backbone of all current chemotherapy for AML is a combination of Ara-C (cytarabine) and an anthracycline [85, 86, 93–96, 102]. There is considerable debate on the best combination, and which anthracycline should be used for induction, and various studies show a variety of results [103, 104]. Current induction therapy uses either 6-tioguanine or etoposide in addition to Ara-C and an anthracyline, but it is unclear if 6-tioguanine is better than etoposide; the medical research

council (MRC) in the United Kingdom compared the two drugs without clear results [85, 86].

Another key aspect of AML therapy to obtain remission is the dose intensity. A study by the Children's Cancer Group (CCG), CCG 2891, compared the timing of chemotherapy [94, 105]. Half of the patients were allowed to have count recovery before receiving a second round of a five-drug DCTER [dexamethasone, cytarabine, tioguanine, etoposide, Rubidomycin (daunorubicin)] regimen, and half received the second round of chemotherapy at day 15 regardless of count recovery. While there was increased toxicity and toxic deaths in the intensively timed group, the remission rates were also significantly better, and overall and event-free survival was also better.

Similarly to ALL therapy, children with AML are at risk of primary CNS disease or CNS relapses. With current chemotherapy, the CNS relapse rate is less than 5% [85, 86, 93–96, 102]. Most treatment protocols include intrathecal Ara-C with each cycle of chemotherapy, with very favorable results. One exception to this standard approach is the German BFM protocols that include 1200 cGy of CNS radiation. The role of radiation with current chemotherapy is unclear, especially with high-dose Ara-C, which is known to have good CNS penetration, and therefore the need to give radiation may be protocol dependent.

The post-remission therapy of AML is still under major debate, and several approaches are employed today. For patients who do not go on to stem cell transplantation, most current COG protocols employ three additional cycles of very high dose chemotherapy after the two cycles of induction chemotherapy. There is also debate over the need for the fifth cycle (depending on the nature of the cycle), as studies have shown that, while there is an increase in disease-free survival, overall survival is not significantly different due to potential toxicity associated with the last course of chemotherapy [85, 86]. In contrast, the BFM group employs a different approach to post-remission therapy, which includes several cycles of high-dose chemotherapy followed by maintenance chemotherapy for one year that is similar to that used in ALL [95]. Both approaches are valid, and the final outcomes are similar: approximately 60% five-year EFS and 65% five-year overall survival.

The biggest debate in the AML therapy today is which patients will benefit from an allogeneic stem cell transplantation. Previous protocols have evaluated the role of autologous stem cell transplant with or without purging of potential leukemia cells, and show improvement of the EFS but not in the overall survival [86, 105, 106]. The current results from the British Medical Research Council (MRC) have shown an overall survival advantage of allogeneic transplantation for patients with high risk of relapse, but not for patients with low risk [85, 86].

With current protocols, children with AML at diagnosis can expect 60% five-year EFS. While this is a considerable improvement over the last 40 years, it is not nearly good enough. As the biology of AML is understood, there is potential to develop

Table 18.4. Therapeutic drugs commonly used in acute myeloid leukemias.

Class of drug/therapy	Drugs	Mechanism of action	Phase of therapy normally used	Short- and long-term toxicity
Anthracyclines	Daunorubicin, Mitoxantrone, Idarubicin	Inhibition of DNA and RNA synthesis by intercalating between DNA base pairs, uncoiling of the helix, and by steric obstruction; may cause free radical damage to DNA	Induction Consolidation	Cardiovascular toxicity, short- and long-term Myelosuppression: thrombocytopenia, leukopenia, neutropenia, mild anemia Mucositis
Protein synthesis inhibitors	L-asparaginase (*E. coli*)	Inhibits protein synthesis by deaminating asparagine and depriving tumor cells of this essential amino acid	Consolidation with high-dose cytarabine	Transient diabetes Hematologic toxicities: leukopenia, hemorrhage Coagulation abnormalities: prolonged thrombin, prothrombin, and partial thromboplastin times, hypofibrinogenemia; thrombosis
Nucleoside analogues	Cytarabine 6-Tioguanine Clofarabine	Converted intracellularly to the active metabolite cytarabine triphosphate; inhibits DNA polymerase by competing with deoxycytidine triphosphate, resulting in inhibition of DNA synthesis; incorporated into DNA chain, resulting in termination of chain elongation; cell cycle-specific for the S-phase of cell division	In all phases for cytarabine In the relapsed setting for clofarabine, but being moved upfront	Myelosuppression: leukopenia, anemia, thrombocytopenia With high doses: fevers, respiratory distress
Antibodies	Gemtuzumab Ozogamicin	Antibody to CD33 antigen which is expressed on leukemic blasts in >80% of AML patients, as well as normal myeloid cells; binding results in internalization of the antibody–antigen complex, leading to the release of the calicheamicin derivative inside the myeloid cell; the calicheamicin derivative binds to DNA, resulting in double-strand breaks and cell death; pluripotent stem cells and non-hematopoietic cells are not affected	Induction Consolidation	Hepatic: hyperbilirubinemia, LDH, ALT, AST, and alkaline phosphatase elevated; veno-occlusive disease – higher incidence in patients with prior history of hematopoietic stem cell transplant; hepatic failure, jaundice, ascites, hepatosplenomegaly, portal vein thrombosis Hematologic: anemia, leukopenia, lymphopenia, neutropenia (neutropenic fever, neutropenic sepsis), thrombocytopenia, bleeding, disseminated intravascular coagulation, PT and PTT elevated
Tyrosine kinase inhibitors	Lestaurtinib	Blocks the signaling of BCR-ABL	Lestaurtinib in early trials for patients with abnormalities at 11q23 or *FLT3*	To be determined
Topoisomerase II inhibitors	Etoposide	Inhibits mitotic activity; inhibits DNA type II topoisomerase producing single- and double-strand DNA breaks	Induction	Myelosuppression: anemia, granulocyte nadir at ~7–14 days, platelet nadir at ~9–16 days Therapy-related t-AML/t-MDS, with 11q23 (*MLL*) rearrangements Therapy-related ALL

much better therapies, because we are probably at the limit of what we can do with traditional cytotoxic chemotherapy. Even with advances in supportive care, treatment-related mortality is still significant, and with current, very high doses of anthracyclines, long-term cardiac toxicity is a major concern. One of the best examples of biology-directed therapy is the use of ATRA in AML M3, and the success with this group of patients. In addition to manipulating the biology of the leukemia, other exciting approaches will develop as we learn to harness the immune system. The benefits of stem cell transplantation have been shown, and they are largely due to the graft versus leukemia effects. New approaches, including utilizing NK-cells, have shown very

exciting initial results, and if used in conjunction with reduced intensity stem cell transplantation to minimize toxicity, can potentially offer additional options [107, 108].

In summary, there has been considerable progress in the therapy of both AML and ALL over the last 40 years. However, progress still needs to be made, particularly in the detection of MRD in order to direct the chemotherapy better, in learning about the biology and developing new more specific therapeutic agents, and understanding how to harness the immune system to fight off cancer. There is optimism on all fronts that progress will continue and more and more patients will be cured to live healthy, active lives.

References

1. **Jemal A, Tiwari RC, Murray T**, *et al.* Cancer statistics, 2004. *CA: a Cancer Journal for Clinicians.* 2004;**54**:8–29.

2. **Shu XO, Potter JD, Linet MS**, *et al.* Diagnostic X-rays and ultrasound exposure and risk of childhood acute lymphoblastic leukemia by immunophenotype. *Cancer Epidemiology, Biomarkers & Prevention.* 2002;**11**:177–185.

3. **Pui C-H, Relling MV, Downing JR.** Acute lymphoblastic leukemia. *New England Journal of Medicine.* 2004;**350**:1535–1548.

4. **Schrappe M.** Evolution of BFM trials for childhood ALL. *Annals of Hematology.* 2004;**83**(Suppl 1): S121–S123.

5. **Chessells JM.** Recent advances in management of acute leukaemia. *Archives of Disease in Childhood.* 2000;**82**:438–442.

6. **Saarinen-Pihkala UM, Gustafsson G, Carlsen N**, *et al.* Outcome of children with high-risk acute lymphoblastic leukemia (HR-ALL): Nordic results on an intensive regimen with restricted central nervous system irradiation. *Pediatric Blood and Cancer.* 2004;**42**: 8–23.

7. **Zuelzer WW.** Pediatric hematology in historical perspective. In Nathan DG, Orkin SH, Oski FH, eds. *Nathan and Oski's Hematology of Infancy and Childhood* (5th edn.). Philadelphia, PA: WB Saunders; 1998, 3–16.

8. **Pollock BH, DeBaun MR, Camitta BM**, *et al.* Racial differences in the survival of childhood B-precursor acute lymphoblastic leukemia: a Pediatric Oncology Group Study. *Journal of Clinical Oncology.* 2000;**18**:813–823.

9. **Bhatia S, Sather HN, Heerema NA**, *et al.* Racial and ethnic differences in survival of children with acute lymphoblastic leukemia. *Blood.* 2002;**100**:1957–1964.

10. **Carroll WL.** Race and outcome in childhood acute lymphoblastic leukemia. *JAMA.* 2003;**290**:2061–2063.

11. **Kadan-Lottick NS, Ness KK, Bhatia S**, *et al.* Survival variability by race and ethnicity in childhood acute lymphoblastic leukemia. *JAMA.* 2003;**290**:2008–2014.

12. **Neglia JP, Robison LL.** Epidemiology of the childhood acute leukemias. *Pediatric Clinics of North America.* 1988;**35**:675–692.

13. **Pui C-H, Boyett JM, Relling MV**, *et al.* Sex differences in prognosis for children with acute lymphoblastic leukemia. *Journal of Clinical Oncology.* 1999;**17**:818–824.

14. **Greaves MF, Colman SM, Beard ME**, *et al.* Geographical distribution of acute lymphoblastic leukaemia subtypes: second report of the collaborative group study. *Leukemia.* 1993;**7**:27–34.

15. **Ramot B, Magrath I.** Hypothesis: the environment is a major determinant of the immunological sub-type of lymphoma and acute lymphoblastic leukaemia in children. *British Journal of Haematology.* 1982;**50**:183–189.

16. **Dordelmann M, Schrappe M, Reiter A**, *et al.* Down's syndrome in childhood acute lymphoblastic leukemia: clinical characteristics and treatment outcome in four consecutive BFM trials. Berlin-Frankfurt-Munster Group. *Leukemia.* 1998;**12**:645–651.

17. **Horwitz M.** The genetics of familial leukemia. *Leukemia.* 1997;**11**:1347–1359.

18. **Yamada Y, Inoue R, Fukao T**, *et al.* Ataxia telangiectasia associated with B-cell lymphoma: the effect of a half-dose of the drugs administered according to the acute lymphoblastic leukemia standard risk protocol. *Pediatric Hematology and Oncology.* 1998;**15**:425–429.

19. **Moloney WC.** Leukemia in survivors of atomic bombing. *New England Journal of Medicine.* 1955;**253**:88–90.

20. **Wald N.** Leukemia in Hiroshima City atomic bomb survivors. *Science.* 1958; **127**:699–700.

21. **Evans JS, Wennberg JE, McNeil BJ.** The influence of diagnostic radiography on the incidence of breast cancer and leukemia. *New England Journal of Medicine.* 1986;**315**:810–815.

22. **Tucker MA, Meadows AT**, Boice JD Jr., *et al.* Leukemia after therapy with alkylating agents for childhood cancer. *Journal of the National Cancer Institute.* 1987;**78**:459–464.

23. **Margolin JF, Steuber CP, Poplack DG.** Acute lymphoblastic leukemia. In Pizzo PA, Poplack DG, eds. *Principles and Practice of Pediatric Oncology* (5th edn.). Philadelphia, PA: Lippincott, Williams & Wilkins; 2006, 538–590.

24. **Crist WM, Shuster JJ, Falletta J**, *et al.* Clinical features and outcome in childhood T-cell leukemia-lymphoma according to stage of thymocyte differentiation: a Pediatric Oncology Group Study. *Blood.* 1988;**72**:1891–1897.

25. **Pui C-H, Behm FG, Singh B**, *et al.* Heterogeneity of presenting features and their relation to treatment outcome in 120 children with T-cell acute lymphoblastic leukemia. *Blood.* 1990; **75**:174–179.

26. **Santana VM, Dodge RK, Crist WM**, *et al.* Presenting features and treatment outcome of adolescents with acute lymphoblastic leukemia. *Leukemia.* 1990;**4**:87–90.

27. **Simone JV, Verzosa MS, Rudy JA.** Initial features and prognosis in 363 children with acute lymphocytic leukemia. *Cancer.* 1975;**36**:2099–2108.

28. **Silverman LB, Sallan SE.** Newly diagnosed childhood acute lymphoblastic leukemia: update on prognostic factors and treatment. *Current Opinion in Hematology.* 2003; **10**:290–296.

29. **Smith M, Arthur D, Camitta B**, *et al.* Uniform approach to risk classification and treatment assignment for children with acute lymphoblastic leukemia. *Journal of Clinical Oncology.* 1996;**14**: 18–24.

30. **Steinherz PG, Gaynon PS, Breneman JC**, *et al.* Cytoreduction and prognosis in acute lymphoblastic leukemia – the importance of early marrow response: report from the Children's Cancer Group. *Journal of Clinical Oncology.* 1996;**14**:389–398.

31. **Schrappe M, Reiter A, Ludwig WD**, *et al.* Improved outcome in childhood acute lymphoblastic leukemia despite reduced use of anthracyclines and cranial radiotherapy: results of trial ALL-BFM 90. German-Austrian-Swiss ALL-BFM Study Group. *Blood.* 2000; **95**:3310–3322.

32. **Gaynon PS, Bleyer WA, Steinherz PG**, *et al.* Day 7 marrow response and outcome for children with acute lymphoblastic leukemia and unfavorable presenting features. *Medical and Pediatric Oncology.* 1990; **18**:273–279.

33. **Nachman JB, Sather HN, Sensel MG**, *et al.* Augmented post-induction therapy for children with high-risk

acute lymphoblastic leukemia and a slow response to initial therapy. *New England Journal of Medicine*. 1998;**338**: 1663–1671.

34. **Nachman J, Sather HN, Cherlow JM,** *et al.* Response of children with high-risk acute lymphoblastic leukemia treated with and without cranial irradiation: a report from the Children's Cancer Group. *Journal of Clinical Oncology*. 1998;**16**:920–930.

35. **Borowitz MJ, Devidas M, Hunger SP,** *et al.* Clinical significance of minimal residual disease in childhood acute lymphoblastic leukemia and its relationship to other prognostic factors: a Children's Oncology Group study. *Blood*. 2008;**111**:5477–5485.

36. **Campana D.** Determination of minimal residual disease in leukaemia patients. *British Journal of Haematology*. 2003;**121**:823–838.

37. **Coustan-Smith E, Sancho J, Hancock ML,** *et al.* Clinical importance of minimal residual disease in childhood acute lymphoblastic leukemia. *Blood*. 2000;**96**:2691–2696.

38. **Ciudad J, San Miguel JF, Lopez-Berges MC,** *et al.* Prognostic value of immunophenotypic detection of minimal residual disease in acute lymphoblastic leukemia. *Journal of Clinical Oncology*. 1998;**16**:3774–3781.

39. **Pui C-H, Robison LL, Look AT.** Acute lymphoblastic leukemia. *Lancet*. 2008; **371**:1030–1043.

40. **Silverman LB, Gelber RD, Young ML,** *et al.* Induction failure in acute lymphoblastic leukemia of childhood. *Cancer*. 1999;**85**:1395–1404.

41. **Ito C, Evans WE, McNinch L,** *et al.* Comparative cytotoxicity of dexamethasone and prednisolone in childhood acute lymphoblastic leukemia. *Journal of Clinical Oncology*. 1996;**14**:2370–2376.

42. **Gaynon PS, Desai AA, Bostrom BC,** *et al.* Early response to therapy and outcome in childhood acute lymphoblastic leukemia: a review. *Cancer*. 1997;**80**:1717–1726.

43. **Aur RJ, Simone JV, Hustu HO,** *et al.* A comparative study of central nervous system irradiation and intensive chemotherapy early in remission of childhood acute lymphocytic leukemia. *Cancer*. 1972;**29**:381–391.

44. **Meadows AT, Gordon J, Massari DJ,** *et al.* Declines in IQ scores and cognitive dysfunctions in children with acute lymphocytic leukaemia treated with cranial irradiation. *Lancet*. 1981;**2**: 1015–1018.

45. **Tubergen DG, Gilchrist GS, O'Brien RT,** *et al.* Prevention of CNS disease in intermediate-risk acute lymphoblastic leukemia: comparison of cranial radiation and intrathecal methotrexate and the importance of systemic therapy: a Childrens Cancer Group report. *Journal of Clinical Oncology*. 1993;**11**:520–526.

46. **Conter V, Arico M, Valsecchi MG,** *et al.* Extended intrathecal methotrexate may replace cranial irradiation for prevention of CNS relapse in children with intermediate-risk acute lymphoblastic leukemia treated with Berlin-Frankfurt-Munster-based intensive chemotherapy. The Associazione Italiana di Ematologia ed Oncologia Pediatrica. *Journal of Clinical Oncology*. 1995;**13**:2497–2502.

47. **Rivera GK, Raimondi SC, Hancock ML,** *et al.* Improved outcome in childhood acute lymphoblastic leukaemia with reinforced early treatment and rotational combination chemotherapy. *Lancet*. 1991;**337**: 61–66.

48. **Chessells JM, Harrison G, Lilleyman JS,** *et al.* Continuing (maintenance) therapy in lymphoblastic leukaemia: lessons from MRC UKALL X. Medical Research Council Working Party in Childhood Leukaemia. *British Journal of Haematology*. 1997;**98**:945–951.

49. **Lennard L, Lilleyman JS.** Variable mercaptopurine metabolism and treatment outcome in childhood lymphoblastic leukaemia. *Journal of Clinical Oncology*. 1989;**7**:1816–1823.

50. **Schmiegelow K, Pulczynska MK.** Maintenance chemotherapy for childhood acute lymphoblastic leukaemia: should dosage be guided by white blood cell counts? *The American Journal of Pediatric Hematology/ Oncology*. 1990;**12**:462–467.

51. **Balduzzi A, Valsecchi MG, Uderzo C.** Chemotherapy versus allogeneic transplantation for very-high-risk childhood acute lymphoblastic leukaemia in first complete remission: comparison by genetic randomisation in an international prospective study. *Lancet*. 2005;**366**:635–642.

52. **Johnson FL, Thomas ED, Clark BS,** *et al.* A comparison of marrow transplantation with chemotherapy for children with acute lymphoblastic leukemia in second or subsequent remission. *New England Journal of Medicine*. 1981;**305**:846–851.

53. **Barrett AJ, Horowitz MM, Pollock BH,** *et al.* Bone marrow transplants from HLA-identical siblings as compared with chemotherapy for children with acute lymphoblastic leukemia in a second remission. *New England Journal of Medicine*. 1994;**331**:1253–1258.

54. **Eden OB.** Acute lymphoblastic leukaemia: whom and when should we transplant? *Pediatric Transplantation*. 1999;**3**(Suppl 1): 108–115.

55. **Smith MA, Gloeckler-Ries LA, Gurney JG, Ross JA.** Leukemia. In Ries LAG, Smith MA, Gurney JG, *et al.*, eds. *Cancer Incidence and Survival among Children and Adolescents: United States SEER Program 1975–1995* (NIH Pub No. 99–4649). Bethesda, MD: National Cancer Institute; 1999, 17–34.

56. **Gurney JG, Severson RK, Davis S, Robison LL.** Incidence of cancer in children in the United States. Sex, race, and 1 year age-specific rates by histologic type. *Cancer*. 1995;**75**:2186–2195.

57. **Sandoval C, Pui C-H, Bowman LC,** *et al.* Secondary acute myeloid leukemia in children previously treated with alkylating agents, intercalating topoisomerase II inhibitors, and irradiation. *Journal of Clinical Oncology*. 1993;**11**:1039–1045.

58. **Pui C-H, Ribeiro RC, Hancock ML,** *et al.* Acute myeloid leukemia in children treated with epipodophyllotoxins for acute lymphoblastic leukemia. *New England Journal of Medicine*. 1991;**325**:1682–1687.

59. **Fong CT, Brodeur GM.** Down's syndrome and leukemia: epidemiology, genetics, cytogenetics and mechanisms of leukemogenesis. *Cancer Genetics and Cytogenetics*. 1987;**28**:55–76.

60. **Freedman MH.** Congenital marrow failure syndromes and malignant hematopoietic transformation. *Oncologist*. 1996;**1**:354–360.

61. **Auerbach AD.** Fanconi anemia and leukemia: tracking the genes. *Leukemia*. 1992;**6**:1–4.

62. **Woods CG.** DNA repair disorders. *Archives of Disease in Childhood*. 1998; **78**:178–184.

63. **Crispino JD**. GATA1 mutations in Down syndrome: implications for biology and diagnosis of children with transient myeloproliferative disorder and acute megakaryoblastic leukemia. *Pediatric Blood and Cancer*. 2005;**44**: 40–44.

64. **Doyle JJ, Thorner P, Poon A**, *et al*. Transient leukemia followed by megakaryoblastic leukemia in a child with mosaic Down syndrome. *Leukemia & Lymphoma*. 1995;**17**:345–350.

65. **Jablon S, Kato H**. Childhood cancer in relation to prenatal exposure to atomic-bomb radiation. *Lancet*. 1970;**7681**:1000–1003.

66. **Shimizu Y, Schull WI, Kato H**. Cancer risk among atomic bomb survivors: the RERF Life Span Study. *JAMA*. 1990;**264**:601–604.

67. **Robison LL, Buckley JD, Daigle AE**, *et al*. Maternal drug use and risk of childhood nonlymphoblastic leukemia among offspring. An epidemiologic investigation implicating marijuana (a report from the Children's Cancer Study Group). *Cancer*. 1989;**63**:1904–1911.

68. **Brondum J, Shu XO, Steinbuch M**, *et al*. Parental cigarette smoking and the risk of acute leukemia in children. *Cancer*. 1999;**85**:1380–1388.

69. **McBride ML**. Childhood cancer and environmental contaminants. *Canadian Journal of Public Health*. 1998;**89**(Suppl 89): S53–S62,S58–S68.

70. **Choi SI, Simone JV**. Acute nonlymphocytic leukemia in 171 children. *Medical and Pediatric Oncology*. 1976;**2**:119–146.

71. **Frohna BJ, Quint DJ**. Granulocytic sarcoma (chloroma) causing spinal cord compression. *Neuroradiology*. 1993;**35**:509–511.

72. **Brown LM, Daeschner CD, Timms J, Crow W**. Granulocytic sarcoma in childhood acute myelogenous leukemia. *Pediatric Neurology*. 1989;**5**:173–178.

73. **Bulas RB, Laine FJ, Das Narla L**. Bilateral orbital granulocytic sarcoma (chloroma) preceding the blast phase of acute myelogenous leukemia: CT findings. *Pediatric Radiology*. 1995;**25**: 488–489.

74. **Creutzig U, Ritter J, Budde M, Sutor A, Schellong G**. Early deaths due to hemorrhage and leukostasis in childhood acute myelogenous leukemia. Associations with hyperleukocytosis and acute monocytic leukemia. *Cancer*. 1987;**60**:3071–3079.

75. **Menell JS, Cesarman GM, Jacovina AT**, *et al*. Annexin II and bleeding in acute promyelocytic leukemia. *New England Journal of Medicine*. 1999;**340**: 994–1004.

76. **Tallman MS, Kwaan HC**. Reassessing the hemostatic disorder associated with acute promyelocytic leukemia. *Blood*. 1992;**79**:543–553.

77. **Rowe JM, Lichtman MA**. Hyperleukocytosis and leukostasis: common features of childhood chronic myelogenous leukemia. *Blood*. 1984;**63**: 1230–1234.

78. **Bloom R, Taveira Da Silva AM, Bracey A**. Reversible respiratory failure due to intravascular leukostasis in chronic myelogenous leukemia. Relationship of oxygen transfer to leukocyte count. *The American Journal of Medicine*. 1979;**67**: 679–683.

79. **Vardiman JW, Thiele J, Arber DA**, *et al*. The 2008 revision of the World Health Organization (WHO) classification of myeloid neoplasms and acute leukemia: rationale and important changes. *Blood*. 2009;**114**: 937–951.

80. **Wells RJ, Woods WG, Buckley JD**, *et al*. Treatment of newly diagnosed children and adolescents with acute myeloid leukemia: a Children's Cancer Group study. *Journal of Clinical Oncology*. 1994;**12**:2367–2377.

81. **Tallman MS, Neuberg D, Bennett JM**, *et al*. Acute megakaryocytic leukemia: the Eastern Cooperative Oncology Group experience. *Blood*. 2000;**96**: 2405–2411.

82. **Hurwitz CA, Schell MJ, Pui CH**, *et al*. Adverse prognostic features in 251 children treated for acute myeloid leukemia. *Medical and Pediatric Oncology*. 1993;**21**:1–7.

83. **Gamis AS, Woods WG, Alonzo TA**, *et al*. Increased age at diagnosis has a significantly negative effect on outcome in children with Down syndrome and acute myeloid leukemia: a report from the Children's Cancer Group Study 2891. *Journal of Clinical Oncology*. 2003;**21**:3415–3422.

84. **Mrozek K, Heinonen K, de la Chapelle A, Bloomfield CD**. Clinical significance of cytogenetics in acute myeloid leukemia. *Seminars in Oncology*. 1997;**24**:17–31.

85. **Webb D, Harrison G, Stevens R**, *et al*. Relationships between age at diagnosis, clinical features, and outcome of therapy in children treated in the Medical Research Council AML10 and 12 trials for acute myeloid leukemia. *Blood*. 2001;**98**:1714–1720.

86. **Burnett AK, Goldstone AH, Stevens RM**, *et al*. Randomised comparison of addition of autologous bone-marrow transplantation to intensive chemotherapy for acute myeloid leukaemia in first remission: results of MRC AML10 trial. UK Medical Research Council Adult and Children's Leukaemia Working Parties. *Lancet*. 1998;**351**:700–708.

87. **Tallman MS, Andersen JW, Schiffer CA**, *et al*. All-trans-retinoic acid in acute promyelocytic leukemia. *New England Journal of Medicine*. 1997;**337**: 1021–1028.

88. **Fenaux P, Chastang C, Chevret S**, *et al*. A randomized comparison of all transretinoic acid (ATRA) followed by chemotherapy and ATRA plus chemotherapy and the role of maintenance therapy in newly diagnosed acute promyelocytic leukemia. The European APL Group. *Blood*. 1999;**94**:1192–1200.

89. **Hasle H, Arico M, Basso G**, *et al*. Myelodysplastic syndrome, juvenile myelomonocytic leukemia, and acute myeloid leukemia associated with complete or partial monosomy 7. European Working Group on MDS in Childhood (EWOG-MDS). *Leukemia*. 1999;**13**:376–385.

90. **Meshinchi S, Stirewalt DL, Alonzo TA**, *et al*. Activating mutations of RTK/ras signal transduction pathway in pediatric acute myeloid leukemia. *Blood*. 2003;**102**:1474–1479.

91. **Meshinchi S, Woods WG, Stirewalt DL**, *et al*. Prevalence and prognostic significance of Flt3 internal tandem duplication in pediatric acute myeloid leukemia. *Blood*. 2001;**97**:89–94.

92. **Kiyoi H, Naoe T, Nakano Y**, *et al*. Prognostic implication of FLT3 and N-RAS gene mutations in acute myeloid leukemia. *Blood*. 1999;**93**: 3074–3080.

93. **Hann IM, Stevens RF, Goldstone AH**, *et al*. Randomized comparison of DAT versus ADE as induction chemotherapy

in children and younger adults with acute myeloid leukemia. Results of the Medical Research Council's 10th AML trial (MRC AML10). Adult and Childhood Leukaemia Working Parties of the Medical Research Council. *Blood.* 1997;**89**:2311–2318.

94. **Woods WG, Kobrinsky N, Buckley JD,** *et al.* Timed-sequential induction therapy improves postremission outcome in acute myeloid leukemia: a report from the Children's Cancer Group. *Blood.* 1996;**87**:4979–4989.

95. **Creutzig U, Ritter J, Zimmermann M,** *et al.* Improved treatment results in high-risk pediatric acute myeloid leukemia patients after intensification with high-dose cytarabine and mitoxantrone: results of study Acute Myeloid Leukemia–Berlin-Frankfurt-Munster 93. *Journal of Clinical Oncology.* 2001;**19**:2705–2713.

96. **Woods WG, Neudorf S, Gold S,** *et al.* A comparison of allogeneic bone marrow transplantation, autologous bone marrow transplantation, and aggressive chemotherapy in children with acute myeloid leukemia in remission: a report from the Children's Cancer Group. *Blood.* 2001;**97**:56–62.

97. **Langebrake C, Creutzig U, Dworzak M,** *et al.* Residual disease monitoring in childhood acute myeloid leukemia: the MRD-AML-BFM Study group. *Journal of Clinical Oncology.* 2006;**24**:3686–3692.

98. **Leroy H, de Button S, Grardel-Duflos N,** *et al.* Prognostic value of real-time quantitative PCR (RQ-PCR) in AML with t(8;21). *Leukemia.* 2005;**19**:367–372.

99. **Perea G, Lasa A, Aventin A,** *et al.* Prognostic value of minimal residual disease (MRD) in acute myeloid leukemia (AML) with favorable cytogenetics [t(8;21) and inv(16)]. *Leukemia.* 2006;**20**:87–94.

100. **Martino R, Subira M, Domingo-Albos A,** *et al.* Low-dose amphotericin B lipid complex for the treatment of persistent fever of unknown origin in patients with hematologic malignancies and prolonged neutropenia. *Chemotherapy.* 1999;**45**:205–212.

101. **Hospenthal DR, Byrd JC, Weiss RB.** Successful treatment of invasive aspergillosis complicating prolonged treatment-related neutropenia in acute myelogenous leukemia with amphotericin B lipid complex. *Medical and Pediatric Oncology.* 1995;**25**:119–122.

102. **Lie SO, Abrahamsson J, Clausen N,** *et al.* Treatment stratification based on initial in vivo response in acute myeloid leukaemia in children without Down's syndrome: results of NOPHO-AML trials. *British Journal of Haematology.* 2003;**122**:217–225.

103. **Wheatley K.** Meta-analysis of randomized trials of idarubicin (IDAR) or metozantrone (Mito) versus daunorubicin (DNR) as induction therapy for acute myeloid leukaemia (AML). *Blood.* 1995;**86**:43A.

104. **Vogler WR, Velez-Garcia E, Weiner RS,** *et al.* A phase III trial comparing idarubicin and daunorubicin in combination with cytarabine in acute myelogenous leukemia: a Southeastern Cancer Study Group Study. *Journal of Clinical Oncology.* 1992;**10**:1103–1111.

105. **Woods WG, Neudorf S, Gold S,** *et al.* A comparison of allogeneic bone marrow transplantation, autologous bone marrow transplantation, and aggressive chemotherapy in children with acute myeloid leukemia in remission: a report from the Children's Cancer Group. *Blood.* 2001;**97**:56–62.

106. **Ball ED, Wilson J, Phelps V, Neudorf S.** Autologous bone marrow transplantation for acute myeloid leukemia in remission or first relapse using monoclonal antibody-purged marrow: results of phase II studies with long-term follow-up. *Bone Marrow Transplant.* 2000;**25**:823–829.

107. **Leung W, Iyengar R, Turner V,** *et al.* Determinants of antileukemia effects of allogeneic NK cells. *Journal of Immunology.* 2004;**172**:644–650.

108. **Ruggeri L, Capanni M, Casucci M,** *et al.* Role of natural killer cell alloreactivity in HLA-mismatched hematopoietic stem cell transplantation. *Blood.* 1999;**94**: 333–339.

The effect of chemotherapy, detection of minimal residual disease, and hematopoietic stem cell transplantation

Maria A. Proytcheva

Introduction

As a result of combination chemotherapy administered from several months to 2–3 years, depending upon the type of malignancy and risk stratification, the cure rate in children with acute lymphoblastic leukemia (ALL) who are younger than 15 years of age has risen from less than 10% in the pre-chemotherapy era to 88% presently [1]. Moreover, the cure rate for acute myeloid leukemia (AML), although not as successful, has also markedly improved. This success came mostly as a result of randomized clinical trials conducted by the Children's Oncology Group (COG), the St. Jude Children's Research Hospital, the Medical Research Council in the United Kingdom, and the German Berlin–Frankfurt–Münster clinical trials group. However, while the chemotherapy is necessary for a cure, most of the chemotherapeutic agents have serious myelosuppressive effects resulting in short- and long-term abnormalities in the peripheral blood and bone marrow. Knowledge of these changes is essential for the proper evaluation of such specimens in children undergoing chemotherapy.

Factors affecting treatment response

The treatment response and leukemia clearance differ depending on multiple factors associated with the host response to chemotherapy. Recent studies have shown that these differences in response to drugs are due to individual genomic variations such as single nucleotide polymorphisms (SNPs), insertion, inversions, copy-number variations, epigenetic variants, or loss of heterozygosity that are able to influence the absorption, distribution, metabolism, and excretion of chemotherapeutic agents [2] (Table 19.1 [3]).

Currently, the best recognized example of genetic polymorphisms that influence antileukemic drug response and adverse effects is thiopurine S-methyltransferase (TPMT). The TPMT pathway is the main mechanism for intracellular inactivation of thiopurine antimetabolites – mercaptopurine, azathioprine, and thioguanine (tioguanine), all key components of the childhood acute leukemia regimens – in hematopoietic tissue [4].

TPMT-deficient individuals treated with conventional doses of thiopurines are predisposed to increased toxicity and profound myelosuppression as a result of the accumulation of excessive intracellular concentrations of the drug in hematopoietic tissues. In addition, TPMT deficiency has been linked to a higher risk of developing a second malignancy in patients with ALL, including etoposide inhibitor-induced AML and radiation-induced brain tumors [5].

The loss of activity of TPMT has been attributed to a single nucleotide polymorphism (SNP) in the human TPMT gene. This polymorphism is frequent in Caucasians, where 1 in 300 individuals has no functional alleles and no detectable activity, and about 11% are heterozygotes with one wild-type allele and intermediate activity [6]. In patients with a lack of, or reduced, TPMT activity, dose adjustment is required in order to ameliorate myelosuppression and other adverse effects. Thus, knowledge of a patient's genotype status allows individualized dosing, resulting in a decreased risk of acute toxicity from chemotherapy, thereby lowering morbidity and mortality. What is more, studies in Europe have shown that genetic testing for TPMT in patients with ALL is cost effective and should be seriously considered as an integral test prior to administration of thiopurine drugs [7].

Other factors that can predict the toxic effect of chemotherapy include age, sex, race, constitutional syndromes, and pharmacogenetic factors. Children older than 10 and in adolescence are at increased risk of developing osteonecrosis, hypercalcemia, mucositis, typhlitis, and death from infection [8]. Furthermore, some genetic variations such as vitamin D receptor FokI polymorphism, TYMS low activity, and PAI-1 polymorphism may contribute to the risk of osteonecrosis [9].

An example of a drug target mechanism that is associated with genetic alterations in AML is the expression of multidrug-resistance-associated protein 1 (MDR1 or P-glycoprotein), which results in a functional cyclosporine A-inhibited drug efflux [10]. The expression of MDR1 has been associated with unfavorable cytogenetic profiles, such as −5/5q, −7/7q, inv(3), or abnormalities at 17p, and poor response to therapy [11].

Table 19.1. Effect of genetic polymorphisms of drug-metabolizing enzymes on treatment response.

Gene product	Polymorphism (s)	Drug affected	Effect of mutations
Thiopurine S-methyltransferase (TPMT)	Non-synonymous single nucleotide polymorphisms (SNPs) that lead to unstable protein	6-Mercaptopurine Azathioprine 6-Tioguanine	Myelosuppression Increased risk of therapy-related cancer
Glutathione S-transferase (GST)	Completion deletions or point mutations	Alkylators Glucocorticoids Epipodophyllotoxins Anthracyclines	Increased sensitivity to antileukemic drugs, increased risk of therapy-related leukemia
Cytochrome P450 3A4 (CYP3A4)	SNPs that lead to non-functional enzyme	Vincristine Anthracyclines Epipodophyllotoxins Glucocorticoids Alkylators	Decreased risk of therapy-related leukemia
Methylene tetrahydrofolate reductase (MTHFR)	Point mutations that lead to protein instability	Methotrexate Leucovorin Reduced folates	Increased risk of mucositis Decreased risk of de novo ALL
NAD(P)H:quinone oxidoreductase 1 (NQO1)	SNPs that lead to non-functional enzyme	Alkylators Mitomycin C	Increased risk of infant and childhood ALL, adult AML and therapy-related leukemia, possibly poorer outcome of ALL

Reproduced with permission from Pui et al. [3].

Table 19.2. Morphologic findings in the bone marrow of children on chemotherapy for acute leukemia.

Early changes (second to third weeks of chemotherapy)
  Cellular depletion with progressive reduction of blasts
  Marrow edema
  Dilated sinuses filled with fibrin
  Focal or diffuse stromal hemorrhage
  Eosinophilic granular stroma due to stromal damage

Stromal reconstitution (third to fourth weeks of chemotherapy)
  Dilated sinuses and fat cell regeneration
  Macrophages containing abundant nuclear debris

Restoration of the normal hematopoiesis (fourth to sixth weeks)
  Minute foci of immature cells, paratrabecularly
  Sequence of erythroid and myeloid recovery depends of the type of leukemia
    Acute lymphoblastic leukemia at the end of induction
      Marked erythroid hyperplasia and myeloid hypoplasia
    Acute myeloid leukemia after the first cycle of therapy
      Erythroid and myeloid regeneration more or less synchronous
  Megakaryocytes recover last and form clusters
  Transient dyspoiesis, particularly dyserythropoiesis
  Marked osteoblastic activity
  Restoration of the bone marrow cellularity and hematopoietic progenitor frequency

While this mechanism of drug resistance is important, it is more pertinent for the adult population. It is seen only in a minority of children or young adults with AML.

Genomic variability is another important determinant of drug disposition and effects in children with ALL. For this reason, an understanding of pharmacogenomics, and applying the knowledge to an individual patient has great potential to improve the use of antileukemic drugs. It does so by reducing the toxicity, enhancing the efficacy of therapy, and guiding the optimal treatment selection through dose individualization [2].

Effect of chemotherapy on the bone marrow

While the chemotherapeutic drugs used to treat leukemia are effective in inducing leukemic cell death by various mechanisms, their effect extends beyond the neoplastic component to other rapidly proliferating cells such as the normal hematopoietic progenitors and bone marrow stroma. As a result, varying degrees of cellular depletion, stromal damage, fibrosis, and bony changes occur in the BM, and the severity of these abnormalities depends upon the type of therapy and underlying malignancy [12–15].

In children and adolescents on chemotherapy for acute leukemia, the changes in the bone marrow are similar to the changes in adults (Table 19.2; Figs. 19.1–19.4) [14]. During the first one to two weeks of induction chemotherapy, there is a progressive reduction of blasts that often begins at the paratrabecular areas, leaving the marrow edematous, with numerous widely dilated vascular sinuses filled with erythrocytes and fibrin. Focal or diffuse stromal hemorrhage may also be present. By the third to fourth week, there is a stromal reconstitution manifested by regenerating fat cells, collagen, and bone. Serous fat atrophy can also be present. The stromal regeneration is followed by restoration of the normal hematopoiesis by the fourth to sixth week of the initiation of chemotherapy. The changes reflect the intensity of chemotherapy and susceptibility of the neoplastic cells to the drugs.

Bone marrow fibrosis is present at diagnosis of childhood ALL and appears to be a significant part of the neoplastic process. The fibrosis disappears when the patient enters remission, but reappears with relapse; most often it is even more prominent than at initial diagnosis [14]. New findings suggest that BM fibrosis determined by reticulin fiber density (RFD) correlates with biological factors, treatment response, and outcomes, and may be a valuable prognostic marker in childhood ALL

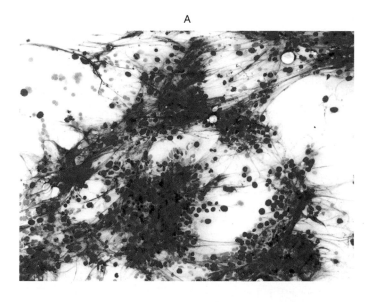

A

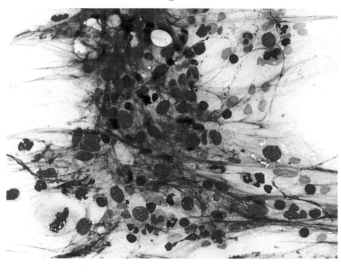

B

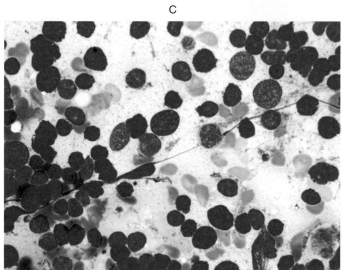

C

Fig. 19.1. Bone marrow from a two-year-old boy with precursor B-cell ALL, day eight of induction chemotherapy (Wright–Giemsa stain). (A) Marked cytoreduction and stromal injury. (B) Eosinophilic bone marrow stroma, emerging multiloculated fat cells. (C) Rare blasts intermixed with naked nuclei.

[16]. In a retrospective study of the diagnostic significance of RFD at diagnosis of precursor B-cell ALL, in correlation with the level of MRD, as determined by flow cytometry on day 29 of induction chemotherapy, patients with low level of fibrosis at diagnosis and rapid reduction by day 29 had favorable outcomes, as compared to patients with slow reduction of reticular fiber density. While this study demonstrates the possibility of a noteworthy trend, a larger prospective study will be necessary to confirm these findings. However, since most current pediatric acute lymphoblastic leukemia COG studies do not require a BM biopsy, data on the degree of BM fibrosis in children may be difficult to collect. This study, as well as other studies, suggests the necessity of a routine BM biopsy at diagnosis and during follow-up in children with acute leukemia, since the information provided by the BM aspirates and peripheral blood may be limited.

In adults, variable plasmacytosis is also present. However, in one small study, young patients below 25 years of age had less pronounced plasmacytosis, regardless of the type of leukemia or therapeutic regimen used [13]. In our experience, plasma cells, although not frequent, can be present in recovering marrow, particularly in older children (Fig. 19.5A). Excessive amounts of hemosiderin are present in the BM after several months of repetitive blood transfusions during the course of chemotherapy (Fig. 19.5B).

The *bone marrow regeneration* after myeloablative chemotherapy starts with recovery of the erythropoiesis and myelopoiesis, followed by a recovery of the megakaryopoiesis. The order in which cell lines recover first in children may depend on the type of leukemia and respective therapy. For example, at the end of induction for precursor B-cell acute lymphoblastic leukemia, there is pronounced erythroid hyperplasia and the myeloid regeneration follows (Fig. 19.6). On the other hand, after the first cycle of chemotherapy for AML, the myeloid regeneration is more pronounced and is followed by erythroid regeneration (Fig. 19.7). This observation is in

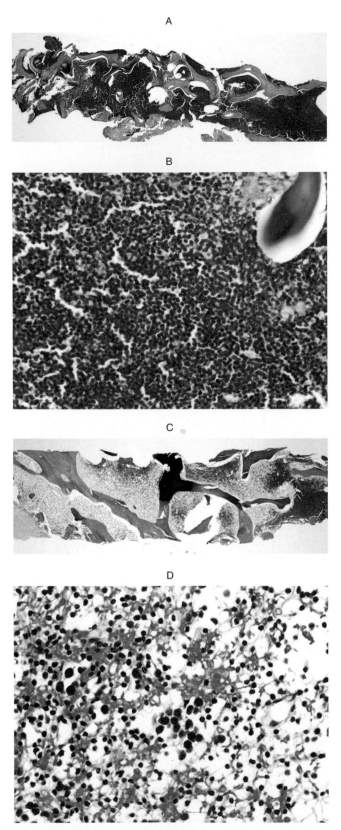

Fig. 19.2. Bone marrow from a nine-year-old boy with precursor B-cell ALL, a comparison of the diagnostic and day eight of induction chemotherapy marrow (H&E stain). A and B show markedly hypercellular marrow infiltrated by blasts, and virtually absent hematopoiesis. (C) Dramatic cytoreduction, stromal damage, and focal hemorrhage. (D) A few residual clusters of blasts.

contrast to studies in adult acute leukemias, where no significant differences in the bone marrow re-growth between AML and ALL were present [17].

During recovery, there is a shift to immaturity and dysplasia that have to be distinguished from the presence of residual leukemia. While it is still not entirely clear how the regeneration originates (whether from circulating stem cells or mesenchymal endosteal cells that either serve as precursors of stem cells or induce the proliferation and differentiation of the near-inactive stem cells), two weeks after the completion of chemotherapy for AML, the regenerating erythroid progenitors are present closely adjacent to bony trabeculae. A week later, clusters of regenerating hematopoietic cells migrate to the intertrabecular space and are present in association with the fat cells far away from the bony trabeculae [18]. The presence of a large number of immature cells along the bony trabeculae is consistent with regeneration rather than residual leukemia, since the leukemic cells are usually present as foci in the interfollicular areas. Furthermore, the regenerating hematopoietic progenitors show both morphologic and immunophenotypic heterogeneity. Flow cytometric studies are helpful in demonstrating some degree of maturation and a gradual increase in the number of more mature forms in regenerating marrow. A comparison with the initial diagnostic immunophenotype is very helpful as well, since the immunophenotypic profile of the leukemic cells is stable.

Chemotherapy for childhood ALL and AML results in dysplasia and abnormalities of spatial organization of the marrow [19]. These changes are most significant in the erythropoietic progenitors, and less pronounced in the megakaryocytes and granulocytes (Fig. 19.8). Relative erythroid hyperplasia with a lack of normal heterogeneity of red cell maturation is usually present at the end of induction chemotherapy. The BM aspirate smears show normocytic erythropoiesis with an excess of early progenitors. After chemotherapy, the erythroid regeneration is accompanied by abundant mitosis and dyserythropoiesis. However, unlike dyserythropoiesis associated with leukemia or therapy-related myelodysplastic syndrome (t-MDS), here the erythropoiesis is effective. This is manifested by the presence of marked polychromasia, reticulocytosis, and various numbers of circulating nucleated red cells in the peripheral blood. This stands in contrast to the presence of macrocytic anemia and a lack of polychromasia and reticulocytosis seen in t-MDS. Under long-term chemotherapy, there is marked myeloid hypoplasia with minimal dysgranulopoiesis.

In the BM biopsy, early erythroid regeneration occurs paratrabecularly rather than in the intertrabecular space. This initial finding is temporal. With the reappearance of the granulopoiesis, the erythroid progenitors migrate into the intertrabecular areas. The BM biopsy shows paratrabecular granulopoiesis shifted to immaturity and, unlike MDS or residual AML, after chemotherapy, there is no abnormal localization of myeloid progenitors present. Monocytes are absent from the bone marrow for a long time.

Post-chemotherapy, megakaryocytes are dysplastic, and the dysplasia may persist for a long time. However, neither

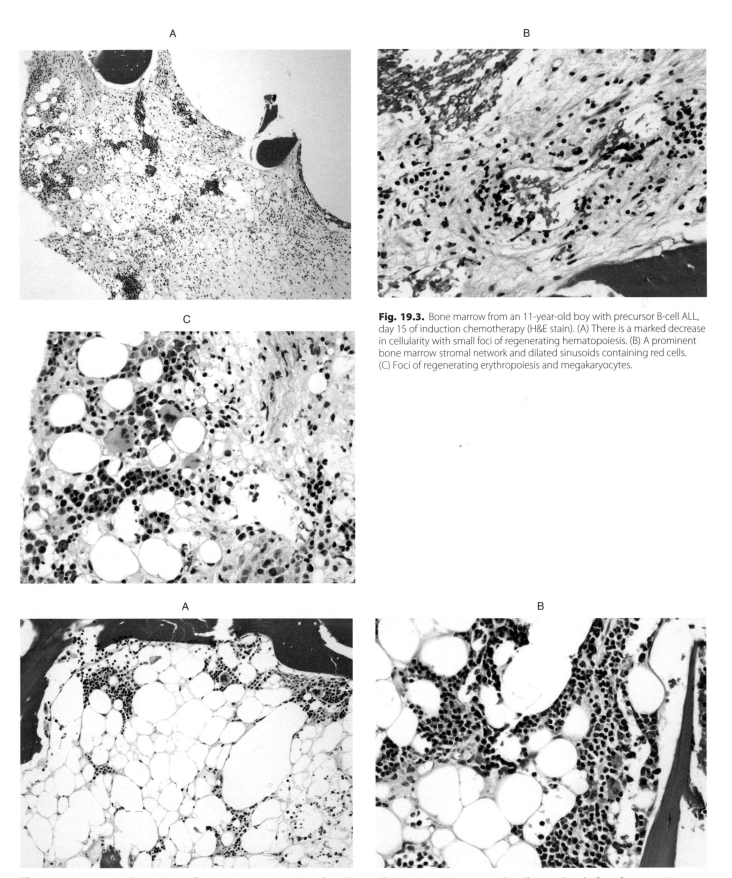

Fig. 19.3. Bone marrow from an 11-year-old boy with precursor B-cell ALL, day 15 of induction chemotherapy (H&E stain). (A) There is a marked decrease in cellularity with small foci of regenerating hematopoiesis. (B) A prominent bone marrow stromal network and dilated sinusoids containing red cells. (C) Foci of regenerating erythropoiesis and megakaryocytes.

Fig. 19.4. Precursor B-cell ALL, day 29 of induction (H&E stain). (A) Profound hypocellularity, stromal damage, and small paratrabecular foci of regenerating hematopoiesis. (B) Erythroid progenitors and megakaryocytes.

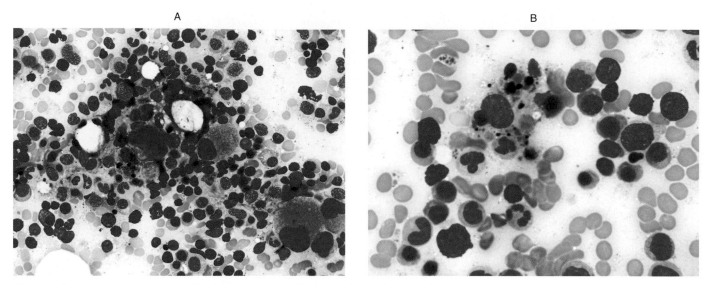

Fig. 19.5. Bone marrow from a 15-year-old girl with acute myeloid leukemia after the first cycle of chemotherapy (Wright–Giemsa stain). (A) Regeneration of the erythroid and myeloid progenitors and megakaryocytes. Mild dyspoiesis is present. Notice several macrophages containing cellular debris and hemosiderin. A few plasma cells are also seen. (B) There is mild dyserythropoiesis.

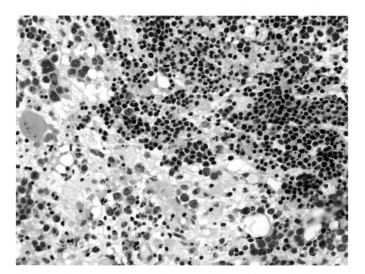

Fig. 19.6. Bone marrow from an eight-year-old boy with precursor B-cell ALL, day 29, end of induction. There is marked erythroid hyperplasia. Notice the increased number of early forms (Wright–Giemsa stain).

Fig. 19.7. Bone marrow aspirate from a two-year-old boy with acute myeloid leukemia after the first cycle of chemotherapy. Notice the multilineage hematopoiesis (Wright–Giemsa stain).

the degree of dysplasia nor the number of megakaryocytes consistently correlates with the platelet count and/or platelet morphology.

Long-term chemotherapy for pediatric acute leukemia induces significant *BM stroma damage*, resulting in defective stromal function and abnormalities in bone marrow regeneration, contributing to the pathogenesis of post-chemotherapy anemia (Table 19.3). This has been demonstrated also in *in vitro* experiments where, as compared to normal stroma, post-chemotherapy BM stromal cells are able to support a low number of burst-forming units – erythroid (BFU-Es) and, to a lesser degree, colony forming units – granulocytic monocytic (CFU-GMs) [15]. While the mechanisms of this chemotherapy-induced stromal injury are not well understood, an increase

in c-β, an erythropoiesis growth inhibitory factor, along with a decrease in the chemoprotective factor MIP-1α, have been shown to contribute to the pathogenesis. These findings support the hypothesis that inhibitors produced by the bone marrow stroma are responsible for the development of anemia in children on chemotherapy. It has been shown that such anemia is strongly correlated with decreased erythropoietic pools, as indicated by a low level of soluble transferrin receptor, despite an adequate increase in the erythropoietin production in response to anemia [20].

Similar severe functional defects of the marrow stroma and abnormal *in vitro* growth of primitive hematopoietic progenitors have been observed in pediatric and adult patients with AML treated with specific chemotherapeutic protocols

A

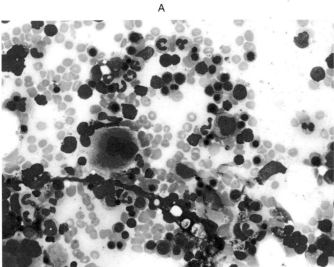

B

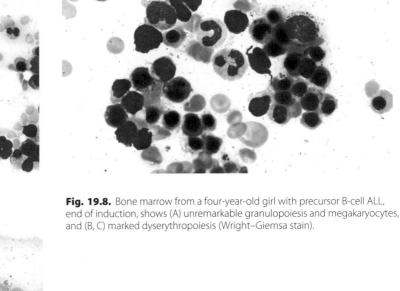

C

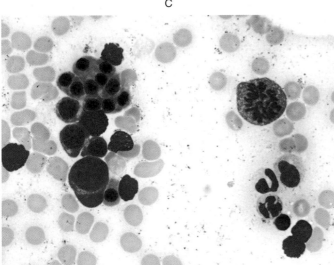

Fig. 19.8. Bone marrow from a four-year-old girl with precursor B-cell ALL, end of induction, shows (A) unremarkable granulopoiesis and megakaryocytes, and (B, C) marked dyserythropoiesis (Wright–Giemsa stain).

Table 19.3. Long-term chemotherapy effect on the bone marrow stroma of children with acute lymphoblastic leukemia [15].

Prolonged injury to the bone marrow stroma, persisting several years after the end of therapy

Defective ability of the BM stroma to sustain hematopoiesis in long-term bone marrow culture experiments
   Reduced burst-forming unit – erythroid (BFU-E) and colony
      forming unit – granulocytic monocytic (CFU-GM) generation
   Quantitative and qualitative defects of hematopoietic stem cells
   Increase in the growth-inhibitory factor TGF-β1, leading to
      functional deregulation within the BM stroma

Defective erythropoiesis despite adequate erythropoietin production   Anemia

Polymorphonuclear cell abnormalities
   Accelerated apoptosis
   Depressed microbicidal activity against Gram-positive and
      Gram-negative microorganisms

[21]. Such stromal damage may play an important role in the subsequent bone marrow regeneration and/or engraftment after an allogeneic hematopoietic stem cell transplant.

Bone marrow studies to monitor the response to therapy in pediatric acute leukemia

The therapeutic regimens and length of chemotherapy vary depending on the type of leukemia, as discussed in Chapter 18. Most ALL treatment protocols require bone marrow evaluation at day 8 and day 29 of induction chemotherapy. If the patient has more than 5% blasts at the day 8 examination, an additional BM study at day 15 is usually performed. If residual disease persists and is present at day 29, the end of the induction chemotherapy, the patient receives an additional chemotherapy until a complete remission is achieved. Thus, BM evaluation to determine the response to therapy is an integral part of the treatment protocols for children with ALL. Subsequent bone marrow evaluations are performed when recurrent/residual disease is suspected or when there is an interruption of treatment regimen due to infections or other reasons.

The initial goal of the AML therapy is to achieve complete remission, which is the most important indication of potential cure. The standard BM evaluation of response to therapy includes marrow studies performed 7–10 days after completing the last dose of the initial course [22]. If the results are inconclusive and do not exclude residual leukemia, a repeat BM is performed in a week.

Bone marrow studies to monitor the response to therapy and detect residual disease require proper sampling. However, frequently BM aspirate smears from children who are on chemotherapy are paucicellular and hemodiluted, and alone they may not represent the true bone marrow content. Furthermore, the BM biopsy may be negative as well, since the residual disease may be focal. For instance, comparing BM aspirates with BM biopsies for detecting the presence of residual disease and cellularity of 45 children with ALL at day 7 and day 14 of induction chemotherapy, Kidd and colleagues found that BM aspirates were negative due to poor sampling or focal disease in 20% of patients who had residual leukemia [23]. To ensure proper sampling, the BM aspirate smears should contain marrow particles and at least 200 nucleated blood cells. A BM biopsy should be obtained if the aspirate smears lack particles.

Minimal residual disease

With our improving abilities to detect the presence of residual disease, the definition of residual leukemia and its prognostic significance have changed. *Morphologic remission* applies to bone marrows having fewer than 5% blasts, without specifying whether these blasts are neoplastic or a result of robust repopulation of the marrow after myeloablative chemotherapy. Morphologically, the blasts look alike, whether neoplastic or non-neoplastic, and cannot be distinguished reliably. Furthermore, multiple studies have shown that the BM of patients in morphologic remission (<5% blasts) may contain a low number of neoplastic cells that can be detected only with more sensitive techniques, such as flow cytometry or genetic studies. The presence of disease at levels below the morphologic recognition is defined as *minimal residual disease (MRD)*.

Clinical implications of MRD

Presence of MRD has serious prognostic implications. Extensive studies of the prognostic impact of MRD in pediatric precursor B-cell ALL show that presence of more than 0.01% (10^{-4}) blasts at the end of induction in the bone marrow determined by flow cytometry is associated with a shorter event-free survival in all risk groups [24, 25]. This includes even children with ALL with favorable cytogenetics, such as *ETV6-RUNX1* (*TEL-AML1*) and hyperdiploidy: they fair poorly if there is presence of MRD in the marrow at day 29 [24]. The presence of MRD at the end of consolidation is associated with an especially poor prognosis.

By contrast, a lack of MRD in the peripheral blood at day eight of induction chemotherapy defines a subset of ALL patients at low risk of relapse, curable with limited chemotherapy that does not include alkylating agents or anthracyclines [24]. Thus, the absence of MRD can be used to stratify patients based upon their response to the initial chemotherapy. In such patients, the same outcome can be achieved using lower doses or less toxic drugs, thereby avoiding the high risk of serious toxicities associated with chemotherapy.

Determination of MRD is important in timing a hematopoietic stem cell transplant, as well. In a prospective blinded study using multivariable analysis of the prognostic impact of MRD, Bader *et al.* found that patients with an MRD load of more than 10^{-4} leukemic cells before an allogeneic stem cell transplant have a higher risk of relapse and lower event-free survival as compared to patients with an MRD load of less fewer 10^{-4} leukemic cells [26].

Detection techniques

The detection of MRD is based on the unique differences – phenotypic or genetic – of the leukemic blasts as compared to the normal cells. These differences can be detected by various techniques including multiparameter flow cytometry, immunoglobulin and *TCR* gene rearrangements by PCR, detection of fusion gene transcripts by RT-PCR, or expression of surrogate genes (*WT1*). Each technique has its advantages and disadvantages and level of sensitivity of detection, which are summarized in Table 19.4.

Multiparameter flow cytometry

Multiparameter flow cytometry is a rapid and sensitive technique for the detection of a small number of neoplastic cells with a distinctive immunophenotype when a high number of cellular events (100 000 or more) are analyzed. The level of detection depends upon the type of leukemia and uniqueness of the neoplastic cells, as well as on the number of cells available for analysis. In almost all cases of ALL, the leukemic blasts have a characteristic immunophenotype that allows the detection of one neoplastic cell in 10 000 normal cells (sensitivity of 0.01% or 10^{-4}) (Fig. 19.9) [30, 31]. While distinctive markers are also present in AML, the level of detection for a significant proportion of cases is lower – one in 1000 normal cells (sensitivity of 0.1% or 10^{-3}) [32].

Flow cytometry for MRD can be performed within 24–48 hours of collecting the specimen. The analysis is rapid. It can provide information within hours and, in addition to detection of MRD, it provides useful information about the normal cells. The disadvantages of this technique for detection of MRD include the need for a sufficient number of viable cells for analysis, proper equipment, and skilled staff with additional expertise that goes beyond simply defining the immunophenotype of the leukemic cells.

This is particularly important, since an abrupt cessation of chemotherapy is sufficient to induce a significant regeneration

Table 19.4. Methods for monitoring minimal residual disease in childhood leukemia.

	ALL		AML	
Method	Reproducible sensitivity	Frequency[a] (%)	Reproducible sensitivity	Frequency[a] (%)
Flow cytometry detecting abnormal phenotype	10^{-4}	98[b]	10^{-3}–10^{-4}	93[b]
PCR amplifications of genes encoding Ig and TCR	10^{-4}–10^{-5}	85[c]	N/A	<10[b]
RT-PCR amplification of fusion transcripts	10^{-3}–10^{-5}	<50[b]	10^{-3}–10^{-5}	<20[d]

[a] Frequency for which the indicated reproducibility can be obtained.
[b] Campana [27].
[c] van der Velden et al. [28].
[d] Boeckx et al. [29].
Abbreviations: ALL, acute lymphoblastic leukemia; AML, acute myeloid leukemia; Ig, immunoglobulin; TCR, T-cell receptor.

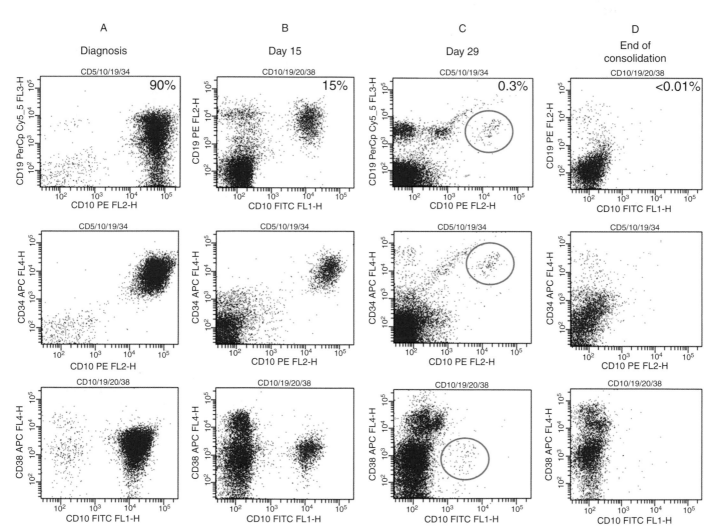

Fig. 19.9. Multiparameter flow cytometry of the bone marrow of a 15-year-old girl with precursor B-cell ALL with minimal residual disease at the end of induction. (A) Diagnostic marrow shows a significant number of CD10, CD19, CD34, and CD38-positive precursor B-lymphoblasts. Notice the bright expression of CD10. (B) Day 15 marrow shows 15% residual leukemia. (C) Day 29 shows a small population (circled) of immature B-cells that have the same immunophenotypic signature as the leukemic blasts. More than 100 000 cellular events were acquired to detect this low number of blasts. (D) End of consolidation. There is no evidence of residual leukemia. The number of immature cells is below the threshold of detection (<0.01%).

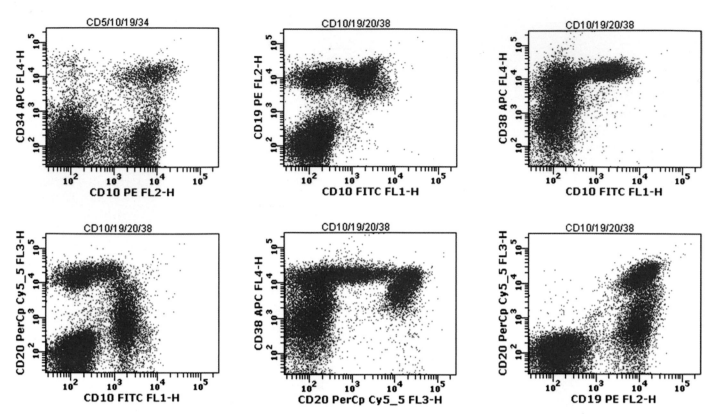

Fig. 19.10. Flow cytometry of the bone marrow of an eight-year-old girl with acute myeloid leukemia, post-hematopoietic stem cell transplant. Notice a significant number of precursor B-cells that show progressive maturation, a pattern characteristic for hematogones.

of normal B-cell progenitors, hematogones [33–35]. While hematogones are naturally present in high numbers in the bone marrow of young children, their number is even higher in those treated with chemotherapy. For instance, after cessation of maintenance chemotherapy, as many as 30% of all mononuclear cells in the marrow are reported to be CD10+ B-cells [34]. The number of hematogones can remain elevated for more than three years post-treatment, as has been shown in long-term follow-up studies. In the setting of autologous and allogeneic hematopoietic stem cell transplants, the number of hematogones is also elevated as part of the normal hematopoietic recovery (Fig. 19.10) [36, 37].

A key characteristic feature of hematogones is their heterogeneity, both immunophenotypic and morphologic. The hematogone population includes early forms that express TdT and CD34 along with early B-cell markers, intermediate forms, and mature B-cells that express surface Ig. This immunophenotypic heterogeneity can be demonstrated by multiparameter flow cytometry using an appropriate combination of antibodies that will allow the recognition of the B-cells at various stages of maturation. In our experience, CD34, CD10, CD19, CD20, and CD38 are very informative in respect to B-cell maturation, but any combination of early and late B-cell markers can be used for that purpose. Based on the degree of maturation, the hematogones can be divided into three stages (I–III). However, even within each stage, some heterogeneity exists (Table 19.5; Figs. 19.11 and 19.12).

Table 19.5. Phenotypic profiles of subsets of normal B-cell progenitors, hematogones.

Antigen expression	Stage I		Stage II	Stage III
	A	B		
TdT	+	+	−	−
CD34	+	+	−	−
CD10	+^{lo}	+^{hi}	+	+^{lo}/−
CD19	+/−	+	+	+
CD20	−	−	Variable from negative to +^{hi}	+^{hi}
cμ	−	−	+	N/A
sμ	−	−	−/minority +	+
CD45 RA	+^{lo}	+^{lo}	+^{lo} to intermediate	+^{hi}

Abbreviations: N/A, not applicable; cμ, cytoplasmic μ heavy chain immunoglobulins; sμ, surface μ heavy chain immunoglobulins.

The least mature hematogones, *stage I*, express CD34/CD10 and TdT. Based on the intensity of CD10 expression (low versus high), these cells can be further subdivided into stage IA (CD10+^{lo}/CD34+) and stage IB (CD10+^{hi}/CD34+). While CD19 is expressed by all hematogones, a small subset of the stage IA hematogones express only CD10 and CD34 and they lack CD19. However, these cells express cytoplasmic CD22 and

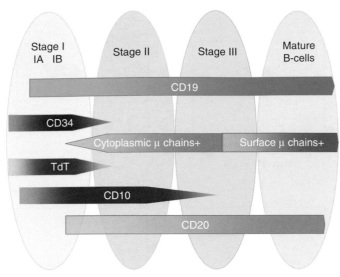

Fig. 19.11. Schematic representation of B-cell maturation sequence and antigen expression present at various stages of maturation. The least mature hematogones, stage I, express CD34 and TdT. A small subset of them express CD10 but are CD19 negative. These cells express cytoplasmic CD22 and PAX-5, B-cell markers that are expressed prior to CD19.

CD79a, early B-cell lineage-specific markers [38]. Thus, finding a lack of CD19 expression of these early, least-mature B-cells reflects the normal B-cell maturation rather than aberrant loss of pan-B-cell marker. On the other hand, more mature subsets of stage I hematogones express cytoplasmic μ heavy chain Ig, but none express surface μ. Lastly, CD20 is expressed at low to intermediate density on a considerable proportion of stage I cells.

Stage II hematogones are more mature and lose CD34 and TdT but retain a lower intensity of CD10 expression as compared to stage I cells. CD20 is variably expressed, from negative to intermediate levels, and these cells have a homogeneous cytoplasmic μ chain expression.

With the transition from stage II to *stage III*, further changes are observed in the antigenic expression, signifying progressive maturation. The most mature forms show decreasing expression of CD10 and bright expression of CD45RA, CD20, and surface μ chains. The degree of expression of CD10 varies and yet, despite the maturation, a significant number of stage III hematogones express CD10.

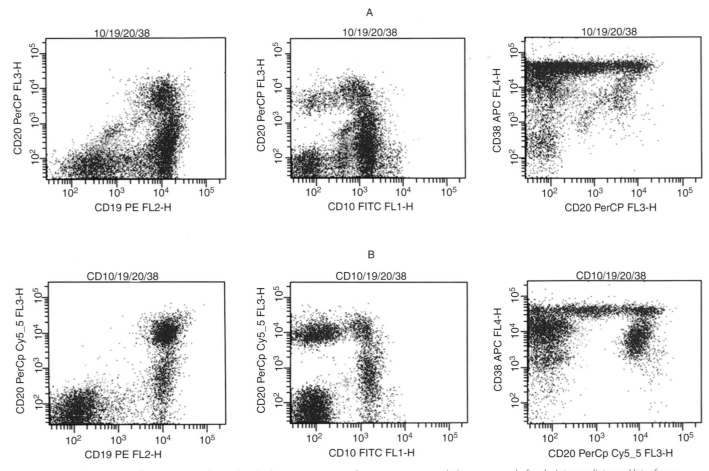

Fig. 19.12. Multiparameter flow cytometry shows that the hematogones are a heterogeneous population composed of early, intermediate, and later forms. (A) Less mature hematogones that are mostly CD10 positive and CD20 negative. This population shows bright CD38 expression and the characteristic progressive maturation of CD20. (B) An example of more mature hematogones. While CD10 is expressed on a substantial number of these cells, most hematogones are CD20 positive. The combination of CD10, CD20, and CD38 is very helpful to demonstrate this maturation.

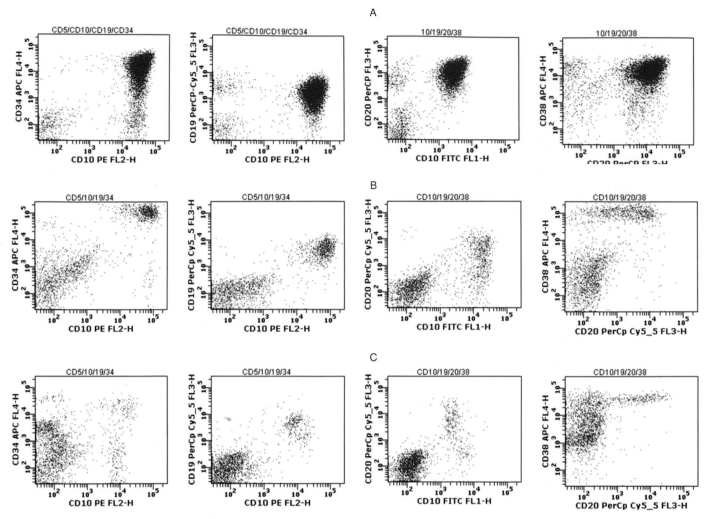

Fig. 19.13. Multiparameter flow cytometry of bone marrow from a five-year-old girl with hyperdiploid precursor B-cell ALL who relapsed two years after the initial diagnosis. (A) Diagnostic bone marrow. There is a significant number of CD10+, CD19+, CD20+, CD34+, and CD38+ B-lymphoblasts. Notice the bright CD10 expression and uniformity in the expression of CD20 and CD38. (B) Bone marrow at relapse. Notice that the immunophenotype of the neoplastic cells at relapse is very similar to the diagnostic blasts. (C) Bone marrow at end of second induction demonstrates a small number of immature B-cells with different intensity of CD10, CD20, CD34, and CD38 expression, consistent with hematogones. CD34/CD10 demonstrates nicely the heterogeneity of this population. No residual leukemia was identified in this sample.

The proportion of stage I, II, and III hematogones varies in individual patients depending upon the intensity of their previous therapy. Following a high-intensity induction chemotherapy for ALL, the least mature stage I hematogones predominate, while stages II and III are more numerous in patients where the preceding block is less intensive, such as the patients on maintenance chemotherapy [34, 35].

Hematogones uniformly express PAX-5 which, along with CD20 and TdT, is very helpful in evaluation of bone marrow biopsies. Unlike leukemic blasts, hematogones are found scattered throughout the bone marrow. Immunohistochemical staining is limited and less sensitive, and does not distinguish between the various stages of hematogones.

Since hematogones share immunophenotypic features with leukemic B-lymphoblasts, their presence in the BM of patients on therapy for precursor B-cell ALL or patients with a history of hematopoietic stem cell transplant (HSCT) for such leukemia may pose a serious diagnostic challenge (Fig. 19.13). The recognition of the maturation patterns of hematogones, and knowledge of the immunophenotype of the neoplastic cells at diagnosis are essential for the proper distinction of the two.

Molecular techniques

While flow cytometry detects neoplastic cells by identifying their abnormal phenotype, molecular techniques detect the characteristic genetic signatures of these cells that also can be used to detect MRD. Various approaches such as detection of gene rearrangements, fusion gene transcripts, or overexpression of surrogate genes can identify neoplastic cells at very low frequency [39, 40].

Table 19.6. Granulocyte colony stimulating factor (G-CSF) and granulocyte/monocyte colony stimulating factor (GM-CSF).

	Generic name	Trade name	Mechanism of action
G-CSF	Filgrastim (*E. coli* derived) Lenograstim (CHO cell derived)	Neupogen® (Amgen Inc.) Granocyte™ (Chugai-Rhone Poulenc)	Expands circulating pools of neutrophils by increasing their production, maturation, and activation Activates neutrophils to increase both their migration and cytotoxicity *Effect on other target cells* – macrophages, fibroblasts, endothelial cells, bone marrow stromal cells
GM-CSF	Sargramostim (yeast derived) Molgramostim (*E. coli* derived)	Leukine (Immunex) Leukomax (Gentaur)	Stimulates proliferation, differentiation, and functional activity of neutrophils, eosinophils, monocytes, and macrophages *Effect on other target cells* – macrophages, endothelial cells, fibroblasts, BM stromal cells, T- and B-lymphocytes, mast cells, eosinophils

Abbreviations: *E. coli, Escherichia coli*; CHO, Chinese hamster ovary cell line.

Immunoglobulin and T-cell receptor (*TCR*) gene rearrangement studies

Quantitative polymerase chain reaction (PCR) can be used to determine clonal immunoglobulin (*IG*) and T-cell receptor (*TCR*) gene rearrangements in order to detect MRD. These studies are most useful in ALL, since clonal gene rearrangements are detected in the majority of such cases [39], but only in fewer than 10% of the cases of AML [29]. This approach allows a routine detection reproducibly of one leukemic cell in 10 000–100 000 normal cells (sensitivity 0.01% to 0.001% or 10^{-4} to 10^{-5}) in about 85% of the patients with ALL, and is not limited by the number of cells available for analysis [28]. While monitoring of gene rearrangements is a sensitive and objective technique for detecting MRD, this approach also has its downsides. Its reliability is affected by the presence of multiple gene rearrangements in the same leukemic cell population. For example, a minor clone may not have been identified at diagnosis but later can become prominent as a residual disease. Such a clone might not be detected because of the decision to follow a major clone that was present at diagnosis [41]. The use of sets of probes matching two or more different rearrangements is helpful to avoid such pitfalls [42]. However, this requires an extensive workup to detect specific rearrangements at the time of diagnosis, which is both time consuming and requires proper equipment and resources that may not be readily available. Furthermore, the follow-up is restricted to the laboratory performing the initial workup. Lastly, for reliable results, there is a need for standardization and regular quality control of this technique [43].

Fusion gene transcript detection

Targeting of fusion gene transcripts such as *E2A-PBX1, MLL-AF4, RUNX1-ETO, BCR-ABL, ETV6-RUNX1, PML-RARA, RUNX1-RUNX1T1*, and *CBFB-MYH11* is probably the most sensitive molecular approach [40]. However, this approach is applicable only in a subset of acute leukemias with recurrent cytogenetic abnormalities (35–45% of ALL and AML) and 90% of CML cases [44]. Real-time quantitative PCR provides an accurate measure of such transcripts, allowing detection of one leukemic cell in up to 100 000 cells (0.001%; 10^{-5}). Another advantage of following MRD by fusion transcript is the strong association between the molecular abnormality and the leukemic clone irrespective of the presence of clonal evolution

or acquired additional abnormalities. However, the number of transcripts per leukemic cell may vary from patient to patient and may be affected by therapy, thus making precise quantitation difficult [44]. Similarly to gene rearrangements, this technique also requires proper standardization and regular quality control. Furthermore, different laboratories may report their results in various units, that is, per mL, per number of white blood cells, and so forth, that may make comparing results between different laboratories challenging.

Detection of surrogate genes

Another approach for detecting MRD is quantitation of surrogate genes such as *WT1*, which is overexpressed in most patients with AML but is not expressed in maturing BM progenitors [45]. The challenges in using such an approach come from the normal expression of *WT1* in CD34+ cells, with the result that a threshold higher than the normal background is needed to determine the presence of MRD and to distinguish between neoplastic and normal CD34+ progenitors.

Comparison of techniques to detect MRD

Which is the best of the techniques to detect MRD in children? The answer is still to be determined. A comparative analysis of four-color flow cytometry and gene rearrangement studies shows a detection level of 0.01% residual disease by flow cytometry in 91% of the samples studied, and the same level or better in only 84% of the patients studied by PCR [46]. However, when MRD was detected using both techniques, all patients were found to be positive. Thus, to improve the sensitivity of detection of MRD, multiple approaches may be necessary. Other studies are needed to confirm this observation.

Effect of growth factors

Two recombinant colony stimulating factors – granulocyte colony stimulating factor (G-CSF) and granulocyte/monocyte colony stimulating factor (GM-CSF) – are used widely for treatment of therapy-induced neutropenia in children [47]. Administration of these factors causes expansion of the circulating pool of granulocytes by mobilization of mature neutrophils from the BM reserve, as well as accelerated proliferation and maturation of myeloid progenitors (Table 19.6). In addition to the granulocytes, GM-CSF increases the production of

Table 19.7. Clinical application of hematopoietic growth factors in children.

To reduce the duration of neutropenia and the associated risk of infection in children with malignancies receiving myelosuppressive chemotherapeutic regimens associated with a significant incidence of severe neutropenia with fever (secondary prophylaxis)

For mobilization of peripheral blood progenitor cells into the peripheral blood for collection by leukapheresis

To accelerate the myeloid recovery in patients undergoing autologous or allogeneic hematopoietic stem cell transplant

In severe chronic neutropenia, which includes patients with congenital neutropenia, cyclic neutropenia, or idiopathic neutropenia, Shwachman syndrome, and neonatal neutropenia

Short-term (<3 months) use in patients with aplastic anemia

Possible immunomodulatory effect (GM-CSF only)

Note: Growth factors *are not recommended* for routine primary prophylaxis in patients on chemotherapy

References: Levine, Boxer [51], and Lehrnbecher, Welte [53].

monocytes and eosinophils. The effect of these growth factors is reversible, so that when the drug is discontinued, the white blood cell count and the number of neutrophils returns to normal, baseline.

The use of G-CSF and GM-CSF in children is reserved for those for whom there is expected incidence of febrile neutropenia, such as children following dose-intensive therapy for high-risk ALL, AML, non-Hodgkin lymphomas, or neuroblastoma (Table 19.7) [48]. However, routine prophylactic administration is not recommended. While such therapy has been shown to decrease the incidence of febrile neutropenia, and shortens the duration of the neutropenia as well as the duration of antibiotic administration, it does not decrease the incidence of infections or lead to an improved outcome [48–50]. Additional utilities of

G-CSF and GM-CSF in children include effective mobilization of hematopoietic stem cells for transplantation, and enhancement of neutrophil engraftment after hematopoietic stem cell transplantation [51]. Administration of G-CSF prior to bone marrow harvesting for allogeneic stem cell transplants has been shown to facilitate the neutrophil and platelet engraftment in the recipients without a discernable increase of the risk of graft versus host disease, and it is safe for the donor [52].

G-CSF is also a standard therapy in children with severe congenital neutropenia [53, 54]. As a result of such therapy, the myeloid progenitors mature successfully to neutrophil stage.

In children on G-CSF, the number of WBCs increases with or without the presence of circulating nucleated red blood cells (NRBCs). The total WBC count may exceed 50×10^9/L, and the peripheral blood finding may resemble a leukemoid reaction or leukoerythroblastic reaction. The number of NRBCs is usually below 5 per 100 WBCs. Most of the white blood cells are neutrophils and, while mature forms predominate, promyelocytes and blasts can also be seen. The number of blasts can rise to 3–5%, but it rarely exceeds 10%. These blasts are heterogeneous, and their number in the peripheral blood is usually higher than the number of blasts in the bone marrow. G-CSF induces acceleration of the granulopoiesis in the bone marrow. As a result, many of the neutrophils have hypo- or hypersegmented nuclei, prominent cytoplasmic granularity, vacuolization, and presence of Döhle bodies (Fig. 19.14) [55].

The bone marrow findings depend on the bone marrow reserves prior to starting G-CSF, the length of therapy, and the degree of BM stromal damage. In children with stromal damage, the G-CSF response may be blunt. Initially, while there is an increase in the myeloid component with a marked granulocytic shift to immaturity and an increased number of early forms such as promyelocytes and myelocytes, the number of

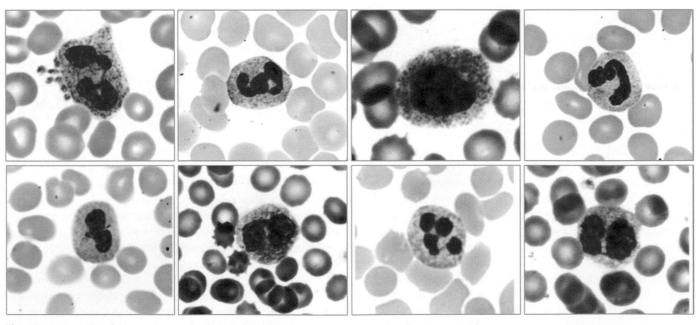

Fig. 19.14. Examples of dysgranulopoiesis in the peripheral blood of children on G-CSF (Wright–Giemsa stain).

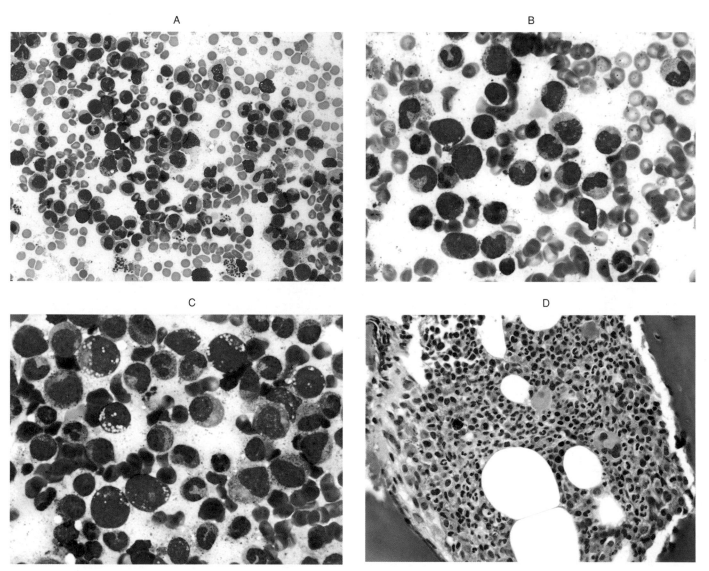

Fig. 19.15. Bone marrow from a child with precursor B-cell ALL receiving G-CSF. Notice the accelerated myeloid hyperplasia and granulocytic shift to immaturity. (A–C) Bone marrow aspirates (Wright–Giemsa stain). (D) Bone marrow biopsy (H&E stain).

blasts may be increased only slightly [56]. Morphologic changes reflecting the accelerated maturation of the myelopoiesis are also present (Fig. 19.15). These include nuclear/cytoplasmic asynchrony; increased number and retained azurophilic granules in more mature forms indicating cytoplasmic immaturity; and abnormal nuclear segmentation such as pseudo-Pelger–Huët, hypersegmented, or ring forms. After the G-CSF is discontinued, the cellularity, myeloid predominance, and myeloid maturation return to normal.

Hematopoietic stem cell transplant

A hematopoietic stem cell transplant (HSCT), either autologous or allogeneic, is ultimately the most intensified treatment modality for otherwise incurable hematologic malignancies.

Children with leukemias with certain cytogenetic abnormalities such as *BCR-ABL*, *MLL-AF4*, hypodiploidy (<45 chromosomes), induction failure (≥5% leukemic blasts at the end of induction), and presence of minimal residual disease of more than 1% after four to six weeks of first line therapy, have a very high risk of relapse and benefit from HSCT. A majority of the transplants in children are performed in the second complete remission, since survival with chemotherapy alone is only in the range of 10–40% [57]. Furthermore, HSCT is used for ultimate therapy in children with congenital hematologic diseases, severe congenital immune deficiencies, or non-hematologic malignancies (Table 19.8) [57–63].

Only pluripotent hematopoietic progenitor cells are capable of reconstituting hematopoiesis by generating multilineage hematopoiesis and hematopoietic cells capable of cell renewal. Such progenitor cells can be obtained from the bone marrow,

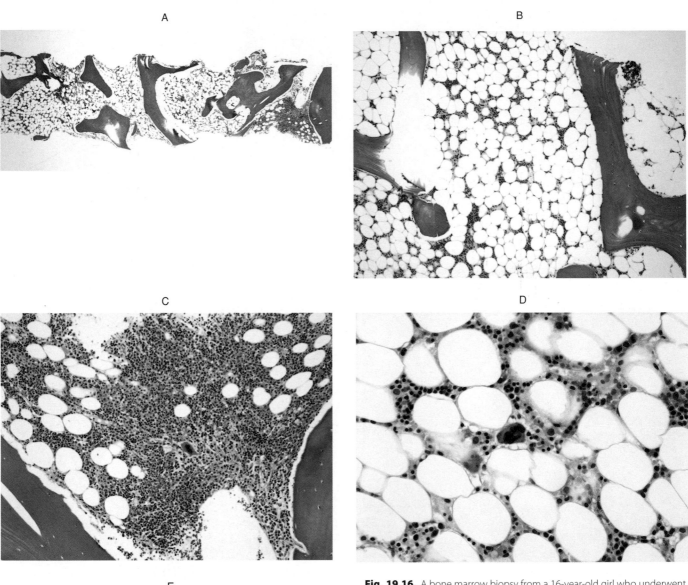

Fig. 19.16. A bone marrow biopsy from a 16-year-old girl who underwent myeloablative hematopoietic stem cell transplant for EBV+ T-cell lymphoproliferative disorder, day 68+ (H&E stain). (A) Markedly hypocellular bone marrow with variable cellularity ranging from 60% in a small subcortical area to less than 5% in the rest of the biopsy. (B) Small foci of regenerating hematopoiesis in the intertrabecular areas and a lack of paratrabecular regeneration. (C) Focal restoration of multilineage hematopoiesis in the subcortical area. (D) Stromal damage, hemosiderin, and a regenerating megakaryocyte with large hyperchromatic nucleus. (E) Erythroid progenitors and hemosiderin present at the bony trabeculae. There is a paucity of myeloid progenitors.

Table 19.8. Indications for hematopoietic stem cell transplant in children.

Acute lymphoblastic leukemia
t(9;22)(q34;q11.2); *BCR-ABL1*
t(4;11)(q21;q23); *MLL-AF4*
Hypodiploidy
Induction failure
Persistent minimal residual disease
Acute myeloid leukemia
Relapsed AML
Myelodysplastic syndrome
Children younger than two years
Refractory anemia with excess blasts
Therapy-related myelodysplastic syndrome/acute myeloid leukemia
Chronic myeloid leukemia t(9;22)(q34;q11.2); *BCR-ABL1*
Children with lymphomas or solid tumors (autologous and allogeneic)
Relapsed or refractory Hodgkin or non-Hodgkin lymphoma
Metastatic or relapsed neuroblastoma, Ewing sarcoma, Wilms tumor
Severe congenital immune deficiencies
Hemoglobinopathies
Sickle cell patients with frequent vaso-occlusive pain crises, acute chest syndrome, or cerebrovascular accidents
Metabolic diseases
Malignant infantile osteopetrosis

Source: Handgretinger *et al.* [57].

Table 19.9. Major and minor incompatibilities between the HSCT donor and recipient in relation to their blood groups.

Recipient blood group	Donor blood group			
	O	A	B	AB
O	Compatible	Major	Major	Major
A	Minor	Compatible	Major/minor	Major
B	Minor	Minor/major	Compatible	Major
AB	Minor	Minor	Minor	Compatible

Major incompatibility – the recipient has antibodies directed against the donor red cells. Minor incompatibility – the donor has antibodies directed to the recipient red blood cells.
Adapted from Kruskall [70].

peripheral blood after G-CSF mobilization, or umbilical cord blood. While the bone marrow was the main source of progenitor cells in the early years of transplantation, G-CSF stimulated peripheral blood progenitor cells are currently more widely used. The donors include HLA-matched siblings or other family members, or unrelated HLA-matched individuals.

The speed and quality of bone marrow regeneration depend on the type of underlying disease, pre-transplant chemotherapy, type and intensity of myeloablative therapy in the preparation for a transplant, and the source of the hematopoietic progenitors. For example, patients with non-myeloablative therapy recover faster than patients with full intensity myeloablative therapy. Earlier engraftment and improved immune reconstitution is present in recipients of peripheral blood progenitor cells compared to recipients of bone marrow-derived progenitor cell transplants. Furthermore, the recovery of the hematopoiesis after a cord blood progenitor cell transplant shows the slowest recovery.

Bone marrow evaluation is usually not performed in the early post-transplant period, and most of the knowledge of the early stages of hematopoietic recovery is limited to observations in post-mortem bone marrows. Early in the first week post-transplant, the changes in the bone marrow resemble those seen in radiation- and/or drug-induced aplasia. This includes a marked decrease in the cellularity, extensive cell necrosis,

edema, and expansion of the adipose tissue [64]. *In vitro* studies show that CD34+ progenitor cells adhere to the stromal cells within one hour of contact [65, 66], and the engrafted CD34+ progenitor cells serve as precursors for both hematopoietic cells and stromal cells [67].

The engrafting progenitor cells are non-randomly distributed in the marrow and, after initial accumulation in the periosteal region, they migrate to the central, highly vascularized areas of the marrow. At the end of the first week after transplant, there is an emergence of small erythroid islands which have a centrally located macrophage that plays a central role in restoring the bone marrow microenvironment and in the regulation and differentiation of the progenitors of all lineages [68, 69]. The erythroid regeneration is followed by the appearance of megakaryocytes and a small number of myeloid progenitors in the paratrabecular areas (Fig. 19.16). From the third week post-transplant onwards, erythroid and myeloid colonies and a patchy regeneration of megakaryocytes are seen. Normalization of the size of the megakaryocytes and their cytologic appearance is an indication of successful engraftment. The bone marrow cellularity increases to at least 50% of the normal cellularity after three weeks, and reaches normal levels in the second month post transplant [64]. The number of lymphocytes varies and is higher in those patients with graft versus host disease. Most of these lymphocytes are normal B-cell progenitors.

In the peripheral blood, the hematopoietic recovery is manifested by recovery of the granulocytes and platelets. Granulocyte recovery is defined as the first of three successive days when the absolute neutrophil count is above 0.5×10^9/L, or the first of three successive days when the total WBC count exceeds 1×10^9/L. The first day that the platelet count reaches and remains above 20×10^9/L without transfusion is an indication of platelet recovery. Red blood cell recovery can be monitored by the degree of reticulocytosis. An ABO and Rh mismatch between the donor and recipient results in delayed red cell engraftment and in various degrees of hemolytic anemia depending upon whether the discrepancy is major or minor (Table 19.9). A complete conversion to the donor blood group occurs after engraftment.

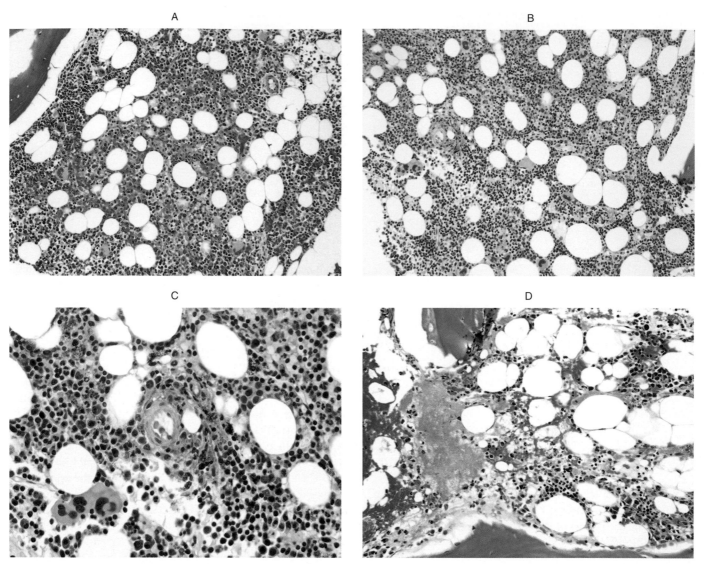

Fig. 19.17. A bone marrow biopsy post-hematopoietic stem cell transplant, day 100+ (H&E stain). (A, B) Examples of restored bone marrow cellularity. (C) Residual stromal damage and numerous hemosiderin-laden macrophages indicating iron overload. (D) Hypocellular marrow with stromal injury worrisome for graft failure.

The number of hematopoietic stem cells in cord blood and their adhesion potential is lower as compared to BM or peripheral stem cells, which limits the use of cord blood to children. A comparison of the BM cellularity, presence of fibrosis, number of CD34+ stem cells, and CD42b+ megakaryocytes at various time points after umbilical cord blood and bone marrow transplant shows delayed engraftment and hematopoietic reconstitution, decreased cellularity, lower number of CD34+ cells and CD42b-positive cells, and increased fibrosis in the early period (day 29), when cord blood is used as source of hematopoietic cells [71]. Furthermore, the cord blood stem cells seem to have a lower adhesion potential as compared to the BM stem cells. After an umbilical cord blood transplantation, the hematopoietic foci are exclusively single lineage and consist of clusters of synchronized cells.

Spatial distribution of the hematopoietic cells is non-random – in the early engraftment phase – and donor stem cells are located in the highly vascularized intertrabecular areas of the bone marrow and adjacent to the bony trabeculae. Gradually the paratrabecular cellularity decreases and the number of hematopoietic cells in the central regions increases – a pattern of migration and retention of cells in distinct marrow sites. Bone marrow cellularity drops up to day 30. There is a transient increase in the reticulin fibrosis which most likely reflects the healing process of the damaged BM microenvironment. Donor megakaryocytes seem to be capable of cytokine production promoting bone marrow fibrosis. The marrow after a cord blood transplant shows gradual recovery and, after day 100 post-transplant, there is no essential difference between a cord blood or bone marrow transplant.

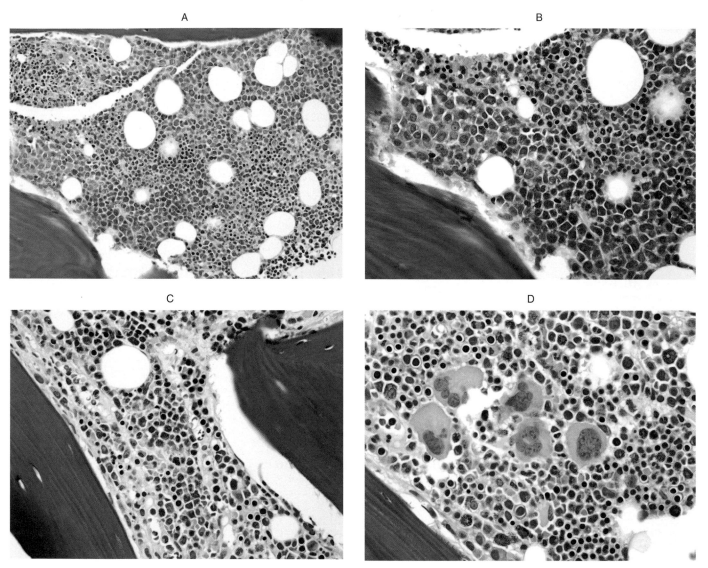

Fig. 19.18. Bone marrow biopsy from an eight-year-old girl after hematopoietic stem cell transplant for relapsed precursor B-cell ALL, day 200+ (H&E stain). (A) Notice restored cellularity and multilineage hematopoiesis. (B) Marked granulocytic shift to immaturity. (C) Erythroid progenitors adjacent to the bony trabeculae. (D) Clusters of megakaryocytes.

Multiple factors can affect bone marrow recovery after HSCT in children. Bone marrow evaluation is routinely performed at day 100 after the hematopoietic stem cell transplant, and the restoration of hematopoiesis is considered to be evidence of long-term engraftment (Figs. 19.17 and 19.18). Factors contributing to graft failure include a low dose of hematopoietic stem cells or significant bone marrow stromal damage. In primary graft failure, the allograph does not resume its function, and the patient remains aplastic after the myeloablative preparative regimen. Rejection or secondary graft failure denotes the loss of allograft after initial engraftment. The risk of rejection is higher in patients with HLA mismatch.

References

1. **Seibel NL**. Treatment of acute lymphoblastic leukemia in children and adolescents: peaks and pitfalls. *Hematology/the Education Program of the American Society of Hematology.* 2008:374–380.

2. **Evans WE, Relling MV**. Moving towards individualized medicine with pharmacogenomics. *Nature.* 2004;**429**: 464–468.

3. **Pui C-H, Relling MV, Evans WE**. Role of pharmacogenomics and pharmacodynamics in the treatment of acute lymphoblastic leukaemia. *Best Practice & Research Clinical Haematology.* 2002;**15**:741–756.

4. **Lennard L, Lilleyman JS, Van Loon J, Weinshilboum RM**. Genetic variation in response to 6-mercaptopurine for childhood acute lymphoblastic leukaemia. *Lancet.* 1990;**336**:225–229.

5. **McLeod HL, Yu J**. Cancer pharmacogenomics: SNPs, chips, and the individual patient. *Cancer Investigation.* 2003;**21**:630–640.

6. **Coulthard SA, Matheson EC, Hall AG, Hogarth LA.** The clinical impact of thiopurine methyltransferase polymorphisms on thiopurine treatment. *Nucleosides, Nucleotides & Nucleic Acids.* 2004;**23**:1385–1391.

7. **Van Den Akker-van Marle ME, Gurwitz D, Detmar SB**, *et al.* Cost-effectiveness of pharmacogenomics in clinical practice: a case study of thiopurine methyltransferase genotyping in acute lymphoblastic leukemia in Europe. *Pharmacogenomics.* 2006;**7**:783–792.

8. **Pui C-H, Evans WE.** Treatment of acute lymphoblastic leukemia. *New England Journal of Medicine.* 2006;**354**:166–178.

9. **Cheok MH, Pottier N, Kager L, Evans WE.** Pharmacogenetics in acute lymphoblastic leukemia. *Seminars in Hematology.* 2009;**46**:39–51.

10. **Leith CP, Kopecky KJ, Chen IM**, *et al.* Frequency and clinical significance of the expression of the multidrug resistance proteins MDR1/P-glycoprotein, MRP1, and LRP in acute myeloid leukemia: a Southwest Oncology Group Study. *Blood.* 1999;**94**:1086–1099.

11. **Leith CP, Kopecky KJ, Godwin J**, *et al.* Acute myeloid leukemia in the elderly: assessment of multidrug resistance (MDR1) and cytogenetics distinguishes biologic subgroups with remarkably distinct responses to standard chemotherapy. A Southwest Oncology Group study. *Blood.* 1997;**89**:3323–3329.

12. **Foucar K.** Effects of therapy and transplantation, and detection of minimal residual disease. In Foucar K, ed. *Bone Marrow Pathology* (2nd edn.). Chicago: ASCP Press; 2001, 655–681.

13. **Brody JP, Krause JR, Penchansky L.** Bone marrow response to chemotherapy in acute lymphocytic leukaemia and acute non-lymphocytic leukaemia. *Scandinavian Journal of Haematology.* 1985;**35**:240–245.

14. **Muretto P, Izzi T, Grianti C, Moretti L.** Histomorphologic study of bone marrow in acute leukemia following chemotherapy and autologous bone marrow transplantation. *Tumori.* 1983;**69**:239–248.

15. **Corazza F, Hermans C, Ferster A**, *et al.* Bone marrow stroma damage induced by chemotherapy for acute lymphoblastic leukemia in children. *Pediatric Research.* 2004;**55**:152–158.

16. **Noren-Nystrom U, Roos G, Bergh A**, *et al.* Bone marrow fibrosis in childhood acute lymphoblastic leukemia correlates to biological factors, treatment response and outcome. *Leukemia.* 2007;**22**:504–510.

17. **Wittels B.** Bone marrow biopsy changes following chemotherapy for acute leukemia. *American Journal of Surgical Pathology.* 1980;**4**:135–142.

18. **Islam A.** Pattern of bone marrow regeneration following chemotherapy for acute myeloid leukemia. *Journal of Medicine.* 1987;**18**:108–122.

19. **Wilkins BS, Bostanci AG, Ryan MF, Jones DB.** Haemopoietic regrowth after chemotherapy for acute leukaemia: an immunohistochemical study of bone marrow trephine biopsy specimens. *Journal of Clinical Pathology.* 1993;**46**:915–921.

20. **Corazza F, Beguin Y, Bergmann P**, *et al.* Anemia in children with cancer is associated with decreased erythropoietic activity and not with inadequate erythropoietin production. *Blood.* 1998;**92**:1793–1798.

21. **Carlo-Stella C, Tabilio A, Regazzi E**, *et al.* Effect of chemotherapy for acute myelogenous leukemia on hematopoietic and fibroblast marrow progenitors. *Bone Marrow Transplantation.* 1997;**20**:465–471.

22. **Cheson BD, Bennett JM, Kopecky KJ**, *et al.* Revised recommendations of the International Working Group for Diagnosis, Standardization of Response Criteria, Treatment Outcomes, and Reporting Standards for Therapeutic Trials in Acute Myeloid Leukemia. *Journal of Clinical Oncology.* 2003;**21**:4642–4649.

23. **Kidd PG, Saminathan T, Drachtman RA, Ettinger LJ.** Comparison of the cellularity and presence of residual leukemia in bone marrow aspirate and biopsy specimens in pediatric patients with acute lymphoblastic leukemia (ALL) at day 7–14 of chemotherapy. *Medical and Pediatric Oncology.* 1997;**29**:541–543.

24. **Borowitz MJ, Devidas M, Hunger SP**, *et al.* Clinical significance of minimal residual disease in childhood acute lymphoblastic leukemia and its relationship to other prognostic factors: a Children's Oncology Group study. *Blood.* 2008;**111**:5477–5485.

25. **Campana D.** Minimal residual disease in acute lymphoblastic leukemia. *Seminars in Hematology.* 2009;**46**:100–106.

26. **Bader P, Kreyenberg H, Henze GH**, *et al.* Prognostic value of minimal residual disease quantification before allogeneic stem-cell transplantation in relapsed childhood acute lymphoblastic leukemia: the ALL-REZ BFM Study Group. *Journal of Clinical Oncology.* 2009;**27**:377–384.

27. **Campana D.** Status of minimal residual disease testing in childhood haematological malignancies. *British Journal of Haematology.* 2008;**143**(4):481–489.

28. **van Der Velden VHJ, Hochhaus A, Cazzaniga G**, *et al.* Detection of minimal residual disease in hematologic malignancies by real-time quantitative PCR: principles, approaches, and laboratory aspects. *Leukemia.* 2003;**17**:1013–1034.

29. **Boeckx N, Willemse MJ, Szczepanski T**, *et al.* Fusion gene transcripts and Ig/TCR gene rearrangements are complementary but infrequent targets for PCR-based detection of minimal residual disease in acute myeloid leukemia. *Leukemia.* 2002;**16**:368–375.

30. **Campana D, Coustan-Smith E.** Detection of minimal residual disease in acute leukemia by flow cytometry. *Cytometry.* 1999;**38**:139–152.

31. **Borowitz MJ, Pullen DJ, Shuster JJ**, *et al.* Minimal residual disease detection in childhood precursor-B-cell acute lymphoblastic leukemia: relation to other risk factors. A Children's Oncology Group study. *Leukemia.* 2003;**17**:1566–1572.

32. **Coustan-Smith E, Ribeiro RC, Rubnitz JE**, *et al.* Clinical significance of residual disease during treatment in childhood acute myeloid leukaemia. *British Journal of Haematology.* 2003;**123**:243–252.

33. **Longacre TA, Foucar K, Crago S**, *et al.* Hematogones: a multiparameter analysis of bone marrow precursor cells. *Blood.* 1989;**73**:543–552.

34. **van Lochem EG, Wiegers YM, Van Den Beemd R**, *et al.* Regeneration pattern of precursor-B-cells in bone marrow of acute lymphoblastic leukemia patients depends on the type

of preceding chemotherapy. *Leukemia*. 2000;**14**:688–695.

35. **Dworzak MN, Fritsch G, Fleischer C,** *et al.* Multiparameter phenotype mapping of normal and post-chemotherapy B lymphopoiesis in pediatric bone marrow. *Leukemia*. 1997;**11**:1266–1273.

36. **Smedmyr B, Bengtsson M, Jakobsson A,** *et al.* Regeneration of CALLA (CD10+), TdT+ and double-positive cells in the bone marrow and blood after autologous bone marrow transplantation. *European Journal of Haematology*. 1991;**46**:146–151.

37. **Leitenberg D, Rappeport JM, Smith BR.** B-cell precursor bone marrow reconstitution after bone marrow transplantation. *American Journal of Clinical Pathology*. 1994;**102**:231–236.

38. **Dworzak MN, Fritsch G, Froschl G, Printz D, Gadner H.** Four-color flow cytometric investigation of terminal deoxynucleotidyl transferase-positive lymphoid precursors in pediatric bone marrow: CD79a expression precedes CD19 in early B-cell ontogeny. *Blood*. 1998;**92**:3203–3209.

39. **Pongers-Willemse MJ, Seriu T, Stolz F,** *et al.* Primers and protocols for standardized detection of minimal residual disease in acute lymphoblastic leukemia using immunoglobulin and T cell receptor gene rearrangements and TAL1 deletions as PCR targets: report of the BIOMED-1 Concerted Action: investigation of minimal residual disease in acute leukemia. *Leukemia*. 1999;**13**:110–118.

40. **van Dongen JJ, Macintyre EA, Gabert JA,** *et al.* Standardized RT-PCR analysis of fusion gene transcripts from chromosome aberrations in acute leukemia for detection of minimal residual disease. Report of the BIOMED-1 Concerted Action: investigation of minimal residual disease in acute leukemia. *Leukemia*. 1999;**13**:1901–1928.

41. **van Der Velden VHJ, Boeckx N, van Wering ER, van Dongen JJM.** Detection of minimal residual disease in acute leukemia. *Journal of Biological Regulators & Homeostatic Agents*. 2004;**18**:146–154.

42. **Flohr T, Schrauder A, Cazzaniga G,** *et al.* Minimal residual disease-directed risk stratification using real-time quantitative PCR analysis of immunoglobulin and T-cell receptor gene rearrangements in the international multicenter trial AIEOP-BFM ALL 2000 for childhood acute lymphoblastic leukemia. *Leukemia*. 2008;**22**:771–782.

43. **van Der Velden VHJ, Panzer-Grumayer ER, Cazzaniga G,** *et al.* Optimization of PCR-based minimal residual disease diagnostics for childhood acute lymphoblastic leukemia in a multi-center setting. *Leukemia*. 2007;**21**:706–713.

44. **Gabert J, Beillard E, van Der Velden VHJ,** *et al.* Standardization and quality control studies of 'real-time' quantitative reverse transcriptase polymerase chain reaction of fusion gene transcripts for residual disease detection in leukemia – a Europe Against Cancer program. *Leukemia*. 2003;**17**:2318–2357.

45. **Cilloni D, Renneville A, Hermitte F,** *et al.* Real-time quantitative polymerase chain reaction detection of minimal residual disease by standardized WT1 assay to enhance risk stratification in acute myeloid leukemia: a European LeukemiaNet study. *Journal of Clinical Oncology*. 2009;**27**:5195–5201.

46. **Kerst G, Kreyenberg H, Roth C,** *et al.* Concurrent detection of minimal residual disease (MRD) in childhood acute lymphoblastic leukaemia by flow cytometry and real-time PCR. *British Journal of Haematology*. 2005;**128**:774–782.

47. **Duhrsen U, Villeval JL, Boyd J,** *et al.* Effects of recombinant human granulocyte colony-stimulating factor on hematopoietic progenitor cells in cancer patients. *Blood*. 1988;**72**:2074–2081.

48. **Lehrnbecher T, Zimmermann M, Reinhardt D,** *et al.* Prophylactic human granulocyte colony-stimulating factor after induction therapy in pediatric acute myeloid leukemia. *Blood*. 2007;**109**:936–943.

49. **Wittman B, Horan J, Lyman GH.** Prophylactic colony-stimulating factors in children receiving myelosuppressive chemotherapy: a meta-analysis of randomized controlled trials. *Cancer Treatment Reviews*. 2006;**32**:289–303.

50. **Heath JA, Steinherz PG, Altman A,** *et al.* Human granulocyte colony-stimulating factor in children with high-risk acute lymphoblastic leukemia: a Children's Cancer Group study. *Journal of Clinical Oncology*. 2003;**21**:1612–1617.

51. **Levine JE, Boxer LA.** Clinical applications of hematopoietic growth factors in pediatric oncology. *Current Opinion in Hematology*. 2002;**9**:222–227.

52. **Frangoul H, Nemecek ER, Billheimer D,** *et al.* A prospective study of G-CSF primed bone marrow as a stem-cell source for allogeneic bone marrow transplantation in children: a Pediatric Blood and Marrow Transplant Consortium (PBMTC) study. *Blood*. 2007;**110**:4584–4587.

53. **Lehrnbecher T, Welte K.** Haematopoietic growth factors in children with neutropenia. *British Journal of Haematology*. 2002;**116**: 28–56.

54. **Bonilla MA, Gillio AP, Ruggeiro M,** *et al.* Effects of recombinant human granulocyte colony-stimulating factor on neutropenia in patients with congenital agranulocytosis. *New England Journal of Medicine*. 1989;**320**: 1574–1580.

55. **Kerrigan DP, Castillo A, Foucar K, Townsend K, Neidhart J.** Peripheral blood morphologic changes after high-dose antineoplastic chemotherapy and recombinant human granulocyte colony-stimulating factor administration. *American Journal of Clinical Pathology*. 1989;**92**:280–285.

56. **Harris AC, Todd WM, Hackney MH, Ben-Ezra J.** Bone marrow changes associated with recombinant granulocyte-macrophage and granulocyte colony-stimulating factors. Discrimination of granulocytic regeneration. *Archives of Pathology & Laboratory Medicine*. 1994;**118**:624–629.

57. **Handgretinger R, Turner V, Barfield R.** Hematopoietic stem cell transplantation. In Pui C-H, ed. *Childhood Leukemias* (2nd edn.). New York: Cambridge University Press; 2006, 599–624.

58. **Barfield RC, Kasow KA, Hale GA.** Advances in pediatric hematopoietic stem cell transplantation. *Cancer Biology & Therapy*. 2008;**7**:1533–1539.

59. **Buckley RH, Schiff SE, Schiff RI,** *et al.* Hematopoietic stem-cell transplantation for the treatment of severe combined immunodeficiency.

New England Journal of Medicine. 1999;**340**:508–516.

60. **Lawson SE, Roberts IAG, Amrolia P,** *et al.* Bone marrow transplantation for beta-thalassaemia major: the UK experience in two paediatric centres. *British Journal of Haematology.* 2003; **120**:289–295.

61. **Vermylen C.** Hematopoietic stem cell transplantation in sickle cell disease. *Blood Reviews.* 2003;**17**:163–166.

62. **Willasch A, Hoelle W, Kreyenberg H,** *et al.* Outcome of allogeneic stem cell transplantation in children with non-malignant diseases. *Haematologica.* 2006;**91**:788–794.

63. **Kletzel M, Katzenstein HM, Haut PR,** *et al.* Treatment of high-risk neuroblastoma with triple-tandem high-dose therapy and stem-cell rescue: results of the Chicago Pilot II study.

64. **van Marion AMW, Thiele J, Kvasnicka HM, Van Den Tweel JG.** Morphology of the bone marrow after stem cell transplantation. *Histopathology.* 2006; **48**:329–342.

65. **Frimberger AE, Stering AI, Quesenberry PJ.** An in vitro model of hematopoietic stem cell homing demonstrates rapid homing and maintenance of engraftable stem cells. *Blood.* 2001;**98**:1012–1018.

66. **Whetton AD, Graham GJ.** Homing and mobilization in the stem cell niche. *Trends in Cell Biology.* 1999;**9**:233–238.

67. **Choi K, Kennedy M, Kazarov A, Papadimitriou JC, Keller G.** A common precursor for hematopoietic and endothelial cells. *Development.* 1998;**125**:725–732.

68. **Chasis JA.** Erythroblastic islands: specialized microenvironmental niches for erythropoiesis. *Current Opinion in Hematology.* 2006;**13**:137–141.

69. **Thiele J, Kvasnicka HM, Beelen DW,** *et al.* Macrophages and their subpopulations following allogeneic bone marrow transplantation for chronic myeloid leukaemia. *Virchows Archiv.* 2000;**437**:160–166.

70. **Kruskall MS.** Transfusion support for the oncology patients. In Simon TL, Dzik WH, Snyder EL, Stowell CP, Stausss RG, eds. *Rossi's Principles of Transfusion Medicine* (3rd edn.). Philadelphia, PA: Lippincott, Williams & Wilkins; 2002, 498–513.

71. **Maeda T, Shiozawa E, Mayumi H,** *et al.* Histopathology of bone marrow reconstitution after umbilical cord blood transplantation for hematological diseases. *Pathology International.* 2008; **58**:126–132.

20 Pediatric small blue cell tumors metastatic to the bone marrow

Maria A. Proytcheva

Introduction

Bone marrow (BM) studies are often performed in children with solid tumors for initial diagnosis, for staging of disease, for monitoring of response to therapy, and for detecting recurrent diseases. In general, the presence of BM metastasis indicates high-stage disease and is associated with inferior outcome. Different pediatric solid tumors, however, metastasize with variable frequency depending on the tumor type. While neuroblastoma and alveolar rhabdomyosarcoma frequently present with BM metastases, other tumors such as pediatric brain tumors, non-rhabdomyosarcoma soft tissue sarcomas, and retinoblastoma metastasize less often. Some tumors, such as Wilms tumor, almost never metastasize to the BM and seldom require bone marrow evaluation. There is no single clinical finding that can predict the presence of BM metastasis in a child with a solid tumor. Bone pain, spinal cord compression, or pathologic fractures, although frequently reported, are non-specific and unreliable in confirming BM metastasis.

The standard for staging BM evaluation for solid tumors requires bilateral aspirates and biopsies with at least 1 cm of BM, not including the bone cortex or cartilage. BM biopsy may not be feasible in young infants, and a combination of MRI scans, BM aspirates, and ancillary studies may be acceptable for proper diagnosis. This approach, while sufficient for the diagnosis of metastasis, is limited in monitoring response to therapy and further follow-up. Thus, staging BM biopsy should be attempted when possible to overcome this limitation.

Changes in the peripheral blood of patients with pediatric solid tumors

Abnormalities in the peripheral blood in children with solid tumors are frequent, but non-specific. Children with metastatic solid tumors often present with a leukoerythroblastic picture manifested by leukocytosis with granulocytic shift to immaturity and circulating nucleated red blood cells. Less often there is pancytopenia. The cause of the leukoerythroblastic reaction is not completely understood. The mechanistic explanation suggesting that hematopoietic cells are being "squeezed out" of the

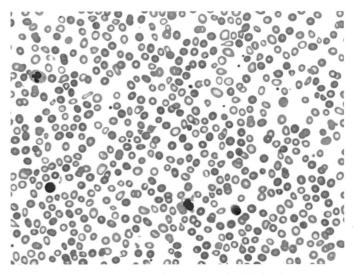

Fig. 20.1. A peripheral blood film from a 17-month-old girl with stage IV neuroblastoma shows marked anisopoikilocytosis and rare circulating nucleated red blood cells. WBC count 6.12 × 10^9/L; Hb 8.2 g/dL; Hct 25.3%; MCV 74.8 fL; RDW 25.2%; platelets 69 × 10^9/L (Wright–Giemsa stain).

bone marrow space due to fibrosis does not account for the fact that a leukoerythroblastic reaction can be present in patients without BM metastases or when there is only minimal or no marrow fibrosis. New evidence suggests that leukoerythroblastic reaction is most likely driven by cytokines produced by the tumor cells [1]. For example, some tumors secrete granulocyte colony stimulating factor (G-CSF), resulting in mobilization of progenitor cells to the peripheral blood with resultant leukocytosis and shift to immaturity.

Normochromic, normocytic or microcytic anemia is frequent in children with solid tumors (Fig. 20.1). However, neither the sole presence of anemia nor its degree is helpful to discriminate between children with and without BM metastases. Other potential causes for anemia include BM suppression secondary to inflammation, and hemorrhage within the primary tumor. Less frequently, increased peripheral destruction occurs due to disseminated intravascular coagulation (DIC) or hypersplenism [2].

The morphologic examination of the peripheral blood film of a child with solid tumor may demonstrate marked anisopoikilocytosis including teardrop-shaped erythrocytes and the presence of variable numbers of nucleated red cells on a background of minimal polychromasia and low reticulocyte count. In cases of tumors complicated by DIC, microangiopathic changes with increased numbers of schistocytes and thrombocytopenia are present.

Children with solid tumors may also present with thrombocytosis. While the underlying mechanisms are still unclear, tumor-derived thrombopoietic-like substances released by the megakaryocytes, platelet-derived microparticles, and factors secreted by the bone marrow endothelial cells have all been postulated to play a role in this process [3].

Rarely, children with extensive BM involvement may present with pancytopenia with or without circulating tumor cells in the peripheral blood. The tumor cells may mimic leukemic blasts. Thus, in cases with unknown primary diagnosis, flow cytometric studies, or other forms of immunophenotyping to rule out leukemia, may be the initial workup. In children, acute leukemia is far more frequent than solid tumors.

Bone marrow aspirate changes in patients with pediatric solid tumors

There is a general agreement that examination of both BM aspirate and biopsy is more sensitive than either aspirate or biopsy alone to detect metastatic disease, regardless of whether the purpose is for initial staging, monitoring of response to therapy, or initial diagnosis in children with an occult malignancy [4]. Even when positive, the BM aspirate smears have limited use in determining the degree of BM involvement by tumor and in monitoring the response to therapy. In addition, they may be negative for tumor in the presence of metastatic disease detected by BM biopsy.

On BM aspirate smears, metastatic pediatric solid tumors look similar to one another. Some tumors manifest as large clumps that tend to be more numerous at the edges than in other parts of the smear (Fig. 20.2). However, when the tumor clumps are rare, the metastases may be hard to find and/or to distinguish from the normal hematopoietic cells such as erythroid progenitors, which in the settings of erythroid hyperplasia may form small clusters (Fig. 20.3). Thorough examination of the entire spread surface and of all available slides at low magnification (4× or 10×) is required in order to detect such tumors. Other, less differentiated tumors, appear as single cells. These cases are particularly challenging, as the tumor cells may mimic leukemic blasts. Individual solid tumor cells may have a high nuclear cytoplasmic ratio, open "blastic" chromatin, nucleoli, and scant to moderate cytoplasm. The distinction between the tumor cells and leukemic blasts may require additional studies, such as immunophenotyping by flow cytometry. The appearance of

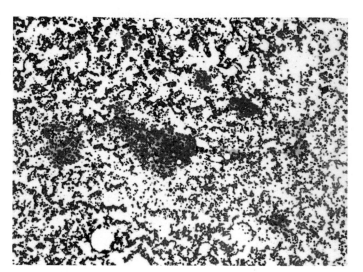

Fig. 20.2. A bone marrow aspirate smear shows large clumps of cohesive non-hematopoietic cells and a small number of single hematopoietic cells (Wright stain).

the most common pediatric solid tumors will be discussed below.

Undifferentiated pediatric solid tumor cells may also share morphologic similarities with the normal bone marrow B-cell progenitors, hematogones [5, 6]. The distinction between the two can be challenging since, in young children with metastatic tumors, both cell types may coexist. Shared features between the two include a similar chromatin pattern, inconspicuous nucleoli, and somewhat scant cytoplasm. The tumor cells, however, are relatively larger and comprise a monotonous population devoid of hematopoietic progenitors. In contrast, hematogones are smaller and are surrounded by intermediate cells sharing features of immature forms and lymphocytes that are easily recognizable as being lymphoid (Fig. 20.4). When the metastatic solid tumor cells are few, they may be obscured by a predominance of hematogones (Fig. 20.5). If the primary diagnosis is unrecognized, this may result in an erroneous diagnosis of acute leukemia. It is therefore critical to be aware of the settings in which increased numbers of hematogones occur, and to know their morphologic and antigenic characteristics, as discussed further below.

Immunophenotyping

Immunophenotyping is an indispensable tool in the characterization of normal bone marrow progenitors and in the diagnosis of hematologic malignancies. The use of this approach has been expanded to include pediatric solid tumors. Based on the observation that some of these tumors express CD56 (a membrane glycoprotein present on neural and muscle tissue), and are negative for CD45, a leukocyte common antigen, new flow cytometric assays for detection of malignant cells have been developed. A specific combination of CD56 and CD45 – coupled with

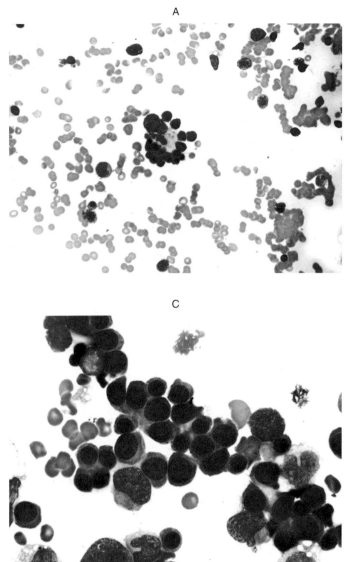

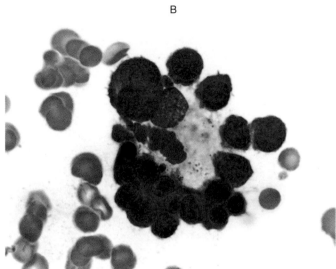

Fig. 20.3. Bone marrow aspirate smears from a patient with a history of neuroblastoma, status post-chemotherapy, who underwent bone marrow evaluation prior to hematopoietic stem cell transplantation. (A) At low magnification there is a small clump of somewhat cohesive cells with a central macrophage, resembling metastatic tumor. (B) The higher magnification reveals that these are immature erythroid progenitors with hemoglobinizing cytoplasm. (C) After intensive chemotherapy the erythroid hyperplasia with a shift to immaturity can be prominent, as shown here (Wright stain).

tumor-specific antibodies such as neuronal-specific antigens GD2 and NB84, muscle-specific antigens such as myogenin, or CD90 and CD99 – is used for the identification of neuroblastoma, rhabdomyosarcoma, or Ewing sarcoma, respectively, when present in bone marrow aspirate or peripheral blood [7–10]. This approach can be used in detecting tumors in limited samples and in monitoring disease persistence or recurrence in patients with previously diagnosed solid tumors. However, its utility in the detection of primary metastatic tumors is relatively limited.

The flow cytometric assay applied routinely for the diagnosis of hematologic malignancies will be of little help in detecting pediatric solid tumors. However, immunophenotyping is very valuable to distinguish between normal B-cell progenitors, hematogones, that can be a differential diagnostic consideration

in the settings of solid tumors, and leukemic blasts. Hematogones, unlike the leukemic blasts, constitute a heterogeneous group of B-cells and show a range of maturation from blasts to mature B-lymphocytes. A proper combination of antibodies such as CD10 and CD20, or other mature B-cell markers, will demonstrate this heterogeneity.

This approach is particularly helpful in cases of young children with pancytopenia and unknown primary tumors, where the marrow aspirate smears are paucicellular and are the only materials available for diagnosis. In such cases, rare tumor clumps may be overlooked and single tumor cells with "blastic" chromatin might be counted as blasts, thus bringing the total number of immature cells to more than 20%. Flow cytometry with a proper panel of antibodies (such as CD10 and a mature B-cell marker) will demonstrate the maturation pattern

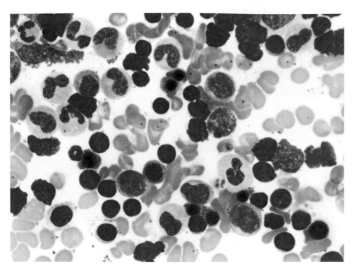

Fig. 20.4. Bone marrow aspirate smear from a child with stage I neuroblastoma illustrates normal B-cell progenitors, hematogones. No tumor cells are present (Wright stain).

characteristic of hematogones or a lack of maturation characteristic of leukemic blasts.

Bone marrow biopsy changes in patients with pediatric solid tumors

The sensitivity of the BM studies is highly enhanced by adding a BM biopsy. Examination at low magnification is very helpful in detection of metastatic cells infiltrating the marrow. Variable metastatic patterns may be present, including diffuse infiltration, well-defined tumor nests, or single neoplastic cells intermixed with the surrounding normal hematopoietic progenitors. The degree of fibrosis also varies, and while in some cases it is prominent, in others, fibrosis is absent.

The degree of differentiation of the pediatric small cell tumors metastatic to the BM varies. In poorly differentiated tumors, the morphologic examination alone may be limited and additional immunohistochemical studies are required to clarify the nature of the process. Immunohistochemistry with lineage-specific antibodies, such as desmin, myogenin, synaptophysin, chromogranin, to name a few, will help to resolve the diagnostic dilemma. Of note, while these antibodies work well on primary tumors, the decalcification process performed on BM biopsy may render the staining suboptimal. Initial workup will help to resolve these technical issues.

To exclude the diagnosis of lymphoblastic leukemia in a bone marrow infiltrated by individual undifferentiated cells, TdT, CD45, and early B- and T-cell markers are helpful. However, one should bear in mind that lymphoblastic leukemias can be CD45 negative, and TdT positivity has been reported in rare cases of rhabdomyosarcoma [11]. Similarly, CD99 by itself has limited use, since it is expressed in a variety of pediatric small blue cell tumors as well as in precursor B- and T-lymphoblastic leukemia/lymphoma, and in a subset of acute

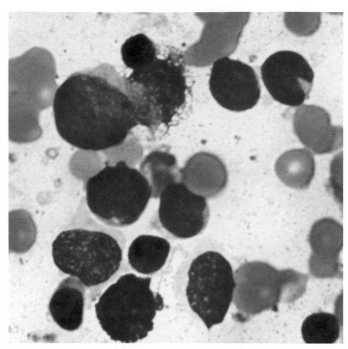

Fig. 20.5. A bone marrow aspirate smear. A single tumor cell and several normal bone marrow B-cell progenitors, hematogones. Note the larger size of the tumor cell, and relatively abundant cytoplasm (Wright stain).

myeloid leukemia, and its expression does not always correlate with the TdT positivity [12].

Recognizing pediatric solid tumors in the bone marrow

Neuroblastoma

Neuroblastoma, a childhood neoplasm arising from the neural crest, is the most common extra-cranial solid tumor, and the leading cause of death in children from one to four years of age [13]. The tumor is characterized by variable clinical behaviors, from spontaneous remission to rapid progression and death. The outcome of the disease depends on multiple factors including stage, age, histologic category, tumor differentiation, status of *NMYC* oncogene, status of chromosomes 1p, 3p, 4p and 11q, and DNA ploidy. Of these factors, stage is one of the most consistent and highly significant prognostic factors in event-free survival [14]. Patients with stage IV disease, defined as having distant metastasis to the bone marrow, have a particularly poor prognosis. One exception is stage IV-S disease, which is seen in children less than 18 months of age who present with metastasis to the skin, liver, and bone marrow, but without osseous involvement. Such children have a favorable prognosis.

Bone marrow evaluation of patients with neuroblastoma is part of the routine initial workup. According to the recommendation of the International Neuroblastoma staging system, bilateral BM aspirates and biopsies are required in children older than six months of age at diagnosis [13, 15]. For the younger children, bilateral aspirates alone are sufficient. While bilateral studies are recommended, only a single positive result is sufficient to document marrow involvement. In the absence of obvious disease, immunohistochemical and/or molecular studies should be performed; however, the results of such studies should not be used for staging. The current standard requires morphologic evidence of metastatic tumor in the BM by routine H&E. In addition to initial staging, bone marrow evaluation is pivotal in following the patient's response to therapy, residual disease, or relapse.

There are a variety of morphologic patterns of metastatic neuroblastoma seen on BM aspirate smears (Fig. 20.6) and biopsies (Fig. 20.7) [16]. The BM aspirate smears most frequently show large, irregular clumps of cohesive tumor cells randomly distributed among the hematopoietic cells. The tumor clumps may be rare or present at the edge of the smear. The clumps are somewhat three-dimensional, and the tumor cells may show molding or form small, compact ball-like aggregates resembling rosettes. Less frequently, the neuroblastoma cells are mostly single. In such cases, tumor clusters may be rare or even absent, so immunophenotyping will be required to rule out leukemia.

The tumor cells may show varying degrees of maturation from mostly single, undifferentiated neuroblasts with scant cytoplasm resembling leukemic blasts, to cells with more pronounced neuroendocrine differentiation embedded in neuropil. Mature ganglion cells may be present in well-differentiated tumors. While these cells are difficult to identify on bone marrow aspirate smears and may be confused with megakaryocytes, they are easily detected on bone marrow biopsy.

The bone marrow biopsies may show various patterns. Diffuse infiltration by large neoplastic cells with various degrees of differentiation may be present. Secondary myelofibrosis is often seen on BM biopsy, resulting in distorted cords of metastatic small cells with hyperchromatic nuclei and scant cytoplasm compressed by the surrounding stromal desmoplastic reaction [16]. In such cases, an increase in reticulin fibers may be seen. Other patterns seen on BM biopsy include discrete islands of small round blue cells in the intertrabecular space, readily identifiable at low magnification as single or multiple foci. Large irregular sheets of tumor cells, spread throughout the intertrabecular or paratrabecular spaces merging with the surrounding hematopoietic cells without sharp demarcation, may also be seen. Lastly, a mixture of focal and interstitial patterns may be present. Various amounts of neuropil, depending on the degree of differentiation of the tumor, and ganglion cells may be present.

Bone marrow biopsies are not used to determine the mitotic/karyorrhectic index (MKI) or to determine whether the neuroblastoma has favorable or unfavorable histology. However, BM aspirates and biopsies can be used as a source of DNA to determine the status of NMYC.

Neuroblastoma-specific monoclonal antibodies are more sensitive than morphologic examination alone in the detection of metastatic tumor in aspirate smears or bone marrow biopsies (Fig. 20.8) [17]. In a study of 197 patients with newly diagnosed neuroblastoma, immunohistochemical stains detected metastatic tumor in 34% of the patients who had previously been considered to have localized disease (stage I–III). A variety of antibodies, such as synaptophysin, cell-surface ganglioside GD2, and chromogranin, have been reported to be useful in bone marrow assessment [10, 17, 18]. Flow cytometry can also be used to detect metastatic cells in BM aspirates or peripheral blood. Using a cocktail of CD45, CD56, CD81, and ganglioside GD2, non-hematopoietic cells with neuroendocrine differentiation can be detected even in patient samples to a level of 0.002% [10]. While this assay is very sensitive (100% sensitivity), it is relatively less specific (83% specificity), and the clinical significance of this information is unclear. Detection of isolated metastatic neuroblastoma cells in the bone marrow may predict the persistence of disease but does not affect overall survival. Therefore, the utility of such studies in the current clinical practice is limited.

Post-treatment bone marrow

After therapy, minimal residual disease may be difficult to detect since small clusters or single cells may not be seen on the marrow aspirate smears and/or a biopsy. Furthermore, therapy may induce differentiation to ganglion cells (Fig. 20.9). While immunohistochemical stains are helpful in detection of even a few residual tumor cells, significance of a single or small number of ganglion cells present in the post-treatment bone marrow has not yet been determined. Similarly, the significance of BM fibrosis after therapy has not been determined. Fibrosis can be associated with residual tumor, healed, negative for tumor, previous metastatic site, or previous bone marrow biopsy site. While the pathophysiology of the BM fibrosis in neuroblastoma is still unclear, some studies suggest that it may be tumor specific, since fibrosis is more frequently present in BM biopsies of patients with neuroblastoma as compared to specimens from patients treated for acute leukemia [19].

Rhabdomyosarcoma

Rhabdomyosarcoma (RMS) is a heterogeneous group of tumors originating from the primitive mesenchyme committed to skeletal muscle differentiation. In children, it is the most common soft tissue sarcoma and, after neuroblastoma, the second most frequent non-hematopoietic tumor to metastasize to the bone marrow [20]. The tumor cells are arrested in the process of muscle differentiation and can be demonstrated by morphology, immunophenotyping, molecular analysis, or electron microscopy. The RMS classification has evolved over many years, and the latest international classification of RMS with overall survival is presented in Table 20.1. Two major histologic subtypes – embryonal and alveolar – have been identified. These two types appear to be histogenetically unrelated in terms of underlying genetic abnormalities, biologic courses, and five-year survival rates. Furthermore, the two types have different prevalence in children. While more than 50% of embryonal or

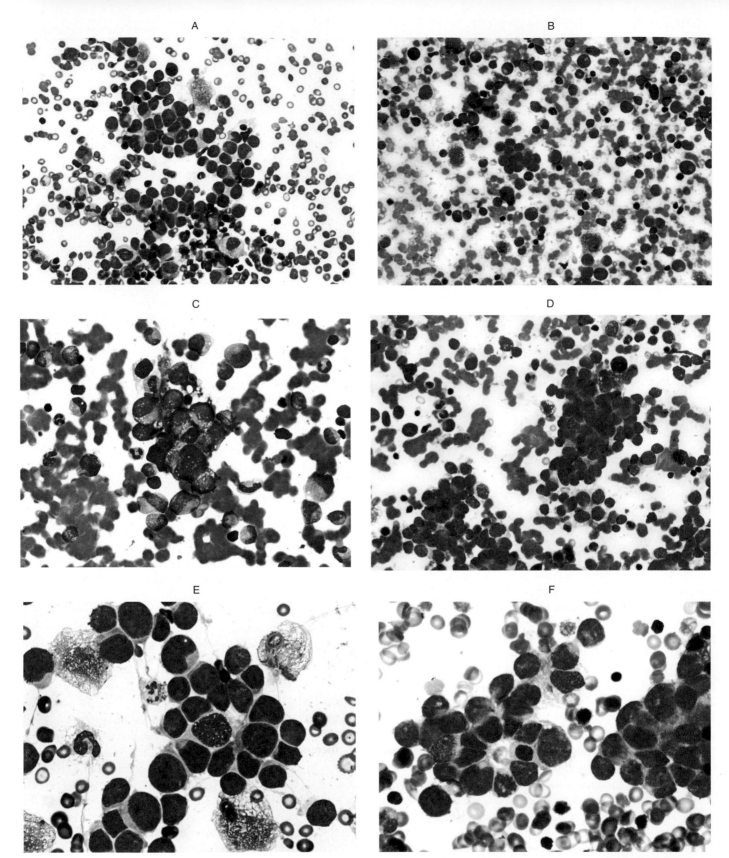

Fig. 20.6. Bone marrow aspirate smear reveals various patterns of metastatic neuroblastoma (Wright stain). (A) Large, conspicuous clusters of cohesive cells. (B) Small clusters that are more conspicuous at low magnification and can be overlooked if the smears are not carefully examined. (C–E) Tumor clusters with various appearance. (F) A cluster of tumor cells forming a classical Homer Wright rosette, characteristic of neuroblastoma. (G) Predominance of single tumor cells. (H) When the single tumor cells are minimally differentiated, they may resemble leukemic blasts or other small blue cell tumor. (I) Neuroblastoma cells embedded in neuropil.

G

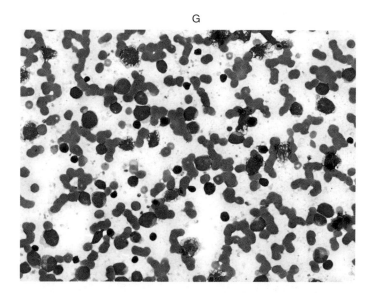

H

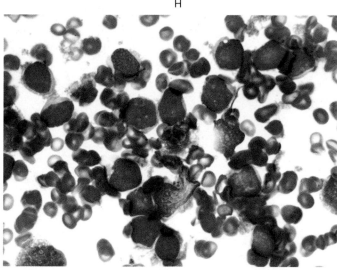

Fig. 20.6. (cont.)

I

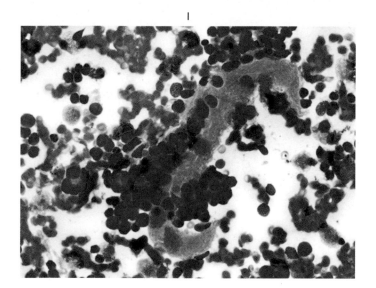

Table 20.1. International classification of rhabdomyosarcoma.

Diagnosis	Histology	Incidence (%)	Five-year survival (%)
Embryonal, botryoid	Favorable	6	95
Embryonal, spindle cell	Favorable	3	88
Embryonal, NOS	Favorable	40	66
Alveolar, NOS or solid variant	Unfavorable	31	53
Anaplastic, diffuse	Unfavorable	2	45
Undifferentiated	Unfavorable	3	44

Adapted from Qualman *et al.* [20].
NOS = not otherwise specified.

botryoid variants occur in the first decade of life, the alveolar type of RMS occurs during adolescence.

Different underlying genetic abnormalities play roles in the pathogenesis of the two types of RMS. This has allowed an increased diagnostic accuracy of discrimination between the two. The hallmark of embryonal RMS is recurrent loss of heterozygosity, loss of imprinting, or paternal disomy at the 11p15 locus which leads to overexpression of the *IGFII* gene. In addition, amplification of 15q25–26 encompassing the *IGFR1* locus, is often seen, thus suggesting a role of the IGF pathway in development of embryonal RMS [21]. In contrast, alveolar RMS is characterized by translocations involving different *PAX* genes and the *FOXO1a* (*FKHR*) gene. Seventy percent of these tumors harbor t(2;13)(q35;q14), which results in the fusion of the *PAX3* gene and *FOXO1a* [21]. Another 10% are associated with t(1;13)(p36;q14) and the fusion of *PAX7* and *FOXO1a*. The remaining 20% have no detectable fusion genes by routine

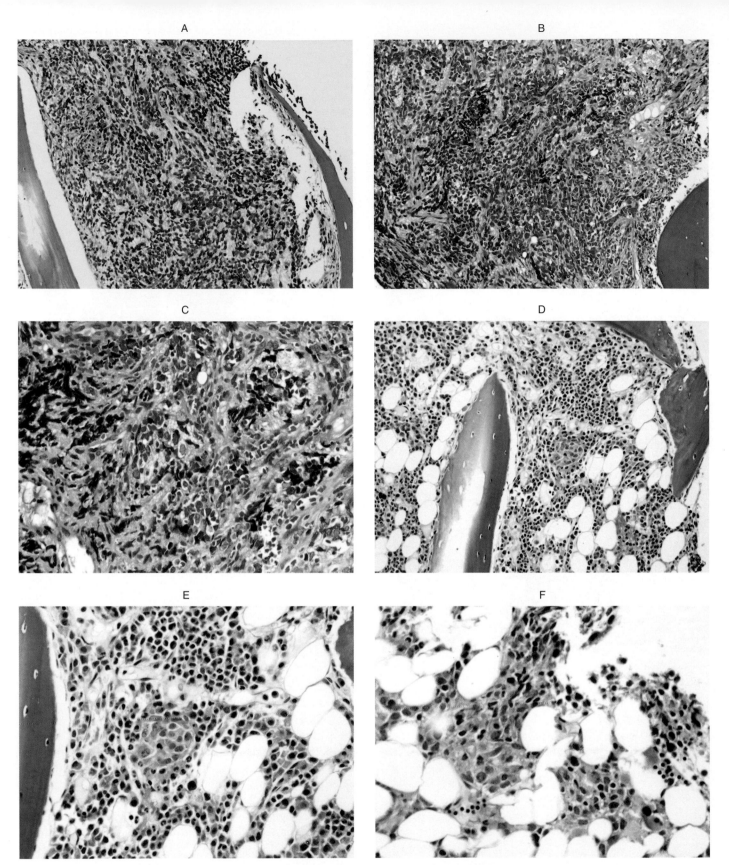

Fig. 20.7. Bone marrow biopsies with various patterns of metastatic neuroblastoma. (A, B) A characteristic diffuse proliferation of large, undifferentiated neoplastic cells forming irregular nests surrounded by stroma (H&E stain). (C) Crush artifact and molding of the neoplastic cells (H&E stain). (D, E) Focal sinusoidal pattern (H&E stain). (F, G) Foci of neuroblastoma merging with the surrounding hematopoietic cells (H&E stain). (H–M). Various degrees of differentiation: from poorly differentiated neuroblastoma (H) to more differentiated tumors demonstrating rare ganglion cells (M) (H&E stain).

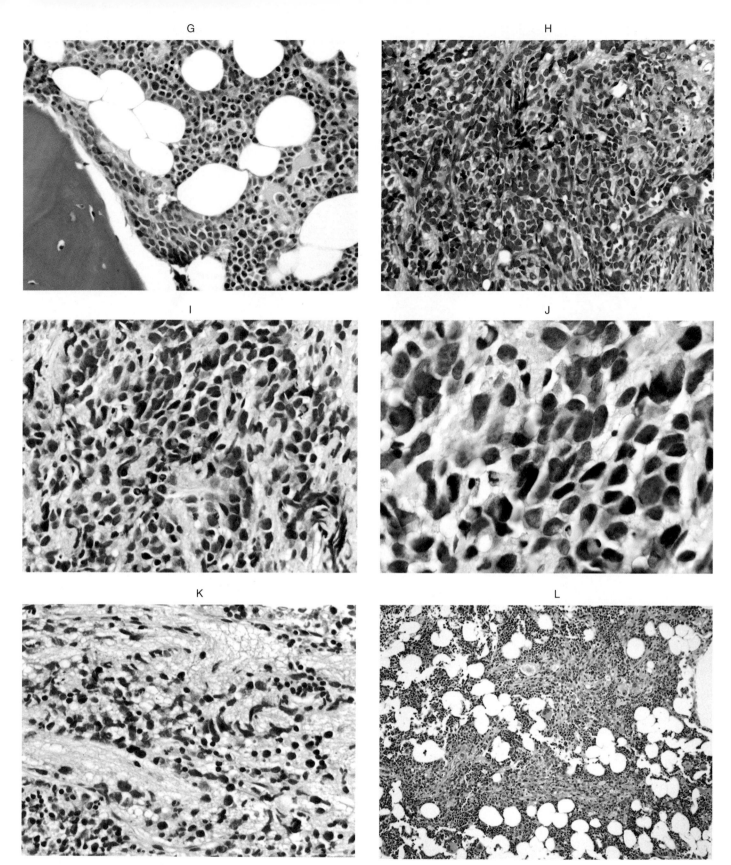

Fig. 20.7. (cont.)

M

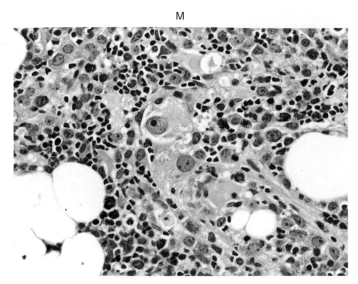

Fig. 20.7. (cont.)

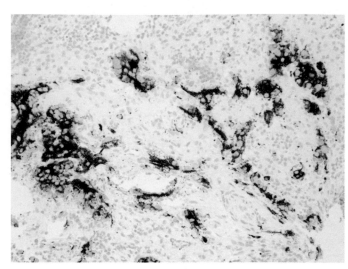

Fig. 20.8. Neuroblastoma. Bone marrow biopsy showing patches of synaptophysin-positive tumor clusters (H&E stain).

A

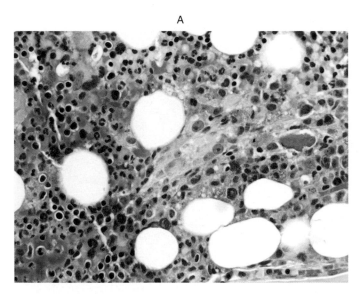

B

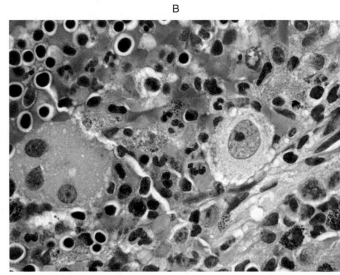

Fig. 20.9. Neuroblastoma, bone marrow biopsy with post-therapy changes. (A, B) Small foci of ganglion cells (H&E stain). (C) Synaptophysin highlighting a ganglion cell. Note numerous hemosiderin-laden macrophages, a frequent finding in post-chemotherapy marrow, that may make the detection of single cells by immunohistochemical stains difficult (immunoperoxidase).

C

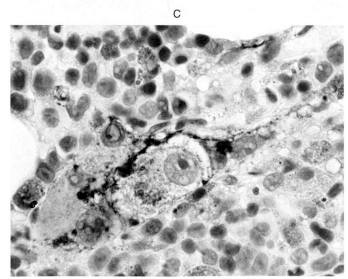

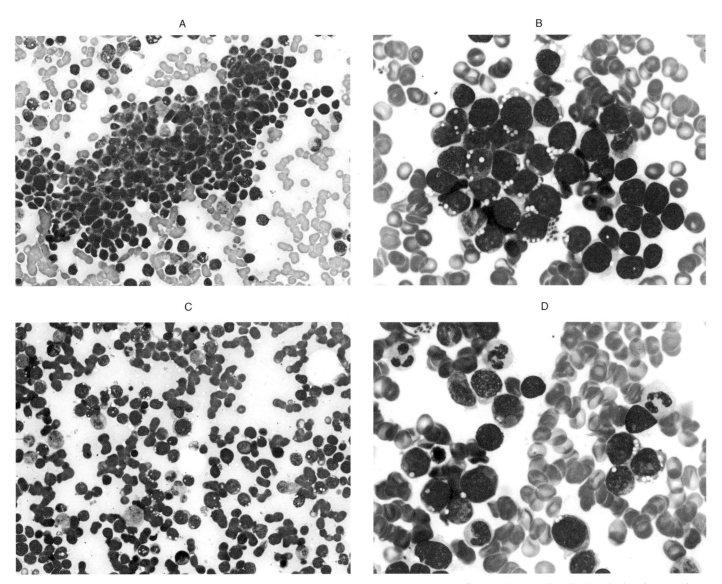

Fig. 20.10. Rhabdomyosarcoma, bone marrow aspirate smears (Wright stain). (A) Characteristic clumps of large, cohesive cells with relatively abundant cytoplasm. (B) A single-layer tumor clump composed of large cells with finely speckled chromatin, several conspicuous nucleoli, and abundant, basophilic vacuolated cytoplasm. Note the well-defined cytoplasmic borders. (C) Mostly single, undifferentiated tumor cells resembling leukemia. (D) The tumor cells display hemophagocytosis.

RT-PCR. While the type of fusion is diagnostically relevant, it does not correlate with the histologic features of particular alveolar RMSs [22].

The alveolar and embryonal RMSs have been reported to have similar potential to metastasize to the bone marrow [23]. However, in our own institution's experience, as well as in almost all reported cases, bone marrow involvement is present exclusively in the alveolar type. On BM aspirate smears, metastatic alveolar RMS appears as single cells or clusters of non-hematopoietic tumor cells with abundant, frequently vacuolated cytoplasm (Fig. 20.10). The neoplastic cells have a regular nuclear contour, fine, "blastic" chromatin with several inconspicuous nucleoli, and an abundant amount of cytoplasm. The

borders of the cytoplasm are conspicuous and the cells are less cohesive when compared to neuroblastoma cells. The tumor clusters are two-dimensional and somewhat flatter as compared to tumor clumps of metastatic neuroblastoma. However, mostly single tumor cells can be present in some tumors. The tumor cells can display hemophagocytosis.

On BM biopsy, patches of RMS cells are more frequently observed, while diffuse infiltration is less frequent (Fig. 20.11). The tumor foci vary in size and may be embedded in fibrosis or intermixed with the hematopoietic progenitors without significant fibrosis. When the fibrosis is minimal, the metastatic tumor may be inconspicuous on morphologic examination. In such cases, immunohistochemical studies demonstrating

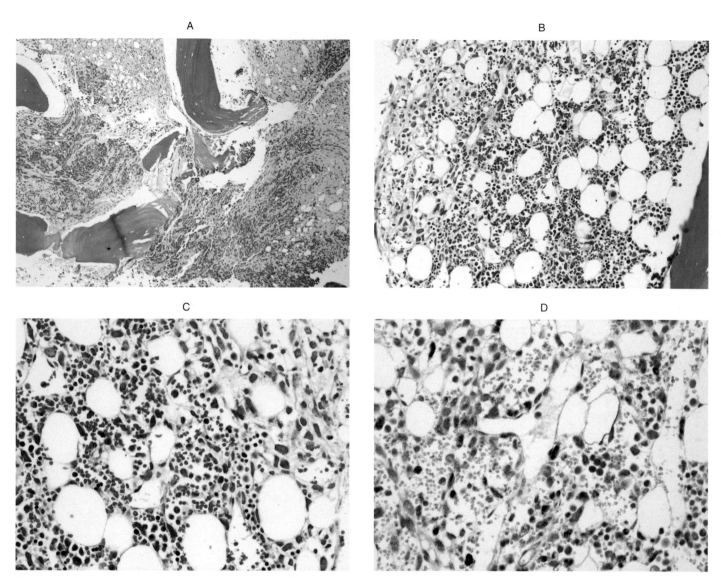

Fig. 20.11. Rhabdomyosarcoma, bone marrow biopsies. (A) Diffuse infiltration of the marrow by tumor easily recognizable as non-hematopoietic. Note prominent stroma and fibrosis that can be associated with some tumors (H&E stain). (B, C) Metastatic tumor with minimal fibrosis. The large tumor cells blend with the hematopoietic cells and are inconspicuous on morphologic examination (H&E stain). (D) Immunohistochemical stains such as myogenin, shown here, are helpful to highlight the neoplastic cells (immunoperoxidase).

muscle-specific differentiation of the tumor cells are very helpful, first in determining the presence of RMS, and second in determining the degree of tumor burden. This initial information can be used further to monitor the response to therapy.

Less frequently, RMS may completely infiltrate and replace the bone marrow (Fig. 20.12). Depending on the degree of differentiation, the tumor cells may be relatively small and have round nuclear contour, single or multiple inconspicuous nucleoli, and moderate eosinophilic cytoplasm, or they may be large, single or multinucleated, and have abundant eosinophilic cytoplasm. Extensive necrosis may occur (Fig. 20.13).

Due to these morphologic features, alveolar RMS has been confused with hematopoietic malignancy, particularly undifferentiated leukemias, as attested to by multiple reports in the literature [24–27]. Immunophenotyping demonstrating muscle differentiation, and/or genetic studies will assist in the proper identification of the neoplastic cells (Fig. 20.14).

Post-treatment bone marrow

Chemotherapy may induced myogenic differentiation within primary, as well as metastatic, rhabdomyosarcoma, known as cytodifferentiation (Fig. 20.15). In primary tumors, cytodifferentiation is associated with a better outcome and is more frequent in the embryonal and botryoid types. In the alveolar RMS, cytodifferentiation is mostly focal [28]. It is still unclear whether the presence of extensive cytodifferentiation is an independent factor regardless of the histologic type, or is related to

A

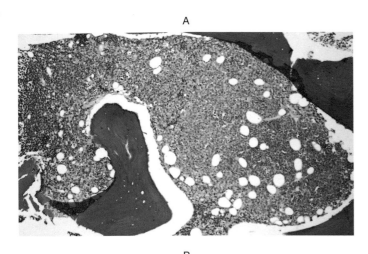

B

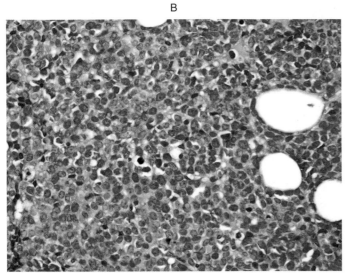

C

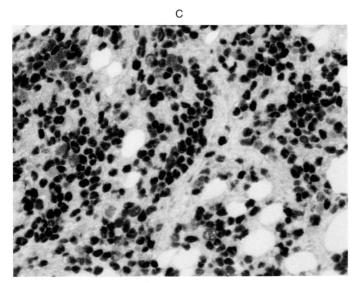

Fig. 20.12. Rhabdomyosarcoma, bone marrow biopsies. (A, B) Diffuse infiltration by poorly differentiated tumor. Note the cellular features of the tumor: medium to large cells with finely speckled chromatin, several inconspicuous nucleoli, and scant to moderate cytoplasm that resemble leukemic blasts (H&E stain). (C) Immunohistochemical stains show that the cells express markers of muscle differentiation (Myogenin, immunoperoxidase).

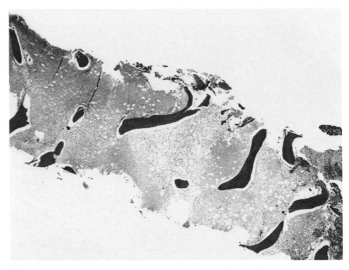

Fig. 20.13. Rhabdomyosarcoma, a bone marrow biopsy shows extensive necrosis (H&E stain).

the fundamental difference between the embryonal and alveolar RMS.

Ewing sarcoma family of tumors

Ewing sarcoma is the second most common bone malignancy in patients younger than 20 years of age [29]. In general, Ewing sarcoma is more prevalent after that age, and only 20–30% of the cases are diagnosed in the first decade of life. Most Ewing sarcomas arise in the bones, particularly pelvic bones, the long bones of the lower extremities, or the chest wall bones, and pain is the most common presenting sign. No single blood, serum, or urine test is diagnostic of Ewing sarcoma. The Ewing sarcoma family of tumors comprises a spectrum of histologic appearances from classical Ewing sarcoma, first described by James Ewing, composed of a monotonous population of small, round cells, to more differentiated tumors such as a peripheral primitive neuroectodermal tumor (PNET). These are recognized as a single family of tumors by their recurrent cytogenetic abnormality, resulting in translocation of the *FLI1* gene on chromosome 11 to the *EWS* gene on chromosome 22, t(11;22)(q24;q12). Fluorescent *in situ* hybridization (FISH) with an *EWS*-specific probe, or RT-PCR, detect this or other variant translocations in approximately 95% of tumors [30].

Strong CD99 expression has been found to correlate with the presence of this translocation [31]. Ewing sarcomas strongly express CD99 in a characteristic, but not specific, membrane pattern. CD99 is also found in precursor T-lymphoblastic lymphomas, immature TdT-positive T-cells, in a small group of precursor cells in the bone marrow, and other TdT-positive hematologic malignancies [32]. Thus, CD99 positivity, particularly in the bone marrow, must be evaluated very carefully along with other markers. The more differentiated PNETs express neuron-specific enolase (NSE), S100, Leu7, and/or PgP 9.5.

At diagnosis, about 25% of the patients present with metastatic Ewing sarcoma, and most often the sites of

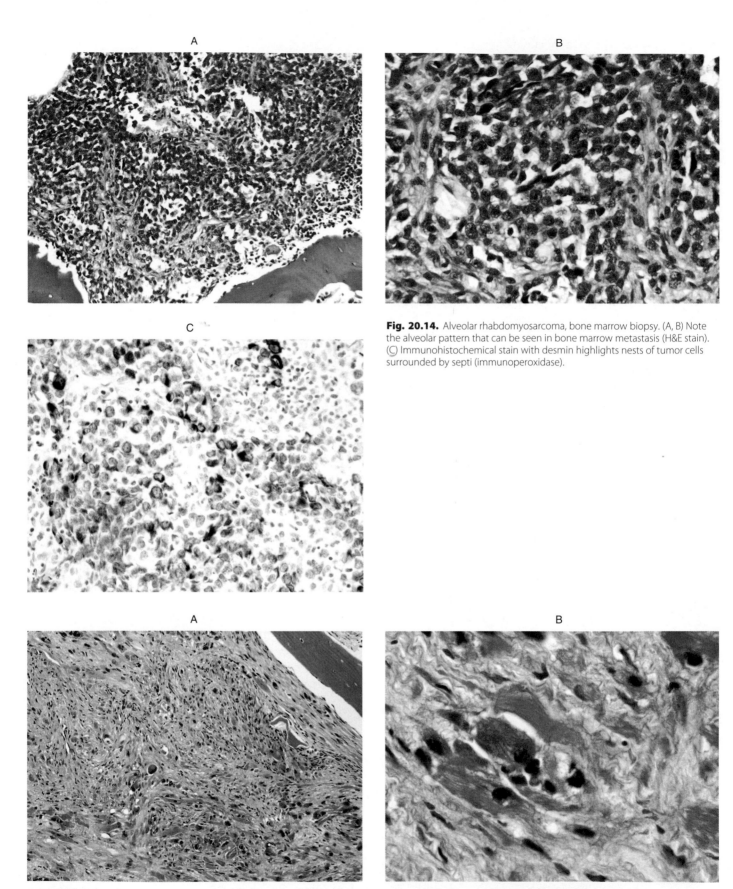

Fig. 20.14. Alveolar rhabdomyosarcoma, bone marrow biopsy. (A, B) Note the alveolar pattern that can be seen in bone marrow metastasis (H&E stain). (C) Immunohistochemical stain with desmin highlights nests of tumor cells surrounded by septi (immunoperoxidase).

Fig. 20.15. Rhabdomyosarcoma. (A, B) A bone marrow biopsy shows marked cytodifferentiation after chemotherapy (H&E stain).

metastases include lungs and pleural space, the skeletal system, and bone marrow, or some combination of them [29]. In one study, more than a half of the patients with widespread disease presented with bone marrow metastases [33]. Overall, microscopic detection of BM metastasis is seen in less than 10% of the patients with Ewing sarcoma and is associated with poor prognosis [34, 35]. Immunohistochemical studies can be helpful for some patients with focal tumor that cannot be detected on H&E stain alone. The clinical implication of such detection of bone marrow involvement, as well as detecting tumor by RT-PCR in lack of tumor clumps, has not been fully determined.

Non-rhabdomyosarcoma soft tissue sarcomas

Soft tissue sarcomas other than rhabdomyosarcomas or Ewing group family represent a heterogeneous group of disorders and comprise about 4% of childhood cancers [36, 37]. Bone marrow involvement is extremely rare in this group of tumors and is associated with advanced stages of disease and with an unfavorable prognosis. The morphologic appearance is similar to the other metastatic tumors to the marrow.

Summary

The metastatic potential of pediatric solid tumors to the bone marrow varies. While neuroblastoma and rhabdomyosarcoma metastasize frequently, the rest of the tumors are seen in the marrow rarely, mostly in children with widespread disease. The morphologic examination remains the gold standard for diagnosis of metastatic disease. Bilateral BM aspirates and biopsies have higher sensitivity in detecting such metastatic disease than either aspirates or biopsies alone. The morphologic patterns of bone marrow metastases are variable and non-specific to discriminate between different tumors. Neuroblastoma and rhabdomyosarcoma may present as single cells and have to be differentiated from leukemias. Another diagnostic challenge is to distinguish metastatic tumor from the normal B-cell progenitors, a frequent finding in patients with tumor. Supplementary evaluations such as immunophenotyping and cytogenetic studies can confirm the cell of origin of the neoplastic cells.

Acknowledgments: I extend great appreciation to Elizabeth Perlman for critical reading of the manuscript and her meaningful suggestions, and Ms. Susan C. Winslow for her editorial help.

References

1. Cotta CV, Konoplev S, Medeiros LJ, Bueso-Ramos CE. Metastatic tumors in bone marrow: histopathology and advances in the biology of the tumor cells and bone marrow environment. *Annals of Diagnostic Pathology*. 2006; **10**:169–192.

2. Scott JP, Morgan E. Coagulopathy of disseminated neuroblastoma. *Journal of Pediatrics*. 1983;**103**:219–222.

3. Sierko E, Wojtukiewicz MZ. Platelets and angiogenesis in malignancy. *Seminars in Thrombosis & Hemostasis*. 2004;**30**:95–108.

4. Aronica PA, Pirrotta VT, Yunis EJ, Penchansky L. Detection of neuroblastoma in the bone marrow: biopsy versus aspiration. *Journal of Pediatric Hematology/Oncology*. 1998;**20**:330–334.

5. Longacre TA, Foucar K, Crago S, et al. Hematogones: a multiparameter analysis of bone marrow precursor cells. *Blood*. 1989;**73**:543–552.

6. Evans AE, Hummeler K. The significance of primitive cells in marrow aspirates of children with neuroblastoma. *Cancer*. 1973;**32**:906–912.

7. Chang A, Benda PM, Wood BL, Kussick SJ. Lineage-specific identification of nonhematopoietic neoplasms by flow cytometry. *American Journal of Clinical Pathology*. 2003;**119**:643–655.

8. Bozzi F, Gambirasio F, Luksch R, et al. Detecting CD56+/NB84+/CD45-immunophenotype in the bone marrow of patients with metastatic neuroblastoma using flow cytometry. *Anticancer Research*. 2006;**26**:3281–3287.

9. Nagai J, Ishida Y, Koga N, et al. A new sensitive and specific combination of CD81/CD56/CD45 monoclonal antibodies for detecting circulating neuroblastoma cells in peripheral blood using flow cytometry. *Journal of Pediatric Hematology/Oncology*. 2000;**22**:20–26.

10. Warzynski MJ, Graham DM, Axtell RA, Higgins JV, Hammers YA. Flow cytometric immunophenotyping test for staging/monitoring neuroblastoma patients. *Cytometry*. 2002;**50**:298–304.

11. Mathewson RC, Kjeldsberg CR, Perkins SL. Detection of terminal deoxynucleotidyl transferase (TdT) in nonhematopoietic small round cell tumors of children. *Pediatric Pathology & Laboratory Medicine*. 1997;**17**:835–844.

12. Kang LC, Dunphy CH. Immunoreactivity of MIC2 (CD99) and terminal deoxynucleotidyl transferase in bone marrow clot and core specimens of acute myeloid leukemias and myelodysplastic syndromes. *Archives of Pathology & Laboratory Medicine*. 2006;**130**:153–157.

13. Monclair T, Brodeur GM, Ambros PF, et al. The International Neuroblastoma Risk Group (INRG) staging system: an INRG Task Force report. *Journal of Clinical Oncology*. 2009;**27**:298–303.

14. Cohn SL, Pearson ADJ, London WB, et al. The International Neuroblastoma Risk Group (INRG) classification system: an INRG Task Force report. *Journal of Clinical Oncology*. 2009;**27**:289–297.

15. Brodeur GM, Pritchard J, Berthold F, et al. Revisions of the international criteria for neuroblastoma diagnosis, staging, and response to treatment. *Journal of Clinical Oncology*. 1993;**11**:1466–1477.

16. Mills AE, Bird AR. Bone marrow changes in neuroblastoma. *Pediatric Pathology*. 1986;**5**:225–234.

17. Moss TJ, Reynolds CP, Sather HN, et al. Prognostic value of immunocytologic detection of bone marrow metastases in neuroblastoma. *New England Journal of Medicine*. 1991;**324**:219–226.

18. Swerts K, Ambros PF, Brouzes C, et al. Standardization of the immunocytochemical detection of neuroblastoma cells in bone marrow.

The Journal of Histochemistry and Cytochemistry. 2005;**53**:1433–1440.

19. **Turner GE, Reid MM.** What is marrow fibrosis after treatment of neuroblastoma? *Journal of Clinical Pathology.* 1993;**46**:61–63.

20. **Qualman SJ, Coffin CM, Newton WA,** *et al.* Intergroup Rhabdomyosarcoma Study: update for pathologists. *Pediatric and Developmental Pathology.* 1998;**1**: 550–561.

21. **Slater O, Shipley J.** Clinical relevance of molecular genetics to paediatric sarcomas. *Journal of Clinical Pathology.* 2007;**60**:1187–1194.

22. **Parham DM, Qualman SJ, Teot L,** *et al.* Correlation between histology and PAX/FKHR fusion status in alveolar rhabdomyosarcoma: a report from the Children's Oncology Group. *American Journal of Surgical Pathology.* 2007;**31**: 895–901.

23. **de la Monte SM, Hutchins GM, Moore GW.** Metastatic behavior of rhabdomyosarcoma. *Pathology, Research & Practice.* 1986;**181**:148–152.

24. **Shinkoda Y, Nagatoshi Y, Fukano R, Nishiyama K, Okamura J.** Rhabdomyosarcoma masquerading as acute leukemia. *Pediatric Blood & Cancer.* 2009;**52**:286–287.

25. **Sandberg AA, Stone JF, Czarnecki L, Cohen JD.** Hematologic masquerade of rhabdomyosarcoma. *American Journal of Hematology.* 2001;**68**:51–57.

26. **Miyoshi I, Uemura Y, Muneishi H, Miyazaki J, Taguchi H.** Bone marrow metastasis of alveolar rhabdomyosarcoma. *Internal Medicine.* 2005;**44**:677–678.

27. **Schwartz S, Menssen HD, Thiel E.** Haemophagocytosis in bone marrow rhabdomyosarcoma. *British Journal of Haematology.* 1999;**105**:573.

28. **Smith LM, Anderson JR, Coffin CM.** Cytodifferentiation and clinical outcome after chemotherapy and radiation therapy for rhabdomyosarcoma (RMS). *Medical & Pediatric Oncology.* 2002;**38**:398–404.

29. **Bernstein M, Kovar H, Paulussen M,** *et al.* Ewing's sarcoma family of tumors: current management. *Oncologist.* 2006; **11**:503–519.

30. **Ladanyi M, Bridge JA.** Contribution of molecular genetic data to the classification of sarcomas. *Human Pathology.* 2000;**31**:532–538.

31. **Ladanyi M, Lewis R, Garin-Chesa P,** *et al.* EWS rearrangement in Ewing's sarcoma and peripheral neuroectodermal tumor. Molecular detection and correlation with cytogenetic analysis and MIC2 expression. *Diagnostic Molecular Pathology.* 1993;**2**:141–146.

32. **Robertson PB, Neiman RS, Worapongpaiboon S, John K, Orazi A.** 013 (CD99) positivity in hematologic proliferations correlates with TdT positivity. *Modern Pathology.* 1997;**10**: 277–282.

33. **Oberlin O, Bayle C, Hartmann O, Terrier-Lacombe MJ, Lemerle J.** Incidence of bone marrow involvement in Ewing's sarcoma: value of extensive investigation of the bone marrow. *Medical & Pediatric Oncology.* 1995;**24**: 343–346.

34. **Lazda EJ, Berry PJ.** Bone marrow metastasis in Ewing's sarcoma and peripheral primitive neuroectodermal tumor: an immunohistochemical study. *Pediatric & Developmental Pathology.* 1998;**1**:125–130.

35. **Madhumathi DS, Premalata CS, Devi VL,** *et al.* Bone marrow involvement at presentation in pediatric non-haematological small round cell tumours. *Indian Journal of Pathology & Microbiology.* 2007;**50**:886–889.

36. **Spunt SL, Skapek SX, Coffin CM.** Pediatric nonrhabdomyosarcoma soft tissue sarcomas. *Oncologist.* 2008;**13**: 668–678.

37. **Pappo AS, Rao BN, Jenkins JJ,** *et al.* Metastatic nonrhabdomyosarcomatous soft-tissue sarcomas in children and adolescents: the St. Jude Children's Research Hospital experience. *Medical & Pediatric Oncology.* 1999;**33**:76–82.

Pediatric mature B-cell non-Hodgkin lymphomas

Sherrie L. Perkins

Non-Hodgkin lymphomas (NHLs) comprise approximately 10% of all childhood cancers and are a diverse collection of malignant neoplasms of lymphoreticular cells [1]. Pediatric NHL includes a varied group of neoplasms that derive from both mature and immature (blastic) cells of both B-cell and T-cell origin (Table 21.1). NHLs in children are typically intermediate to high-grade (clinically aggressive) tumors. This is in direct contrast to NHL in adults, in which more than two-thirds of the tumors are indolent, low-grade malignancies [2–5]. Pediatric NHL also appears very different from adult lymphomas in that nearly all of the tumors are diffuse neoplasms, and follicular (nodular) lymphomas are exceedingly rare. Pediatric NHL is nearly evenly split between B-cell and T-cell neoplasms, whereas in adults nearly 80% of NHLs are of B-cell phenotype. In addition, pediatric populations have a high incidence of precursor (lymphoblastic) lymphomas, whereas nearly all adult lymphomas arise from mature B- and T-cells [3–4, 6–8].

Diagnosis of pediatric NHL requires similar approaches to those used in adults. Pediatric NHLs are usually aggressive, fast-growing neoplasms that require efficient and appropriate handling of pathologic materials to ensure that a diagnosis can be established (Table 21.2) [9–10]. Morphology and immunophenotype provide the cornerstones of diagnosis, with some problematic cases requiring additional diagnostic ancillary testing, including cytogenetics (to identify specific recurrent cytogenetic abnormalities) or molecular studies (to determine clonality or specific translocations). However, it should be noted that immunophenotypic, cytogenetic, and molecular data often provide important prognostic and treatment data, making the ability to perform these tests extremely important beyond initial diagnosis [11–17]. Optimally, sufficient tissue to allow for morphologic analysis and appropriate ancillary testing will be collected, usually requiring an open tissue biopsy. In some cases, cytologic preparations may be sufficient to allow for diagnosis of a pediatric NHL, particularly if handled appropriately to allow for immunophenotypic studies by flow cytometry or immunohistochemistry [18–22].

In order to assure that all the information and ancillary studies that are necessary are able to be performed, it is usually preferable that biopsy specimens be collected and provided to the pathologist as fresh tissue, so that it may be appropriately handled and divided for ancillary studies (Table 21.2). Many ancillary investigations, including flow cytometry and cytogenetic studies, require fresh tissue. Immunophenotypic analysis and limited cytogenetic analysis by fluorescent *in situ* hybridization (FISH) studies may be performed on fixed tissues, if no fresh tissue is available. Many molecular studies may be performed on fixed or fresh/frozen tissues [2, 14–15, 23–26]. However, despite the wide variety of ancillary studies that are available and that are helpful in making a diagnosis of NHL, morphology remains the cornerstone, and sufficient care must be taken that adequate biopsy materials are adequately fixed, processed and sectioned to allow for appropriate evaluation of morphologic features [2].

Classification of mature B-cell non-Hodgkin lymphoma

Classification of the mature B-cell NHL in current pathology practice is usually done using the World Health Organization (WHO) classification [11]. This approach integrates clinical presentation, and morphology, as well as immunophenotypic, molecular, and cytogenetic features to classify NHL entities. Use of ancillary testing techniques is integral to making a definitive diagnosis, and use of the data generated by these tests helps to increase the reliability and reproducibility of diagnosis. However, many of the entities seen in children have overlapping immunophenotypic and molecular features; hence morphology remains an essential component of diagnosis [2]. Despite use of phenotypic, molecular, and cytogenetic testing, some of the diagnoses seen frequently in children and adolescents remain difficult, in particular distinguishing some cases of Burkitt lymphoma from diffuse large B-cell lymphoma and recognizing low-grade lymphomas in children [27–29].

Diagnostic Pediatric Hematopathology, ed. Maria A. Proytcheva. Published by Cambridge University Press.
© Cambridge University Press 2011.

Table 21.1. Common non-Hodgkin lymphoma in children.

Subtype	Incidence (%)	Immunophenotype	Primary sites
Burkitt lymphoma	40	B-cell	Abdomen, head and neck, central nervous system, marrow
Lymphoblastic lymphoma	30	Precursor T – 90% Precursor B – 10%	Mediastinum, nodes Skin, nodes
Diffuse large B-cell lymphoma	20	B-cell	Nodes, abdomen, mediastinum
Anaplastic large cell lymphoma, ALK positive	10	T-cell	Extranodal sites, lymph nodes, mediastinum

Table 21.2. Workup of pediatric mature B-cell non-Hodgkin lymphoma.

Approach	Utility	Tissue requirement
Morphology	Required for diagnosis	Fixed
Immunophenotypic analysis	Very helpful, usually required	Fixed, fresh
Cytogenetics	May provide diagnostic or prognostic information	Fresh
Molecular analysis	May provide diagnostic or prognostic information	Fresh, fixed
FISH for specific translocations	May provide diagnostic or prognostic information	Fresh, fixed
Immunoglobulin gene arrangements	May help in diagnosis	Fresh, frozen, fixed

Table 21.3. WHO histological classification of mature B-cell neoplasms.

Chronic lymphocytic leukemia/small lymphocytic lymphoma
B-cell prolymphocytic leukemia
Lymphoplasmacytic lymphoma
Splenic marginal zone lymphoma
Hairy cell leukemia
Splenic lymphoma/leukemia, unclassifiable
Plasma cell neoplasms
Heavy chain diseases
Extranodal marginal zone B-cell lymphoma of mucosa-associated tissue (MALT-lymphoma)
Nodal marginal zone lymphoma
Follicular lymphoma
Primary cutaneous follicle center lymphoma
Mantle cell lymphoma
Diffuse large B-cell lymphoma (DLBCL), NOS
T-cell/histiocyte-rich large B-cell lymphoma
Primary DLBCL of the CNS
Primary cutaneous DLBCL, leg type
EBV-positive DLBCL of the elderly
DLBCL associated with chronic inflammation
Lymphomatoid granulomatosis
Primary mediastinal (thymic) large B-cell lymphoma
Intravascular large B-cell lymphoma
ALK-positive large B-cell lymphoma
Plasmablastic lymphoma
Large B-cell lymphoma arising in HHV-8-associated multicentric Castleman disease
Primary effusion lymphoma
Burkitt lymphoma
B-cell lymphoma, unclassifiable, with features intermediate between DLBCL and Burkitt lymphoma
B-cell lymphoma, unclassifiable, with features intermediate between DLBCL and classical Hodgkin lymphoma
NOS = not otherwise specified.

The WHO classification recognizes a large spectrum of mature B-cell NHL (Table 21.3) that includes a range of clinical presentations including primarily nodal lymphomas, lymphomas that present primarily with extranodal disease, and those that are primarily leukemic in presentation (Table 21.4). The distribution of diseases varies widely between the pediatric population and adults, with a more limited subset of mature B-cell NHL subtypes seen in children and adolescents (Table 21.5). Most pediatric mature B-cell NHLs present as nodal or extranodal disease, and leukemic presentations are very infrequent, with the exception of Burkitt leukemia [2, 4, 11].

Mature B-cell NHLs in children are most typically Burkitt lymphoma (BL) and diffuse large B-cell lymphoma (DLBCL). Burkitt lymphoma is relatively common in children and much more rarely seen in adults, particularly in immunocompetent adults. Other aggressive neoplasms, such as B-prolymphocytic lymphoma, are not seen in children [7]. Many of the low-grade neoplasms that are seen in adults, such as follicular lymphomas and marginal zone lymphomas (MZLs) are seen infrequently in children but have been recently recognized as distinct disease entities in children by the current WHO classification [6, 11, 30]. A few low-grade B-cell lymphoproliferative disorders seen in adults, such as chronic lymphocytic leukemia/small lymphocytic lymphoma (CLL/SLL), plasmacytomas, and the more aggressive mantle cell lymphoma are very rare in children, and others, such as hairy cell leukemia, have not been reported in children.

One feature of pediatric mature B-cell NHL is the relatively high proportion of follicular-center-cell-derived neoplasms compared to adults, where there is more of a split between follicular and post-follicular neoplasms [7, 11]. This

Table 21.4. Primary presentation of mature B-cell lymphomas.

Nodal
    Diffuse large B-cell lymphoma (may also be extranodal)
    Small lymphocytic lymphoma
    Nodal marginal zone lymphoma
    Follicular lymphoma
    Mantle cell lymphoma (may also be extranodal)

Extranodal
    Splenic marginal zone lymphoma
    Extranodal marginal zone lymphoma
    Burkitt lymphoma (may also be nodal or leukemic)
    Plasmacytoma

Leukemic/bone marrow disease
    Chronic lymphocytic leukemia
    B-prolymphocytic leukemia
    Hairy cell leukemia
    Plasma cell myeloma
    Lymphoplasmacytic lymphoma (may also be nodal or extranodal disease)

Table 21.5. Mature B-cell lymphomas seen in pediatric populations.

Type of lymphoma	Incidence
Burkitt lymphoma	Common
Diffuse large B-cell lymphoma	Less common
Primary mediastinal (thymic) large B-cell lymphoma	Uncommon
T-cell/histiocyte-rich large B-cell lymphoma	Rare
Follicular lymphoma	Rare
Nodal and extranodal marginal zone lymphoma	Rare
Chronic lymphocytic leukemia/small lymphocytic lymphoma	Very rare
Lymphomatoid granulomatosis	Very rare
Plasmacytoma	Extremely rare
Mantle cell lymphoma	Extremely rare

Table 21.6. Immunophenotypic markers useful in workup of pediatric mature B-cell lymphomas.

Marker	Utility	Tissue
CD20	Mature B-cells, absent in precursor B-cells and plasma cells	Fixed, fresh
CD19	Mature and immature B-cells, absent in plasma cells	Fixed, fresh
CD22	Mature and immature B-cells	Fixed, fresh
CD79a	Mature and immature B-cells, plasma cells	Fixed, fresh
PAX-5	B-cells	Fixed
Oct-2	B-cell transcription factor useful in distinguishing NHL from Hodgkin lymphoma	Fixed
BOB.1	B-cell transcription factor useful in distinguishing NHL from Hodgkin lymphoma	Fixed
CD10	Germinal center marker	Fixed, fresh
BCL6	Germinal center marker	Fixed
MUM-1	Marker of post-germinal center, activated B-cells	Fixed
CD138	Plasma cells	Fixed, fresh
Ig heavy chain	Identify neoplastic clones	Fixed, fresh
Kappa, lambda	Identify clonal B-cell populations	Fixed, fresh
TdT	Exclude precursor (lymphoblastic) lesions	Fixed, fresh
CD30	Activation marker positive in some DLBCL (especially primary mediastinal large B-cell lymphoma), Hodgkin lymphoma, or ALCL	Fixed, fresh

may, in part, be due to the developing immune system and primary responses to antigens in the pediatric age group. This may also help to explain the relatively uniform response to therapy for children, where short, intense therapy achieves a very high likelihood of cure for most patients [31, 32]. In addition, as discussed below, many of the pediatric B-cell NHLs have a high proliferation rate and overexpression of pro-proliferative proteins (such as cMYC), suggesting that the mechanism of lymphomagenesis is due to abnormal proliferation rather than the defective apoptosis seen in many adult B-cell lymphomas [33].

Workup of mature B-cell non-Hodgkin lymphoma

As noted above, ancillary testing is considered integral to the workup and diagnosis of most mature B-cell NHL in the WHO classification [11, 30, 34]. Immunophenotypic analysis may be achieved by either flow cytometry or immunohistochemistry [2]. A wide variety of immunoperoxidase stains that may be utilized on paraffin-embedded tissues and identify mature B-cell neoplasms are now available, facilitating immunopheno-

typic analysis on routine pathology biopsies. A limited listing of the most useful immunophenotypic markers for the workup of pediatric mature B-cell NHLs is presented in Table 21.6.

Several of the mature B-cell NHLs seen in the pediatric age group are associated with specific cytogenetic and molecular characteristics. Translocations of the *cMYC* oncogene are used to define BL, but it should be noted that abnormalities in the *cMYC* locus are also seen in many cases of DLBCL [12]. Conversely, the t(14;18) translocation seen in many adult DLBCLs is not seen in pediatric DLBCL and is usually not seen in those rare cases of pediatric follicular lymphoma [6, 12, 35].

Molecular approaches will usually identify B-cell immunoglobulin gene rearrangements, similar to adults, in most cases of pediatric B-cell NHL [15, 17, 26, 36]. Analysis of pediatric tumors by standard cytogenetics or FISH identifies diagnostic information as well as providing insights into possible mechanisms of pediatric lymphomagenesis. Chromosomal translocations are frequently seen in pediatric mature B-cell NHL, and are associated with two possible mechanisms of transformation. In some cases, translocations may fuse sequences from one chromosome (often encoding either a transcription factor, receptor or cytoplasmic tyrosine kinase) to those of an unrelated gene to produce a chimeric gene or protein that possesses oncogenic capabilities. Another mechanism whereby

Table 21.7. St. Jude staging system of pediatric non-Hodgkin lymphoma.

Stage	Definition
I	A single tumor (extranodal) or single anatomic area (nodal) with the exclusion of mediastinum or abdomen
II	A single tumor (extranodal) with regional node involvement Two or more nodal areas on the same side of the diaphragm Two single (extranodal) tumors with or without regional node involvement on the same side of the diaphragm Primary gastrointestinal tract tumor, usually in the ileocecal area, with or without involvement of associated mesenteric nodes only
II R	Completely resected abdominal disease
III	Two single tumors (extranodal) on opposite sites of the diaphragm Two or more nodal areas above and below the diaphragm All primary intrathoracic tumors (mediastinal, pleural, thymic) All paraspinal or epidural tumors, regardless of other tumor site(s) All extensive primary intraabdominal disease
III A	Localized but non-resectable abdominal disease
III B	Widespread multi-organ abdominal disease
IV	Any of the above with initial CNS and/or bone marrow involvement

Table 21.8. Comparison of endemic and sporadic Burkitt lymphoma.

Feature	Endemic	Sporadic
Clinical features	5–10 years at presentation Males > females	6–12 years at presentation Males > females
Most common distribution of disease	Equatorial Africa, New Guinea, Amazonian Brazil, Turkey	North America, Europe most common
Annual incidence	10 in 100 000	0.2 in 100 000
Common tumor sites	Jaw, abdomen, central nervous system, cerebrospinal fluid	Abdomen, marrow, lymph nodes, ovaries
Histopathologic features	Diffuse growth pattern, monomorphic intermediate-sized cell, starry-sky pattern	Same
Immunologic features	CD20+, usually IgM, κ or λ, CD10+, BCL2−	CD20+, usually IgM, κ or λ, CD10+, BCL2−
Presence of Epstein–Barr virus DNA in tumor cells	95%	15%
Presence of t(8;14), t(2;8), or t(8;22)	Yes	Yes
Chromosome 8 breakpoints	Upstream of cMYC gene	Within cMYC gene

translocations may deregulate gene function is by the relocation of a gene to the vicinity of highly active promoters or enhancers that drive the overexpression of the gene product. In mature B-cell NHL, this often involves the immunoglobulin gene loci. These chimeric genes are unique to lymphoma, allowing FISH or reverse transcriptase polymerase chain reaction (RT-PCR) to detect the translocation [37–39]. Overexpression of the gene often leads to increased protein expression, detectable by immunohistochemical methods [40].

Another important function of the pathologist in diagnosis and treatment of pediatric NHL is in helping to establish the stage of disease in conjunction with radiologic studies and physical examination. As pediatric patients tend to have a higher incidence of extranodal disease, the staging system used differs slightly from that used in adults (Table 21.7) [41]. However, features such as determination of involvement of the bone marrow or cerebrospinal fluid and the extent of disease remain essential to clinical staging and will ultimately impact upon therapy [42–44].

Burkitt lymphomas

Burkitt lymphomas (BLs), including the atypical Burkitt lymphomas (aBLs), comprise approximately 40–50% of pediatric NHL and are the main subtype of mature B-cell NHL seen in this population [2–4]. Although most patients will present with extranodal disease in a variety of sites, nodal and leukemic presentations are also seen. The extranodal sites involved by BL vary in different populations [45].

Burkitt lymphoma was first recognized as a distinct disease process by Dr. Denis Burkitt, who described an unusual tumor of the jaw in children from equatorial Africa, where this tumor is endemic [46]. BL occurs worldwide, although there are clinicopathologic differences observed between the endemic (African) and the sporadic (non-African) forms (Table 21.8) [45]. Sporadic and endemic cases are morphologically indistinguishable, although endemic BL tends to have a high propensity for involvement of the bones of the face (particularly the jaw and maxilla) and occurs in younger children [47, 48]. The sporadic form of BL also tends to involve extranodal sites, but is more common in the GI tract (particularly the ileocecal area), as well as in the kidneys and ovaries, but involvement of the bones of the face is unusual [45, 47]. Extensive involvement of the bone marrow is not frequently seen at diagnosis, but may be prominent in late-stage progressive disease [1, 46]. A small cohort, 1–2% of patients, may present with disseminated disease including extensive peripheral blood and bone marrow involvement. Previously termed ALL L3, this is not an acute leukemia but rather a leukemic phase of BL, and is preferably termed Burkitt leukemia [11]. CNS involvement may also be seen in BL, especially with disseminated disease [1, 46]. Burkitt lymphoma is also common in HIV-infected or other immunocompromised individuals [10, 48–50].

Morphology

Morphologically, BLs are characterized by intermediate-sized homogeneous cells with round to oval nuclei containing multiple, variably prominent basophilic nucleoli (Fig. 21.1). The cells have a modest amount of somewhat basophilic cytoplasm, which will appear vacuolated, due to lipid droplets, on cytologic preparations (Fig. 21.2). These tumors have very high mitotic activity, and tissue sections will often show a "starry sky"

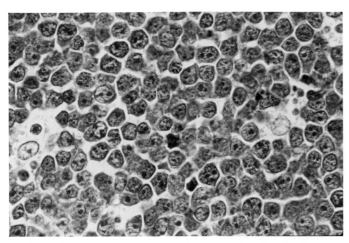

Fig. 21.1. High power depiction of Burkitt lymphoma demonstrating relative uniformity of the neoplastic cell population with relatively inconspicuous nuclei and modest amounts of cytoplasm. Admixed with the neoplastic cells are tingible body macrophages ingesting apoptotic debris (H&E stain).

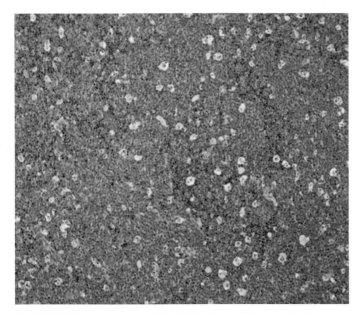

Fig. 21.3. A lower power view of Burkitt lymphoma demonstrating the starry-sky pattern imparted by admixed tingible body macrophages that ingest apoptotic debris. The overall pattern is of diffuse effacement of the lymph node architecture by a monomorphous infiltrate (H&E stain).

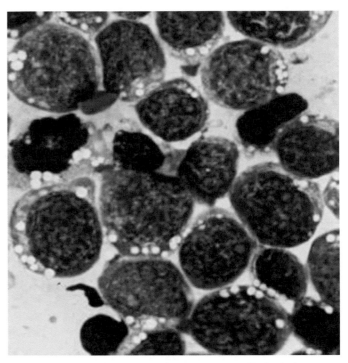

Fig. 21.2. Wright–Giemsa stain cytologic preparation of Burkitt leukemia demonstrating the uniform cells with basophilic cytoplasm and cytoplasmic vacuoles. The nuclei show relatively mature chromatin features, helping to distinguish them from acute lymphoblastic leukemia (Wright–Giemsa stain).

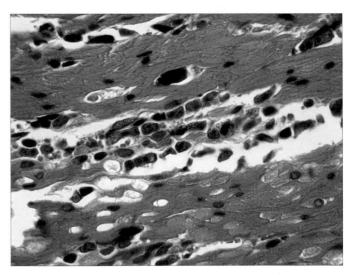

Fig. 21.4. The tumor cells of Burkitt lymphoma can occasionally show a syncytial appearance with molding of the nuclear membranes to a more squared–off appearance. This may occasionally be confused with a carcinoma or other tumor (H&E stain).

appearance which results from reactive macrophages scattered among the malignant lymphoid cells that are engulfing apoptotic debris from the rapidly dividing tumor cells (Fig. 21.3) [11]. It should be noted that the "starry sky" appearance is not specific for BL, but can be seen in any rapidly dividing NHL [2]. Mitoses are numerous, and the neoplastic cells often appear to form syncytial masses with molding of the cell membranes (Fig. 21.4). In some areas, the tumor cells may preferentially invade germinal centers [47]. Burkitt lymphomas in current classifications are noted to have somewhat more morphologic diversity and include cases previously termed non-Burkitt, or Burkitt-like, lymphoma [51], high-grade mature B-cell lymphomas (REAL classification) [52], or atypical Burkitt

lymphoma (aBL) in the previous WHO classification [53]. Although aBLs have many features that are similar to classical BL (Table 21.9), they are characterized by more cellular pleomorphism, variable nuclear irregularities, and more variable numbers of nucleoli that may be more prominent than are typically seen in classic BL (Fig. 21.5). In tissue sections, aBL may not have the typical "starry sky" pattern and may show a slightly less elevated mitotic rate [11, 54–56].

Table 21.9. Features of pediatric lymphoma (BL) compared with atypical Burkitt lymphoma (aBL).

	BL	aBL
Morphologic features	Diffuse effacement Prominent starry-sky pattern More likely to be extranodal disease	Diffuse effacement Variable starry-sky pattern More likely to involve lymph nodes
Cytologic features	Monomorphic Inconspicuous nucleoli Smooth nuclear contours	More pleomorphic Variable nucleoli Smooth to irregular nuclear contours
Immunophenotypic features	CD20+, CD10+ IgM with light chain restriction MIB-1 proliferative rate > 99% BCL6 positive BCL2 negative	CD20+, variable CD10 Variable IgM or IgG with light chain restriction MIB-1 rate 90–99% BCL6 expression may be higher BCL2 negative
Cytogenetic features	cMYC translocation in all May have additional abnormalities Usually <3 abnormalities	cMYC translocations in 85% of cases Usually additional cytogenetic abnormalities Usually complex (>3 abnormalities)

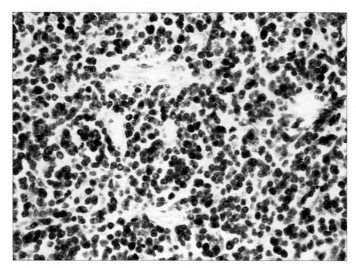

Fig. 21.6. Immunohistochemical stain for Ki-67 (MIB-1), demonstrating the extremely high mitotic activity of Burkitt lymphoma (> 99% of cells staining positively) (MIB-1 immunohistochemical stain).

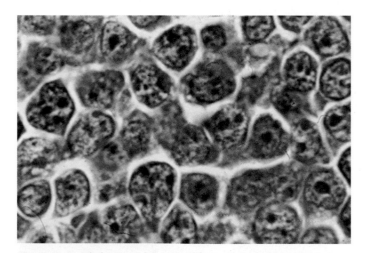

Fig. 21.5. Morphologic variability in Burkitt lymphoma (previously called atypical Burkitt lymphoma) shows an intermediate-sized neoplastic cell population with increased cellular heterogeneity when compared to classical Burkitt lymphoma. The neoplastic cells show a moderate degree of pleomorphism with somewhat irregular nuclear contours and variably prominent nuclei (H&E stain).

The inclusion of aBL in the BL category reflects the WHO philosophy that the diagnosis of BL requires integration of morphologic, cytogenetic/molecular, and immunophenotypic features [11]. Most pediatric cases of aBL had features of BL with the exception of morphology, and it has been shown that ability to reproducibly distinguish BL from aBL strictly on the basis of morphology is very unreliable, with poor intra-observer consensus shown in numerous studies between pathologists [28, 56], and quality of tissue fixation and sectioning greatly impacting diagnostic reproducibility [56, 57]. Furthermore, in children, these two entities were clinically very similar, and the value of making this distinction in pediatric populations, other than for descriptive purposes, has not been conclusively demonstrated, as the approach to therapy for these entities is the same and outcome appears identical [31, 32].

Immunophenotype

Immunophenotypic features of BL demonstrate mature B-cell phenotype with expression of cell-surface CD19, CD20, CD22, CD10, and cell-surface immunoglobulin. Usually the immunoglobulin is IgM heavy chain with light chain restriction [2, 11, 47]. Atypical Burkitt lymphomas tend to have more variability in cell-surface antigen expression, with variable CD10 or expression of cell-surface IgG [55, 58]. The expression profile of a mature B-cell (cell-surface CD20 and immunoglobulin expression) phenotype with co-expression of CD10 suggests that BL is derived from a follicular center cell [59]. BL will not express significant levels of the anti-apoptotic protein BCL2. This can be very helpful in distinguishing BL from DLBCL, where BCL2 expression is more commonly seen [9, 10, 60]. Immunohistochemical staining for cMYC protein is positive in BL and aBL [58, 60], but may also be seen in DLBCL [60].

BL is one of the most rapidly proliferating human tumors, with a doubling time of approximately 12–24 hours [61]. Immunohistochemical staining with proliferation markers, such as Ki-67 or MIB-1 (Fig. 21.6), will show staining in excess of 99% of the tumor cells, and this has been used as a defining immunophenotypic feature in the WHO classification [11].

Table 21.10. Translocations of *cMYC* seen in pediatric Burkitt lymphoma.

Translocation	Partner gene	Incidence
t(8;14)(q24;q32)	Immunoglobulin heavy chain gene	80% of cases, most common
t(8;22)(q23;q11)	Lambda light chain gene	5%
t(2;8)(p12;q24)	Kappa light chain gene	15%

Table 21.11. Additional cytogenetics seen in pediatric Burkitt lymphoma.

Cytogenetic abnormality	Prognostic impact
Deletion (13q)	Poor
Duplication (7q)	Poor
Derivative (3q)	Poor
Duplication (1q)	Poor – variable between studies
High complexity (>3 abnormalities)	Poor

Cytogenetics and oncogenesis

Cytogenetic analysis of BL will demonstrate characteristic translocations, involving the *cMYC* oncogene locus at chromosome 8q24 in most cases (Table 21.10) [62–65]. Roughly 80% of BLs contain a t(8;14)(q24;q32) rearrangement in which there is translocation of one allele of the transcription factor gene *cMYC*, on chromosome 8, to the immunoglobulin heavy chain gene locus on chromosome 14. The remaining cases have either a t(2;8)(p12;q24) (found in 15% of cases) or a t(8;22)(q24;q11) (5% of cases) involving *cMYC* and either the kappa or lambda immunoglobulin light chain gene loci on chromosomes 2 or 22, respectively [49, 64]. Despite large variation in the breakpoints on chromosome 8 in these translocations, the coding regions of the cMYC protein remain intact, allowing for the constitutive overexpression of cMYC protein that is driven by the immunoglobulin gene promoters [25, 26, 36, 49, 66, 67]. Differences in the chromosome 8 breakpoint location also exist between endemic and sporadic BL (Table 21.9). Most endemic BLs possess breakpoints upstream of *cMYC*, whereas sporadic tumors almost always have breakpoints within or very near to the *cMYC* locus [25, 47, 68]. Translocations of *cMYC* are most reliably identified by karyotyping of metaphase chromosomes or FISH on either metaphase or interphase nuclei in intact cells or paraffin sections [25, 64, 69].

In addition to *cMYC* translocations, more than half of children with BL will have additional cytogenetic abnormalities (Tables 21.11 and 21.12). The most commonly seen additional chromosomal changes include deletion 13q, duplication 1q, and deletion 6q that may impact upon prognosis [12, 62, 70, 71]. Study of the translocations seen in neoplasms previously classified as aBL in adults showed much more heterogeneity, and revealed *cMYC* translocations and translocations involving the *BCL2* locus, more commonly associated with follicular lymphomas or DLBCL [62]. In children, the *cMYC* translocation

Table 21.12. Comparative features of Burkitt lymphoma and diffuse large B-cell lymphoma.

	DLBCL	Burkitt lymphoma
Morphology		
Cell size	Large	Intermediate
Nuclear chromatin	Clumped, vesicular	Coarse
Nucleoli	Variable – single, prominent, or inconspicuous	Variable – multiple, inconspicuous
Cytoplasm	Moderate to abundant	Moderate to scanty with prominent vacuoles
Nodal effacement	Diffuse	Diffuse, starry-sky pattern
Molecular genetics	Ig gene rearrangement	Ig gene rearrangements
Cytogenetics	t(8;14) may be seen in 30% of cases. Complex cytogenetics, multiple abnormalities	t(8;14), t(8;22), t(2;8) Additional abnormalities including derl (13q), −1q, +7q common

in aBL appears to be much more common, and is seen in more than 85% of cases [11, 63, 71, 72]. The remaining cases often display complex cytogenetic abnormalities, and those cases with *cMYC* translocation invariably have multiple additional cytogenetic aberrations, similar to those seen in BL [12]. Translocations involving the *BCL2* locus are distinctly uncommon in children [12, 63, 71].

The cMYC protein is a transcription factor that promotes cell cycle progression and cell transformation, as well as inhibiting differentiation and apoptosis [67, 73–76]. Overexpression of cMYC in growth factor-deprived cells is sufficient to overcome cell cycle arrest and initiate S-phase [77–79], whereas removal of cMYC blocks cellular entry into S-phase [73]. Transgenic mice engineered to overexpress cMYC in lymphocytes develop a polyclonal pre-B-cell hyperplasia that progresses within a short period of time to a monoclonal malignancy [80, 81].

Overexpression and deregulation of cMYC appears to affect multiple cell pathways that impact on cell cycle progression, differentiation, metabolism, apoptosis, cell immortalization, and adhesion [67, 76]. Terminal differentiation requires exit from the cell cycle; however, cMYC promotes constant cycling. A number of metabolic pathways are also affected by cMYC, allowing lymphoma cells to participate in aerobic glycolysis and grow under hypoxic conditions [82, 83]. The cMYC protein may also be able to maintain the expression of telomerase, which contributes to the immortalization of cells by inhibiting the normal shortening of the chromosomal ends or telomeres. Telomeric shortening is associated with cellular senescence, and lack of telomerase activity is associated with higher susceptibility to oncogenic transformation [84].

Recent work with genetic profiling has identified a specific BL molecular signature that differentiates BL from other aggressive mature B-cell lymphomas [5, 13, 25, 26, 29, 85–87]. These studies suggested that molecular characterization may be a highly reproducible means whereby BL may be diagnosed, and was superior to diagnosis based on morphologic

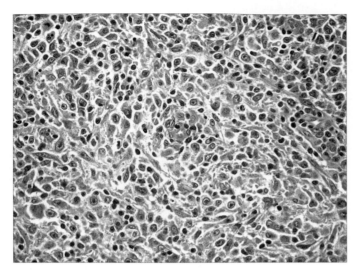

Fig. 21.7. Medium-power view of diffuse large B-cell lymphoma demonstrating diffuse effacement of lymph node architecture by large non-cleaved cells that are admixed with occasional reactive small cells (H&E stain).

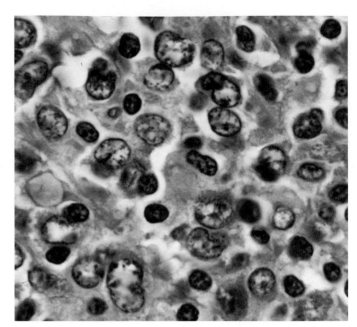

Fig. 21.8. High-powered view of diffuse large B-cell lymphoma demonstrating large non-cleaved morphology. The large neoplastic cells are two to three times the size of the admixed small reactive lymphocytes and have moderate amounts of granular, eosinophilic cytoplasm (H&E stain).

and immunophenotypic features. Unfortunately, the utility of molecular profiling as a diagnostic tool remains controversial, particularly with the good clinical response of pediatric mature B-cell lymphomas, independent of subtype [5, 8, 13, 29].

In endemic BL, approximately 95% of tumors contain clonal Epstein–Barr virus (EBV) DNA, whereas only some 15% of pediatric sporadic tumors in the United States and Europe are EBV associated [47, 48, 88, 89]. The role of EBV in development of BL is not clear [48, 90]. EBV is capable of immortalizing B-lymphocytes *in vitro* [89]. EBV-encoded proteins drive polyclonal lymphoid proliferation, which may be followed by development of a monoclonal tumor once the *cMYC* gene overexpression is established. Epstein–Barr nuclear antigen 1 (EBNA-1) has been shown to induce B-cell lymphomas in transgenic mice [91], and the latently expressed EBV-encoded RNA (*EBER*)-1 and *EBER-2* transcripts exhibit oncogenic potential in cell lines [92].

Therapy and prognosis

Treatment of BL and aBL is by short, intensive multiagent chemotherapy [8, 31, 32]. The outcome for either BL is highly related to stage, with outcomes ranging from >90% cure rates in limited stage disease [32] to 50–60% for disseminated disease involving bone and/or bone marrow [31].

Diffuse large B-cell lymphomas

Diffuse large B-cell lymphomas (DLBCLs) make up approximately 20% of pediatric NHL [1, 3, 4]. DLBCL tends to occur in slightly older age groups and is the most common histology of NHL seen in children older than 10 years of age, and teenagers. Diffuse large B-cell histology is also strongly associated with immunodeficiency states (inherited or iatrogenic) and

is the most common subtype of immunodeficiency-associated lymphoma seen in childhood [1, 50, 93].

Morphology and diagnostic subtypes

DLBCL frequently occurs at a single site, with mediastinal and abdominal disease being most common [3, 94]. Nodal disease is the most frequent presentation, although extranodal disease may also be seen, in contrast to the more frequent extranodal presentation seen in BL [10, 95]. DLBCL will diffusely efface lymph node architecture (Fig. 21.7), and may display a variety of morphologic and cytologic appearances including tumors composed of large non-cleaved cells (Fig. 21.8), large cleaved cells, polylobated or multilobated cells (Fig. 21.9), and immunoblasts (exhibiting a single prominent eosinophilic nucleolus; Fig. 21.10) [2, 9, 10, 96]. All morphologic subtypes of DLBCL are considered to be of similar clinical aggressiveness [10, 11, 96, 97]. The neoplastic lymphoid cells are large and have a nucleus that is at least the size of a tissue histiocyte or twice the size of a small, reactive lymphocyte. The cytoplasm in DLBCL is variable in appearance and may range from pale to plasmacytoid or granular appearing. The cytoplasm may also vary in volume, but is always significantly more abundant than that seen in BL (Table 21.12). The overall growth pattern is diffuse, although tissue components such as vessels or fibrosis may impart a vaguely nodular appearance in some cases [2, 9, 11].

Several diagnostic subtypes of DLBCL have been described in the pediatric population, including T-cell/histiocyte-rich large B-cell lymphomas (THRLBCLs), consisting of tumors

Table 21.13. Diagnosis of CD30+ large cell processes by immunohistochemistry.

	CD30	CD20/CD79A	T-cell antigens CD2, CD7	CD45	CD15
Primary mediastinal large B-cell lymphoma	+ may be weak	+	−	+	−
Hodgkin lymphoma	+	− / + (may be variably CD20 + in 20–30% of cases)	−	−	+
Anaplastic large cell lymphoma, ALK positive	+	−	+	+	−
B-cell lymphoma, unclassifiable, with features intermediate between diffuse large B-cell lymphoma and classical Hodgkin lymphoma	+	Variable expression, usually positive but may be negative	−	+	+

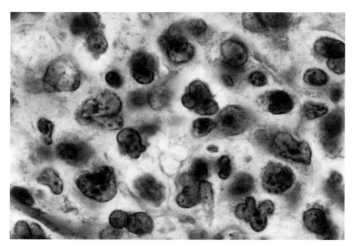

Fig. 21.9. Multilobated or polylobated morphologic variant of diffuse large B-cell lymphoma demonstrating polylobated neoplastic cells due to marked nuclear irregularities and infoldings (H&E stain).

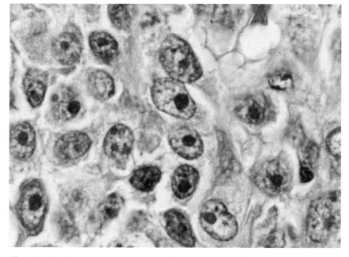

Fig. 21.10. Morphologic variant of diffuse large B-cell lymphoma showing immunoblastic features. The neoplastic cells are large, have moderately abundant eosinophilic cytoplasm and very prominent, centrally placed, eosinophilic nucleoli (H&E stain).

with relatively small numbers of neoplastic large B-cells and an abundant infiltrate of small reactive T-cells that may obscure the malignant large B-lymphocytes (Fig. 21.11) [56, 98, 99]. Primary mediastinal (thymic) large B-cell lymphomas (PMB-CLs) are also seen in the pediatric population, predominantly in older adolescents. These tumors arise in the mediastinum from thymic B-cells and show a diffuse large cell proliferation with relatively abundant pale cytoplasm, with a variable amount of dense, compartmentalizing sclerosis that surrounds neoplastic cells (Fig. 21.12) [5, 8, 11, 100–102]. This type of lymphoma may be difficult to clinically and morphologically distinguish from Hodgkin lymphoma in small mediastinal biopsies because of extensive sclerosis and necrosis, although immunophenotypic analysis will reliably separate these entities (Table 21.13) [11, 103]. In the current WHO classification, PMBCLs are identified as a clinically and pathologically distinct subtype of DLBCL [11]. Clinically, PMBCL tends to present with extensive mediastinal disease and associated sequelae such as superior vena cava syndrome. Dissemination is often by extension to adjacent sites or to other extranodal sites such as kidney, adrenal or liver [100, 101, 104].

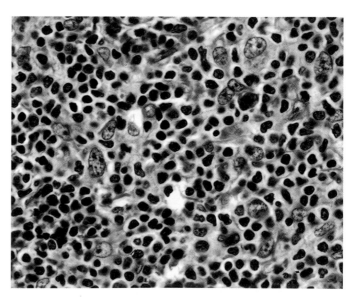

Fig. 21.11. T-cell/histiocyte-rich large B-cell lymphoma demonstrating relatively rare large, neoplastic B-cells admixed with many small, reactive T-cells (H&E stain).

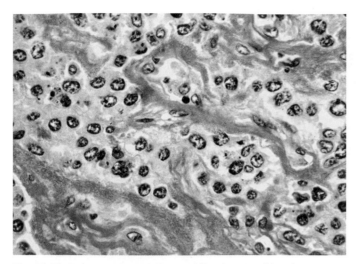

Fig. 21.12. Primary mediastinal (thymic) diffuse large B-cell lymphoma demonstrating the large neoplastic B-cells with abundant clear cytoplasm, and surrounding compartmentalizing sclerosis (H&E stain).

Immunophenotyping

Immunophenotypic characterization of DLBCL demonstrates a mature B-cell phenotype with expression of cell-surface immunoglobulin and B-cell-specific lineage markers such as CD19, CD20, CD22, CD79a, and PAX-5 (Fig. 21.13A) [2, 10, 11, 34, 99]. Most DLBCL will express monoclonal cell-surface immunoglobulin light chains. PMBCL may lack cell-surface immunoglobulin expression, but will display cytoplasmic immunoglobulins [8, 11, 103]. CD30 expression may be seen in some cases of DLBCL, and is most commonly expressed in PMBCL, but may also be seen in more typical DLBCL where it represents a non-specific activation marker [105]. The expres-

sion of CD30 may create a differential diagnostic consideration of Hodgkin lymphoma (HL) (Table 21.13), but HL should also express CD15 (Leu M1) and lack expression of all B-cell markers such as CD79a and PAX-5, as well as B-cell transcription factors Oct-2 or BOB.1 [106]. Approximately 20–30% of Hodgkin lymphomas may express variable levels of CD20, although this is usually more variable than the uniform, strong expression typically seen in DLBCL [11, 107, 108]. Careful attention to the surrounding cellular components may also be helpful, as DLBCL will typically not have associated infiltrates of reactive plasma cells, eosinophils, small lymphocytes, and histiocytes that are associated with HL [108]. If a PMBCL shows strong expression of CD15 or variable expression of CD20 or CD79a, a diagnosis of B-cell lymphoma, unclassifiable, with features intermediate between diffuse large B-cell lymphoma and classical Hodgkin lymphoma or "gray zone" lymphoma (discussed further below) may be considered (Table 21.13). Expression of CD30 may also lead to inclusion of anaplastic large cell lymphoma (ALCL) in the differential diagnostic considerations (Table 21.13). However, ALCL is a T-cell neoplasm, and inclusion of appropriate T- and B-cell markers should allow for these entities to be easily distinguished from each other [103, 108].

Pediatric DLBCL tends to have a high mitotic rate as determined by staining with Ki-67 or MIB-1, although this is usually lower than that seen in BL (Fig. 21.13B) [33]. In contrast to adult DLBCL, pediatric cases tend to have high expression of cMYC protein and lower expression levels of BCL2 [60]. As cMYC is known to stimulate lymphoid proliferation, this may be important in the pathogenesis of pediatric DLBCL [33, 73]. In addition, as discussed further below, pediatric DLBCL has high levels of expression of the germinal center markers BCL6 and CD10, although these are not seen in PMBCL. Expression

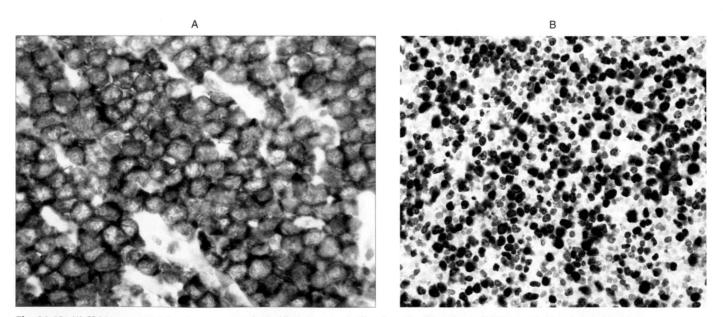

Fig. 21.13. (A) CD20 immunostaining demonstrating the B-cell phenotype of diffuse large B-cell lymphoma (CD20 immunohistochemical stain). (B) Immunohistochemical staining of Ki-67 (MIB-1) demonstrating relatively low number (approximately 70%) of positive neoplastic cells as compared to BL (MIB-1 immunohistochemical stain).

Table 21.14. Cytogenetic abnormalities associated with pediatric DLBCL.

	Incidence (%)
High frequency	
Complex karyotype (> 3 abnormalities)	>80
Aneuploidy	78–80
del (6q)	50
Intermediate frequency	
cMYC abnormalities	**20–30**
+(12q)	15–20
der (11q)	25
+(7q)	25–30
Low frequency	
t(14;18)	**Very low (<5%)**

Bolded findings significantly different from adult DLBCL.

of CD10 is variable, but can be seen in approximately half of the cases of pediatric DLBCL [60, 33]. BCL6 expression may be seen in 50–80% of pediatric DLBCL [33, 60, 109]. CD5 co-expression is not commonly seen in pediatric cases.

Cytogenetics and molecular genetics

There are no specific, highly recurrent characteristic cytogenetic abnormalities associated with DLBCL in children and adolescents [12, 110]. Unlike adults, where 20–40% of cases will demonstrate a *BCL2* translocation, such as the t(14;18)(q32;q21) that is also associated with follicular lymphoma, *BCL2* translocation is extremely rare in children [12, 109, 110]. It should also be noted that translocations associated with the *cMYC* oncogene, such as t(8;14), are much more frequently seen in pediatric DLBCL, being reported in 20–40% of cases in some studies, suggesting a possible relationship with BL [12, 110]. The prominence of *cMYC* abnormalities in contrast to *BCL2* abnormalities suggests that stimulation of proliferation may be an important pathogenetic mechanism for development of DLBCL in children and adolescents, in contrast to the *BCL2* abnormalities that function to inhibit apoptosis, most commonly seen in adults. Despite the lack of defining recurrent abnormalities, nearly all of the pediatric DLBCL studied will contain detectable karyotypic aberrations [12]. Cytogenetic abnormalities described in pediatric DLBCL include structural abnormalities (seen in nearly all cases) and numeric abnormalities (seen in over half of the cases studied). Most cases will contain three or more cytogenetic aberrations, typically creating more complex karyotypes than are usual in BL (Tables 21.12 and 21.14) [12, 110, 111].

Analysis of adult cases of DLBCL has identified cytogenetically detectable chromosomal abnormalities affecting band 3q27, encoding the *BCL6* transcription factor, in 10 to 12% of cases; these are usually reciprocal translocations of 3q27 with a variety of partner chromosomes, but most commonly the immunoglobulin heavy or light chain genes [97, 112]. Normal BCL6 protein expression is tightly regulated during B-cell development, being expressed in mature B-cells but not in B-lymphoblasts, immunoblasts or plasma cells [113, 114]. In

lymph nodes, BCL6 protein expression is present only within the germinal center [115], and is thought to be important for germinal center-associated functions including regulation of BCL2 apoptotic activity and transcription factors [116–119].

The frequency of *BCL6* gene rearrangement detected by molecular techniques significantly exceeds that detected by cytogenetic studies, suggesting that cryptic chromosomal abnormalities are important in development of adult DLBCL [112, 117, 120–122]. Approximately one-third of adult DLBCLs have molecular *BCL6* gene rearrangements identified by Southern blot hybridization analysis. These tend to occur exclusive of *BCL2* rearrangement, suggesting that *BCL6* is specifically involved in the pathogenesis of *de novo* large cell lymphoma [114, 117, 123]. Rearrangement of *BCL6* has been associated with primary extranodal DLBCL, tumors that lack bone marrow involvement [124, 125], and lymphomas that have a favorable prognosis after chemotherapy in adults [112–114]. The *BCL6* translocations that have been fully characterized have been shown to result in dysregulated expression of a normal BCL6 protein and loss of normal BCL6 downregulation occurring during terminal plasma cell differentiation [114, 117].

The incidence of *BCL6* translocations and mutations in pediatric DLBCL is unknown; however, karyotypic abnormalities involving 3q27 have been reported in <10% of cases [12, 110]. Molecular analysis for non-translocation-related *BCL6* mutations in pediatric DLBCL has not been well described. Thus, it is uncertain what molecular mechanisms may lead to development of pediatric DLBCL, and this is an important area for future investigation.

PMBCL often shows gains in chromosome 9p with amplification of the *REL* gene, which distinguishes it from other subtypes of DLBCL [126]. Overexpression of the *MAL* gene has also been described in PMBCL, and these cases typically lack *BCL2*, *BCL6*, and *cMYC* translocations [102, 127, 128]. Gene expression profiling studies of PMBCL lymphoma have shown significant overlap of the gene expression profiles with classical Hodgkin lymphoma, suggesting that this particular subtype of DLBCL may share features with that disorder [129–131]. In addition, studies have shown PMBCL to have significant dysregulation of the NFκB signaling pathway [100–102].

Three major gene expression profiling (microarray) studies have addressed the biological and clinical heterogeneity of adult DLBCL [132–134]. In the initial DLBCL gene expression profiling study, lymph node biopsy samples from previously untreated adult patients were analyzed [132]. Genes that define the germinal center stage of B-cell differentiation were used to define two prominent DLBCL subgroups. The "germinal center B-cell-like" DLBCL subgroup (GCB DLBCL) expressed genes characteristic of normal germinal center B-cells (e.g., *CD10*, *BCL6*, *A-myb*), whereas the "activated B-cell-like" DLBCL subgroup (ABC DLBCL) expressed genes that are induced during mitogenic activation of peripheral blood B-cells (e.g., *BCL2*, *IRF-4*, *cyclin D2*). A larger gene expression profiling study of DLBCL cases confirmed the existence of these two DLBCL subgroups, but also identified another set of cases, termed "type 3"

DLBCLs, that do not resemble GCB or ABC DLBCL and may represent an additional molecular subgroup of DLBCL [133].

These studies raised the possibility that the DLBCL subgroups represent pathogenetically distinct entities that are derived from cells at different stages of B-lymphoid differentiation. Support for this hypothesis has come from analysis of immunoglobulin gene mutations in the DLBCL subgroups. Although DLBCLs in both the GCB and ABC subgroups were found to have mutated immunoglobulin genes, only GCB DLBCLs had ongoing somatic hypermutation [135, 136]. Since somatic hypermutation of immunoglobulin genes is a hallmark of germinal center B-cells, this suggests that the GCB DLBCL tumors retain some of the biological characteristics of normal germinal center B-cells [136, 137].

Two recurrent chromosomal alterations in DLBCL were detected exclusively in the GCB DLBCL subgroup. The t(14;18)(q32;q21) translocation involving the anti-apoptosis BCL2 gene was detected in 23–35% of GCB DLBCL cases but never in ABC or type 3 DLBCL cases. Similarly, amplification of the cREL locus on chromosome 2p was detected in 15% of GCB DLBCLs but not in the other subgroups [133, 136, 138]. By contrast, ABC DLBCLs were found to have constitutive activity of the NFκB pathway, which is not a feature of GCB DLBCL [135, 139]. These findings suggest that the DLBCL subgroups utilize distinct oncogenic mechanisms, and may have future implications for specific diagnosis-directed therapy.

The DLBCL gene expression subgroups have distinctly different overall survival rates following anthracycline-based multiagent chemotherapy (e.g., the CHOP regimen) [132, 133]. The five-year survival rates for the GCB, ABC, and type 3 DLBCL subgroups were 60%, 35%, and 39%, respectively [133]. Unfortunately, only limited genetic array studies of pediatric DLBCL are currently published to document if pediatric DLBCL is similarly heterogeneous or demonstrates more homogeneous gene expression profiles [13]. It has been suggested that immunoperoxidase staining with specific germinal center markers, such as BCL6 or CD10, may help to identify DLBCL of germinal center origin, while other post-germinal center proteins, such as CD138 or MUM-1, will identify ABC tumors [124, 140–142]. When this approach is applied to pediatric DLBCL, it appears that the pediatric cases have a much higher incidence of germinal center phenotype than is seen in adult populations, with >85–90% of DLBCL in two large pediatric studies displaying a germinal center phenotype [33, 109]. The predominance of a germinal center phenotype in light of the lack of BCL2 rearrangements in children and adolescents suggests a different pathogenetic mechanism of lymphomagenesis in the pediatric population [109].

Treatment and prognosis

Treatment of DLBCL is usually by short, intensive multiagent chemotherapy similar to the approach for BL [31, 32]. To date, immune-based therapy with agents like anti-CD20 (rituximab) is not widely used in pediatrics, although it forms the corner-stone of adult DLBCL therapy [143, 144]. Patients have high response and cure rates of >90% for most cases of DLBCL. One subtype of DLBCL, PMBCL, appears to have an inferior response and cure rate in children and adolescents and may require alternative approaches to treatment, although cure rates are similar to those seen in adults [31, 32, 145]. This may require development of new therapeutic approaches and disease-specific pathways, such as NFκB, for targeted therapy [100, 102].

Pediatric follicular lymphomas

Follicular lymphomas (FLs) are rare in children and adolescents, in contrast to their relatively high frequency in older adults, where they comprise approximately one-quarter to one-third of all adult NHLs [7]. Pediatric FLs have mostly been described in several small series of patients, and overall appear to comprise fewer than 5% of pediatric NHL [2–4, 146]. Pediatric FL appears to differ from adult FL in several important features, including that they are more likely to be localized disease, may present at extranodal sites, often lack BCL2 protein overexpression in the neoplastic cells, and lack characteristic BCL2 translocations. A higher proportion of pediatric FLs are grade 3 (follicular large cell lymphoma) than in adults [6, 35, 146–151]. Often the differential diagnostic consideration in pediatric cases of FL is with reactive follicular hyperplasia [6]. This has led to pediatric follicular lymphoma being recognized as a distinct clinicopathologic variant of FL in the newest WHO classification [11], with a more favorable prognosis with respect to adult-type FL [11, 30]. However, due to overlap with reactive processes, a diagnosis of pediatric FL must have clear-cut morphologic evidence of malignancy [11].

Most of the studies of FL in pediatric patients have demonstrated a male predominance (M : F between 2 and 4 : 1), and broad age range of three years to adolescents with a median age ranging between 7 and 12 years, depending on the study [35, 146–148, 151]. The most common site of involvement is the head and neck, involving cervical lymph nodes and tonsils. In addition, there are several reports of presentation in extranodal sites such as testis, kidney, gastrointestinal tract, and parotid [6, 35, 147–149]. Most often the tumors were localized (stage I), in contrast to adults, where FL usually presents as disseminated disease [11, 35]. A few older adolescents may present with higher clinical stage disease and pathologic features, more similar to adult-type FL [6].

Morphology

The morphologic features seen in pediatric FL are identical to those seen in adults. FL is characterized by effacement of lymph node architecture by a nodular proliferation of neoplastic lymphocytes that recapitulates the normal follicle structure (Fig. 21.14) [11]. Because of the architectural and morphologic resemblance of the tumor to reactive germinal centers, most often, diagnostic difficulties arise in distinguishing FL from reactive follicular hyperplasia, particularly in children and

Table 21.15. Morphologic features of follicular hyperplasia vs. follicular lymphoma.

Follicular hyperplasia	Follicular lymphoma
Architectural features	
(1) Overall preservation of architecture	Effacement of architecture
(2) Marked variation in size and shape of follicles	Slight to moderate variation in follicular size and shape
(3) No capsular infiltration	Extension beyond nodal capsule
(4) Follicles have intervening lymphoid tissue	Back-to-back follicular pattern
(5) Low density of follicles	High density of follicles
(6) Well-defined follicle and definite mantle zone and polarization	Ill-defined follicle with absent mantle zone and polarization
Cytologic features	
(1) Polymorphic cells in germinal center	Monomorphic cells in follicle
(2) Moderate to pronounced mitotic activity	Relatively low number of mitoses
(3) Prominent phagocytosis	Relative lack of phagocytosis
(4) Reactive cells in interfollicular areas	Neoplastic cells in interfollicular areas

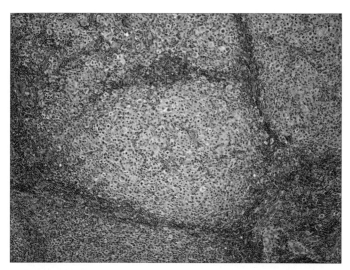

Fig. 21.15. Medium-powered view of a neoplastic follicle in pediatric follicular lymphoma, demonstrating relatively homogeneous infiltration by large neoplastic cells (grade 3A morphology) and lack of an intact mantle zone. The large cell infiltrate is associated with more mitotic figures than is typical in lower grades of follicular lymphoma, and occasional tingible body macrophages are seen (H&E stain).

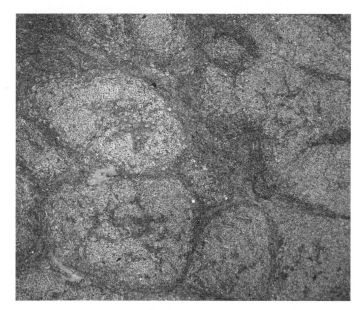

Fig. 21.14. Low-power magnification of pediatric follicular lymphoma demonstrating high-density, back-to-back follicles with relatively homogeneous composition with the neoplastic follicles. This is a grade 3A (predominantly large cell) follicular lymphoma. Several large-sized follicles are present (H&E stain).

adolescents, where reactive follicular hyperplasia is very common [6]. Several morphologic features have been identified that are characteristic of follicular lymphomas and are particularly useful in differentiating between follicular hyperplasia and follicular lymphoma (summarized in Table 21.15 and below).

Most pediatric FLs display a primarily follicular growth pattern, although mixed follicular and diffuse patterns have been noted [11, 149]. Morphologic features that are helpful in distinguishing FL from a reactive process include follicular distribution and density. Follicular lymphomas will tend to have an even

distribution of follicles with back-to-back follicles, as compared to the typical paracortical distribution with intervening T-cell areas in reactive processes. However, it has been noted that up to 15% of adult FLs do not demonstrate a back-to-back follicular pattern. Another helpful feature is the extension of malignant follicles or neoplastic cells outside of the nodal capsule, if it is present [152]. Neoplastic follicles may range in size from that of a primary (unstimulated) follicle up to much larger than a typical reactive follicle [11], and in pediatric populations neoplastic follicles are more likely to be larger in size (Fig. 21.14) [6]. Although usually round to oval in shape, they may become irregular and serpiginous. In most cases of FL, the follicles will appear relatively uniform and monotonous in size and shape, although many pediatric cases may display wide variation in follicle morphology [11, 153]. Variation in follicle size and shape is more commonly associated with reactive processes. Another useful feature in distinguishing reactive from neoplastic follicles is the lack of an intact mantle zone (Fig. 21.15) surrounding the follicle and loss of germinal center polarization (Fig. 21.16) in FL [153–155]. Other morphologic patterns include a reverse pattern with darker nodules against the lighter interfollicular background [156], or mottled follicles creating a so-called "floral" variant that resembles progressive transformation of germinal centers [157].

The cytologic composition of the follicle may also be useful in distinguishing between a lymphoma and a reactive process, particularly when the neoplastic follicle is composed primarily of small cleaved (grade 1) or large cells (grade 3) (Fig. 21.15). However, the so-called mixed small cleaved cell (grade 2) lymphomas may be more difficult to distinguish from follicular hyperplasia due to their diversity of cellular cytology. The presence of mitotic activity and phagocytic histiocytes (tingible body macrophages) is more commonly seen in reactive

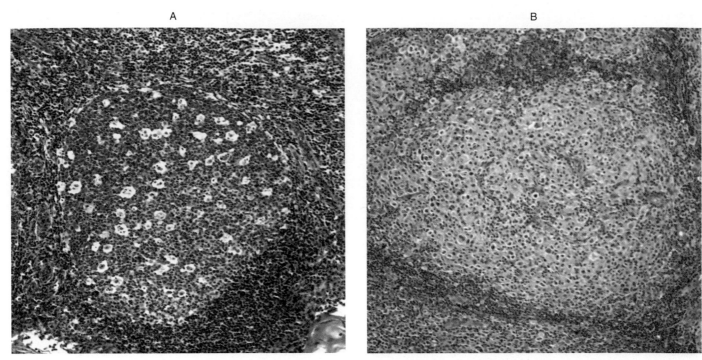

Fig. 21.16. (A) High-powered demonstration of follicular polarization in a reactive follicle. The larger cells tend to cluster at one pole of the follicle showing a light and dark zone of the follicle. Also note the prominent numbers of tingible body macrophages (H&E stain). (B) Neoplastic follicle from follicular lymphoma lacking the light and dark zone created by follicular polarization (H&E stain).

follicular hyperplasia when compared to follicular lymphoma [11, 155, 158]. Follicular hyperplasia often has prominent mitotic activity, whereas mitotic activity in follicular lymphomas is less prominent. The average reported number of mitotic figures per 5 follicles was 50 in reactive follicles as compared to 25 in FL [153]. However, the number of mitoses in FL increases with the proportion of large cells, and increased mitotic activity may be seen in follicular large cell lymphomas, which are more common in pediatric patients [11, 35, 146, 151].

Grading

Follicular lymphoma is graded by determination of the proportion of centroblasts or large cells present within the neoplastic follicle. Histologic grading can help predict clinical outcome, but there is wide diversity and controversy about the optimal grading method, clinical significance, and reproducibility [159, 160]. The WHO classification recommends using a three-grade system (grade 1–3) based on counting the absolute number of centroblasts in 10 neoplastic follicles per 40× high-powered microscopic field (Table 21.16). Grade 1 cases will have 0–5 centroblasts/high-powered field; grade 2 cases will have 6–15 centroblasts/high-powered field; grade 3 cases will have >15 centroblasts/high-powered field (Table 21.16). Those cases that are grade 1 or grade 2 are considered low grade [11, 161]. When doing the counts, selection of 10 high-power fields should be at random, to include a variety of follicles, and should not be selected for those having the largest number of

Table 21.16. Grading of follicular lymphoma by the WHO classification.

Grading	Definition
Grade 1–2 (low grade)	0–15 centroblasts per hpf[a]
Grade 1	0–5 centroblasts per hpf[a]
Grade 2	6–15 centroblasts per hpf[a]
Grade 3	>15 centroblasts per hpf[a]
3A	Centrocytes present
3B	Solid sheets of centroblasts
Reporting of pattern	Proportion follicular (%)
Follicular	>75
Follicular and diffuse	25–75[b]
Focally follicular	<25[b]
Diffuse	0[b]

[a] hpf = high-power field of 0.159 mm^2 (40× objective, 18 mm field of view ocular; count 10 hpf and divide by 10).
[b] Give approximate % of each in report.

large cells. If a discreet area of grade 3 follicular lymphoma is present in an otherwise grade 1 process, a separate diagnosis should be made indicating the predominant histologic pattern as well as the presence of a grade 3 lesion, with estimates of the approximate amounts of each grade present. Under the WHO classification, grade 3 FL can be further divided according to the number of centroblasts, with grade 3A being greater than 15 centroblasts per high-powered field but still having centrocytes present, whereas grade 3B has solid sheets of centroblasts present within the neoplastic follicle [11]. In

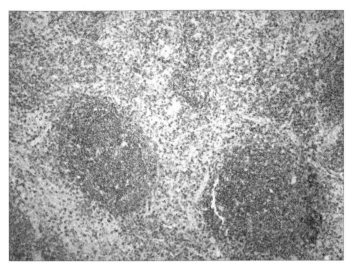

Fig. 21.17. Pediatric follicular lymphoma immunostained with CD20, demonstrating highlighting of the neoplastic follicles with extension into the interfollicular zones (immunohistochemical stain for CD20).

addition, the pattern or amount of follicular pattern identified should be stated, and includes follicular (>75% follicular) to diffuse (0% follicular) (Table 21.16) [11, 162].

One of the controversial problems with grading of follicular lymphomas is use of a standardized ocular, where one high-powered field equal to 0.159 mm^2 (40× objective with a 18 mm field of view ocular) is required for uniformity [11]. Unfortunately, there is a wide variety of oculars, and use of wide-field microscopes is increasingly more common. If one is using an ocular with a 20 mm diameter of field of view, it will give a 0.196 mm^2 high-powered field, or 1.2 times as large as the standardized 0.159 mm^2 field. Thus, one must know the ocular field dimensions of the microscope that is being used to make the counts, and adjust counts by a correction factor based on the ocular field size of that particular scope [11].

Immunophenotype

FLs are derived from follicular center cells and are mature B-cell monoclonal processes. In paraffin-embedded tissues, the specific B-cell antibodies available (CD20, CD45RA, CD79A, CD22, PAX-5) stain reactive and neoplastic follicles similarly and may not be helpful in distinguishing between these processes (Fig. 21.17) [154, 155, 158, 163, 164]. Both reactive and neoplastic follicles may also have interspersed T-cells which stain positively with T-cell markers such as CD3, CD43, and CD45RO. FL in adults will overexpress the BCL6 protein, although this feature is often lacking in pediatric cases, and when present is associated with more disseminated disease [35, 151, 154]. Both CD10 and BCL6 staining will be seen in both FL as well as reactive germinal centers, and is not helpful in distinguishing between these two processes [154, 155, 164–166]. FL will be monoclonal, which is often seen by flow cytometry, but this may be difficult to demonstrate in paraffin-embedded materials by immunohistochemistry

[154, 167]. In addition, small CD10-positive monoclonal clones may be detected in some cases of reactive follicular hyperplasia, so definitive diagnosis of FL will require morphologic features of lymphoma in addition to detection of a CD10-positive clonal population [11, 168, 169]. In adults, FL is characterized by overexpression of BCL2 protein in germinal centers, allowing it to be distinguished from follicular hyperplasia where BCL2 protein is absent (Fig. 21.18A). In contrast, pediatric FLs do not have overexpression of BCL2 (Fig. 21.18B) [11].

As noted above, FL tends to have a lower mitotic rate than follicular hyperplasia. Staining with markers such as Ki-67 (MIB-1) will demonstrate this, with lower levels of staining than in follicular hyperplasia [153, 155, 163]. However, it must be noted that a high proliferative fraction does not exclude a diagnosis of lymphoma, and that a low proliferative index does not exclude a reactive process [155]. Because pediatric FL tends to be grade 3 (follicular large cell), mitotic activity is often higher than seen in lower grade lymphomas [6, 11, 35, 149], and the proliferation index must be interpreted with other available morphologic and immunophenotypic data. In addition, the MIB-1 staining will highlight polarization of the follicle in reactive processes, with most proliferative cells being located at one pole of the follicle. In contrast, MIB-1 staining in FL will tend to be evenly distributed across the follicle, without polarization (Fig. 21.19) [155, 170].

Genetics

Molecular genetic analysis of follicular lymphoma by Southern blot analysis or RT-PCR will demonstrate immunoglobulin heavy and light chain rearrangements, confirming the monoclonality of FL [11, 25, 161, 163]. This may be quite helpful in delineating between follicular hyperplasia and lymphoma in pediatric cases. It should be noted that the immunoglobulin variable region often shows extensive somatic hypermutation with abundant intraclonal heterogeneity in FL, which may decrease the sensitivity of immunoglobulin gene rearrangements using RT-PCR approaches [163], although some reported cases of pediatric FL have detectable immunoglobulin gene rearrangements [11, 35].

Virtually all cases of adult FL will have cytogenetic abnormalities. The most common abnormality seen in adults is the rearrangement of the *BCL2* gene associated with the t(14;18)(q32;q21), which is seen in 70–95% of cases [11, 25, 161]. This leads to overexpression of BCL2 protein (Fig. 21.18A) that confers the survival advantage of neoplastic B-cells *in vitro* by preventing apoptosis under conditions of growth factor deprivation [171]. Pediatric cases are much less likely to have *BCL2* rearrangements or overexpression of BCL2 protein (Fig. 21.18B), suggesting an alternative mechanism of lymphomagenesis in children and adolescents, perhaps involving the *BCL6* gene [148]. Abnormalities including *BCL6* rearrangements and isochromosome (17q) have been described in pediatric FL [148, 149]. In adult studies, a small number of cases of follicular lymphoma that lack *BCL2* rearrangements have been

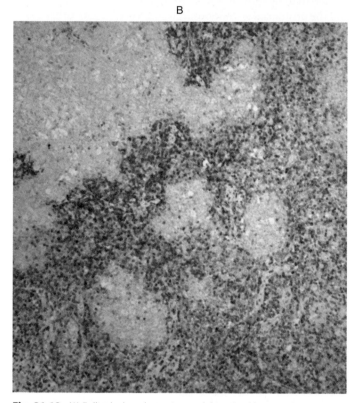

A

B

Fig. 21.18. (A) Follicular lymphoma in an adult, stained by immunoperoxidase methods with BCL2, demonstrating overexpression of BCL2 within the neoplastic follicle. The neoplastic follicular cells stain slightly less intensely than the reactive T-cells (BCL2 immunohistochemical stain). (B) Follicular lymphoma in a pediatric patient with prominent, large neoplastic follicles stained with BCL2 lacks overexpression of BCL2 in the neoplastic follicle, although reactive T-cells in the interfollicular area stain positively, providing an internal control (BCL2 immunohistochemical stain).

studied and shown to have mutations of *BCL6*, or *BCL6* translocations [11, 25, 161].

Clinically, FL in children and adolescents is usually indolent, despite being mostly of grade 3 histology [6]. Treatment is variable; some patients have been treated by local excision while others are treated with chemotherapy or radiotherapy. Patients usually achieve durable remissions [6, 11, 30, 35].

Pediatric marginal zone lymphoma

Extranodal marginal zone lymphoma (EMZL) or lymphomas of mucosa-associated lymphoid tissues (MALT) make up 6–8% of NHL in adults [7, 95, 172–174]. Patients tend to be older (mean age 61 years), with a slight female predominance [11, 172]. EMZLs also are seen in children, although with much lower frequency (reported as 0.1% of cases in one large series of pediatric NHL) [175]. Most pediatric cases of EMZL are found in case reports or small series and reviews [175–182]. In pediatric populations, almost half of the reported cases arise in children with immunodeficiency, most commonly secondary to HIV infection [179]. The reported range of ages is 5–18 years, with approximately equal numbers of males and females [6, 179].

Extranodal sites of involvement in children are similar to those seen in adults but show some differences depending on underlying immunodeficiency. Patients with HIV infection or other immunodeficiency most commonly show involvement of the parotid gland or lung, whereas patients without underlying immunodeficiency have had localized tumors reported in the stomach, orbit and ocular adnexa, tonsils and adenoids, submandibular gland, nasal sinus, skin, and lip [176–178, 180–183]. There are also several case reports of primary cutaneous marginal zone lymphomas in children [181, 184, 185].

Nodal marginal zone lymphoma (NMZL) is also reported in children [6, 176, 186], but there do not appear to be any cases of splenic marginal zone lymphoma reported. Reported ages of patients with NMZL ranged from 2 to 19 years and it appeared more frequently in males (M : F ratio of 20 : 1). Most patients presented with localized lymphadenopathy (usually clinical stage I) in the head and neck, and there was no clear association with immunodeficiency [176]. Because of unique clinical and morphologic features of NMZL in the pediatric age group, they have been recognized as a unique diagnostic category in the WHO classification [11].

Morphology

Morphologically and immunophenotypically, pediatric EMZL and NMZL appear similar to adult cases, although some morphologic features vary [11]. EMZLs are believed to be derived from mucosal lymphocytes of marginal zone derivation, and are closely related to NMZLs, which are postulated to arise from nodal marginal zone cells [158, 187–190]. Both NMZLs and EMZLs are characterized by morphologic diversity that is in part due to morphologic plasticity of the neoplastic component, and in part due to the presence of admixed reactive components [172–174, 189, 191]. The neoplastic cellular component consists of small to medium lymphocytes with a moderate amount of cytoplasm and irregular nuclear contours which resemble small cleaved lymphocytes (termed centrocyte-like cells), small lymphocytes, large centroblasts, monocytoid B-cells, and

A

B

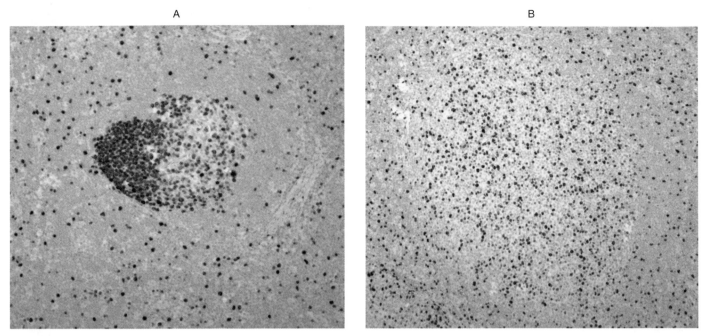

Fig. 21.19. (A) Reactive follicle stained by immunohistochemical staining with MIB-1, demonstrating follicular polarization with MIB-1 staining concentrated at one pole of the reactive follicle (MIB-1 immunohistochemical stain). (B) Pediatric follicular lymphoma stained by immunohistochemical staining for MIB-1 to demonstrate the lower than expected proliferative rate, with lack of polarization, resulting in relatively uniform distribution of MIB-1 staining in the neoplastic follicle (MIB-1 immunohistochemical stain).

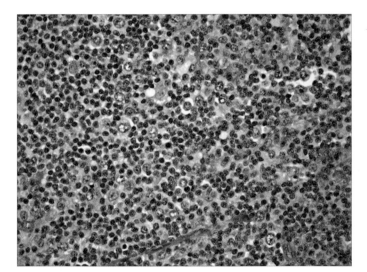

Fig. 21.20. High-powered view of a nodal marginal zone lymphoma demonstrating the diversity of cell types in the neoplastic infiltrate. The neoplastic infiltrate includes small cells, small cleaved cells, admixed large cells, rare plasma cells, and monocytoid B-cells (H&E stain).

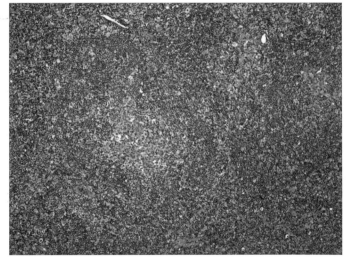

Fig. 21.21. Demonstration of reactive germinal centers admixed with neoplastic infiltrate in nodal marginal zone lymphoma. There is infiltration of neoplastic cells (follicular colonization) into the reactive germinal center (H&E stain).

monotypic plasma cells (Fig. 21.20). Because of the varying amounts of the different cellular elements in the neoplastic cellular component, there is wide diversity often present within areas of the same neoplasm, as well as between different cases of NMZL or EMZL. Often there are reactive components admixed with the neoplasm, including germinal centers (Fig. 21.21) and reactive (polyclonal) plasma cells [11, 172, 174]. The neoplastic cells infiltrate around reactive follicles, often infiltrating into the follicle (follicular colonization) (Fig. 21.21). In EMZL,

the neoplastic lymphoid cells will infiltrate mucosal epithelium to create characteristic lymphoepithelial lesions (Fig. 21.22) [172, 174, 191]. Lymphoepithelial lesions are highly suggestive, although not diagnostic, of lymphoma. For example, in the stomach lymphoepithelial lesions may also be seen in some cases of gastritis, particularly in the presence of *Helicobacter pylori* infection [174, 192]. Plasma cell differentiation is present to varying degrees, and is often most prominent under the luminal epithelium in EMZL. In some cases, the plasma cell

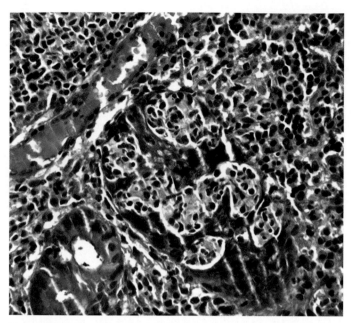

Fig. 21.22. Extranodal marginal zone lymphoma in the colon demonstrating infiltration of neoplastic cells into the glandular epithelium to form characteristic lymphoepithelial lesions. The neoplastic infiltrate is an admixture of small lymphocytes, centrocyte-like cells, plasma cells, large cells, and monocytoid B-cells (H&E stain).

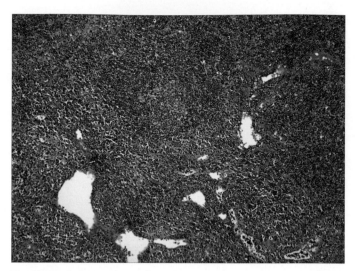

Fig. 21.23. Progressively transformed germinal centers in a pediatric patient with nodal marginal zone lymphoma. This pattern is unusual in adult nodal marginal zone lymphomas (H&E stain).

differentiation may be so marked as to allow the diagnosis of plasmacytoma to enter into the differential [173, 191]. In pediatric NMZL, follicles resembling progressively transformed germinal centers are frequently seen (Fig. 21.23), and this feature has not been described in adult NMZL [6, 11, 176, 193]. This is the primary morphologic feature that has led to identification of pediatric NMZL as a unique entity in the WHO classification [11].

EMZL or NMZL may have areas of large-cell transformation, with increased numbers of large cells, forming sheets or clusters of transformed large, non-cleaved cells, often appearing as a diffuse large B-cell lymphoma [194]. Usually there is a clearly identifiable focus of lower-grade marginal zone lymphoma, which allows for the diagnosis of transformation to a high-grade lesion to be made. The WHO classification recommends that cases with large-cell clusters of greater than 20 cells be referred to as DLBCL in EMZL, but no well-defined criteria are set for NMZL [11]. One must be careful to exclude reactive germinal centers when considering large-cell sheets, and use of immunohistochemical staining with follicular dendritic markers such as CD21 or CD23 may be required [11, 158, 195].

In children, the primary differential diagnostic consideration is reactive lymphoid hyperplasia. In the gut, where diagnosis is attempted on small endoscopic biopsies, differentiating between reactive conditions and EMZL may be particularly difficult. Crush artifact and the presence of reactive components often complicate the evaluation of biopsy material [158]. In some cases, ancillary studies to determine monoclonality may be required. The presence of a very dense infiltrate with sheets of centrocyte-like cells and well-formed lymphoepithe-

lial lesions with degeneration of the epithelium are extremely useful in arriving at a diagnosis of lymphoma [172]. In children, there is a rather unique form of reactive hyperplasia, termed atypical marginal zone hyperplasia of MALT, that shows lambda light chain restriction by immunoperoxidase staining. This entity occurs primarily in the tonsils and appendices of children between 2 and 11 years of age, and appears to represent a localized extranodal hyperplasia that must be distinguished from true EMZL [6, 196]. The hyperplasia is characterized by markedly hyperplastic follicles with prominent marginal zones. There is a prominent population of centrocyte-like cells that may extend into overlying epithelial structures. The B-cell marginal zone expansion often shows co-expression of CD43 [196], a feature often associated with malignancy but also seen in a restricted population of reactive B-cells [197]. The presence of an apparently monoclonal population by immunostaining is not confirmed by molecular studies, which demonstrate a polytypic pattern and non-mutated immunoglobulins. All the patients described have done well without lymphoma therapy [196].

Immunophenotype

NMZL and EMZL are mature B-cell neoplasms that will express pan-B-cell markers such as CD20, CD19, CD22, CD79a, and PAX-5 (Figs. 21.24 and 21.25). There is usually no co-expression of CD10 or CD5 in the neoplastic B-cells [158, 172, 195]. Monoclonality may often be demonstrated in the plasma cell population in those tumors that show extensive plasma cell differentiation, or the plasma cells may be polyclonal if they are primarily a reactive component. Reactive germinal centers are polyclonal, and should be negative for BCL2 expression, although BCL2 staining may highlight follicle colonization (Fig. 21.25) [158, 195]. An extensive T-cell infiltrate may be admixed with the neoplastic infiltrate, again reflecting normal

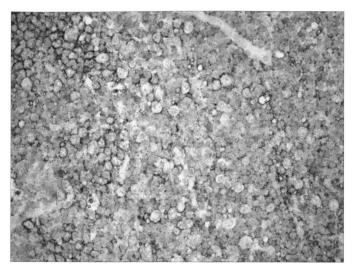

Fig. 21.24. Immunohistochemical stain demonstrating the diffuse staining for the B-cell marker CD20 in nodal marginal zone lymphoma. The CD20 staining highlights the diversity of cell sizes in the neoplastic infiltrate (CD20 immunohistochemical stain).

reactive components within the tumor. Keratin stains may be helpful in highlighting lymphoepithelial lesions, especially in cases where there is marked epithelial destruction [172].

Genetics

Molecular analysis of NMZL and EMZL demonstrates the presence of both heavy and light chain immunoglobulin rearrangements, by Southern blot or PCR analysis [172, 198]. Several recurrent cytogenetic translocations have been described in adults with marginal zone lymphomas, including t(11;18)(q21;q21), t(1;14)(p22;q32), t(14;18)(q32;q21), and t(3;14)(q27;q32), as well as trisomies of chromosome 3 and 18 [198, 199]. There is no available information on cytogenetic abnormalities in pediatric EMZL or NMZL.

Treatment and prognosis

Treatment of marginal zone lymphomas is variable, with some cases treated conservatively with antibiotic therapy (cases of *Helicobacter pylori*-associated gastric EMZL), local excision, local radiotherapy, or more aggressive approaches of systemic chemotherapy. Despite the variety of therapies used, patients appear to do well with few recurrences or development of more extensive disease, suggesting that conservative therapy may be preferable [173, 174, 176, 179, 186, 193, 195].

Other pediatric mature B-cell lymphomas

Other subtypes of pediatric mature B-cell lymphoma are extremely rare and appear mostly as individual case reports in the literature when children or adolescents are affected. These appear to represent unusual presentations of typical adult diseases in children or adolescents in most cases.

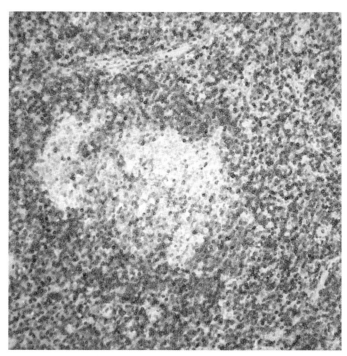

Fig. 21.25. BCL2 immunostaining demonstrating follicular colonization in nodal marginal zone lymphoma. The BCL2 highlights the neoplastic B-cells that are infiltrating into the reactive follicle, which is BCL2 negative (BCL2 immunohistochemical stain).

Small lymphocytic lymphoma

Small lymphocytic lymphoma/chronic lymphocytic leukemia (SLL/CLL) is usually a disease of older adults, with cases occurring in patients less than 30 years of age being very rare [200, 201]. A few cases in the literature have described SLL/CLL occurring in patients in their late teens to early twenties. These cases have the same morphologic (Fig. 21.26) and immunophenotypic features seen in older adults (summarized in Table 21.17) and are a neoplasm of mature, small B-cells that co-express the T-cell marker CD5 [11, 200]. In general, CLL/SLL in younger patients tends to be associated with a more aggressive clinical course.

Mantle cell lymphoma

Another CD5-positive B-cell lymphoma, mantle cell lymphoma (Table 21.18), has been described in a single case report in an 18-year-old woman [202]. This case was of interest as the initial presentation was with a large-cell variant of mantle cell lymphoma (Fig. 21.27) that was diagnosed as DLBCL and not initially recognized as mantle cell lymphoma until relapse revealed a more classic morphologic appearance with widespread involvement of gut and bone marrow (Fig. 21.28). The typical morphology of mantle cell lymphoma is a small, mature-appearing lymphocyte with slightly irregular nuclear contours, although blastic and large-cell variants are well recognized [11, 158, 203]. Mantle cell lymphomas have a classic molecular cytogenetic abnormality, the t(11;14)(q13;q32), that transposes the immunoglobulin heavy chain gene with the *BCL1* (also known as *CCND1*

Table 21.17. Features of SLL/CLL.

Clinical	Blood involvement common, may have lymph adenopathy, splenomegaly tissue involvement
Morphology	Diffuse effacement; small, mature lymphocytes; pseudoproliferation centers
Immunophenotype	CD20+ with co-expression of CD5 CD23+ BCL1 (cyclin D1) negative Dim cell-surface immunoglobulins
Cytogenetics – common abnormalities	Trisomy 12 13q deletion

Table 21.18. Clinical and pathologic features of mantle cell lymphoma.

Clinical	Lymph nodes most commonly involved Gut, spleen, bone marrow, and blood also frequently involved Stage IV disease common
Morphology	Usually diffuse to nodular effacement Proliferation of benign histiocytes is common No pseudoproliferation centers Hyalinized vessels common
Cytology	Usually small to intermediate-sized lymphocytes with variably irregular nuclear contours (centrocyte like) May have variant blastoid or large-cell morphology
Immunophenotype	Mature B-cell (CD19+, CD20+) with co-expression of CD5 CD10, BCL6, CD23 negative Cyclin D1 nuclear staining Bright cell-surface immunoglobulins
Molecular/cytogenetics	Monoclonal gene rearrangement studies t(11;14)(q13;q32) translocation

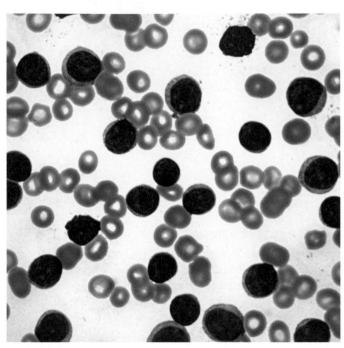

Fig. 21.26. Peripheral blood smear demonstrating the small, mature-appearing neoplastic lymphocytes and occasional smudge cells seen in chronic lymphocytic leukemia (Wright–Giemsa stain).

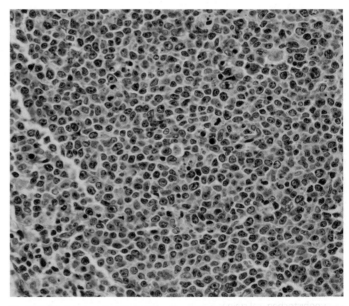

Fig. 21.27. Large-cell variant of mantle cell lymphoma seen in an 18-year-old patient, which was initially not recognized as mantle cell lymphoma. The tumor was later found to co-express CD5 and cyclin D1 and to have a t(11;14), by FISH (H&E stain).

or *PRAD1*) gene, leading to overexpression of cyclin D1 protein, and is considered essential for diagnosis [15, 25]. Detection of the abnormality may be by either cytogenetics, FISH (Fig. 21.29), or cyclin D1 protein staining by immunoperoxidase (Fig. 21.30), with FISH and immunoperoxidase staining being the most sensitive methods [11]. This tumor has a deceptively small, mature B-cell appearance with few mitotic figures, no large cells, and lack of pseudoproliferation centers, but is relatively resistant to chemotherapy, making it a clinically aggressive lymphoma. In young patients, aggressive chemotherapy followed by bone marrow transplant is usually attempted as therapy [204–206].

Plasma cell neoplasms

Although most subtypes of plasma cell neoplasms, in particular multiple myeloma, have not been described in children or adolescents, rare case reports of plasmacytomas

of bone [207, 208], adenoids [209], or other tissues [210] have been reported. These are usually collections of mature-appearing, but light chain restricted plasma cells (Fig. 21.31) [207, 209], although less mature plasma cell neoplasms have also been described [210]. Bone lesions are usually seen in older adolescents, and patients appear to respond to local therapy with no reports of progression to disseminated disease [207, 208]. It should be noted that some marginal zone lymphomas may have extensive plasma cell differentiation, and it is not clear if the reported non-osseous plasmacytomas may

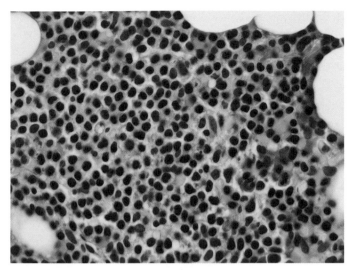

Fig. 21.28. Relapse of the large-cell process seen in Figure 21.27, in the bone marrow as a typical mantle cell lymphoma showing an infiltrate of small-to-intermediate-sized cells with mature chromatin and slightly irregular nuclear contours, characteristic of mantle cell lymphoma. The tumor had a classic mantle cell phenotype with co-expression of CD5 and cyclin D1. (H&E stain.)

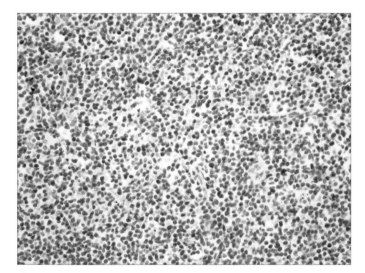

Fig. 21.30. Immunohistochemical staining for cyclin D1 protein overexpression seen in mantle cell lymphoma. Cyclin D1 immunostaining shows a characteristic nuclear staining pattern. (Cyclin D1 immunohistochemical stain.)

represent extranodal marginal zone lymphomas [11, 211]. A single pediatric case of a plasma cell neoplasm resembling multiple myeloma has been describe in the post-transplant setting [212].

Lymphomatoid granulomatosis

A rare subtype of NHL that is associated with EBV, and which is most commonly seen in middle-aged men but has been reported in children is lymphomatoid granulomatosis (LYG) [213–219]. This tumor predominantly involves extranodal sites and is characteristically angiocentric and angiodestructive (Fig. 21.32). The tumor cells are large B-cells that are EBV positive, which are admixed with reactive small T-cells

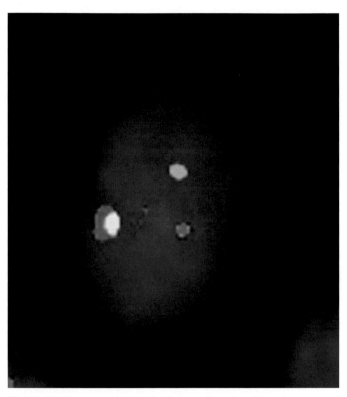

Fig. 21.29. Fluorescent *in situ* hybridization of mantle cell lymphoma demonstrating the characteristic translocation of BCL1, the t(11;14). The probe labels the 14 and 11 chromosomes with red and green fluorochromes that are separated in absence of a translocation. When the t(11;14) translocation is present there is fusion of the signals, giving rise to an orange or yellow fusion signal (fluorescent staining).

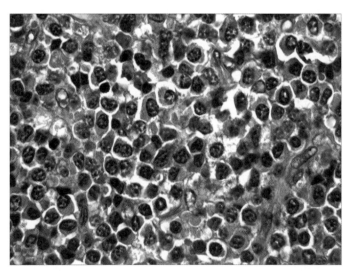

Fig. 21.31. Plasmacytoma of bone comprised of mature-appearing monoclonal plasma cells that created a solitary, lytic lesion in the femur of a child (H&E stain).

as well as histiocytes and plasma cells, giving the overall impression of a T-cell rich, large B-cell lymphoma (Fig. 21.33). There may be variable numbers of large B-cells present. A lymphocytic vasculitis with infiltration of vascular walls and associated necrosis is usually seen. LYG affects males more frequently than

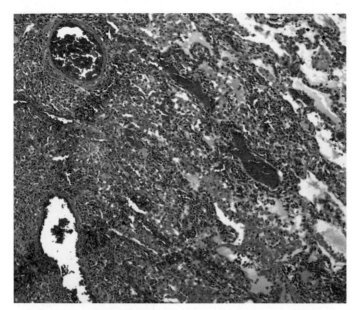

Fig. 21.32. Low-power histology of lymphomatoid granulomatosis in the lung, showing the mixed cellular morphology, angiocentric and angiodestructive infiltrate (H&E stain).

females (M : F ratio of 2 : 1), and has been seen in immunodeficient as well as immunocompetent patients [11, 213, 215]. The most common disease site is the lungs, although brain, kidney, skin, liver, and gastrointestinal tract may also be involved. Involvement of lymph nodes or spleen is unusual. Presentation is usually due to respiratory symptoms such as dyspnea, cough, or chest pain, but patients often experience non-specific symptoms of fever, weight loss, and malaise [213, 220]. The chest X-ray will usually show pulmonary nodules of varying sizes bilaterally in the mid to lower lung fields, with central necrosis [219, 221]. Similar lesions will be seen in other organs, with prominent central necrosis [213, 215].

In children and adolescents, LYG is a very rare but recognized entity with cases reported in children as young as 13 months [222]. Case reports of pediatric LYG include immunocompetent patients [216, 217], as well as in presumably immunosuppressed patients following therapy for AML or ALL [218, 219, 223], or in a patient with Wiscott–Aldrich syndrome [224]. Although most pediatric patients present with lung disease [220, 225], unusual presentations in skin [224, 226], limited neurologic disease [217, 227], and lymph node [228] as well as widespread disease are also seen. Treatment may be by systemic chemotherapy with or without addition of anti-CD20 (rituximab) [229].

B-cell lymphoma, unclassifiable

The new WHO classification has recognized two subtypes of B-cell lymphoma that have previously been difficult to classify. These include B-cell lymphoma, unclassifiable, with features intermediate between diffuse large B-cell lymphoma and Hodgkin lymphoma, as well as B-cell lymphoma, unclassifiable, with features intermediate between diffuse large B-cell lymphoma and Burkitt lymphoma [11, 230]. It is not clear how prevalent the disease entities are in pediatric populations.

B-cell lymphoma, unclassifiable, with features intermediate between diffuse large B-cell lymphoma and Hodgkin lymphoma

This represents a B-cell lineage neoplasm that has features overlapping that of classical Hodgkin lymphoma (cHL) and primary mediastinal (thymic) large B-cell lymphoma (PMBCL) [11]. Previously these were referred to as "gray zone" lymphomas. They are typically described as anterior mediastinal tumors in young men presenting between the ages of 20 and 40 years, although some pediatric cases are included in reported series. Rarely, peripheral nodes are involved. This group includes patients which have tumors with morphologic and immunophenotypic overlap between cHL and PMBCL, as well as patients with disease that appears as composite tumors with distinct presentation of both entities, or as sequential transformation between entities at one site [11, 231, 232].

These lymphomas show sheets of pleomorphic large cells within a fibrotic stoma. Often the cells are more pleomorphic than in typical PMBCL and may resemble Reed–Sternberg cells or lacunar cells. Usually there is a broad spectrum of morphologic appearance within the tumor. Unlike cHL, there is usually a sparse or absent inflammatory infiltrate of eosinophils, lymphocytes and histiocytes. Necrosis is common. The neoplastic cells will display an immunophenotype that is between that expected for PMBCL and cHL, with expression of CD45, CD15, and CD30 (Table 21.13). B-cell markers, such as CD20 and CD79a, are frequently strongly expressed in the majority of cells. B-cell transcription factors, such as PAX-5, Oct-2, and BOB.1, are expressed with variable expression of BCL6 but absent CD10. EBV staining may be positive [11, 231].

Molecular studies have suggested a close relationship between cHL and PMBCL, and the identification of tumors that have characteristics of both tumor types further highlights the close relationship of the neoplasms [11, 129, 230]. No recurrent cytogenetic abnormalities have been identified [11].

B-cell lymphoma, unclassifiable with features intermediate between diffuse large B-cell lymphoma and Hodgkin lymphoma appears to have a more aggressive clinical course than either cHL or PMBCL. There is no consensus as to the best approach to therapy, with both NHL and cHL protocols reported [231, 232].

B-cell lymphoma, unclassifiable, with features intermediate between diffuse large B-cell lymphoma and Burkitt lymphoma

This subtype of NHL, recognized in the most recent WHO classification, is an aggressive, mature B-cell lymphoma that has morphologic and immunophenotypic features that overlap between diffuse large B-cell lymphoma (DLBCL) and Burkitt

A

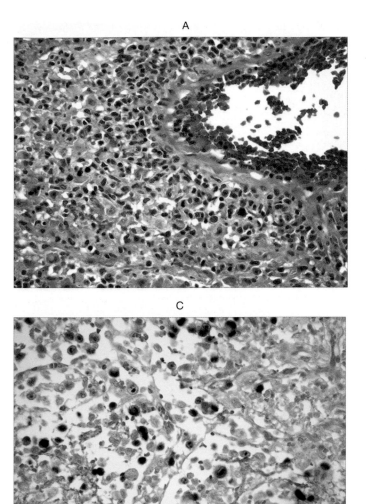

C

B

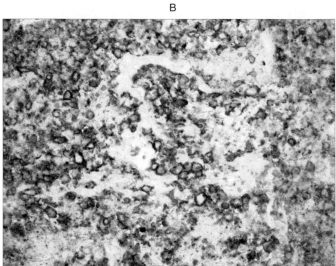

Fig. 21.33. (A) Hematoxylin and eosin stain demonstrating the mixed infiltrates of lymphomatoid granulomatosis surrounding the vessels composed of small lymphocytes, larger transformed cells, and reactive histiocytes (H&E stain). (B) CD20 immunostaining highlighting the large neoplastic B-cells in the mixed infiltrate (CD20 immunoperoxidase stain). (C) Epstein–Barr virus *in situ* hybridization demonstrating EBV positivity in the neoplastic large B-cells (EBER-1 *in situ* hybridization stain).

lymphoma (BL) [11, 230]. Some of these lymphomas were probably classified as Burkitt-like lymphoma previously. These are considered to be rare tumors that occur primarily in adults, and it is unclear if true pediatric cases exist, as most pediatric cases of Burkitt-like lymphoma appear to be closely related to BL, as discussed above. Most of the cases included in this subtype of NHL will have morphologic features that are between DLBCL and BL, with a spectrum of cell size, a high proliferation rate, starry-sky pattern, and an immunophenotype most consistent with BL (CD20, CD22, CD10 positive, BCL2 negative with proliferation rate >95%). Other cases will resemble BL morphologically but lack molecular evidence of a *MYC* rearrangement or have an abnormal phenotype (such as moderate-to-strong BCL2 expression or proliferation rate varying between 50 and 100%) [11, 232–234].

In adults, these tumors appear to have a high frequency of extranodal disease or leukemic presentation. All cases will show clonal immunoglobulin rearrangements. Up to 50% of cases may have a *MYC* translocation, often with unusual translocation partners, and 15% of cases may also have a *BCL2* translocation ("double hit" lymphoma) and/or *BCL6* translocation ("triple hit" lymphoma). Often there is a very complex cytogenetic pattern [11, 235, 236].

The biologic behavior of B-cell lymphoma, unclassifiable with features intermediate between diffuse large B-cell lymphoma and Burkitt lymphoma is aggressive, and a unified approach to therapy has not been established [237, 238].

Immunodeficiency-related lymphoproliferative disorders

Post-transplant lymphoproliferative disorders

With the advent of more accessible solid organ transplantation in the pediatric population, immunosuppression-related

417

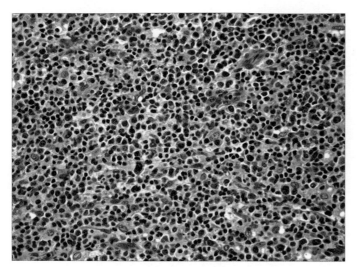

Fig. 21.34. Post-transplant lymphoproliferative disorder arising in a child following solid organ transplant. The post-transplant lymphoproliferative disorder is a relatively monomorphic proliferation that was monoclonal, resembling diffuse large B-cell lymphoma (H&E stain).

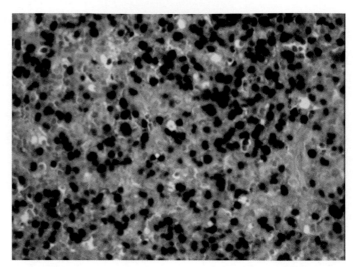

Fig. 21.35. Epstein–Barr virus *in situ* hybridization demonstrates high expression of Epstein–Barr virus in a pediatric post-transplant lymphoproliferative disorder. (EBER-1 *in situ* hybridization staining.)

post-transplant lymphoproliferative disorders (PTLDs) are now recognized in this population [239–244]. Although T-cell PTLDs are rarely seen, the majority of PTLDs are mature B-cell proliferations [11, 245, 246], and most are driven by EBV [241, 245, 247, 248]. In children, because they may not harbor EBV at the time of transplant, acute EBV infections and polymorphic/polyclonal B-cell proliferations, particularly involving the tonsils or gut, may be the initial presentation of PTLD [50, 245, 249–251]. As in adults, many pediatric patients will present with an EBV-driven large-cell proliferation that is monoclonal and resembles DLBCL (Fig. 21.34) [240, 245], although unusual presentations, such as a child presenting with an EBV-positive plasma cell proliferation resembling multiple myeloma, have also been described [212]. Although PTLD following autologous bone marrow transplant is well described in adults, it appears to be rare in children [252, 253], and is associated with T-cell depletion of the allograft.

The risk of development of PTLD in children is associated with intensity, duration, and type of immunosuppression, and age of the graft recipient, as well as if an organ that is EBV positive is transplanted into a seronegative recipient [241, 250, 254]. Often PTLD involves extranodal or unusual sites, including presentation in the gastrointestinal tract or allograft [255, 256]. The tumors are usually positive with B-cell markers, such as CD20, and will usually show evidence of EBV by *in-situ* hybridization (Fig. 21.35), although a small proportion of cases may be EBV negative [11, 245].

Treatment of mature B-cell PTLD is usually aimed at reducing immunosuppression, although this may not be feasible in many pediatric transplants, where loss of the transplanted organ by rejection is not compatible with life. Many pediatric patients are treated with low-dose chemotherapy alone or in conjunction with anti-CD20 (rituximab) with good outcomes [241, 254, 257].

Table 21.19. Pediatric HIV-associated non-Hodgkin lymphoma.

Subtype of NHL	Clinical behavior
Burkitt lymphoma	Aggressive
Diffuse large B-cell lymphoma	Aggressive
Marginal zone lymphoma	Indolent

HIV-associated lymphomas

Pediatric patients with either congenital or acquired childhood/adolescent HIV (human immunodeficiency virus) infection are at a greatly increased risk for development of NHL, estimated to be 50–500× over that of the non-infected population, and occurring in approximately 2% of pediatric HIV patients [258–261]. The median time to development of NHL in pediatric patients is 14 months after infection [259]. As in adults, these lymphomas are primarily aggressive B-cell neoplasms (DLBCL or BL), but pediatric HIV patients also have an increase in development of clinically indolent extranodal marginal zone lymphomas (Table 21.19) [176, 179, 259]. BL appears to be the most common aggressive NHL in the pediatric age group [259]. HIV-associated NHL has a markedly increased propensity to arise in unusual sites such as the central nervous system, gastrointestinal tract, and other extranodal sites, with primary brain lymphomas being seen in children that survive several years with HIV infection [11, 258, 259, 262].

The NHL seen in HIV patients may be associated with EBV or human herpesvirus 8 (HHV-8) in some, but not all, cases [11]. In children, EBV appears to be the associated with most reported cases of NHL [50, 262]. It has been postulated that chronic immune stimulation due to the immunodeficiency status of the patient may lead to benign lymphoid expansion, which then progresses to a lymphoid malignancy when genetic alterations in *BCL6*, *cMYC*, or other genes occur

[258]. The NHLs that arise in HIV patients appear morphologically and immunophenotypically similar to those seen in the non-immunosuppressed population [11]. A few subtypes of HIV-associated lymphomas: primary effusion lymphoma and plasmablastic lymphoma of the oral cavity or other extranodal sites, are much more commonly seen in adult HIV patients, and are extremely rare in children and adolescents with HIV [50, 259]. Clinical behavior is variable and is dependent on the subtype of lymphoma as well as the patient's underlying performance status and degree of immunocompromise, and patients may respond poorly to therapy due to immunosuppression [11, 50]. Rare patients have been treated with high-dose chemotherapy and autologous bone marrow transplant with good results [263].

Primary immunodeficiency-associated lymphomas

In addition to iatrogenic or infection-associated immunodeficiencies, several primary or hereditary immunodeficiencies are associated with the development of lymphoproliferative disorders [50, 261, 264, 265]. As in post-transplant and HIV patients, these are usually mature B-cell neoplasms. The risk of developing a lymphoproliferative process varies with the type and severity of the underlying immunodeficiency, but in most cases patients with primary immunodeficiency will have a 10–300-fold increase in the incidence of lymphoproliferative disorders, and most of these will occur in pediatric patients under the age of 10 years [264, 265]. Often these lymphoproliferative processes arise in extranodal sites, including the gastrointestinal tract and central nervous system. As many are associated with X-linked genes, the lymphomas occur more frequently in males [50, 266]. Diverse types of lymphoma are seen, although DLBCL is the most common [50, 261, 264]. Some patients present with a LYG appearance [224], and other presentations such as fatal infectious mononucleosis or polymorphic lymphoproliferations may also be seen. Hodgkin lymphoma may also be seen in some patients [267]. The proliferations may be clonal or polyclonal [11, 261].

Some of the primary immunodeficiencies associated with an increased risk of developing a lymphoproliferative disorder include chromosomal breakage syndromes such as ataxia telangiectasia (AT) or Nijmegen breakage syndrome, as well as other immunodeficient states including Wiscott–Aldrich syndrome (WAS), common variable immunodeficiency (CVID), severe combined immunodeficiency (SCID), X-linked lymphoproliferative disorder (XLP), hyper-IgM syndrome, and autoimmune lymphoproliferative syndrome (ALPS) (Table 21.20).

The chromosomal breakage syndromes are associated with a very high incidence of development of leukemia and lymphoma, and these are often clinically aggressive. These disorders are not usually associated with EBV. In ataxia telangiectasia there is a broad range of tumors seen, including a predominance of T-cell NHL and carcinomas. In Nijmegen breakage syndrome, DLBCL is the most commonly seen tumor [11, 50, 261, 268, 269].

Table 21.20. Congenital immunodeficiencies associated with B-lymphoproliferative disorders.

Disorder	Risk	Pathogenesis
Nijmegen breakage syndrome	High	Genetic damage
Ataxia telangiectasia	High	Genetic damage
X-linked lymphoproliferative syndrome	High	EBV
Wiscott–Aldrich syndrome	Moderate	EBV
Severe combined immunodeficiency	Moderate	EBV
Hyper-IgM syndrome	Moderate	CD40 ligand
Autoimmune lymphoproliferative syndrome	Moderate	*FAS* gene
Common variable immunodeficiency	Low	EBV

The majority of the other primary immunodeficiencies are associated with development of EBV-associated lymphoproliferative disorders, similar to those seen in the post-transplant setting [264]. This is thought to be secondary to derangement of T-cell-based immunity, allowing for uncontrolled EBV expansion [267, 270]. In hyper-IgM syndrome there are mutations in the CD40 ligand, which interferes with normal B- and T-cell interactions and differentiation of antigen-stimulated B-cells into plasma cells [264]. In ALPS, there is a mutation of the *FAS* gene that allows for accumulation of lymphoid cells due to an abnormality in apoptosis [271–273].

As noted above, lymphoproliferative disorders associated with primary immunodeficiencies are often clinically aggressive, with the exception of CVID where there is often more indolent disease and later onset. Unlike the post-transplant setting, modulation of immunosuppression is not possible as a therapeutic approach, and the degree of immune suppression may impact clinical response and increase toxicity of chemotherapy [268, 274, 275]. Allogeneic bone marrow transplant may be used to treat the patients and will also restore more normal immune function [264].

Conclusions

Mature B-cell NHL, in particular Burkitt lymphoma and diffuse large B-cell lymphoma, are common subtypes of lymphoma seen in children and adolescents. These are aggressive neoplasms that are treated by intense, short-duration chemotherapy, and immune-based therapies, such as use of anti-CD20 (rituximab) are currently not widely utilized. Both BL and DLBCL in the pediatric population appear to be highly associated with a follicular center phenotype and high levels of proliferation, suggesting that dysregulation of proliferation may be an important pathogenetic mechanism in development of these lymphomas. Unlike adults, where a large variety of indolent or low-grade mature B-cell lymphomas are seen, NHLs such as follicular lymphoma and marginal zone lymphoma are rare in children and may have clinicopathologic features that differ from adults. Other subtypes of mature B-cell NHL are not seen in children or exist as only as very rare, reportable cases.

References

1. **Cairo MS, Raetz E, Perkins SL.** Non-Hodgkin lymphoma in children. In Kufe D, Pollock RE, Weishelbaum RR, *et al.*, eds. *Cancer Medicine* (6th edn.). London: BC Decker Inc.; 2003, 2337–2348.

2. **Perkins SL,** Work-up and diagnosis of pediatric non-Hodgkin's lymphomas. *Pediatric and Developmental Pathology.* 2000;**3**(4):374–390.

3. **Sandlund JT, Downing JR, Crist WM.** Non-Hodgkin's lymphoma in childhood. *New England Journal of Medicine.* 1996;**334**(19):1238–1248.

4. **Gross TG, Termuhlen AM.** Pediatric non-Hodgkin's lymphoma. *Current Oncology Reports.* 2007;**9**(6):459–465.

5. **Reiter A, Klapper W.** Recent advances in the understanding and management of diffuse large B-cell lymphoma in children. *British Journal of Haematology.* 2008;**142**(3):329–347.

6. **Swerdlow SH.** Pediatric follicular lymphomas, marginal zone lymphomas, and marginal zone hyperplasia. *American Journal of Clinical Pathology.* 2004;**122**(Suppl): S98–S109.

7. Effect of age on the characteristics and clinical behavior of non-Hodgkin's lymphoma patients. The Non-Hodgkin's Lymphoma Classification Project. *Annals of Oncology.* 1997; 8:973–978.

8. **Hochberg J, Waxman IM, Kelly KM, Morris E, Cairo MS.** Adolescent non-Hodgkin lymphoma and Hodgkin lymphoma: state of the science. *British Journal of Haematology.* 2009;**144**(1): 24–40.

9. **Said J.** Diffuse aggressive B-cell lymphomas. *Advances in Anatomic Pathology.* 2009;**16**(4):216–235.

10. **de Leval L, Hasserjian RP.** Diffuse large B-cell lymphomas and Burkitt lymphoma. *Hematology/Oncology Clinics of North America.* 2009;**23**(4): 791–827.

11. **Swerdlow SH, Campo E, Harris NL,** *et al.* *WHO Classification of Tumours of Haematopoietic and Lymphoid Tissues* (4th edn.). Lyon: IARC Press; 2008.

12. **Poirel HA, Cairo MS, Heerema NA.** Specific cytogenetic abnormalities are associated with a significantly inferior outcome in children and adolescents with mature B-cell non-Hodgkin's

lymphoma: results of the FAB/LMB 96 international study. *Leukemia.* 2009; **23**(2):323–331.

13. **Klapper W, Szczepanowski M, Burkhardt B,** *et al.* Molecular profiling of pediatric mature B-cell lymphoma treated in population-based prospective clinical trials. *Blood.* 2008;**112**(4):1374–1381.

14. **Craig FE, Foon KA.** Flow cytometric immunophenotyping for hematologic neoplasms. *Blood.* 2008;**111**(8): 3941–3967.

15. **Bagg A.** Molecular diagnosis in lymphoma. *Current Hematology Reports.* 2005;**4**(4):313–323.

16. **Leonard JP, Martin P, Barrientos J, Elstrom R.** Targeted treatment and new agents in diffuse large B-cell lymphoma. *Seminars in Hematology.* 2008; **45**(3 Suppl 2):S11–S16.

17. **Kwong YL.** Predicting the outcome in non-Hodgkin lymphoma with molecular markers. *British Journal of Haematology.* 2007;**137**(4):273–287.

18. **Casimiro Onofre AS, Pomjanski N, Buckstegge B, Böcking A.** Immunocytochemical typing of primary tumors on fine-needle aspiration cytologies of lymph nodes. *Diagnostic Cytopathology.* 2008;**36**(4): 207–215.

19. **Maroto A, Martinez M, Martinez MA, de Agustin P, Rodriguez- Peralto JL.** Comparative analysis of immunoglobulin polymerase chain reaction and flow cytometry in fine needle aspiration biopsy differential diagnosis of non-Hodgkin B-cell lymphoid malignancies. *Diagnostic Cytopathology.* 2009;**37**(9):647–653.

20. **Gautam, U, Srinivasan R, Rajwanshi A, Bansal D, Marwaha RK.** Comparative evaluation of flow-cytometric immunophenotyping and immunocytochemistry in the categorization of malignant small round cell tumors in fine-needle aspiration cytologic specimens. *Cancer.* 2008;**114**(6):494–503.

21. **Muzzafar T, Srinivasan R, Rajwanshi A, Bansal D, Marwaha RK.** Flow cytometric immunophenotyping of anaplastic large cell lymphoma. *Archives of Pathology and Laboratory Medicine.* 2009;**133**(1):49–56.

22. **Dey P.** Role of ancillary techniques in diagnosing and subclassifying non-Hodgkin's lymphomas on

fine needle aspiration cytology. *Cytopathology.* 2006;**17**(5):275–287.

23. **Teruya-Feldstein J.** Getting the diagnosis right in NHL: role of immunohistochemistry and molecular diagnostic testing. *Journal of the National Comprehensive Cancer Network.* 2008;**6**(4):422–427.

24. **Cairo MS, Raetz E, Lim MS, Davenport V, Perkins SL.** Childhood and adolescent non-Hodgkin lymphoma: new insights in biology and critical challenges for the future. *Pediatric Blood and Cancer.* 2005;**45**(6): 753–769.

25. **Hartmann EM, Ott G, Rosenwald A.** Molecular biology and genetics of lymphomas. *Hematology/Oncology Clinics of North America.* 2008;**22**(5): 807–823, vii.

26. **Bench AJ, Erber WN, Follows GA, Scott MA.** Molecular genetic analysis of haematological malignancies II: Mature lymphoid neoplasms. *International Journal of Laboratory Hematology.* 2007;**29**(4):229–260.

27. **Lones MA, Cairo MS, Perkins SL.** T-cell-rich large B-cell lymphoma in children and adolescents: a clinicopathologic report of six cases from the Children's Cancer Group Study CCG-5961. *Cancer.* 2000; **88**(10):2378–2386.

28. **Wilson J, Kjeldsberg CR, Sposto R,** *et al.* The pathology of non-Hodgkin's lymphoma of childhood: reproducibility and relevance of the histologic classification of "undifferentiated" lymphomas (Burkitt's versus non-Burkitts). *Human Pathology.* 1987;**18**:1008–1014.

29. **Rosenwald A, Ott G.** Burkitt lymphoma versus diffuse large B-cell lymphoma. *Annals of Oncology.* 2008;**19**(Suppl 4):iv67–iv69.

30. **Ott G, Balague-Ponz O,** de Leval L, *et al.* Commentary on the WHO classification of tumors of lymphoid tissues (2008): indolent B cell lymphomas. *Journal of Hematopathology.* 2009;**2**(2): 77–81.

31. **Cairo MS, Gerrard M, Sposto R,** *et al.* Results of a randomized international study of high-risk central nervous system B non-Hodgkin lymphoma and B acute lymphoblastic leukemia in children and adolescents. *Blood.* 2007; **109**(7):2736–2743.

32. **Patte C, Auperin A, Gerrard M,** *et al.* Results of the randomized international FAB/LMB96 trial for intermediate risk B-cell non-Hodgkin lymphoma in children and adolescents: it is possible to reduce treatment for the early responding patients. *Blood.* 2007; **109**(7):2773–2780.

33. **Miles RR, Raphael M, McCarthy K,** *et al.* Pediatric diffuse large B-cell lymphoma demonstrates a high proliferation index, frequent c-Myc protein expression, and a high incidence of germinal center subtype: Report of the French-American-British (FAB) international study group. *Pediatric Blood and Cancer.* 2008; **51**(3): 369–374.

34. **Balague Ponz O, Ott G, Hasserjian RP,** *et al.* Commentary on the WHO classification of tumors of lymphoid tissues (2008): aggressive B-cell lymphomas. *Journal of Hematopathology.* 2009; **2**(2):83–87.

35. **Lorsbach RB, Shay-Seymore D, Moore J,** *et al.* Clinicopathologic analysis of follicular lymphoma occurring in children. *Blood.* 2002; **99**(6):1959–1964.

36. **Goldsby RE, Carroll WL.** The molecular biology of pediatric lymphomas. *Journal of Pediatric Hematology/Oncology.* 1998; **20**(4): 282–296.

37. **Harris NL, Stein H, Coupland SE,** *et al.* New approaches to lymphoma diagnosis. *Hematology/The Education Program of the American Society of Hematology.* 2001:194–220.

38. **Rowland JM.** Molecular genetic diagnosis of pediatric cancer: current and emerging methods. *Pediatric Clinics of North America.* 2002; **49**(6): 1415–1435.

39. **Sen F, Vega F, Medeiros LJ.** Molecular genetic methods in the diagnosis of hematologic neoplasms. *Seminars in Diagnostic Pathology.* 2002; **19**(2):72–93.

40. **Falini B, Bigerna B, Pasqualucci L,** *et al.* Distinctive expression pattern of the BCL-6 protein in nodular lymphocyte predominance Hodgkin's disease. *Blood.* 1996; **87**(2):465–471.

41. **Murphy S.** Classification, staging and end results of treatment of childhood non-Hodgkinn's lymphomas: Dissimilarities from lymphomas in adults. *Seminars in Oncology.* 1980; **7**: 332–338.

42. **Zhang QY, Foucar K.** Bone marrow involvement by Hodgkin and non-Hodgkin lymphomas. *Hematology/Oncology Clinics of North America.* 2009; **23**(4):873–902.

43. **Talaulikar D, Dahlstrom JE.** Staging bone marrow in diffuse large B-cell lymphoma: the role of ancillary investigations. *Pathology.* 2009; **41**(3): 214–222.

44. **Cheson BD.** Staging and evaluation of the patient with lymphoma. *Hematology/Oncology Clinics of North America.* 2008; **22**(5):825–837, vii–viii.

45. **Diebold J, Raphael M, Prevot S, Audouin J.** Burkitt lymphoma. In Jaffe ES, Harris NL, Stein H, Vardiman J, eds. *World Health Organization Classification of Tumours: Pathology and Genetics of Tumours of Haematopoietic and Lymphoid Tissues.* Lyon: IARC Press; 2001, 181–184.

46. **Burkitt D.** A sarcoma involving the jaws in African children. *British Journal of Surgery.* 1958; **46**:218–223.

47. **Magrath I.** Small noncleaved cell lymphomas (Burkitt and Burkitt-like lymphomas). In Magrath I, ed. *The Non-Hodgkin's Lymphomas* (2nd edn.). New York: Arnold; 1997, 781–811.

48. **Brady G, MacArthur GJ, Farrell PG.** Epstein-Barr virus and Burkitt lymphoma. *Journal of Clinical Pathology.* 2007; **60**(12):1397–1402.

49. **Hecht JL, Aster JC.** Molecular biology of Burkitt's lymphoma. *Journal of Clinical Oncology.* 2000; **18**(21):3707–3721.

50. **van Krieken JH.** Lymphoproliferative disease associated with immune deficiency in children. *American Journal of Clinical Pathology.* 2004; **122**(Suppl):S122–S127.

51. The Non-Hodgkin's Lymphoma Pathologic Classification Project. The National Cancer Institute sponsored study of classification of non-Hodgkin's lymphomas: summary and description of working formulation for clinical usage. *Cancer.* 1982; 49:2112–2135.

52. **Harris AC, Todd WM, Hackney MH, Ben-Ezra J.** Bone marrow changes associated with recombinant granulocyte-macrophage and granulocyte colony-stimulating factors. *Archives of Pathology and Laboratory Medicine.* 1994; **118**:624–629.

53. **Jaffe ES, Harris NL, Stein H,** Vardiman JW (eds.). *World Health Organization Classification of Tumours: Pathology and Genetics of Tumours of Haematopoietic and Lymphoid Tissues.* Lyon: IARC Press; 2001.

54. **Kelly D, Nathwani BN, Griffith RC,** *et al.* A morphologic study of childhood lymphoma of the undifferentiated type. The Pediatric Oncology Group experience. *Cancer.* 1987; **59**:1132–1137.

55. **Spina D, Leoncini L, Megha T,** *et al.* Cellular kinetic and phenotypic heterogeneity in and among Burkitt's and Burkitt-like lymphomas. *Journal of Pathology.* 1997; **182**(2):145–150.

56. **Lones MA, Auperin A, Raphael M,** *et al.* Mature B-cell lymphoma/leukemia in children and adolescents: intergroup pathologist consensus with the revised European-American lymphoma classification. *Annals of Oncology.* 2000; **11**(1):47–51.

57. **Lones MA, Raphael M, Perkins SL,** *et al.* Mature B-cell lymphoma in children and adolescents: international group pathologist consensus correlates with histology technical quality. *Journal of Pediatric Hematology/Oncology.* 2006; **28**(9):568–574.

58. **Hutchison RE, Finch C, Kepner J,** *et al.* Burkitt lymphoma is immunophenotypically different from Burkitt-like lymphoma in young persons. *Annals of Oncology.* 2000; **11**(Suppl 1):35–38.

59. **Mann R, Jaffe ES, Braylan RC,** *et al.* Non-edemic Burkitt's lymphoma: a B-cell tumor related to germinal centers. *New England Journal of Medicine.* 1976; **295**:685–691.

60. **Frost M, Newell J, Lones MA,** *et al.* Comparative immunohistochemical analysis of pediatric Burkitt lymphoma and diffuse large B-cell lymphoma. *American Journal of Clinical Pathology.* 2004; **121**:384–392.

61. **Iverson O, Iversen U, Ziegler JL, Bluming AZ.** Cell kinetics in Burkitt's lymphoma. *European Journal of Cancer.* 1974; **10**:1507–1512.

62. **Macpherson N, Lesack D, Klasa R,** *et al.* Small noncleaved, non-Burkitt's (Burkitt-like) lymphoma: cytogenetics predict outcome and reflect clinical presentation. *Journal of Clinical Oncology.* 1999; **17**:1558–1567.

63. **Sanger W.** Primary (8q24) and secondary chromosome abnormalities (1q, 6q, 13q, & 17p) are similar in

pediatric Burkitt lymphoma/Burkitt leukemia & Burkitt-like lymphoma: a report of the International Pediatric B-cell Non-Hodgkin Lymphoma study. *Blood*. 2003;**102**(11):845a.

64. **Heerema NA, Bernheim A, Lim MS,** *et al.* State of the art and future needs in cytogenetic/molecular genetics/arrays in childhood lymphoma: summary report of workshop at the First International Symposium on Childhood and Adolescent non-Hodgkin Lymphoma, April 9, 2003, New York City, NY. *Pediatric Blood and Cancer*. 2005;**45**(5):616–622.

65. **Boerma EG, Siebert R, Kluin PM, Baudis M.** Translocations involving 8q24 in Burkitt lymphoma and other malignant lymphomas: a historical review of cytogenetics in the light of todays knowledge. *Leukemia*. 2009;**23**(2):225–234.

66. **Yustein JT, Dang CV.** Biology and treatment of Burkitt's lymphoma. *Current Opinion in Hematology*. 2007;**14**(4):375–381.

67. **O' Neil J, Look AT.** Mechanisms of transcription factor deregulation in lymphoid cell transformation. *Oncogene*. 2007;**26**(47):6838–6849.

68. **Pelicci PG, Knowles DM, Magrath I, Dalla-Favera R.** Chromosomal breakpoints and structural alterations of the c-myc locus differ in endemic and sporadic forms of Burkitt lymphoma. *Proceedings of the National Academy of Sciences of the United States of America*. 1986;**83**(9):2984–2988.

69. **Haralambieva E, Banham AH, Bastard C,** *et al.* Detection by the fluorescence in situ hybridization technique of MYC translocations in paraffin-embedded lymphoma biopsy samples. *British Journal of Haematology*. 2003;**121**(1):49–56.

70. **Garcia JL, Hernandez JM, Gutiérrez NC,** *et al.* Abnormalities on 1q and 7q are associated with poor outcome in sporadic Burkitt's lymphoma. A cytogenetic and comparative genomic hybridization study. *Leukemia*. 2003;**17**(10):2016–2024.

71. **Lones MA, Sanger WG, LeBeau MM,** *et al.* Chromosome abnormalities may correlate with prognosis in Burkitt/Burkitt-like lymphomas of children and adolescents. *Journal of Pediatric Hematology/Oncology*. 2004;**26**(3):169–178.

72. **Jaffe ES, Harris NL, Stein H,** Vardiman JW (eds.). *World Health Organization Classification of Tumours: Pathology and Genetics of Tumours of Haematopoietic and Lymphoid Tissues*. Lyon: IARC Press; 2001.

73. **Dang CV.** c-Myc target genes involved in cell growth, apoptosis, and metabolism. *Molecular and Cellular Biology*. 1999;**19**(1):1–11.

74. **Gartel AL, Shchors K.** Mechanisms of c-myc-mediated transcriptional repression of growth arrest genes. *Experimental Cell Research*. 2003;**283**(1):17–21.

75. **Packham G, Cleveland JL.** c-Myc and apoptosis. *Biochimica et Biophysica Acta*. 1995;**1242**(1):11–28.

76. **Wierstra I, Alves J.** The c-myc promoter: still MysterY and Challenge. *Advances in Cancer Research*. 2008;**99**:113–333.

77. **Eilers M, Schirm S, Bishop JM.** The MYC protein activates transcription of the alpha-prothymosin gene. *EMBO Journal*. 1991;**10**(1):133–141.

78. **Askew DS, Ashmun RA, Simmons BC, Cleveland JL.** Constitutive c-myc expression in an IL-3-dependent myeloid cell line suppresses cell cycle arrest and accelerates apoptosis. *Oncogene*. 1991;**6**(10):1915–1922.

79. **Evan GI, Wyllie AH, Gilbert CS,** *et al.* Induction of apoptosis in fibroblasts by c-myc protein. *Cell*. 1992;**69**(1):119–128.

80. **Langdon WY, Harris AW, Cory S, Adams JM.** The c-myc oncogene perturbs B lymphocyte development in E-mu-myc transgenic mice. *Cell*. 1986;**47**(1):11–18.

81. **Adams JA, Barrett AJ.** Haematopoietic stimulators in the serum of patients with severe aplastic anaemia. *British Journal of Haematology*. 1982;**52**:327–335.

82. **Hayashi Y.** The molecular genetics of recurring chromosome abnormalities in acute myeloid leukemia. *Seminars in Hematology*. 2000;**37**(4):368–380.

83. **Shim H, Dolde C, Lewis BC,** *et al.* c-Myc transactivation of LDH-A: implications for tumor metabolism and growth. *Proceedings of the National Academy of Sciences of the United States of America*. 1997;**94**(13):6658–6663.

84. **Wick M, Zubov D, Hagen G.** Genomic organization and promoter characterization of the gene encoding the human telomerase reverse transcriptase (hTERT). *Gene*. 1999;**232**(1):97–106.

85. **Martin-Subero JI, Kreuz M, Bibikova M,** *et al.* New insights into the biology and origin of mature aggressive B-cell lymphomas by combined epigenomic, genomic, and transcriptional profiling. *Blood*. 2009;**113**(11):2488–2497.

86. **Dave SS, Fu K, Wright GW,** *et al.* Molecular diagnosis of Burkitt's lymphoma. *New England Journal of Medicine*. 2006;**354**(23):2431–2442.

87. **Hummel M, Bentink S, Berger H,** *et al.* A biologic definition of Burkitt's lymphoma from transcriptional and genomic profiling. *New England Journal of Medicine*. 2006;**354**(23):2419–2430.

88. **Young L, Alfieri C, Hennessy K,** *et al.* Expression of Epstein-Barr virus transformation-associated genes in tissues of patients with EBV lymphoproliferative disease. *New England Journal of Medicine*. 1989;**321**(16):1080–1085.

89. **Lyons SF, Liebowitz DN.** The roles of human viruses in the pathogenesis of lymphoma. *Seminars in Oncology*. 1998;**25**(4):461–475.

90. **Bornkamm GW.** Epstein-Barr virus and the pathogenesis of Burkitt's lymphoma: more questions than answers. *International Journal of Cancer*. 2009;**124**(8):1745–1755.

91. **Wilson JB, Bell JL, Levine AJ.** Expression of Epstein-Barr virus nuclear antigen-1 induces B cell neoplasia in transgenic mice. *EMBO Journal*. 1996;**15**(12):3117–3126.

92. **Komano J, Maruo S, Kurozumi K, Oda T, Takada K.** Oncogenic role of Epstein-Barr virus-encoded RNAs in Burkitt's lymphoma cell line Akata. *Journal of Virology*. 1999;**73**(12):9827–9831.

93. **Preciado MV, Fallo A, Chabay P, Calcagno L, De Matteo E.** Epstein Barr virus-associated lymphoma in HIV-infected children. *Pathology, Research and Practice*. 2002;**98**(5):327–332.

94. **Cairo MS.** Current advances and future strategies of B large cell lymphoma in children and adolescents. *Proceedings of the American Society of Oncology*. 2002;**21**:512–519.

95. **Ferry JA.** Extranodal lymphoma. *Archives of Pathology and Laboratory Medicine*. 2008;**132**(4):565–578.

96. **Hunt KE, Reichard KK.** Diffuse large B-cell lymphoma. *Archives of Pathology and Laboratory Medicine.* 2008;**132**(1): 118–124.

97. **Friedberg JW, Fisher RI.** Diffuse large B-cell lymphoma. *Hematology/ Oncology Clinics of North America.* 2008;**22**(5):941–952, ix.

98. **El Weshi A, Akhtar S, Mourad WA,** *et al.* T-cell/histiocyte-rich B-cell lymphoma: Clinical presentation, management and prognostic factors: report on 61 patients and review of literature. *Leukemia and Lymphoma.* 2007;**48**(9):1764–1773.

99. **Gurbuxani S, Anastasi J, Hyjek E.** Diffuse large B-cell lymphoma–more than a diffuse collection of large B cells: an entity in search of a meaningful classification. *Archives of Pathology and Laboratory Medicine.* 2009;**133**(7): 1121–1134.

100. **Rodriguez J, Gutierrez A, Piris M.** Primary mediastinal B-cell lymphoma: treatment and therapeutic targets. *Leukemia and Lymphoma.* 2008; **49**(6):1050–1061.

101. **Boleti E, Johnson PW.** Primary mediastinal B-cell lymphoma. *Hematological Oncology.* 2007; **25**(4):157–163.

102. **Martelli M, Ferreri AJ, Johnson P.** Primary mediastinal large B-cell lymphoma. *Critical Reviews in Oncology/Hematology.* 2008;**68**(3): 256–263.

103. **Chadburn A, Frizzera G.** Mediastinal large B-cell lymphoma versus classic Hodgkin lymphoma. *American Journal of Clinical Pathology.* 1999;**112**:155–158.

104. **Savage KJ.** Primary mediastinal large B-cell lymphoma. *Oncologist.* 2006; **11**(5):488–495.

105. **Higgin JP, Warnke RA.** CD30 expression is common in mediastinal large B-cell lymphoma. *American Journal of Clinical Pathology.* 1999; **112**:241–247.

106. **Browne P, Petrosyan K, Hernandez A, Chan JA.** The B-cell transcription factors BSAP, Oct-2, and BOB.1 and the pan-B-cell markers CD20, CD22, and CD79a are useful in the differential diagnosis of classic Hodgkin lymphoma. *American Journal of Clinical Pathology.* 2003;**120**(5):767–777.

107. **Watanabe K, Yamashita Y, Nakayama A,** *et al.* Varied B-cell immunophenotypes of Hodgkin/Reed-Sternberg cells in classic Hodgkin's disease. *Histopathology.* 2000;**36**(4): 353–361.

108. **Elgin J, Phillips JG, Reddy VV, Gibbs PO, Listinsky CM.** Hodgkin's and non-Hodgkin's lymphoma: spectrum of morphologic and immunophenotypic overlap. *Annals of Diagnostic Pathology.* 1999;**3**(5):263–275.

109. **Oschlies I, Klapper W, Zimmermann M,** *et al.* Diffuse large B-cell lymphoma in pediatric patients belongs predominantly to the germinal-center type B-cell lymphomas: a clinicopathologic analysis of cases included in the German BFM (Berlin-Frankfurt-Munster) multicenter trial. *Blood.* 2006; **107**(10):4047–4052.

110. **Heerema N, Poirel H, Swansbury J,** *et al.* Chromosomal abnormalities of pediatric (ped) and adult diffuse large B-cell lymphoma (DLBCL) differ and may reflect potential differences in oncogenesis. An international pediatric mature B-cell non-Hodgkin lymphoma study (FAB/LMB96). *Blood.* 2003;**102**: 3139.

111. **Nanjangud G, Rao PH, Hegde A,** *et al.* Spectral karyotyping identifies new rearrangements, translocations, and clinical associations in diffuse large B-cell lymphoma. *Blood.* 2002;**99**(7): 2554–2561.

112. **Tibiletti MG, Martin V, Bernasconi B,** *et al.* BCL2, BCL6, MYC, MALT 1, and BCL10 rearrangements in nodal diffuse large B-cell lymphomas: a multicenter evaluation of a new set of fluorescent in situ hybridization probes and correlation with clinical outcome. *Human Pathology.* 2009;**40**(5):645–652.

113. **Tzankov A, Schneider A, Hoeller S, Dirnhofer S.** Prognostic importance of BCL6 rearrangements in diffuse large B-cell lymphoma with respect to Bcl6 protein levels and primary lymphoma site. *Human Pathology.* 2009;**40**(7): 1055–1056.

114. **Morton LM, Purdue MP, Zheng T,** *et al.* Risk of non-Hodgkin lymphoma associated with germline variation in genes that regulate the cell cycle, apoptosis, and lymphocyte development. *Cancer Epidemiology Biomarkers and Prevention.* 2009;**18**(4): 1259–1270.

115. **Flenghi L, Ye BH, Fizzotti M,** *et al.* A specific monoclonal antibody (PG-B6) detects expression of the BCL-6 protein in germinal center B cells. *American Journal of Pathology.* 1995;**147**(2):405–411.

116. **Saito M, Novak U, Piovan E,** *et al.* BCL6 suppression of BCL2 via Miz1 and its disruption in diffuse large B cell lymphoma. *Proceedings of the National Academy of Sciences of the United States of America.* 2009;**106**(27):11294–11299.

117. **Ci W, Polo JM, Cerchietti L,** *et al.* The BCL6 transcriptional program features repression of multiple oncogenes in primary B cells and is deregulated in DLBCL. *Blood.* 2009;**113**(22):5536–5548.

118. **Perez-Rosado A, Artiga M, Vargiu P,** *et al.* BCL6 represses NFkappaB activity in diffuse large B-cell lymphomas. *Journal of Pathology.* 2008;**214**(4): 498–507.

119. **Parekh S, Polo JM, Shaknovich R,** *et al.* BCL6 programs lymphoma cells for survival and differentiation through distinct biochemical mechanisms. *Blood.* 2007;**110**(6):2067–2074.

120. **Jardin F, Ruminy P, Kerckaert JP,** *et al.* Detection of somatic quantitative genetic alterations by multiplex polymerase chain reaction for the prediction of outcome in diffuse large B-cell lymphomas. *Haematologica.* 2008;**93**(4):543–550.

121. **Iqbal J, Greiner TC, Patel K,** *et al.* Distinctive patterns of BCL6 molecular alterations and their functional consequences in different subgroups of diffuse large B-cell lymphoma. *Leukemia.* 2007;**21**(11):2332–2343.

122. **Bernicot I, Douet-Guilbert N, Le Bris MJ,** *et al.* Molecular cytogenetics of IGH rearrangements in non-Hodgkin B-cell lymphoma. *Cytogenetic and Genome Research.* 2007;**118**(2-4):345–352.

123. **Dalla-Favera R, Ye BH, Cattoretti G,** *et al.* BCL-6 in diffuse large-cell lymphomas. *Important Advances in Oncology.* 1996:139–148.

124. **Veelken H, Vik Dannheim S, Schulte Moenting J,** *et al.* Immunophenotype as prognostic factor for diffuse large B-cell lymphoma in patients undergoing clinical risk-adapted therapy. *Annals of Oncology.* 2007;**18**(5):931–939.

125. **van Imhoff GW, Boerma EJ, van der Holt B,** *et al.* Prognostic impact of

germinal center-associated proteins and chromosomal breakpoints in poor-risk diffuse large B-cell lymphoma. *Journal of Clinical Oncology.* 2006;**24**(25):4135–4142.

126. **Rodig SJ, Savage KJ, LaCasce AS,** *et al.* Expression of TRAF1 and nuclear c-Rel distinguishes primary mediastinal large cell lymphoma from other types of diffuse large B-cell lymphoma. *American Journal of Surgical Pathology.* 2007;**31**(1):106–112.

127. **van Besien K, Kelta M, Bahaguna P.** Primary mediastinal B-cell lymphoma: a review of pathology and management. *Journal of Clinical Oncology.* 2001; **19**(6):1855–1864.

128. **Weniger MA, Gesk S, Ehrlich S,** *et al.* Gains of REL in primary mediastinal B-cell lymphoma coincide with nuclear accumulation of REL protein. *Genes, Chromosomes and Cancer.* 2007;**46**(4): 406–415.

129. **Calvo KR, Traverse-Glehen A, Pittaluga S, Jaffe ES.** Molecular profiling provides evidence of primary mediastinal large B-cell lymphoma as a distinct entity related to classic Hodgkin lymphoma: implications for mediastinal gray zone lymphomas as an intermediate form of B-cell lymphoma. *Advances in Anatomic Pathology.* 2004; **11**(5):227–238.

130. **Marafioti T, Pozzobon M, Hansmann ML,** *et al.* Expression pattern of intracellular leukocyte-associated proteins in primary mediastinal B cell lymphoma. *Leukemia.* 2005;**19**(5): 856–861.

131. **Pileri SA, Dirnhofer S, Went P,** *et al.* Diffuse large B-cell lymphoma: one or more entities? Present controversies and possible tools for its subclassification. *Histopathology.* 2002;**41**(6):482–509.

132. **Alizadeh AA, Eisen MB, Davis RE,** *et al.* Distinct types of diffuse large B-cell lymphoma identified by gene expression profiling. *Nature* 2000;**403** (6769):503–511.

133. **Rosenwald A, Wright G, Chan WC,** *et al.* The use of molecular profiling to predict survival after chemotherapy for diffuse large-B-cell lymphoma. *New England Journal of Medicine.* 2002;**346** (25):1937–1947.

134. **Shipp MA, Ross KN, Tamayo P,** *et al.* Diffuse large B-cell lymphoma outcome prediction by gene-expression profiling

and supervised machine learning. *Nature Medicine.* 2002;**8**(1):68–74.

135. **Lenz G, Wright GW, Emre NC,** *et al.* Molecular subtypes of diffuse large B-cell lymphoma arise by distinct genetic pathways. *Proceedings of the National Academy of Sciences of the United States of America.* 2008;**105**(36): 13520–13525.

136. **Leich E, Hartmann EM, Burek C, Ott G, Rosenwald A.** Diagnostic and prognostic significance of gene expression profiling in lymphomas. *Acta Pathologica, Microbiologica et Immunologica Scandinavica.* 2007; **115**(10):1135–1146.

137. **Lossos IS, Alizadeh AA, Eisen MB,** *et al.* Ongoing immunoglobulin somatic mutation in germinal center B cell-like but not in activated B cell-like diffuse large cell lymphomas. *Proceedings of the National Academy of Sciences of the United States of America.* 2000;**97**(18):10209–10213.

138. **Huang JZ, Sanger WG, Greiner TC,** *et al.* The t(14;18) defines a unique subset of diffuse large B-cell lymphoma with a germinal center B-cell gene expression profile. *Blood.* 2002;**99**(7): 2285–2290.

139. **Davis RE, Brown KD, Siebenlist U, Staudt LM.** Constitutive nuclear factor kappaB activity is required for survival of activated B cell-like diffuse large B cell lymphoma cells. *Journal of Experimental Medicine.* 2001;**194**(12): 1861–1874.

140. **Hans CP, Weisenburger DD, Greiner TC,** *et al.* Confirmation of the molecular classification of diffuse large B-cell lymphoma by immunohisto-chemistry using a tissue microarray. *Blood.* 2004;**103**(1):275–282.

141. **Chang CC, McClintock S, Cleveland RP,** *et al.* Immunohistochemical expression patterns of germinal center and activation B-cell markers correlate with prognosis in diffuse large B-cell lymphoma. *American Journal of Surgical Pathology.* 2004;**28**(4):464–470.

142. **Haarer CF, Roberts RA, Frutiger YM, Grogan TM, Rimsza LM.** Immunohistochemical classification of de novo, transformed, and relapsed diffuse large B-cell lymphoma into germinal center B-cell and nongerminal center B-cell subtypes correlates with gene expression profile and patient survival. *Archives of*

Pathology and Laboratory Medicine. 2006;**130**(12):1819–1824.

143. **Brusamolino E, Rusconi C, Montalbetti L,** *et al.* Dose-dense R-CHOP-14 supported by pegfilgrastim in patients with diffuse large B-cell lymphoma: a phase II study of feasibility and toxicity. *Haematologica.* 2006;**91**(4):496–502.

144. **Coiffier B.** Treatment of diffuse large B-cell lymphoma. *Current Hematology Reports.* 2005;**4**(1):7–14.

145. **Attias D, Hodgson D, Weitzman S.** Primary mediastinal B-cell lymphoma in the pediatric patient: Can a rational approach to therapy be based on adult studies? *Pediatric Blood and Cancer.* 2009;**52**(5):566–570.

146. **Ribeiro R, Pui CH, Murphy SB,** *et al.* Childhood malignant non-Hodgkin's lymphomas of uncommon histology. *Leukemia.* 1992;**6**:761–765.

147. **Pakzad K, MacLennan GT, Elder JS,** *et al.* Follicular large cell lymphoma localized to the testis in children. *Journal of Urology.* 2002;**168**(1):225–228.

148. **Finn LS, Viswanatha DS, Belasco JB,** *et al.* Primary follicular lymphoma of the testis in childhood. *Cancer.* 1999; **85**(7):1626–1635.

149. **Pinto A, Hutchison RE, Grant LH, Trevenen CL, Berard CW.** Follicular lymphomas in pediatric patients. *Modern Pathology.* 1990;**3**(3):308–313.

150. **Winberg CD, Nathwani BN, Bearman RM, Rappaport H.** Follicular (nodular) lymphoma during the first two decades of life: a clinicopathologic study of 12 patients. *Cancer.* 1981;**48**(10):2223–2235.

151. **Agrawal R, Wang J.** Pediatric follicular lymphoma: a rare clinicopathologic entity. *Archives of Pathology and Laboratory Medicine.* 2009;**133**(1): 142–146.

152. **Nathwani BN, Winberg CD, Diamond LW, Bearman RM, Kim H.** Morphologic criteria for the differentiation of follicular lymphoma from florid reactive follicular hyperplasia: a study of 80 cases. *Cancer.* 1981;**48**(8):1794–1806.

153. **Nathwani B, Diamond LW, Winberg CD,** *et al.* Lymphoblastic lymphoma: a clinicopathologic study of 95 patients. *Cancer.* 1981;**48**:2347–2357.

154. **Swerdlow SH**. Small B-cell lymphomas of the lymph nodes and spleen: practical insights to diagnosis and pathogenesis. *Modern Pathology*. 1999; **12**(2):125–140.

155. **Good DJ, Gascoyne RD**. Atypical lymphoid hyperplasia mimicking lymphoma. *Hematology/Oncology Clinics of North America*. 2009;**23**(4): 729–745.

156. **Chan JK, Ng CS, Hui PK**. An unusual morphological variant of follicular lymphoma. Report of two cases. *Histopathology*. 1988;**12**(6):649–658.

157. **Goates JJ, Kamel OW, LeBrun DP, Benharroch D, Dorfman RF**. Floral variant of follicular lymphoma. Immunological and molecular studies support a neoplastic process. *American Journal of Surgical Pathology*. 1994; **18**(1):37–47.

158. **Kurtin PJ**. Indolent lymphomas of mature B lymphocytes. *Hematology/Oncology Clinics of North America*. 2009;**23**(4):769–790.

159. **Metter GE, Nathwani BN, Burke JS, *et al*.** Morphological subclassification of follicular lymphoma: variability of diagnoses among hematopathologists, a collaborative study between the Repository Center and Pathology Panel for Lymphoma Clinical Studies. *Journal of Clinical Oncology*. 1985;**3**(1):25–38.

160. **Martin AR, Weisenburger DD, Chan WC, *et al*.** Prognostic value of cellular proliferation and histologic grade in follicular lymphoma. *Blood*. 1995; **85**(12):3671–3678.

161. **Vitolo U, Ferreri AJ, Montoto S**. Follicular lymphomas. *Critical Reviews in Oncology/Hematology*. 2008;**66**(3): 248–261.

162. **Martinez AE, Lin L, Dunphy CH**. Grading of follicular lymphoma: comparison of routine histology with immunohistochemistry. *Archives of Pathology and Laboratory Medicine*. 2007;**131**(7):1084–1088.

163. **Ashton-Key M, Diss TC, Isaacson PG, Smith ME**. A comparative study of the value of immunohistochemistry and the polymerase chain reaction in the diagnosis of follicular lymphoma. *Histopathology*. 1995;**27**(6):501–508.

164. **Tan LH**. A practical approach to the understanding and diagnosis of lymphoma: an assessment of the WHO classification based on immunoarchitecture and immuno-ontogenic principles. *Pathology*. 2009;**41**(4):305–326.

165. **Jack A, Barrans S, Blythe D, Rawstron A**. Demonstration of a germinal center immunophenotype in lymphomas by immunocytochemistry and flow cytometry. *Methods in Molecular Medicine*. 2005;**115**:65–91.

166. **Dogan A, Bagdi E, Munson P, Isaacson PG**. CD10 and BCL-6 expression in paraffin sections of normal lymphoid tissue and B-cell lymphomas. *American Journal of Surgical Pathology*. 2000;**24**(6):846–852.

167. **Olejniczak SH, Stewart CC, Donohue K, Czuczman MS**. A quantitative exploration of surface antigen expression in common B-cell malignancies using flow cytometry. *Immunological Investigations*. 2006; **35**(1):93–114.

168. **Nam-Cha SH, San-Millán B, Mollejo M, *et al*.** Light-chain-restricted germinal centres in reactive lymphadenitis: report of eight cases. *Histopathology*. 2008;**52**(4):436–444.

169. **Kussick SJ, Kalnoski M, Braziel RM, Wood BL**. Prominent clonal B-cell populations identified by flow cytometry in histologically reactive lymphoid proliferations. *American Journal of Clinical Pathology*. 2004; **121**(4):464–472.

170. **Bryant RJ, Banks PM, O'Malley DP**. Ki67 staining pattern as a diagnostic tool in the evaluation of lymphoproliferative disorders. *Histopathology*. 2006;**48**(5):505–515.

171. **Cory S, Adams JM**. Killing cancer cells by flipping the Bcl-2/Bax switch. *Cancer Cell*. 2005;**8**(1):5–6.

172. **Bacon CM, Du MQ, Dogan A**. Mucosa-associated lymphoid tissue (MALT) lymphoma: a practical guide for pathologists. *Journal of Clinical Pathology*. 2007;**60**(4):361–372.

173. **Peinert S, Seymour JF**. Indolent lymphomas other than follicular and marginal zone lymphomas. *Hematology/Oncology Clinics of North America*. 2008;**22**(5):903–940, viii.

174. **Zucca E, Bertoni F, Stathis A, *et al*.** Marginal zone lymphomas. *Hematology/Oncology Clinics of North America*. 2008;**22**(5):883–901, viii.

175. **Claviez A, Meyer U, Dominick C, *et al*.** MALT lymphoma in children: a report from the NHL-BFM Study Group. *Pediatric Blood and Cancer*. 2006;**47**(2): 210–214.

176. **Taddesse-Heath L, Pittaluga S, Sorbara L, *et al*.** Marginal zone B-cell lymphoma in children and young adults. *American Journal of Surgical Pathology*. 2003;**27**(4):522–531.

177. **Aghamohammadi A, Parvaneh N, Tirgari F, *et al*.** Lymphoma of mucosa-associated lymphoid tissue in common variable immunodeficiency. *Leukemia and Lymphoma*. 2006;**47**(2): 343–346.

178. **Tiemann M, Häring S, Heidemann M, Reichelt J, Claviez A**. Mucosa-associated lymphoid tissue lymphoma in the conjunctiva of a child. *Virchows Archiv*. 2004;**444**(2):198–201.

179. **Mo JQ, Dimashkieh H, Mallery SR, Swerdlow SH, Bove KE**. MALT lymphoma in children: Case report and review of the literature. *Pediatric and Developmental Pathology*. 2004; **7**(4):407–413.

180. **Liang X, Stork LC, Albano EA**. Primary ocular adnexal lymphoma in pediatric patients: report of two cases and review of the literature. *Pediatric and Developmental Pathology*. 2003; **6**(5):458–463.

181. **Sharon V, Mecca PS, Steinherz PG, Trippett TM, Myskowski PL**. Two pediatric cases of primary cutaneous B-cell lymphoma and review of the literature. *Pediatric Dermatology*. 2009; **26**(1):34–39.

182. **Ryu M, Han S, Che Z, *et al*.** Pediatric mucosa-associated lymphoid tissue (MALT) lymphoma of lip: a case report and literature review. *Oral surgery, Oral Medicine, Oral Pathology, Oral Radiology and Endodontics*. 2009; **107**(3):393–397.

183. **Dargent JL, Ferster A, Andry G, *et al*.** Marginal zone B-cell lymphoma of the sinonasal tract in an eleven-year-old girl. *Medical and Pediatric Oncology*. 2003;**40**(6):393–395.

184. **Sroa N, Magro CM**. Pediatric primary cutaneous marginal zone lymphoma: in association with chronic antihistamine use. *Journal of Cutaneous Pathology*. 2006;**33**(Suppl) 2:1–5.

185. **Dargent JL, Devalck C, De Mey A, *et al*.** Primary cutaneous marginal zone B-cell lymphoma of MALT type in a child. *Pediatric and Developmental Pathology*. 2006;**9**(6):468–473.

186. **Arcaini L, Lucioni M, Boveri E, Paulli M**. Nodal marginal zone lymphoma: current knowledge and future directions of an heterogeneous disease. *European Journal of Haematology.* 2009;**83**(3):165–174.

187. **Spencer J, Finn T, Pulford KA, Mason DY, Isaacson PG**. The human gut contains a novel population of B lymphocytes which resemble marginal zone cells. *Clinical and Experimental Immunology.* 1985;**62**(3):607–612.

188. **Dierlamm J, Pittaluga S, Wlodarska I,** *et al.* Marginal zone B-cell lymphomas of different sites share similar cytogenetic and morphologic features. *Blood.* 1996;**87**(1):299–307.

189. **Jaffe ES, Harris NL, Stein H, Isaacson PG**. Classification of lymphoid neoplasms: the microscope as a tool for disease discovery. *Blood.* 2008;**112**(12): 4384–4399.

190. **Roulland S, Suarez F, Hermine O, Nadel B**. Pathophysiological aspects of memory B-cell development. *Trends in Immunology.* 2008;**29**(1):25–33.

191. **Shaye OS, Levine AM**. Marginal zone lymphoma. *Journal of the National Comprehensive Cancer Network.* 2006; **4**(3):311–318.

192. **Wotherspoon AC, Ortiz-Hidalgo C, Falzon MR, Isaacson PG**. *Helicobacter pylori*-associated gastritis and primary B-cell gastric lymphoma. *Lancet.* 1991; **338**(8776):1175–1176.

193. **Thieblemont C**. Non-MALT marginal zone lymphomas. *Annals of Oncology.* 2008;**19**(Suppl 4):iv70–73.

194. **Ghesquières H, Berger F, Felman P,** *et al.* Clinicopathologic characteristics and outcome of diffuse large B-cell lymphomas presenting with an associated low-grade component at diagnosis. *Journal of Clinical Oncology.* 2006;**24**(33):5234–5241.

195. **Landgren O, Tilly H**. Epidemiology, pathology and treatment of non-follicular indolent lymphomas. *Leukemia and Lymphoma.* 2008; **49**(Suppl 1):35–42.

196. **Attygalle AD, Liu H, Shirali S,** *et al.* Atypical marginal zone hyperplasia of mucosa-associated lymphoid tissue: a reactive condition of childhood showing immunoglobulin lambda light-chain restriction. *Blood.* 2004; **104**(10):3343–3348.

197. **Lynch EF, Jones PA, Swerdlow SH**. CD43 and CD5 antibodies define four normal and neoplastic B-cell subsets: a three-color flow cytometric study. *Cytometry.* 1995;**22**(3):223–231.

198. **Du MQ**. MALT lymphoma: recent advances in aetiology and molecular genetics. *Journal of Clinical and Experimental Hematopathology.* 2007;**47**(2):31–42.

199. **Farinha P, Gascoyne RD**. Molecular pathogenesis of mucosa-associated lymphoid tissue lymphoma. *Journal of Clinical Oncology.* 2005;**23**(26): 6370–6378.

200. **Inamdar KV, Bueso-Ramos CE**. Pathology of chronic lymphocytic leukemia: an update. *Annals of Diagnostic Pathology.* 2007;**11**(5): 363–389.

201. **Zent CS, Kay NE**. Chronic lymphocytic leukemia: biology and current treatment. *Current Oncology Reports.* 2007;**9**(5):345–352.

202. **Smock K, Yaish HM, Cairo MS,** *et al.* Mantle cell lymphoma presenting with unusual morphology in an adolescent female: A case report and review of the literature. *Pediatric and Developmental Pathology,* 2007;**10** (5):403–408.

203. **Bertoni F, Zucca E, Cavalli F**. Mantle cell lymphoma. *Current Opinion in Hematology.* 2004;**11**(6):411–418.

204. **Ghielmini M, Zucca E**. How I treat mantle cell lymphoma. *Blood.* 2009; **114**(8):1469–1476.

205. **Schmidt C, Dreyling M**. Therapy of mantle cell lymphoma: current standards and future strategies. *Hematology/Oncology Clinics of North America.* 2008;**22**(5):953–963, ix.

206. **Smith MR**. Mantle cell lymphoma: advances in biology and therapy. *Current Opinion in Hematology.* 2008; **15**(4):415–421.

207. **Dumesnil C, Schneider P, Dolgopolov I,** *et al.* Solitary bone plasmocytoma of the spine in an adolescent. *Pediatric Blood and Cancer.* 2006;**47**(3):335–338.

208. **Bertoni-Salateo R, de Camargo B, Soares F, Chojniak R, Penna V**. Solitary plasmocytoma of bone in an adolescent. *Journal of Pediatric Hematology/Oncology.* 1998;**20**(6): 574–576.

209. **Mann G, Trebo MM, Minkov M,** *et al.* Extramedullary plasmacytoma of the adenoids. *Pediatric Blood and Cancer.* 2007;**48**(3):361–362.

210. **Dannenberg C, Haupt R, Mantovani L, Skuballa A, Körholz D**. Primary high-grade non-Hodgkin lymphoma of the trachea in an adolescent. *Pediatric Hematological Oncology.* 2003;**20**(5): 399–402.

211. **Rawal A, Finn WG, Schnitzer B, Valdez R**. Site-specific morphologic differences in extranodal marginal zone B-cell lymphomas. *Archives of Pathology and Laboratory Medicine.* 2007;**131**(11):1673–1678.

212. **Tcheng WY, Said J, Hall T,** *et al.* Post-transplant multiple myeloma in a pediatric renal transplant patient. *Pediatric Blood and Cancer.* 2006; **47**(2):218–223.

213. **Gitelson E, Al-Saleem T, Smith MR**. Review: lymphomatoid granulomatosis: challenges in diagnosis and treatment. *Clinical Advances in Hematology and Oncology.* 2009;**7**(1):68–70.

214. **Kendi AT, McKinney AM, Clark HB, Kieffer SA**. A pediatric case of low-grade lymphomatoid granulomatosis presenting with a cerebellar mass. *American Journal of Neuroradiology.* 2007;**28**(9):1803–1805.

215. **Rezk SA, Weiss LM**. Epstein-Barr virus-associated lymphoproliferative disorders. *Human Pathology.* 2007; **38**(9):1293–1304.

216. **Mazzie JP, Price AP, Khullar P,** *et al.* Lymphomatoid granulomatosis in a pediatric patient. *Clinical Imaging.* 2004;**28**(3):209–213.

217. **Hareema A**. Lymphomatoid granulomatosis: unusual presentation in a pediatric patient. *Pediatric and Developmental Pathology.* 2003;**6**(2): 106–107.

218. **Oren H, Irken G, Kargi A,** *et al.* A pediatric case of lymphomatoid granulomatosis with onset after completion of chemotherapy for acute myeloid leukemia. *Journal of Pediatric Hematology/Oncology.* 2003;**25**(2): 163–166.

219. **Erdur B, Yilmaz S, Oren H,** *et al.* Evaluating pulmonary complications in childhood acute leukemias. *Journal of Pediatric Hematology/Oncology.* 2008; **30**(7):522–526.

220. **Hu X, Selbs E, Drexler S**. An 18-year-old man with persistent cough and bilateral lower lung infiltration. Epstein-Barr virus-positive lymphoproliferative disorder consistent with lymphomatoid granulomatosis.

Archives of Pathology and Laboratory Medicine. 2006;**130**(3):e44–e46.

221. **Lee JS, Tuder R, Lynch DA.** Lymphomatoid granulomatosis: radiologic features and pathologic correlations. *American Journal of Roentgenology*. 2000;**175**(5):1335–1339.

222. **Lehman TJ, Church JA, Isaacs H.** Lymphomatoid granulomatosis in a 13-month-old infant. *Journal of Roentgenology*. 1989;**16**(2):235–238.

223. **Moertel CL, Carlson-Green B, Watterson J, Simonton SC.** Lymphomatoid granulomatosis after childhood acute lymphoblastic leukemia: report of effective therapy. *Pediatrics*. 2001;**107**(5):E82.

224. **Sebire NJ, Haselden S, Malone M, Davies EG, Ramsay AD.** Isolated EBV lymphoproliferative disease in a child with Wiskott-Aldrich syndrome manifesting as cutaneous lymphomatoid granulomatosis and responsive to anti-CD20 immunotherapy. *Journal of Clinical Pathology*. 2003;**56**(7):555–557.

225. **Karnak I, Ciftci AO, Talim B, Kale G, Senocak ME.** Pulmonary lymphomatoid granulomatosis in a 4 year old. *Journal of Pediatric Surgery*. 1999;**34**(6):1033–1035.

226. **LeSueur BW, Ellsworth L, Bangert JL, Hansen RC.** Lymphomatoid granulomatosis in a 4-year-old boy. *Pediatric Dermatology*. 2000;**17**(5):369–372.

227. **Kleinschmidt-DeMasters BK, Filley CM, Bitter MA.** Central nervous system angiocentric, angiodestructive T-cell lymphoma (lymphomatoid granulomatosis). *Surgical Neurology*. 1992;**37**(2):130–137.

228. **Drut R, Drut RM.** Angiocentric immunoproliferative lesion and angiocentric lymphoma of lymph node in children. A report of two cases. *Journal of Clinical Pathology*. 2005;**58**(5):550–552.

229. **Hu YH, Liu CY, Chiu CH, Hsiao LT.** Successful treatment of elderly advanced lymphomatoid granulomatosis with rituximab-CVP combination therapy. *European Journal of Haematology*. 2007;**78**(2):176–177.

230. **Hasserjian RP, Ott G, Elenitoba-Johnson KS,** *et al.* Commentary on the WHO classification of tumors of lymphoid tissues (2008): "Gray zone" lymphomas overlapping with Burkitt lymphoma or classical Hodgkin lymphoma. *Journal of Hematopathology*. 2009; 2(2):89–95.

231. **Traverse-Glehen A, Pittaluga S, Gaulard P,** *et al.* Mediastinal gray zone lymphoma: the missing link between classic Hodgkin's lymphoma and mediastinal large B-cell lymphoma. *American Journal of Surgical Pathology*. 2005;**29**(11):1411–1421.

232. **Dogan A.** Gray zone lymphomas. *Hematology*. 2005;**10**(Suppl 1):190–192.

233. **Haralambieva E, Boerma EJ, van Imhoff GW,** *et al.* Clinical, immunophenotypic, and genetic analysis of adult lymphomas with morphologic features of Burkitt lymphoma. *American Journal of Surgical Pathology*. 2005;**29**(8):1086–1094.

234. **Rodig SJ, Vergilio JA, Shahsafaei A, Dorfman DM.** Characteristic expression patterns of TCL1, CD38, and CD44 identify aggressive lymphomas harboring a MYC translocation. *American Journal of Surgical Pathology*. 2008;**32**(1):113–122.

235. **Dunphy C, Tang W.** Usefulness of routine conventional cytogenetic analysis in tissues submitted for "lymphoma work-up". *Leukemia and Lymphoma*. 2008;**49**(1):75–80.

236. **Zhao XF, Hassan A, Perry A,** *et al.* C-MYC rearrangements are frequent in aggressive mature B-cell lymphoma with atypical morphology. *International Journal of Clinical and Experimental Pathology*. 2008;**1**(1):65–74.

237. **McClure RF, Remstein ED, Macon WR,** *et al.* Adult B-cell lymphomas with Burkitt-like morphology are phenotypically and genotypically heterogeneous with aggressive clinical behavior. *American Journal of Surgical Pathology*. 2005;**29**(12):1652–1660.

238. **Kanungo A, Medeiros LJ, Abruzzo LV, Lin P.** Lymphoid neoplasms associated with concurrent t(14;18) and 8q24/c-MYC translocation generally have a poor prognosis. *Modern Pathology*. 2006;**19**(1):25–33.

239. **Waite E, Laraque D.** Pediatric organ transplant patients and long-term care: a review. *The Mount Sinai Journal of Medicine, New York*. 2006;**73**(8):1148–1155.

240. **Buell JF, Gross TG, Thomas MJ,** *et al.* Malignancy in pediatric transplant recipients. *Seminars in Pediatric Surgery*. 2006;**15**(3):179–187.

241. **Gross TG.** Treatment for Epstein-Barr virus-associated PTLD. *Herpes*. 2009; **5**(3):64–67.

242. **Schubert S, Abdul-Khaliq H, Lehmkuhl HB,** *et al.* Diagnosis and treatment of post-transplantation lymphoproliferative disorder in pediatric heart transplant patients. *Pediatric Transplantation*. 2009;**13**(1): 54–62.

243. **Fernandez MC, Bes D, De Dávila M,** *et al.* Post-transplant lymphoproliferative disorder after pediatric liver transplantation: characteristics and outcome. *Pediatric Transplantation*. 2009;**13**(3):307–310.

244. **Dharnidharka VR, Araya CE.** Post-transplant lymphoproliferative disease. *Pediatric Nephrology*. 2009; **24**(4):731–736.

245. **Nalesnik MA.** Clinicopathologic characteristics of post-transplant lymphoproliferative disorders. *Recent Results in Cancer Research*. 2002;**159**: 9–18.

246. **Yang F, Li Y, Braylan R, Hunger SP, Yang LJ.** Pediatric T-cell post-transplant lymphoproliferative disorder after solid organ transplantation. *Pediatric Blood and Cancer*. 2008;**50**(2): 415–418.

247. **LaCasce AS.** Post-transplant lymphoproliferative disorders. *Oncologist*. 2006;**11**(6):674–680.

248. **Green M, Michaels MG, Webber SA, Rowe D, Reyes J.** The management of Epstein-Barr virus associated post-transplant lymphoproliferative disorders in pediatric solid-organ transplant recipients. *Pediatric Transplantation*. 1999;**3**(4):271–281.

249. **Smets F, Sokal EM.** Epstein-Barr virus-related lymphoproliferation in children after liver transplant: role of immunity, diagnosis, and management. *Pediatric Transplantation*. 2002;**6**(4): 280–287.

250. **Holmes RD, Sokol RJ.** Epstein-Barr virus and post-transplant lymphoproliferative disease. *Pediatric Transplantation*. 2002;**6**(6):456–464.

251. **Mowry SE, Strocker AM, Chan J,** *et al.* Immunohistochemical analysis and Epstein-Barr virus in the tonsils of transplant recipients and healthy controls. *Archives of Otolaryngology,*

Head and Neck Surgery. 2008;**134**(9): 936–939.

252. **Lones MA, Kirov I, Said JW, Shintaku IP, Neudorf S.** Post-transplant lymphoproliferative disorder after autologous peripheral stem cell transplantation in a pediatric patient. *Bone Marrow Transplant.* 2000;**26**(9): 1021–1024.

253. **Ocheni S, Kroeger N, Zabelina T,** *et al.* EBV reactivation and post transplant lymphoproliferative disorders following allogeneic SCT. *Bone Marrow Transplant.* 2008;**42**(3):181–186.

254. **Faye A, Vilmer E.** Post-transplant lymphoproliferative disorder in children: incidence, prognosis, and treatment options. *Paediatric Drugs.* 2005;**7**(1):55–65.

255. **Bakker NA, van Imhoff GW, Verschuuren EA, van Son WJ.** Presentation and early detection of post-transplant lymphoproliferative disorder after solid organ transplantation. *Transplant International.* 2007;**20**(3):207–218.

256. **Taylor AL, Marcus R, Bradley JA.** Post-transplant lymphoproliferative disorders (PTLD) after solid organ transplantation. *Critical Reviews in Oncology/Hematology.* 2005;**56**(1): 155–167.

257. **Pescovitz MD.** The use of rituximab, anti-CD20 monoclonal antibody, in pediatric transplantation. *Pediatric Transplantation.* 2004;**8**(1):9–21.

258. **Oertel SH, Riess H.** Immunosurveillance, immunodeficiency and lymphoproliferations. *Recent Results in Cancer Research.* 2002;**159**:1–8.

259. **Biggar RJ, Frisch M, Goedert JJ.** Risk of cancer in children with AIDS. AIDS-Cancer Match Registry Study Group. *Journal of the American Medical Society.* 2000;**284**(2):205–209.

260. **Sinfield RL, Molyneux EM, Banda K,** *et al.* Spectrum and presentation of pediatric malignancies in the HIV era: experience from Blantyre, Malawi, 1998–2003. *Pediatric Blood and Cancer.* 2007;**48**(5):515–20.

261. **Tran H, Nourse J, Hall S,** *et al.* Immunodeficiency-associated lymphomas. *Blood Reviews.* 2008;**22**(5): 261–281.

262. **Nadal D, Caduff R, Frey E,** *et al.* Non-Hodgkin's lymphoma in four children infected with the human immunodeficiency virus. Association with Epstein-Barr virus and treatment. *Cancer.* 1994;**73**(1):224–230.

263. **Fluri S, Ammann R, Lüthy AR,** *et al.* High-dose therapy and autologous stem cell transplantation for children with HIV-associated non-Hodgkin lymphoma. *Pediatric Blood and Cancer.* 2007;**49**(7):984–987.

264. **Elenitoba-Johnson KS, Jaffe ES.** Lymphoproliferative disorders associated with congenital immunodeficiencies. *Seminars in Diagnostic Pathology.* 1997;**14**(1):35–47.

265. **Paller AS.** Immunodeficiency syndromes. X-linked agammaglobulinemia, common variable immunodeficiency, Chediak-Higashi syndrome, Wiskott-Aldrich syndrome, and X-linked lymphoproliferative disorder. *Dermatological Clinics.* 1995;**13**(1): 65–71.

266. **Nichols KE.** X-linked lymphoproliferative disease: genetics and biochemistry. *Reviews in Immunogenetics.* 2000;**2**(2):256–266.

267. **Filipovich AH, Mathur A, Kamat D, Kersey JH, Shapiro RS.** Lymphoproliferative disorders and other tumors complicating immunodeficiencies. *Immunodeficiency.* 1994;**5**(2):91–112.

268. **Dembowska-Baginska B, Perek D, Brozyna A,** *et al.* Non-Hodgkin lymphoma (NHL) in children with Nijmegen Breakage syndrome (NBS). *Pediatric Blood and Cancer.* 2009;**52**(2): 186–190.

269. **Gladkowska-Dura M, Dzierzanowska-Fangrat K, Dura WT,** *et al.* Unique morphological spectrum of lymphomas in Nijmegen breakage syndrome (NBS) patients with high frequency of consecutive lymphoma formation. *Journal of Pathology.* 2008;**216**(3): 337–344.

270. **Okano M, Gross TG.** A review of Epstein-Barr virus infection in patients with immunodeficiency disorders. *American Journal of the Medical Sciences.* 2000;**319**(6):392–396.

271. **Poppema S, Maggio E, Van Den Berg A.** Development of lymphoma in Autoimmune Lymphoproliferative Syndrome (ALPS) and its relationship to Fas gene mutations. *Leukemia and Lymphoma.* 2004;**45**(3):423–431.

272. **Straus SE, Jaffe ES, Puck JM,** *et al.* The development of lymphomas in families with autoimmune lymphoproliferative syndrome with germline Fas mutations and defective lymphocyte apoptosis. *Blood.* 2001;**98**(1):194–200.

273. **Fleisher TA.** The autoimmune lymphoproliferative syndrome: an experiment of nature involving lymphocyte apoptosis. *Immunologic Research.* 2008;**40**(1):87–92.

274. **Canioni D, Jabado N, MacIntyre E,** *et al.* Lymphoproliferative disorders in children with primary immunodeficiencies: immunological status may be more predictive of the outcome than other criteria. *Histopathology.* 2001;**38**(2):146–159.

275. **Shabbat S, Aharoni J, Sarid L, Ben-Harush M, Kapelushnik J.** Rituximab as monotherapy and in addition to reduced CHOP in children with primary immunodeficiency and non-Hodgkin lymphoma. *Pediatric Blood and Cancer.* 2009;**52**(5):664–666.

22 Pediatric mature T-cell and NK-cell non-Hodgkin lymphomas

Sherrie L. Perkins

Mature T-cell lymphomas in children and adolescents comprise about 10–15% of the non-Hodgkin lymphomas (NHLs) observed. Unlike adults, where there is a broad spectrum of T-cell neoplasms, most mature T-cell disease in this age group is ALK (anaplastic lymphoma kinase)-positive anaplastic large cell lymphoma (ALCL, ALK positive), with other subtypes of T-cell lymphomas being much more rarely observed (Tables 22.1 and 22.2). Similarly, although NK-cell neoplasms are rare in adults, comprising approximately 1–2% of NHL (although with higher frequency in Asia and Latin America), these neoplasms are extremely rare in children and most appear in the literature as single case reports or small series. As in adults, mature T- and NK-cell lymphomas tend to present with a broad spectrum of clinical disease including nodal, extranodal, and leukemic diseases, and are frequently associated with paraneoplastic phenomena such as hemophagocytosis, fevers, rashes, and other manifestations that may be, in part, attributable to cytokines produced by the neoplastic cells [1, 2].

Epidemiology

Mature T- and NK-cell lymphomas are rarer than B-cell disease in North American and European populations. However, there are significant differences in geographic distribution, with higher incidences of T/NK-cell lymphoma in adults in Asia and Latin American populations than are seen in the United States and Europe. In Asia, T-cell lymphomas in adults make up 30–70% of all NHLs, whereas in the pediatric population they make up about 37% of cases [3, 4]. Mature T-cell lymphomas are relatively uncommon in adults, and (with the exception of ALCL, ALK positive) extremely rare in pediatric populations. In several subtypes of T/NK-cell lymphoma, Epstein–Barr virus (EBV) activation appears to play a role, and this appears to be especially true in pediatric populations (Table 22.3). In addition, the activation of EBV influences the clinical presentation of these tumors by inducing chemokines and cytokines [5–8].

Mature T-cell NHL, primarily represented by ALCL, ALK positive, makes up approximately 10–15% of the NHLs seen in children and adolescents, and 30–40% of the large cell lymphomas. Although ALCL, ALK positive has been described in

very young patients [9], most patients are above the age of 10 years [4, 8]. Males are slightly more affected than females. Other subtypes of peripheral T-cell NHL are rarely seen in children and make up <1% of the reported cases of NHL, and appear to encompass all age groups. Interestingly, mature T-cell lymphomas in children have a high proportion of T/NK-cell tumors that are derived from cytotoxic T-cells, including NK-cells and γδ T-cells [1, 3]. These cells are components of the innate immune system rather than the antigen-driven immune system, and do not require antigen sensitization for activation. This is also considered a more primitive or early component of the immune system that may be more functionally active in children. It does appear that the innate immune system is more susceptible to development of lymphoma in children, whereas tumors arising from the more mature, antigen-driven or adaptive immune system are very rare in the pediatric population and more common in adults [3].

NK-cell lymphomas and leukemias are very rare in children and adolescents, comprising much fewer than 1% of reported cases. No clear sex predominance is noted, reflecting the relative paucity of cases. Most patients are adolescents or young adults, and there is a strong association with EBV in these disorders (Table 22.3) [1, 10].

The distribution of mature T/NK-cell lymphomas seen in children includes nodal disease, extranodal disease, and primary cutaneous lymphomas (see Table 22.1). Although some diseases may involve the blood, as a part of the disease spectrum, the primary blood and bone marrow diseases seen in adults (adult T-cell leukemia/lymphoma, T-cell prolymphocytic lymphoma, and NK-cell or T-cell large granular lymphocyte leukemias) have not been described or represent very rare case reports in children. The primary blood diseases seen in children and adolescents are aggressive NK-cell leukemia, and systemic EBV-positive lymphoproliferative disease of childhood [1, 7, 10–13].

Classification of mature T- and NK-cell NHL

Specific subtypes of mature T-cell and NK-cell NHL have been recognized and defined by the WHO classification (Table 22.1)

Diagnostic Pediatric Hematopathology, ed. Maria A. Proytcheva. Published by Cambridge University Press.
© Cambridge University Press 2011.

Table 22.1. Mature T-cell and NK-cell neoplasms in the WHO classification [1].

Leukemic or disseminated
   T-cell prolymphocytic leukemia
   T-cell large granular lymphocytic leukemia
   Aggressive NK-cell leukemia
   Adult T-cell lymphoma/leukemia
   Systemic EBV-positive lymphoproliferative disease of childhood

Extranodal
   Extranodal NK/T-cell lymphoma, nasal type
   Enteropathy-type T-cell lymphoma
   Hepatosplenic T-cell lymphoma
   Subcutaneous panniculitis-like T-cell lymphoma

Cutaneous
   Mycosis fungoides/Sézary syndrome
   Primary cutaneous CD30-positive lymphoproliferative disorders
   Hydroa vacciniforme-like lymphoma
   Primary cutaneous gamma delta T-cell lymphoma

Nodal
   Peripheral T-call lymphoma, unspecified
   Angioimmunoblastic T-cell lymphoma
   Anaplastic large cell lymphoma, ALK positive[a] (often extranodal)
   Anaplastic large cell lymphoma, ALK negative

Bolded diseases have been described in children and adolescents.
[a] Common in children and adolescents.

Table 22.2. Mature T- and NK-cell neoplasms seen in pediatric patients.

Lymphoproliferative disorder	Frequency
Systemic anaplastic large cell lymphoma, ALK positive	Common
Peripheral T-cell lymphoma, not otherwise specified	Less common
Aggressive NK-cell leukemia	Less common
Hepatosplenic T-cell lymphoma	Less common
Subcutaneous panniculitis-like T-cell lymphoma	Uncommon
Extranodal NK/T-cell lymphoma, nasal type	Uncommon
Primary cutaneous anaplastic large cell lymphoma	Uncommon
Systemic EBV-positive T-cell lymphoproliferative disease of childhood	Uncommon
Hydroa vacciniforme-like lymphoma	Rare
Mycosis fungoides/Sézary syndrome	Rare
Enteropathy-type T-cell lymphoma	Very rare
T-cell large granular lymphocytic leukemia	Very rare
Adult T-cell lymphoma/leukemia (HTLV 1+)	Very rare
Angioimmunoblastic T-cell lymphoma	Very rare

[1]. There is a broad distribution of mature T-cell diseases seen in adult populations, but in children almost all of the mature T-cell NHL is ALCL, ALK positive (Table 22.2). The WHO classification defines each mature T- and NK-cell neoplasm on the basis of clinical features, immunophenotype, and cytogenetic/molecular features (see below for descriptions of each entity). Most T- and NK-cell NHLs are clinically aggressive diseases, although some of the primary cutaneous presentations may act in a more indolent manner [2]. The WHO/EORTC (World Health Organization/European Organisation for Research and Treatment of Cancer) have provided clinical, immunophenotypic and genetic characterization of the primary cutaneous T-cell lymphomas, incorporating aspects of the WHO classification used by hematopathologists and oncol-

ogists with that of the EORTC classification that was more widely used in Europe and by dermatologists. Aspects of the WHO/EORTC classification have been incorporated into the most current WHO classification (Table 22.4) [1, 2, 14].

Clinically and morphologically, mature extranodal T/NK-cell lymphomas share many features, as outlined in Table 22.5. Often the tumors display a broad cytologic spectrum rather than the monomorphism that often characterizes mature B-cell lymphomas. Because of the cytokines produced by the tumor cells, there may be extensive infiltration of benign inflammatory cells or a hemophagocytic component within the tumor. Often T/NK-cell lymphomas are defined by their clinical, molecular, and immunophenotypic features rather than their morphology, reflecting the extreme morphologic overlap. Mature T/NK-cell lymphomas also have a high incidence of extranodal presentations, and in children are strongly associated with either a cytotoxic T-cell or NK-cell phenotype. In addition, many of the mature T/NK-cell neoplasms seen in children are linked with

Table 22.3. EBV-associated T-cell and NK-cell neoplasms seen in children.

	Extranodal NK/T-cell lymphoma, nasal type	Aggressive NK-cell leukemia	Hydroa vacciniforme-like lymphoma	Systemic EBV-positive T-cell lymphoproliferative disease of childhood
Ethnic predisposition	Yes	Yes	Yes	Yes
Clonal	Yes	Yes	Usually	Yes
Primary age group	Rare in children	Adolescents	Children/adolescents	Children and adolescents
Clinical features	Extranodal	Systemic	Cutaneous, rarely systemic	Systemic
Course	Aggressive	Aggressive	Aggressive	Aggressive
Primary lineage	NK-cell	NK-cell	T- or NK-cell	T-cell

Adapted from Jaffe [3].

Table 22.4. WHO/EORTC classification of mature T/NK-cell lymphomas with primary cutaneous manifestations.

Cutaneous T-cell and NK-cell lymphomas
Mycosis fungoides (MF)[a]
MF variants and subtypes
Folliculotropic MF
Pagetoid reticulosis
Granulomatous slack skin
Sézary syndrome
Adult T-cell leukemia/lymphoma
Primary cutaneous CD30+ lymphoproliferative disorders[a]
Primary cutaneous anaplastic large cell lymphoma
Lymphomatoid papulosis
Subcutaneous panniculitis-like T-cell lymphoma[a]
Extranodal NK/T-cell lymphoma, nasal type[a]
Primary cutaneous peripheral T-cell lymphoma, unspecified
Primary cutaneous aggressive epidermotropic CD8+ T-cell lymphoma (provisional)
Cutaneous γδ T-cell lymphoma (provisional)
Primary cutaneous CD4+ small/medium-sized pleomorphic T-cell lymphoma (provisional)

[a] Indicates disorders well described in children.

Table 22.5. Frequent features of mature T/NK-cell lymphomas in children.

Disease definition is heavily dependent upon clinical, molecular, and immunophenotypic features, not morphology
High incidence of extranodal disease
Frequent apoptosis and/or necrosis, with or without angioinvasion
Increased incidence of a hemophagocytic syndrome or other symptoms associated with cytokine release
Broad cytologic spectrum in neoplastic cells
May have extensive infiltration of benign inflammatory cells
Cytotoxic T-cell or NK-cell phenotype
Presence of EBV often correlates with both anatomic site and ethnic factors (Hispanic or Asian ethnicity)

Table 22.6. Antigens commonly used to classify T-cell NHL.

Antigen	Cellular distribution
CD1	Immature T-cells (common thymocyte stage); Langerhans granule histiocytes and other dendritic cells
CD2	Pan-T-cell; NK-cells
CD3	Pan-T-cell; cytoplasmic expression may be seen in NK cells
CD4	Helper T-cell subset; monocytes; histiocytes
CD5	Pan-T-cell; B-cell subsets
CD7	Pan-T-cell; NK-cells; subset of granulocyte precursors
CD8	Suppressor T-cells; NK-cells
CD25	Activated T-cells (IL-2 receptor); activated B-cells and macrophages
CD30	Activated T-cells; subset of activated B-cells; Reed–Sternberg cells
CD43	T-cells; granulocyte precursors; B-cell subset
CD45RO	T-cells; histiocytes
CD56	NK-cells
CD57	NK-cells
TCRβF1	T-cells (framework antigen of TCRα/β protein)
TIA-1	Cytotoxic granules of T/NK-cells
Granzyme B	Cytotoxic granules of T/NK-cells
Perforin	Cytotoxic granules of T/NK-cells
EMA	Neoplastic cells in ALCL, especially ALK+ variant
ALK-1	Neoplastic cells in most pediatric ALCL
LMP-1	EBV latent membrane protein indicating EBV infection

Abbreviations: IL-2, interleukin-2; NK, natural killer; TCR, T-cell receptor; EMA, epithelial membrane antigen; ALCL, anaplastic large cell lymphoma; ALK, anaplastic lymphoma kinase.

the presence of EBV. The EBV-driven T/NK-cell neoplasms are highly associated with specific anatomic sites, as well as ethnic features (as they tend to be much more common in patients of Asian or Central and South American ethnicity) (Table 22.3). Because molecular, immunophenotypic, and clinical information is essential in making a diagnosis, it is important that the pathologist correctly handles all biopsy materials to allow for appropriate morphologic analysis, immunophenotypic analysis by either flow cytometry or immunoperoxidase staining, and molecular or cytogenetic studies, and correlates with clinical information [1–2, 15, 16].

In general, mature T-cell lymphomas have immunophenotypic and molecular features of a mature (post-thymic) T-lymphocyte [1, 15, 17]. T-cells include two major molecularly defined groups, the αβ and γδ subtypes, based on the configuration of the T-cell receptor [18]. Each subtype is associated with specific subtypes of disease, as discussed below [2]. Although antigen deletion is frequently seen in mature T-cell lymphomas, they will express T-cell antigens such as CD2, CD3,

CD5, and CD7, but lack markers of immaturity such as CD1a and TdT. The αβ subtype of T-cells will express either CD4 or CD8, with CD4 or helper phenotypes predominating in adults. The γδ subtypes will lack expression of either CD4 or CD8 [1, 19]. Unlike B-cell lymphomas, T-cell neoplasms do not have readily assessable immunophenotypic markers of clonality, and a neoplasm is often identified by aberrant antigen expression patterns or by molecular demonstration of a T-cell receptor gene rearrangement [1, 18]. There is variable expression of cytotoxic proteins such as perforin, TIA-1 and granzyme B [1, 20]. A listing of immunophenotypic markers useful in the workup and diagnosis of T/NK-cell neoplasms is presented in Table 22.6.

The NK/T-cell lymphomas are vanishingly rare in children. These disorders arise from the NK (natural killer) subset of T-cells that express CD2, CD7, CD8, CD16, CD56, CD57, and cytotoxic proteins. The cells may express cytoplasmic CD3, as they only express the ε chain of CD3, preventing translocation of the CD3 molecule to the cell surface. These neoplasms are often associated with clonal EBV infection and lack clonal TCR gene rearrangements, as they do not have a complete T-cell receptor complex. In children and adolescents, both a leukemic form, aggressive NK-cell leukemia (also termed aggressive NK leukemia/lymphoma), and lymphomatous forms (NK/T-cell lymphoma, nasal type) are seen [1, 3, 5, 7, 16]. Although the prognosis may be variable, these are often clinically aggressive neoplasms.

Primary nodal mature T-cell lymphomas

Anaplastic large cell lymphoma

ALCL is a peripheral T-cell lymphoma characterized by expression of CD30 that includes two broad categories of disease: systemic ALCL and primary cutaneous ALCL (C-ALCL), with slightly different pathologic features. C-ALCL (limited to the skin only) is not commonly seen in the pediatric population, but when present typically occurs in older adolescents, and will be further discussed below [21, 22]. Systemic ALCL patients are most commonly male and older than 10 years of age. Most patients will present with advanced stage (stage III or IV) disease. CNS involvement, although rare, is more commonly seen in children than adults [4, 23–26].

The current WHO classification subdivides systemic ALCL into two distinct disease entities based on expression of ALK (anaplastic lymphoma kinase) protein by the tumor cells. Almost all cases of systemic ALCL seen in children and adolescents are the ALK-positive subtype (>90%) [1, 4, 27].

ALCL, ALK positive is the most common subtype of mature T-cell lymphoma in the pediatric age group, comprising >95% of the mature T-cell NHL, and 10–15% of all pediatric NHL [4, 24, 28–30]. Clinically, ALCL, ALK positive has a variety of presentations including nodal disease and extranodal disease. There is a high propensity of ALCL, ALK positive for involvement of extranodal tissues (bowel, bone, soft tissues) either as the only sites of disease or, more commonly, in association with nodal disease [17, 24, 31, 32]. Rare cases of ALCL, ALK positive may present with leukemic blood involvement, a high propensity for CNS involvement, and an extremely poor prognosis [21, 33, 34]. Secondary involvement of skin is also common and must be distinguished from C-ALCL [21, 22, 35].

Morphology

The first pathologic descriptions of ALCL were based on identification of large neoplastic cells with significant anaplasia and cytologic atypia with strong expression of the CD30 (Ki-1) antigen in a Golgi and membranous staining pattern, leading to initial designation as a Ki-1-positive lymphoma [36]. However, with further study it has been found that ALCL, ALK positive shows a broad morphologic spectrum, and several morphologic variants have been recognized in the WHO classification (Table 22.7) [1]. However, all of the morphologic subtypes described will contain at least some proportion of the characteristic large, pleomorphic, multinucleated cells, or cells with eccentric horseshoe-shaped nuclei and abundant, clear to basophilic cytoplasm with an area of eosinophilia near the nucleus (termed "hallmark cells") (Fig. 22.1) [37–39]. These

Table 22.7. Morphologic variants of anaplastic large cell lymphoma, ALK positive.

Variant	Incidence
Anaplastic (common) variant	Common, > 75% of cases
Anaplastic type	More common
Monomorphic type	Relatively rare
Lymphohistiocytic variant	Infrequent, ~10% of cases
Small cell variant	Infrequent, ~5–10% of cases
Hodgkin-like variant	Rare

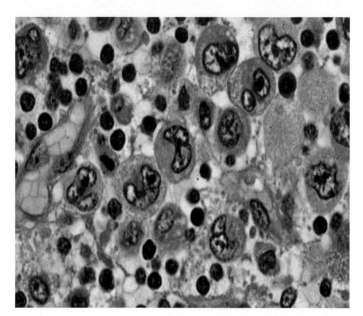

Fig. 22.1. Common type of anaplastic large cell lymphoma, ALK positive demonstrating characteristic hallmark cells which are large and pleomorphic with eccentric horseshoe-shaped nuclei and abundant clear to slightly basophilic cytoplasm. Occasional hallmark cells are multinucleated (H&E stain).

cells may resemble Reed–Sternberg cells of classical Hodgkin lymphoma, although hallmark cells tend to have less conspicuous nucleoli [40].

The most common ALCL morphologic subtype is the anaplastic or common variant (>75% of ALCL, ALK positive) that is composed primarily of large anaplastic cells and hallmark cells. This subtype of ALCL shows a sinusoidal (Fig. 22.2) to diffuse (Fig. 22.3) infiltrate of large cells showing varying degrees of cellular anaplasia. The variable anaplasia implies that some tumors may show a wide variability of cell size, multinuclearity, and atypical nuclear features, whereas some tumors may be comprised of a more monomorphic population of large cells with rare hallmark or anaplastic cells admixed [21, 36]. The sinusoidal infiltration pattern may be subtle and confused with a reactive histiocytic proliferation or involvement by metastatic disease [36, 41].

The lymphohistiocytic variant (approximately 10% of ALCL, ALK positive) is more rarely seen in children and is characterized by a large number of benign histiocytes obscuring the relatively fewer, larger neoplastic cells (Fig. 22.4). This may be confused with a reactive disorder or classical Hodgkin

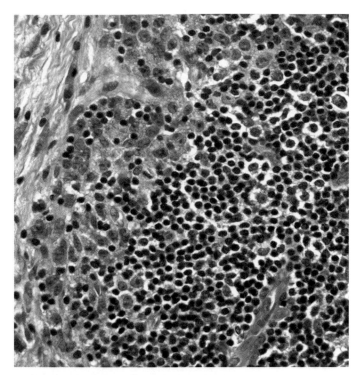

Fig. 22.2. Sinusoidal invasion of anaplastic large cell lymphoma, ALK positive. The tumor cells invade along the sinuses, slightly distending them, which may be confused with metastatic carcinoma (H&E stain).

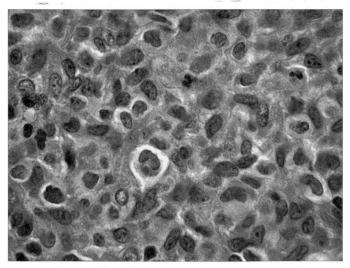

Fig. 22.4. Lymphohistiocytic variant of anaplastic large cell lymphoma, ALK positive. Large numbers of benign-appearing histiocytes are admixed with scattered large neoplastic cells of anaplastic large cell lymphoma. The extensive histiocytic infiltrate may mask the tumor cells and lead to confusion with either Hodgkin lymphoma or a reactive process. (H&E stain.)

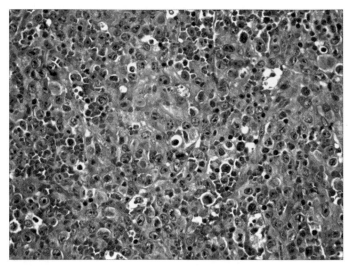

Fig. 22.3. Anaplastic large cell lymphoma, ALK positive infiltrating in a diffuse pattern. The neoplastic large cells show diffuse effacement of nodal architecture. There is marked pleomorphism of the tumor cells (H&E stain).

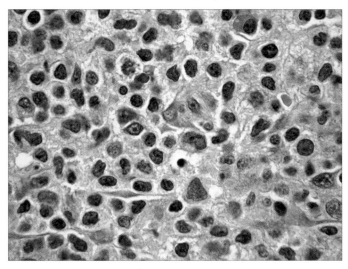

Fig. 22.5. Small cell variant of anaplastic large cell lymphoma, ALK positive. Only occasional larger anaplastic cells are seen admixed with many small but morphologically atypical cells. The small cells show the same phenotype as the larger cells and represent part of the morphologic spectrum of the neoplastic clone (H&E stain).

lymphoma [38, 42, 43]. The small cell variant (approximately 5–10% of ALCL, ALK positive), characterized by a predominance of small neoplastic cells and only scattered hallmark cells, is also seen in children (Fig. 22.5) [37, 42]. The small cell variant tends to have a variable predominance of smaller-sized tumor cells (ranging in size from one- to two-times the size of a small, reactive lymphocyte nucleus) with relatively rare larger and classic hallmark cells admixed [37, 42–44]. These tumors often cause diffuse effacement of lymph node architecture, but, when there is partial nodal involvement, the tumor cells tend to cluster along vascular structures and may invade vessels (Fig. 22.6). The neoplastic infiltrate may be subtle, and easily missed, or confused with reactive processes [1, 44]. The rare larger cells tend to be most prominent closer to the vessels (Fig. 22.6) [44]. In extranodal sites or skin lesions, the neoplastic infiltrate is also variable and may show a perivascular distribution or a sheet-like pattern of growth with few interspersed inflammatory cells and a relatively high mitotic rate [42]. Rarely, the small cell variant may transform to a common type morphology or vice versa [21]. It should be noted that the small cell variant is more commonly associated with high-stage disease, and blood and

433

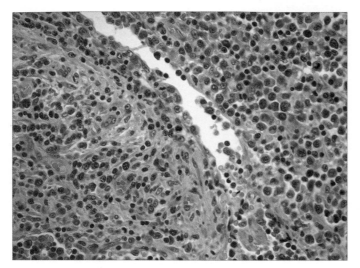

Fig. 22.6. Small cell variant of anaplastic large cell lymphoma, ALK positive, showing clustering of the neoplastic cells along a vessel with vascular invasion. The larger cells tend to cluster along the vessel, and the smaller neoplastic cells extend away from the vessel. (H&E stain.)

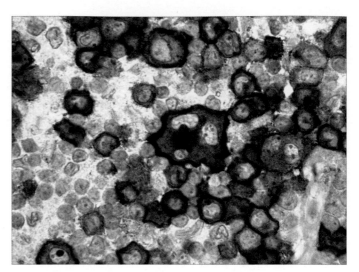

Fig. 22.7. CD30+ immunostaining of anaplastic large cell lymphoma, ALK positive. CD30 immunostaining highlights the neoplastic cells of anaplastic large cell lymphoma and shows the wide diversity of cells in the tumor, including large, multinucleated cells as well as smaller cells. (CD30 immunohistochemical stain.)

Table 22.8. Immunophenotypic features of anaplastic large cell lymphomas.

Antibody	Staining
CD30	Positive, strong expression

T-cell antigens
  CD2
  CD3
  CD4
  CD5
  CD7
  CD8
  CD43
	Variable expression
	  Often positive
	  Often negative
	  Usually positive
	  Variably positive
	  Often negative
	  Negative
	  Usually positive

Cytotoxic granules (TIA-1, perforin, granzyme)	Usually positive
CD45	Usually positive (variable intensity)
CD15	Usually negative (rare weak expression)
ALK-1	Positive in >90% of pediatric cases
EMA	Usually positive
Clusterin	Usually positive
Epstein–Barr virus (LMP-1)	Rarely positive in pediatric cases

Table 22.9. Expression of CD30 in large lymphoid cells.

Anaplastic large cell lymphoma	Uniform tumor cell expression, all cases
Classical Hodgkin lymphoma	Positive in Reed–Sternberg cells and variants, all cases
Diffuse large B-cell lymphoma	Variable (strong to weak) positivity in minority of cases. May be present in a subset of tumor cells
Peripheral T-cell lymphomas	Variable (strong to weak) positivity in minority of cases. May be present in a subset of tumor cells
Benign immunoblasts (e.g., Epstein–Barr infection)	Variable positivity, usually in a subset of cells

CNS involvement [38, 42]. Another rare but well-described variant of ALCL, ALK positive is the Hodgkin-like variant (Table 22.7) [37, 38, 45, 46]. This subtype may be difficult to distinguish from classic Hodgkin lymphoma, and it has been suggested that with extensive workup many cases may actually represent Hodgkin lymphoma [47].

Immunophenotype

Despite the relatively broad morphologic diversity, all subtypes of ALCL, ALK positive have similar immunophenotypic features (Table 22.8) [1, 37, 42]. Thus, ALCL, ALK positive will consistently show expression of CD30 by immunohistochemistry (Fig. 22.7). CD30 is an activation marker that is found in the tumor necrosis factor superfamily [48, 49]. It should be noted that expression of CD30 is not diagnostic of ALCL, as CD30 is also expressed in classical Hodgkin lymphomas, in a subset of diffuse B-large cell lymphoma, and in other subtypes of mature T-cell lymphoma, as well as in benign lymphocytes (in its role as an activation marker) (Table 22.9) [20, 47, 50–52]. CD45 expression may vary from strong to weak or absent, and it may be focally expressed [47], which should be kept in mind when considering the differential diagnosis of classic Hodgkin lymphoma (Table 22.10), where Reed–Sternberg cells are typically CD45 negative and CD30 positive. In most cases, classic Hodgkin lymphoma will be CD15 (Leu M1) positive, although up to 20% of cases may lack CD15 expression, and rare cases of ALCL may express weak and patchy CD15 in some of the neoplastic cells, necessitating additional analysis [40]. EBV is seen in a small proportion of cases of ALCL, and expression of EBV-associated genes has varied between 5 and 40% in a variety of studies [42, 53]. In most pediatric cases, EBV expression appears to be infrequent or absent [53–55].

Table 22.10. Comparative immunophenotype for anaplastic large cell lymphoma (ALCL) and classical Hodgkin lymphoma (cHL).

Antibody	ALCL	cHL
CD30	+	+
CD15	−[a]	+[b]
CD20	−	+ (20–30%)
CD45	+	−
CD43	+	−
T-cell markers (CD2, CD3, CD4, CD5, CD7)	+[c]	−
Cytotoxic markers (TIA-1, granzyme, perforin)	+	−
Clusterin	+	−
ALK-1	+[d]	−

[a] Rare cases may have weak, patchy staining.
[b] 20–30% of cases may lack CD15 staining.
[c] Often have extensive deletion of T-cell antigens.
[d] >90% of pediatric cases are positive.

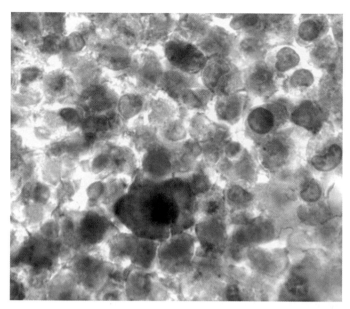

Fig. 22.9. Epithelial membrane antigen (EMA) immunohistochemical stain of anaplastic large cell lymphoma, ALK positive. EMA highlights the neoplastic large anaplastic cells. Staining with EMA may raise the differential of a metastatic carcinoma. (Epithelial membrane antigen immunostain.)

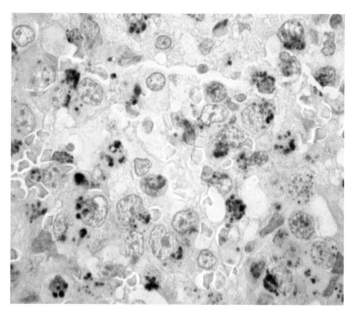

Fig. 22.8. TIA-1 immunostaining of anaplastic large cell lymphoma, ALK positive demonstrates the presence of cytotoxic granular proteins in the neoplastic cells. There is a characteristic granular, cytoplasmic staining pattern in the large and intermediate-sized neoplastic cells. (TIA-1 immunohistochemical stain.)

The majority of ALCLs have been shown to be of T-cell phenotype by molecular studies, although immunophenotypic analysis may either show staining with T-cell markers (CD2, CD3, CD5, CD7, CD45RO, CD43) or may fail to demonstrate staining with either T- or B-cell markers (null cell). Antigenic deletion, especially of CD3, CD5 and/or CD7, is very common [37, 56, 57]. Previous studies, using much more limited T-cell antigen panels, reported 20–30% of ALCL as being "null cell" (expressing neither B- nor T-cell-specific antigens) [23]. With an expanded T-cell panel, >80% of cases will stain for a T-cell in paraffin-embedded tissues, allowing for most ALCL to be clearly identified to be of T-cell origin [1, 23]. Most tumors will express CD4 and/or CD2 as well as the less-specific CD43 [23, 45, 56]. Expression of cytotoxic antigens, such as TIA-1 or granzyme-B, is also very commonly seen and may be useful, particularly when most of the T-cell antigens are deleted (Fig. 22.8). A somewhat unique feature of ALCL is the frequent co-expression of epithelial membrane antigen (EMA) by the neoplastic T-cells (Fig. 22.9). Weak cytokeratin expression has been described in rare cases of ALCL, which may complicate resolution of a differential diagnosis that includes metastatic tumor. Another marker, identified by gene expression profiling of ALCL, is clusterin. This marker appears relatively specific for ALCL, although staining has been seen in some carcinomas [58]. It should be noted, despite early reports, that clusterin does not reliably distinguish systemic ALCL from C-ALCL [59]. CD56 is also expressed in some cases of pediatric ALCL, and appears to be associated with a poorer prognosis [60, 61].

ALK (anaplastic lymphoma kinase) antibodies detect the fusion protein generated by translocations characterizing the ALK-positive subtype of ALCL (see below and Table 22.11). It is frequently expressed in pediatric cases (Figure 22.10) [22, 27, 62, 63]. ALK staining is very specific for ALCL, ALK positive, and is otherwise only noted in brain cells, some rhabdomyosarcomas, and inflammatory myofibroblastic tumors. ALK staining is characteristically absent or very rarely seen in C-ALCL, and if observed in a skin presentation, indicates the likelihood that systemic disease is present.

Anti-ALK immunohistochemical staining of most ALCL cases shows a typical staining pattern, in which the chimeric protein is present in both the cytoplasm and the nucleus of the tumor cells and is associated with the most frequently observed nucleophosmin (*NPM*) translocation partner

A

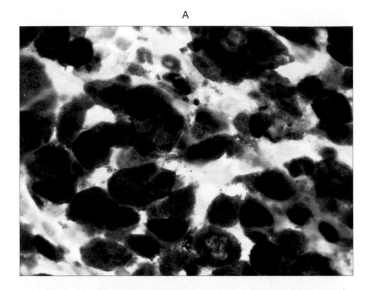

B

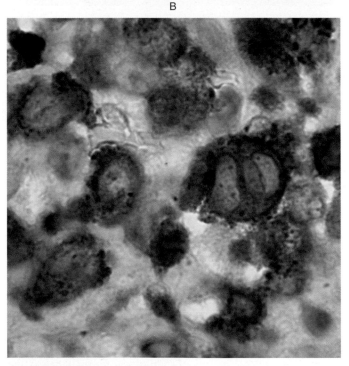

Fig. 22.10. ALK-1 immunostain of anaplastic large cell lymphoma. Panel A shows the characteristic nuclear and cytoplasmic staining that is associated with the t(2;5) translocation in anaplastic large cell lymphoma. Panel B shows a cytoplasmic ALK staining that is associated with the less common, alternative translocations in anaplastic large cell lymphoma. (ALK immunostain.)

(Fig. 22.10A) [64]. However, approximately 20–25% of ALCLs exhibit anti-ALK staining in the cytoplasm of the tumor cells only (Fig. 22.10B), and these cases have been shown to possess variant chromosomal translocations involving the *ALK* gene locus 2p23 but not the *NPM* gene. These other, less common, translocations include rearrangements of *ALK* to partner genes on chromosomes 1, 2, 3, 17, 19, 22, and X (Table 22.11) [1, 57, 65–67].

Table 22.11. Common ALK translocations in anaplastic large cell lymphoma.

Translocation partner		Frequency (%)	ALK localization[a]
5q35	Nucleophosmin (*NPM*)	90	N/C
1q25	Non-muscle tropomyosin 3 (*TPM3*)	3–5	C – diffuse
3q23	Trk fusion gene (*TFG*)	~2–3	C – diffuse
2q35	5-aminoimidazole-4-carboxamide ribonucleotide formyltransferase/ IMP cyclohydrolase (*ATIC*)	~2	C – diffuse
17q11	Clathrin heavy chain (*CLTC*)	~1	C – granular
19p13	Non-muscle tropomyosin 4 (*TPM4*)	<1	C – diffuse
Xq11–12	Moesin (*MSN*)	<1	M
2q11–13	Ran binding protein 2 (*Ran BP2*)	<1	N/M
22q11.2	Myosin heavy chain 9	<1	C
17q25	ALK protein oligomerization partner on chromosome 17	<1	C

[a] Abbreviations: C, cytoplasmic; N, nuclear; M, membrane.

The small cell variant shows distinctive immunohistochemical staining patterns, with CD30 and ALK expression being stronger nearer to the vessels and attenuated in the smaller cells away from the vessel (Figs. 22.11 and 22.12) [37, 43, 44]. CD30 staining tends to be in a diffuse cytoplasmic pattern rather than the classic Golgi and membrane pattern described above (see Fig. 22.11). A CD68 or lysozyme immunostain will highlight increased numbers of histiocytes in the lymphohistiocytic variant (Fig. 22.13) [42, 43].

As noted above, it is important to recognize that ALCL, ALK positive often occurs in the context of large numbers of benign reactive cells (histiocytes, neutrophils) or fibrosis. Thus, it is important to consider ALCL in the differential diagnosis when there is an atypical infiltrate with inflammatory features. This is particularly important when there is morphologic atypia, tissue destruction, and effacement of normal architectural features. Use of appropriate immunostaining with CD30 and ALK may help to identify a subtle large cell population in the background [37, 40, 42]. In rare pediatric cases, immune responses initiated by the tumor may lead to a lymphocyte-depleted or hypocellular appearance [68].

Staging of ALCL may occasionally be problematic, as bone marrow involvement may be morphologically subtle with single

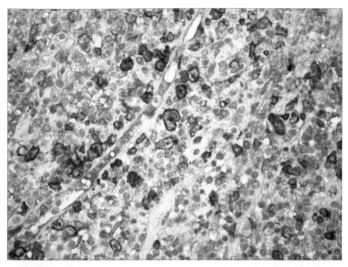

Fig. 22.11. Small cell variant of anaplastic large cell lymphoma, ALK positive immunostained with CD30. CD30 highlights the larger neoplastic cells in a typical membrane and Golgi pattern. Smaller neoplastic cells are also positive but tend to have a diffuse cytoplasmic pattern. (CD30 immunostain.)

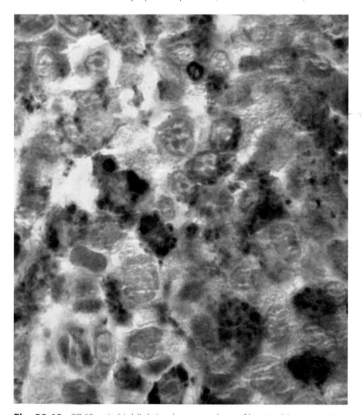

Fig. 22.13. CD68 stain highlighting large numbers of benign histiocytes in a lymphohistiocytic variant of anaplastic large cell lymphoma, ALK positive. The large numbers of benign histiocytes may obscure the smaller numbers of neoplastic cells. (CD68 immunostain.)

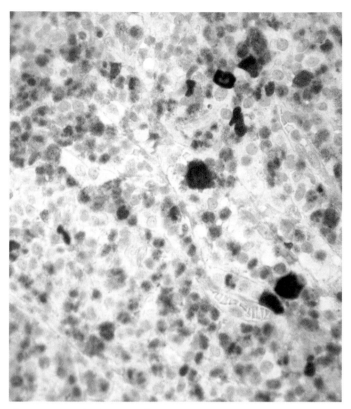

Fig. 22.12. Small cell variant of anaplastic large cell lymphoma immunostained with ALK. ALK highlights the larger neoplastic cells, but is also expressed in the smaller cells that resemble mature lymphocytes. The ALK stain appears darker in the larger anaplastic cells and shows a weaker staining pattern in the small neoplastic cells. (ALK immunostains.)

cell interstitial infiltrates rather than clearly definable nodules or clusters of neoplastic cells. This necessitates immunostaining with CD30 and/or ALK to identify rare tumor cells (Fig. 22.14) [69]. It must be kept in mind that CD30 may stain plasma cells, and the immunostaining must be in morphologically appropriate cells to allow for correct identification of bone marrow involvement. Molecular testing, such as RT-PCR analysis for T-cell gene arrangements or ALK rearrangements, may also be useful adjunct tests to identify low levels of bone marrow involvement [70]. Recent studies have shown that persistence of disease in the bone marrow (minimal residual disease) or detection of circulating tumor cells in blood is associated with a higher risk of relapse [70–72]. Other markers that may be useful in monitoring disease progression or response to therapy include serum soluble CD30 and soluble interleukin-2 receptor levels. These serum proteins are increased in patients with *de novo* or relapsed ALCL, and will decrease with response to therapy [73, 74].

Molecular genetics

Nearly all ALCL, ALK positive will demonstrate T-cell receptor gene rearrangements, even when immunophenotypic analysis fails to demonstrate expression of T-cell antigens [55, 75]. Cytogenetic and molecular analyses very often demonstrate characteristic genetic alterations involving the *ALK* gene locus on chromosome 2, with >90% of pediatric cases having a detectable ALK rearrangement [1, 27, 32, 63]. Classically, this has been manifested as a t(2;5)(p23;q35) translocation which comprises approximately 90% of the ALK translocations seen in ALCL [45, 57, 76, 77]. The molecular cloning of the t(2;5) in 1994 revealed that this chromosomal rearrangement

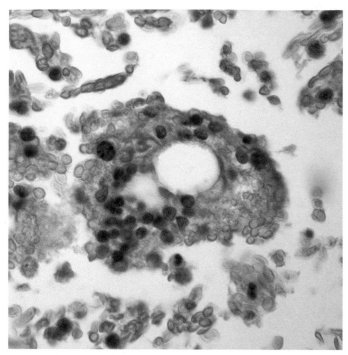

Fig. 22.14. Bone marrow aspirate stained with an ALK immunostain to identify rare metastatic tumor cells. Often the bone marrow involvement in anaplastic large cell lymphoma, ALK positive is manifested as widely scattered single cells that may be difficult to identify by morphology alone. Staining with either CD30 or ALK immunostaining helps to highlight the rare, isolated neoplastic cells. (ALK immunostains.)

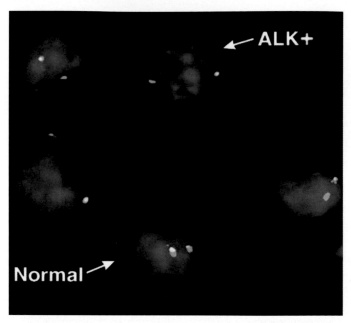

Fig. 22.15. Fluorescence *in situ* hybridization (FISH) of anaplastic large cell lymphoma using an ALK break-apart probe. Normally the probe will show a fused red and green or yellow fusion pattern. When an ALK translocation is present, the ALK probe sequence is disrupted by the translocation process, giving rise to separated red and green signals, identifying that an ALK translocation is present. (ALK break-apart probe FISH.)

produces a fusion gene, *NPM-ALK*, encoding the amino-terminal portion of nucleophosmin (NPM), a nucleolar phosphoprotein encoded on chromosome 5, that is linked to the cytoplasmic part of anaplastic lymphoma kinase (ALK), a receptor tyrosine kinase of the insulin receptor superfamily encoded on chromosome 2 (Table 22.11) [67, 78, 79].

Less common or variant translocations comprise the remaining 10% of pediatric cases, and include translocations of ALK to partner genes on chromosomes 1, 2, 3, 17, and X, also resulting in upregulation of ALK expression (Table 22.11). Over the past five years, these variant-specific *ALK* rearrangements have been molecularly cloned, and the *ALK* fusion partners identified. Genes that form the ALK fusion protein in the variant translocations include *TPM3* (non-muscle tropomyosin 3), *ATIC* (5-aminoimidazole-4-carboxamide ribonucleotide formyltransferase/IMP cyclohydrolase), *CLTC* (clathrin heavy chain), *TFG* (TRK-fused gene), and *MSN* (moesin) [45, 65, 79].

ALK translocations may be detected by conventional cytogenetics, RT-PCR, or fluorescent *in situ* hybridization (FISH) using ALK-specific probes (Fig. 22.15) [27, 80–82]. The fusion protein product of these translocations is detected by immunohistochemistry using ALK antibodies. The pattern of ALK staining is usually nuclear with or without cytoplasmic staining for the t(2;5) (Fig. 22.10B), but is localized only to the cytoplasm for many of the alternative translocations (see Fig. 22.10B) (Table 22.11) [1, 77]. There does not appear to be strong corre-

lation between specific translocations and disease presentation, clinical outcome, or morphologic subtype of ALCL.

There is a high incidence of ALK translocations in pediatric ALCL: in excess of 90% of cases in most studies, when a combination of ALK immunostaining, cytogenetics, and FISH is employed [27, 32, 63, 77]. ALK translocations are typically absent in C-ALCL and seen with lower frequency in adults, resulting in a much higher incidence of ALK-negative staining (23–30% of cases) [37, 45, 65]. The presence of an ALK translocation or ALK protein expression appears to be associated with a better prognosis in adults, but this association has not been observed in pediatric patients, reflecting the small numbers of ALK-negative cases available for study [45, 83–85].

Work on the ALK translocation has provided interesting insights into the pathophysiology of ALCL. NPM is a highly conserved, ubiquitously expressed, 38 kDa, non-ribosomal RNA-binding shuttle protein that transports ribonucleoproteins between the nucleolus and the cytoplasm [86–88]. NPM has also recently been reported to control centrosome duplication initiated by CDK2/cyclin E-mediated phosphorylation, which is critical for normal progression through mitosis [89], and to enhance p53 activity by preventing the proteolytic degradation [90, 91]. It is presently unclear whether any of these NPM functions play a significant role in the development of ALCL [57, 67]. ALK is normally expressed mainly in the central and peripheral nervous systems [79, 92, 93], but understanding of the normal functions of this receptor tyrosine kinase is incomplete. Mice with ALK genes "knocked out" have a normal lifespan and no grossly evident abnormalities [65, 79].

As a result of the t(2;5), transcription of the ALK kinase domain is driven by the strong *NPM* gene promoter, leading to its inappropriate overexpression in lymphoid cells [78]. This causes the ALK kinase catalytic function to be constitutively activated, and activates mitogenic signaling by protein phosphorylation, leading to oncogenic transformation [65, 79, 94]. Lethally irradiated mice rescued by transplantation with bone marrow that expresses high levels of NPM-ALK protein have been demonstrated to develop lymphomas after a three- to four-month latency period [95], and transgenic mice engineered to express NPM-ALK in their lymphoid cells develop both T- and B-cell malignancies that are rapidly fatal [67, 96].

A similar transforming mechanism appears to be operative for the variant ALK fusions. The N-terminal portion of each ALK partner protein will initiate ALK kinase catalytic domain activation. Because the fusion proteins are constantly kinase-active, they transmit unremitting mitogenic signals, resulting in uncontrolled cellular proliferation [67, 78, 79]. The ability of ALK fusion proteins to oncogenically transform cells is not limited to lymphocytes. ALK has been shown to participate in the pathogenesis of a non-hematopoietic malignancy, inflammatory myofibroblastic tumor (IMT), with some of the same ALK fusion proteins seen in ALCL, ALK positive also contributing to the development of IMT. A recent study of IMTs has shown 44 of 73 cases (60%) to aberrantly express ALK proteins [97].

Genetic profiling (microarray analysis) of ALCL shows differential gene expression between ALK-positive and ALK-negative tumors, suggesting different mechanisms of lymphomagenesis in ALK-negative systemic ALCL [98]. Similarly, comparison of common type ALCL with small cell variant shows differential expression of genes involved in transcription and proliferation [99]. There are also significant gene expression differences between ALCL, ALK positive and other types of peripheral T-cell lymphoma [100]. This suggests that the specific genetic expression profiles may, in part, explain different clinical, morphologic, and immunophenotypic features seen in these diverse tumors.

Treatment and prognosis

Therapy of ALCL in children is with systemic chemotherapy using either a short, intensive approach for up to six months, or a longer-term lymphoblastic leukemia type of approach with therapy lasting 12 to 36 months. Event-free survivals range from 56–76% [32, 37, 45, 84, 85]. Approximately 30–40% of ALK-positive ALCL patients fail to remain in remission using conventional multiagent chemotherapy and late (up to four years after therapy) relapses may be seen [101, 102]. Poor prognostic factors include organ involvement, mediastinal disease, extensive skin disease and systemic symptoms. Children with refractory or relapsed ALCL are often treated with allogeneic bone marrow transplant [103]. ALK-specific targeted therapies including ATP-competitive small molecule inhibitors, and antibodies against CD30 are under development and are likely to be beneficial in the future management of patients refractory to currently available treatments [104–106].

Peripheral T-cell lymphoma, not otherwise specified

Peripheral T-cell lymphoma, not otherwise specified (PTCL-NOS), is relatively infrequently seen in pediatric populations, although it represents the most common type of T-cell lymphomas in adults. Most series of large cell lymphomas in pediatric populations describe 1–5% PTCL-NOS and represent small series or case reports, representing wide diversity in workup, morphologic descriptions, and therapeutic approaches. Many of the cases reported in the older literature have been classified as large cell lymphoma, most likely as ALCL, but without appropriate immunophenotyping and molecular analysis may be better subclassified under the WHO classification as PTCL-NOS [107–114]. Most pediatric PTCL-NOS described arises as mediastinal masses or nodal disease rather than extranodal disease, although extranodal disease including involvement of skin, organs, bone, bone marrow, and blood may rarely occur. The main unifying feature of PTCL-NOS is that these lymphomas do not appear to belong to any of the other, better-defined subtypes of T/NK-cell lymphoma described in the WHO classification [1, 17, 115]. Most patients will present with advanced-stage disease or systemic (B) symptoms of fever or weight loss. Paraneoplastic features, such as hemophagocytosis, pruritus, or eosinophilia, are also common [107, 111]. By the case reports available, pediatric PTCL-NOS appears more frequently in Asian and Central or South American populations, similar to adults [116].

Morphology

Morphologically, PTCL-NOS is somewhat variable, although most reported pediatric cases present as diffuse large cell lymphoma (Fig. 22.16) [111–114]. The tumor cells typically efface normal lymph node architecture or show infiltration into normal structures, but some cases will present with expansion of the interfollicular (T-zone) area of the lymph node, with preservation of reactive follicles. There may be a wide diversity in tumor cell size, ranging from small to large-sized cells. Most tumors will show a medium to large cell size with variably prominent nucleoli, variably irregular nuclear contours, and variable amounts of clear to basophilic cytoplasm (Fig. 22.17). Some cases will demonstrate variable cell sizes or a small cell neoplastic infiltrate (Fig. 22.18), and these may be confused with reactive T-cell infiltrates. It is also common to have an inflammatory background of plasma cells, eosinophils, and small lymphocytes associated with PTCL-NOS. Occasionally, clusters of benign epithelioid histiocytes may also be present [1, 115, 117, 118].

Immunophenotype

Ancillary testing is usually essential in making a diagnosis of PTCL-NOS. The immunophenotype, as determined by either flow cytometric analysis or immunoperoxidase staining, will usually show deletion or aberrant expression levels of one or more of the normally observed T-cell antigens (CD2, CD3,

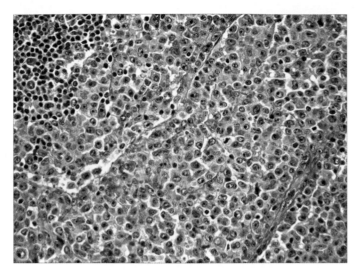

Fig. 22.16. Peripheral T-cell lymphoma, not otherwise specified. This peripheral T-cell lymphoma has the appearance of a diffuse large cell lymphoma with diffuse effacement of nodal architecture. The neoplastic cells are two to three times the size of the small lymphocytes admixed with the tumor cells, and have relatively abundant, slightly basophilic cytoplasm. (H&E stain.)

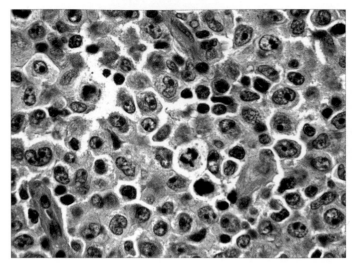

Fig. 22.17. High-powered view of peripheral T-cell lymphoma, not otherwise specified, showing the moderately prominent pleomorphism of the large tumor cells with relatively abundant cytoplasm. The neoplastic cells have variably prominent nucleoli, and atypical mitotic figures are present. The cytoplasm is somewhat basophilic and granular in appearance. (H&E stain.)

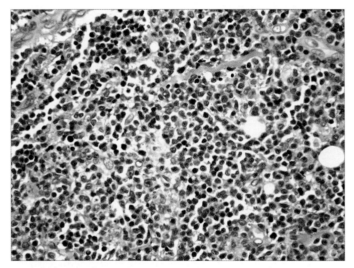

Fig. 22.18. Peripheral T-cell lymphoma, not otherwise specified, small cell variant. This peripheral cell lymphoma is comprised of small to intermediate-sized lymphocytes with somewhat finer chromatin than the admixed reactive lymphocytes. The nuclear contours show irregularity. Occasional reactive plasma cells and eosinophils are admixed with the tumor cells (H&E stain).

CD5, or CD7). The cells will typically express either CD4 or CD8, although some neoplasms will show co-expression of CD4 and CD8 or lack expression of either molecule. PTCL-NOS will express cytotoxic granule proteins in about 50–60% of cases. The tumor will lack the antigens associated with immaturity (CD1a and TdT). CD30 may be expressed in some cases of PTCL-NOS, particularly in large cell types. Usually CD30 expression is weaker and less consistent than seen in ALCL. Distinction of ALK-negative ALCL from CD30-positive PTCL-NOS is often problematic and based on somewhat subjective criteria, such as lack of anaplasia in tumor cells or the lack of expression of cytotoxic proteins (TIA-1 and granzyme A) being more consistent with PTCL-NOS, but this remains highly controversial, both in current classification systems and clinical practice [1, 17, 47]. CD56 may be expressed in some cases. EBV is usually absent in adult cases of PTCL-NOS but appears more prominently in pediatric cases [1, 113–115, 119, 120].

Molecular genetics

Molecular analysis of PTCL-NOS will detect T-cell receptor gene rearrangements by either RT-PCR or Southern blot analysis [55, 119, 120]. The Southern blot analysis is more sensitive in detection of gene rearrangements, but requires fresh or frozen tissue. RT-PCR sensitivity is variable between laboratories, and is dependent on the number and types of PCR primers utilized and the quality of the nucleic acids analyzed from either fixed or fresh tissue. Assays making use of fewer primers may have a sensitivity of only 50%, whereas those using primers that utilize all of the T-cell receptor frameworks have a sensitivity of >85% in many studies [121]. Cytogenetic abnormalities are common and usually are complex in nature. No recurrent cytogenetic abnormalities are described for PTCL-NOS [119, 120, 122].

Treatment of PTCL-NOS is variable in pediatric populations, and some patients have been treated with adult-type regimes or regimes used for treatment of ALCL, while other patients have been treated with a T-lymphoblastic type of approach, with prolonged therapy extending over one year or longer, or bone marrow transplant [114, 123–125]. Most clinicians approach treatment as an aggressive lymphoma [117]. Because of low numbers of patients in pediatric age groups, response and survival data are not well defined.

A B

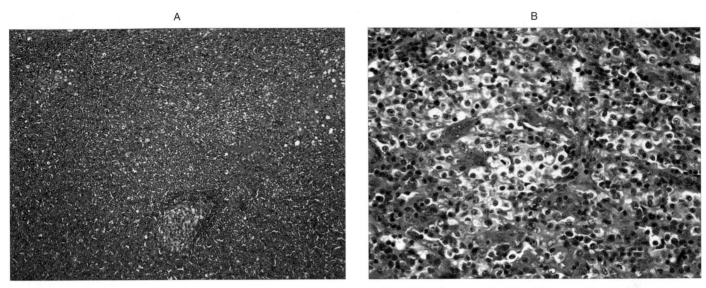

Fig. 22.19. Angioimmunoblastic T-cell lymphoma. Panel A shows a low power view of the diffuse effacement of nodal architecture with residual, regressed germinal centers and proliferation of high endothelial venules. Panel B shows prominent clear cell change that may be seen, reflecting retraction of relatively abundant cytoplasm in a subset of the neoplastic cells. (H&E stain.)

Angioimmunoblastic T-cell lymphoma

Angioimmunoblastic T-cell lymphoma (AILT) is one of the more common types of T-cell lymphoma in adults, but is very rare in children, with only a few, older cases reported in the literature, many of which do not have extensive immunophenotypic or molecular characterization [111, 126–131]. AILT is associated with systemic disease including skin rashes, pruritus, edema, pleural effusions, arthritis, and ascites. Patients will often have polyclonal hypergammaglobulinemia with circulating immune complexes, cold agglutinins, and other autoantibodies. In most cases there is extensive, widespread lymphadenopathy [132–135]. AILT in the past was thought to be an atypical immune reaction with an increased incidence of progression to lymphoma, though currently most investigators believe that it represents a true T-cell lymphoma [1, 132, 135, 136].

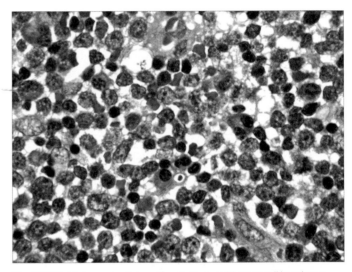

Fig. 22.20. High-powered view of angioimmunoblastic T-cell lymphoma showing admixed plasma cells and occasional eosinophils with the tumor cells. Most of the tumor cells show somewhat vesicular chromatin and are intermediate in size, although occasional larger cells (representing transformed B-cells) are present. Some of the cells show clear cell change of the cytoplasm. There is moderate variation in cell size and lobulation. (H&E stain.)

Morphology

Morphologically, lymph nodes will have partial effacement of architecture, with retention of non-neoplastic follicles that are usually regressed but may rarely be hyperplastic in appearance (Fig. 22.19A). There is expansion of the interfollicular areas and paracortex, with a polymorphous infiltrate of small to intermediate-sized lymphocytes with pale cytoplasm and distinct cellular membranes (Fig. 22.19B). There are usually minimal cytologic atypia, making it difficult to clearly identify this as a lymphomatous process. Often numerous small lymphocytes, plasma cells, eosinophils, and follicular dendritic cells are admixed with the neoplastic T-cells (Fig. 22.20). Small to moderate numbers of larger, transformed-appearing B-cells may also be present. Increased vascularity, in particular high endothelial venules, is prominent, and these may branch (arborizing vessels; Fig. 22.21). Higher-grade disease is usu-

ally associated with increased numbers of large B-cells or large T-cells [1, 132–134]. Extranodal disease may occur, involving skin, blood, bone marrow, spleen, and liver [137, 138].

Immunophenotype

The T-cell infiltrate is usually a mixture of CD4+ and CD8+ cells, with predominant CD4 positivity. T-cell antigen deletion or modulation may be seen, and the neoplastic cells characteristically co-express CD10 by either immunohistochemistry or flow cytometry (Fig. 22.22) [139, 140]. The increased dendritic cells are best appreciated by staining with CD21 that shows

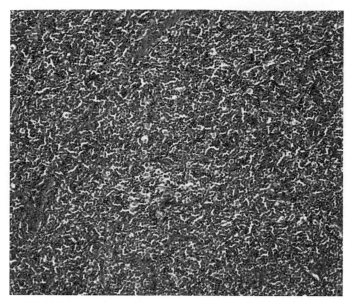

Fig. 22.21. Angioimmunoblastic T-cell lymphoma showing diffuse effacement and the prominent arborizing vasculature that characterizes this neoplasm (H&E stain).

malities, most frequently trisomy 3, trisomy 5, and additional X [1, 132].

Clinical course

AILT is usually an aggressive lymphoma with a complicated clinical course due to the associated immune abnormalities [135, 138, 142]. Differential diagnostic considerations include atypical reactive processes including drug reactions and viral infections, especially EBV infection [133].

Primary extranodal T-cell lymphomas

Hepatosplenic T-cell lymphoma

Hepatosplenic T-cell lymphomas are rare disorders in children, but have been described in adolescent patients and recently in a group of young patients with Crohn disease being treated with infliximab, a monoclonal antibody against tumor necrosis factor, or other types of immunosuppression [143–151]. However, some may arise as *de novo* cases in children [151–155]. There is a marked male predominance. There is no association with EBV or other viruses [156]. This is a neoplasm of cytotoxic T-cells, usually of $\gamma\delta$ subtype, that is usually systemic at the time of presentation with involvement of the spleen, liver, and bone marrow [1, 151, 156, 157].

a characteristic pattern where they are displaced towards the periphery of the node [139, 141]. The B-cells are also displaced peripherally, with the exception of the admixed large transformed B-cells. Occasional cells will express CD30. The large B-cells will be positive for EBV by either immunohistochemistry or *in situ* hybridization [132, 141]. Molecular analysis will show T-cell receptor gene rearrangements in about 75–90% of cases, but clonal B-cell rearrangements will be seen in 10% of cases and may represent detection of the large, EBV-positive B-cell expansion [133, 134, 141]. Cytogenetics often shows abnor-

Patients usually present with hepatosplenomegaly, marked thrombocytopenia, and anemia and/or leukopenia. Blood involvement is usually minimal and manifested as a minor population of atypical lymphocytes. Often there is leukocytosis but minimal or no lymphadenopathy [151, 157]. Patients often have systemic (B) symptoms [156]. The tumor cells infiltrate in a sinusoidal pattern in the red pulp of the spleen and liver, without discrete mass lesions (Fig. 22.23). The bone marrow is always involved, and this usually manifests as sinusoidal

A

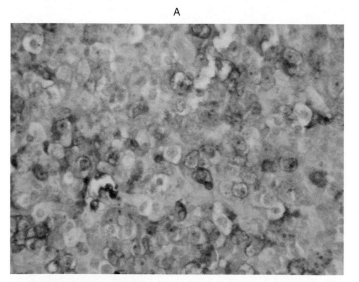

B

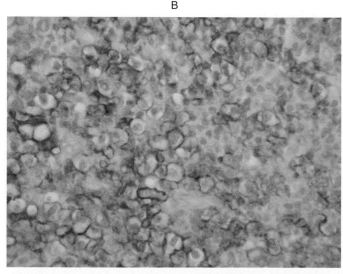

Fig. 22.22. Angioimmunoblastic T-cell lymphoma immunostaining. Panel A shows immunostaining with the T-cell marker CD2 highlighting the somewhat polymorphic T-cell infiltrate that includes larger cells with abundant cytoplasm, and smaller cells (CD2 immunostain). Panel B shows co-expression of CD10 in the neoplastic cells, which is a characteristic feature of angioimmunoblastic T-cell lymphoma (CD10 immunostain).

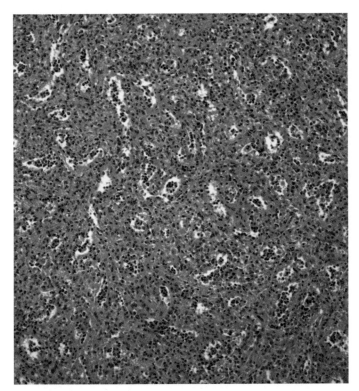

Fig. 22.23. Low-power view of a gamma delta hepatosplenic T-cell lymphoma showing neoplastic cells infiltrating primarily in the hepatic sinusoids. At low power, the neoplastic cells are intermediate in size with relatively abundant cytoplasms and round nuclear contours (H&E stain).

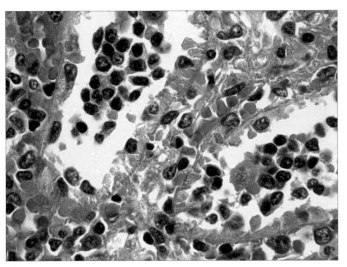

Fig. 22.24. High-powered view of gamma delta hepatosplenic T-cell lymphoma showing the neoplastic cells infiltrating in the hepatic sinusoids. The neoplastic cells show an intermediate size with moderately condensed chromatin and variable nuclear contours. Occasional cells show prominent nucleoli. Most cells show relatively abundant cytoplasm. (H&E stain.)

infiltration that may be subtle. The disease tends to remain confined to spleen, liver, and marrow, with only rare reports of involvement of other sites [149, 156].

Morphology

The neoplastic cells are medium in size, with loosely condensed nuclear chromatin and a thin rim of pale cytoplasm. The nuclear contours are usually slightly irregular, but in most cases cytologic atypia is not marked (Fig. 22.24). The neoplastic cells are usually positive with CD3, but lack staining for EBV, CD4, CD5, and CD8, and most, but not all, cases will be negative for βF-1, reflecting derivation from γδ T-cells. CD7 is variably positive. CD56 is usually positive, but CD16 is variably expressed and CD57 is negative. Most cases will express the cytotoxic granule protein TIA-1 but will be negative for perforin [1, 151, 158]. CD30 is negative.

Molecular genetics

Most of the cases will show rearrangement of T-cell receptor γ genes, but δ genes may be germline or rearranged [159]. It should be noted that most hepatosplenic T-cell lymphomas are thought to be of γδ T-cell derivation, but cases with similar morphologic and clinical features have been found to be of αβ phenotype, and these are considered a variant of this disease [158]. A specific, recurrent cytogenetic abnormality, isochromosome 7q, is present and may be associated with other cytogenetic abnormalities, in particular trisomy 8 [152, 153, 158–162].

Clinical course

The clinical course of hepatosplenic T-cell lymphoma is aggressive, with median survivals of less than two years despite aggressive multiagent chemotherapy [149–151, 163]. Patients often develop liver failure [149]. A few reported pediatric patients have had long-term survival following allogeneic bone marrow transplantation [154]. Immunotherapy with alemtuzumab, targeting the CD52 epitope, has also been used [164, 165].

Enteropathy-associated T-cell lymphoma

Enteropathy-associated T-cell lymphoma (EATL), or intestinal T-cell lymphoma, is a tumor arising from intraepithelial T-cells and has been associated with celiac disease [1, 166–168]. EATL has a higher incidence in populations where celiac disease occurs, as well as association with HLA DQ7/8 [166, 169]. Most often the tumor arises in the jejunum or ileum. Presentation in other gastrointestinal sites is rare. Most patients do not have a preceding clinical history of celiac disease, but histologic evidence may be seen at the diagnosis of lymphoma [167, 168, 170, 171]. Patients usually present with abdominal pain or perforation. This lymphoma occurs primarily in adults, with a mean age of presentation of 60 years, although there is a single case report of a child responding to the gluten-free diet that developed an aggressive intestinal lymphoma. Other rare cases have been described in young adults [172].

The lymphoma usually presents as multiple ulcerated mucosal masses, but may also present as mucosal ulceration, intestinal perforation, or an exophytic mass causing obstruction. The tumor most commonly arises in the proximal jejunum, but may be seen more rarely in other sites in the small intestine, stomach, or colon [168, 173]. At the time of presentation, about two-thirds of cases are limited to the gastrointestinal

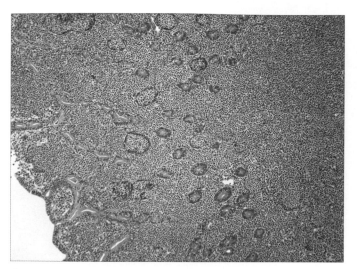

Fig. 22.25. Low-power view of enteropathy-associated T-cell lymphoma involving the small intestine. The neoplastic infiltrate extends through the intestinal wall, and the mucosal surface shows extensive infiltration and focal ulceration. The neoplastic cells focally invade into the deeper epithelial structures. In this particular case, the neoplastic cells are small to intermediate and are relatively monomorphic in appearance (H&E stain).

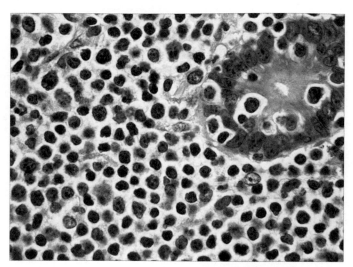

Fig. 22.26. High-powered view of enteropathy-associated T-cell lymphoma showing the relatively monomorphic small cell neoplastic infiltrate. The cells are the same size or slightly larger than a small lymphocyte and show condensed nuclear chromatin features with moderate nuclear irregularity and atypia. Occasional cells show chromocenters. The retraction of cytoplasms give a clear cell appearance to the neoplasm. The neoplastic cells are invading granular structures. Reactive lymphocytes and occasional eosinophils and histiocytes are admixed with the neoplastic infiltrate. (H&E stain.)

tract and mesenteric nodes, although dissemination may occur to liver, spleen, skin, and other sites [1, 173].

Morphology

Morphologically, the tumor shows invasion of the tumor cells into the intestinal wall, often extending through the bowel wall (Fig. 22.25). The neoplastic cells are variable in appearance, ranging in size from small to large, with approximately 20% of cases having small to intermediate-sized, monomorphic-appearing cells (Fig. 22.26), and 80% of cases having larger and more pleomorphic cells that resemble large cell lymphoma [1, 173]. Some authors have advocated subtyping into small and large cell subtypes, although this has not been shown to have prognostic value. Cytologic atypia is also variable, and some tumors will show nuclear irregularities or angulation, variably prominent nucleoli, and moderate to abundant clear or pale-staining cytoplasm. A subset of tumors may show more marked pleomorphism. Admixed inflammatory cells, especially histiocytes and eosinophils, may be prominent. The adjacent intestinal mucosa usually shows evidence of coexistent enteropathy, with villous atrophy, crypt hyperplasia, increased lymphocytes and plasma cells in the lamina propria, and increased numbers of intraepithelial lymphocytes, even if there is no clinical history of enteropathy or malabsorption [1, 171].

Immunophenotype

The tumor cells will be positive for CD3, CD7, and CD103, with variable CD8 positivity, and will also stain for cytotoxic granular proteins. CD56 is variably positive [1, 174]. EATL is negative for CD5 and CD4. Variable numbers of cells will stain for CD30 [1]. The small cell variant is typically positive for CD8 and usually expresses CD56, but is less likely to be associated with distinct enteropathy changes, whereas the large cell vari-

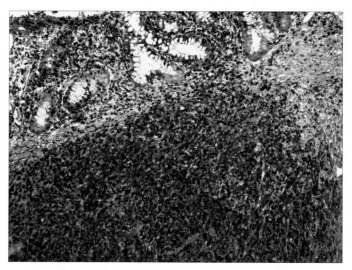

Fig. 22.27. CD8 immunostain demonstrating the extensive CD8 neoplastic infiltrate in the small cell variant of enteropathy-associated T-cell lymphoma (CD8 immunostain).

ant is usually CD8 and CD56 negative, and highly associated with enteropathy changes (Fig. 22.27) [173]. The intraepithelial lymphocytes associated with celiac disease are typically CD3+, CD5−, CD8−, and CD4−, similar to the phenotype seen in the lymphoma, suggesting that they are the neoplastic cell of origin [175]. Phenotypic atypia of intraepithelial lymphocytes has been suggested as a precursor to development of EATL [175].

Molecular genetics

Tumors will show T-cell receptor gene rearrangements [1, 176, 177]. Comparative genomic hybridization studies have shown

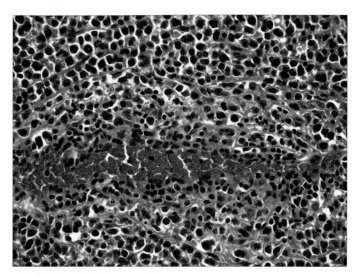

Fig. 22.28. Extranodal NK/T-cell lymphoma showing a prominent angiocentric and angiodestructive infiltrate. The neoplastic cells invade into the vascular structure, obliterating the normal vascular wall. The neoplastic cells range from small to intermediate in size with relatively abundant cytoplasm and condensed chromatin (H&E stain).

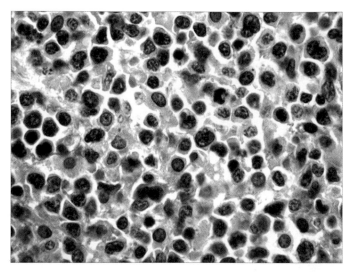

Fig. 22.29. High-powered view demonstrating the cytology of an extranodal NK/T-cell lymphoma. These cells are small to intermediate in size, with abundant, slightly basophilic cytoplasm which may appear granular in some cases. The nuclear contours range from round to slightly irregular. The chromatin of the cells is mature, with prominent chromocenters, but distinct nucleoli are relatively infrequent. Some cells show a hyperchromatic appearance, and atypical mitotic figures are present. (H&E stain.)

consistent gains in 9q, 7q, 5q, and 1q, and losses of 8p, 13q, and 9p in EATL, with gains of 9q33–q34 being most common [173]. EBV staining is usually negative [178], although it has been reported as positive in limited Mexican and Central American cases [179]. Often a differential diagnosis exists between EATL and T/NK-cell lymphomas, which may also involve the intestine [3, 180]. The T/NK-cell lymphomas typically express EBV and do not demonstrate evidence of enteropathy [1].

Clinical course

Enteropathy-associated T-cell lymphoma is an aggressive disorder, and many patients die from complications from intestinal perforation and malabsorption. Cures have occurred, but recurrences are frequent, and bone marrow transplant may be useful [181, 182].

Extranodal NK/T-cell lymphoma, nasal type

This subtype of lymphoma is very rarely seen in children, but its incidence is increased in immunosuppressed patients and patients from Asia, as well as Central and South America [3, 114, 116, 183]. Males are more frequently affected [5, 184]. In the past, this process was referred to as polymorphic reticulosis, reflecting the mixed cellular component that is often associated with these lymphomas. Extranodal NK/T-cell lymphomas, as the name implies, arise predominantly in extranodal sites, with the nasal cavity being the most common site, but tumors are also seen in the nasopharynx, palate, skin, soft tissues, gastrointestinal tract, and testis [5, 156, 185]. Unlike adults, pediatric presentations appear to be primarily gastrointestinal or cutaneous [1, 114, 186, 187]. Presenting symptoms are usually due to tumor mass effect, bleeding, or perforation. Although often localized at diagnosis, the tumor may rapidly disseminate to bone marrow, blood, lymph nodes, or other extra-

nodal sites [5]. Some patients may also have hemophagocytosis, or systemic symptoms, such as fever and weight loss, may be present, perhaps reflecting the effect of secretion of cytokines and chemokines from neoplastic cells that is associated with this disorder. There is a strong association with EBV [1, 3, 5].

Morphology

Morphologically, extranodal T/NK-cell lymphomas are characterized by a broad spectrum of appearances. Most of the tumors have an extensive angiocentric/angiodestructive component that is associated with ulceration, necrosis, and hemorrhage (Fig. 22.28) [5, 115]. There is usually a diffuse infiltrate of atypical lymphoid cells that may be small, intermediate, or large in size. Usually the cells are medium to large in size, or there may be a mixture of cell sizes. The cells often have irregular nuclear contours and granular to vesicular chromatin with inconspicuous nucleoli (Fig. 22.29). There is usually a moderate to abundant amount of clear to pale cytoplasm. Often the tumor cells are accompanied by a moderate to dense infiltrate of benign inflammatory cells including plasma cells, small lymphocytes, eosinophils, and histiocytes, and may raise the differential diagnostic consideration of an inflammatory lesion [1, 5, 188].

Immunophenotype

The immunophenotype of the tumor cells is variable (hence the designation of NK/T-cell lymphoma). Most lesions will display a phenotype of CD2+, CD56+, surface CD3−, and cytoplasmic CD3+, as well as being positive for cytotoxic granular proteins such as TIA-1, granzyme B, and perforin (Fig. 22.30). CD43, CD45RO, interleukin-2 receptor, CD95 (Fas), and Fas ligand may be positive. Other T/NK antigens including CD4,

A

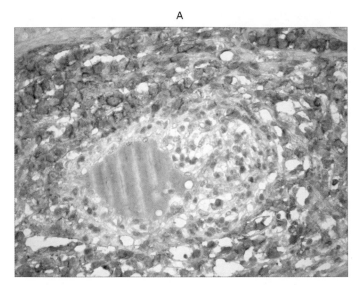

B

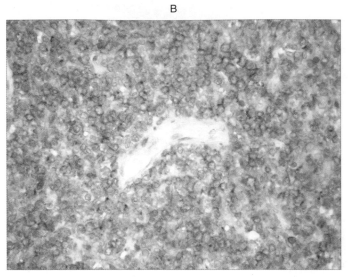

Fig. 22.30. Immunophenotypic analysis of T/NK-cell lymphoma. (A) Immunostaining with the T-cell marker CD2 demonstrates extensive staining of the neoplastic infiltrate. The staining with CD2 is in a membranous and cytoplasmic pattern. This tumor also showed staining with CD3 in a weaker pattern without membranous staining, and was positive for CD8 but lacked CD4 (CD2 immunostain). (B) CD56 staining in T/NK-cell lymphoma showing uniform staining of the neoplastic infiltrate (CD56 immunostain).

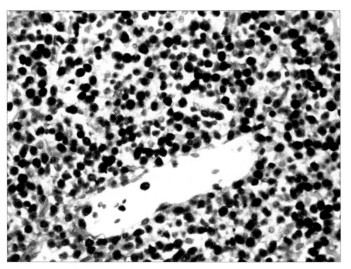

Fig. 22.31. Epstein–Barr virus *in situ* hybridization in T/NK-cell lymphoma demonstrates a strong positivity for Epstein–Barr virus in all the neoplastic cells (Epstein–Barr virus *in situ* hybridization).

CD5, CD8, βF-1, CD16, and CD57 are usually negative. CD7 and CD30 may show variable positivity. Stains for EBV by either immunoperoxidase or *in situ* hybridization are positive (Fig. 22.31). The WHO classification also accepts what appears to be a related phenotypic variant that lacks CD56 but will express cytoplasmic CD3 and cytotoxic granules as well as EBV. In these cases, demonstration of EBV and cytotoxic granule staining is considered essential for diagnosis [1, 5, 115, 183].

Molecular genetics

Molecular analysis will show germline B- and T-cell gene rearrangements in most cases. Molecular analysis of EBV will show a clonal, episomal form. Although cytogenetic abnormalities are common, no consistent, recurrent cytogenetic findings are associated with this disorder [1, 5, 183].

Clinical course

Most patients with extranodal T/NK-cell lymphoma will be treated with systemic chemotherapy. The outcome is somewhat variable, with some patients having good responses while others have aggressive disease. In general, children may have a more favorable outcome [184, 189], although, in general, those tumors occurring outside of the nasal cavity appear to have a more aggressive course. In children and younger patients, bone marrow transplant may be curative [184].

Cutaneous mature T/NK-cell lymphomas

Primary cutaneous CD30-positive T-cell lymphoproliferative disorders

Primary cutaneous ALCL (C-ALCL) is a CD30-positive lymphoproliferative disorder of the skin, a morphologic and histopathologic spectrum that also includes lymphomatoid papulosis (LyP). These are tumors of activated T-cells that express CD30 [190, 191] and have a tendency for spontaneous regression. C-ALCL is a relatively rare disorder in the pediatric population, and most cases thought to represent C-ALCL are often found, with further study and staging, to represent the much more common systemic ALCL. C-ALCL in children will usually occur in adolescents, although cases have been described in younger patients [192–195].

C-ALCL typically occurs in older patients, with a median age of 60 years, and approximately 25% of these cases spontaneously undergo either partial or complete regression

A

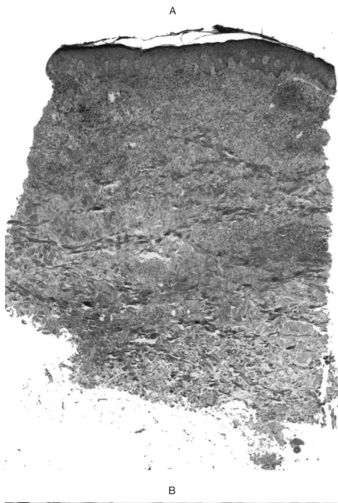

B

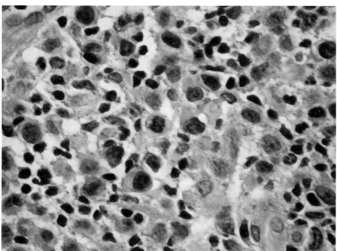

Fig. 22.32. Cutaneous anaplastic large cell lymphoma. Panel A shows the low-power appearance with a neoplastic infiltrate that extends from the basal layer deep into the dermis (H&E stain). Panel B is a high-power view demonstrating the neoplastic large, anaplastic cells that stain positively with CD30 (H&E stain).

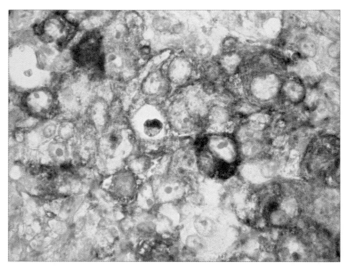

Fig. 22.33. CD30 immunostain of cutaneous anaplastic large cell lymphoma demonstrating positive staining of the anaplastic large cells present in the dermal infiltrate (CD30 immunostain).

without treatment, in contrast to the aggressive clinical course typical of untreated systemic ALCL [196]. Except for those patients with generalized skin involvement, who appear to be at greater risk of developing extracutaneous involvement and may benefit from multiagent systemic chemotherapy, C-ALCL patients can be treated by excision of their lesions, with or without radiation [197]. Thus, it is important, if possible, to discriminate between systemic ALCL with cutaneous involvement, and primary C-ALCL, which may appear essentially identical histologically. ALK staining is rarely, if ever, seen in C-ALCL, and ALK expression is highly associated with a diagnosis of systemic ALCL in children and adolescents [1, 196, 198].

Morphology

Clinically, C-ALCL presents as one or more tumor nodules that are usually >2 cm in diameter. The nodules may arise in adjacent or distant sites and may coalesce or ulcerate [197, 199]. The tumors are composed of sheets of large, anaplastic-appearing cells that often display prominent nucleoli and abundant, pale cytoplasm. The nuclear contours may be round to oval and often appear indented (doughnut cells; Fig. 22.32) [41]. Multinucleated or classic hallmark cells may be rare. The tumor cells near the surface may appear smaller and more convoluted, resembling the cells of primary cutaneous T-cell lymphoma (mycosis fungoides), and clinical correlation (i.e., lack of typical plaques and patches) is often required to distinguish between these entities [196–198]. Inflammatory cells, especially eosinophils and neutrophils, may be prominent and resemble an inflammatory infiltrate [200, 201].

Immunophenotype

Immunohistochemical analysis will demonstrate strong expression of CD30 (Fig. 22.33) and T-cell antigens, although there is frequent deletion of CD3 and other pan-T-cell markers. Most tumors will express CD4. EMA is frequently negative [192].

ALK expression should be absent in most C-ALCL, although rare cases limited to the skin and expressing ALK have been described [1, 196]. Another antigen, clusterin, was originally described as being specific for systemic forms of ALCL, but it has been also seen in up to 50% of C-ALCL and is not a useful discriminator between these processes [59, 192, 202]. The ALK-negative, EMA-negative phenotype for an ALCL in the skin of a child appears to be a strong predictor of C-ALCL, but significant immunophenotypic overlap occurs [192]. A majority of C-ALCLs will demonstrate T-cell receptor gene rearrangements [203], but diagnosis may need to be made on clinical and morphologic features if no clonal population is identified [1]. There are no recurrent cytogenetic abnormalities associated with this disorder, and detection of a t(2;5) or other ALK translocation will strongly favor the diagnosis of skin involvement by systemic ALCL, ALK positive [1, 35].

Differential diagnosis

Differential diagnostic considerations also include LyP, which presents clinically as a papulonodular eruption with spontaneous regression of nodules, usually over four to six weeks. The nodules are usually smaller in size (ranging from a few millimeters to <2 cm in diameter) and will develop central necrosis prior to regression. The lesions often appear erythematous with a paler, surrounding halo. The lesions may occur in all areas of the skin, but do not involve mucous membranes. Often lesions will cluster [204].

Pathologically, LyP and C-ALCL may have significant overlap, although C-ALCL typically has a higher density of large, CD30-positive cells in clusters or sheets [198, 205]. The early lesions of LyP will have a perivascular to wedge-shaped lymphoid infiltrate with intravascular accumulation of neutrophils. The epidermis will often show central necrosis. The lymphoid cells range from small to larger in size. The larger cells will have prominent nucleoli and abundant, pale cytoplasm, and may be present in varying numbers, but are usually less frequent and more likely to be seen as individual cells. Smaller atypical lymphocytes are admixed, and there may be a prominent infiltrate of reactive lymphocytes, eosinophils, and neutrophils. The cells will stain with CD30 and T-cell antigens, including CD4. Often, one or more T-cell antigens is deleted and occasional cases may express CD8 or show co-expression of CD4 and CD8 [1, 206]. Clonal T-cell receptor gene rearrangements will be seen in many cases [203]. Subsequent lymphomas are often clonally related [203, 207]. These lesions often demonstrate structural and numerical cytogenetic abnormalities, but are not associated with recurrent abnormalities [208].

LyP is usually seen in adults, with a peak incidence between 40 and 50 years, although cases have been described in children as young as 1 year of age [209]. There does not seem to be a preferential sex distribution. It has been reported that up to 20% of patients with LyP will develop lymphoma, usually a systemic form of ALCL or Hodgkin lymphoma, sometime during their lives [205, 210]. It has been suggested in one study that children

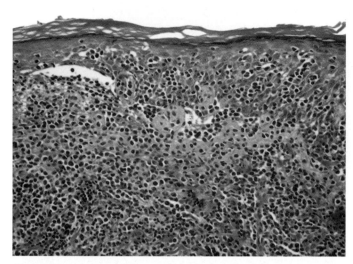

Fig. 22.34. Primary cutaneous T-cell lymphoma (mycoses fungoides) demonstrating a band-like infiltrate of atypical cells with epidermatropism into the epidermal layer. The cells are small to intermediate in size and appear slightly more hypochromatic than typical lymphocytes. There is a distinct lack of spongiotic change at the dermal–epidermal junction, and the cells tend to align along the junction with mild papillary fibrosis (H&E stain).

with LyP may have an even higher risk for development of lymphoma [211].

Primary cutaneous T-cell lymphoma/ mycosis fungoides

Cutaneous T-cell lymphomas, most notably mycosis fungoides (MF), have been rarely described in pediatric patients, with small series describing patients presenting as early as infancy, but most occurring in the teens and early twenties [212–214]. As in adults, there appears to be a male predominance of 1.6–2 : 1. These patients present with typical skin findings of a skin rash or eruption that resembles eczema, and non-neoplastic causes such as parapsoriasis, chronic or atopic dermatitis, hypersensitivity reactions, eczema, psoriasis, or systemic lupus erythematosus must be excluded [215–217]. Hypopigmented and poikilodermatous lesions are more frequently seen in pediatric patients [212–213, 218], but occasionally the lesions may be pigmented [219]. Often the presentation is of waxing and waning skin findings over several years before a diagnosis is made, with an average time to diagnosis of five years from the onset of skin lesions in the pediatric age group [212, 213]. The lesions are often patch stage at diagnosis, but may thicken and form plaques and tumors [217, 218].

Morphology

MF in pediatric populations has a similar pathologic appearance to that seen in adults. There is a variably thick band-like infiltrate of atypical lymphocytes in the upper dermis and at the dermal–epidermal junction (Fig. 22.34). The atypical lymphocytes may infiltrate into the basal layer of the epidermis and may form collections in the mid to upper epidermis (Pautrier

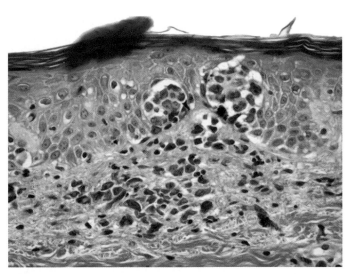

Fig. 22.35. Primary cutaneous T-cell lymphoma (mycoses fungoides) demonstrating characteristic protease microabscesses in the epithelium. The neoplastic cells have formed an intraepithelial collection. The neoplastic cells are slightly larger than a reactive lymphocyte and show distinctly convoluted nuclear contours, characteristic of this neoplasm (H&E stain).

microabscesses; Fig. 22.35). The atypical lymphocytes will have convoluted nuclear features and often appear hyperchromatic; There may be fibrosis of the papillary dermis, but this is not a specific feature [191, 220]. As the disease progresses, there may be loss of epidermotropism, and large cell transformation (defined as greater than 20% large neoplastic cells or clusters of large cells with mitotic activity) may occur [198, 221]. Lymphadenopathy is often seen with more advanced disease, and may be secondary to involvement by the tumor, or dermatopathic lymphadenopathy with expansion of interfollicular T-zones by melanin-containing histiocytes [222].

Immunophenotype

Because of the broad clinical and histologic differential diagnosis, ancillary studies such as immunophenotyping and molecular T-cell receptor gene rearrangements are often required for diagnosis [191, 220]. The availability of a large number of specific T-cell antigens has helped to make immunophenotypic analysis of MF in fixed and paraffin-embedded tissues achievable. Features that suggest MF are deletion of pan-T-cell antigens, such as CD2, CD3, or CD5, in the tumor cells. CD7 is often partially or completely deleted in MF, but this may also be seen in inflammatory processes and lacks specificity for diagnosis of MF [220, 223]. Most adult MF is CD4 positive, with about 5–10% showing a CD8-positive phenotype, although the small, published studies suggest that CD8-positive disease may be more common in pediatric patients, occurring in 30–38% of patients in some studies [212, 218]. Clonal T-cell receptor gene rearrangements are seen in >75% of cases of MF, and are useful in confirming a diagnosis of MF [1]. No specific cytogenetic abnormalities have been identified [224].

Clinical course

Treatment and prognosis of MF is similar in children and adolescents to that seen in adults. The prognosis is based on the stage of disease, and all reported pediatric patients to date have had limited-stage disease (stage IA or IB) [212, 213]. Focal patches are treated with topical steroids or retinoids, while more extensive disease is treated with ultraviolet A phototherapy following sensitization with psoralen (PUVA). Resistant cases may require localized electron beam radiotherapy [215, 217]. Most children appear to have a good response to therapy with no, or slow, progression of disease [213, 218].

Subcutaneous panniculitis-like T-cell lymphoma

Subcutaneous panniculitis-like T-cell lymphoma (SPTCL) is a rare lymphoma arising from CD8-positive cytotoxic T-cells that invade the subcutaneous tissue with extension into the dermis [1, 225]. SPTCL has a broad age range. Most cases occur in young to middle-aged adults, but cases have been reported in children and adolescents, with some cases occurring in children less than two years of age [114, 226–229].

Patients present with erythematous to violaceous nodules and plaques with ulceration, that range from 0.5 to several centimeters in size. The most common site of involvement is the lower extremities and trunk, but many children and adolescents present with head and neck disease [226, 230]. Children often present with septic symptoms of fever and malaise. There is frequent association with hemophagocytic syndrome, with associated pancytopenia, fever, and hepatosplenomegaly [1, 226]. Children seem to have a high incidence of hemophagocytic syndrome (nearly half of the patients). Hemophagocytosis is associated with rapid clinical deterioration, with most patients dying within 3–11 months of initial diagnosis [226, 231].

Morphology

The tumor is comprised of a diffuse infiltrate of lymphoid cells extending through the subcutaneous tissues and fat without sparing of septae. The dermis and epidermis are usually not involved, but the infiltrate may extend into these structures in the γδ subtype of this tumor. The neoplastic cells range in size from small, to larger transformed cells, with hyperchromatic nuclei and moderate, pale cytoplasm. Characteristically, the tumor cells will surround individual fat cells (Fig. 22.36). There is often an increased number of histiocytes, some of which may contain vacuoles or show hemophagocytosis (Fig. 22.37). Vascular invasion, karyorrhexis, and necrosis are often prominent [1, 225, 232].

Immunophenotype

The neoplastic cells are CD8 positive and express cytotoxic granular proteins such as granzyme B, perforin, and TIA-1. Most cases are αβ T-cells and will stain with βF-1 antibodies. Approximately 25% of cases will be of γδ derivation, and these cases will be negative for CD4 and CD8 and will express CD56

449

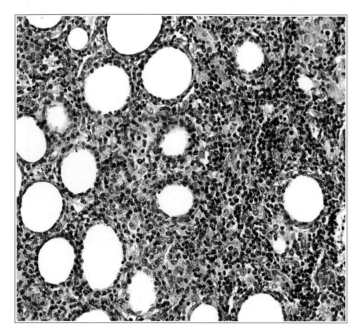

Fig. 22.36. Subcutaneous panniculitis-like T-cell lymphoma demonstrating invasion of the neoplastic infiltrate into the panniculitic fat. The infiltrate surrounds the fat lobules and is comprised of small to intermediate neoplastic cells with moderate cytologic atypia. Immunophenotypic analysis may be required to distinguish this from lupus profundus, which may have a similar histologic appearance, but the subcutaneous panniculitis-like T-cell lymphoma is more likely to have antigenic deletion, characteristic of lymphoma. (H&E stain.)

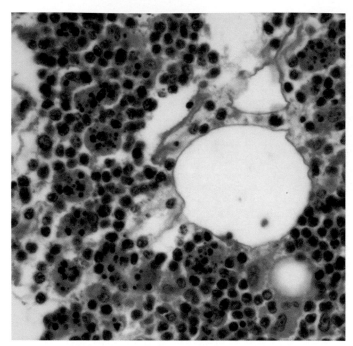

Fig. 22.37. High-powered view of subcutaneous panniculitis-like T-cell lymphoma demonstrating the small to intermediate-sized neoplastic cells with slightly irregular nuclear contours and nuclear atypia. Admixed with the neoplastic cells are numerous benign histiocytes showing hemophagocytosis. Hemophagocytosis may be associated with many different subtypes of T/NK-cell lymphoma. (H&E stain.)

[225, 231, 233, 234]. The γδ cases often have a more aggressive clinical course and are uniquely classified in the WHO classification [1, 191, 225, 231, 235]. The neoplastic cells show T-cell gene rearrangements and lack Epstein–Barr virus [225, 232, 233]. The differential diagnosis considerations include panniculitis, particularly in association with systemic lupus erythematosus [236, 237].

Clinical course

The clinical course of SPTCL is variable, ranging from indolent with spontaneous remission to an aggressive lymphomatous process. In children, systemic chemotherapy is usually used [225, 235]. Patients with widespread disease, constitutional symptom, or hemophagocytosis usually have a more aggressive clinical course, but treatment with cyclosporine to block cytokines may be of benefit [226].

Leukemic T/NK-cell disorders

Aggressive NK-cell leukemia

Aggressive NK-cell leukemia (ANKL) in children has been described in several small series and is most commonly seen in children and adolescents of Asian descent [1, 5, 238–243]. A few sporadic cases have also been described in other populations [5, 244]. This is the most likely mature T/NK-cell lymphoma to present as a leukemic process in children, but clinically patients usually have widespread disease, with extensive lymphadenopa-

thy, hepatosplenomegaly, and patchy bone marrow involvement. Rarely, patients may present with extensive adenopathy and minimal blood or marrow involvement. Patients often have extensive systemic symptoms including fever, malaise, hemophagocytic syndrome, or multi-organ failure. There may be a slight male predominance [5, 239, 242, 245–247]. This disorder is an aggressive disorder and is distinctly different clinically from the indolent NK-lymphoproliferative disorder that is most typically seen in adults and is characterized by persistent circulating large granular lymphocytes in patients that are usually asymptomatic [1, 243].

Morphology

Morphologically, in the blood there may be variable numbers of circulating tumor cells and there is often associated anemia, neutropenia, and thrombocytopenia. The tumor cells are slightly larger than normal, large granular lymphocytes. The nuclei may be round to slightly irregular and may appear hyperchromatic or have slightly dispersed chromatin. Nucleoli are variably present. There is abundant pale to slightly basophilic cytoplasm that contains variable numbers of fine to coarse azurophilic granules (Fig. 22.38) [1, 242]. Characteristically, the bone marrow shows patchy involvement, suggesting that the marrow may not be the site of transformation in this disorder (Fig. 22.39) [5]. Marrow involvement may vary from a subtle interstitial infiltrate to extensive involvement. Often histiocytes demonstrating hemophagocytosis are intermingled. In tissues, the cells may show patchy to massive infiltration with tissue

A

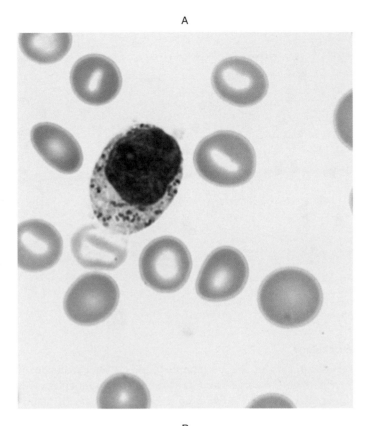

B

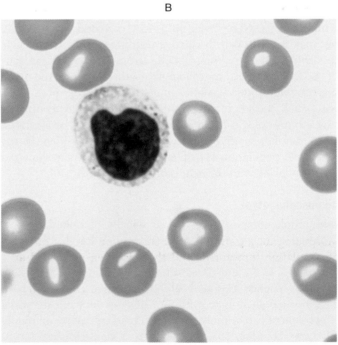

Fig. 22.38. Aggressive NK-cell leukemia demonstrating circulating neoplastic NK-cells. There is variable morphology of the neoplastic cells. Panel A shows a cell with course azurophilic granules and a somewhat irregular nucleolus with finer chromatin than is seen in reactive NK-cells (Wright–Giemsa stain). Panel B demonstrates another neoplastic cell with fewer granules, markedly irregular nuclear contours and somewhat finer chromatin than is seen in a reactive NK-cell (Wright–Giemsa stain).

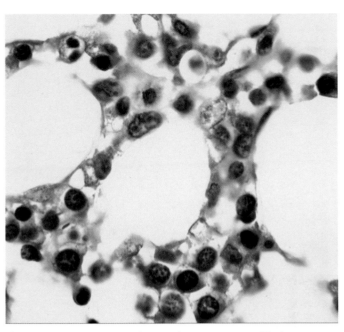

Fig. 22.39. Bone marrow involvement by aggressive NK-cell leukemia showing an interstitial infiltrate of neoplastic cells with variable, medium to large size. The neoplastic cells have variable nuclear contours ranging from round to irregular, and chromatin varies from condensed to relatively fine with prominent nucleoli. The neoplastic cells tend to have relatively abundant, granular-appearing cytoplasm. (H&E stain.)

destruction. The cells appear intermediate to large in size and relatively monotonous, with round to slightly irregular nuclei, condensed chromatin, small to prominent nucleoli, and relatively abundant, pale cytoplasm. Necrosis is common and apoptosis is frequently observed. Angioinvasion may be seen but is not a consistent feature [1].

Immunophenotype

The immunophenotype of the tumor cells demonstrates a NK-cell phenotype that is CD2+, surface CD3−, cytoplasmic CD3+, CD56+, CD57−, and positive for cytotoxic granular proteins (Fig. 22.40). The tumors will lack T-cell receptor gene rearrangements and are positive for EBV (Fig. 22.41), which is in a clonal episomal form [1, 5, 11, 238, 239, 242]. This phenotype is similar to that seen in extranodal NK/T-cell lymphomas of nasal type, and suggests that there may be overlap in these two entities, although blood and marrow involvement are rare in the extranodal NK/T-cell lymphomas of nasal type, which are more likely to be localized extranodal disease [5]. There may also be some overlap in children with other clinically aggressive EBV-associated T/NK-lymphoproliferative processes of childhood, including systemic EBV-positive T-cell lymphoproliferative disease of childhood [1, 11, 242]. Cytogenetic studies have shown deletions at the 6q16–q27 and 13q14–q34 loci in some, but not all cases [11, 242, 245, 248]. It has been suggested that gene methylation patterns may also be important in this disorder, leading to inactivation of the p53 tumor suppressor gene [249].

451

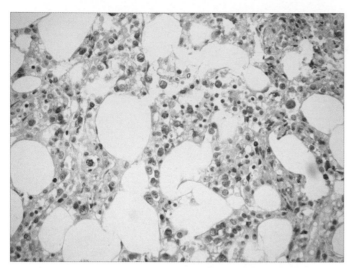

Fig. 22.40. CD2 immunostain of aggressive NK-cell leukemia demonstrating CD2 expression in the neoplastic cells. Neoplastic cells were also positive for CD8 but lacked expression of CD3, CD4, and CD7. The cells were also positive for CD56. (CD2 immunostain.)

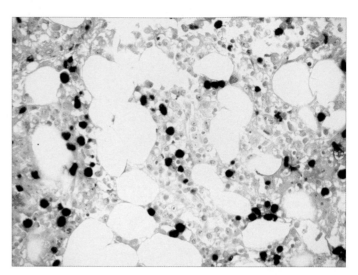

Fig. 22.41. Epstein–Barr virus *in situ* hybridization of aggressive NK-cell leukemia demonstrating EBV expression in the majority of the tumor cells. The tumor cells are seen in an interstitial infiltration pattern within the marrow. (Epstein–Barr virus *in situ* hybridization.)

Clinical course

Clinically, ANKL is usually an aggressive disorder that responds poorly to therapy [5, 11, 239, 244, 250]. A few cases with a preceding subacute or chronic phase that progressed to more aggressive disease have been described [11, 239], but many patients die within weeks to months of diagnosis. Patients may require bone marrow transplant or aggressive chemotherapy with L-asparaginase to achieve remission [251, 252].

T-cell large granular leukemia

T-cell large granular leukemia (T-LGL) is a neoplastic proliferation of CD8-positive cytotoxic lymphocytes that typically occurs in older patients, with an average age of onset of 60 years, although rare cases have been described in children, often associated with immune dysfunction [253–257] and in association with Turner syndrome [258]. Most patients present with fever, recurrent bacterial infections, fatigue, and weight loss. Splenomegaly is seen in about half of the patients, and hepatomegaly may be seen in up to 20% [257]. The most uniform presenting feature is neutropenia, often severe, that is seen in 60–85% of patients at presentation. Many patients are diagnosed with T-LGL during workup of asymptomatic cytopenias, neutropenia, or lymphocytosis [255].

T-LGL usually presents with lymphocytosis, usually in the range of 2000–20 000/μL (2–20 × 10⁹/L) that is sustained for at least six months [1, 256, 257]. It should be noted that benign or reactive expansions of large granular lymphocytes may be seen in infections, autoimmune disorders, post-transplantation and in viral infections [255]. Hematologic manifestations include neutropenia in most patients, anemia in approximately half of patients, and thrombocytopenia in about 20% [1, 255, 257]. Rare patients may present with aplastic anemia [259].

Morphology

T-LGL appears in the peripheral blood as an expansion of intermediate- to large-sized (15–18 μm) lymphocytes with abundant cytoplasm containing variable numbers of azurophilic granules and round to slightly indented nuclei with mature chromatin (Fig. 22.42). Normally, large granular lymphocytes (LGLs) make up 5–15% of blood lymphocytes, but may be expanded in reactive conditions. It is not possible to distinguish the clonal T-LGLs from reactive expansions of LGLs based on morphologic features [255]. The bone marrow will show a subtle, interstitial infiltrate of T-LGLs with small clusters of neoplastic cells. Usually this is difficult to see morphologically in bone marrow sections or aspirates, and immunophenotypic analysis may help to identify the neoplastic population [1]. Splenic involvement may show red pulp expansion with the neoplastic cells [260].

Immunophenotype

Immunophenotypically, T-LGL is usually identified by flow cytometric analysis that demonstrates an atypical phenotype. Benign T-LGLs characteristically express CD2, cytoplasmic CD3, CD5, CD7, and CD8, but are negative for surface CD3, CD4, CD16, and CD56 [261–263]. All cases of T-LGL will have an abnormal phenotype, with 80% of cases showing abnormal expression of two or more pan-T-cell markers, most commonly CD5 or CD7 [262, 263]. Usually this is manifested as dim to absent expression of the antigen. CD16 and CD57 (natural killer antigens) are expressed in nearly all cases [261, 262, 264].

By molecular analysis, nearly all cases will demonstrate αβ T-cell receptor gene rearrangements, although some more clinically aggressive cases will demonstrate γδ T-cell receptor gene rearrangements [256, 257]. Analysis of Vβ T-cell receptor epitopes or killer cell immunoglobulin-like receptors (KIRs) expression patterns on the cell surface of lymphoid expansions

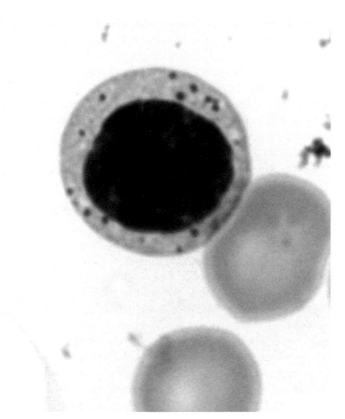

Fig. 22.42. Large granular lymphocyte seen in T-cell large granular lymphocytic leukemia. The large granular lymphocyte is characterized by mature chromatin features and relatively smooth nuclear contours. Variable numbers of fine to coarse azurophilic granules are seen in the cytoplasm (Wright–Giemsa stain).

by flow cytometry may also indicate whether a clonal expansion of T-LGL is present, as a clonal expansion will display a single Vβ or KIR epitope rather than the polymorphic expression seen in reactive proliferations [262, 265]. Cytogenetic abnormalities are relatively rare in T-LGL, and are reported in approximately 20% of adult cases. Reported abnormalities include inversion of chromosome 7 and deletion of 6q [255, 266].

Clinical course

Because of the relatively indolent clinical nature of T-LGL, many patients may be observed or treated with cytokine therapy for neutropenia. Single agent therapy with methotrexate, steroids, or other agents may be used in more severely symptomatic cases to try to improve cytopenias [256, 257].

EBV-positive T-cell lymphoproliferative disorders of childhood

EBV-positive T-cell lymphoproliferative disorders of childhood include a systemic disorder (also referred to as fatal infectious mononucleosis) as well as a cutaneous lymphoma termed hydroa vacciniforme-like lymphoma [1].

Systemic EBV-positive T-cell lymphoproliferative disease of childhood

Systemic EBV-positive T-cell lymphoproliferative disease of childhood is a clonal and clinically aggressive proliferation of cytotoxic T-cells that are infected by EBV. Most occur after primary acute infection [1, 7]. This may show overlap with aggressive NK-cell leukemia [1, 267]. A few cases have been associated with reactivation of preceding chronic EBV infection [11, 12, 268, 269]. The patients are children and young adults, but infants are also affected. Presenting symptoms include fever, skin rashes, hepatosplenomegaly, lymphadenopathy, and pancytopenia. There is often associated hemophagocytic syndrome and multi-organ failure. In the blood there may be an increased number of activated-appearing lymphocytes. The spleen, liver, and lymph nodes will show infiltration of atypical mononuclear cells in the sinusoids and portal areas. The atypical cells are usually positive for CD3, CD8, βF-1, TIA-1, and EBV by EBER, but negative for CD56. Those cases arising from a chronic-active EBV infection may be CD4+ [1, 13]. Molecular analysis will demonstrate a clonal T-cell population, but no recurrent cytogenetic abnormalities have been described. Usually patients have a fulminant course with death within days to months [1, 7, 12]. The patients show defective immune responses to EBV, as evidenced by low increases in EBV serologic titers during the course of the disease [3].

Hydroa vacciniforme-like lymphoma

Hydroa vacciniforme (HV) is a papulovesicular eruption that proceeds to blistering or ulcers and scarring that occurs on sun-exposed skin in children and adolescents of Asian and Latin American ethnicity. Most lesions occur on the face, and less frequently in the extremities [270]. In some cases it may resemble lymphomatoid papulosis [271], and patients often develop hypersensitivity reactions to insect bites preceding development of the eruption. The skin lesions often show infiltration of the skin with a T-cell infiltrate with angiocentric features that may extend into the subcutis [270, 272]. Clonal T-cell populations may arise in this setting [273].

A small number of children developed HV-like skin lesions with necrosis, ulceration, and progression to a lymphoma with systemic involvement including splenomegaly, lymphadenopathy, and hemophagocytosis that has been recognized as a part of the spectrum of EBV-positive T-cell lymphoproliferative disorders of childhood [1, 3, 272]. Several small series of pediatric patients developing this unusual type of HV-like lymphoma have been described in Japan, China, Korea, Mexico, and Peru [238, 274–279]. The neoplastic infiltrate in skin and other organs often shows angiocentric infiltration and invasion with extensive necrosis. The infiltrate may extend into the subcutis, imparting the appearance of a vasculitic panniculitis. The neoplastic cells are usually intermediate in size with dense, hyperchromatic nuclei, inconspicuous nucleoli, and infrequent mitoses. A variable inflammatory background of neutrophils and eosinophils is often seen [1, 274, 277].

The immunophenotype is that of an EBV-positive T/NK-cell with a CD8-positive cytotoxic phenotype. The NK markers CD56 and CD57 are usually positive. CD30 may be positive in a subset of cells [1, 3, 274, 277]. Studies of EBV show a type II latency pattern and monoclonal EBV genomes [238, 276]. T-cell receptor gene rearrangements have been positive in those cases studied [274]. Differential diagnostic considerations include inflammatory processes, and other cutaneous T-cell lymphomas, but the CD8-positive, EBV-positive phenotype and preceding blistering skin disease help to identify this peculiar type of lymphoma [1, 272, 278].

Treatment of HV-like lymphoma is by chemotherapy or radiotherapy, but the disease usually has an aggressive course with poor overall survival and response to therapy [238, 274, 278].

T-cell post-transplant lymphoproliferative disorders

Although the majority of post-transplant lymphoproliferative disorders (PTLDs) seen after solid organ transplant are of B-cell origin, rare cases may be of T-cell origin [280–283]. T-cell PTLDs in children are often associated with hemophagocytic

syndrome and more aggressive behavior. EBV may be present or absent [115, 283]. Most T-cell PTLDs have the appearance of a peripheral T-cell lymphoma, unspecified, although a few cases may have the appearance of ALCL, hepatosplenic gamma delta lymphoma, or NK-cell neoplasms [283–286]. T-cell PTLD appears to act aggressively, and those cases without EBV may not respond as well to reduction of immunosuppression, but clinical behavior can vary [282, 286]. It is interesting to note that many of the T/NK-cell PTLDs are of cytotoxic phenotype and occur in extranodal sites [115, 280, 282].

Summary

Mature T/NK-cell lymphomas represent a minority of the NHLs seen in children. S-ALCL comprises the majority of cases, with other subtypes of disease being extremely rare. T/NK-cell lymphomas are characterized by a wide spectrum of disease presentations, including nodal and extranodal sites of disease. The tumors are often associated with paraneoplastic syndromes such as hemophagocytosis. Marked morphologic diversity and infiltrates of benign inflammatory cells may make initial recognition of a neoplastic process difficult, but use of appropriate immunophenotypic, molecular, and cytogenetic analysis will aid in making a diagnosis. Often, mature T/NK-cell lymphomas in children are clinically aggressive.

References

1. **Swerdlow SH, Campo E, Harris NL,** *et al. WHO Classification of Tumours of Haematopoietic and Lymphoid Tissues* (4th edn.). Lyon: IARC Press; 2008.

2. **Lim MS, de Leval L, Quintanilla-Martinez L.** Commentary on the 2008 WHO classification of mature T- and NK-cell neoplasms. *Journal of Hematopathology.* 2009;2(2):65–73.

3. **Jaffe ES.** Mature T-cell and NK-cell lymphomas in the pediatric age group. *American Journal of Clinical Pathology.* 2004;122(Suppl):S110–S121.

4. **Gross TG, Termuhlen AM.** Pediatric non-Hodgkin's lymphoma. *Current Oncology Reports.* 2007;9(6):459–465.

5. **Nava VE, Jaffe ES.** The pathology of NK-cell lymphomas and leukemias. *Advances in Anatomic Pathology.* 2005;12(1):27–34.

6. **Raziuddin S, Abu-Eshy S, Sheikha A.** Peripheral T-cell lymphomas. Immunoregulatory cytokine (interleukin-2, interleukin-4, and interferon-gamma) abnormalities and autologous mixed lymphocyte reaction. *Cancer.* 1994;74(10):2843–2849.

7. **Rezk SA, Weiss LM.** Epstein-Barr virus-associated lymphoproliferative disorders. *Human Pathology.* 2007; 38(9):1293–1304.

8. **Good DJ, Gascoyne RD.** Classification of non-Hodgkin's lymphoma. *Hematology/Oncology Clinics of North America.* 2008;22(5):781–805, vii.

9. **Ben Barak A, Elhasid R, Ben Itzhak O,** *et al.* Infant anaplastic lymphoma: case report and review of the literature. *Pediatr Hematological Oncology.* 2007;24(5):379–385.

10. **Ohshima K, Kimura H, Yoshino T,** *et al.* Proposed categorization of pathological states of EBV-associated T/natural killer-cell lymphoproliferative disorder (LPD) in children and young adults: overlap with chronic active EBV infection and infantile fulminant EBV T-LPD. *Pathology International.* 2008;58(4):209–217.

11. **Suzuki K, Ohshima K, Karube K,** *et al.* Clinicopathological states of Epstein-Barr virus-associated T/NK-cell lymphoproliferative disorders (severe chronic active EBV infection) of children and young adults.

International Journal of Oncology. 2004; 24(5):1165–1174.

12. **Quintanilla-Martinez L, Kumar S, Fend F,** *et al.* Fulminant EBV(+) T-cell lymphoproliferative disorder following acute/chronic EBV infection: a distinct clinicopathologic syndrome. *Blood.* 2000;96(2):443–451.

13. **Imashuku S.** Systemic type Epstein-Barr virus-related lymphoproliferative diseases in children and young adults: challenges for pediatric hemato-oncologists and infectious disease specialists. *Pediatric Hematological Oncology.* 2007;24(8):563–568.

14. **Burg G, Kempf W, Cozzio A,** *et al.* WHO/EORTC classification of cutaneous lymphomas 2005: histological and molecular aspects. *Journal of Cutaneous Pathology.* 2005; 32(10):647–674.

15. **Rodriguez-Abreu D, Filho VB, Zucca E.** Peripheral T-cell lymphomas, unspecified (or not otherwise specified): a review. *Hematological Oncology.* 2008;26(1):8–20.

16. **Suzuki R, Takeuchi K, Ohshima K, Nakamura S.** Extranodal NK/T-cell lymphoma: diagnosis and treatment

cues. *Hematological Oncology.* 2008; **26**(2):66–72.

17. **Savage KJ**. Peripheral T-cell lymphomas. *Blood Reviews.* 2007;**21**(4): 201–216.

18. **Macintyre EA, Delabesse E**. Molecular approaches to the diagnosis and evaluation of lymphoid malignancies. *Seminars in Hematology.* 1999;**36**(4): 373–389.

19. **Jones D, Dorfman DM**. Phenotypic characterization of subsets of T cell lymphoma: towards a functional classification of T cell lymphoma. *Leukemia and Lymphoma.* 2001; **40**(5–6):449–459.

20. **Kanavaros P, Boulland ML, Petit B, Arnulf B, Gaulard P**. Expression of cytotoxic proteins in peripheral T-cell and natural killer-cell (NK) lymphomas: association with extranodal site, NK or Tgammadelta phenotype, anaplastic morphology and CD30 expression. *Leukemia and Lymphoma.* 2000;**38**(3–4):317–326.

21. **Hodges VM, Molloy GY, Wickramasinghe SN**. Genetic heterogeneity of congenital dyserythropoietic anemia type I. *Blood.* 1999;**94**(3):1139–1140.

22. **Hochberg J, Waxman IM, Kelly KM, Morris E, Cairo MS**. Adolescent non-Hodgkin lymphoma and Hodgkin lymphoma: state of the science. *British Journal of Haematology.* 2009;**144**(1): 24–40.

23. **Perkins SL**. Work-up and diagnosis of pediatric non-Hodgkin's lymphomas. *Pediatric and Developmental Pathology.* 2000;**3**(4):374–390.

24. **Alessandri AJ, Pritchard SL, Schultz KR, Massing BG**. A population-based study of pediatric anaplastic large cell lymphoma. *Cancer.* 2002;**94**(6):1830–1835.

25. **Sandlund JT, Downing JR, Christ WM**. Non-Hodgkin's lymphoma in childhood. *New England Journal of Medicine.* 1996;**334**:1238–1248.

26. **Cairo MS, Raetz E, Perkins SL**. Non-Hodgkin lymphoma in children. In Kufe D, Pollock RE, Weishelbaum RR, *et al.*, eds. *Cancer Medicine* (6th edn.). London: BC Decker Inc.; 2003, 2337–2348.

27. **Perkins SL, Pickering D, Lowe EJ, et al.** Childhood anaplastic large cell lymphoma has a high incidence of ALK gene rearrangement as determined by immunohistochemical staining and fluorescent in situ hybridisation: a genetic and pathological correlation. *British Journal of Haematology.* 2005; **131**(5):624–627.

28. **Jaffe ES, Krenacs L, Raffeld M**. Classification of cytotoxic T-cell and natural killer cell lymphomas. *Seminars in Hematology.* 2003;**40**(3):175–184.

29. **Burkhardt B, Zimmermann M, Oschlies I, et al.** The impact of age and gender on biology, clinical features and treatment outcome of non-Hodgkin lymphoma in childhood and adolescence. *British Journal of Haematology.* 2005;**131**(1):39–49.

30. **Kodama K, Hokama M, Kawaguchi K, Tanaka Y, Hongo K**. Primary ALK-1-negative anaplastic large cell lymphoma of the brain: case report and review of the literature. *Neuropathology.* 2009;**29**(2):166–171.

31. **Bakshi NA, Ross CW, Finn WG, et al.** ALK-positive anaplastic large cell lymphoma with primary bone involvement in children. *American Journal of Clinical Pathology.* 2006; **125**(1):57–63.

32. **Brugieres L, Deley MC, Pacquement H, et al.** CD30(+) anaplastic large-cell lymphoma in children: analysis of 82 patients enrolled in two consecutive studies of the French Society of Pediatric Oncology. *Blood.* 1998;**92**(10): 3591–3598.

33. **Grewal JS, Smith LB, Winegarden JD, et al.** Highly aggressive ALK-positive anaplastic large cell lymphoma with a leukemic phase and multi-organ involvement: a report of three cases and a review of the literature. *Annals of Hematology.* 2007;**86**(7):499–508.

34. **Takahashi D, Nagatoshi Y, Nagayama J, et al.** Anaplastic large cell lymphoma in leukemic presentation: a case report and a review of the literature. *Journal of Pediatric Hematology/Oncology.* 2008; **30**(9):696–700.

35. **Hinshaw M, Trowers AB, Kodish E, et al.** Three children with CD30 cutaneous anaplastic large cell lymphomas bearing the t(2;5)(p23;q35) translocation. *Pediatric Dermatology.* 2004;**21**(3):212–217.

36. **Stein H, Mason DY, Gerdes J, et al.** The expression of the Hodgkin's disease associated antigen Ki-1 in reactive and neoplastic lymphoid tissue: evidence that Reed-Sternberg cells and histiocytic malignancies are derived from activated lymphoid cells. *Blood.* 1985;**66**(4):848–858.

37. **Stein H, Foss HD, Dürkop H, et al.** CD30(+) anaplastic large cell lymphoma: a review of its histopathologic, genetic, and clinical features. *Blood.* 2000;**96**(12):3681–3695.

38. **Kadin M**. Anaplastic large cell lymphoma and its morphologic variants. *Cancer Surveys.* 1997;**30**:77–86.

39. **Benharroch D, Meguerian-Bedoyan Z, Lamant L, et al.** ALK-positive lymphoma: a single disease with a broad spectrum of morphology. *Blood.* 1998;**91**(6):2076–2084.

40. **Vassallo J, Lamant L, Brugieres L, et al.** ALK-positive anaplastic large cell lymphoma mimicking nodular sclerosis Hodgkin's lymphoma: report of 10 cases. *American Journal of Surgical Pathology.* 2006;**30**(2):223–229.

41. **Agnarrson B, Kadin M**. Ki-1 positive large cell lymphoma. A morphologic and immunologic study of 19 cases. *American Journal of Surgical Pathology.* 1988;**12**:264–274.

42. **Kinney MC, Kadin ME**. The pathologic and clinical spectrum of anaplastic large cell lymphoma and correlation with ALK gene dysregulation. *American Journal of Clinical Pathology.* 1999;**111**(1 Suppl 1):S56–S67.

43. **Pileri S, Falini B, Delsol G, et al.** Lymphohistiocytic T-cell lymphoma (anaplastic large cell lymphoma CD30+/Ki-1 + with a high content of reactive histiocytes). *Histopathology.* 1990;**16**(4):383–391.

44. **Kinney M, Collins RD, Greer JP, et al.** A small-cell-predominant varaint of primary Ki-1 (CD30)+ T-cell lymphoma. *American Journal of Surgical Pathology.* 1993;**17**:859–868.

45. **Falini B**. Anaplastic large cell lymphoma: pathological, molecular and clinical features. *British Journal of Haematology.* 2001;**114**(4):741–760.

46. **Falini B, Bigerna B, Fizzotti M, et al.** ALK expression defines a distinct group of T/null lymphomas ("ALK lymphomas") with a wide morphological spectrum. *American Journal of Pathology.* 1998;**153**(3):875–886.

47. **Medeiros LJ, Elenitoba-Johnson KS**. Anaplastic large cell lymphoma.

American Journal of Clinical Pathology. 2007;**127**(5):707–722.

48. **Chiarle R, Podda A, Prolla G**, *et al.* CD30 in normal and neoplastic cells. *Clin Immunol.* 1999;**90**(2):157–164.

49. **So T, Lee SW, Croft M.** Tumor necrosis factor/tumor necrosis factor receptor family members that positively regulate immunity. *International Journal of Hematology.* 2006;**83**(1):1–11.

50. **Higgin JP, Warnke RA.** CD30 expression is common in mediastinal large B-cell lymphoma. *American Journal of Clinical Pathology.* 1999; **112**:241–247.

51. **Pileri SA, Zinzani PL, Gaidano G**, *et al.* Pathobiology of primary mediastinal B-cell lymphoma. *Leukemia and Lymphoma.* 2003;**44**(Suppl 3):S21–S26.

52. **Gardner LJ, Polski JM, Evans HL, Perkins SL, Dunphy CH.** CD30 expression in follicular lymphoma. *Archives of Pathology and Laboratory Medicine.* 2001;**125**(8):1036–1041.

53. **Nakagawa A, Nakamura S, Ito M**, *et al.* CD30-positive anaplastic large cell lymphoma in childhood: expression of p80 npm/alk and absence of Epstein-Barr virus. *Modern Pathology.* 1997; **10**(3):210–215.

54. **Herling M, Rassidakis GZ, Jones D**, *et al.* Absence of Epstein-Barr virus in anaplastic large cell lymphoma: a study of 64 cases classified according to World Health Organization criteria. *Human Pathology.* 2004;**35**(4):455–459.

55. **Tan BT, Seo K, Warnke RA, Arber DA.** The frequency of immunoglobulin heavy chain gene and T-cell receptor gamma-chain gene rearrangements and Epstein-Barr virus in ALK+ and ALK- anaplastic large cell lymphoma and other peripheral T-cell lymphomas. *Journal of Molecular Diagnostics.* 2008; **10**(6):502–512.

56. **Chu PG, Chang KL, Arber DA, Weiss LM.** Practical applications of immunohistochemistry in hematolymphoid neoplasms. *Annals of Diagnostic Pathology.* 1999;**3**:104–133.

57. **Amin HM, Lai R.** Pathobiology of ALK + anaplastic large-cell lymphoma. *Blood.* 2007;**110**(7):2259–2267.

58. **Nascimento AF, Pinkus JL, Pinkus GS.** Clusterin, a marker for anaplastic large cell lymphoma immunohistochemical profile in hematopoietic and nonhematopoietic malignant neoplasms. *American Journal of Clinical Pathology.* 2004;**121**(5):709–717.

59. **Lae ME, Ahmed I, Macon WR.** Clusterin is widely expressed in systemic anaplastic large cell lymphoma but fails to differentiate primary from secondary cutaneous anaplastic large cell lymphoma. *American Journal of Clinical Pathology.* 2002;**118**(5):773–779.

60. **Dunphy CH, DeMello DE, Gale GB.** Pediatric CD56+ anaplastic large cell lymphoma: a review of the literature. *Archives of Pathology and Laboratory Medicine.* 2006;**130**(12):1859–1864.

61. **Suzuki R, Kagami Y, Takeuchi K**, *et al.* Prognostic significance of CD56 expression for ALK-positive and ALK-negative anaplastic large-cell lymphoma of T/null cell phenotype. *Blood.* 2000;**96**(9):2993–3000.

62. **Pulford K, Morris SW, Mason DY.** Anaplastic lymphoma kinase proteins and malignancy. *Current Opinion in Hematology.* 2001;**8**(4):231–236.

63. **Sherman CG, Zielenska M, Lorenzana AN**, *et al.* Morphological and phenotypic features in pediatric large cell lymphoma and their correlation with ALK expression and the t(2;5)(p23;q35) translocation. *Pediatric and Developmental Pathology.* 2001; **4**(2):129–137.

64. **Pulford K, Lamant L, Morris SW**, *et al.* Detection of anaplastic lymphoma kinase (ALK) and nucleolar protein nucleophosmin (NPM)-ALK proteins in normal and neoplastic cells with the monoclonal antibody ALK1. *Blood.* 1997;**89**(4):1394–1404.

65. **Duyster J, Bai RY, Morris SW.** Translocations involving anaplastic lymphoma kinase (ALK). *Oncogene.* 2001;**20**(40):5623–5637.

66. **Oertel J, Huhn D.** Immunocytochemical methods in haematology and oncology. *Journal of Cancer Research and Clinical Oncology.* 2000;**126**(8):425–440.

67. **Chiarle R, Voena C, Ambrogio C, Piva R, Inghirami G.** The anaplastic lymphoma kinase in the pathogenesis of cancer. *Nature Reviews, Cancer.* 2008; **8**(1):11–23.

68. **Borisch B, Yerly S, Cerato Ch**, *et al.* ALK-positive anaplastic large-cell lymphoma: strong T and B anti-tumour responses may cause hypocellular aspects of lymph nodes mimicking inflammatory lesions. *European Journal of Haematology.* 2003;**71**(4):243–249.

69. **Kremer M, Quintanilla-Martínez L, Nährig J, von Schilling C, Fend F.** Immunohistochemistry in bone marrow pathology: a useful adjunct for morphologic diagnosis. *Virchows Archiv.* 2005;**447**(6):920–937.

70. **Mussolin L, Pillon M, d'Amore ES**, *et al.* Prevalence and clinical implications of bone marrow involvement in pediatric anaplastic large cell lymphoma. *Leukemia.* 2005; **19**(9):1643–1647.

71. **Kalinova M, Krskova L, Brizova H**, *et al.* Quantitative PCR detection of NPM/ALK fusion gene and CD30 gene expression in patients with anaplastic large cell lymphoma – residual disease monitoring and a correlation with the disease status. *Leukemia Research.* 2008;**32**(1):25–32.

72. **Damm-Welk C, Busch K, Burkhardt B**, *et al.* Prognostic significance of circulating tumor cells in bone marrow or peripheral blood as detected by qualitative and quantitative PCR in pediatric NPM-ALK-positive anaplastic large-cell lymphoma. *Blood.* 2007; **110**(2):670–677.

73. **Janik JE, Morris JC, Pittaluga S**, *et al.* Elevated serum soluble interleukin-2 receptor levels in patients with anaplastic large cell lymphoma. *Blood.* 2004;**104** (10):3355–3357.

74. **Zinzani PL, Pileri S, Bendandi M**, *et al.* Clinical implications of serum levels of soluble CD30 in 70 adult anaplastic large-cell lymphoma patients. *Journal of Clinical Oncology.* 1998;**16**(4):1532–1537.

75. **Goldsby RE, Carroll WL.** The molecular biology of pediatric lymphomas. *Journal of Pediatric Hematology/Oncology.* 1998;**20**(4):282–296.

76. **Drexler HG, Gignac SM, von Wasielewski R, Werner M, Dirks WG.** Pathobiology of NPM-ALK and variant fusion genes in anaplastic large cell lymphoma and other lymphomas. *Leukemia.* 2000;**14**(9):1533–1559.

77. **Damm-Welk C, Klapper W, Oschlies I**, *et al.* Distribution of NPM1-ALK and X-ALK fusion transcripts in paediatric anaplastic large cell lymphoma: a molecular-histological correlation. *British Journal of Haematology.* 2009; **146**:306–309.

78. Morris SW, Kirstein MN, Valentine MB, *et al.* Fusion of a kinase gene, ALK, to a nucleolar protein gene, NPM, in non-Hodgkin's lymphoma. *Science.* 1994;**263**(5151):1281–1284.

79. Pulford K, Lamant L, Espinos E, *et al.* The emerging normal and disease-related roles of anaplastic lymphoma kinase. *Cellular and Molecular Life Sciences.* 2004;**61**(23):2939–2953.

80. Cataldo KA, Jalal SM, Law ME, *et al.* Detection of t(2;5) in anaplastic large cell lymphoma: comparison of immunohistochemical studies, FISH, and RT-PCR in paraffin-embedded tissue. *American Journal of Surgical Pathology.* 1999;**23**(11):1386–1392.

81. Mathew P, Sanger WG, Weisenburger DD, *et al.* Detection of the t(2;5)(p23;q35) and NPM-ALK fusion in non-Hodgkin's lymphoma by two-color fluorescence in situ hybridization. *Blood.* 1997;**89**(5):1678–1685.

82. Waggott W, Lo YM, Bastard C, *et al.* Detection of NPM-ALK DNA rearrangement in CD30 positive anaplastic large cell lymphoma. *British Journal of Haematology.* 1995;**89**(4):905–907.

83. Gascoyne RD, Aoun P, Wu D, *et al.* Prognostic significance of anaplastic lymphoma kinase (ALK) protein expression in adults with anaplastic large cell lymphoma. *Blood.* 1999;**93**(11):3913–3921.

84. Brugieres L, Le Deley MC, Rosolen A, *et al.* Impact of the methotrexate administration dose on the need for intrathecal treatment in children and adolescents with anaplastic large-cell lymphoma: results of a randomized trial of the EICNHL Group. *Journal of Clinical Oncology.* 2009;**27**(6):897–903.

85. Lowe EJ, Sposto R, Perkins SL, *et al.* Intensive chemotherapy for systemic anaplastic large cell lymphoma in children and adolescents: final results of Children's Cancer Group Study 5941. *Pediatric Blood and Cancer.* 2009;**52**(3):335–339.

86. Borer RA, Lehner CF, Eppenberger HM, Nigg EA. Major nucleolar proteins shuttle between nucleus and cytoplasm. *Cell.* 1989;**56**(3):379–90.

87. Schmidt-Zachmann MS, Franke WW. DNA cloning and amino acid sequence determination of a major constituent protein of mammalian nucleoli. Correspondence of the nucleoplasmin-related protein NO38 to mammalian protein B23. *Chromosoma.* 1988;**96**(6):417–426.

88. Schmidt-Zachmann MS, Hugle-Dorr B, Franke WW. A constitutive nucleolar protein identified as a member of the nucleoplasmin family. *EMBO Journal.* 1987;**6**(7):1881–1890.

89. Okuda M, Horn HF, Tarapore P, *et al.* Nucleophosmin/B23 is a target of CDK2/cyclin E in centrosome duplication. *Cell.* 2000;**103**(1):127–140.

90. Colombo E, Marine JC, Danovi D, Falini B, Pelicci PG. Nucleophosmin regulates the stability and transcriptional activity of p53. *Nature Cell Biology.* 2002;**4**(7):529–533.

91. Kurki S, Peltonen K, Latonen L, *et al.* Nucleolar protein NPM interacts with HDM2 and protects tumor suppressor protein p53 from HDM2-mediated degradation. *Cancer Cell.* 2004;**5**(5):465–75.

92. Iwatsubo T. The gamma-secretase complex: machinery for intramembrane proteolysis. *Current Opinion in Neurobiology.* 2004;**14**(3):379–383.

93. Morris SW, Naeve C, Mathew P, *et al.* ALK, the chromosome 2 gene locus altered by the t(2;5) in non-Hodgkin's lymphoma, encodes a novel neural receptor tyrosine kinase that is highly related to leukocyte tyrosine kinase (LTK). *Oncogene.* 1997;**14**(18):2175–2188.

94. Fujimoto J, Shiota M, Iwahara T, *et al.* Characterization of the transforming activity of p80, a hyperphosphorylated protein in a Ki-1 lymphoma cell line with chromosomal translocation t(2;5). *Proceedings of the National Academy of Sciences of the United States of America.* 1996;**93**(9):4181–4186.

95. Kuefer MU, Look AT, Pulford K, *et al.* Retrovirus-mediated gene transfer of NPM-ALK causes lymphoid malignancy in mice. *Blood.* 1997;**90**(8):2901–2910.

96. Chiarle R, Gong JZ, Guasparri I, *et al.* NPM-ALK transgenic mice spontaneously develop T-cell lymphomas and plasma cell tumors. *Blood.* 2003;**101**(5):1919–1927.

97. Cook JR, Dehner LP, Collins MH, *et al.* Anaplastic lymphoma kinase (ALK) expression in the inflammatory myofibroblastic tumor: a comparative immunohistochemical study. *American Journal of Surgical Pathology.* 2001;**25**(11):1364–1371.

98. Thompson MA, Stumph J, Henrickson SE, *et al.* Differential gene expression in anaplastic lymphoma kinase-positive and anaplastic lymphoma kinase-negative anaplastic large cell lymphomas. *Human Pathology.* 2005;**36**(5):494–504.

99. Lamant L, de Reyniès A, Duplantier MM, *et al.* Gene-expression profiling of systemic anaplastic large-cell lymphoma reveals differences based on ALK status and two distinct morphologic ALK+ subtypes. *Blood.* 2007;**109**(5):2156–2164.

100. Zettl A, Rüdiger T, Konrad MA, *et al.* Genomic profiling of peripheral T-cell lymphoma, unspecified, and anaplastic large T-cell lymphoma delineates novel recurrent chromosomal alterations. *American Journal of Pathology.* 2004;**164**(5):1837–1848.

101. Seidemann K, Tiemann M, Schrappe M, *et al.* Short-pulse B-non-Hodgkin lymphoma-type chemotherapy is efficacious treatment for pediatric anaplastic large cell lymphoma: a report of the Berlin-Frankfurt-Munster Group Trial NHL-BFM 90. *Blood.* 2001;**97**(12):3699–3706.

102. Rosolen A, Pillon M, Garaventa A, *et al.* Anaplastic large cell lymphoma treated with a leukemia-like therapy: report of the Italian Association of Pediatric Hematology and Oncology (AIEOP) LNH-92 protocol. *Cancer.* 2005;**104**(10):2133–2140.

103. Woessmann W, Peters C, Lenhard M, *et al.* Allogeneic haematopoietic stem cell transplantation in relapsed or refractory anaplastic large cell lymphoma of children and adolescents – a Berlin-Frankfurt-Munster group report. *British Journal of Haematology.* 2006;**133**(2):176–182.

104. Zhang M, Yao Z, Zhang Z, *et al.* Effective therapy for a murine model of human anaplastic large-cell lymphoma with the anti-CD30 monoclonal antibody, HeFi-1, does not require activating Fc receptors. *Blood.* 2006;**108**(2):705–710.

105. Galkin AV, Melnick JS, Kim S, *et al.* Identification of NVP-TAE684, a potent, selective, and efficacious inhibitor of NPM-ALK. *Proceedings of*

the National Academy of Sciences of the United States of America. 2007;**104**(1): 270–275.

106. **Li R, Morris SW.** Development of anaplastic lymphoma kinase (ALK) small-molecule inhibitors for cancer therapy. *Medicinal Research Reviews.* 2008;**28**(3):372–412.

107. **Lin KH, Su IJ, Chen RL,** *et al.* Peripheral T-cell lymphoma in childhood: a report of five cases in Taiwan. *Medical and Pediatric Oncology.* 1994;**23**(1):26–35.

108. **Leake J, Kellie SJ, Pritchard J, Chessells JM, Risdon RA.** Peripheral T-cell lymphoma in childhood: a clinicopathologic study of six cases. *Histopathology.* 1989;**14**:255–268.

109. **Schulz L, Twite M, Liang X, Lovell M, Stork L.** A case of childhood peripheral T-cell lymphoma with massive cardiac infiltration. *Journal of Pediatric Hematology/Oncology.* 2004;**26**(1): 48–51.

110. **Massimino M, Perotti D, Spreafico F,** *et al.* Non-ALC peripheral T-cell lymphomas in children: report on two cases and review of the literature. *Haematologica.* 2000;**85**(10):1109–1111.

111. **Agnarsson B, Kadin M.** Peripheral T-cell lymphomas in children. *Seminars in Diagnostic Pathology.* 1995;**12**:314–324.

112. **Gordon BG, Weisenburger DD, Warkentin PI,** *et al.* Peripheral T-cell lymphoma in childhood and adolescence. A clinicopathologic study of 22 patients. *Cancer.* 1993;**71**(1):257–263.

113. **Lee SH, Su IJ, Chen RL,** *et al.* A pathologic study of childhood lymphoma in Taiwan with special reference to peripheral T-cell lymphoma and the association with Epstein-Barr viral infection. *Cancer.* 1991;**68**(9):1954–1962.

114. **Hutchison RE, Laver JH, Chang M,** *et al.* Non-anaplastic peripheral T-cell lymphoma in childhood and adolescence: a Children's Oncology Group study. *Pediatric Blood and Cancer.* 2008;**51**(1):29–33.

115. **Kluin PM, Feller A, Gaulard P,** *et al.* Peripheral T/NK-cell lymphoma: a report of the IXth Workshop of the European Association for Haematopathology. *Histopathology.* 2001;**38**(3):250–270.

116. **Anderson JR, Armitage JO, Weisenburger DD.** Epidemiology of the non-Hodgkin's lymphomas: distributions of the major subtypes differ by geographic locations. Non-Hodgkin's Lymphoma Classification Project. *Annals of Oncology.* 1998;**9**(7):717–720.

117. **Reiser M, Josting A, Soltani M,** *et al.* T-cell non-Hodgkin's lymphoma in adults: clinicopathological characteristics, response to treatment and prognostic factors. *Leukemia and Lymphoma.* 2002;**43**(4):805–811.

118. **Rudiger T, Gascoyne RD, Jaffe ES,** *et al.* Workshop on the relationship between nodular lymphocyte predominant Hodgkin's lymphoma and T cell/histiocyte-rich B cell lymphoma. *Annals of Oncology.* 2002;**13**(Suppl 1): 44–51.

119. **Zucca E, Zinzani PL.** Understanding the group of peripheral T-cell lymphomas, unspecified. *Current Hematology Reports.* 2005;**4**(1):23–30.

120. **Dearden CE, Foss FM.** Peripheral T-cell lymphomas: diagnosis and management. *Hematology/Oncology Clinics of North America.* 2003;**17**(6): 1351–1366.

121. **van Dongen JJ, Langerak AW, Brüggemann M,** *et al.* Design and standardization of PCR primers and protocols for detection of clonal immunoglobulin and T-cell receptor gene recombinations in suspect lymphoproliferations: report of the BIOMED-2 Concerted Action BMH4-CT98-3936. *Leukemia.* 2003;**17**(12):2257–2317.

122. **Smith JL, Hodges E, Howell WM, Jones DB.** Genotypic heterogeneity of node based peripheral T-cell lymphoma. *Leukemia and Lymphoma.* 1993;**10**(4–5):273–279.

123. **Gordon BG, Weisenburger DD, Sanger WG, Armitage JO, Coccia PF.** Peripheral T-cell lymphoma in children and adolescents: role of bone marrow transplantation. *Leukemia and Lymphoma.* 1994;**14**(1–2):1–10.

124. **Laver JH, Kraveka JM, Hutchison RE,** *et al.* Advanced-stage large-cell lymphoma in children and adolescents: results of a randomized trial incorporating intermediate-dose methotrexate and high-dose cytarabine in the maintenance phase of the APO regimen: a Pediatric Oncology Group phase III trial. *Journal of Clinical Oncology.* 2005;**23**(3):541–547.

125. **Mora J, Filippa DA, Thaler HT,** *et al.* Large cell non-Hodgkin lymphoma of childhood: Analysis of 78 consecutive patients enrolled in 2 consecutive protocols at the Memorial Sloan-Kettering Cancer Center. *Cancer.* 2000; **88**(1):186–197.

126. **Geha RS, Perez Atayde AR, Griscom T, Vawter GF.** A 10-year-old boy with progressive lymphadenopathy, fever, and rash. *Annals of Allergy.* 1984;**53**(5): 381–389.

127. **Howarth CB, Bird CC.** Immunoblastic sarcoma arising in child with immunoblastic lymphadenopathy. *Lancet.* 1976;**2**(7988):747–748.

128. **Kissane JM, Gephardt GN.** Lymphadenopathy in childhood: long term follow-up in patients with nondiagnostic lymph node biopsies. *Human Pathology.* 1974;**5**(4):431–439.

129. **Nakazono S, Kitahara T, Takezaki T,** *et al.* Immunoblastic lymphadenopathy (IBL)-like T-cell lymphoma in a child. *Acta Paediatrica Japonica.* 1991;**33**(3): 398–407.

130. **Nezelof C, Virelizier JL.** Long lasting lymphadenopathy in childhood as an expression of a severe hyperimmune B lymphocyte disorder. *Hematological Oncology.* 1983;**1**(3):227–242.

131. **Stensvold K, Brandtzaeg P, Kvaløy S, Seip M, Lie SO.** Immunoblastic lymphadenopathy with early onset in two boys: immunohistochemical study and indication of decreased proportion of circulating T-helper cells. *British Journal of Haematology.* 1984;**56**(3): 417–430.

132. **Dogan A, Isaacson PG.** Splenic marginal zone lymphoma. *Seminars in Diagnostic Pathology.* 2003;**20**(2):121–127.

133. **Ferry JA.** Angioimmunoblastic T-cell lymphoma. *Advances in Anatomic Pathology.* 2002;**9**(5):273–279.

134. **Iannitto E, Ferreri AJ, Minardi V, Tripodo C, Kreipe HH.** Angioimmunoblastic T-cell lymphoma. *Critical Reviews in Oncology/Hematology.* 2008;**68**(3):264–271.

135. **Dunleavy K, Wilson WH.** Angioimmunoblastic T-cell lymphoma: immune modulation as a therapeutic strategy. *Leukemia and Lymphoma.* 2007;**48**(3):449–451.

136. Cotta CV, Hsi ED. Pathobiology of mature T-cell lymphomas. *Clinical Lymphoma and Myeloma.* 2008; 8(Suppl 5):S168–S179.

137. Attygalle AD, Liu H, Shirali S, *et al.* Atypical marginal zone hyperplasia of mucosa-associated lymphoid tissue: a reactive condition of childhood showing immunoglobulin lambda light-chain restriction. *Blood.* 2004; 104(10):3343–3348.

138. Alizadeh AA, Advani RH. Evaluation and management of angioimmunoblastic T-cell lymphoma: a review of current approaches and future strategies. *Clinical Advances in Hematology and Oncology.* 2008;6(12): 899–909.

139. Merchant SH, Amin MB, Viswanatha DS. Morphologic and immunophenotypic analysis of angioimmunoblastic T-cell lymphoma: Emphasis on phenotypic aberrancies for early diagnosis. *American Journal of Clinical Pathology.* 2006;126(1):29–38.

140. Attygalle A, Al-Jehani R, Diss TC, *et al.* Neoplastic T cells in angioimmunoblastic T-cell lymphoma express CD10. *Blood.* 2002;99(2):627–633.

141. Attygalle AD, Chuang SS, Diss TC, *et al.* Distinguishing angioimmunoblastic T-cell lymphoma from peripheral T-cell lymphoma, unspecified, using morphology, immunophenotype and molecular genetics. *Histopathology.* 2007;50(4): 498–508.

142. Sonnen R, Schmidt WP, Müller-Hermelink HK, Schmitz N. The International Prognostic Index determines the outcome of patients with nodal mature T-cell lymphomas. *British Journal of Haematology.* 2005; 129(3):366–372.

143. Mackey AC, Green L, Liang LC, Dinndorf P, Avigan M. Hepatosplenic T cell lymphoma associated with infliximab use in young patients treated for inflammatory bowel disease. *Journal of Pediatric Gastroenterology and Nutrition.* 2007;44(2):265–267.

144. Thayu M, Markowitz JE, Mamula P, *et al.* Hepatosplenic T-cell lymphoma in an adolescent patient after immunomodulator and biologic therapy for Crohn disease. *Journal of Pediatric Gastroenterology and Nutrition.* 2005;40(2):220–222.

145. Mackey AC, Green L, Leptak C, Avigan M. Hepatosplenic T cell lymphoma associated with infliximab use in young patients treated for inflammatory bowel disease: update. *Journal of Pediatric Gastroenterology and Nutrition.* 2009;48(3):386–388.

146. Shale M, Kanfer E, Panaccione R, Ghosh S. Hepatosplenic T cell lymphoma in inflammatory bowel disease. *Gut.* 2008;57(12):1639–1641.

147. Veres G, Baldassano RN, Mamula P. Infliximab therapy for pediatric Crohn's disease. *Expert Opinion on Biological Therapy.* 2007;7(12):1869–1880.

148. Khan WA, Yu L, Eisenbrey AB, *et al.* Hepatosplenic gamma/delta T-cell lymphoma in immunocompromised patients. Report of two cases and review of literature. *American Journal of Clinical Pathology.* 2001;116(1):41–50.

149. Belhadj K, Reyes F, Farcet JP, *et al.* Hepatosplenic gammadelta T-cell lymphoma is a rare clinicopathologic entity with poor outcome: report on a series of 21 patients. *Blood.* 2003; 102(13):4261–4269.

150. Weidmann E. Hepatosplenic T cell lymphoma. A review on 45 cases since the first report describing the disease as a distinct lymphoma entity in 1990. *Leukemia.* 2000;14(6):991–997.

151. Falchook GS, Vega F, Dang NH, *et al.* Hepatosplenic gamma-delta T-cell lymphoma: clinicopathological features and treatment. *Annals of Oncology.* 2009;20(6):1080–1085.

152. Coventry S, Punnett HH, Tomczak EZ, *et al.* Consistency of isochromosome 7q and trisomy 8 in hepatosplenic gammadelta T-cell lymphoma: detection by fluorescence in situ hybridization of a splenic touch-preparation from a pediatric patient. *Pediatric and Developmental Pathology.* 1999;2(5):478–483.

153. Rossbach HC, Chamizo W, Dumont DP, Barbosa JL, Sutcliffe MJ. Hepatosplenic gamma/delta T-cell lymphoma with isochromosome 7q, translocation t(7;21), and tetrasomy 8 in a 9-year-old girl. *Journal of Pediatric Hematology/Oncology.* 2002;24(2): 154–157.

154. Domm JA, Thompson M, Kuttesch JF, Acra S, Frangoul H. Allogeneic bone marrow transplantation for chemotherapy-refractory hepatosplenic

gammadelta T-cell lymphoma: case report and review of the literature. *Journal of Pediatric Hematology/Oncology.* 2005;27(11):607–610.

155. Garcia-Sanchez F, Menárguez J, Cristobal E, *et al.* Hepatosplenic gamma-delta T-cell malignant lymphoma: report of the first case in childhood, including molecular minimal residual disease follow-up. *British Journal of Haematology.* 1995;90(4):943–946.

156. Vega F, Medeiros LJ, Gaulard P. Hepatosplenic and other gammadelta T-cell lymphomas. *American Journal of Clinical Pathology.* 2007;127(6):869–880.

157. Cooke CB, Krenacs L, Stetler-Stevenson M, *et al.* Hepatosplenic T-cell lymphoma: a distinct clinicopathologic entity of cytotoxic gamma delta T-cell origin. *Blood.* 1996;88(11):4265–4274.

158. Macon WR, Levy NB, Kurtin PJ, *et al.* Hepatosplenic alpha beta T-cell lymphomas: a report of 14 cases and comparison with hepatosplenic gamma delta T-cell lymphomas. *American Journal of Surgical Pathology.* 2001;25(3):285–296.

159. Feldman AL, Law M, Grogg KL, *et al.* Incidence of TCR and TCL1 gene translocations and isochromosome 7q in peripheral T-cell lymphomas using fluorescence in situ hybridization. *American Journal of Clinical Pathology.* 2008;130(2):178–185.

160. Wang CC, Tien HF, Lin MT, *et al.* Consistent presence of isochromosome 7q in hepatosplenic T gamma/delta lymphoma: a new cytogenetic-clinicopathologic entity. *Genes, Chromosomes and Cancer.* 1995;12(3): 161–164.

161. Shetty S, Mansoor A, Roland B. Ring chromosome 7 with amplification of 7q sequences in a pediatric case of hepatosplenic T-cell lymphoma. *Cancer Genetics and Cytogenetics.* 2006;167(2): 161–163.

162. Leich E, Haralambieva E, Zettl A, *et al.* Tissue microarray-based screening for chromosomal breakpoints affecting the T-cell receptor gene loci in mature T-cell lymphomas. *Journal of Pathology.* 2007;213(1):99–105.

163. Humphreys MR, Cino M, Quirt I, Barth D, Kukreti V. Long-term survival in two patients with

hepatosplenic T cell lymphoma treated with interferon-alpha. *Leukemia and Lymphoma.* 2008;**49**(7):1420–1423.

164. Jiang L, Yuan CM, Hubacheck J, *et al.* Variable CD52 expression in mature T cell and NK cell malignancies: implications for alemtuzumab therapy. *British Journal of Haematology.* 2009; **145**(2):173–179.

165. Jaeger G, Bauer F, Brezinschek R, *et al.* Hepatosplenic gamma delta T-cell lymphoma successfully treated with a combination of alemtuzumab and cladribine. *Annals of Oncology.* 2008; **19**(5):1025–1026.

166. Meresse B, Ripoche J, Heyman M, Cerf-Bensussan N. Celiac disease: from oral tolerance to intestinal inflammation, autoimmunity and lymphomagenesis. *Mucosal Immunology.* 2009;**2**(1):8–23.

167. Li B, Shi YK, He XH, *et al.* Primary non-Hodgkin lymphomas in the small and large intestine: clinicopathological characteristics and management of 40 patients. *International Journal of Hematology.* 2008;**87**(4):375–381.

168. Di Sabatino A, Corazza GR. Coeliac disease. *Lancet.* 2009;**373**(9673): 1480–1493.

169. Howell WM, Leung ST, Jones DB, *et al.* HLA-DRB, -DQA, and -DQB polymorphism in celiac disease and enteropathy-associated T-cell lymphoma. Common features and additional risk factors for malignancy. *Human Immunology.* 1995;**43**(1):29–37.

170. Chott A, Vesely M, Simonitsch I, Mosberger I, Hanak H. Classification of intestinal T-cell neoplasms and their differential diagnosis. *American Journal of Clinical Pathology.* 1999; **111**(1 Suppl 1):S68–S74.

171. Catassi C, Bearzi I, Holmes GK. Association of celiac disease and intestinal lymphomas and other cancers. *Gastroenterology.* 2005; **128**(4 Suppl 1):S79–S86.

172. Arnaud-Battandier F, Schmitz J, Ricour C, Rey J. Intestinal malignant lymphoma in a child with familial celiac disease. *Journal of Pediatric Gastroenterology and Nutrition.* 1983;**2**(2):320–323.

173. Zettl A, deLeeuw R, Haralambieva E, Mueller-Hermelink H-K. Enteropathy-type T-cell lymphoma. *American Journal of Clinical Pathology.* 2007; **127**(5):701–706.

174. Muram-Zborovski T, Loeb D, Sun T. Primary intestinal intraepithelial natural killer-like T-cell lymphoma: case report of a distinct clinicopathologic entity. *Archives of Pathology and Laboratory Medicine.* 2009;**133**(1):133–137.

175. Verbeek WH, von Blomberg BM, Scholten PE, *et al.* The presence of small intestinal intraepithelial gamma/delta T-lymphocytes is inversely correlated with lymphoma development in refractory celiac disease. *American Journal of Gastroenterology.* 2008;**103**(12): 3152–3158.

176. Murray A, Cuevas EC, Jones DB, Wright DH. Study of the immunohistochemistry and T cell clonality of enteropathy-associated T cell lymphoma. *American Journal of Pathology.* 1995;**146**(2):509–519.

177. Isaacson PG, Du MQ. Gastrointestinal lymphoma: where morphology meets molecular biology. *Journal of Pathology.* 2005;**205**(2):255–274.

178. Ilyas M, Niedobitek G, Agathanggelou A, *et al.* Non-Hodgkin's lymphoma, coeliac disease, and Epstein-Barr virus: a study of 13 cases of enteropathy-associated T- and B-cell lymphoma. *Journal of Pathology.* 1995;**177**(2): 115–122.

179. Quintanilla-Martinez L, Lome-Maldonado C, Ott G, *et al.* Primary intestinal non-Hodgkin's lymphoma and Epstein-Barr virus: high frequency of EBV-infection in T-cell lymphomas of Mexican origin. *Leukemia and Lymphoma.* 1998; **30**(1–2):111–121.

180. Foss HD, Stein H. Pathology of intestinal lymphomas. *Recent Results in Cancer Research.* 2000;**156**:33–41.

181. Bishton MJ, Haynes AP. Combination chemotherapy followed by autologous stem cell transplant for enteropathy-associated T cell lymphoma. *British Journal of Haematology.* 2007;**136**(1): 111–113.

182. Molina AM, Horwitz SM. Rare T-cell lymphomas. *Cancer Treatment and Research,* 2008;**142**:331–347.

183. Jaffe ES, Chan JK, Su IJ, *et al.* Report of the Workshop on Nasal and Related Extranodal Angiocentric T/Natural Killer Cell Lymphomas. Definitions, differential diagnosis, and epidemiology. *American Journal of Surgical Pathology.* 1996;**20**(1):103–111.

184. Shaw PH, Cohn SL, Morgan ER, *et al.* Natural killer cell lymphoma: report of two pediatric cases, therapeutic options, and review of the literature. *Cancer.* 2001;**91**(4):642–646.

185. Kwong YL. Natural killer-cell malignancies: diagnosis and treatment. *Leukemia.* 2005;**19**(12):2186–2194.

186. Drut R, Drut RM. Primary angiocentric T-cell intestinal lymphoma with Epstein-Barr virus in a 5-year-old boy. *International Journal of Surgical Pathology.* 2001;**9**(2):163–168.

187. Weiss RL, Lazarus KH, Macon WR, Gulley ML, Kjeldsberg CR. Natural killer-like T-cell lymphoma in the small intestine of a child without evidence of enteropathy. *American Journal of Surgical Pathology.* 1997;**21**:964–969.

188. Chan JK, Sin VC, Wong KF, *et al.* Nonnasal lymphoma expressing the natural killer cell marker CD56: a clinicopathologic study of 49 cases of an uncommon aggressive neoplasm. *Blood.* 1997;**89**(12):4501–4513.

189. Di Cataldo A, Bertuna G, Mirabile E, *et al.* Natural killer lymphoma/leukemia: an uncommon pediatric case with indolent course. *Leukemia and Lymphoma.* 2004;**45**(8):1687–1689.

190. Willemze R, Beljaards RC. Spectrum of primary cutaneous CD30 (Ki-1)-positive lymphoproliferative disorders. A proposal for classification and guidelines for management and treatment. *Journal of the American Academy of Dermatology.* 1993;**28**(6): 973–980.

191. Willemze R, Jaffe ES, Burg G. WHO-EORTC classification for cutaneous lymphomas. *Blood.* 2005;**105**(10):3768–3785.

192. Kumar S, Pittaluga S, Raffeld M, *et al.* Primary cutaneous CD30-positive anaplastic large cell lymphoma in childhood: report of 4 cases and review of the literature. *Pediatric and Developmental Pathology.* 2005;**8**(1): 52–60.

193. Tomaszewski MM, Moad JC, Lupton GP. Primary cutaneous Ki-1(CD30) positive anaplastic large cell lymphoma in childhood. *Journal of the American Academy of Dermatology.* 1999; **40**(5 Pt 2):857–861.

194. **Hazneci E, Aydin NE, Dogan G, Turhan IO.** Primary cutaneous anaplastic large cell lymphoma in a young girl. *Journal of the European Academy of Dermatology and Venereology.* 2001;**15**(4):366–367.

195. **Hung TY, Lin YC, Sun HL, Liu MC.** Primary cutaneous anaplastic large cell lymphoma in a young child. *European Journal of Pediatrics.* 2008;**167**(1): 111–113.

196. **Kadin ME, Carpenter C.** Systemic and primary cutaneous anaplastic large cell lymphomas. *Seminars in Hematology.* 2003;**40**(3):244–256.

197. **Willemze R, Meijer CJ.** Primary cutaneous CD30-positive lymphoproliferative disorders. *Hematology/Oncology Clinics of North America.* 2003;**17**(6):1319–1332, vii–viii.

198. **Kinney MC, Jones D.** Cutaneous T-cell and NK-cell lymphomas: the WHO-EORTC classification and the increasing recognition of specialized tumor types. *American Journal of Clinical Pathology.* 2007;**127**(5): 670–686.

199. **Querfeld C, Kuzel TM, Guitart J, Rosen ST.** Primary cutaneous CD30+lymphoproliferative disorders: new insights into biology and therapy. *Oncology (Williston Park).* 2007;**21**(6):689–696; discussion 699–700.

200. **Burg G, Kempf W, Kazakov DV,** *et al.* Pyogenic lymphoma of the skin: a peculiar variant of primary cutaneous neutrophil-rich CD30+ anaplastic large-cell lymphoma. Clinicopathological study of four cases and review of the literature. *British Journal of Dermatology.* 2003;**148**(3):580–586.

201. **Massone C, El-Shabrawi-Caelen L, Kerl H, Cerroni L.** The morphologic spectrum of primary cutaneous anaplastic large T-cell lymphoma: a histopathologic study on 66 biopsy specimens from 47 patients with report of rare variants. *Journal of Cutaneous Pathology.* 2008;**35**(1):46–53.

202. **Wellmann A, Thieblemont C, Pittaluga S,** *et al.* Detection of differentially expressed genes in lymphomas using cDNA arrays: identification of clusterin as a new diagnostic marker for anaplastic large-cell lymphomas. *Blood.* 2000; **96**(2):398–404.

203. **Greisser J, Palmedo G, Sander C,** *et al.* Detection of clonal rearrangement of T-cell receptor genes in the diagnosis of primary cutaneous CD30 lymphoproliferative disorders. *Journal of Cutaneous Pathology.* 2006;**33**(11): 711–715.

204. **Liu HL, Hoppe RT, Kohler S,** *et al.* CD30+ cutaneous lymphoproliferative disorders: the Stanford experience in lymphomatoid papulosis and primary cutaneous anaplastic large cell lymphoma. *Journal of the American Academy of Dermatology.* 2003;**49**(6): 1049–1058.

205. **Kunishige JH, McDonald H, Alvarez G,** *et al.* Lymphomatoid papulosis and associated lymphomas: a retrospective case series of 84 patients. *Clinical and Experimental Dermatology.* 2009;**34**(5): 576–581.

206. **El Shabrawi-Caelen L, Kerl H, Cerroni L.** Lymphomatoid papulosis: reappraisal of clinicopathologic presentation and classification into subtypes A, B, and C. *Archives of Dermatology.* 2004;**140**(4):441–447.

207. **Chott A, Vonderheid EC, Olbricht S,** *et al.* The dominant T cell clone is present in multiple regressing skin lesions and associated T cell lymphomas of patients with lymphomatoid papulosis. *Journal of Investigative Dermatology.* 1996;**106**(4): 696–700.

208. **Peters K, Knoll JH, Kadin ME.** Cytogenetic findings in regressing skin lesions of lymphomatoid papulosis. *Cancer Genetics and Cytogenetics.* 1995;**80**(1):13–16.

209. **Nijsten T, Curiel-Lewandrowski C, Kadin ME.** Lymphomatoid papulosis in children: a retrospective cohort study of 35 cases. *Archives of Dermatology.* 2004;**140**(3):306–312.

210. **Bekkenk MW, Geelen FA, van Voorst Vader PC,** *et al.* Primary and secondary cutaneous CD30(+) lymphoproliferative disorders: a report from the Dutch Cutaneous Lymphoma Group on the long-term follow-up data of 219 patients and guidelines for diagnosis and treatment. *Blood.* 2000;**95**(12):3653–3661.

211. **Cabanillas F, Armitage J, Pugh WC, Weisenburger D, Duvic M.** Lymphomatoid papulosis: a T-cell dyscrasia with a propensity to

transform into malignant lymphoma. *Annals of Internal Medicine.* 1995; **122**(3):210–217.

212. **Wain EM, Orchard GE, Whittaker SJ,** *et al.* Outcome in 34 patients with juvenile-onset mycosis fungoides: a clinical, immunophenotypic, and molecular study. *Cancer.* 2003;**98**(10): 2282–2290.

213. **Tsianakas A, Kienast AK, Hoeger PH.** Infantile-onset cutaneous T-cell lymphoma. *British Journal of Dermatology.* 2008;**159**(6):1338–1341.

214. **Fink-Puches R, Chott A, Ardigó M,** *et al.* The spectrum of cutaneous lymphomas in patients less than 20 years of age. *Pediatric Dermatology.* 2004;**21**(5):525–533.

215. **Lansigan F, Choi J, Foss FM.** Cutaneous T-cell lymphoma. *Hematology/Oncology Clinics of North America.* 2008;**22**(5):979–996, x.

216. **Smoller BR.** Mycosis fungoides: what do/do not we know? *Journal of Cutaneous Pathology.* 2008;**35**(Suppl 2): 35–39.

217. **Zinzani PL, Ferreri AJ, Cerroni L.** Mycosis fungoides. *Critical Reviews in Oncology/Hematology.* 2008;**65**(2):172–182.

218. **Ben-Amitai D, Michael D, Feinmesser M, Hodak E.** Juvenile mycosis fungoides diagnosed before 18 years of age. *Acta Dermato-Venereologica.* 2003;**83**(6):451–456.

219. **Hanna S, Walsh N, D'Intino Y, Langley RG.** Mycosis fungoides presenting as pigmented purpuric dermatitis. *Pediatric Dermatology.* 2006;**23**(4):350–354.

220. **Robson A.** The pathology of cutaneous T-cell lymphoma. *Oncology (Williston Park).* 2007;**21**(2 Suppl 1):9–12.

221. **Diamandidou E, Colome-Grimmer M, Fayad L, Duvic M, Kurzrock R.** Transformation of mycosis fungoides/Sezary syndrome: clinical characteristics and prognosis. *Blood.* 1998;**92**(4):1150–1159.

222. **Scheffer E, Meijer CJ, van Vloten WA, Willemze R.** A histologic study of lymph nodes from patients with the Sezary syndrome. *Cancer.* 1986;**57**(12): 2375–2380.

223. **Florell SR, Cessna M, Lundell RB,** *et al.* Usefulness (or lack thereof) of immunophenotyping in atypical cutaneous T-cell infiltrates. *American*

Journal of Clinical Pathology. 2006; **125**(5):727–736.

224. **Karenko L, Hahtola S, Ranki A.** Molecular cytogenetics in the study of cutaneous T-cell lymphomas (CTCL). *Cytogenetic and Genome Research.* 2007;**118**(2–4):353–361.

225. **Parveen Z, Thompson K.** Subcutaneous panniculitis-like T-cell lymphoma: redefinition of diagnostic criteria in the recent World Health Organization-European Organization for Research and Treatment of Cancer classification for cutaneous lymphomas. *Archives of Pathology and Laboratory Medicine.* 2009;**133**(2):303–308.

226. **Shani-Adir A, Lucky AW, Prendiville J,** *et al.* Subcutaneous panniculitic T-cell lymphoma in children: response to combination therapy with cyclosporine and chemotherapy. *Journal of the American Academy of Dermatology.* 2004;**50**(2 Suppl): S18–S22.

227. **Imaizumi M, Ichinohasama R, Sato A,** *et al.* Primary cutaneous T-cell lymphoma involving the cheek: an infant case with a unique clinicopathologic feature. *Leukemia and Lymphoma.* 1998;**31**(1–2):225–229.

228. **Yim JH, Kim MY, Kim HO,** *et al.* Subcutaneous panniculitis-like T-cell lymphoma in a 26-month-old child with a review of the literature. *Pediatric Dermatology.* 2006;**23**(6):537–540.

229. **Windsor R, Stiller C, Webb D.** Peripheral T-cell lymphoma in childhood: population-based experience in the United Kingdom over 20 years. *Pediatric Blood and Cancer.* 2008;**50**(4):784–787.

230. **Hung IJ, Kuo TT, Sun CF.** Subcutaneous panniculitic T-cell lymphoma developing in a child with idiopathic myelofibrosis. *Journal of Pediatric Hematology/Oncology.* 1999;**21**:38–41.

231. **Willemze R, Jansen PM, Cerroni L,** *et al.* Subcutaneous panniculitis-like T-cell lymphoma: definition, classification, and prognostic factors: an EORTC Cutaneous Lymphoma Group Study of 83 cases. *Blood.* 2008;**111**(2): 838–845.

232. **Kong YY, Dai B, Kong JC,** *et al.* Subcutaneous panniculitis-like T-cell lymphoma: a clinicopathologic, immunophenotypic, and molecular study of 22 Asian cases according to

WHO-EORTC classification. *American Journal of Surgical Pathology.* 2008; **32**(10):1495–1502.

233. **Hoque SR, Child FJ, Whittaker SJ,** *et al.* Subcutaneous panniculitis-like T-cell lymphoma: a clinicopathological, immunophenotypic and molecular analysis of six patients. *British Journal of Dermatology.* 2003;**148**(3):516–525.

234. **Massone C, Chott A, Metze D,** *et al.* Subcutaneous, blastic natural killer (NK), NK/T-cell, and other cytotoxic lymphomas of the skin: a morphologic, immunophenotypic, and molecular study of 50 patients. *American Journal of Surgical Pathology.* 2004;**28**(6):719–735.

235. **Kao GF, Resh B, McMahon C,** *et al.* Fatal subcutaneous panniculitis-like T-cell lymphoma gamma/delta subtype (cutaneous gamma/delta T-cell lymphoma): report of a case and review of the literature. *American Journal of Dermatopathology.* 2008;**30**(6): 593–599.

236. **Gonzalez EG, Selvi E, Lorenzini S,** *et al.* Subcutaneous panniculitis-like T-cell lymphoma misdiagnosed as lupus erythematosus panniculitis. *Clinical Rheumatology.* 2007;**26**(2): 244–246.

237. **Fraga J, Garcia-Diez A.** Lupus erythematosus panniculitis. *Dermatological Clinics.* 2008;**26**(4):453–463, vi.

238. **Kim D, Ko Y, Suh Y,** *et al.* Characteristics of Epstein-Barr virus associated childhood non-Hodgkin's lymphoma in the Republic of Korea. *Virchows Archiv.* 2005;**447**(3):593–596.

239. **Ohnuma K, Toyoda Y, Nishihira H,** *et al.* Aggressive natural killer (NK) cell lymphoma: report of a pediatric case and review of the literature. *Leukemia and Lymphoma.* 1997;**25**(3–4):387–392.

240. **Chou WC, Chiang IP, Tang JL,** *et al.* Clonal disease of natural killer large granular lymphocytes in Taiwan. *British Journal of Haematology.* 1998;**103**(4): 1124–1128.

241. **Mori N, Yamashita Y, Tsuzuki T,** *et al.* Lymphomatous features of aggressive NK cell leukaemia/lymphoma with massive necrosis, haemophagocytosis and EB virus infection. *Histopathology.* 2000;**37**(4):363–371.

242. **Liang X, Graham DK.** Natural killer cell neoplasms. *Cancer.* 2008;**112**(7): 1425–1436.

243. **Alekshun TJ, Sokol L.** Diseases of large granular lymphocytes. *Cancer Control.* 2007;**14**(2):141–150.

244. **Macon WR, Williams ME, Greer JP,** *et al.* Natural killer-like T-cell lymphomas: aggressive lymphomas of T-large granular lymphocytes. *Blood.* 1996;**87**(4):1474–1483.

245. **Siu LL, Chan V, Chan JK,** *et al.* Consistent patterns of allelic loss in natural killer cell lymphoma. *American Journal of Pathology.* 2000;**157**(6): 1803–1809.

246. **Petterson TE, Bosco AA, Cohn RJ.** Aggressive natural killer cell leukemia presenting with hemophagocytic lymphohistiocytosis. *Pediatric Blood and Cancer.* 2008;**50**(3):654–657.

247. **Ryder J, Wang X, Bao L,** *et al.* Aggressive natural killer cell leukemia: report of a Chinese series and review of the literature. *International Journal of Hematology.* 2007;**85**(1):18–25.

248. **Siu LL, Wong KF, Chan JK, Kwong YL.** Comparative genomic hybridization analysis of natural killer cell lymphoma/ leukemia. Recognition of consistent patterns of genetic alterations. *American Journal of Pathology.* 1999; **155**(5):1419–1425.

249. **Siu LL, Chan JK, Kwong YL.** Natural killer cell malignancies: clinicopathologic and molecular features. *Histology and Histopathology.* 2002;**17**(2):539–554.

250. **Kwong YL, Wong KF, Chan LC,** *et al.* Large granular lymphocyte leukemia. A study of nine cases in a Chinese population. *American Journal of Clinical Pathology.* 1995;**103**(1): 76–81.

251. **Ito T, Makishima H, Nakazawa H,** *et al.* Promising approach for aggressive NK cell leukaemia with allogeneic haematopoietic cell transplantation. *European Journal of Haematology.* 2008;**81**(2):107–111.

252. **Jaccard A, Petit B, Girault S,** *et al.* L-asparaginase-based treatment of 15 western patients with extranodal NK/T-cell lymphoma and leukemia and a review of the literature. *Annals of Oncology.* 2009;**20**(1):110–116.

253. **Boztug K, Baumann U, Ballmaier M,** *et al.* Large granular lymphocyte proliferation and revertant mosaicism: two rare events in a Wiskott-Aldrich syndrome patient. *Haematologica.* 2007;**92**(3):e43–e45.

254. Kitchen BJ, Boxer LA. Large granular lymphocyte leukemia (LGL) in a child with hyper IgM syndrome and autoimmune hemolytic anemia. *Pediatric Blood and Cancer.* 2008; **50**(1):142–145.

255. O'Malley DP. T-cell large granular leukemia and related proliferations. *American Journal of Clinical Pathology.* 2007;**127**(6):850–859.

256. Rose MG, Berliner N. T-cell large granular lymphocyte leukemia and related disorders. *Oncologist.* 2004;**9**(3): 247–258.

257. Lamy T, Loughran TP Jr. Clinical features of large granular lymphocyte leukemia. *Seminars in Hematology.* 2003;**40**(3):185–195.

258. Manola KN, Sambani C, Karakasis D, *et al.* Leukemias associated with Turner syndrome: report of three cases and review of the literature. *Leukemia Research.* 2008;**32**(3):481–486.

259. Dhodapkar MV, Li CY, Lust JA, Tefferi A, Phyliky RL. Clinical spectrum of clonal proliferations of T-large granular lymphocytes: a T-cell clonopathy of undetermined significance? *Blood.* 1994;**84**(5):1620–1627.

260. Osuji N, Matutes E, Catovsky D, Lampert I, Wotherspoon A. Histopathology of the spleen in T-cell large granular lymphocyte leukemia and T-cell prolymphocytic leukemia: a comparative review. *American Journal of Surgical Pathology.* 2005;**29**(7): 935–941.

261. Morice WG, Kurtin PJ, Leibson PJ, Tefferi A, Hanson CA. Demonstration of aberrant T-cell and natural killer-cell antigen expression in all cases of granular lymphocytic leukaemia. *British Journal of Haematology.* 2003; **120**(6):1026–1036.

262. Morice WG. The immunophenotypic attributes of NK cells and NK-cell lineage lymphoproliferative disorders. *American Journal of Clinical Pathology.* 2007;**127**(6):881–886.

263. Lundell R, Hartung L, Hill S, Perkins SL, Bahler DW. T-cell large granular lymphocyte leukemias have multiple phenotypic abnormalities involving pan-T-cell antigens and receptors for MHC molecules. *American Journal of Clinical Pathology.* 2005;**124**(6): 937–946.

264. Gorczyca W, Weisberger J, Liu Z, *et al.* An approach to diagnosis of T-cell lymphoproliferative disorders by flow cytometry. *Cytometry.* 2002;**50**(3): 177–190.

265. Morice WG, Kimlinger T, Katzmann JA, *et al.* Flow cytometric assessment of TCR-Vbeta expression in the evaluation of peripheral blood involvement by T-cell lymphoproliferative disorders: a comparison with conventional T-cell immunophenotyping and molecular genetic techniques. *American Journal of Clinical Pathology.* 2004;**121**(3):373–383.

266. Man C, Au WY, Pang A, Kwong YL. Deletion 6q as a recurrent chromosomal aberration in T-cell large granular lymphocyte leukemia. *Cancer Genetics and Cytogenetics.* 2002;**139**(1): 71–74.

267. Ohtsuka R, Abe Y, Sada E, *et al.* Adult patient with Epstein-Barr virus (EBV)-associated lymphoproliferative disorder: chronic active EBV infection or de novo extranodal natural killer (NK)/T-cell lymphoma, nasal type? *Internal Medicine.* 2009;**48**(6):471–474.

268. Tazawa Y, Nishinomiya F, Noguchi H, *et al.* A case of fatal infectious mononucleosis presenting with fulminant hepatic failure associated with an extensive CD8-positive lymphocyte infiltration in the liver. *Human Pathology.* 1993;**24**(10): 1135–1139.

269. Su IJ, Hsieh HC, Lin KH, *et al.* Aggressive peripheral T-cell lymphomas containing Epstein-Barr viral DNA: a clinicopathologic and molecular analysis. *Blood.* 1991;**77**(4): 799–808.

270. Millard TP, Hawk JL. Photosensitivity disorders: cause, effect and management. *American Journal of Clinical Dermatology.* 2002;**3**(4): 239–246.

271. Tabata N, Aiba S, Ichinohazama R, *et al.* Hydroa vacciniforme-like lymphomatoid papulosis in a Japanese child: a new subset. *Journal of the American Academy of Dermatology.* 1995;**32**(2 Pt 2):378–381.

272. Kazakov DV, Burg G, Dummer R, Kempf W. Cutaneous lymphomas and pseudolymphomas: newly described entities. *Recent Results in Cancer Research.* 2002;**160**:283–293.

273. Wu YH, Chen HC, Hsiao PF, *et al.* Hydroa vacciniforme-like Epstein-Barr virus-associated monoclonal T-lymphoproliferative disorder in a child. *International Journal of Dermatology.* 2007;**46**(10):1081–1086.

274. Barrionuevo C, Anderson VM, Zevallos-Giampietri E, *et al.* Hydroa-like cutaneous T-cell lymphoma: a clinicopathologic and molecular genetic study of 16 pediatric cases from Peru. *Applied Immunohistochemistry and Molecular Morphology.* 2002;**10**(1):7–14.

275. Chen HH, Hsiao CH, Chiu HC. Hydroa vacciniforme-like primary cutaneous CD8-positive T-cell lymphoma. *British Journal of Dermatology.* 2002;**147**(3):587–591.

276. Zhang Y, Nagata H, Ikeuchi T, *et al.* Common cytological and cytogenetic features of Epstein-Barr virus (EBV)-positive natural killer (NK) cells and cell lines derived from patients with nasal T/NK-cell lymphomas, chronic active EBV infection and hydroa vacciniforme-like eruptions. *British Journal of Haematology.* 2003;**121**(5):805–814.

277. Magaña M, Sangüeza P, Gil-Beristain J, *et al.* Angiocentric cutaneous T-cell lymphoma of childhood (hydroa-like lymphoma): a distinctive type of cutaneous T-cell lymphoma. *Journal of the American Academy of Dermatology.* 1998;**38**(4):574–579.

278. Park S, Kim K, Kim WS, *et al.* Systemic EBV+ T-cell lymphoma in elderly patients: comparison with children and young adult patients. *Virchows Archiv.* 2008;**453**(2):155–163.

279. Feng S, Jin P, Zeng X. Hydroa vacciniforme-like primary cutaneous CD8-positive T-cell lymphoma. *European Journal of Dermatology.* 2008; **18**(3):364–365.

280. Swerdlow SH. T-cell and NK-cell posttransplantation lymphoproliferative disorders. *American Journal of Clinical Pathology.* 2007;**127**(6):887–895.

281. Carbone A, Gloghini A, Dotti G. EBV-associated lymphoproliferative disorders: classification and treatment. *Oncologist.* 2008;**13**(5):577–585.

282. Jamali FR, Otrock ZK, Soweid AM, *et al.* An overview of the pathogenesis and natural history of post-transplant T-cell lymphoma (corrected and republished article originally printed in *Leukemia and Lymphoma,* June 2007;

48(6): 1237–1241). *Leukemia and Lymphoma*. 2007;**48**(9):1780–1784.

283. **Yang F, Li Y, Braylan R, Hunger SP, Yang LJ**. Pediatric T-cell post-transplant lymphoproliferative disorder after solid organ transplantation. *Pediatric Blood and Cancer*. 2008;**50**(2):415–418.

284. **Salama S**. Primary "cutaneous" T-cell anaplastic large cell lymphoma,

CD30+, neutrophil-rich variant with subcutaneous panniculitic lesions, in a post-renal transplant patient: report of unusual case and literature review. *American Journal of Dermatopathology*. 2005;**27**(3):217–223.

285. **Coyne JD, Banerjee SS, Bromley M**, *et al*. Post-transplant T-cell lymphoproliferative disorder/T-cell lymphoma: a report of three cases of

T-anaplastic large-cell lymphoma with cutaneous presentation and a review of the literature. *Histopathology*. 2004; **44**(4):387–393.

286. **Costes-Martineau V, Delfour C, Obled S**, *et al*. Anaplastic lymphoma kinase (ALK) protein expressing lymphoma after liver transplantation: case report and literature review. *Journal of Clinical Pathology*. 2002;**55**(11):868–871.

Hodgkin lymphoma

Mihaela Onciu

Definition

Hodgkin lymphomas (HLs) encompass at least two morphologically, biologically, and clinically distinct subtypes of germinal center-derived B-lineage lymphoma [1]. Morphologically, these lymphomas are characterized by a small number of large atypical malignant cells (Hodgkin, Reed–Sternberg, and lymphocytic and histiocytic, or L&H, cells) set in the background of benign inflammatory elements, with or without associated fibrosis, that make up the bulk of the tumoral tissue. The neoplastic cells are typically surrounded by rosettes of T-lymphocytes. In the nodular lymphocyte-predominant type of HL (NLPHL), the neoplastic cells exhibit overt B-lineage differentiation. In the classical type of HL (cHL), these cells exhibit an aberrant differentiation program, and have a characteristic, CD15-positive, CD30-positive, CD45 (leukocyte common antigen)-negative immunophenotype. Classical HL is further subclassified according to the growth pattern and cellular milieu, into the lymphocyte-rich (LR), nodular sclerosis (NS), mixed cellularity (MC), and lymphocyte-depleted (LD) subtypes.

Epidemiology

HL has a bimodal age distribution throughout the world, with a peak of incidence at 15–34 years and a second peak after the age of 60 years [2]. A significant proportion of cases occurs in the pediatric age group, the majority of which present in adolescents, with only a minority of cases seen in patients under the age of 10 years [3, 4]. In the United States and Western European countries, the incidence of HL is <1 per million in children under 10 years of age, and approximately 29 per million in adolescents (10–19 years of age) [3, 4]. The same case distribution is seen in developing countries, where a slightly higher incidence is seen in patients younger than 10 years [5]. Children younger than 6 years of age represent 11–18% of all pediatric HL patients [4, 6]. The age of the youngest HL patient reported is seven months [4]. All histologic subtypes of HL may be encountered in this very young age group; however, the mixed cellularity subtype appears to be significantly more common

than in other age groups, as it represents 35–40% of the cases [4, 6]. Some studies suggest that cases occurring in this age group may also have a distinct pattern of chromosomal alterations (see below) [7]. HL shows a slight male predominance in adolescents (male : female ratio 1–1.5 : 1), and a marked male predominance in younger children (male : female ratio 3–4 : 1) [4, 6]. There is no race predilection [3, 4].

Both genetic and environmental factors appear to play a role in the predisposition to HL. A genetic predisposition for HL is suggested by cases with familial aggregation, some occurring in monozygotic twins [8]. This association has been described for both classical and nodular lymphocyte-predominant types. Associations with certain HLA subtypes have been suggested in the context of familial HL, such as with class II HLA subtypes DR16, Drw51, and DQ5, and with a haplotype consisting of DRB*1501-DQA1*0102-DQB1*0602, the TAP1 allele encoding Ile at residue 333, and DRB5*0101 allele [8]. Data suggesting an increased risk of HL associated with long-standing smoking and environmental chemicals, such as benzene and various herbicides and pesticides, has remained conflicting [2].

Hodgkin lymphoma occurs with increased frequency in the setting of immunodeficiency, both congenital (primary) and acquired immunodeficiencies. Hodgkin lymphoma is one of the lymphomas encountered in common variable immunodeficiency, hyper-IgM syndrome, Wiscott–Aldrich syndrome, ataxia telangiectasia, and Nijmegen breakage syndrome, as well as in HIV infection, and as a post-transplant lymphoproliferative disorder. The subtype of HL lymphoma typically seen in this setting is cHL [1]. Hodgkin lymphoma of both lymphocyte-predominant and classical types also occurs with increased frequency in the autoimmune lymphoproliferative syndrome (Canale–Smith syndrome), associated with immune dysregulation [1]. A strong association with the Epstein–Barr virus has been well documented in cHL (see below).

Clinical presentation and staging

The typical clinical presentation of HL includes lymphadenopathy (usually cervical or supraclavicular), a mediastinal mass which may be associated with symptoms of airway

Table 23.1. The Ann Arbor staging system for Hodgkin lymphoma.

Stage	Definition

I
(A or B)[a]
	Involvement of a single site:
	    Single lymph node region (I)
	    Single extranodal/extralymphatic site (I$_E$)

II
(A or B)[a]
	Involvement of >1 site on the same side of the diaphragm:
	    Involvement of two or more lymph node regions (II)
	    Involvement of an extranodal/extralymphatic site and of
	    one or more lymph node regions (II$_E$)

III
(A or B)[a]
	Involvement of several sites on both sides of the diaphragm:
	    Involvement of lymph node regions (III)
	    Involvement of the spleen (III$_S$)
	    Involvement of extranodal/extralymphatic site (III$_E$)

IV (A or B)[a]	Diffuse/disseminated involvement of one or more extranodal/extralymphatic sites, with/without lymph node involvement

[a] Each stage is additionally designated as A or B depending on the absence or presence, respectively, of high fever (>38 °C for three consecutive days), drenching night sweats, or unexplained weight loss of at least 10% of body weight in the preceding six months.

compression, and a variety of systemic symptoms [9]. Some of these systemic symptoms (so-called B symptoms), including fever (exceeding 38 °C), weight loss (greater than 10% within six months), and drenching night sweats, are associated with prognosis in HL. Other classical symptoms include pruritus (often associated with advanced-stage disease) and pain that occurs immediately following alcohol ingestion and is localized to the areas of lymphadenopathy or to the chest [9]. Laboratory abnormalities are usually non-specific, and may include leukocytosis with neutrophilia, eosinophilia, monocytosis, and/or lymphopenia. In addition, a variety of autoimmune cytopenias, most commonly hemolytic anemia and immune thrombocytopenia, may be found in this setting. Finally, a variety of immune system abnormalities, including anergy to delayed sensitivity skin tests, decreased mitogen-induced T-cell proliferation, and a decreased CD4 : CD8 ratio, may be found in HL patients at diagnosis, and during and after therapy [9].

The extent of disease (translated into the disease staging) and the presence or absence of B-symptoms are the most important determinants of outcome in HL, especially in classical HL [9]. Hodgkin lymphoma is currently staged according to the Ann Arbor system adopted in 1971, that was developed based on the initial observation that this lymphoma spreads to lymph node stations in a contiguous fashion [10] (see Table 23.1). While in the 1970s staging laparotomy with splenectomy was undertaken in order to ensure accurate pathologic staging, the current imaging technology has allowed for less-invasive and equally accurate staging, while preserving splenic function in HL patients [9].

The biology and genetics of Hodgkin lymphoma

This section will focus on the essential biological aspects underlying the pathology, immunophenotype, and clinical presenta-

tion of this lymphoma, which should allow for better understanding of the remaining material covered in this chapter. In-depth coverage of this topic is beyond the scope of this textbook.

Histogenesis

The origin of the neoplastic cells of HL had remained enigmatic for a long period of time. By *in situ* immunophenotypic studies, these cells expressed markers of dendritic cells, granulocytes, and T- and B-lymphocytes. In addition, the characteristic composition of the HL tumor tissue, including a minority of neoplastic cells (less than 1%) "diluted" in a mass of benign polyclonal inflammatory cells, often with associated fibrosis, precluded accurate studies of the neoplastic cells by conventional molecular techniques. The availability of tissue microdissection techniques, that allowed for selective analysis of these cells, led to the discovery that the malignant cells of HL are in fact clonal B-lineage lymphocytes with abnormal differentiation programs [11].

Extensive research, employing microdissected HL cells, has demonstrated three distinct origins for these cells [12].

(1) In the NLPHL, the tumor cells, named "lymphocytic and histiocytic" (L&H) derive from germinal center (GC) or post-GC B-cells [showing rearranged immunoglobulin variable (IgV) genes]. The presence of intraclonal IgV gene diversity further shows that they originate in mutated and selected GC B-cells (selection due to affinity with the cognate antigen). These neoplastic cells retain expression of all B-cell-specific molecules, including CD19, CD20, CD79a, J chain, PAX-5, Ig (with light chain restriction), Oct-2, BOB.1, and PU-1, although at reduced levels of expression.

(2) In cHL, the tumor cells, named Hodgkin and Reed–Sternberg (HRS) cells, are also GC B-cells, but they additionally show crippling mutations that destroy the coding capacity of their previously functional IgV gene rearrangements. In the normal GC, such cells are typically targeted for apoptosis. Therefore, HRS cells appear to originate in preapoptotic GC B-cells that escape apoptosis through various mechanisms. The inhibition of apoptosis in these cells has been attributed to a variety of molecular and genetic alterations found in the cells, including constitutive activation of the NFκB pathway, activation of NOTCH-1, aberrant activities of multiple receptor tyrosine kinases (some of which may constitute attractive therapeutic targets), and activation of STAT (STAT 3, 5 and 6) and AP-1 transcription factors. Notably, the CD30 molecule, highly expressed by HRS cells, appears to play an important role in at least two of these altered signaling pathways, including NFκB and AP-1.

The HRS cells show an aberrant differentiation program that includes the profound downregulation of most B-cell-specific genes (including those for CD19, CD20, CD79a, Ig, and the transcription factors Oct-2, BOB.1, and

PU-1), although they surprisingly retain typically weak expression of PAX-5/BSAP, a B-lineage commitment and maintenance factor. They also retain molecules important in B–T-cell interactions, such as CD80, CD86, and MHC class II, and often express molecules typically upregulated in plasma cells (CD138 and MUM-1) [13, 14].

(3) Last, in a minority of cHL cases (2%), the HRS cells show a cytotoxic T-lymphoid immunophenotype, that may be associated with a B-cell genotype or harbor T-cell receptor beta gene rearrangements [12, 15].

Cytokines and chemokines

The inflammatory background of HL suggests that this disease is characterized by an extensive but, nevertheless, ineffective immune response, that allows the neoplastic cells to escape immune surveillance. This inflammatory response, along with the systemic symptoms present in a significant proportion of HL patients, appears to be initiated and maintained by a rich network of cytokines and chemokines produced by the HRS cells and the inflammatory cells and fibroblasts in their immediate vicinity. Some of these factors are responsible for attracting various subtypes of inflammatory cells at the sites of disease. Furthermore, the neoplastic cells appear to have receptors for some of these factors, leading to self-maintained autocrine loops.

The profile of chemokines and cytokines produced by the tumor cells appears to determine the disease subtype and clinical manifestations of disease. Among the cytokines identified in HRS cells, their cellular environment, and the serum of HL patients are interleukin-5 (IL-5), IL-8, IL-10, IL-13, IL-17, and IL-18 [16–20]. Interleukin-8 elevation appears to correlate with granulocyte infiltration in cHL tumors [16]. Additional cytokines and cytokine receptors elevated in the serum of HL patients and shown to correlate with clinical symptoms, disease activity, and outcome include soluble IL-2 receptor (sIL-2R), IL-6, IL-7, IL-8, and granulocyte colony stimulating factor (G-CSF) [21]. Numerous chemokines have been shown to be produced in the HRS cells, some of which are also elevated in the serum of HL patients. These include: chemokine (C-C motif) ligand 17 (CCL 17) and CCL22, as well as CCL2, CCL3, CCL5 (RANTES), CCL11, CCL28, chemokine (CXC motif) ligand 8 (CXCL8), CXCL9, and CXCL10 [18, 22]. Some of these factors show interesting correlations. For instance, CCL17 (TARC) has been shown to be specific for cHL (and not expressed in NLPHL or non-Hodgkin lymphoma) [23–25]. CCL17 and CCL22, elevated in the serum of HL patients, more often in the NS subtype than in the MC subtype, also correlate with high-stage disease and disease activity [18]. Both of these chemokines interact with specific receptors that attract T-helper type 2 (Th2) cells to the sites of disease, which may contribute to the defects in immune surveillance observed in HL. Lastly, it has been shown that HRS cells can induce adjacent fibroblasts to produce eotaxin, which is an eosinophil and T-lymphocyte attractant [26].

HL and the Epstein–Barr virus (EBV)

The association between HL and EBV has been long documented through identification of EBV in the serum and neoplastic tissues of patients with HL [27, 28]. Epstein–Barr virus is present in a high proportion of cHL cases, with a frequency that depends on the histologic subtype (see below). By contrast it is found only extremely rarely in NLPHL [29]. In addition, EBV occurs with increased frequency in patients with congenital or acquired immunodeficiency states (see above), as well as in children and older adults [30]. It appears to be more frequent in males of Asian or Hispanic descent [30]. EBV-positive HL is also more likely to occur in individuals carrying the HLA-A*01 genotype, and less likely to affect individuals with HLA-A*02 [31]. The frequency of EBV+ HL is also increased in developing countries [30].

Genotyping studies have shown that, as opposed to reactive EBV-related conditions, EBV is monoclonal or oligoclonal in HL, suggesting that it is present in the B-lymphocytes before malignant transformation and potentially plays a role in lymphomagenesis [28]. Similar to the gene expression pattern of EBV infecting normal germinal center B-cells, the transformed HRS cells show a type II EBV latency pattern, with only partial expression of the latency genes/antigens, including EBNA-1, LMP-1, and LMP-2 [30]. Also, similar to infected B-lymphocytes of all stages of maturation, HRS cells express the EBV-encoded RNAs EBER-1 and EBER-2, which are non-polyadenylated RNAs expressed in the nuclei of these cells [30]. While not essential for malignant transformation, these RNAs (EBERs) are easily detectable in paraffin-embedded tissue sections using in situ hybridization techniques, allowing for rapid identification of EBV+ cases in the clinical setting. Epstein–Barr virus-positive cases of HL remain as such at relapse. Also, patients with EBV+ HL (much like other EBV+ neoplasms) have elevated levels of EBV in their serum, which correlate well with their disease burden, response to therapy, and relapse [32, 33]. It has been postulated that EBV infection may play a role in malignant transformation by rescuing the germinal center B-cells otherwise destined for apoptosis, as viral proteins expressed in the infected HRS cells may mimic constitutively active receptors (e.g., LMP-1 for CD40, and LMP2A for BCR) [12, 30], and may inhibit apoptosis by upregulating BCL2 expression and the NFκB signaling pathway [30].

Genetics

Nodular lymphocyte-predominant Hodgkin lymphoma

Conventional cytogenetics, fluorescence in situ hybridization (FISH), and gene expression profiling studies show NLPHL to be genetically closer to B-cell non-Hodgkin lymphoma than to cHL. Conventional cytogenetics, typically successful in only limited series of cases [7, 34], shows predominantly complex diploid, hypodiploid, or tetraploid karyotypes. Recurrent abnormalities include additional material on chromosome 1q, isochromosome and other rearrangements of 7q, rearrangements involving 3q27 (harboring the BCL6 locus), monosomy 4 and deletion 4q28, monosomy 13 and deletion 13q, and rearrangements of 14q32 (harboring the immunoglobulin heavy chain gene, IGH locus). FISH combined with immunohistochemical staining for CD20 (FICTION technique: fluorescence immunophenotyping and interphase FISH as a tool for the investigation of neoplasms) has been applied to study rearrangements of the BCL6 gene in the L&H cells [35–37]. These studies demonstrated that 38–48% of NLPHL cases contain translocations that juxtapose the BCL6 gene to immunoglobulin gene loci. The most common translocation involves the BCL6 and IGH genes, as t(3;14)(q27;q32). Other less common partners/rearrangement mechanisms for the BCL6 rearrangements include the immunoglobulin lambda light chain gene (at 22q11), loci on chromosomes 4 and 9, and internal deletions of BCL6.

Comparative genomic hybridization (CGH) studies performed on microdissected L&H cells from a small series of NLPHLs [7] found chromosomal imbalances in all cases and outlined several patterns of genomic alterations: a pattern characterized predominantly by chromosomal gains, a second pattern with balanced gains and losses, and a third, least frequent pattern (seen in two patients of 10 and 11 years of age) with complex (17 or more) genomic changes. Recurrent affected chromosomal regions were similar to those found by conventional cytogenetics and were also largely similar in all of the three patterns observed. Additional abnormalities, not previously identified by conventional cytogenetics, included gains of 5q, 6, 20p, partial Xq, and loss of partial Xp. Gene expression profiling studies of microdissected L&H cells [38] have shown NLPHL to resemble a normal B-cell in transition between the GC and memory B-cell stages. The overall gene expression pattern was closest to that of T-cell rich large B-cell lymphoma and of a subset of diffuse large B-cell lymphomas, and it was different from that of cHL cells. Similar to GC B-cells, NLPHL showed downregulation of some B-cell-specific genes (such as CD22, CD79B, PAX5, BCL6, BOB1), although not to the extent seen in cHL. However, in spite of their resemblance to GC B-cells, these lymphomas were found to be quite different in their patterns of gene expression from other GC-derived lymphomas, such as the follicular and Burkitt types. Finally, these studies have found NLPHL to show activation of genes in the NFκB pathway, similar to cHL cells, although likely through different mechanisms.

Classical Hodgkin lymphoma

Conventional cytogenetics is typically successful in only a small proportion of cHL cases [39]. The abnormal karyotypes may be hypodiploid or hyperdiploid and often show complex aberrancies. The recurrent cytogenetic abnormalities found in these cases overlap with those seen in NLPHL and other B-cell lymphomas. They include abnormalities of 1q, 1p, 4q35, 5q, 6q,

9p, monosomy 7, and trisomy 13. FISH and FICTION studies have demonstrated that HRS cells only rarely harbor BCL6 rearrangements [36, 40]. In 15–19% of the cases they show rearrangements of IGH, and, in rare cases (1–3%), also rearrangements of IGK or IGL [40]. Additionally, these studies showed that a significant proportion of cHL cases have amplifications and gains at the REL (54%) and JAK2 (43%) gene loci [40–42]. CGH studies performed on microdissected HRS cells have demonstrated recurrent abnormalities as gains affecting 2p12–16, 5q15–23, 6p22, 8q13, 8q24, 9p21–24, 9q34, 12q13–14, 17q12, 19p13, 19q13, and 20q11, and losses at Xp21, 6q23–24, and 13q22 [41, 43].

Diagnostic features

Nodular lymphocyte-predominant Hodgkin lymphoma

NLPHL represents only approximately 5% of HL, and likely an even lower percentage in the pediatric age group. Its typical clinical presentation includes localized peripheral lymphadenopathy with low-stage (I or II) disease, and only rare splenic or bone marrow involvement [1].

Morphology

Morphologically, this subtype of HL is characterized by complete or subtotal effacement of the underlying lymph node architecture by the neoplastic infiltrate, most often without associated capsular or interstitial fibrosis. Fibrosis with a pattern similar to that of NS type of cHL may be seen in about 20% of the cases [44]. The neoplastic infiltrate may have an entirely nodular, or a nodular and diffuse growth pattern (Fig. 23.1A). Nodularity may be only very focal in rare cases. Therefore, since this component is crucial in the differential diagnosis with T-cell-rich large B-cell lymphoma, obtaining large excisional biopsies is of high importance in such cases. The neoplastic nodules are typically large, with smooth, pushing borders, and are composed predominantly of small, mature lymphocytes with monotonous appearance. The nodules also contain variable (usually low) numbers of large neoplastic cells, and associated epithelioid histiocytes with eosinophilic cytoplasm, that may form small aggregates (Fig. 23.1B). The neoplastic L&H cells, also termed "popcorn" cells, are very large and are characterized by marked nuclear lobulation, a vesicular chromatin, and multiple, often peripherally located small, amphophilic nucleoli (Fig. 23.2). Most cases also contain occasional Hodgkin and Reed–Sternberg cells (see below under Classical Hodgkin lymphoma). Examination at high power may also show enlarged, binucleated cells, with the two nuclei flattened against each other and small central nucleoli, which typically represent follicular dendritic cells. These should not be confused with the neoplastic cells. A subset of NLPHL may present with a combination of nodular and diffuse patterns [44]. In this subset, the neoplastic cells may be found scattered among small lymphocytes in the diffuse areas, sometimes outside of the nodules. The

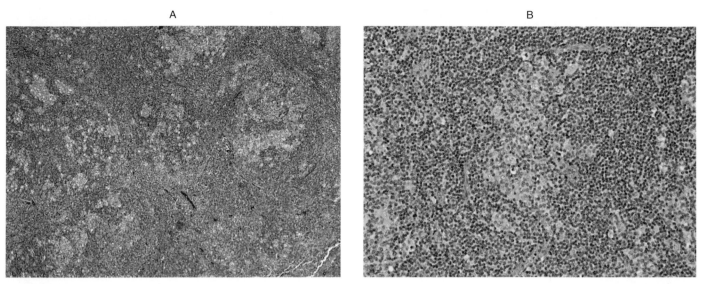

Fig. 23.1. (A) Nodular lymphocyte-predominant Hodgkin lymphoma demonstrating a predominantly nodular growth pattern, with a mottled appearance of the nodules (H&E stain). (B) At higher magnification, the pale areas of the nodules consist of large neoplastic cells and epithelioid histiocytes (H&E stain).

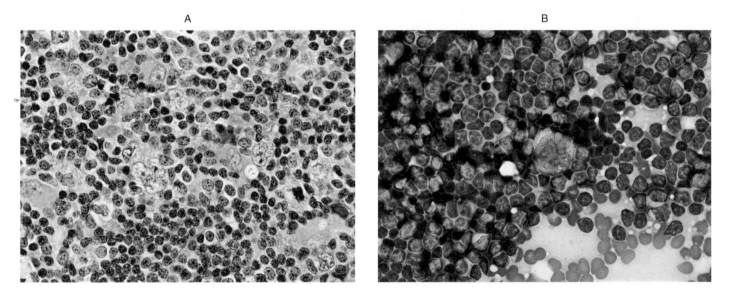

Fig. 23.2. (A) L&H cells seen in paraffin-embedded tissue sections (H&E stain). (B) L&H cells seen in cytologic preparations (touch imprints). (Wright–Giemsa stain.) Both images show prominent nuclear lobulation and small peripheral nucleoli.

latter distribution is particularly common in the IgD-positive cases of NLPHL [45]. Approximately 15% of the cases may also contain small atretic germinal centers present within or around the large neoplastic nodules [44].

Immunophenotype

The immunophenotype of L&H cells overlaps with that of the neoplastic cells of diffuse large B-cell lymphoma (Fig. 23.3). They typically express CD20, CD79a, PAX-5, Oct-2, BOB.1, and PU.1, as well as CD45, and are negative for CD15 and CD30. In addition, they often express epithelial membrane antigen (EMA). The B-lineage markers typically highlight a background rich in normal B-lymphocytes that have a mantle zone immunophenotype, with expression of IgD and IgM. Stains for

CD3 are positive in the small T-lymphocytes that form distinct rosettes around the L&H cells (easily seen as negative cells on staining for B-lineage antigens). In a subset of cases, the T-lymphocytes forming rosettes are also positive for CD57. There are also increased numbers of CD57-positive cells within the neoplastic nodules, and in the diffuse areas (if the neoplasm presents with diffuse growth patterns). Stains for follicular dendritic reticulum cells (CD21, CD35) typically highlight irregularly expanded meshworks of cells that underlie the neoplastic nodules, as well as the diffuse areas that contain L&H cells.

When combining the morphologic and immunophenotypic features, several growth patterns may be observed in lymph nodes involved by NLPHL, occurring as the single pattern in

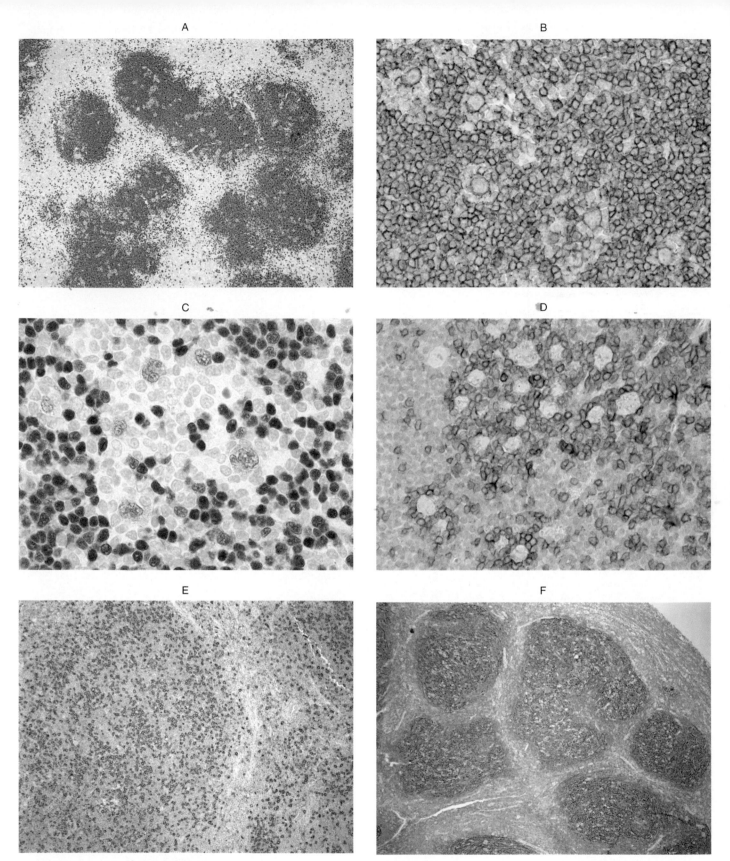

Fig. 23.3. The immunophenotype of L&H cells, as seen on immunohistochemical staining, is characterized by expression of CD20 and PAX-5, which is also seen in the small lymphocytes composing the neoplastic nodules. The L&H cells are surrounded by rosettes of CD20−, PAX-5−, CD3+, and sometimes CD57+ T-cells. These T-cells may be markedly increased in the nodules, which are set on an underlying expanded network of CD21+ dendritic cells. (A, B) CD20; (C) PAX-5; (D) CD3; (E) CD57; (F) CD21. (All slides avidin–biotin–peroxidase technique, hematoxylin counterstain.)

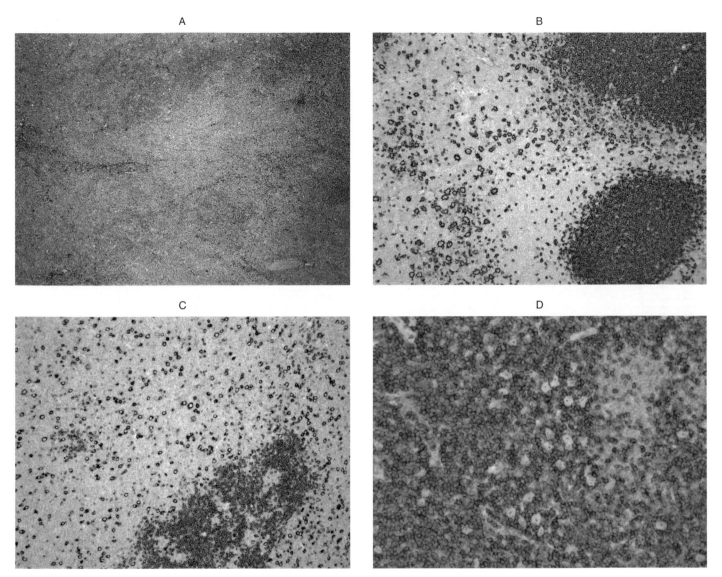

Fig. 23.4. IgD+ NLPHL may show a predominance of L&H cells in an extranodal location, where they reside in T-cell-rich areas ("Pattern C" described by Fan *et al.* [44]). (A) The tumor shows a mixture of nodular and expanded interfollicular areas on low-magnification (H&E stain). Immunostaining for CD20 (B) and IgD (C) demonstrates the predominant extranodal location of the L&H cells, surrounded by a predominance of CD3+ T-cells (D). (Hematoxylin counterstain.)

at least half of the cases, and as a mixture of two to four patterns in the remainder [44]. These patterns were described by Fan *et al.* [44]. *Pattern A*, "classical" B-cell-rich nodular, is the pattern described above, and the most common. *Pattern B*, serpiginous/interconnected nodular, consists of nodules similar to those of pattern A, but taking on serpiginous interconnected shapes (a growth pattern unique to this type of lymphoma). *Pattern C*, nodular with prominent extranodal L&H cells, includes less well-defined nodules, containing increased numbers of T-lymphocytes, and has numerous L&H cells located in perinodal areas or in diffuse areas. The L&H cells are typically set in a T-cell-rich background, lacking CD57+ T-cell rosettes. This subtype is often associated with the IgD+ subtype [45] (Fig. 23.4). *Pattern D*, nodular with T-cell-rich background, is characterized by a predominantly nodular growth pattern, but the immune architecture of the nod-

ules includes decreased numbers of B-lymphocytes, with a predominance of T-lymphocytes, as well as frequently attenuated meshworks of CD21+ dendritic cells. These nodules contain the L&H cells with classic immunophenotype, often surrounded by the CD57+ T-cell rosettes. *Pattern E* is a diffuse pattern, T-cell-rich B-cell lymphoma-like, that is composed predominantly of diffuse areas containing predominantly T-cells, with scattered L&H cells. Essentially, identification of at least one nodule is required to differentiate this pattern from T-cell-rich diffuse large B-cell lymphoma. Finally, *pattern F*, diffuse "moth eaten," with B-cell-rich background, has the immune composition of a massively expanded nodule. The diffuse areas are composed predominantly of small B-lymphocytes, with an underlying dendritic cell meshwork and rosettes of T-lymphocytes surrounding the L&H cells, and imparting a "moth eaten" appearance on staining for CD20. It appears that the presence

A B

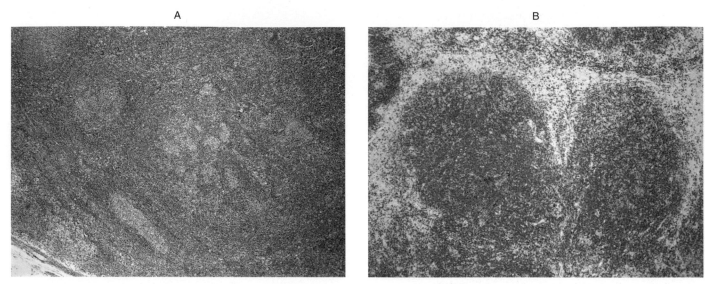

Fig. 23.5. Progressive transformation of germinal centers. (A) The nodules of PTGC contain pale fragments of residual germinal center and are admixed with reactive germinal centers (H&E stain). (B) CD20 immunostaining highlights well-demarcated nodules lacking the mottled appearance seen in NLPHL (hematoxylin counterstain).

of diffuse areas, especially as a predominant growth pattern, is more often associated with disease recurrence [44].

Differential diagnosis

Progressive transformation of germinal centers (PTGC), a pattern of recurrent benign lymphoid hyperplasia, may precede, be associated with, or follow the clinical presentation of NLPHL [46]. The majority of the patients presenting with florid PTGC are adolescent boys and young men, and most of these patients will *not* develop HL [46]. The characteristic appearance of PTGC consists of markedly enlarged nodules (two- to three-times the diameter of a reactive follicle) with smooth, expansile borders (Fig. 23.5A) composed predominantly of small B-lymphocytes of mantle cell origin. They are often admixed with reactive follicles. These nodules contain residual, large transformed lymphocytes (centroblasts) occurring singly or in small clusters, as well as dendritic cells, but no clusters of epithelioid histiocytes. By contrast, the nodules of NLPHL grow in a back-to-back fashion, with no intervening reactive follicles, which are more often compressed at the periphery of the area replaced by lymphoma. On immunohistochemical staining, these nodules consist of confluent sheets of CD20+ B-lymphocytes and centroblasts (Fig. 23.5B), with only scattered single CD3+ and CD57+ T-cells, and tightly-woven, well-circumscribed meshworks of CD21+ dendritic cells. The centroblasts are always negative for epithelial membrane antigen (EMA). These centroblasts may only rarely be surrounded by T-cell rosettes, with only few (up to four) rosettes present in each nodule. The rosettes are never formed of CD57+ lymphocytes. These morphologic and immunophenotypic features are typically sufficient to differentiate between the two entities,

although this differential diagnosis may occasionally be quite challenging.

T-cell-rich large B-cell lymphoma (TCRLBCL) is included in the differential diagnosis of cases with an extensive, diffuse, T-cell-rich component, especially in small samples. This distinction is critical, as the therapeutic approach and prognosis for these two lymphomas is quite different. The clinical presentation of the two entities is different, with TCRLBCL presenting more often with disseminated, high-stage disease, while NLPHL tends to present as localized lymphadenopathy. Features that suggest the possibility of NLPHL in an otherwise diffuse process include: the presence of any nodularity, even if focal; the presence of large aggregates of small B-lymphocytes surrounding the large neoplastic cells (even if without nodularity); the presence of underlying expanded and disorganized dendritic cell meshworks; and IgD expression by the large neoplastic cells, which appears to be unique to NLPHL [45].

Classical Hodgkin lymphoma, lymphocyte rich (cHL-LR) overlaps closely in clinical presentation and immune architecture with NLPHL (see below). The most helpful feature in the differential diagnosis is the immunophenotype of the large neoplastic cells. In addition, the presence of EBV in the latter cells would favor cHL-LR.

Follicular lymphoma is less likely to enter the differential diagnosis of pediatric NLPHL. The neoplastic follicles are usually smaller than those of NLPHL and have a distinct cellular composition, consisting of CD10+ CD20+ centrocytes and centroblasts that typically form confluent sheets. In particular, in the pediatric subtype of follicular lymphoma, which tends to also present as localized, low-stage disease, the neoplastic nodules may be large and irregular, with disrupted underlying

Table 23.2. Clinical features of the main histologic subtypes of Hodgkin lymphoma.

Histologic subtype	Proportion of all HL (%)	M : F ratio	Age (years)	Stage[a]	Sites involved	B symptoms	EBV positive (%)
Nodular lymphocyte predominant	5	1 (74% male)	30–50	I/II	Peripheral LNs (cervical, axillary, inguinal)	Rare (10%)	<1
Nodular sclerosis	60–80	~1	15–34 (median, 28)	II	Mediastinum (80%) Peripheral LNs Spleen (10%) Lung (10%) BM (3%)	Frequent (40%)	10–40
Mixed cellularity	20–25 (35–40 in patients under 6 years of age)	>1 (70% male)	Median 37	III/IV	Peripheral LNs Spleen (30%) BM (10%) Liver (3%)	Frequent (35%)	75
Lymphocyte rich	5	>1 (70% male)		I/II	Peripheral LNs (cervical) Mediastinum (15%)	Rare (11%)	47 (61 in diffuse and interfollicular)
Lymphocyte depleted	<1 (strong association with HIV infection)	>1 (60–75% male)	Median 30–37	III/IV	Retroperitoneal LNs Spleen Liver BM	Frequent	~100%

[a] Stage at presentation in over 50% of the patients.
Abbreviations: LN, lymph node; BM, bone marrow.

meshworks of dendritic cells, but they are typically formed predominantly of centroblasts, which should allow for easy differentiation from NLPHL [47, 48].

Classical Hodgkin lymphoma

Morphology

Classical HL includes several histologic subtypes that correlate with distinct clinical features but are not used in patient risk stratification at the present time. The clinical features of these subtypes are summarized in Table 23.2.

All of these histologic subtypes share the same morphologic and immunophenotypic features of their malignant cells, but differ in growth pattern and composition of the inflammatory cell background.

The neoplastic cells of the cHL are the Hodgkin and Reed–Sternberg cells and lacunar cells (Fig. 23.6). The *classic Reed–Sternberg (RS) cells* are giant cells that may have lobulated nuclei or be binucleated or multinucleated. At least two macronucleoli (sometimes resembling inclusions) are present in their separate nuclei or nuclear lobes. These cells typically have ample amphophilic or eosinophilic cytoplasm. *Hodgkin cells* are mononuclear variants of the RS cells. *Lacunar cells* derive their name from the observation that, in formalin-fixed tissues, the retraction artifact that occurs around these cells gives the appearance of a space surrounding them. The lacunar appearance is not seen in tissues fixed using precipitating agents (such as B5 or zinc formalin). The lacunar cells are giant cells with ample, pale-eosinophilic cytoplasm and often lobulated or anaplastic nuclei, containing single prominent nucleoli which

are smaller than those seen in the RS cells. Finally, *mummified cells* are apoptotic RS cells with pyknotic nuclei and retracted, sometimes eosinophilic cytoplasm.

Immunophenotype

All of the morphologic subtypes of neoplastic (HRS) cells show a similar immunophenotype (Fig. 23.7), characterized by consistent expression of CD30 and fascin, frequent expression of CD15 (75–85%), and lack of CD45 expression. CD15 and CD30 typically show a membrane and Golgi-type expression pattern. Of note, CD15 expression may only be seen in a very small fraction of the neoplastic cells, sometimes only in a Golgi pattern. The HRS cells also show variable expression of some B-lymphoid antigens, including PAX-5 (95% of cases, often weaker than the surrounding normal lymphocytes), CD20 (30–40% of cases), IRF4/MUM (>90% of cases), and rarely CD79a. However, they are consistently negative for PU-1, and negative for at least one of the other B-cell-specific transcription factors Oct-2 and BOB.1. These features are very useful in the differential diagnosis with NLPHL and diffuse large B-cell lymphoma. EBV expression (tested using either immunohistochemistry for LMP-1 and EBNA-1, or *in situ* hybridization for EBER) (Fig. 23.8) may be seen in a variable percentage of cases, depending on the clinical setting (e.g., immunodeficiency, geographic area) and histologic subtype (see Table 23.2).

Nodular sclerosis (NS) subtype

The hallmark features of this subtype include a nodular growth pattern (associated with a patchy distribution of the neoplastic cells) and the presence of associated dense fibrosis

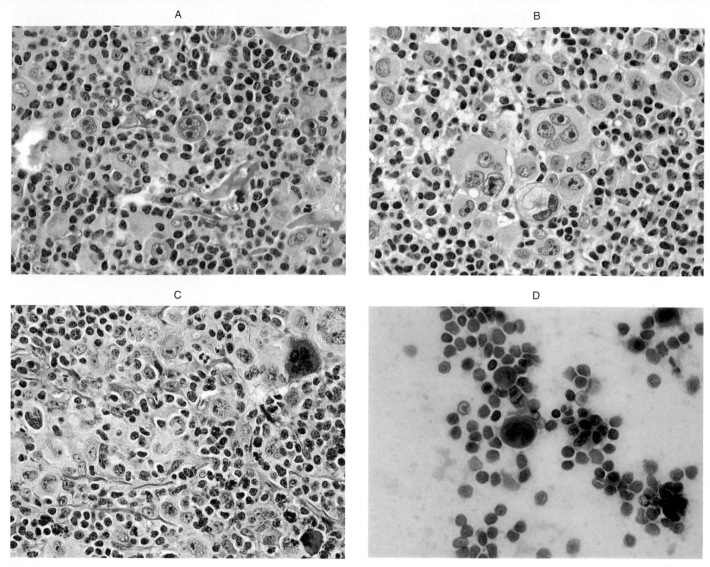

Fig. 23.6. The neoplastic cells of cHL. (A) Classic Reed–Sternberg cell and several mononucleated Hodgkin cells. (B) Multinucleated Reed–Sternberg cells and Hodgkin cells. (C) Hodgkin cells, lacunar cells, and several mummified cells. (D) Cytologic appearance of Reed–Sternberg cells, as seen on touch imprints. (H&E stain.)

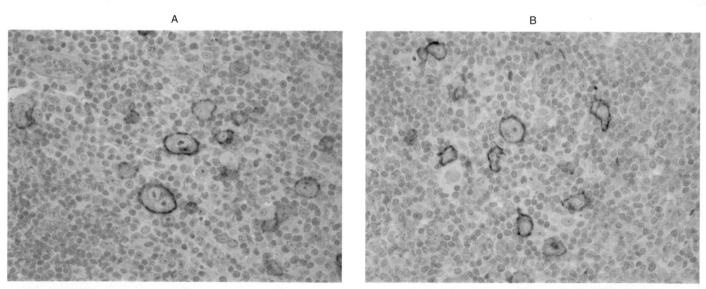

Fig. 23.7. The immunophenotype of HRS cells. On immunostaining, there is membrane-associated and cytoplasmic (Golgi-type) expression of CD30 (A) and CD15 (B). (Hematoxylin counterstain.)

A

B

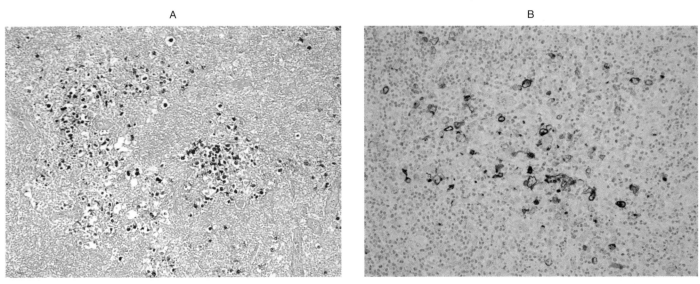

Fig. 23.8. (A) Nuclear EBV expression seen in the HRS cells by *in situ* hybridization for EBER, in a case of NS cHL. (B) Cytoplasmic and membrane LMP-1 expression seen by immunostaining in a case of cHL.

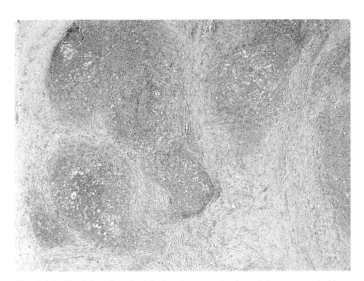

Fig. 23.9. Nodular sclerosis cHL showing neoplastic nodules surrounded by broad bands of sclerosis (H&E stain).

(or sclerosis) forming bands that surround completely at least one nodule (Fig. 23.9). In some cases, the sclerotic bands are so prominent that they can be identified grossly on a cut section of the involved lymph node. Frequently, there is also marked capsular fibrosis. The neoplastic cells most often associated with this pattern consist predominantly of lacunar cells, with fewer HRS cells and mummified forms. The inflammatory background of the nodules includes a predominance of small T-lymphocytes, with a minority of small B-lymphocytes, as well as dendritic cells, fibroblasts, epithelioid histiocytes, and variable numbers of granulocytes, predominantly eosinophils. The presence of numerous eosinophils, especially when forming clusters, has been shown to correlate with an adverse prognosis in NS cHL [49, 50]. In some cases, the lacunar cells may form large syncytial aggregates, sometimes with associated cen-

tral coagulative or suppurative eosinophilic necrosis, imparting a pseudo-granulomatous appearance. True necrotizing or non-necrotizing granulomata may also be seen adjacent to the neoplasm or between the neoplastic nodules. Cases with a predominance of lacunar cells and a relative lack of intervening inflammatory cells have been designated as the "syncytial variant" of NS cHL (Fig. 23.10). Last, cases with a vaguely nodular pattern, and patchy distribution of the HRS/lacunar cells, but no fibrous bands have been designated as "the cellular phase of NS cHL." This latter pattern may correlate with a classic NS pattern when other anatomic sites of disease are sampled. Various histologic grading systems have been devised for NS cHL [1, 50]. None of these systems is currently sanctioned by the clinical risk stratification schemas. All of these systems rely on the observation that lymphocyte depletion, the presence of syncytial aggregates of HRS/lacunar cells, especially when very pleomorphic, and the presence of numerous eosinophils, appear to correlate with a more aggressive clinical course and a higher risk for disease relapse.

Mixed cellularity (MC) subtype

The MC subtype is characterized by a diffuse growth pattern with an even distribution of neoplastic cells, and absence of bands of sclerosis (Fig. 23.11). Some cases may show fine interstitial fibrosis. The predominant neoplastic cells in this subtype are HRS cells, with fewer lacunar cells. The inflammatory background is similar to that seen in the nodules of the NS subtype.

Lymphocyte-rich (LR) subtype

The LR subtype shows considerable clinical and morphologic overlap with NLPHL. The predominant neoplastic cells are HRS cells with only occasional L&H cells. The inflammatory background consists predominantly of mantle zone-type, small

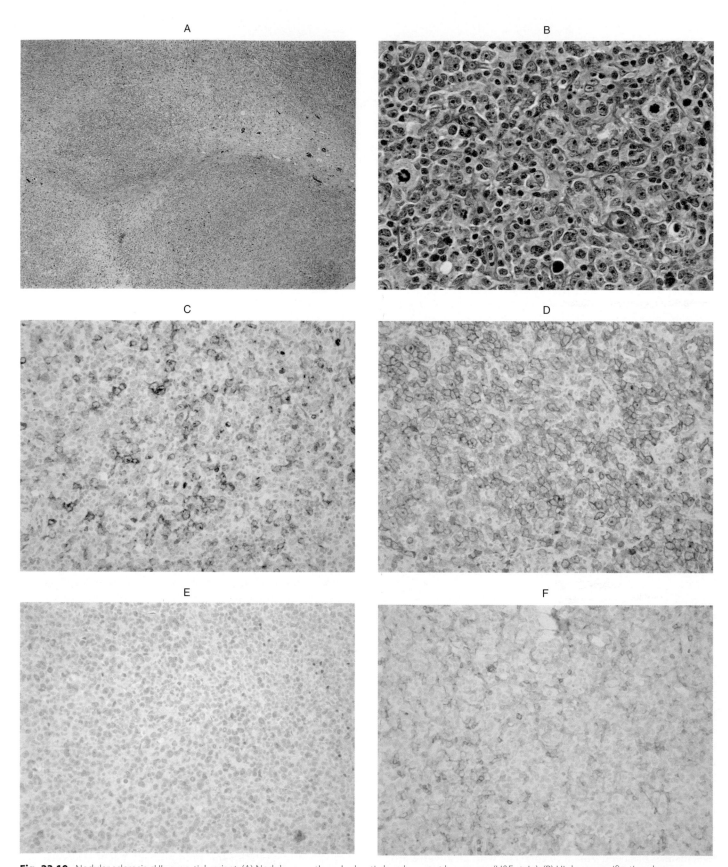

Fig. 23.10. Nodular sclerosis cHL, syncytial variant. (A) Nodular growth and sclerotic bands seen at low power (H&E stain). (B) Higher magnification shows a predominance of large neoplastic cells (H&E stain). On immunostaining, the neoplastic cells are positive for CD15 (C), CD30 (D), and PAX-5 (E), and negative for CD45 (F).

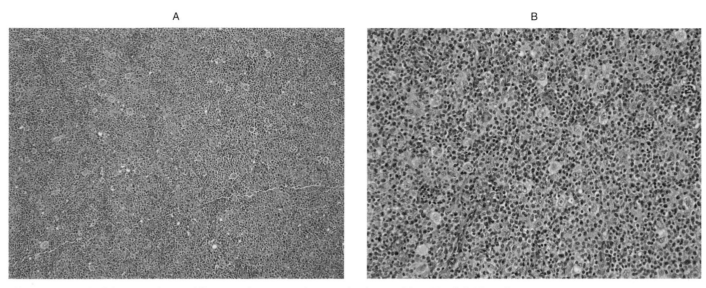

Fig. 23.11. Mixed cellularity cHL shows a diffuse growth pattern and an even distribution of the HRS cells (H&E stain).

B-lymphocytes expressing IgD and IgM, with absent or only rare granulocytes and eosinophils. The predominant subtype is nodular (also designated previously as the follicular subtype of HL), with many of the nodules containing residual small, benign germinal centers, while the neoplastic cells are found within or at the margin of the mantle zone of these follicles (Fig. 23.12). Much more rarely, LR cHL may show a diffuse architecture with a similar cellular composition. This diagnosis requires large samples, as needle biopsies may only partially sample large nodules, giving the appearance of diffuse growth.

Lymphocyte-depleted (LD) subtype

This subtype has a diffuse growth pattern and a cellular composition characterized by a predominance of malignant, typically HRS cells, over lymphocytes. The morphologic appearance may be variable, ranging from a MC-type appearance with markedly increased numbers of neoplastic cells, to a sarcomatoid appearance due to large numbers of pleomorphic HRS cells, to a diffusely fibrotic process containing scattered HRS cells and only rare lymphocytes (Fig. 23.13). This subtype is most often associated with immunosuppression, such as HIV infection, and is typically EBV positive.

Interfollicular cHL

In rare cases, cHL with a cellular composition similar to that of NS cHL may involve only the interfollicular areas of the lymph nodes (Fig. 23.14). These cases are designated as "interfollicular HL," without further subclassification. In many of these cases, sampling of other sites of disease will typically show NS or MC types of cHL.

Classical HL as a post-transplant lymphoproliferative disorder (PTLD)

Classical HL may occur in the post-organ-transplant setting and is a relatively uncommon form of PTLD. These cases ful-

fill the diagnostic criteria for cHL seen in immunocompetent patients and are typically EBV positive, with the EBV expression restricted to the HRS cells. They are designated as cHL-type PTLD. The main differential diagnosis in this setting is with Hodgkin-like PTLD, typically characterized by a monomorphous or polymorphous lymphoid proliferation containing increased numbers of RS-like cells. The RS-like cells usually have an activated B-cell immunophenotype (CD15−, CD20+, CD30+, CD45+, CD79a+) and are EBV (LMP-1)+ [51]. In addition, EBV expression is usually seen not only in the latter cells, but also in other small and intermediate-sized lymphoid cells present in the background [52]. It also appears that EBV shows different patterns of expression of latency genes in the two entities, with a latency type III (all EBV-associated latency proteins expressed) in HL-like PTLD, and a latency type II (only EBNA-1, LMP-1, and LMP-2 expressed) in cHL-type PTLD [53]. A high proportion of these cases may show clonal immunoglobulin gene rearrangements when examined by conventional techniques [54]. The distinction between these two entities is clinically important, as HL-like PTLD may be managed solely with withdrawal of immunosuppression and rituximab therapy, while cHL-type PTLD typically requires a standard therapeutic approach [55, 56].

Differential diagnosis of cHL

A variety of malignant hematopoietic and non-hematopoietic disorders, as well as benign reactive conditions, enter the differential diagnosis of cHL, due to its unique combination of neoplastic cells and heterogeneous inflammatory background. In most cases, the differential diagnosis rests upon identifying the characteristic immunophenotype of the HRS cells (see Table 23.3).

Diffuse large B-cell lymphoma (DLBCL): the centroblastic and anaplastic variants of this lymphoma enter the differential diagnosis of the syncytial variants of NS cHL, while

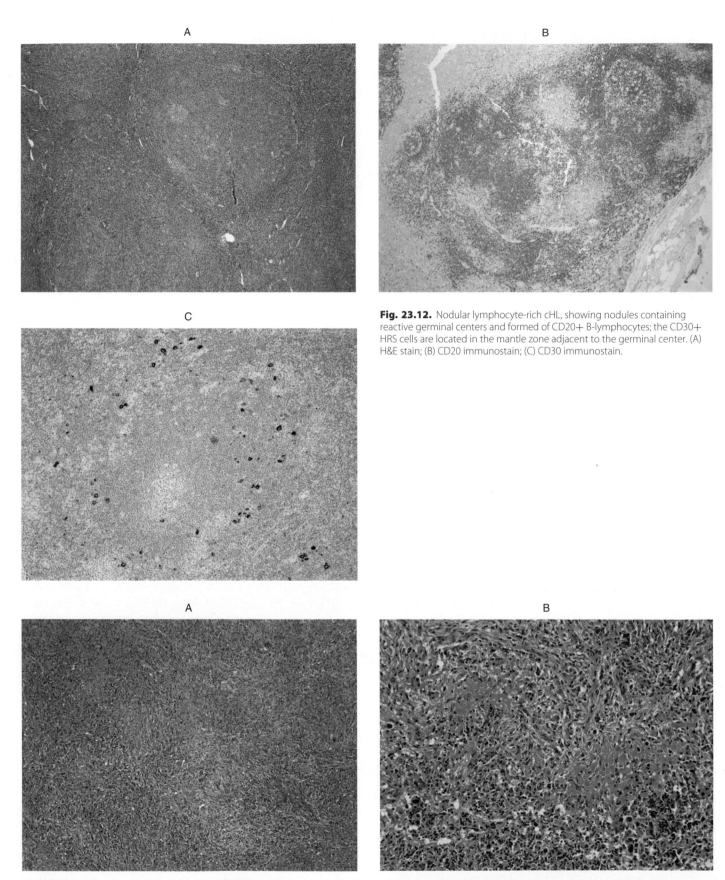

Fig. 23.12. Nodular lymphocyte-rich cHL, showing nodules containing reactive germinal centers and formed of CD20+ B-lymphocytes; the CD30+ HRS cells are located in the mantle zone adjacent to the germinal center. (A) H&E stain; (B) CD20 immunostain; (C) CD30 immunostain.

Fig. 23.13. Lymphocyte-depleted cHL, with diffuse fibrosis, lymphocyte depletion and patchy necrosis (H&E stain).

Table 23.3. Immunophenotypic features of HRS and HRS-like cells in neoplastic and non-neoplastic disorders included in the differential diagnosis of Hodgkin lymphoma.

Disease	CD45	CD3	CD15	CD20	CD30	PAX-5	ALK	PLAP	S100	EBV
cHL	−	−	+/−	+/−	+	+	−	−	−	+/−
NLPHL	+	−	−	+	−	+	−	−	−	−
ALCL	+/−	−/+	−	−	+	−	+/−	−	−	−
DLBCL	+	−	−	+	−/+	+	−/+	−	−	−/+
PTCL	+	+	−	−	−/+	−/+	−	−	−	−/+
GZL	+	−	+/−	+	+	+	−	−	−	−/+
Benign immunoblastic proliferations[a]	+	+/−	−	+/−	+	+/−	−	−	−	+
Germ cell tumors	−	−	−	−	+/−	−	−	+	−	−
Carcinoma, metastatic	−	−	−	−	−	−/+	−	−	−	−/+
Melanoma, metastatic	−	−	−	−	−	−	−	−	+	−
Sarcoma	−	−	−	−	−	−	−/+	−	−/+	−/+

[a] Benign immunoblastic proliferations include infectious mononucleosis, drug-induced hypersensitivity reactions, HL-like methotrexate-associated lymphoproliferative disorders, and granulomatous adenitis.

Abbreviations: ALCL, anaplastic large cell lymphoma; DLBCL, diffuse large B-cell lymphoma (including the T-cell-rich/histiocyte-rich, and primary mediastinal subtypes); PTCL, peripheral T-cell lymphoma; GZL, gray zone lymphoma.

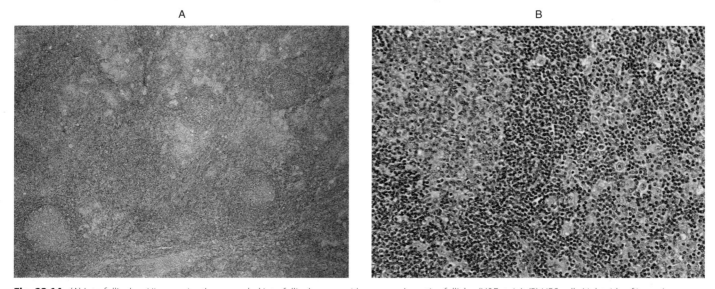

A   B

Fig. 23.14. (A) Interfollicular cHL occupies the expanded interfollicular area, with preserved reactive follicles (H&E stain). (B) HRS cells (right side of image) are present adjacent to the mantle of a reactive follicle (left side of image). (H&E stain.)

diffuse forms with prominent interstitial fibrosis (as often seen in abdominal sites of involvement) may need to be differentiated from the LD subtype. Primary mediastinal large B-cell lymphoma should always be considered in samples obtained from mediastinal masses. T-cell-rich large B-cell lymphoma may resemble the MC subtype or the rare diffuse forms of the LR subtype. In all of these cases, a combination of immunophenotypic features of the large neoplastic cells and of the inflammatory cell background are sufficient. Of note, most large B-cell lymphomas lack significant numbers of infiltrating granulocytes and contain mostly T-lymphocytes in their inflammatory background.

Gray zone lymphomas, also designated as unclassifiable B-cell lymphomas with features intermediate between diffuse large B-cell lymphoma and classical Hodgkin lymphoma [1], may present significant differential diagnostic challenges [57–59]. Typically they present in the mediastinum and show a diffuse growth pattern, with prominent stromal fibrosis, sometimes forming bands, patchy necrosis, and a predominance of pleomorphic, HRS-like neoplastic cells growing in confluent sheets. The inflammatory background is sparse, and lacks significant numbers of granulocytes and eosinophils. Characteristically, some areas resemble cHL, while others DLBCL. Likewise, the immunophenotype of the neoplastic cells has

A

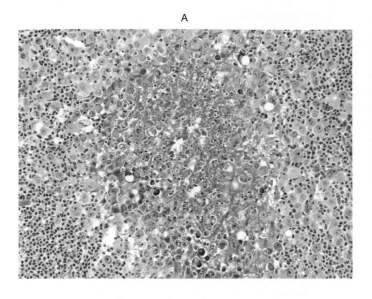

B

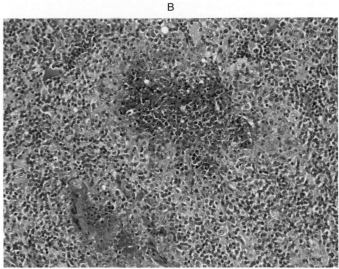

C

Fig. 23.15. Granulomatous inflammation in the differential diagnosis of cHL. (A) Syncytial aggregate of HRS cells with central suppurative necrosis. (B) Suppurative granuloma seen in a case of cHL. (C) Non-necrotizing granuloma seen in a case of cHL. (H&E stain.)

intermediate features between the two entities, with expression of B-cell markers (CD20, CD79a), B-cell-specific transcription factors (PAX-5, Oct-2, BOB.1), but also CD15 and CD30. They consistently lack immunoglobulin expression and are ALK negative. Some cases may show EBV expression [1].

NLPHL is the main entity entering the differential diagnosis of LR cHL. The distinction between the two entities is made primarily based on the immunophenotype of the neoplastic cells.

Anaplastic large cell lymphoma may enter the differential diagnosis of cHL, especially in NS cases with syncytial morphology, and in the LD subtype. Of note, much like cHL, ALCL may present with focal nodularity, band-like or diffuse fibrosis, a predominant inflammatory background (the lymphohistiocytic subtype), or sarcomatoid morphology that may resemble the LD subtype of cHL. In all of these cases, the distinct immunophenotypic features, including ALK expression and the presence of T-cell receptor gene rearrangements, should allow for easy differentiation.

Peripheral T-cell lymphoma, NOS may be considered in the differential diagnosis of the MC and LD subtypes. These lymphomas may show overlapping morphologic features, with large neoplastic cells, sometimes with HRS-like features, and a heterogeneous inflammatory background that may contain granulocytes, eosinophils, and even granulomata. The distinction from cHL is based on the immunophenotypic features of the neoplastic cells, as well as on the finding of clonal T-cell receptor gene rearrangements on molecular testing.

Non-hematopoietic neoplasms may enter the differential diagnosis of cHL, particularly in the mediastinal location, where typically only small biopsy samples, often with significant crush artifact, may be obtained. These neoplasms include mediastinal germ cell tumors and metastatic carcinoma or melanoma. In addition, various sarcomas may be considered in the differential diagnosis of the NS type (syncytial variant), and the LD subtype. The distinction is easily made based on the characteristic immunophenotypic features of each entity.

Granulomatous lymphadenitis may enter the differential diagnosis of CHL in two circumstances: (1) the finding of small benign necrotizing or non-necrotizing granulomata adjacent to the neoplastic areas; (2) the presence of syncytial aggregates of HRS cells with central suppurative necrosis (e.g., cat-scratch disease; Fig. 23.15). A combination of morphologic and immunophenotypic features should help with this distinction. Benign necrotizing granulomata are typically composed of histiocytic cells that express weak CD4, very weak CD15, CD45, CD68, and, variably, S100, and are negative for CD30. It is also important to remember here that, in addition to cHL, other metastatic malignant processes may be associated with granuloma formation in the lymph nodes. The most common include seminoma and nasopharyngeal carcinoma.

Benign proliferations containing HRS-like cells: a variety of non-neoplastic expansions of immunoblasts may contain cells with HRS-like morphology that raise the differential diagnosis with cHL. These include infectious mononucleosis, drug hypersensitivity reactions, such as those related to diphenylhydantoin, and methotrexate-related proliferations. Most of these disorders enter the differential diagnosis of the MC subtype of cHL. The distinction between these entities and MC cHL requires a correlation with the clinical history, serologic studies, and immunophenotypic features of the HRS-like cells. In all of these benign conditions, the large atypical cells are a mixture of CD3+ and CD20+ T- and B-immunoblasts, respectively. These cells express CD45 and CD30, but typically lack CD15 expression. In addition, the cellular background of these entities may include a spectrum of small lymphocytes, plasmacytoid lymphocytes, plasma cells, and more typical immunoblasts, while usually lacking significant numbers of granulocytes and eosinophils.

Prognosis and therapy

The prognosis and optimal therapeutic approach in HL depend largely on the disease stage at presentation, presence of B-symptoms, bulk of disease, and number of involved nodal regions. Typically, combined-modality therapy is employed, including combination chemotherapy and radiation therapy. Most current chemotherapy regimens include a combination of MOPP [mechlorethamine (chlormethine), vincristine, procarbazine, prednisone] and ABVD (doxorubicin, bleomycin, vinblastine, dacarbazine). The rate of event-free survival ranges from 77 to 96%, relapse-free survival from 80 to 95%, and overall survival from 87 to 93% [9]. Relapsed HL, most often occurring within three years from diagnosis [9], typically shows the same histologic subtype as the presenting disease. The salvage rate for patients with relapsed disease ranges from 40 to 50%, using chemotherapy, combined-modality therapy, and hematopoietic stem cell transplantation [9].

Last, a small percentage (2–3%) of NLPHL cases may show transformation into clonally related diffuse large B-cell lymphomas. This may be found in the lymph nodes involved by NLPHL (adjacent to it and sharply demarcated) or in lymph nodes not involved by HL. The large lymphoma cells may resemble the L&H cells, or may have the appearance of centroblasts, immunoblasts, or anaplastic cells. The rare cases of transformation to T-cell-rich large B-cell lymphoma should be evaluated carefully to distinguish from diffuse areas of NLPHL.

References

1. **Swerdlow SH, Campo E, Harris NL,** *et al.* (eds.). *WHO Classification of Tumours of Haematopoietic and Lymphoid Tissues* (4th edn.). Lyon: IARC Press; 2008.

2. **Cartwright RA, Watkins G.** Epidemiology of Hodgkin's disease: a review. *Hematological Oncology.* 2004;**22**:11–26.

3. **Ries LAG, Harkins D, Krapcho M,** *et al.* (eds). Section 9, Hodgkin lymphoma. In *SEER Cancer Statistics Review, 1975-2003.* Bethesda, MD: National Cancer Institute. Available online: http://seer.cancer.gov/csr/1975_2003/results_merged/sect_09_hodgkins.pdf (accessed July 7, 2007).

4. **Clavel J, Steliarova-Foucher E, Berger C,** *et al.* Hodgkin's disease incidence and survival in European children and adolescents (1978–1997): report from the Automated Cancer Information System project. *European Journal of Cancer.* 2006;**42**:2037–2049.

5. **Macfarlane GJ, Evstifeeva T, Boyle P,** *et al.* International patterns in the occurrence of Hodgkin's disease in children and young adult males. *International Journal of Cancer.* 1995;**61**:165–169.

6. **Belgaumi A, Al Kofide A, Joseph N,** *et al.* Hodgkin lymphoma in very young children: clinical characteristics and outcome of treatment. *Leukemia & Lymphoma.* 2008;**49**:910–916.

7. **Franke S, Wlodarska I, Maes B,** *et al.* Lymphocyte predominance Hodgkin disease is characterized by recurrent genomic imbalances. *Blood.* 2001;**97**:1845–1853.

8. **Paltiel O.** Family matters in Hodgkin lymphoma. *Leukemia & Lymphoma.* 2008;**49**:1234–1235.

9. **Hudson MM, Onciu M, Donaldson SS.** Hodgkin lymphoma. In Pizzo PA, Poplack DG, eds. *Principles and Practice of Pediatric Oncology* (5th edn.). Phildelphia, PA: Lippincott, Williams & Wilkins; 2006, 695–721.

10. **Carbone PP, Kaplan HS, Musshoff K,** *et al.* Report of the Committee on Hodgkin's Disease Staging Classification. *Cancer Research.* 1971; **31**:1860–1861.

11. **Kuppers R, Rajewsky K, Zhao M,** *et al.* Hodgkin disease: Hodgkin and Reed-Sternberg cells picked from histological sections show clonal immunoglobulin gene rearrangements and appear to be derived from B cells at various stages of development. *Proceedings of the National Academy of Sciences of the United States of America.* 1994;**91**:10962–10966.

12. **Brauninger A, Schmitz R, Bechtel D,** *et al.* Molecular biology of Hodgkin's and Reed/Sternberg cells in Hodgkin's lymphoma. *International Journal of Cancer.* 2006;**118**:1853–1861.

13. **Kuppers R, Schmitz R, Distler V,** *et al.* Pathogenesis of Hodgkin's lymphoma. *European Journal of Haematology. Supplementum.* 2005; 26–33.

14. **Stein H, Marafioti T, Foss HD**, *et al.* Down-regulation of BOB.1/OBF.1 and Oct2 in classical Hodgkin disease but not in lymphocyte predominant Hodgkin disease correlates with immunoglobulin transcription. *Blood.* 2001;**97**:496–501.

15. **Muschen M, Rajewsky K, Brauninger A**, *et al.* Rare occurrence of classical Hodgkin's disease as a T cell lymphoma. *The Journal of Experimental Medicine.* 2000;**191**:387–394.

16. **Foss HD, Herbst H, Gottstein S**, *et al.* Interleukin-8 in Hodgkin's disease. Preferential expression by reactive cells and association with neutrophil density. *The American Journal of Pathology.* 1996;**148**:1229–1236.

17. **Maggio E, Van Den BA, Diepstra A**, *et al.* Chemokines, cytokines and their receptors in Hodgkin's lymphoma cell lines and tissues. *Annals of Oncology.* 2002;**13**(Suppl 1):52–56.

18. **Niens M, Visser L, Nolte IM**, *et al.* Serum chemokine levels in Hodgkin lymphoma patients: highly increased levels of CCL17 and CCL22. *British Journal of Haematology.* 2008;**140**: 527–536.

19. **Skinnider BF, Kapp U, Mak TW.** The role of interleukin 13 in classical Hodgkin lymphoma. *Leukemia & Lymphoma.* 2002;**43**:1203–1210.

20. **Trumper L, Jung W, Dahl G**, *et al.* Interleukin-7, interleukin-8, soluble TNF receptor, and p53 protein levels are elevated in the serum of patients with Hodgkin's disease. *Annals of Oncology.* 1994;**5**(Suppl 1):93–96.

21. **Gorschluter M, Bohlen H, Hasenclever D**, *et al.* Serum cytokine levels correlate with clinical parameters in Hodgkin's disease. *Annals of Oncology.* 1995;**6**:477–482.

22. **Hanamoto H, Nakayama T, Miyazato H**, *et al.* Expression of CCL28 by Reed-Sternberg cells defines a major subtype of classical Hodgkin's disease with frequent infiltration of eosinophils and/or plasma cells. *The American Journal of Pathology.* 2004;**164**:997–1006.

23. **Maggio EM, Van Den BA, Visser L**, *et al.* Common and differential chemokine expression patterns in rs cells of NLP, EBV positive and negative classical Hodgkin lymphomas. *International Journal of Cancer.* 2002;**99**:665–672.

24. **Peh SC, Kim LH, Poppema S.** TARC, a CC chemokine, is frequently expressed in classic Hodgkin's lymphoma but not in NLP Hodgkin's lymphoma, T-cell-rich B-cell lymphoma, and most cases of anaplastic large cell lymphoma. *The American Journal of Surgical Pathology.* 2001;**25**:925–929.

25. **Van Den BA, Visser L, Poppema S.** High expression of the CC chemokine TARC in Reed-Sternberg cells. A possible explanation for the characteristic T-cell infiltrate in Hodgkin's lymphoma. *The American Journal of Pathology.* 1999;**154**:1685–1691.

26. **Jundt F, Anagnostopoulos I, Bommert K**, *et al.* Hodgkin/Reed-Sternberg cells induce fibroblasts to secrete eotaxin, a potent chemoattractant for T cells and eosinophils. *Blood.* 1999;**94**:2065–2071.

27. **Levine PH, Ablashi DV, Berard CW**, *et al.* Elevated antibody titers to Epstein-Barr virus in Hodgkin's disease. *Cancer.* 1971;**27**:416–421.

28. **Weiss LM, Strickler JG, Warnke RA**, *et al.* Epstein-Barr viral DNA in tissues of Hodgkin's disease. *The American Journal of Pathology.* 1987;**129**:86–91.

29. **Khalidi HS, Lones MA, Zhou Y**, *et al.* Detection of Epstein-Barr virus in the L & H cells of nodular lymphocyte predominance Hodgkin's disease: report of a case documented by immunohistochemical, in situ hybridization, and polymerase chain reaction methods. *American Journal of Clinical Pathology.* 1997;**108**:687–692.

30. **Rezk SA, Weiss LM.** Epstein-Barr virus-associated lymphoproliferative disorders. *Human Pathology.* 2007;**38**:1293–1304.

31. **Niens M, Jarrett RF, Hepkema B**, *et al.* HLA-A*02 is associated with a reduced risk and HLA-A*01 with an increased risk of developing EBV+ Hodgkin lymphoma. *Blood.* 2007;**110**:3310–3315.

32. **Berger C, Day P, Meier G**, *et al.* Dynamics of Epstein-Barr virus DNA levels in serum during EBV-associated disease. *Journal of Medical Virology.* 2001;**64**:505–512.

33. **Wagner HJ, Schlager F, Claviez A**, *et al.* Detection of Epstein-Barr virus DNA in peripheral blood of paediatric patients with Hodgkin's disease by real-time polymerase chain reaction. *European Journal of Cancer.* 2001;**37**:1853–1857.

34. **Stamatoullas A, Picquenot JM, Dumesnil C**, *et al.* Conventional cytogenetics of nodular lymphocyte-predominant Hodgkin's lymphoma. *Leukemia.* 2007;**21**:2064–2067.

35. **Renne C, Martin-Subero JI, Hansmann ML**, *et al.* Molecular cytogenetic analyses of immunoglobulin loci in nodular lymphocyte predominant Hodgkin's lymphoma reveal a recurrent IGH-BCL6 juxtaposition. *The Journal of Molecular Diagnostics: JMD.* 2005;**7**: 352–356.

36. **Wlodarska I, Nooyen P, Maes B**, *et al.* Frequent occurrence of BCL6 rearrangements in nodular lymphocyte predominance Hodgkin lymphoma but not in classical Hodgkin lymphoma. *Blood.* 2003;**101**:706–710.

37. **Wlodarska I, Stul M, Wolf-Peeters C**, *et al.* Heterogeneity of BCL6 rearrangements in nodular lymphocyte predominant Hodgkin's lymphoma. *Haematologica.* 2004;**89**:965–972.

38. **Brune V, Tiacci E, Pfeil I**, *et al.* Origin and pathogenesis of nodular lymphocyte-predominant Hodgkin lymphoma as revealed by global gene expression analysis. *The Journal of Experimental Medicine.* 2008;**205**:2251–2268.

39. **Ladanyi M, Parsa NZ, Offit K**, *et al.* Clonal cytogenetic abnormalities in Hodgkin's disease. *Genes, Chromosomes & Cancer.* 1991;**3**:294–299.

40. **Martin-Subero JI, Klapper W, Sotnikova A**, *et al.* Chromosomal breakpoints affecting immunoglobulin loci are recurrent in Hodgkin and Reed-Sternberg cells of classical Hodgkin lymphoma. *Cancer Research.* 2006;**66**:10332–10338.

41. **Hartmann S, Martin-Subero JI, Gesk S**, *et al.* Detection of genomic imbalances in microdissected Hodgkin and Reed-Sternberg cells of classical Hodgkin's lymphoma by array-based comparative genomic hybridization. *Haematologica.* 2008;**93**:1318–1326.

42. **Martin-Subero JI, Gesk S, Harder L**, *et al.* Recurrent involvement of the REL and BCL11A loci in classical Hodgkin lymphoma. *Blood.* 2002;**99**:1474–1477.

43. **Joos S, Menz CK, Wrobel G**, *et al.* Classical Hodgkin lymphoma is characterized by recurrent copy number gains of the short arm of

chromosome 2. *Blood*. 2002;**99**:1381–1387.

44. **Fan Z, Natkunam Y, Bair E**, *et al*. Characterization of variant patterns of nodular lymphocyte predominant hodgkin lymphoma with immunohistologic and clinical correlation. *The American Journal of Surgical Pathology*. 2003;**27**:1346–1356.

45. **Prakash S, Fountaine T, Raffeld M**, *et al*. IgD positive L&H cells identify a unique subset of nodular lymphocyte predominant Hodgkin lymphoma. *The American Journal of Surgical Pathology*. 2006;**30**:585–592.

46. **Ferry JA, Zukerberg LR, Harris NL**. Florid progressive transformation of germinal centers. A syndrome affecting young men, without early progression to nodular lymphocyte predominance Hodgkin's disease. *The American Journal of Surgical Pathology*. 1992;**16**:252–258.

47. **Lorsbach RB, Shay-Seymore D, Moore J**, *et al*. Clinicopathologic analysis of follicular lymphoma occurring in children. *Blood*. 2002;**99**:1959–1964.

48. **Pileri SA, Sabattini E, Rosito P**, *et al*. Primary follicular lymphoma of the testis in childhood: an entity with peculiar clinical and molecular characteristics. *Journal of Clinical Pathology*. 2002;**55**:684–688.

49. **von Wasielewski R, Seth S, Franklin J**, *et al*. Tissue eosinophilia correlates strongly with poor prognosis in nodular sclerosing Hodgkin's disease, allowing for known prognostic factors. *Blood*. 2000;**95**:1207–1213.

50. **von Wasielewski S, Franklin J, Fischer R**, *et al*. Nodular sclerosing disease: new grading predicts prognosis in intermediate and advanced stages. *Blood*. 2003;**101**:4063–4069.

51. **Chetty R, Biddolph S, Gatter K**. An immunohistochemical analysis of Reed-Sternberg-like cells in posttransplantation lymphoproliferative disorders: the possible pathogenetic relationship to Reed-Sternberg cells in Hodgkin's disease and Reed-Sternberg-like cells in non-Hodgkin's lymphomas and reactive conditions. *Human Pathology*. 1997;**28**:493–498.

52. **Chetty R, Biddolph SC, Kaklamanis L**, *et al*. EBV latent membrane protein (LMP-1) and bcl-2 protein expression in Reed-Sternberg-like cells in post-transplant lymphoproliferative disorders. *Histopathology*. 1996;**28**:257–260.

53. **Rohr JC, Wagner HJ, Lauten M**, *et al*. Differentiation of EBV-induced post-transplant Hodgkin lymphoma from Hodgkin-like post-transplant lymphoproliferative disease. *Pediatric Transplantation*. 2008;**12**:426–431.

54. **Pitman SD, Huang Q, Zuppan CW**, *et al*. Hodgkin lymphoma-like posttransplant lymphoproliferative disorder (HL-like PTLD) simulates monomorphic B-cell PTLD both clinically and pathologically. *The American Journal of Surgical Pathology*. 2006;**30**:470–476.

55. **Ranganathan S, Jaffe R**. Is there a difference between Hodgkin's disease and a Hodgkin's-like post-transplant lymphoproliferative disorder, and why should that be of any interest? *Pediatric Transplantation*. 2004;**8**:6–8.

56. **Ranganathan S, Webber S, Ahuja S**, *et al*. Hodgkin-like posttransplant lymphoproliferative disorder in children: does it differ from posttransplant Hodgkin lymphoma? *Pediatric and Developmental Pathology*. 2004;**7**:348–360.

57. **Poppema S, Kluiver JL, Atayar C**, *et al*. Report: workshop on mediastinal grey zone lymphoma. *European Journal of Haematology. Supplementum*. 2005;45–52.

58. **Stein H, Johrens K, Anagnostopoulos I**. Non-mediastinal grey zone lymphomas and report from the workshop. *European Journal of Haematology. Supplementum*. 2005;42–44.

59. **Traverse-Glehen A, Pittaluga S, Gaulard P**, *et al*. Mediastinal gray zone lymphoma: the missing link between classic Hodgkin's lymphoma and mediastinal large B-cell lymphoma. *The American Journal of Surgical Pathology*. 2005;**29**:1411–1421.

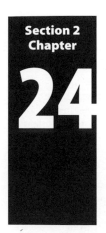

24 Immunodeficiency-associated lymphoproliferative disorders

Congenital immune deficiencies, acquired immune deficiencies, and post-transplant lymphoproliferative disorders

Mihaela Onciu and J. Han van Krieken

Introduction

The immune system encompasses a complex network of cells and signaling molecules crucial to the defense against microorganisms and specific forms of cancer. It includes several different subsystems, and many cell types, such as lymphocytes, macrophages, granulocytes, and dendritic cells, each with their own functional subsets. The normal immune response involves a variety of processes, including cell activation and proliferation in response to a variety of ligands recognized by specific receptors, as well as mechanisms of termination of the response when it is no longer necessary. This complexity results in a large variety of diseases if the function of one or more of these cell types, and one or more of the processes essential to immune homeostasis, is affected. As a result, immunodeficiencies with a wide range of clinical manifestations, from complete inability to mount a proper response to infections, to uncontrolled ongoing immune responses, develop. This chapter addresses lymphoproliferative disorders that are a consequence of immunodeficiency.

Immunodeficiency is associated with an increased risk of benign and malignant lymphoproliferative diseases (LPDs). These may result from aberrant reactions to normal stimuli, the complete inability to terminate an immune response, or accumulation of genetic defects in the immune cells. Biopsies from patients with immunodeficiencies pose a challenge to the pathologist, due to the aberrant make-up of the immune response in this context, the different nature of the lymphoproliferations, and the altered morphology of lymphomas arising in this setting, when compared to immunocompetent hosts. Furthermore, the course of the disease is difficult to predict based on morphology alone. It is therefore important that the pathologist be informed of the underlying condition when evaluating samples from such patients. When there is no knowledge of an underlying immune defect, one should keep in mind that an unusual lymphoproliferation, especially in a child, might be related to immunodeficiency.

Categories of immunodeficiencies

Immunodeficiencies may be primary (congenital), or acquired, which in turn encompasses those caused by human immunodeficiency virus (HIV) infection, solid organ or hematopoietic stem cell transplantation, and other iatrogenic LPDs, typically associated with immunosuppressive therapies.

Primary immunodeficiencies comprise more than 60 diseases associated with a wide variety of distinct genetic defects that affect the function of various immune cell subsets [1] (Table 24.1). While traditionally these have been described as clinically defined syndromes, the enormous increase in knowledge of the human genome has allowed the characterization of increasing numbers of such disorders according to their primary genetic defect. A clinical syndrome may be associated with a single causative genetic defect, or with several distinct defects affecting the same signaling pathway. Classification of the primary immunodeficiencies is most often based on the predominant type of cells that are affected functionally or developmentally. These may represent a well-delineated subset of immune cells, or several components of the immune system. The classification used in this chapter is based on a recent report of the Centers for Disease Control (Atlanta, USA) (Table 24.1; http://bioinf.uta.fi/idr/index.shtml).

Immunodeficiency due to infection with HIV results in a defective T4 (CD4-positive lymphocyte) function, leading to propensity to infections, including infection with the Epstein–Barr virus (see below). A specific problem in this setting is that the historically known course of this disease and its complications have been significantly modified by the use of combination antiretroviral therapy: while initially infections were a leading cause of death, later these were replaced by lymphomas, and, currently, modern therapy has led to long-term survival with normal CD4 counts, adequate T-cell function, and a lack of infectious or malignant complications in patients who have access to adequate management.

Diagnostic Pediatric Hematopathology, ed. Maria A. Proytcheva. Published by Cambridge University Press.
© Cambridge University Press 2011.

Table 24.1. Primary immunodeficiencies [ImmunoDeficiency Resource (IDR) http://bioinf.uta.fi/idr/index.shtml].

Disease	Fact file[a]	OMIM[b]
Combined B- and T-cell immunodeficiencies		
T-B- severe combined immunodeficiency (SCID)		
Reticular dysgenesis	1	OMIM:267500
RAG1 deficiency	2	OMIM:601457, OMIM:179615
RAG2 deficiency	3	OMIM:601457, OMIM:179616
Omenn syndrome	4	OMIM:603554
Artemis deficiency	5	OMIM:602450, OMIM:605988
T-B+ SCID		
X-linked SCID (γc chain deficiency)	8	OMIM:300400, OMIM:308380
JAK3 deficiency	9	OMIM:600802, OMIM:600173
Interleukin 7 receptor deficiency	106	OMIM:600802, OMIM:146661
CD45 deficiency	6	OMIM:202500, OMIM:151460
CD3delta deficiency	111	OMIM:600802, OMIM:186790
T-cell immunodeficiency, congenital alopecia, and nail dystrophy	128	OMIM:601705, OMIM:600838
Deficiencies of purine metabolism		
Adenosine deaminase deficiency	10	OMIM:202500, OMIM:102700
Purine nucleoside phosphorylase deficiency	11	OMIM:202500, OMIM:164050
Major histocompatibility complex class II deficiency		
CIITA, MHCII transactivating protein deficiency	12	OMIM:209920, OMIM:600005
RFX-5, MHCII promoter X box regulatory factor 5 deficiency	13	OMIM:209920, OMIM:601863
Regulatory factor X-associated protein deficiency	14	OMIM:209920, OMIM:601861
RFXANK, Ankyrin repeat containing regulatory factor X-associated protein deficiency	15	OMIM:209920, OMIM:603200
Major histocompatibility complex class I deficiency		
TAP2 deficiency	60	OMIM:604571, OMIM:170261
TAP1 deficiency	107	OMIM:604571, OMIM:170260
Tapasin deficiency	136	OMIM:604571, OMIM:601962
Hyper-IgM syndrome		
X-linked hyper-IgM syndrome (CD40L deficiency)	16	OMIM:308230, OMIM:300386
CD40 deficiency	18	OMIM:606843, OMIM:109535
CD3 deficiency		
CD3ε deficiency	20	OMIM:186830
CD3γ deficiency	21	OMIM:186740
CD3ζ deficiency	149	OMIM:186780
Other		
ZAP-70 deficiency	62	OMIM:600802, OMIM:176947
IL-2 receptor α-chain deficiency (CD25 deficiency)	63	OMIM:606367, OMIM:147730

Table 24.1. (cont.)

Disease	Fact file[a]	OMIM[b]
Combined B- and T-cell immunodeficiencies		
CD8α deficiency	64	OMIM:186910
p56 Lck deficiency	137	OMIM:153390
Schimke immuno-osseous dysplasia	148	OMIM:606622, OMIM:242900
Cernunnos deficiency	152	OMIM:611290
TMEM142 deficiency	147	OMIM:610277
Deficiencies predominantly affecting antibody production		
Agammaglobulinemia		
X-linked agammaglobulinemia	22	OMIM:300310, OMIM:300300
X-linked hypogammaglobulinemia with growth hormone deficiency	23	OMIM:307200
BLNK deficiency	24	OMIM:601495, OMIM:604515
Igα deficiency	25	OMIM:601495, OMIM:112205
μ heavy chain deficiency	26	OMIM:601495, OMIM:147020
λ5 surrogate light chain deficiency	27	OMIM:146770
Non-Bruton type autosomal dominant agammaglobulinemia	151	OMIM:601495, OMIM:608360, OMIM:601495
Light chain deficiency		
κ light chain deficiency	65	OMIM:147200
Selective deficiency of IgG subclass, IgE and/or IgA class or subclass		
γ1 isotype deficiency	28	OMIM:147100
γ2 isotype deficiency	29	OMIM:147110
Partial γ3 isotype deficiency	30	OMIM:147120
γ4 isotype deficiency	31	OMIM:147130
α1 isotype deficiency	32	OMIM:146900
α2 isotype deficiency	33	OMIM:147000
ε isotype deficiency	34	OMIM:147180
IgG subclass deficiency with or without IgA deficiency	35	
IgA deficiency	67	OMIM:137100
Common variable immunodeficiency		
Common variable immunodeficiency of unknown origin	66	OMIM:240500
ICOS deficiency	116	OMIM:607594, OMIM:240500, OMIM:604558
TACI deficiency	153	OMIM:604907, OMIM:240500, OMIM:609529
Other antibody deficiencies		
Antibody deficiency with normal immunoglobulin levels	68	OMIM:240500

[a] Fact files are available at http://bioinf.uta.fi/xml/idr/factfiles.xml. To access an individual fact file directly, type http://bioinf.uta.fi/xml/idr/ff/FF**000**.xml into your web browser, replacing '**000**' with the fact file number.
[b] OMIM files are available at www.ncbi.nlm.nih.gov/omim/. To access an individual record directly, type www.ncbi.nlm.nih.gov/omim**000000** into your web browser, replacing '**000000**' with the record number.

Table 24.1. (*cont.*)

Disease	Fact file[a]	OMIM[b]
Deficiencies predominantly affecting antibody production		
Other antibody deficiencies		
Transient hypogammaglobulinemia of infancy	69	OMIM:240500
CD19 deficiency	150	OMIM:107265
Defects of class-switch recombination and somatic hypermutation (hyper-IgM syndromes) affecting B-cells		
AID deficiency	17	OMIM:605258, OMIM:605257
UNG deficiency	127	OMIM:608106, OMIM:191525
Selective deficiency in Ig class-switch recombination	138	OMIM:608184
Defects in lymphocyte apoptosis		
Autoimmune lymphoproliferative syndrome		
Apoptosis mediator APO-1/Fas defect type Ia	36	OMIM:601859, OMIM:601859, OMIM:134637, OMIM:601762
APO-1 ligand/Fas ligand defect type Ib	37	OMIM:601859, OMIM:134638
Autoimmune lymphoproliferative syndrome type II	109	OMIM:603909, OMIM:601859, OMIM:601762, OMIM:134637, OMIM:605027
Caspase 8 deficiency	110	OMIM:601859, OMIM:607271, OMIM:601763
Other well-defined immunodeficiency syndromes		
Wiskott–Aldrich syndrome and X-linked thrombocytopenia	71	OMIM:301000, OMIM:313900, OMIM:300392
Autoimmune disorders		
Autoimmune polyendocrinopathy with candidiasis and ectodermal dystrophy	72	OMIM:240300, OMIM:607358
X-linked immunodeficiency, polyendocrinopathy, enteropathy (IPEX)	78	OMIM:304790, OMIM:300292
X-linked lymphoproliferative disease (Duncan disease)	73	OMIM:308240, OMIM:300490
DiGeorge anomaly	74	OMIM:188400, OMIM:192430, OMIM:602054
Hyper-IgE recurrent infection syndrome	75	OMIM:147060, OMIM:243700
Chronic mucocutaneous candidiasis	76	OMIM:606415, OMIM:114580, OMIM:212050
Cartilage–hair hypoplasia	77	OMIM:250250, OMIM:157660
Epidermodysplasia verruciformis		
Epidermodysplasia verruciformis type 1	114	OMIM:226400, OMIM:605828
Epidermodysplasia verruciformis type 2	115	OMIM:226400, OMIM:605829

Table 24.1. (*cont.*)

Disease	Fact file[a]	OMIM[b]
Other well-defined immunodeficiency syndromes		
Netherton syndrome	133	OMIM:256500, OMIM:605010
Natural killer deficiency	135	OMIM:146740
Transcobalamin II deficiency	130	OMIM:275350
AR osteopetrosis	157	OMIM:604592, OMIM:259700
Hepatic veno-occlusive disease with immunodeficiency syndrome	158	OMIM:604457, OMIM:235550
Defects of phagocyte function		
Chronic granulomatous disease		
X-linked chronic granulomatous disease	38	OMIM:306400, OMIM:300481
p22^{phox} deficiency	39	OMIM:233690, OMIM:608508
p47^{phox} deficiency	40	OMIM:233700, OMIM:608512
p67^{phox} deficiency	41	OMIM:233710, OMIM:608515
Leukocyte adhesion defects		
Leukocyte adhesion deficiency I	42	OMIM:116920, OMIM:600065
Leukocyte adhesion deficiency II	43	OMIM:266265, OMIM:605881
LAD3 deficiency	139	OMIM:116920
LAD with RAC2 deficiency	123	OMIM:608203, OMIM:602049
Chédiak–Higashi syndrome	79	OMIM:214500, OMIM:606897
Griscelli syndrome		
Griscelli syndrome, type 1	80	OMIM:214450, OMIM:160777
Griscelli syndrome, type 2	122	OMIM:607624, OMIM:604228, OMIM:214450, OMIM:603868
Griscelli syndrome, type 3	156	OMIM:606526, OMIM:609227
Glucose 6-phosphate dehydrogenase deficiency	81	OMIM:305900
Myeloperoxidase deficiency	82	OMIM:254600, OMIM:606989
Glycogen storage disease Ib	83	OMIM:232200, OMIM:232220, OMIM:232240, OMIM:602671
Shwachman syndrome	84	OMIM:260400, OMIM:607444

[a] Fact files are available at http://bioinf.uta.fi/xml/idr/factfiles.xml. To access an individual fact file directly, type http://bioinf.uta.fi/xml/idr/ff/FF**000**.xml into your web browser, replacing '**000**' with the fact file number.
[b] OMIM files are available at www.ncbi.nlm.nih.gov/omim/. To access an individual record directly, type www.ncbi.nlm.nih.gov/omim**000000** into your web browser, replacing '**000000**' with the record number.

Table 24.1. (cont.)

Disease	Fact file[a]	OMIM[b]
Defects of phagocyte function		
Neutropenia		
Severe congenital neutropenias, including Kostmann syndrome	85	OMIM:202700, OMIM:130130, OMIM:138971, OMIM:600871
Cyclic neutropenia	86	OMIM:162800, OMIM:130130
GFI1 deficiency	129	OMIM:202700, OMIM:600871, OMIM:130130
Familial hemophagocytic lymphohistiocytosis		
Familial hemophagocytic lymphohistiocytosis type 1	104	OMIM:267700, OMIM:603552
Familial hemophagocytic lymphohistiocytosis type 2	105	OMIM:267700, OMIM:170280
Familial hemophagocytic lymphohistiocytosis type 3	126	OMIM:608898, OMIM:608897
Familial hemophagocytic lymphohistiocytosis type 4	155	OMIM:267700, OMIM:603552, OMIM:605014
Hoyeraal–Hreidarsson syndrome/dyskeratosis congenita	113	OMIM:300240, OMIM:305000, OMIM:300126
CD64 deficiency	132	OMIM:146760
Hermansky–Pudlak syndrome 2	108	OMIM:608233, OMIM:603401
Barth syndrome	134	OMIM:302060, OMIM:300069, OMIM:300394
Neutrophil-specific granule deficiency	112	OMIM:245480, OMIM:600749
Papillon–Lefèvre syndrome	154	OMIM:602365, OMIM:245000
Defects of innate immune system, receptors and signaling components		
Interferon-γ (IFN-γ) receptor deficiency		
IFN-γ 1 receptor deficiency	44	OMIM:209950, OMIM:107470, OMIM:600263
IFN-γ 2 receptor deficiency	45	OMIM:209950, OMIM:147569
Interleukin-12 receptor β1 deficiency	47	OMIM:209950, OMIM:601604
Interleukin-12 (IL-12) p40 deficiency	46	OMIM:209950, OMIM:161561
STAT1 deficiency	70	OMIM:600555, OMIM:209950
Growth hormone insensitivity with immunodeficiency	125	OMIM:245590, OMIM:604260
IRAK4 deficiency	117	OMIM:607676, OMIM:606883
Autosomal dominant anhidrotic ectodermal dysplasia and T-cell immunodeficiency	121	OMIM:129490, OMIM:164008, OMIM:300291
WHIM syndrome	7	OMIM:193670, OMIM:162643

Table 24.1. (cont.)

Disease	Fact file[a]	OMIM[b]
Defects of innate immune system, receptors and signaling components		
X-linked hyper-IgM syndrome and hypohidrotic ectodermal dysplasia (Nemo deficiency)	19	OMIM:300291, OMIM:300248
DNA-breakage-associated syndromes and DNA epigenetic modification syndromes		
DNA-breakage-associated syndromes		
Ataxia telangiectasia	87	OMIM:208900, OMIM:607585
Nijmegen breakage syndrome	88	OMIM:251260, OMIM:602667
Ataxia telangiectasia-like disorder	120	OMIM:604391, OMIM:600814
DNA ligase deficiency		
DNA ligase I deficiency	131	OMIM:126391
DNA ligase deficiency IV	118	OMIM:606593, OMIM:601837
Bloom syndrome	89	OMIM:210900, OMIM:604610
Immunodeficiency, centromere instability, and facial abnormalities syndrome (ICF)	124	OMIM:242860, OMIM:602900
Defects of the classical complement cascade proteins		
C1q deficiency		
C1q α-polypeptide deficiency	48	OMIM:120550
C1q β-polypeptide deficiency	49	OMIM:120570
C1q γ-polypeptide deficiency	50	OMIM:120575
C1r and C1s deficiency		
C1r deficiency	51	OMIM:216950
C1s deficiency	52	OMIM:120580
C2 deficiency	90	OMIM:217000
C3 deficiency	61	OMIM:120700
C4 deficiency		
C4A deficiency	53	OMIM:120810
C4B deficiency	54	OMIM:120820
C5 deficiency	91	OMIM:120900
C6 deficiency	92	OMIM:217050
C7 deficiency	93	OMIM:217070
C8 deficiency		
C8 α-polypeptide deficiency	55	OMIM:120950
C8 β-polypeptide deficiency	56	OMIM:120960
C8 γ-polypeptide deficiency	57	OMIM:120930
C9 deficiency	94	OMIM:120940
Defects of the alternative complement pathway		
Factor B deficiency	95	OMIM:138470
Factor D deficiency	98	OMIM:134350
Factor H1 deficiency	101	OMIM:134370

[a] Fact files are available at http://bioinf.uta.fi/xml/idr/factfiles.xml. To access an individual fact file directly, type http://bioinf.uta.fi/xml/idr/ff/FF**000**.xml into your web browser, replacing '**000**' with the fact file number.
[b] OMIM files are available at www.ncbi.nlm.nih.gov/omim/. To access an individual record directly, type www.ncbi.nlm.nih.gov/omim**000000** into your web browser, replacing '**000000**' with the record number.

Table 24.1. (cont.)

Disease	Fact file[a]	OMIM[b]
Defects of the alternative complement pathway		
Properdin factor C deficiency	100	OMIM:312060, OMIM:300383
Defects of complement regulatory proteins		
Hereditary angioedema	97	OMIM:106100, OMIM:606860
C4-binding protein deficiency		
C4 binding protein α deficiency	58	OMIM:120830
C4 binding protein β deficiency	59	OMIM:120831
Decay-accelerating factor (CD55) deficiency	102	OMIM:125240
Factor I deficiency	99	OMIM:217030
CD59 deficiency	103	OMIM:107271
Mannose-binding lectin deficiency		
Mannose-binding lectin deficiency	96	OMIM:154545
Mannan-binding lectin-associated serine protease 2 deficiency	119	OMIM:605102
Periodic fever syndromes		
Familial Mediterranean fever	140	OMIM:608107
Hyperimmunoglobulinemia D with periodic fever syndrome	141	OMIM:260920, OMIM:251170
Tumor necrosis factor receptor-associated periodic syndrome	142	OMIM:142680, OMIM:191190
Cold autoinflammatory syndrome		
Familial cold urticaria and Muckle–Wells syndrome	143	OMIM:120100, OMIM:191900, OMIM:606416
Chronic infantile neurological cutaneous and articular syndrome	144	OMIM:607115, OMIM:606416
Granulomatous synovitis with uveitis and cranial neuropathies	145	OMIM:186580, OMIM:605956
Crohn disease	146	OMIM:266600, OMIM:605956

[a] Fact files are available at http://bioinf.uta.fi/xml/idr/factfiles.xml. To access an individual fact file directly, type http://bioinf.uta.fi/xml/idr/ff/FF**000**.xml into your web browser, replacing '**000**' with the fact file number.
[b] OMIM files are available at www.ncbi.nlm.nih.gov/omim/. To access an individual record directly, type www.ncbi.nlm.nih.gov/omim**000000** into your web browser, replacing '**000000**' with the record number.

Post-transplant lymphoproliferative disorders (PTLDs) were recognized as a complication soon after transplantation was introduced as a therapeutic modality. The incidence of PTLDs varies widely with the type of transplantation and the immunosuppressive therapy given. In bone transplantation, the preparatory regimens, for instance the use of T-cell depletion or not, also affect the incidence and severity of these disorders.

Other iatrogenic immunodeficiency-associated LPDs represent an evolving field, due to the continuous introduction of new treatments, including biologic agents. Next to well-

Table 24.2. Diseases associated with the Epstein–Barr virus (EBV).

Infectious mononucleosis

EBV-positive lymphoproliferative disorders
  In primary immunodeficiency
  Iatrogenic
  Of the elderly

Burkitt lymphoma
Lymphomatoid granulomatosis
Extranodal NK/T-cell lymphoma, nasal type
Hodgkin lymphoma (about 50% of cases)
Nasopharyngeal carcinoma
Gastric carcinoma, medullary type

known examples like methotrexate, now infliximab, a monoclonal antibody directed against TNF-α has been increasingly recognized as predisposing to LPD. In these iatrogenic conditions, the prognosis, initially unfavorable, has been significantly improved by anti-CD20 (rituximab) therapy.

This chapter will include a description of the two major pathways leading to LPDs in immunodeficient patients, and will then address the most common primary immunodeficiency syndromes with a short description of their features and the most common types of associated LPDs, with a focus on those entities that may be encountered in the pediatric age group.

Pathogenesis of immunodeficiency-associated LPDs

Immunodeficiency-associated LPDs occur through two major mechanistic pathways: abnormal lymphoproliferations induced by microorganisms, most notably the Epstein–Barr virus (EBV); and defects in DNA repair that lead to accumulation of genetic abnormalities at an increased rate in highly proliferating cells, such as lymphocytes.

Pathogenesis of EBV-related LPDs

Epstein–Barr virus (EBV) belongs to the genus *Lymphocryptovirus*, subfamily *Gammaherpesvirinae*, family *Herpesviridae*. Almost all humans encounter EBV during their lifetime. In most individuals this results in minor illness followed by a lifelong carrier status. The virus is also responsible for a variety of diseases, which occur mostly as a result of the host–virus interaction, with the immune system as a major player (Table 24.2). The most common clinical disorder is infectious mononucleosis, which, in rare instances, may be rapidly fatal, or lead to a chronic syndrome. Several subtypes of neoplasms are related to EBV as well, including Burkitt lymphoma, classical Hodgkin lymphoma, NK/T-cell lymphoma of nasal type, nasopharyngeal carcinoma, some forms of gastric cancer, and, most relevant to this chapter, lymphoproliferative disorders occurring in immunodeficient individuals [2].

EBV enters cells through binding CD21, complement component receptor 2 (CR2), which is present on B-lymphocytes, follicular dendritic cells, and a subset of epithelial cells and T-lymphocytes. After entering the cell, the EBV virus induces the transcription of genes that have similarities to human genes, such as p53, and takes over the control of cell growth processes. *In vitro* culturing of B-cells with EBV results in immortalization of the B-cells, a feature that has also been used to develop lymphoblastoid cell lines. The infected cells express a variety of EBV proteins on their membrane, depending on the stage of infection. These proteins are recognized by the immune system, leading to removal of the infected cells by cytotoxic T-cells in individuals with a normal immune function. In some cells, the EBV will not lead to protein synthesis, resulting in a lack of EBV-specific protein expression on the cell surface. These cells are not removed by the immune system and form a life-long reservoir of EBV. In these cells, EBV replicates at low rates, likely repressed by the competent immune system. Under conditions of immunosuppression, such as HIV infection or post-transplantation, reactivation of EBV proliferation may occur and lead to EBV-induced lymphoproliferative disorders. T-cells are the most important component of the immune system with regards to removal and repression of EBV. Hence, T-cell dysfunction results in a variety of lymphoproliferative diseases, varying from fatal infectious mononucleosis to mild chronic disease, and indolent and aggressive lymphoproliferative disorders. Primary immune deficiencies, depending on the deficient components of the immune system, may be associated with the full range of these EBV-induced diseases, or only with specific entities (see below).

Types of EBV latency

In primary human infection, EBV infects B-lymphocytes, causing them to become proliferating blasts [3], and establishing a latent infection, as those lymphocytes are largely non-permissive for virus replication. Viral gene expression in EBV-associated diseases is limited to one of three latency patterns [4]. In latency type I, which is found in Burkitt lymphoma, only EBV nuclear antigen (EBNA)-1 and EBV-encoded small RNAs (EBERs) are expressed. In latency type II, which is characteristic of classical Hodgkin lymphoma, EBNA-1, latent membrane protein (LMP)-1, LMP-2, and EBERs are expressed. In latency type III, which is associated with lymphoproliferative disorders in immunodeficiency, all of the latency genes (EBNA-1, EBNA-2, EBNA-3A–C, EBNA-LP, LMP-1, LMP-2, and EBERs) are expressed.

Techniques for EBV detection

EBV can be demonstrated in biopsy material by a variety of methods, including immunohistochemistry, DNA- or RNA-*in situ* hybridization, and PCR-based techniques. Monoclonal antibodies against several of the EBV proteins are available, and, by using a combination of these, the latency status of EBV can be determined. This is, however, of scientific value only, and has no practical consequences in the diagnostic workup of patients. Most of the antibodies cannot be used for formalin-fixed and paraffin-embedded tissues, with the antibody against LMP-1

and EBNA-2 as notable exceptions. It is important to remember that LMP-1 and EBNA-2 are useful EBV markers only in lesions associated with viral latency type III. While latency type III is the most common pattern seen in immunodeficiency-associated LPDs, other latency patterns may also occur in this setting, and therefore absence of LMP-1 staining does not exclude EBV-infection in these disorders [4]. The most reliable and feasible method for detecting EBV in tissue sections is *in situ* hybridization for EBER. EBERs are small mRNAs that are transcribed in large amounts in cells infected with EBV, regardless of latency status. The function of the EBERs is unknown, but in practice they allow visualization of EBV-infected cells using labeled probes that bind to these mRNAs, even in formalin-fixed, paraffin-embedded tissues. This method is commercially available and can be used in every laboratory that has the ability to perform immunohistochemistry. Notably, when using this methodology in lymph nodes from normal individuals, one may find occasional EBER-positive cells. Increased numbers of such cells point towards primary infection or immune deficiency. Correlation with the clinical context is necessary [5].

Clinical manifestations of EBV infection in immunocompromised patients

Fatal infectious mononucleosis

Primary infection with EBV can result in overwhelming disease that is fatal, mainly seen in severe primary immunodeficiency [6]. The patients present with high fever and enlargement of the lymph nodes, tonsils, and spleen. Histologically, these organs show highly polymorphic proliferations of B-cells, some of which have features of Hodgkin and even Reed–Sternberg cells. Often there is an associated hemophagocytic syndrome. The course of fatal infectious mononucleosis is so rapid, that the pathologist often encounters such cases at autopsy only. In such patients, especially when they are of young age, the underlying primary immunodeficiency may not have been recognized prior to presentation.

Chronic EBV infection

Patients with a less severe abnormality of T-lymphocytes may develop chronic EBV infections. These patients present with chronic fatigue and mild lymph node enlargement. Upon biopsy, one sees follicular and paracortical hyperplasia, but without the atypical cells characteristic of EBV-infected lymphoid tissues. *In situ* hybridization for EBER shows a significant increase in EBV-infected cells, which are generally of the size and appearance of normal lymphocytes (Fig. 24.1).

EBV-associated lymphoproliferative disorders

The EBV-associated lymphoproliferative disorders form a spectrum ranging from benign-appearing lymphoid infiltrates to processes with morphologic features of lymphoma [7]. Most benign-appearing cases contain large numbers of EBER-positive B-cells, including small and large cells, plasma

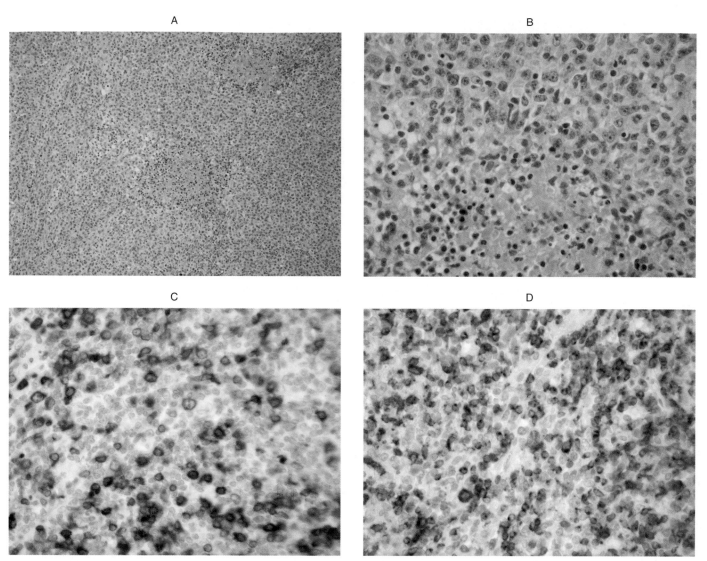

Fig. 24.1. Chronic EBV infection seen in the spleen of a 27-year-old woman with common variable immunodeficiency (CVID). The markedly enlarged spleen (2200 g) showed a polymorphous infiltrate with areas of necrosis, composed of many mildly atypical B- and T-cells of variable size, that were partially EBV positive. Cytogenetics and flow cytometry showed no abnormalities. Molecular analysis showed a predominantly polyclonal pattern with a small T-cell clone and a small B-cell clone. (A, B) H&E stain; (C) CD20 IHC stain; (D) CD2 IHC stain.

cells, and plasmacytoid lymphocytes. These benign-appearing lesions can be difficult to recognize as LPDs without EBER staining, and when no clinical data are available, such cases are likely to be interpreted as reactive lymph nodes. Recognizing such lesion as LPDs is important, however, since if left untreated, they may progress to more aggressive forms. Increasing numbers of large atypical cells can be found in more advanced cases, and the most aggressive forms can very closely resemble malignant lymphomas, especially diffuse large B-cell lymphoma (Fig. 24.2) or Burkitt lymphoma, and more rarely Hodgkin lymphoma. The lymphoma cases often show plasma cell differentiation. The phenotype is most often that of a mature B-cell (CD20+, CD79a+, CD138−) and sometimes of a plasma cell (CD20−, CD79a−, CD138+) type. In many cases, intracytoplasmic immunoglobulin can be detected, allowing for determination of light chain restriction, indicative of monoclonality.

Progression to more aggressive lesions is accompanied by increasing genetic changes, similar to those seen in *de novo* lymphoma, such as the involvement of the *c-MYC* gene in Burkitt lymphoma. These LPDs may evolve from reactive-appearing polyclonal proliferations, to oligoclonal processes, to monoclonal infiltrates when there is progression. Monoclonal LPDs have a more aggressive clinical behavior. It is important to remember that, in this context, there is morphologic overlap between polyclonal, oligoclonal, and monoclonal processes, such that lesions with the appearance of diffuse large B-cell lymphoma may still be poly- or oligoclonal. A surrogate marker for clonality in these disorders that often express significant levels of cytoplasmic immunoglobulin is the demonstration

A

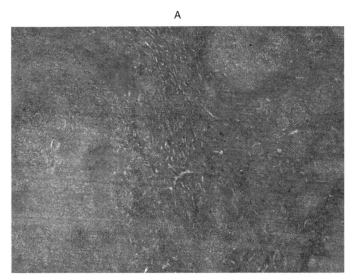

B

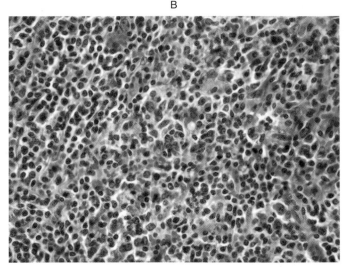

Fig. 24.2. EBV-positive lymphoproliferation, morphologically diffuse large B-cell lymphoma, seen in a cervical lymph node from a five-year-old boy with severe combined immunodeficiency (SCID). (A) At low magnification, the architecture is effaced, with focal areas of necrosis. (B) At high magnification, the abnormal infiltrate consists of large, centroblastic B-cells, which were CD20 positive, with only a minority of the cells EBV positive. Molecular analysis showed a polyclonal pattern with a small dominant clone. (H&E stain.)

of light chain restriction, which can be accomplished by immunohistochemical or *in situ* hybridization analysis for immunoglobulin light chains. However, clonal immunoglobulin-negative cases do occur. Therefore, the most reliable method for clonality assessment is polymerase chain reaction (PCR) for the complete spectrum of possible rearrangements. PCR allows for the detection of even relatively small clones in a reactive background [8]. The course of these LPDs is partially determined by the morphologic aggressiveness and the clonality status, and is mainly determined by the underlying disease. In primary immune deficiencies the cause can rarely be addressed. Most standard treatment regimens for lymphoma are not well tolerated by these patients, and are associated with a high mortality due to infections. It is recommended to treat lymphoma in these patients as mildly as possible, with anti-CD20 antibody (rituximab) treatment as a key element [9].

Pathogenesis of lymphoproliferations associated with DNA metabolism defects

There are several DNA metabolism systems, each specific to certain types of DNA damage, which may occur mostly during DNA replication and mitosis. Some of these systems are affected in specific forms of primary immune deficiencies, such as Nijmegen breakage syndrome, Bloom syndrome, and ataxia telangiectasia. These defects lead to high numbers of DNA alterations in the affected patients. Lymphomas are often associated with chromosomal translocations that bring oncogenes under the influence of the promoter of antigen receptor genes, leading to their overexpression. Therefore, an increased number of lymphomas can be seen in patients with defective DNA repair, both of B-cell and T-cell lineage [10]. Some of the lymphomas presenting in this context are similar to those occurring

in immunocompetent patients, but more often these lesions are difficult to classify (see below).

LPDs associated with specific primary immunodeficiencies

Primary immunodeficiencies have very complex clinical features, due to environmental variability, and variation in (prophylactic) treatment and monitoring that the patients receive (Table 24.3). Therefore, biopsies from these patients may present to pathology laboratories at very different phases of the disease, and sometimes without a clinical diagnosis of immunodeficiency. Lymphoproliferative diseases in these patients pose a great diagnostic challenge to the pathologists. Clues that may raise suspicion for an underlying immunodeficiency include lymphoproliferations that are very difficult to classify as specific subtypes of lymphoma, and unusual histologic reactive patterns. In such cases, especially when the LPD is also EBV positive, contact with the clinician is important to raise the possibility of a (primary) immunodeficiency. It is important to realize in this context that the specific pathologic classification of the lymphoproliferative diseases is of less importance than in immunocompetent individuals, since the severity of the underlying immune deficiency determines the outcome to a large extent, and therapeutic options are limited in these patients [11].

Antibody deficiencies

There are three main types of hypogammaglobulinemia: X-linked hypogammaglobulinemia (XLA), common variable immunodeficiency (CVID), and IgA deficiency. These diseases not only predispose to infection but are also associated with an increased risk of cancer, which generally presents beyond the

Table 24.3. Clinical, genetic, and laboratory features of the primary immunodeficiencies (PIDs) most commonly associated with lymphoproliferative disorders.

Type of primary immunodeficiency	Frequency among all PID (%)[a]	Gene(s) affected	Immunologic abnormalities	Most common clinical and laboratory abnormalities	Most common associated lymphoproliferative disorders
Combined T- and B-cell immunodeficiencies	9–18				
Severe combined immunodeficiency (SCID)	1–5	γ chain of IL-2R, IL-4R, IL-7R, IL-9R, IL15R, IL-21R; JAK3 kinase; IL-7R, CD45, CD3δ or CD3ε; RAG1/2, ARTEMIS, ADA	Markedly ↓circulating T, B (in T-B- subtype), and serum Ig	Recurrent, severe bacterial, fungal, and viral infections, including opportunistic infections; skin rash	Frequency unknown DLBCL, fatal infectious mononucleosis
CD40 ligand and CD40 deficiencies (former hyper-IgM syndrome)	1–2	CD40 ligand (CD40L, CD154) or CD40	Nl T, IgM and IgD B memory cells present, others absent; IgM ↓/↑, other isotypes	Neutropenia, thrombocytopenia, hemolytic anemia, biliary tract and liver disease, opportunistic infections	Incidence unknown DLBCL, Hodgkin lymphoma, large granular lymphocyte leukemia
Predominantly antibody PIDs	53–72				
Common variable immunodeficiency (CVID)	21–31	Unknown	Nl T, B Nl/↓; IgG and IgA↓	Bacterial infections (lung, GI), autoimmune cytopenias, granulomatous disease (lung, liver)	2–7% B-cell lymphomas (DLBCL, extranodal marginal zone lymphoma, small lymphocytic lymphoma, lymphoplasmacytic lymphoma), Hodgkin lymphoma, peripheral T-cell lymphoma (rare)
Other well-defined immunodeficiency syndromes	5–22				
Wiscott–Aldrich syndrome	1–3	WASP	Progressive ↓ of T, IgM↓, Nl B	Thrombocytopenia, small platelets, eczema, autoimmune disease, bacterial infections	Frequency unknown DLBCL, Hodgkin lymphoma, lymphomatoid granulomatosis
Ataxia telangiectasia	2–8	ATM	T↓, Nl B; IgA, IgE, IgG↓; IgM monomers↑; antibodies↓	Ataxia, telangiectasias, increased AFP, increased X-ray sensitivity	10–30% Non-leukemic clonal T-cell proliferations, DLBCL, Burkitt lymphoma, T-PLL, T-ALL, Hodgkin lymphoma
Nijmegen breakage syndrome	1–2	NBS1(nibrin)	T↓, Nl B; IgA, IgE, IgG↓; IgM monomers↑; antibodies↓	Microcephaly, progressive mental retardation, sensitivity to ionizing radiation, predisposition to cancer	28–36% DLBCL, peripheral T-cell lymphoma, T-LBL/ALL, Hodgkin lymphoma
Diseases of immune dysregulation	1–3				
X-linked lymphoproliferative syndrome (XLP)	<1	SH2D1A	Nl T, B, Ig	EBV-triggered abnormalities (fatal IM, hepatitis, aplastic anemia), lymphoma	Frequency unknown Burkitt lymphoma, DLBCL
Autoimmune lymphoproliferative syndrome (ALPS)	<1	TNFRSF6 (CD95, Fas) (type 1a), TNFS6 (CD95L) (type 1b), CASP10 (caspase 10) (type 2a), or CASP8 (caspase 8) (type 2b)	Nl T, B, Ig Increased double-negative T (CD4-CD8-)	Defective lymphocyte apoptosis, splenomegaly, adenopathy, autoimmune cytopenias, recurrent infections	3–10% Hodgkin lymphoma (classical and nodular LP), DLBCL, peripheral T-cell lymphoma (rare)

[a] Data compiled from reports of several national and international registries.
Abbreviations: TCR, T-cell antigen receptor; Nl, normal; ADA, adenosine deaminase; B, B-lymphocytes; T, T-lymphocytes; Ig, serum immunoglobulin; AFP, alpha fetoprotein.

Table 24.4. Severe combined immune deficiencies (SCIDs).

Some of the known forms of SCID	Gene	Lymphocyte phenotype
X-linked SCID (gamma chain gene mutations)	*IL2RG*	T(−) B(+) NK(−)
Autosomal recessive SCID		
Jak3 gene mutations	*JAK3*	T(−) B(+) NK(−)
ADA gene mutations	*ADA*	T(−) B(−) NK(−)
IL-7R alpha chain mutations	IL7R alpha	T(−) B(+) NK(+)
CD3 delta or epsilon mutations	CD3 delta or epsilon	T(-) B(+) NK(+)
RAG1/RAG2 mutations	*RAG1/RAG2*	T(−) B(−) NK(+)
Artemis gene mutations	ARTEMIS	T(−) B(−) NK(+)
CD45 gene mutations	CD45	T(−) B(+) NK(+)

pediatric age. In XLA there is an increased risk for colorectal cancer [12], whereas patients with the CVID have a 50× increased risk for gastric cancer and a 30× increased risk for lymphoma [13]. The risk for lymphoma in CVID is estimated to be between 1.4 and 7% [14–16], with all of these cases presenting at adult age [17].

CVID, the most common form of antibody deficiency, is characterized by decreased (or absent) levels of immunoglobulins, and recurrent bacterial infections of the respiratory and gastrointestinal tracts [18]. Most of the patients also have T-cell abnormalities, including decreased lymphocyte response to mitogens and microbial antigens. A subset of CVID patients harbors polyclonal expansions of large granular lymphocytes (LGLs) with a CD4/CD8 ratio ≤0.9, in some cases due to an increase in CD8+ T-cells expressing CD57 [19, 20]. Non-caseating granulomatous lesions occur in 5.4–10% of CVID patients [21].

Combined B- and T-cell deficiencies

Severe combined immunodeficiency (SCID)

Severe combined immunodeficiency can be caused by different genetic defects, with variable NK-, T-, and B-cell abnormalities (see Table 24.4). A common feature is the lack of T-cell response, resulting in inability to surmount EBV infection. These patients present relatively frequently with rapidly evolving EBV-induced lymphoproliferative disorders, occurring at a very young age and often combined with hemophagocytic lymphohistiocytosis. Such a combination should prompt evaluation for an underlying immune deficiency. Hemophagocytic lymphohistiocytosis presenting in young children should be evaluated using EBV (EBER) staining, to rule out an EBV-related lymphoproliferation as the cause [22]. These lymphoproliferations are particularly difficult to treat, since only repairing the underlying immune defect is truly effective. Approaches such as hematopoietic stem cell transplantation (HSCT) and gene therapy are being considered for these patients.

Wiskott–Aldrich syndrome

Wiskott–Aldrich syndrome (WAS) and X-linked thrombocytopenia (XLT) are rare X-linked genetic disorders caused by mutations of the Wiskott–Aldrich syndrome protein (WASP) gene. Both disorders are characterized by chronic thrombocytopenia and small platelets. Wiskott–Aldrich syndrome is a more severe form of the disorder with immune dysfunction and susceptibility to malignant lymphoma [23]. These patients have an increased risk for EBV-induced lymphoproliferative disease, sometimes associated with hemophagocytosis [24]. EBV-associated lymphoproliferative disease occurring in WAS patients includes two clinicopathologic subsets: one with a relatively benign clinical behavior, despite clonality and aggressive morphology, and a second subset presenting with lymphomatoid granulomatosis [25]. Lymphomatoid granulomatosis is a clonal EBV-positive large B-cell proliferation associated with an exuberant T-lymphocyte proliferation, which typically presents at extranodal sites, most commonly the lung. Although the predominant infiltrating cells are T-cells, the T-cell receptor genes are not clonally rearranged. The large atypical B-cells, which represent a minority of the infiltrate, are EBER positive and, by PCR-methods, are clonal for immunoglobulin gene rearrangements, which support B-cell lymphoma. The course of the disease is generally aggressive despite treatment [26]. Allogeneic HSCT represents a curative approach but remains problematic in light of its severe associated risks and side effects. Recently, gene therapy (*WASP* gene reconstitution) has emerged as an alternative treatment option. The first clinical trial is currently being conducted to assess the feasibility, toxicity, and potential therapeutic benefit of the latter approach [27].

Ataxia telangiectasia (AT)

AT is a relatively rare autosomal recessive disorder caused by mutations in the *ATM* gene, manifested by progressive cerebellar ataxia, oculocutaneous telangiectasia, gonadal sterility, and general growth retardation. Severe disease morbidity also results from immunodeficiency, leading to frequent respiratory infections and significantly increased susceptibility to cancer, particularly to lymphoproliferative diseases [28, 29]. AT patients have an estimated 70- to 250-fold risk increase for both B-cell and T-cell malignancies [30–33]. In contrast to most other immunodeficiencies, the frequency of T-cell neoplasms exceeds that of B-cell malignancies by a factor of four. The vast majority of lymphoid tumors that develop in AT children are T-cell lymphoblastic leukemia/lymphomas, while young adults are mostly predisposed to T-cell prolymphocytic leukemia (T-PLL). Early studies revealed that AT children diagnosed with ALL at older age and with higher tumor burden tend to have a less favorable prognosis. Early childhood T-cell malignancies have an immature or mixed immature/mature phenotype, supporting a thymic origin, while leukemias arising in adult AT patients have a more mature phenotype and are probably of post-thymic origin [34].

Nijmegen breakage syndrome (NBS)

Nijmegen breakage syndrome is an inherited condition that is caused by mutation of the *NBS1* gene located on chromosome 8q21 [35, 36]. The NBS1 protein, also called nibrin, is indirectly involved in double-strand DNA break (DSB) repair, which is also needed during immunoglobulin (Ig) and T-cell receptor (TCR) gene rearrangement [37]. Nijmegen breakage syndrome is characterized by chromosomal instability, cellular and humoral immunodeficiency, sensitivity to ionizing radiation, gonadal failure, and predisposition to lymphoproliferative disease at very young age, largely similar to AT. Chromosomal instability in NBS results in characteristic chromosome rearrangements involving chromosomes 7 and 14, with breakpoints at the Ig and TCR loci. These aberrations are caused by aberrant VDJ recombination and mostly concern so-called Ig/TCR trans-rearrangements. NBS patients are estimated to have a >1000-fold risk of developing lymphoproliferative disease, generally of B-cell origin [25, 38, 39].

Bloom syndrome (BS)

BS is a rare autosomal recessive disorder characterized by prenatal and postnatal growth retardation, immune deficiency, characteristic facial rash, and enormous predisposition to a variety of cancers. The disorder is a consequence of homozygous mutation at *BLM*, a RecQ DNA helicase [40]. The pathogenesis of immune deficiency in BS is still poorly understood. Such individuals present with decreased levels of one or more immunoglobulins and decreased or absent delayed hypersensitivity manifested clinically as diarrhea and respiratory tract infections during infancy and early childhood [41, 42]. Human and animal studies show variable effects of mutated *BLM* on B- and T-cell development, with resultant low levels of immunoglobulin and also abnormal functioning of the $\alpha\beta$ T-cells [43, 44].

Mutation at the *BLM* gene results in chromosome breakage, increased sister chromatid, and, at the molecular level, an excessive amount of somatic recombination [45]. As a result, individuals with BS have a multifold increased risk of developing a variety of malignancies including hematopoietic malignancies, solid tumors, and childhood malignancies. Acute leukemias, both ALL and AML, along with non-Hodgkin and Hodgkin lymphomas, comprise about one-half of the first 100 cancers reported in a cohort of 168 individuals with BS [46]. Similarly to individuals with other congenital immune deficiencies, the non-Hodgkin lymphomas in BS are diffuse, high-grade lesions.

Hyper-IgE syndrome

The hyper-IgE syndrome (or Job syndrome) is an autosomal dominant syndrome, resulting from a *STAT3* gene mutation, and is characterized by the occurrence of bacterial infections, eczema, and increased levels of serum IgE. There is a small increase in the risk for lymphoma which may occasionally develop at pediatric age, especially Hodgkin lymphoma. EBV is not involved in these cases and the mechanism remains unknown. The pathology is similar to lymphomas arising in immunocompetent hosts [47].

T-cell deficiencies

DiGeorge syndrome

DiGeorge syndrome is a clinical entity manifested mainly by thymic hypoplasia that results from a developmental defect in the mesenchyme of the embryologic pharyngeal arches. Most patients with the clinical features of DiGeorge syndrome have a hemizygous deletion of chromosome 22q11.2. Manifestations include thymic hypoplasia or aplasia, parathyroid hypoplasia, cardiac anomalies, and a cleft palate. Thymic hypoplasia is not always directly demonstrated, and a decreased number of T-cells is often used as a surrogate diagnostic feature. While these decreased numbers of T-cells are secondary to decreased production resulting from the thymic hypoplasia, the T-cells that successfully transit the thymus are functionally normal, and there is no intrinsic T-cell defect. As a consequence, these patients develop relatively few infectious and neoplastic complications. Compared with a population of HIV patients with comparable T-cell counts, patients with DiGeorge syndrome only rarely have opportunistic infections, and usually only in the setting of very low T-cell counts. While prolonged viral infections and secondary bacterial infections are reasonably common, death is seldom from infection, and hospitalization is rare outside of infancy. This explains why EBV-driven lymphoproliferative disease is not found in these patients.

Defects in signaling proteins

Auto-immune lymphoproliferative syndrome (ALPS)

Auto-immune lymphoproliferative syndrome is a heritable disorder of lymphocyte apoptosis involving mutations in genes from the Fas/CD95/APO-1 pathway of programmed cell death. Fas (*TNFRSF6*) is a cell-surface receptor in the tumor necrosis factor receptor superfamily, which upon stimulation activates a caspase-mediated apoptosis pathway that controls the homeostasis of mature lymphocytes. ALPS is subdivided into several subtypes according to the underlying genetic defect: type Ia (*Fas* gene mutations); type Ib (Fas ligand gene mutations); type II (mutations in caspase genes); type III (genetic defect not yet defined); type IV (*N-Ras* gene mutations). Most ALPS patients are of type Ia and have heterozygous mutations of *TNFRSF6*. The different subtypes of ALPS share similar clinical manifestation and pathologic findings [48].

Patients with ALPS have chronic, waxing and waning lymphadenopathy and splenomegaly, of childhood onset, often with associated autoimmune manifestations, especially autoimmune cytopenias. There is also an increased risk of B-cell lymphoma, Hodgkin lymphoma (Fig. 24.3), and EBV-driven lymphoproliferative disease (Fig. 24.4). There is significant variation in the severity of the clinical symptoms, even between family members with the same inherited mutation.

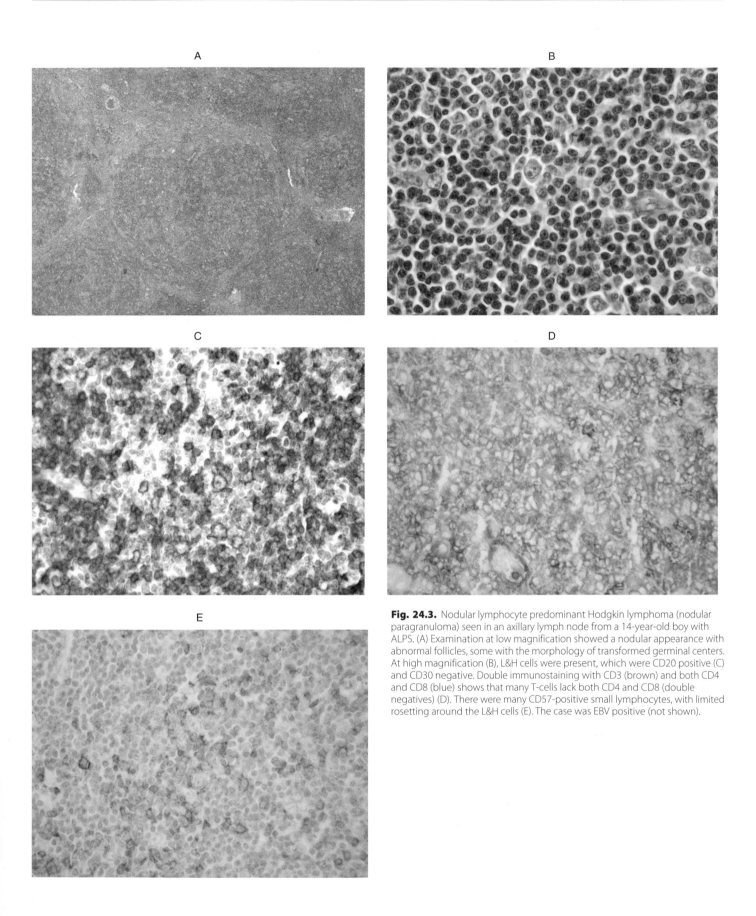

Fig. 24.3. Nodular lymphocyte predominant Hodgkin lymphoma (nodular paragranuloma) seen in an axillary lymph node from a 14-year-old boy with ALPS. (A) Examination at low magnification showed a nodular appearance with abnormal follicles, some with the morphology of transformed germinal centers. At high magnification (B), L&H cells were present, which were CD20 positive (C) and CD30 negative. Double immunostaining with CD3 (brown) and both CD4 and CD8 (blue) shows that many T-cells lack both CD4 and CD8 (double negatives) (D). There were many CD57-positive small lymphocytes, with limited rosetting around the L&H cells (E). The case was EBV positive (not shown).

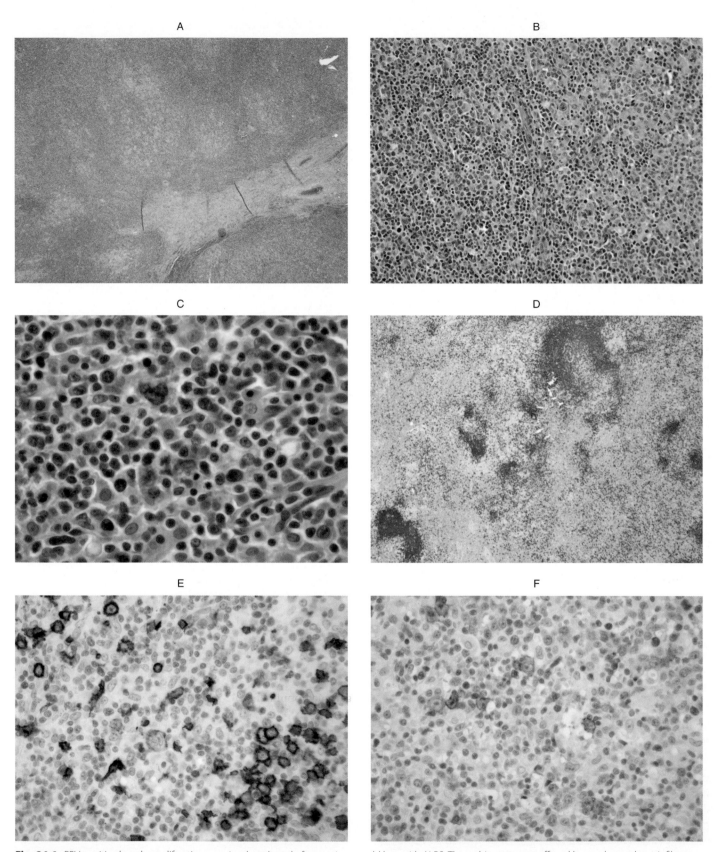

Fig. 24.4. EBV-positive lymphoproliferation seen in a lymph node from a six-year-old boy with ALPS. The architecture was effaced by a polymorphous infiltrate composed of lymphocytes, plasma cells, and eosinophils, admixed with scattered large atypical cells. The large cells were reminiscent of Hodgkin cells but true Reed–Sternberg cells were not seen (A–C, H&E stain). They were positive for CD20 (D, E), sometimes weaker than normal B-cells, CD79A, and CD30 (F). Many cells, both small and large, were positive for EBER (G, H). Flow cytometry showed a population of CD4- and CD8-negative T-cells.

G

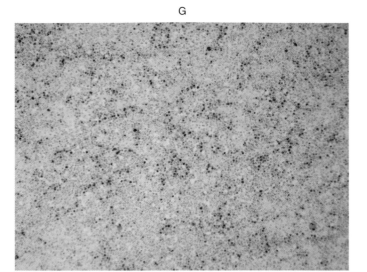

H

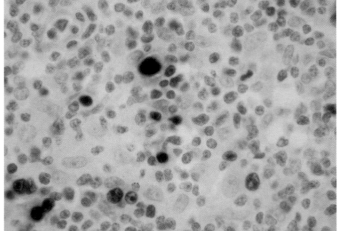

Fig. 24.4. (cont.)

The disease may be difficult to diagnose on clinical grounds and, with increasing awareness of the characteristic lymph node histology seen in ALPS, the pathologist may have an important role in suggesting this diagnosis. A hallmark of the disease is the presence of increased numbers of normally rare CD3+CD4−CD8− or "double-negative αβ T-cells" (DNTs). These cells may be detected by flow cytometry in the peripheral blood or may be seen in lymph node biopsy material (Fig. 24.5). Their accumulation in lymph nodes gives rise to the characteristic histologic pattern that includes a marked expansion of the interfollicular (paracortical) area by large lymphoid cells with abundant pale cytoplasm and often prominent nucleoli. These cells have an aberrant DNT phenotype: T-cell receptor (TCR)αβ+, CD3+, CD4−, CD8−, CD45RO−, CD57+, TIA-1+, CD25−, CD30−. Additional morphologic findings may include follicular hyperplasia with even focal progressive transformation of germinal centers, plasma cell hyperplasia, and Castleman-like changes in areas of the lymph node where the DNTs are less prominent [41]. In the markedly enlarged spleens of ALPS patients, the same DNT population typically expands the red and white pulp, while in liver biopsies, these cells may be infiltrating the portal tracts. Recognizing these abnormalities as a part of ALPS is essential in discriminating it from T-cell non-Hodgkin lymphoma.

Hyper-IgM syndrome

Hyper immunoglobulin (Ig) M syndrome is a term used to describe a heterogeneous group of disorders characterized by normal or elevated concentrations of serum IgM, with markedly decreased IgG, IgA, and IgE. These abnormalities result from the failure of B-cells to complete their normal maturation program, due to defects in Ig isotype class-switch recombination and somatic hypermutation.

X-linked hyper-IgM (XHIM) syndrome is caused by mutations of the CD40 ligand gene located at Xq26, and character-ized by chronic neutropenia, autoimmune disorders, recurrent opportunistic infections, and rarely lymphoma [49, 50]. The functional effect of the mutation is that the CD40 ligand on T-cells cannot interact with the CD40 glycoprotein on the surface of B-cells. This interaction normally mediates Ig synthesis by B-cells. Lymphomas arising in this setting are not associated with EBV and are similar to lymphomas presenting in immuno-competent patients.

X-linked lymphoproliferative syndrome (XLP)

XLP is an X-linked congenital immunodeficiency that is estimated to affect 1 in 1 000 000 males, and may manifest clinically anywhere from childhood to early adulthood [51, 52]. Most (60%) of the patients harbor a mutation in the *SH1D1A* gene, and more rarely a mutation in the X-linked inhibitor of apoptosis (*XIAP*) has been reported. These genetic defects, resulting in increased apoptosis of T-cells, lead to loss of functional T-lymphocytes and an impaired ability to control EBV infections [53–55]. XLP may manifest with one or more of three main phenotypes: inappropriate immune response to EBV with fatal or near-fatal infectious mononucleosis, EBV-driven lymphoproliferative diseases, typically of B-cell origin, and dys-gammaglobulinemia. The defect is severe, and fatal infectious mononucleosis is relatively common, being the presenting feature in two-thirds of the cases.

A less common but important manifestation is EBV-induced hemophagocytic lymphohistiocytosis (HLH) [56–58]. Lymphoproliferation affects approximately one-third of all XLP patients, manifesting at a median age of four to six years [52]. The risk of developing lymphoproliferative disease is higher for patients with XLP than for any other primary immuno-deficiency [54]. Nearly all lesions are EBV associated and of B-cell origin, and approximately half of these can be classified as Burkitt lymphoma. The presentation of these lymphomas is usually extranodal, with the majority localized in the ileocecal

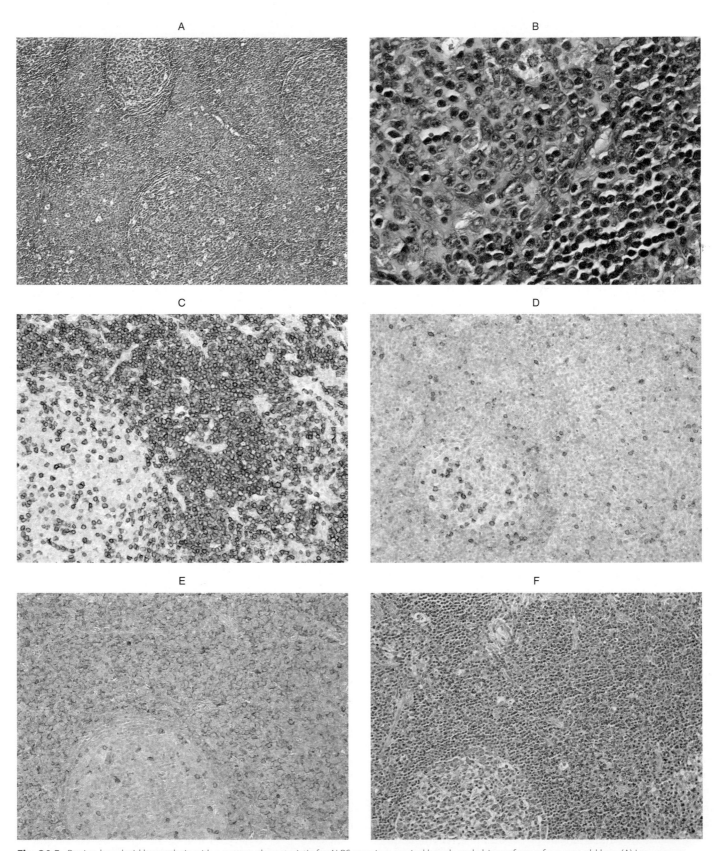

Fig. 24.5. Benign lymphoid hyperplasia with a pattern characteristic for ALPS seen in a cervical lymph node biopsy from a four-year-old boy. (A) Low-power examination shows follicular hyperplasia and paracortical expansion by a population of cells with pale cytoplasm and "starry sky" appearance (H&E stain). (B) At high power, these cells have immunoblastic features with prominent central nucleoli (H&E stain). On immunohistochemical staining, these cells are CD3 positive (C), CD45RO negative (D), CD57 positive (E), and TIA-1 positive (F).

region. A characteristic feature of Burkitt lymphoma in XLP is the tendency of these patients to develop second lymphomas. A history of Burkitt lymphoma in a male child that appears to recur after a long period of remission should prompt the evaluation of that patient for XLP. A similar approach should be considered if a male patient with Burkitt lymphoma has a family history of a similar lymphoma occurring in his male sibling(s).

Lymphoproliferations in HIV infection

Similar to adults with AIDS, the risk of malignancies is increased in HIV-infected children, but the precise incidence of cancer has been difficult to define. Before the introduction of effective antiretroviral therapy there was at least a 100-fold increased risk of malignancy, mainly lymphomas, in HIV-infected children. Exposure to antiretroviral drugs has decreased the risk for lymphoma development substantially [59]. High EBV viral loads and severity of immunosuppression, as reflected by CD4 cell count, were associated with an increased risk of cancer. EBV seroprevalence, while ubiquitous in older adults, is lower in young children. Virtually all HIV-associated lymphomas are associated with EBV, and, as can be expected, subtypes include atypical lymphoproliferations, Burkitt lymphoma, diffuse large B-cell lymphoma, plasmablastic lymphoma, and Hodgkin lymhoma [60, 61]. Occasionally, hemophagocytic syndrome (HS) may complicate the lymphoproliferation [62].

Iatrogenic lymphoproliferative diseases

Post-transplantation lymphoproliferative diseases (PTLDs)

PTLDs comprise a heterogeneous category of disorders that arise in the clinical setting of immunosuppression following solid organ or hematopoietic stem cell transplant. In HSCT patients, the lymphoproliferative disease is generally of donor-derived cells, while in solid organ transplants, of host cells. PTLD is characterized by a proliferation of EBV-transformed B-lymphocytes, including germinal center B-cells, memory B-cells, non-antigen-selected post-germinal center B-cells, and also naïve B-cells [63, 64]. Rare EBV-negative cases [65] and T-lineage PTLDs [66] have been described as well.

PTLD is the paradigm of EBV-associated lymphoproliferations (see above). It represents one of the major complications of transplantation, and occurs more frequently in children than in adults. Its occurrence is strongly dependent on the type and severity of the immunosuppressive drugs used, with the use of tacrolimus being one of the known risk factors. When the lymphoproliferative disease occurs within six months after transplantation the prognosis is very poor. Lowering the dose of immunosuppression can decrease the incidence of PTLD. Monitoring of peripheral blood by quantitative PCR for EBV genome copy numbers may help in identifying patients who are at very high risk of developing PTLD, such that

early treatment may be instituted and prevent the occurrence of clinically detectable lymphoproliferative disease. The prognosis has improved in recent years due to better understanding of the pathogenesis, better recognition, and earlier, less intensive treatment. While most patients who were treated with aggressive chemotherapy followed a fatal course, more recently, less intensively treated patients (receiving anti-CD20 therapy, EBV-specific cytotoxic T-cell infusion), are often cured.

By far the most cases are B-cell lymphoproliferations (Fig. 24.6), but other lymphoma types may occur, including different types of T-cell and Hodgkin lymphomas. These latter types of lymphoma often occur years after the transplantation, and their relationship with this underlying condition is not always clear. Most of them are, however, EBV positive. The prognosis appears to be similar to lymphomas of the same subtype developing in immunocompetent patients. The histopathology of PTLD is complex and evolving, reflecting ongoing changes in the use of immunosuppressive agents, the understanding of their biology, and the therapeutic approach. The spectrum varies from early cases with a polymorphous infiltrate which has features of reactive processes like infection or rejection, to aggressive cases with the morphology of Burkitt lymphoma. When interpreting the pathologic findings, it is crucial to be informed on the clinical data, type, and time of transplantation. The detection of EBV in these cases is important for the diagnosis. The prognosis of PTLD depends on both histological subtype (polymorphic or monomorphic) and clonality of the cell population; monomorphic, monoclonal proliferations are associated with more aggressive disease. Detection of monoclonality may be accomplished by assessing light chain restriction by immunohistochemistry (Fig. 24.6) and/or immunofluorescence for cytoplasmic and cell-surface expression of the immunoglobulin heavy and light chain (κ or λ) proteins. Clonality may be difficult to detect by these techniques in small monoclonal proliferations admixed with a predominant polyclonal background, or when these proliferations lack expression of immunoglobulin (Ig) heavy and/or light chain proteins. Therefore, molecular assays for detecting clonal gene rearrangements of the immunoglobulin heavy and light chain genes, *IGH*, *IGK*, and *IGL*, respectively may be very useful in this context.

Other types of iatrogenic immune suppression

Since a T-cell defect is the prime cause for EBV-associated lymphoproliferative disease in primary immune deficiencies (PIDs), HIV, and PTLD, it is not surprising that such proliferations also occur in association with iatrogenic immunosuppression. Therapy for the inflammatory bowel diseases (IBDs) and other autoimmune disorders employs, to an increasing extent, the use of immune-modifying and other biologic agents. In children this is mainly seen in early and severe inflammatory bowel disease and, to a lesser extent, in rheumatoid arthritis treated with monoclonal antibodies to tumor necrosis factor (TNF), including infliximab. Most of the lymphoproliferative

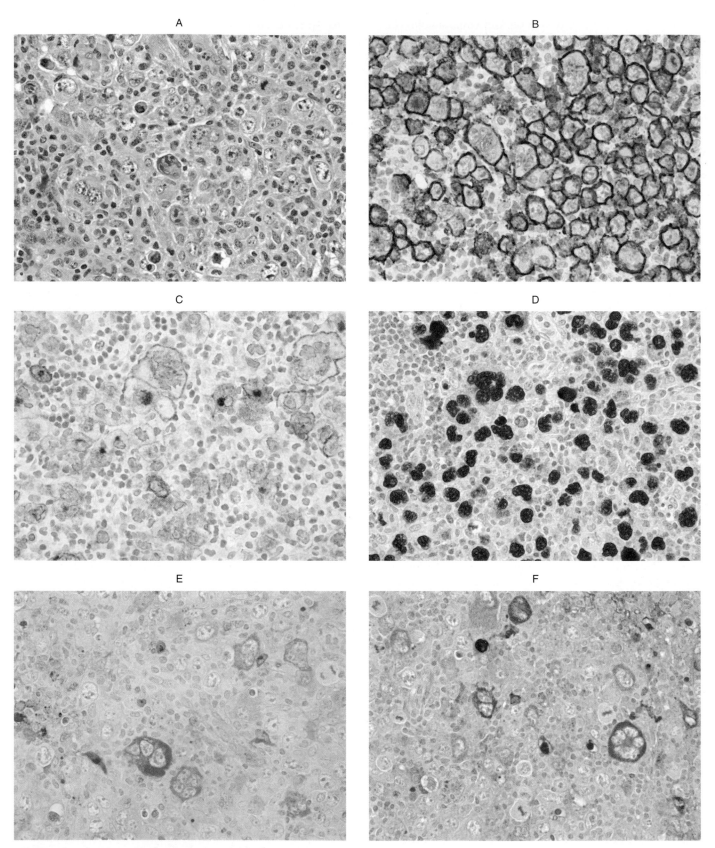

Fig. 24.6. Polymorphic PTLD with Hodgkin lymphoma-like features seen in a cervical lymph node from a four-year-old boy, status post-kidney transplant. The large Hodgkin and Reed–Sternberg-like cells were CD15−, CD20+, CD30+, CD45 partially+, EBER+, and showed polyclonal cytoplasmic expression of immunoglobulin kappa and lambda light chains. (A, H&E stain; B, CD20 IHC; C, CD30 IHC; D, EBER *in situ* hybridization (ISH); E, Ig kappa IHC; F, Ig lambda IHC).

disorders developing in this context are indistinguishable from the other forms of EBV-related lymphoproliferative diseases. The LPDs occurring in this setting seem to include an increased proportion of Hodgkin lymphoma and other proliferations with Hodgkin-like features. Other types of non-Hodgkin lymphoma are similar to lymphomas seen in immunocompetent individuals. There is a four-fold increased risk of lymphoma in this patient population, but it is not certain whether this is a result of the severity of the disease, an effect of therapy, or a combination of both. Recently, in young patients with IBD, an association has been noted between the use of infliximab along with concomitant purine analogues and the development of hepatosplenic T-cell lymphoma (HSTCL), a rare form of non-Hodgkin lymphoma with very poor prognosis [67].

HSTCL is a rare subtype of peripheral T-cell NHL with a propensity to infiltrate sinusoids of spleen, liver, and bone marrow. The cases associated with iatrogenic immunosuppression are similar clinically and pathologically to those presenting in immunocompetent patients. The typical clinical presentation includes hepatosplenomegaly and cytopenias. As with other mature T-cell NHL, and as observed in the first reported cases of HSTCL, prominent erythrophagocytosis may be seen in the spleen and bone marrow, and may occasionally contribute to a very dramatic initial clinical presentation. Histologically, tumor cells infiltrating the liver and spleen have the appearance of normal activated T-cells. Most of the cases involving the bone marrow in pediatric patients have a blastic morphology, with features overlapping with those of acute leukemias. Immunophenotypic characterization by immunohistochemical staining or flow cytometry is therefore essential in correctly classifying these neoplasms. The lymphoma cells are TdT−, CD34−, CD2+, CD3+, CD4−, CD5−, CD7−, often CD16+, rarely CD8+ and CD56+/−, TIA-1+, perforin−, granzyme B−, TCR gamma delta (and more rarely alpha beta)+, and most are negative for EBV.

Several epidemiologic studies have demonstrated that patients with rheumatoid arthritis (RA) develop LPDs at a higher frequency than the general population. Several cases of EBV-associated lymphoproliferative disease have been described in children with rheumatoid arthritis [68]. It has been reported that rheumatic patients have a reduced capacity to control EBV infection; EBV-specific T-cells are not efficient at controlling the outgrowth of EBV-infected B-lymphocytes, and EBV load in peripheral blood is much higher than that in normal individuals. In addition to this already-impaired immunologic state, immunosuppression caused by therapy with methotrexate may further diminish the immune control of EBV-infected cells, leading to the development of LPDs. Lymphoproliferative diseases reported in patients receiving methotrexate (typically following at least six months of therapy) include diffuse large B-cell lymphoma (DLBCL), Hodgkin lymphoma, polymorphic LPD (some with Hodgkin-like features), and peripheral T-cell lymphoma.

The outcome of LPDs associated with iatrogenic immunodeficiencies depends on the type of immunosuppressive therapy and the histologic subtype. A high proportion of the methotrexate-associated EBV-related LPDs, and 30–40% of DLBCLs and Hodgkin lymphomas associated with methotrexate show at least partial regression after withdrawal of the drug. The remainder are likely to require chemotherapy. Lymphoproliferative diseases related to TNF antagonists are not likely to regress with discontinuation of therapy.

References

1. **Samarghitean C, Valiaho J, Vihinen M**. IDR knowledge base for primary immunodeficiencies. *Immunome Research*. 2007;**3**:6.

2. **Klein E, Kis LL, Klein G**. Epstein-Barr virus infection in humans: from harmless to life endangering virus-lymphocyte interactions. *Oncogene*. 2007;**26**:1297–1305.

3. **Thorley-Lawson DA, Gross A**. Persistence of the Epstein-Barr virus and the origins of associated lymphomas. *New England Journal of Medicine*. 2004;**350**:1328–1337.

4. **Hamilton-Dutoit SJ, Rea D, Raphael M**, *et al*. Epstein-Barr virus-latent gene expression and tumor cell phenotype in acquired immunodeficiency syndrome-related non-Hodgkin's lymphoma. Correlation of lymphoma phenotype with three distinct patterns of viral latency. *The American Journal of Pathology*. 1993;**143**:1072–1085.

5. **Ambinder RF, Mann RB**. Detection and characterization of Epstein-Barr virus in clinical specimens. *The American Journal of Pathology*. 1994;**145**:239–252.

6. **Cohen JI**. Benign and malignant Epstein-Barr virus-associated B-cell lymphoproliferative diseases. *Seminars in Hematology*. 2003;**40**:116–123.

7. **Oertel SH, Riess H**. Immunosurveillance, immunodeficiency and lymphoproliferations. *Recent Results in Cancer Research*. 2002;**159**:1–8.

8. **van Krieken JH, Langerak AW, Macintyre EA**, *et al*. Improved reliability of lymphoma diagnostics via PCR-based clonality testing: report of the BIOMED-2 Concerted Action BHM4-CT98-3936. *Leukemia*. 2007;**21**:201–206.

9. **van Dongen JJ, Langerak AW, Bruggemann M**, *et al*. Design and standardization of PCR primers and protocols for detection of clonal immunoglobulin and T-cell receptor gene recombinations in suspect lymphoproliferations: report of the BIOMED-2 Concerted Action BMH4-CT98-3936. *Leukemia*. 2003; **17**:2257–2317.

10. **Franco S, Alt FW, Manis JP**. Pathways that suppress programmed DNA breaks from progressing to chromosomal breaks and translocations. *DNA Repair*. 2006;**5**:1030–1041.

11. **Canioni D, Jabado N, MacIntyre E**, *et al*. Lymphoproliferative disorders in children with primary immunodeficiencies: immunological status may be more predictive of the outcome than other criteria. *Histopathology*. 2001;**38**: 146–159.

12. **Van Der Meer JW, Weening RS, Schellekens PT, Van Munster IP, Nagengast FM**. Colorectal cancer in patients with X-linked

agammaglobulinaemia. *Lancet.* 1993; **341**:1439–1440.

13. **Kinlen LJ, Webster ADB, Bird AG**, *et al.* Prospective study of cancer in patients with hypogammaglobulinaemia. *Lancet.* 1985;**1**:263–266.

14. **Filipovich AH, Heinitz KJ, Robison LL**, *et al.* The immunodeficiency cancer registry. A research resource. *American Journal of Paediatric Hematology/Oncology* 1987;**9**:183–187.

15. **Kersey JH, Shapiro RS, Filipovich AH**. Relationship of immunodeficiency to lymphoid malignancy. *Pediatric Infectious Disease Journal.* 1988;**7**:10–12.

16. **Cunningham-Rundles C, Lieberman P, Hellman G**, *et al.* Non-Hodgkin lymphoma in common variable immunodeficiency. *American Journal of Hematology.* 1991;**37**:69–74.

17. **Gompels MM, Hodges E, Lock RJ**, *et al.* Lymphoproliferative disease in antibody deficiency: a multi-centre study. *Clinical and Experimental Immunology.* 2003;**134**:314–320.

18. **Di Renzo M, Pasqui AL, Auteri A**. Common variable immunodeficiency: a review. *Clinical and Experimental Medicine.* 2004;**3**:211–217.

19. **Holm AM, Tjonnfjord G, Yndestad A**, *et al.* Polyclonal expansion of large granular lymphocytes in common variable immunodeficiency – association with neutropenia. *Clinical and Experimental Immunology.* 2006; **44**:418–424.

20. **Wright JJ, Wagner DK, Blaese RM**, *et al.* Characterization of common variable immunodeficiency: identification of a subset of patients with distinctive immunophenotytic and clinical features. *Blood.* 1990;**76**:2046–2051.

21. **Mechanic LJ, Dikman S, Cunningham-Rumndles C**. Granulomatous disease in common variable immunodeficiency. *Annals of Internal Medicine.* 1997;**127**:613–617.

22. **Schmid I, Reiter K, Schuster F**, *et al.* Allogeneic bone marrow transplantation for active Epstein-Barr virus-related lymphoproliferative disease and hemophagocytic lymphohistiocytosis in an infant with severe combined immunodeficiency syndrome. *Bone Marrow Transplant.* 2002;**29**:519–521.

23. **Andreu N, Matamoros N, Escudero A, Fillat C**. Two novel mutations identified in the Wiskott-Aldrich syndrome protein gene cause Wiskott-Aldrich syndrome and thrombocytopenia. *International Journal of Molecular Medicine.* 2007;**19**:777–782.

24. **Pasic S, Micic D, Kuzmanovic M**. Epstein-Barr virus-associated haemophagocytic lymphohistiocytosis in Wiskott-Aldrich syndrome. *Acta Paediatrica.* 2003;**92**:859–861.

25. **Elenitoba-Johnson KS, Jaffe ES**. Lymphoproliferative disorders associated with congenital immunodeficiencies. *Seminars in Diagnostic Pathology.* 1997;**14**:35–47.

26. **Jaffe ES, Wilson WH**. Lymphomatoid granulomatosis: pathogenesis, pathology and clinical implications. *Cancer Surveys.* 1997;**30**:233–248.

27. **Boztug K, Dewey RA, Klein C**. Development of hematopoietic stem cell gene therapy for Wiskott-Aldrich syndrome. *Current Opinion in Molecular Therapeutics.* 2006;**8**:390–395.

28. **Tauchi H, Kobayashi J, Morishima K**, *et al.* Nbs1 is essential for DNA repair by homologous recombination in higher vertebrate cells. *Nature.* 2002; **420**:93–98.

29. **Wegner RD, Chrzanowska KH, Sperling K, Stumm M**. Ataxia teleangiectasia variants (Nijmegen breakage syndrome). In Ochs HD, Smits CIE, Puck JM, eds. *Primary Immunodeficiencies. A Molecular and Genetic Approach.* Oxford: Oxford University Press; 1999, 324–334.

30. **Morrell D, Cromartie E, Swift M**. Mortality and cancer incidence in 263 patients with ataxia-telangiectasia. *Journal of the National Cancer Institute.* 1986;**77**:89–92.

31. **Filipovich AH, Mathur A, Kamat D, Shapiro RS**. Primary immunodeficiencies: genetic risk factors for lymphoma. *Cancer Research.* 1992;**52**:5465s–5467s.

32. **Taylor AM**. Ataxia telangiectasia genes and predisposition to leukaemia, lymphoma and breast cancer. *British Journal of Cancer.* 1992;**66**:5–9.

33. **Taylor AM, Metcalfe JA, Thick J, Mak YF**. Leukemia and lymphoma in ataxia telangiectasia. *Blood.* 1996;**87**:423–438.

34. **Matei IR, Guidos CJ, Danska JS**. ATM-dependent DNA damage surveillance in T-cell development and leukemogenesis: the DSB connection. *Immunological Reviews.* 2006;**209**:142–158.

35. **Weemaes CM, Hustinx TW, Scheres JM**, *et al.* A new chromosomal instability disorder: the Nijmegen breakage syndrome. *Acta Paediatrica Scandinavica.* 1981;**70**:557–564.

36. **Matsuura S, Tauchi H, Nakamura A**, *et al.* Positional cloning of the gene for Nijmegen breakage syndrome. *Nature Genetics.* 1998;**19**:179–181.

37. **Carney JP, Maser RS, Olivares H**, *et al.* The hMre11/hRad50 protein complex and Nijmegen breakage syndrome: linkage of double-strand break repair to the cellular DNA damage response. *Cell.* 1998;**93**:477–486.

38. **Seidemann K, Henze G, Beck JD**, *et al.* Non-Hodgkin's lymphoma in pediatric patients with chromosomal breakage syndromes (AT and NBS): experience from the BFM trials. *Annals of Oncology.* 2000;**11**(Suppl 1): 141–145.

39. **Gladkowska-Dura MJ, Dzierzanowska-Fangrat K, Langerak AW, Van Dongen JJM**. Immunophenotypic and immunogenotypic profile of NHL in Nijmegen breakage syndrome (NBS) with special emphasis on DLBCL. *Journal of Clinical Pathology.* 2002;**55S**:A15.

40. **Ellis NA, Groden J, Ye TZ**, *et al.* The Bloom's syndrome gene product is homologous to RecQ helicases. *Cell.* 1995;**83**(4): 655–666.

41. **Kondo N, Motoyoshi F, Mori S**, *et al.* Long-term study of the immunodeficiency of Bloom's syndrome. *Acta Paediatrica.* 1992; **81**(1):86–90.

42. **German J**. Bloom syndrome: a mendelian prototype of somatic mutational disease. *Medicine.* 1993;**72**(6):393–406.

43. **Babbe H, Chester N, Leder P, Reizis B**. The Bloom's syndrome helicase is critical for development and function of the alphabeta T-cell lineage. *Molecular and Cellular Biology.* 2007;**27**(5):1947–1959.

44. **Babbe H, McMenamin J, Hobeika E**, *et al.* Genomic instability resulting from Blm deficiency compromises development, maintenance, and function of the B cell lineage. *Journal of Immunology.* 2009;**182**(1): 347–360.

45. **German J, Sanz MM, Ciocci S, Ye TZ, Ellis NA**. Syndrome-causing mutations of the *BLM* gene in persons in the Bloom's Syndrome Registry. *Human Mutation*. 2007;**28**(8):743–753.

46. **German J**. Bloom's syndrome. XX. The first 100 cancers. *Cancer Genetics and Cytogenetics*. 1997;**93**(1): 100–106.

47. **Renner ED, Torgerson TR, Rylaarsdam S,** *et al.* STAT3 mutation in the original patient with Job's syndrome. *New England Journal of Medicine*. 2007;**357**:1667–1668.

48. **Bi LL, Pan G, Atkinson TP,** *et al.* Dominant inhibition of Fas ligand-mediated apoptosis due to a heterozygous mutation associated with autoimmune lymphoproliferative syndrome (ALPS) Type Ib. *BMC Medical Genetics*. 2007;**8**:41.

49. **Korthauer U, Graf D, Mages HW,** *et al.* Defective expression of T-cell CD40 ligand causes X-linked immunodeficiency with hyper-IgM. *Nature*. 1993;**361**:539–541.

50. **Fuentes-Paez G, Saornil MA, Herreras JM,** *et al.* CHARGE association, hyper-immunoglobulin M syndrome, and conjunctival MALT lymphoma. *Cornea*. 2007;**26**:864–867.

51. **Sumegi J, Johnson J, Filipovich A, Zhang K, Marsh R**. Lymphoproliferative disease, X-linked. In Pagon RA, Bird TC, Dolan CR, Stephens K, eds. *GeneReviews* [Internet]. Seattle: University of Washington, Seattle; 2009. Available at: www.ncbi.nlm.nih.gov/bookshelf/br.fcgi?book=gene&part=x-lpd (Accessed June 24, 2010).

52. **Purtilo DT, Cassel CK, Yang JP, Harper R**. X-linked recessive progressive combined variable immunodeficiency (Duncan's disease). *Lancet*. 1975;**1**:935–940.

53. **Schuster V, Kreth HW**. X-linked lymphoproliferative disease is caused by deficiency of a novel SH2-domain containing signal transduction adaptor protein (SH2D1A). *Immunological Reviews*. 2000;**178**:21–28.

54. **Gaspar HB, Sharifi R, Gilmour KC, Thrasher AJ**. X-linked lymphoproliferative disease: clinical, diagnostic and molecular perspective. *British Journal of Haematology*. 2002;**119**:585–595.

55. **Latour S, Veillette A**. Molecular and immunological basis of X-linked lymphoproliferative disease. *Immunological Reviews*. 2003;**192**:212–224.

56. **Ohshima K, Shimazaki K, Sugihara M,** *et al.* Clinicopathological findings of virus-associated hemophagocytic syndrome in bone marrow: association with Epstein-Barr virus and apoptosis. *Pathology International*. 1999;**49**:533–540.

57. **Grierson H, Purtilo DT**. Epstein-Barr virus infections in males with the X-linked lymphoproliferative syndrome. *Annals of Internal Medicine*. 1987;**106**:538–545.

58. **Sumegi J, Huang D, Lanyi A,** *et al.* Correlation of mutations of the SH2D1A gene and Epstein-Barr virus infection with clinical phenotype and outcome in X-linked lymphoproliferative disease. *Blood*. 2003;**96**:3118–3125.

59. **Pollock BH, Jenson HB, Leach CT,** *et al.* Risk factors for pediatric human immunodeficiency virus-related malignancy. *JAMA*. 2003;**289**:2393–2399.

60. **Preciado MV, Fallo A, Chabay P, Calcagno L,** De **Matteo E**. Epstein Barr virus-associated lymphoma in HIV-infected children. *Pathology, Research and Practice*. 2002;**198**:327–332.

61. **Preciado MV, De Matteo E, Fallo A,** *et al.* Plasmablastic lymphoma of the oral cavity in an HIV-positive child. *Oral Surgery, Oral Medicine, Oral Pathology, Oral Radiology, and Endodontics*. 2005;**100**:725–731.

62. **Radhakrishnan R, Suhas S, Kumar RV,** *et al.* EBV-associated Hodgkin's disease in an HIV-infected child presenting with a hemophagocytic syndrome. *Leukemia & Lymphoma*. 2001;**42**:231–234.

63. **Capello D, Cerri M, Muti G,** *et al.* Molecular histogenesis of post-transplant lymphoproliferative disorders. *Blood*. 2003;**102**:3775–3785.

64. **Abed N, Casper JT, Camitta BM,** *et al.* Post-transplant lymphoproliferative disorder. Evaluation of histogenesis of B-lymphocytes in pediatric EBV-related post-transplant lymphoproliferative disorders. *Bone Marrow Transplantation*. 2004;**33**:321–327.

65. **Nelson BP, Nalesnik MA, Bahler DW,** *et al.* Epstein-Barr virus-negative post-transplant lymphoproliferative disorders: a distinct entity? *The American Journal of Surgical Pathology*. 2000;**24**:375–385.

66. **Dockrell DH, Strickler JG, Paya CV**. Epstein-Barr virus-induced T cell lymphoma in solid organ recipients. *Clinical Infectious Diseases*. 1998;**26**:180–182.

67. **Rosh JR, Gross T, Mamula P, Griffiths A, Hyams J**. Hepatosplenic T-cell lymphoma in adolescents and young adults with Crohn's disease: a cautionary tale? *Inflammatory Bowel Diseases*. 2007;**13**:1024–1030.

68. **Takeyama J, Sato A, Nakano K,** *et al.* Epstein-Barr virus associated Hodgkin lymphoma in a 9-year-old girl receiving long-term methotrexate therapy for juvenile idiopathic arthritis. *Journal of Pediatric Hematology/Oncology*. 2006;**28**:622–624.

25

Histiocytic proliferations in childhood

Ronald Jaffe

Definition

The term "histiocyte" (tissue cell) has evolved and is now often used as a collective noun for two related groups of immune regulatory cells, the monocyte/macrophage and the dendritic cell–accessory antigen presenting cells [1, 2]. The histiocytic proliferations of childhood, therefore, encompass the benign and malignant accumulations of monocyte-macrophages and of dendritic cells, though distinguishing the borderline between their reactive and neoplastic states still seems to be elusive [3, 4].

Origins and variety of histiocytes

Macrophages and dendritic histiocytes appear to share origin from a common marrow precursor that gives rise to divergent lines of differentiation [5], although a dendritic cell precursor independent of the myeloid and lymphoid line has been identified [6]. A competing theory is that various cell lines, lymphoid and myeloid, can produce cells that have macrophage and/or dendritic cell features as an adaptive state rather than as separate lineages [7–9]. The macrophages are most important in immediate innate immunity, with rapid response that leads to particulate removal and destruction, whereas dendritic cells preserve the antigenic information for use in adaptive responses [10]. Macrophage-derived pro- and anti-inflammatory cytokines mediate an ongoing process that interacts with the dendritic, antigen-presenting cells and also effects reconstitution of damaged tissues [11]. The distinctions between the monocyte-macrophages and dendritic cells are probably not as rigid as supposed, with a capability for some cross-differentiation until late in the process, and back-and-forth modulation [12, 13].

Local proliferation plays a role in the production of monocyte-macrophages. Some of the "fixed" macrophages and dendritic cells appear to have a low intrinsic turnover rate, while recruitment of inflammatory macrophages and dendritic cells on demand from a circulating pool of "monocytes" is more versatile [14–16].

Inflammatory macrophages are recruited as monocytes to sites of need. In addition, there are "fixed" macrophages at various sites in the body, such as Kupffer cells in the liver;

cordal macrophages in the spleen; paracortical, sinus, and follicular center macrophages in lymph nodes; macrophages and osteoclasts in the bone marrow; and microglia in the brain, among others. The activity and appearance of these various macrophages will be determined by local requirements, and gene expression, phenotype, enzyme content, and physiologic activity will vary in response to needs. Phagocytic activity is just one example of a process that accommodates to local or systemic demand [17].

Similarly, dendritic cells occur at various body sites and respond to changing demands. Epidermal Langerhans cells and dermal/mucosal dendritic cells will become activated by a variety of stimuli, including macrophage-generated ones, and migrate centrally to interact with lymphoid cells [18]. Interstitial dendritic cells are found in soft tissue and in most solid organs [19]. Lymph node interdigitating dendritic cells are derived, in part, from the Langerhans cells of the periphery and from blood-derived precursors [18]. Follicular dendritic cells, on the other hand, are thought to be of mesenchymal, not marrow, origin, and they bind antigen for prolonged periods [20]. Plasmacytoid pre-dendritic cells (plasmacytoid monocytes) are probably also of myeloid origin but can respond with efficient production of interferon [21]. Fibroblast reticular cells in lymph nodes are thought to be of mesenchymal origin, related more closely to myofibroblasts and not part of the dendritic cell family [22].

Identification of macrophages and dendritic cells

As mentioned, the appearance and phenotype of the histiocytes can change with levels of maturation and activation, and only a few markers are truly constitutive. A wide variety of surface and cytoplasmic molecules are informative for these cells by flow cytometry, though many are not unique to these cell lines. Others are more useful for the identification of macrophages, dendritic cells, and their neoplastic counterparts in fixed tissues. Table 25.1 lists some antibodies informative for histiocytes by flow cytometry, only some of which are restricted to macrophages or dendritic cells; many are common to both [23]. Table 25.2 lists the common types of monocyte/macrophage

Diagnostic Pediatric Hematopathology, ed. Maria A. Proytcheva. Published by Cambridge University Press.
© Cambridge University Press 2011.

Table 25.1. Selected antibodies informative for histiocytes.

Cluster	Cell function	Predominant cell
CD1 a, b, c	Non-MHC presentation of lipid-containing antigens	DC
CD4	MHC Class II HIV receptor	M, DC
CD11b	Complement C3B receptor	M
CD11c	CD11/CD18 receptor	M, DC
CD14	Lipopolysaccharide receptor	M
CD25	Interleukin-2 receptor	M
CD31	PECAM-1	M
CD32	Fc IgG receptor, low affinity	M
CD33	Sialoadhesin	M
CD49	Integrin receptors	M
CD52	GP1-anchored glycoprotein	M
CD64	Fc IgG receptor, high affinity	M
CD68	Macrosialin	M, DC
CD83	Immunoglobulin superfamily	DC
CD86	CD28/CD152 ligand	DC
CD91	Low-density lipoprotein related protein 1	M
CD116	Granulocyte/macrophage colony stimulating factor α	M
CD123	Interleukin-3 receptor α	DC
CD163	Hemoglobin/haptoglobin scavenger receptor	M
CD169	Sialoadhesin	M
CD204	Macrophage scavenger receptor	M
CD205	DEC 205	M, DC
CD206	Macrophage-mannose receptor	M
CD207	Langerin	DC
CD208	DC-Lamp	DC
CD209	DC-SIGN	M, DC
CD227	MUC1 Mucin glycoprotein	M, DC
CD284	TLR4 Toll-like receptor 4	M

Abbreviations: DC, dendritic cell; M, monocyte, macrophage. Many of the molecules are not unique to the histiocytes but are expressed as indicated on monocytes, macrophages, and/or dendritic cells as well as other cells.

Table 25.2. Antibodies and enzymes most informative for histiocytes in tissues.

Macrophages	CD14, CD163, acid phosphatase, non-specific esterase
Macrophages and dendritic cells	CD68, HLA-DR, S100
Dermal macrophages	CD163, Factor XIIIa
Dendritic cells: Immature; Langerhans cells Mature dendritic cells	 CD1a, Langerin CD83, DC-LAMP, hi-fascin
Dermal/interstitial dendritic cells	S100, CD68
Plasmacytoid dendritic cells	CD123, CD68
Follicular dendritic cells	CD21, CD35, clusterin

Table 25.3. Immunophenotypic markers of non-neoplastic macrophages and dendritic cells.

Marker	LC	IDC	DM	DID	FDC	PDC	Mø
MHC–class II	+c	++s	+/−	+	−	+	+
Fc receptors	−	−	+/−	+	+	−	+
CD1a	++	−	−	+/−	−	−	−
CD4	+	+	−	+	+	+	+
CD21	−	−	−	−	++	−	−
CD35	−	−	−	−	++	−	−
CD68	+/−	+/−	+	+	−	++	++
CD123	−	−	−	−	−	++	−
CD163	−	−	+	−	−	−	++
Factor 13a	−	−	+	−	+/−	−	−
Fascin	−	++	−	+	+/++	−	-/+
CD207	++	−	−	−	−	−	−
Lysozyme	+/−	−	−	−	−	−	+
S100	++	++	−	+/−	+	−	+/−
TCL1	−	−	−	−	−	+	−

Expression is semiquantitatively graded 0 through ++: +, present; ++, high; +/−, low or varies with cell activity.
Abbreviations: c, cytoplasmic; s, surface; FCR, Fc IgG receptors (include CD16, CD32, CD64 on some cells); LC, Langerhans cell; IDC, interdigitating dendritic cell; FDC, follicular dendritic cell; PDC, plasmacytoid dendritic cell; M, macrophage; DID, dermal/interstitial dendritic cell; DM, dermal macrophage.

and dendritic cells and the markers most useful in their identification in fixed tissues [23]. Table 25.3 presents the immunophenotypic markers of non-neoplastic macrophages and dendritic cells.

Pathologic accumulations of macrophages

Hyperlipidemic states can be associated with the accumulation of xanthomatous macrophages, and, when dermal or tendinous masses of xanthomatous cells are found, hyperlipidemia should be excluded before other causes are sought [24]. Sec-

ondary hyperlipidemic states that include diabetes mellitus, nephrotic syndrome, and cholestatic liver disorders (Alagille syndrome, prominently) can be associated with xanthomatous macrophage collections. Necrobiotic xanthogranulomas in soft tissue and viscera, on the other hand, are more likely to be associated with a paraproteinemia or leukemia [25]. Xanthogranulomatous pyelonephritis or cholecystitis can cause extensive local destruction, and bacteria of various kinds can be recovered, suggesting that this is an exaggerated response with local damage following infection. Xanthomatous macrophages in all the above conditions share the macrophage phenotype CD14+/CD68+/CD163+, but generally have absent to very low expression of Factor 13a, fascin, and S100.

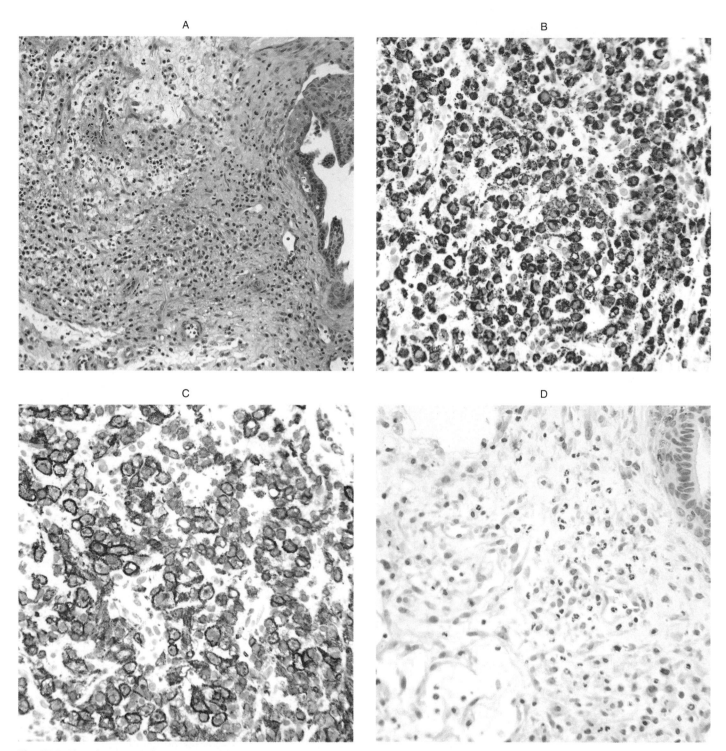

Fig. 25.1. Physiologic macrophage response. (A) Mucocele (H&E stain). (B) CD68 shows the dense granular phagocytic pattern. (C) CD163 has both surface and paranuclear staining. (D) S100 is virtually devoid of staining cells.

Macrophages accumulate at sites of infection as they participate in scavenging and tissue repair, in proportion to the amount of tissue damage (Fig. 25.1). Some organisms, however, have adapted, and subvert the macrophage's defenses in order to find shelter in the macrophage, safe from other immune cells. In other instances, the organisms accumulate by virtue of some form of genetic or acquired immune deficiency or immune depression (such as anti-TNF agents in the host), most commonly atypical mycobacteria or salmonella [26]. Furthermore, in chronic granulomatous diseases, a genetically heterogeneous group of conditions characterized by defects in the NADPH oxidase enzyme complex resulting in an inability to

A

B

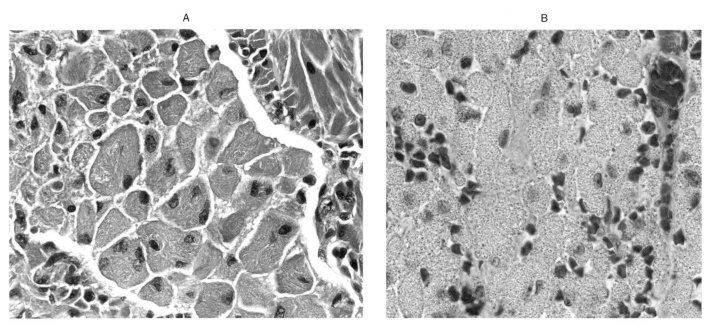

Fig. 25.2. Pathologic accumulation of endogenous or exogenous macrophage content. (A) Crystal-storing histiocytosis (H&E stain). (B) Barium-filled macrophages (H&E stain).

kill ingested organisms, collections of pigmented, lipochrome-filled macrophages in skin and viscera are characteristic [27]. Malakoplakia is a disordered response to *Escherichia coli*, most common in the urinary tract, in which the macrophages (Hansemann cells) accumulate concentric calcified intracytoplasmic Michaelis–Gutman bodies that are typical but not required for diagnosis [28]. Instances of crystal-storing histiocytosis are most commonly Kappa light chain immunoglobulin (Fig. 25.2), but can be associated with Charcot–Leyden crystals [29, 30]; it is common to see intracellular Charcot–Leyden crystals in colonic macrophages, and barium-filled macrophages can be seen in the appropriate context (Fig. 25.2). Drugs or their metabolites can accumulate in macrophages. Red birefringent crystals are noted with clofazimine administration [31].

Epithelioid transformation is a reaction pattern of activated and high-secretory, but poorly phagocytic macrophages most characteristic of the granulomatous response [32]. Nonnecrotizing epithelioid granulomas are more commonly seen in sarcoidosis, Crohn disease, hypersensitivity, as a drug effect, and in immune deficiency states such as "common variable" immune deficiency in which the extensive epithelioid granulomas can mimic sarcoidosis [33]. Blau syndrome caused by NOD2 mutations causes a sarcoid-like granulomatous dermatitis in early infancy [34]. Epithelioid cells appear to lose their monocyte/macrophage attributes and are low in CD14/CD68/CD163 expression but rich in cytoplasmic lysozyme (Fig. 25.3).

A number of tumors are characterized by their high content of histiocytes. Among the childhood lymphomas, the lymphohistiocytic variant of anaplastic large cell lymphoma is probably best known, but Hodgkin disease can also be rich in histiocytes [35]. The high content of histiocytes can be so abundant that they obscure the number of tumor cells in the background (Fig. 25.4).

Macrophages are rich in lysosomes, well shown by their rich content of macrosialin demonstrated by anti-CD68. A number of inherited lysosomal defects lead to deficiency in the macromolecules responsible for lysosomal metabolism, degradation, or transport. Metabolites or substrates can accumulate within the lysosomes leading to the so-called "lysosomal storage disorders." The materials can be recognized by their tinctorial properties, histochemical reactions, or ultrastructure, though specific diagnosis is available for most by assay of the relevant enzymes or by mutation analysis of the relevant genes. The diseases arising from lysosomal defects include the mucopolysaccharidoses (MPS I to VII), glycoproteinoses, glycogenosis type II, sphingolipidoses, lipidoses, multiple enzyme deficiency disorders, and lysosomal transport defects [36]. On rare occasions, discovery of the storage cells in biopsy or even autopsy tissue might provide the first clue to the presence of a lysosomal storage disorder.

Dendritic cells

Like their macrophage counterparts, dendritic cells participate in normal immune functions, and their relative prominence in blood and tissues undergoes age-related and functional physiologic change [37]. Primary lymphoid follicles are devoid of germinal centers in the fetus and unstimulated newborn, and the follicular prominence varies with the relative size of the germinal center [38, 39]. Autoimmune disorders and rheumatic conditions lead to follicular hyperplasia, and the follicular dendritic cells participate proportionately [40]. Follicular dendritic cell (FDC) hyperplasia with cytologically atypical forms and FDC

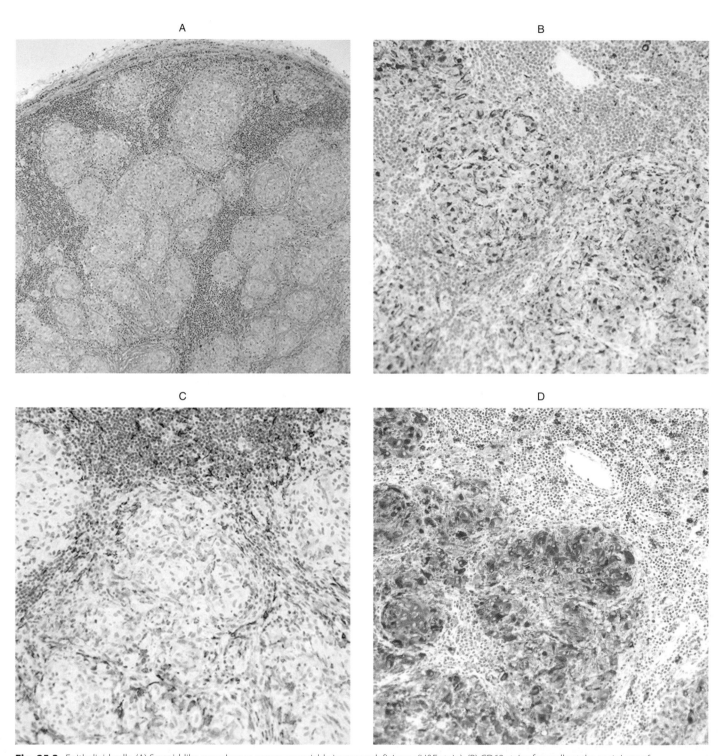

Fig. 25.3. Epithelioid cells. (A) Sarcoid-like granulomas, common variable immune deficiency (H&E stain). (B) CD68 stains few cells at the periphery of micro-nodules. (C) CD163 stains few cells at the periphery of micro-nodules. (D) Lysozyme stain has rich cytoplasmic pattern in the epithelioid cells.

tumors can be seen in some instances of multicentric Castleman disease, hyaline-vascular type, and rarely in the plasma cell variant of Castleman disease [41, 42]. Interestingly, there is some overlap with Hodgkin and Castleman diseases, and follicular dendritic cell hyperplasia is said to be a prognostic feature of nodular lymphocyte-predominant Hodgkin disease [43].

Langerhans cells in the epidermis express both CD1a and Langerin. Increased numbers of dermal dendritic cells that express CD1a but not Langerin are seen in a number of chronic skin conditions. The CD1a-reactive dermal dendritic cells in chronic dermatoses are small and dendriform in shape, and perivascular in distribution, unlike the Langerhans cell

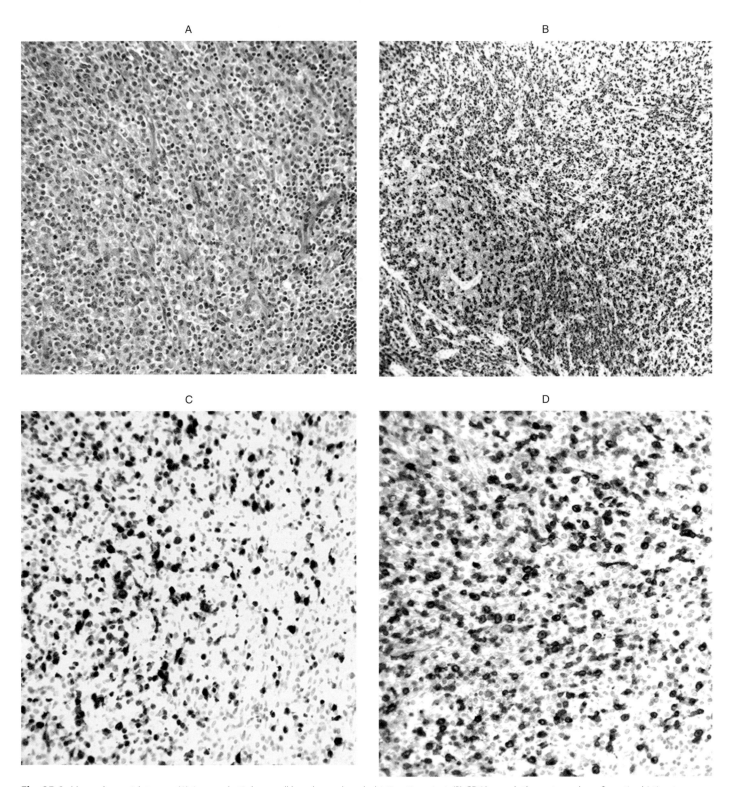

Fig. 25.4. Macrophage-rich tumor. (A) An anaplastic large cell lymphoma, lymphohistiocytic variant. (B) CD68 reveals the vast number of reactive histiocytes. (C) ALK stain picks out the interspersed tumor cells. (D) CD30 stains the tumor cells obscured on the H&E stain.

histiocytosis (LCH) cells, which are large, oval, and not strictly perivascular [44, 45]. Importantly, in the differential diagnosis of LCH, these dermal CD1a+ cells are largely devoid of Langerin.

Discrete lesions simulating Langerhans cell histiocytosis have been found in lymph nodes harboring lymphomas, Hodgkin disease, Rosai–Dorfman disease, and, rarely, other tumors, as well as in the thymus of myasthenia gravis [46].

Christie *et al.* [47] showed by laser capture microdissection that some of these collections are polyclonal, like the pulmonary Langerhans cell lesions in smokers [48] and, hence, more likely to be local Langerhans cell hyperplasias than LCH. No LCH lesions have been found elsewhere, at the time or subsequently, in those patients with incidental collections of Langerhans cells.

In a parody of the normal presence of Langerhans cells in the lymph node paracortex, large numbers of Langerhans cells accumulate in the expanded paracortical nodules of dermatopathic lymphadenopathy [18]. It is likely that they mature into interdigitating dendritic cells that express CD83, DC-Lamp, and have high fascin expression as CD1a and Langerin are lost. By contrast, LCH in lymph nodes has a sinus pattern but may then spill over into the paracortex. Diffuse paracortical dendritic cell hyperplasia of the interdigitating phenotype may be a feature of some forms of immune deficiency, severe combined form or Omenn syndrome [49–51] (Fig. 25.5). Like their macrophage counterparts, dendritic cells can respond to local cytokines and chemokines, and dendritic cell hyperplasia may mask an underlying nodal leukemia, lymphoma, EBV-related lymphoproliferation, or, rarely, carcinoma.

Plasmacytoid dendritic cells can form hyperplastic nodules in association with chronic myeloid or myelomonocytic leukemias, and can occur in lymph nodes, skin, spleen, or bone marrow [52] (Fig. 25.6).

Macrophage activation and the hemophagocytic syndromes

In order to participate actively in the immune and inflammatory repertoire of the body, monocytes respond to extrinsic or intrinsic stimuli that will determine the type of response. Classically activated macrophages (M1) are induced by IFN-γ, LPS, TNF-α, or GM-CSF. M2 or alternatively activated macrophages are stimulated by IL-4, IL-10, or IL-13, immune complexes, or glucocorticoids [53]. The classically activated macrophages are pro-inflammatory, inducing and effecting a Th1 polarized response, killing intracellular organisms and tumors, and producing IL-12, IL-6, and TNF-α. Alternatively activated macrophages are more effective at scavenging, tissue repair, and remodeling and stimulating tumor growth. These cells produce IL-10, IL-1, but little IL-12 or TNF-α [54]. CD163 and Stabilin-1 are upregulated by alternative M2 activation, but do not distinguish between classical and alternative pathways [55, 56]. Macrophage heterogeneity and diversity is more complex, however, and extends beyond this simple categorization [11, 57]. In addition, there is evidence of trans-differentiation between the monocyte–dendritic cell and monocyte-macrophage pathways that can affect the functional and morphologic outcome [58]. The dendritic cells also have Toll-like receptors and receptors for cytokines, chemokines, and danger signals that can respond to macrophage activation. Den-

dritic cells interact with NK-cells and T-cells to regulate the outcome of the immune reaction [59].

Macrophage activation, therefore, sets off a train of inflammatory responses and needs tight autoregulation to avoid excessive systemic effect. All of the various hemophagocytic or macrophage activation syndromes appear to be due to ineffective or defective ability of CD8+ T-regulatory cells to contain the immune responses, leading to persistently high cytokine levels. The clinical picture will vary; some forms of persistent macrophage activation are transient and mild but there is a spectrum of persistent macrophage activation that, at its most severe, is irreversible and lethal [60].

The clinical features of the primary genetic hemophagocytic syndromes (HLH1–5) and those of secondary macrophage activation syndromes are identical, and only the clinical context and molecular testing can distinguish the two [61]. Fevers, hepatosplenomegaly, anemia, and thrombocytopenia are usual [62].

The incidence of HLH varies with the frequency of the responsible genes in various populations. In Japan, where a high incidence of EBV-related secondary HLH is noted, the annual incidence of primary and secondary HLH was estimated at 1 in 800 000 per year [63].

In response to a variety of stimuli, a systemic macrophage activation process can develop; viruses are the most common instigators, but bacterial or protozoal infections, rheumatologic disorders, cancers, lymphoproliferative disorders, multiple organ failure, and intravenous alimentation can do the same thing [64]. NK-cells and cytotoxic T-cells contain cytotoxic and cytolytic granules in vesicles that contain perforin and granzymes that kill the target cells. The activated macrophages may also be killed, or their production inhibited, when the system functions. When there is a defect in perforin itself, its transport, vesicular trafficking, export, cell docking, and granule release, then lymphocyte and macrophage activation may persist [65, 66]. Large numbers of activated macrophages accumulate, produce toxic cytokines, and demonstrate excessive hemophagocytic activity.

The "macrophage activation syndrome" generally refers to the above process, often in the face of an autoimmune disorder such as systemic juvenile rheumatoid arthritis. Virus or drugs can serve as the instigators. NK-cell function is reversibly depressed, perforin expression may be transiently low, and the condition is reversible. The acquired hemophagocytic syndromes (viral-associated and others) are examples of the macrophage activation syndrome of varying severity. By contrast, the genetic hemophagocytic lymphohistiocytoses (HLHs) or familial hemophagocytic lymphohistiocytosis (FHL) are inherent defects in the ability to limit the macrophage-related inflammatory response [67, 68]. Table 25.4 depicts the genetic defects that have been identified to date that involve the ability of NK- and cytotoxic T-cells to make or export perforin or granzyme.

The clinical diagnosis is often very difficult because both the acquired and familial syndromes can be triggered by infectious

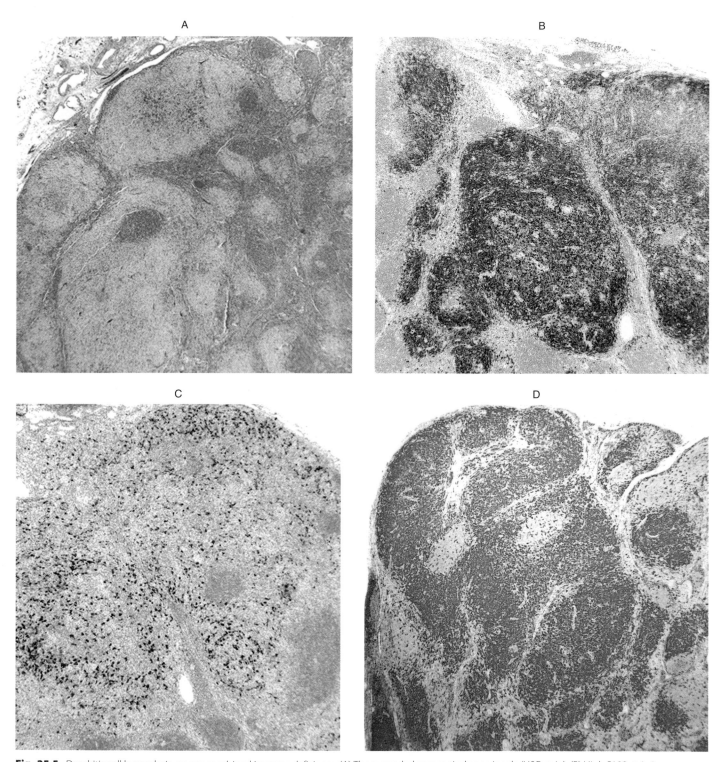

Fig. 25.5. Dendritic cell hyperplasia, severe combined immune deficiency. (A) The expanded paracortical zone is pale (H&E stain). (B) High S100 stain is characteristic of the interdigitating dendritic cell. (C) CD1a reveals an interspersed population like that of the dermatopathic pattern. (D) High fascin stain characteristic of the interdigitating dendritic cell.

organisms. The clinical manifestations of the macrophage activation syndrome often overlap with those of the infection itself, and hemophagocytosis, per se, is neither required for the diagnosis (low specificity) nor diagnostic of it (low sensitivity). Very

high levels of ferritin, over10 000 μg/L, have high sensitivity and specificity for HLH [69].

The updated diagnostic criteria for the hemophagocytic syndromes are given in Table 25.5 [70].

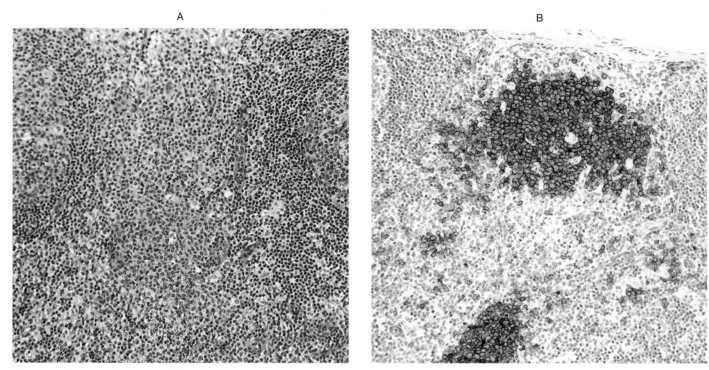

Fig. 25.6. Plasmacytoid dendritic cell hyperplasia, lymph node with myeloid infiltrate. (A) The nodular aggregate simulates a naked follicle (H&E stain). (B) CD123 highlights the nodular aggregates.

Table 25.4. Genetic defects in hemophagocytic lymphohistiocytosis.

Disease	Chromosome location	Associated gene	Gene function
FHLH-1	9q21.3–22	Not known	Not known
FHLH-2	10q21–22	PFR1	Induction of apoptosis
FHLH-3	17q25	UNC13D	Vesicle priming
FHLH-4	6q24	STX11	Vesicle transport
FHLH-5	19p	STXBP2	Vesicle transport
GS-2	15q21	RAB27A	Vesicle docking
CHS-1	1q42.1–42.2	LYST	Vesicle transport
XLP	Xq25	SH2D1A	Signal transduction and activation of lymphocytes

Abbreviations: FHLH, familial hemophagocytic lymphohistiocytosis; GS, Griscelli syndrome; CHS, Chédiak–Higashi syndrome; XLP, X-linked lymphoproliferative disorder.

Table 25.5. Diagnostic criteria for HLH.

(1) Familial disease/known genetic defect

(2) Clinical and laboratory criteria (5/8 criteria)
- Fever
- Splenomegaly
- Cytopenia ≥2 cell lines
    Hemoglobin <90 g/L (below four weeks, <120 g/L)
    Platelets <100 × 10^9/L
    Neutrophils <1 × 10^9/L
- Hypertriglyceridemia and/or hypofibrinogenemia
    Fasting triglycerides ≥3 mmol/L
    Fibrinogen <1.5 g/L
- Ferritin >500 μg/L
- sCD25 ≥2400 U/mL[a]
- Decreased or absent NK-cell activity
- Hemophagocytosis in bone marrow, CSF, or lymph nodes
- High circulating sCD163 (n = 1.8 ± 0.6 mg/L)[b]

Supportive evidence is cerebral symptoms with moderate pleocytosis and/or elevated protein, elevated transaminases, bilirubin, and LDH.
[a] For methods see Schneider et al. [71].
[b] This additional criterion was not included in the eight given by Henter et al. [70].

Histopathology

Hemophagocytic syndromes are poorly named because the sentinel descriptor, hemophagocytosis, is neither sensitive nor specific [72]. False-negative lack of sensitivity occurs because hemophagocytosis can be episodic, often absent or subtle at the onset of the clinical condition, especially on examination of the bone marrow aspirate. False positivity, the find-

ing of hemophagocytosis and, more commonly, erythrophago-cytosis in conditions other than HLH, has been described after minor transfusion reactions, surgical interventions, and immunoglobulin infusion. There is still debate as to whether reactive macrophage activation syndromes and hemophago-cytic lymphohistiocytosis are synonymous and represent an identical pathophysiology [61, 73]. The hallmark of both, how-ever, is the systemic activation of macrophages leading to excessive cytokine release with ineffective shut-down of the process. Histopathologic distinctions have not been clearly validated [74].

Special sites

Bone marrow

In the early stages, marrow aspirate may reveal only a mild increase in the number of enlarged, cytoplasmic-rich macrophages, with little hemophagocytic activity. In the original diagnostic guidelines, Henter wrote "In the bone marrow, histiocytes are initially unevenly distributed but later become more diffuse. In early stages, the bone marrow may only show slight hyperplasia without any diagnostic features. Hemophagocytic activity is rarely found in this stage" [75]. Bone marrow biopsy, stained for macrophages with CD68 (PGM-1 antibody) or CD163, will reveal an increase in macrophage size with abundant cytoplasm (rather than the oval, spindled small, and stellate forms); increased numbers of macrophages in some and hemophagocytic activity is highlighted by the CD163 stain [74] (Fig. 25.7). CD3/CD8-positive T-cells are also increased. Early disease often has generous hematopoiesis with cellular marrow indicating that the cytopenias are not due to replacement but to cytokine effect. Dyserythropoiesis and pseudo-Pelger–Huët change may be an early feature [76]. In late disease, especially following therapy, hematopoiesis may be depleted and macrophages fill the marrow in about half of the children; these macrophages are mostly xanthomatous [77].

Lymph node

Lymph node involvement is mostly sinus in distribution, although some increase in paracortical cells can occur. Sinus histiocytes are enlarged, cytoplasm-rich, and hemophagocytosis can be evident [78]. Fine needle aspiration can reveal the activated and phagocytic macrophages when bone marrow findings are equivocal. As the disease progresses, and with treatment, lymphoid depletion is progressive [77].

Spleen

Splenic enlargement is almost invariable (84–98%) [75] and constitutes one of the major diagnostic criteria. The hemophagocytic macrophages fill red pulp sinuses, and splenic fine needle aspirate has been used in diagnosis [75, 79].

Liver

Liver involvement is common [80]. Hepatomegaly with evidence of tissue damage and increased serum hepatocellular enzymes (SGOT/SGPT, biliary enzymes, GGT, and bilirubin) can be accompanied by evidence of loss of hepatocellular function, prolonged PT/PTT, hypofibrinogenemia, hypoalbuminemia, and hyperferritinemia [81]. The portal lymphohistiocytosis that mimics chronic hepatitis is more prominent in the primary HLH conditions, whereas sinusoidal Kupffer cell involvement is more prominent in reactive macrophage activation syndromes [82]. Hemophagocytosis is best appreciated in the sinusoids. The portal infiltrate is rich in lymphocytes that are CD3+/CD8+. In those children who harbor perforin mutations, the CD8 population generally lacks staining for perforin [82] (Fig. 25.8). Central venulitis with red cell extravasation is common with, the presence of large, cytoplasm-rich intravenous floating macrophages in some [80]. Biliary epithelial damage is uncommon but documented [83]. Hepatic presentation of hemophagocytic lymphohistiocytosis in the newborn can mimic neonatal hemochromatosis [84, 85].

Skin

Skin rash is generally non-specific, and the biopsy findings are non-diagnostic in HLH. The presence of perivascular hemophagocytosis is not specific to HLH [86].

Central nervous system

Central nervous system involvement is common [87], with neurologic symptoms in 37% and CSF abnormality in 52% [88]. MRI findings are described, and spinal fluid involvement is one of the diagnostic features. A cell count of 50×10^6/L with a pleocytosis that includes cytoplasm-rich activated macrophages and, on occasion, hemophagocytic cells can be found [88, 89] (Fig. 25.9). A staging system quantifies the extent of spinal, perivascular, and intraparenchymal involvement [89]. CNS involvement can precede other manifestations and be the dominant clinical feature [90, 91].

The systemic histiocytoses

These are a restricted group of histiocytic disorders that have common features: all are identified by the unique features of the specific dominant histiocyte, and each can manifest as a focal lesion, multiple lesions at different sites, or as a widespread multisystem disorder with organ involvement. Langerhans cell histiocytosis, juvenile xanthogranuloma, and, to a lesser extent, Rosai–Dorfman disease and multicentric reticulohistiocytosis share these features.

Langerhans cell histiocytosis (LCH)

Ascertainment of the incidence of LCH is best in countries that have a national registry. LCH occurs at a rate of 4–5 cases/million/year, with a 3.7 : 1.0 male–female preponderance [92] decreasing with age. About 75% of cases are solitary, usually in bone, formerly described as eosinophilic granuloma. About 25% have multiple lesions often involving more than one tissue, formerly described as Hand–Schüller–Christian disease. About 10% of patients who have multifocal disease have involvement of high-risk organs such as liver, lung, spleen, or bone marrow [93]. These cases were formerly described as disseminated or Letterer–Siwe disease. Mortality is restricted to this last, high "risk" category and still stands at about 20% and is characterized by fevers, hepatosplenomegaly, hematopoietic failure, and liver dysfunction. "CNS risk" patients have a head/neck primary site

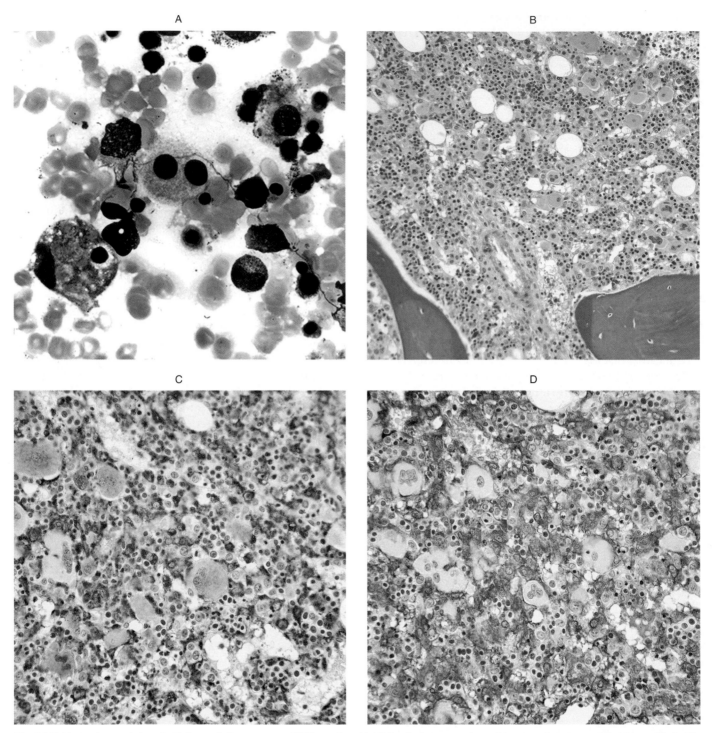

Fig. 25.7. Hemophagocytic lymphohistiocytosis, bone marrow. (A) The aspirate highlights the large, cytoplasm-rich macrophages, some of which are filled with blood cells (Wright–Giemsa stain). (B) The marrow is cellular and the histiocytic content is not obvious (H&E stain). (C) CD68, PGM-1 antibody. The high content of histiocytes is apparent. (D) CD163 stains the cytoplasm and the hemophagocytosis is more apparent.

with high likelihood of diabetes insipidus. A late neurodegenerative cerebellar syndrome in some of these children appears to be paraneoplastic and not LCH infiltration.

LCH is protean in clinical manifestation, and is defined by the presence of the LCH cell, a cell that shares the phenotype of the epidermal Langerhans cell, S100+/CD1a+/

Langerin+/Birbeck granule+, but is large and oval in shape. This represents an immature dendritic cell phenotype that can show some maturation in the lymph node, but fails to mature to a central instructive-type dendritic cell [94, 95]. Whether the LCH cell is truly neoplastic or represents a dysregulation is not universally agreed upon, though the clonal nature of most LCH

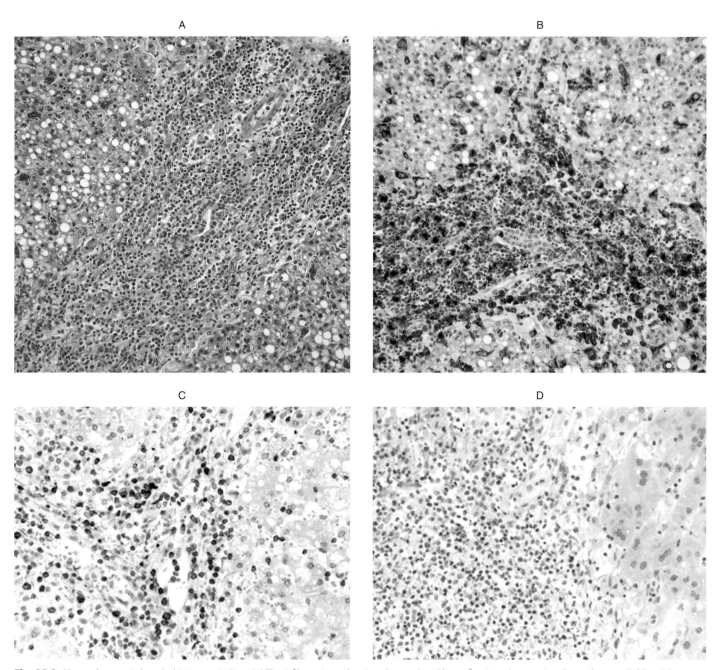

Fig. 25.8. Hemophagocytic lymphohistiocytosis, liver. (A) The infiltrate is predominantly portal, and large, floating phagocytic cells can be seen (H&E stain). (B) CD68 reveals the high macrophage content in the portal area, with a lymphocytic background. (C) Lymphocytes stain for perforin when there is no mutation. (D) In HLH-2, with a perforin mutation, the high CD3/CD8+ lymphoid content is devoid of perforin staining.

lesions, loss of heterozygosity, and telomeric changes suggest a neoplasm [96–99].

The disorder has traditionally been thought of as a childhood disease, but increasing adult involvement is being documented.

Special sites

Bone

Bone involvement is the most frequent site, presenting with pain, pathologic fractures, vertebral collapse, and local soft

tissue extension. Early and expanding lesions have more "aggressive" imaging features, with active bone destruction mimicking a high-grade malignant process [100, 101]. In this phase, diagnosis is relatively easy because biopsy or needle aspirate will reveal sheets of LCH cells that can be recognized by their cytologic features and confirmed by immunohistochemistry on tissue, or immunocytology on the aspirated cells. Bone and its adjacent soft tissue lesions are commonly rich in osteoclast-like giant cells, but the LCH cells have distinctive cytologic features, with complex angular nuclear folds

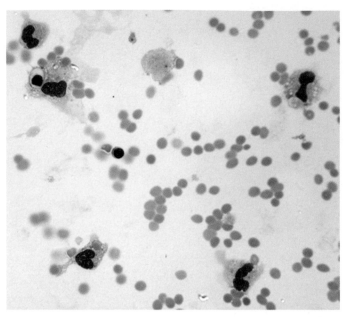

Fig. 25.9. Hemophagocytic lymphohistiocytosis, spinal fluid. The large, cytoplasm-rich activated macrophages may have some hemophagocytosis (Wright–Giemsa stain).

and grooves, and the phenotype is S100+/CD1a+/Langerin+ (Fig. 25.10). The presence of Birbeck granules is not required for diagnosis once the other criteria have been satisfied. Plasma cells are unusual in LCH lesions, though they may participate in the lymphoid reaction around LCH nodules, and any prominence of plasma cells in a bone lesion should move the diagnostic consideration to osteomyelitis.

Late lesions may be more difficult to diagnose with certainty. Because the LCH component regresses, leaving behind a fibrosing and scarring process that eventually remodels, there may come a time when the LCH cells are sparse or have even totally regressed. Imaging at this time reveals more sclerotic and low-grade changes, and the differential diagnosis shifts to the fibrosing lesions of bone [101]. Extensive search may be required to find any residual clusters of LCH cells identified by their classical phenotype. A bone aspirate is less likely to yield a firm diagnosis in this setting.

Skin

Skin involvement in LCH can take a wide variety of clinical forms but the principle is similar; the diagnosis is made by identification of LCH cells in the appropriate context. Congenital lesions may be large, papular, or ulcerating. Some papular dermal-only LCH infiltrates may regress spontaneously (Hashimoto–Pritzker disease), but the clinical course cannot be predicted from the histopathology, and no clear prognostic features are validated [102–104]. Skin involvement commonly involved flexures, the scalp, and groin, with a petechial seborrheic rash. There is a wide clinical differential diagnosis, but the histopathologic diagnosis rests on identifying clusters of oval LCH cells in the papillary and/or deeper dermis that have the classical S100+/CD1a+/Langerin+ phenotype

(Fig. 25.11). Eosinophils and giant cells are not commonly seen in any abundance. The major differential difficulty is encountered with some of the chronic dermatitides, mostly notably chronic scabies, in which large numbers of dermal dendritic cells accumulate [105–107]. While these dermal dendritic cells are CD1a+, they are not oval like the LCH cell, they are dispersed in a perivascular fashion, and lack Langerin. A less common mimicker is Langerhans cell sarcoma (generally in adults) that has the same phenotypic features but is cytologically high grade [108]. Rare myelodysplastic or myelomonocytic leukemic infiltrates can express CD1a in their dermal infiltrates even when the marrow cells do not [109].

Lymph nodes

Lymph node involvement is commonly the only site of LCH, but can also be seen as part of more generalized multivisceral disease and sometimes in the immediate vicinity of a bone lesion [110, 111]. The few examples of ostensible LCH that occur in lymph nodes occupied by other lesions such as lymphomas are probably not true LCH, because no other disease is identified in these patients, and the phenomenon is best regarded as a local benign site of involvement of Langerhans cell hyperplasia [47].

The pattern of nodal involvement is strictly or predominantly sinus in pattern, though this may not be obvious when paracortical infiltration obscures the landmarks. The sinus pattern is important, however, in differentiating LCH from its prime mimicker, dermatopathic lymphadenopathy, and the dendritic cell hyperplasias of immune deficiency [111, 112]. LCH in the lymph node demonstrates high S100 expression uniformly, but the CD1a and Langerin positivity may be confined to the intrasinus component almost exclusively, with the paracortical LCH cells being relatively unstained [94] (Fig. 25.12). There is some suggestion that LCH cells in the lymph node retain a limited capacity to differentiate, further exemplified by their loss of Langerin and CD1a in the paracortex, in conjunction with upregulation of HLA-DR from the cytoplasm to the surface, and increase in fascin expression [95]. Maturation is limited though, and no CD83 or DC-LAMP is demonstrable. As a word of caution, Langerin expression is noted on a population of normal medullary sinus cells in the normal lymph node [113] (Fig. 25.12E). Dermatopathic lymphadenopathy can have high CD1a/Langerin content but lacks the filled sinuses, and the fascin content is vastly increased [18]. This differential diagnosis needs to be taken into account when diagnosis is made by fine needle cytology [114].

Liver

Langerhans cell involvement of the liver is of two types. During an active phase of bone or skin disease, there may be hepatomegaly and hypoalbuminemia. This is regarded as a cytokine effect that does not, by itself, indicate LCH infiltration, and is evanescent. Because of the unusually strong affiliation of LCH cells for the bile ducts, both intra- and extrahepatic, the gamma glutamyl transpeptidase (GGT) is a better indicator of LCH

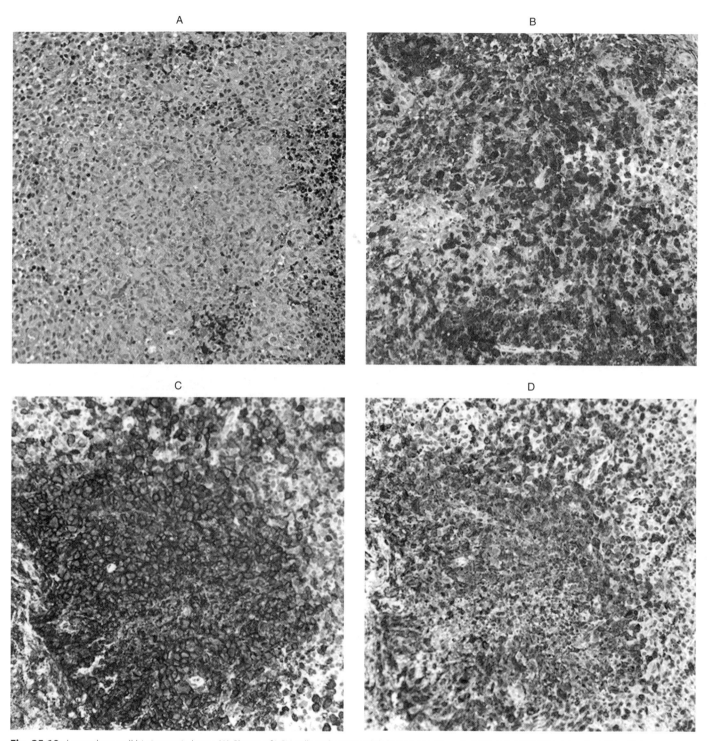

Fig. 25.10. Langerhans cell histiocytosis, bone. (A) Sheets of LCH cells with eosinophils but no plasma cells (H&E stain). (B) S100 stains the LCH cells in a nuclear/cytoplasmic fashion. (C) CD1a is strongly represented on the cell membrane. (D) Langerin stains the LCH cells.

infiltration and damage [82] (Fig. 25.13). LCH can involve the major bile ducts, and the LCH cells migrate more peripherally within the basement membrane of the bile ducts, leading to a clinical and pathologic picture of sclerosing cholangitis that is only rarely reversible [115, 116]. LCH infiltration can be subtle within the bile ducts on biopsy, and the LCH cells are demonstrable with S100, CD1a, and Langerin [82].

Often the features of biliary obstruction overwhelm the portal areas, and LCH infiltration may be hard to demonstrate. Also, as the disease regresses, leaving behind a sclerosing cholangitis that leads to biliary cirrhosis, the inciting LCH process may no longer be demonstrable. Occasionally, though, LCH in the active phase will produce larger peribiliary aggregates, or even visible parenchymal nodules [117].

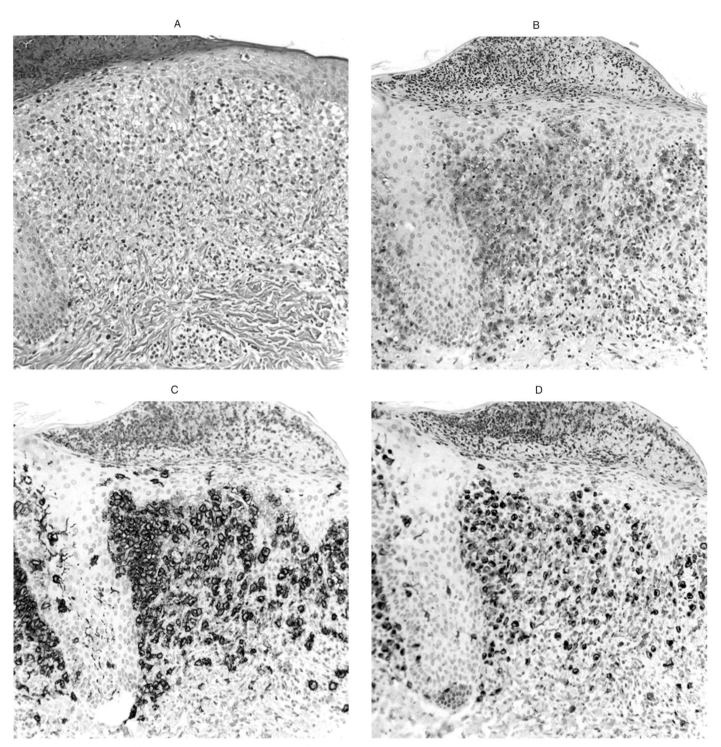

Fig. 25.11. Langerhans cell histiocytosis, skin. (A) LCH cells with interspersed eosinophils fill the papillary dermis (H&E stain). (B) LCH cells stain for S100. (C) The same population and endogenous branched Langerhans cells stain for surface CD1a. (D) Langerin stains much of the same population.

Bone marrow

Verification of bone marrow involvement is important because it is one of the major high-risk sites in small children. The key confounder to the diagnosis is the sporadic distribution of the clusters of CD1a cells, and the high content of other macrophages in the marrow. Under normal circumstances, there are very few, if any, CD1a+ cells in the bone marrow, and these are small and single cells only [118]. S100 is not acceptable as a marker since there is a population of S100+ marrow cells, fat cells, and some S100+ macrophages. Bone marrow involvement can be documented by finding clusters or aggregates of CD1a+ cells on aspirate or biopsy, and

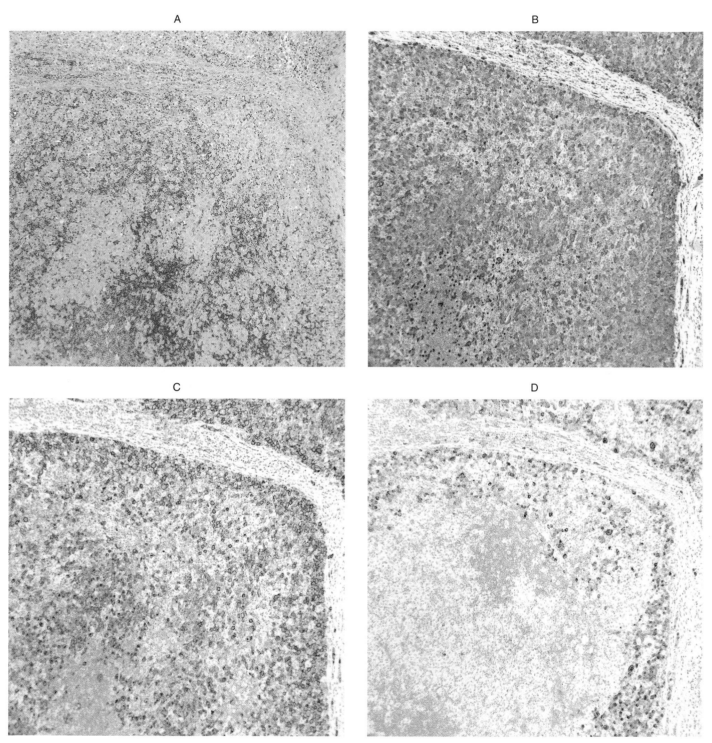

Fig. 25.12. Langerhans cell histiocytosis, lymph node. (A) The node appears to be diffusely replaced by pale histiocytes. (B) S100 stains all the sinus and paracortical histiocytes. (C) CD1a stain, by contrast, is most strongly represented in the sinus component. (D) Langerin stains the sinus population with little in the paracortex. (E) Medullary sinuses of the node, and in normal nodes, stain for Langerin, a potential distracter. (F) High-power view of the complex nuclear folds characteristic of the LCH cells (H&E stain).

these can be distinguished from the macrophages by use of CD163 or CD68 (PGM-1 antibody) [94] (Fig. 25.14). Like HLH, early marrow involvement by LCH is usually set in a cellular hematopoietic marrow, and cytopenias are attributed to cytokine effects, not to marrow replacement. The macrophage content can increase substantially with treatment, and sheets of xanthomatous and hemosiderin-filled macrophages can be confounding.

E

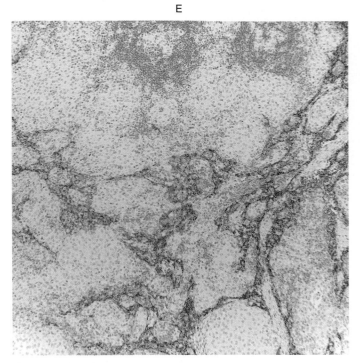

F

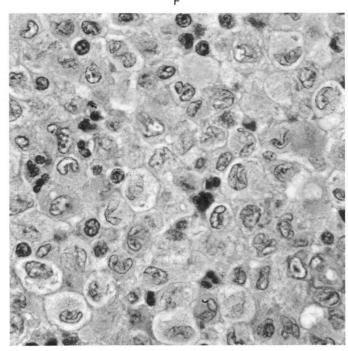

Fig. 25.12. (cont.)

Lung

Lung involvement in children appears to be a different process from that in adults. Solitary lung involvement is very rare in childhood, whereas it is a more common event in adult smokers [119]. Most children who have lung involvement with LCH have other visceral sites [120]. Clonality studies have shown that lung lesions in children, like those at other sites, are generally clonal, while the lesions from adult smokers are non-clonal in 70% of those examined [48]. Diagnosis rests on identifying the oval CD1a- and Langerin-positive cells on biopsy, or on bronchoalveolar lavage, in which more than 5% of CD1a+ large cells is suggestive of lung involvement in a child with LCH elsewhere [121]. The high content of CD1a+ cells in lavage from adult interstitial lung diseases is interpreted as Langerhans cell hyperplasia, not LCH, though the addition of Langerin to the diagnostic panel can increase the diagnostic sensitivity [122, 123]. As in other sites, progressive pulmonary fibrosis with loss of the diagnostic LCH cells can handicap late diagnosis.

Central nervous system

Three forms of involvement have been documented [124, 125]. Most common is LCH that involves the meninges or choroid plexus with a space-occupying process. Diagnosis rests on identifying the CD1a+/Langerin+ LCH cell, but in the regressing phase, these may be rare, and reactive xanthomatous macrophages predominate, mimicking juvenile xanthogranuloma [124]. LCH may occur as a leptomeningeal-based lesion with contiguous brain parenchymal involvement, and, much more rarely, without the meningeal connection. Neurodegenerative lesions, most commonly bilateral cerebellar or brainstem lesions in patients who have active LCH elsewhere in the body, are more akin to a paraneoplastic inflammatory process, and LCH cells are not demonstrable within the lesions [125]. The imaging findings in the cerebellum and basal ganglia are progressive but do not correlate well with neurologic deterioration [126].

Spleen

Splenomegaly may be a manifestation of the macrophage activation that commonly accompanies multifocal and disseminated LCH (Fig. 25.15). True infiltration is either subtle and diffuse, or nodular and tumoral. Since needle aspiration is not commonly used, splenic involvement is documented only at splenectomy or autopsy.

Gastrointestinal tract

It is rare for LCH to present in the intestine or for it to be the only site, but gastrointestinal infiltration is usually part of a multivisceral process [127, 128]. Diarrhea and protein-losing enteropathy can signal intestinal infiltration that is documented by finding infiltration of the mucosal lamina propria with LCH cells [129].

Thymus and thyroid

Both may be the site of solitary LCH involvement. Hyperplastic Langerhans cell foci have been described in patients with myasthenia gravis and other autoimmune conditions. Thymic

A

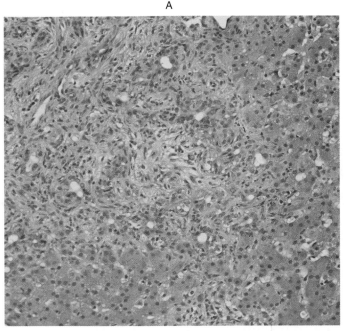

B

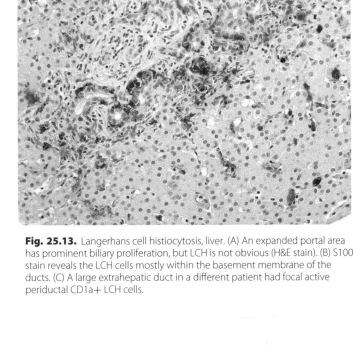

Fig. 25.13. Langerhans cell histiocytosis, liver. (A) An expanded portal area has prominent biliary proliferation, but LCH is not obvious (H&E stain). (B) S100 stain reveals the LCH cells mostly within the basement membrane of the ducts. (C) A large extrahepatic duct in a different patient had focal active periductal CD1a+ LCH cells.

C

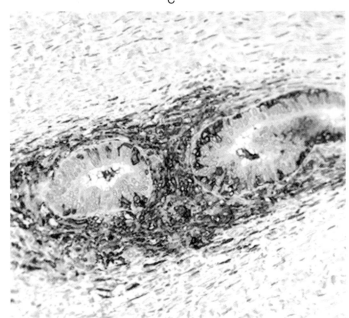

infiltration usually leads to cystic transformation of the gland [130]. Thyroid involvement spills into surrounding soft tissue, obscuring its origin [131].

LCH and macrophage activation

LCH, most notably active multifocal disease or disseminated visceral involvement, can be accompanied by a cytokine-driven state of macrophage activation with variable clinical expression. In mild instances, the component of activated macrophages in marrow may act as a confounder to diagnosis. In severe instances of hemophagocytic syndrome, the condition can be life threatening [62]. The diagnosis of LCH in organs such

as spleen and lymph node can be more difficult due to the macrophage presence (Fig. 25.15), and severe macrophage activation syndrome accounts for some of the mortality in LCH.

Langerhans cell-related histiocytoses that do not meet the diagnostic criteria for LCH

Two prototypic groups have been identified. The first resembles LCH on morphological grounds, but the principal cells are CD1a negative and Langerin negative. For lack of a better term, these have been described as "dendritic cell histiocytosis,

A

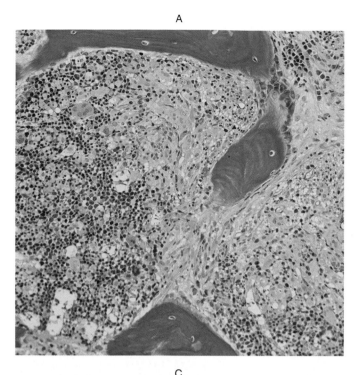

B

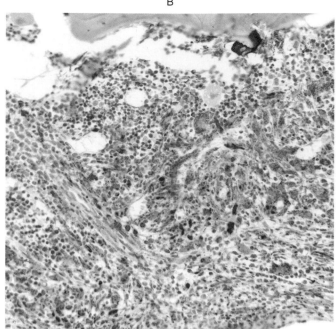

C

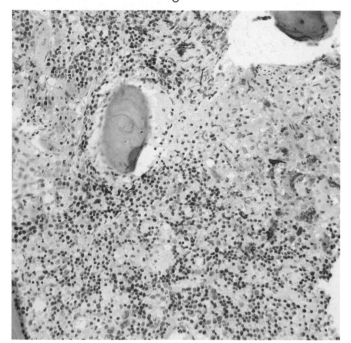

Fig. 25.14. Langerhans cell histiocytosis, bone marrow. (A) A pale area of hematopoietic replacement in a child with systemic LCH (H&E stain). (B) CD68 (PGM-1) reveals that most of the pale cells react. (C) CD1a, on the other hand, reveals only a minority of cells, a common finding.

NOS" (Fig. 25.16). The clinical behavior and response to therapy is similar to LCH, and one was a late local recurrence following classical LCH. A higher incidence of intradural lesions (both cranial and spinal) has been noted, and local soft tissue recurrence is also higher than would be expected for usual LCH [132].

The second, more common in adults, is the indeterminate cell histiocytosis defined as being CD1a positive but without Birbeck granules on electron microscopy. The lack of Langerin staining can now serve as a surrogate (Fig. 25.17). The clinical behavior in childhood, and response to therapy has generally been that of similarly staged LCH [133].

The juvenile xanthogranuloma (JXG) family of disorders

In many ways, the JXG family is very similar to LCH, in that there are solitary, multifocal, and systemic variants confounded by a wide variety of clinical terms. What they all have in common is a similar cell type that shares morphologic and

A

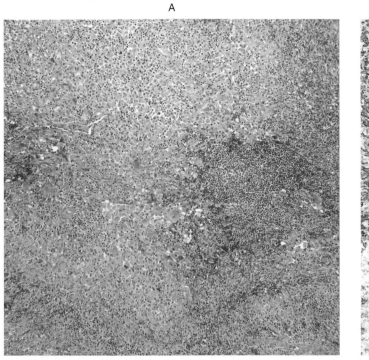

B

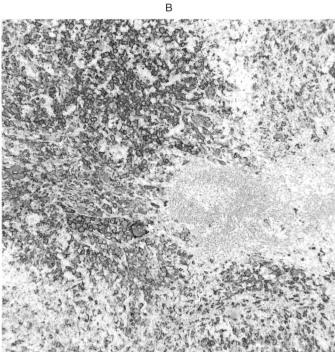

C

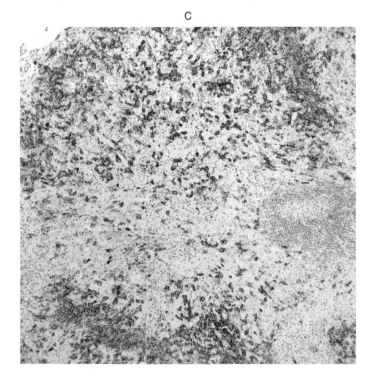

Fig. 25.15. Langerhans cell histiocytosis with macrophage activation syndrome, spleen. (A) The red pulp is filled with pale histiocytes (H&E stain). (B) CD163 stains vast numbers of cells in this child who has symptomatic macrophage activation syndrome. (C) CD1a reveals the LCH infiltrate almost obscured by the macrophages.

phenotypic features across the spectrum [134]. JXG lesions are rarely found in lymph nodes, even in systemic disease.

Like LCH, multiple JXGs, and especially the disseminated and systemic variants, can be associated with a macrophage activation syndrome that can be severe or even life threatening. Table 25.6 lists the clinical variants of the JXG family.

The incidence of juvenile xanthogranulomas has not been ascertained; solitary skin lesions are relatively common in diagnostic practice. Deep and systemic lesions however, are rare: 3.9% of all JXGs in one registry report, less common than LCH. The registry data indicate a M : F ratio of 1.4 : 1, and over 70% are diagnosed within the first year [135].

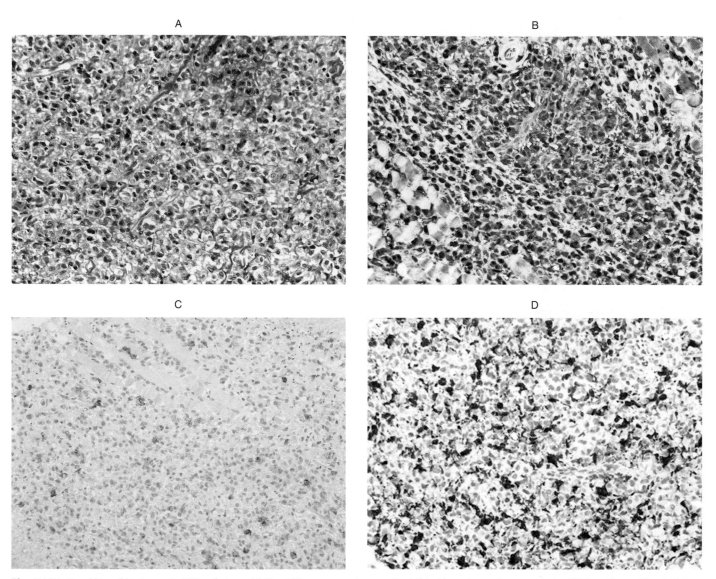

Fig. 25.16. Dendritic cell histiocytosis, NOS, soft tissue. (A) The H&E appearance is not unlike LCH without the nuclear complexity. (B) The cells are diffusely S100 positive. (C) CD1a (and Langerin) was represented by few cells only. (D) Factor 13a was thought to stain the interspersed dermal-interstitial cells but not the lesional cells.

Table 25.6. Juvenile xanthogranuloma family of disorders.

Clinical nomenclature	Mean age
Solitary dermal JXG	0–18 years, median 2
Multiple dermal JXGs	<6 months
Systemic JXG	<3 months
Deep (and giant) JXG	0–18 years
Xanthoma disseminatum	10–30 years
Generalized non-lipidemic eruptive xanthoma	Infants–young adults
Benign cephalic histiocytosis	10–30 years
Progressive nodular histiocytosis	Young adults
Erdheim–Chester disease	7–84 years, mean 53

The common histopathologic features include a dominant histiocyte that is generally small and bland, with an oval or folded nucleus that is much less complex than that of the LCH cell. Early lesions have pale-pink cytoplasm on H&E, but accumulate intracytoplasmic lipid in vacuoles until the lesions are largely xanthomatous. A short spindle cell component is not unusual, and rare lesions are totally spindle in shape. A characteristic but not essential accompaniment is the Touton-type giant cell that most classically has a wreath of nuclei that surround an inner eosinophilic core, while the peripheral cytoplasm is clear or frankly xanthomatous. An inflammatory component of interspersed T-cells and eosinophils can vary from sparse to very prominent. The lesional cells may vary in their

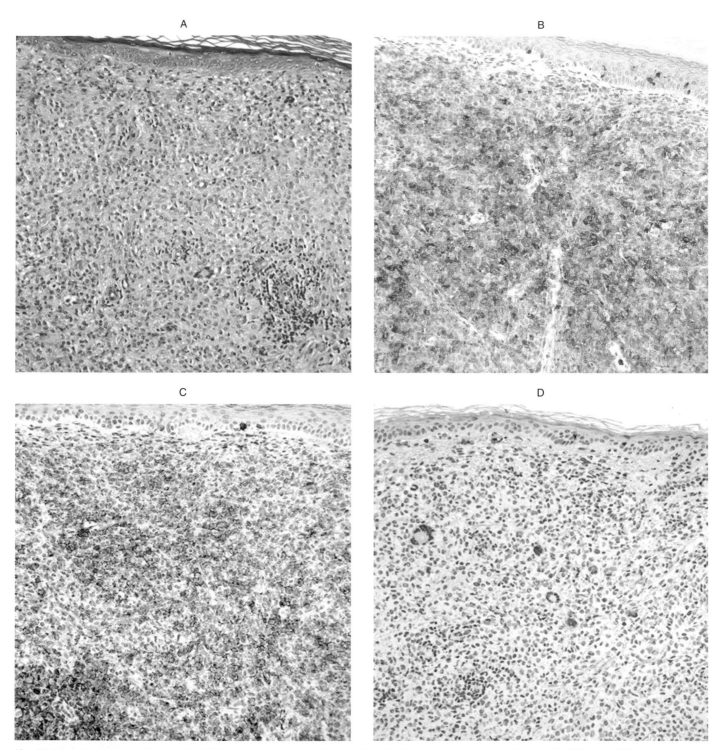

Fig. 25.17. Indeterminate cell lesion, skin. (A) The appearance is not unlike the JXG, with Touton-type giant cells in this example (H&E stain). (B) S100 staining was diffusely positive. (C) CD1a stains the surface of lesional cells. (D) Langerin, however, is negative.

phenotype depending on the age of the lesion; more recent cells at the periphery often mark more consistently. The cells stain as monocyte/macrophages for CD14 in a strong membrane fashion; CD68 (both KP-1 and PGM-1) has a coarse granular cytoplasmic pattern, and CD163 is generally strongly expressed on the cell surface. More specifically for this group of lesions and in addition to the above, the cells stain for Factor 13a, and have high fascin expression. CD1a and Langerin expression is absent, though variable levels of cytoplasmic S100 can be demonstrated in about 30% (Fig. 25.18).

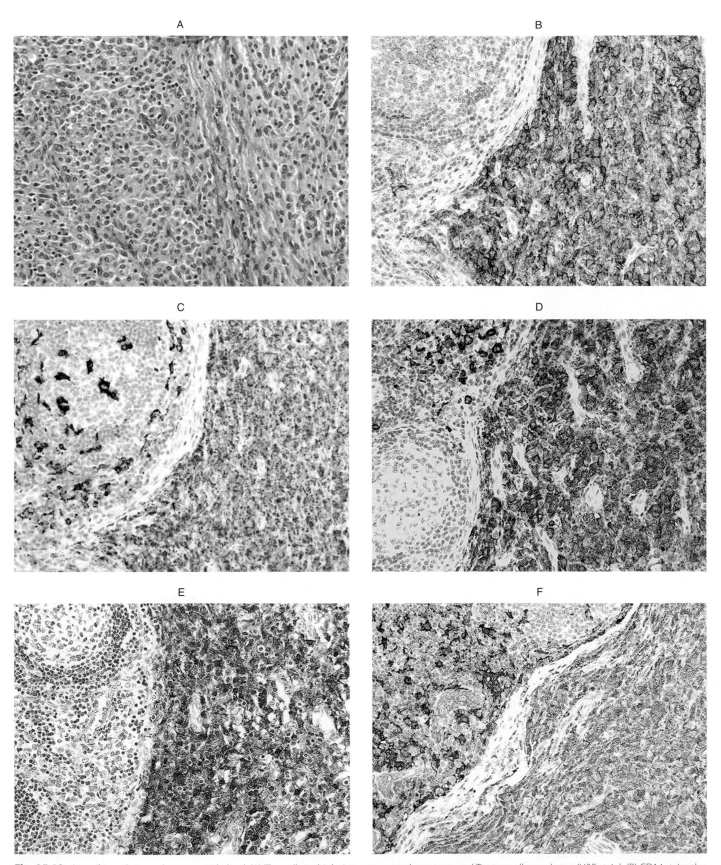

A

B

C

D

E

F

Fig. 25.18. Juvenile xanthogranuloma, parotid gland. (A) The cells in this lesion are not xanthomatous, and Touton cells are absent (H&E stain). (B) CD14 stains the surface. (C) CD68 has a coarse, granular appearance. (D) CD163 stains the cell surface. (E) Factor 13a is cytoplasmic in distribution. (F) Fascin stains the cytoplasm.

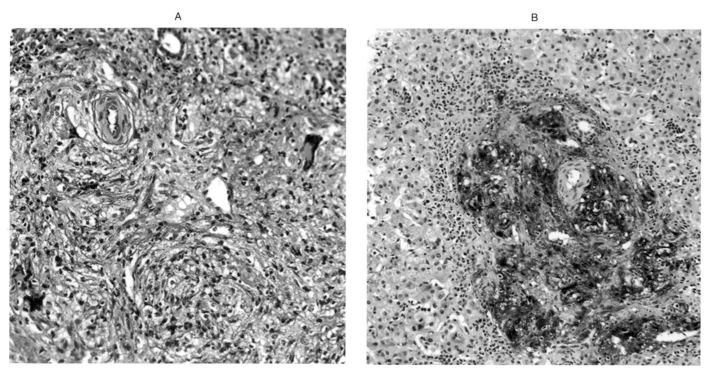

Fig. 25.19. Juvenile xanthogranuloma, liver. (A) The portal area is filled with JXG including Touton cells (H&E stain). (B) Factor 13a stains the JXG cells but not sinusoidal cells.

Skin and systemic involvement

Nodules or papules of JXG can be present at birth or develop later, generally regressing slowly over years. Multiple dermal xanthogranulomas may occur; some of these patients have systemic involvement that can include liver, lung, central nervous system, bone marrow, and spleen [135–139]. These too can regress, but in some instances fatality has been described with hepatic necrosis or CNS damage. Ocular involvement, particularly of the iris, can lead to glaucoma [140]. When there are myriads of dermal lesions in association with mucosal lesions, especially the upper aerodigestive tract, the condition is referred to as xanthoma disseminatum [141]. A presumed adult disseminated form is Erdheim–Chester disease (ECD) [142, 143]. The most distinctive distribution of lesions includes bilateral, symmetric long bone involvement, lung, retroperitoneal, and cardiac lesions. Posterior pituitary involvement can lead to diabetes insipidus, further mimicking LCH. The ECD phenotype is consistently identical to that of the JXG: CD14/CD68/CD163/Factor 13a/fascin positive, but CD1a and S100 negative.

In addition to the dermal and systemic forms, there are a number of tumoral-type lesions that share the JXG morphology phenotype. These include deep soft tissue JXG, which can occur at any site including the retroperitoneum, a preferred site, and intracranial, usually dural-based [144]. Small lesions on the face and head have been termed "benign cephalic histiocytosis", more commonly seen in younger children [145], while "progressive nodular histiocytosis" in older patients may be larger disfiguring nodules on the face and head [146, 147].

Some instances of "generalized eruptive histiocytoma of childhood" are also JXGs, though hyperlipidemic states must always be excluded [148].

Special sites
Liver

JXG involving liver is generally a portal-based infiltrate that can spill over into the adjacent lobule. The lesions are morphologically and phenotypically characteristic, though Touton cells can be sparse (Fig. 25.19). Unlike LCH, JXG has no specific tropism for the bile ducts, and progressive biliary damage is not described [80, 82]. Liver lesions, if few, can resolve. There is a rare description of JXG that involves the liver, leading to massive hepatic necrosis, presumably on the basis of cytokine-mediated cytotoxicity [149].

Central nervous system

JXG-type lesions can occur in the CNS as solitary masses or as part of systemic JXG, including xanthoma disseminatum [135, 138, 150]. Morphology and phenotype are classical of JXG; the critical determinant of prognosis appears to be the site of the lesions [151]. Healing LCH lesions in the CNS are often highly xanthomatous and can confound.

ALK-positive histiocytosis

An unusual systemic histiocytosis of infancy had features of the juvenile xanthogranuloma and was ALK+ in a membranous and cytoplasmic pattern, one of which revealed TPM3–ALK fusion. Two of the three cases resolved slowly with treatment [152].

Rosai–Dorfman disease

Originally described as sinus histiocytosis with massive lymphadenopathy after its most common clinicopathologic manifestation, Rosai-Dorfman disease (RDD) may have local, multifocal, and even systemic forms [41, 153]. The classical presentation is that of very large, painless cervical lymph nodes in a child with fever, raised sedimentation rate, hyperglobulinemia, and, uncommonly, autoimmune hemolytic anemia. Other local sites of disease can occur in the presence or absence of nodal involvement, most commonly skin or subcutaneous tissues, the orbit, bone, leptomeninges, and virtually any other site or organ [154]. Extranodal disease most commonly presents as a mass lesion without systemic effects, and instances of multifocal disease, some with organ involvement, are described, mostly in the head and neck, but liver, kidney, and respiratory tract involvement occurs [41]. Familial aggregation is rare.

Diagnosis is made by recognizing the distinctive Rosai-Dorfman cell, a very large macrophage with abundant, clear (or foamy) eosinophilic cytoplasm, and a large vesicular nucleus and prominent nucleolus. The large nucleus is distinctive, being larger than those of most other monocyte/macrophages. Within lymph nodes, the presence of emperipolesis, intact blood cells, mostly lymphocytes, monocytes, and eosinophils, in the RDD cell cytoplasm is the hallmark, but at extranodal sites emperipolesis may be sparse. Plasma cells are commonly abundant around local venules. The phenotype of the RDD cell is consistently positive for S100, CD68, and fascin, and variably for CD14 and CD163 (Fig. 25.20). CD1a is absent.

Lymph nodes

The sinus pattern is commonly overwhelming, so that it may not be clearly evident when the disease is long standing. Capsular thickening is usual, and nodal architecture with some preservation of follicles is seen. The classical RDD cells with large, pale nuclei, abundant cytoplasm, and emperipolesis are the hallmark. Necrosis and clusters of neutrophils occur. The distinction between a reactive sinus histiocytosis in a draining node, and Rosai–Dorfman disease, should not be difficult. Rosai–Dorfman foci are described in other processes such as lymph nodes with autoimmune lymphoproliferative syndrome (ALPS) [155], and LCH [156].

Skin and soft tissues, bone

The diagnosis is sometimes difficult because the lymph node context is lost, but the RDD cells in other sites have the same large nuclei, abundant pale cytoplasm, and consistent phenotype. Emperipolesis can be relatively sparse at extranodal sites, and stromal fibrosis (with or without plasma cells) can be more extensive. Like the LCH and JXG cell, RDD cells can involute and eventually disappear, and making a diagnosis when a lesion is involuting can be challenging. There is a wide differential in soft tissues, but, in bone, the presence of histiocytes and plasma cells mimics osteomyelitis.

Multicentric reticulohistiocytosis (MR)

Much like the other histiocytoses, JXG, LCH, and Rosai–Dorfman disease, multicentric reticulohistiocytosis has examples that are local (reticulohistiocytoma), multifocal, or clinically more widespread – all unified by the identification of a common cell type [157]. The purely dermal form can be seen in newborns; there is a dermal form in adult males, and the systemic form with predilection for joints is seen mostly in older woman.

The dermal nodule (solitary epithelioid histiocytoma) is benign and can regress, and does not recur after excision. All body sites, central, peripheral, and head and neck, are represented. The diagnosis rests largely on the involved cell: a large histiocyte with one to three oval, grooved nuclei and abundant, eosinophilic ("epithelioid") glassy cytoplasm without significant emperipolesis. The H&E appearance of the cell is the major distinction from the Rosai–Dorfman cell, which has more abundant, clear cytoplasm and a large, pale nucleus unlike the MR cell. PAS stain is lightly positive even after diastase digestion. The cells stain for CD68, CD163, and lysozyme, negative or lightly and variably for F13a and S100, and the major differential diagnosis is the Rosai–Dorfman cell [158], though the phenotype is indistinguishable from the JXG cell (Fig. 25.21).

The systemic condition is characterized by an arthropathy with infiltration by the MR cells. In more than half of the patients, there is an underlying malignancy, autoimmune disorder, or hyperlipidemia [159, 160].

Post-leukemic histiocytic disorders

There is an increasing awareness of histiocytic lesions that occur after acute lymphoblastic leukemia in childhood and adults. In the compiled examples and those seen by the author, T-cell leukemias are generally followed by LCH-like lesions, and B-cell lymphoblastic leukemias by JXG-type lesions. The lesions are generally more pleomorphic and cytologically more "atypical" than their usual LCH or JXG counterparts, and some have been called "histiocytic sarcomas" on the basis of their high-grade cytologic features (Fig. 25.22). The lesions display more aggressive biologic features with recurrence and progression. Most interestingly, whenever it has been sought, the molecular genetic signature of the original leukemia has been present in the histiocytic lesion. By virtue of their more aggressive behavior, this group deserves special recognition [2, 161–165].

Other histiocytic neoplasms

Langerhans cell sarcoma

Langerhans cell sarcoma is more commonly seen in adults; only rare examples in childhood exist [108, 166]. The

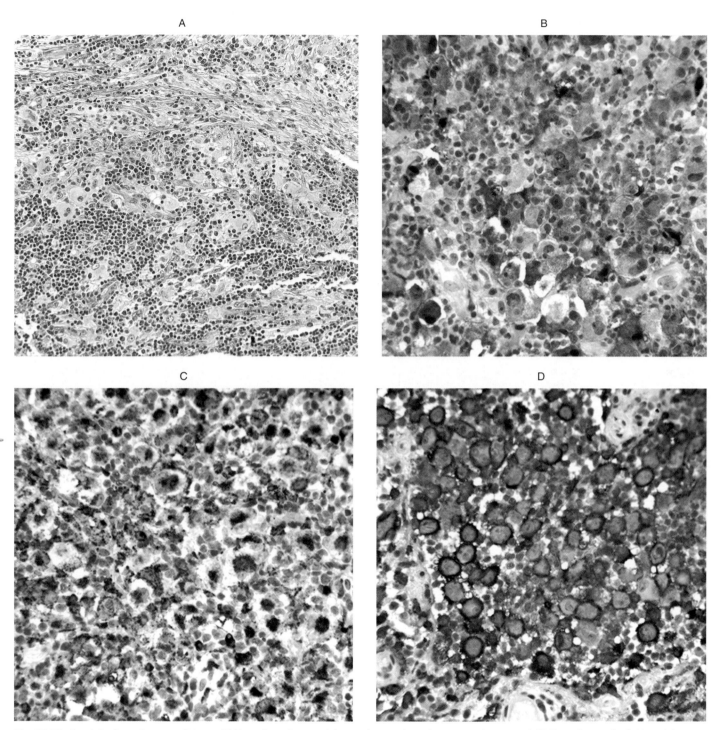

Fig. 25.20. Rosai–Dorfman disease, soft tissue. (A) The cells are large and the very large, pale nucleus is typical (H&E stain). (B) The cells stain for S100, and the cytoplasmic blush makes emperipolesis more obvious. (C) CD68 has a granular intracytoplasmic and paranuclear pattern. (D) CD163 is generally strongly represented.

condition develops *de novo*, and not as a progression from prior LCH [108, 166]. Most present as a soft tissue mass or, less commonly, lymph node, and progression to lung, liver, spleen, and bone marrow occurs.

The histopathology may not be distinctive, generally having oval to poorly spindled cells, with high-grade cytologic anaplasia that includes atypical mitoses, and while the complex nuclear grooves may be reminiscent of those of the LCH, there are few morphologic clues. The diagnosis is made by demonstrating the Langerhans cell phenotype: S100+, though more variable than in LCH, CD1a+, Langerin+, and Birbeck granules can be found on extensive ultrastructural search, but are

Table 25.7. Immunohistochemical features of the histiocytic/dendritic sarcomas.

	LCA	CD14	CD68	CD163	Lysozyme	S100	CD1a	Langerin	Fascin	CD21	CD35	Clusterin	Factor XIIIa
HS[a]	+	++	++	++	++	+/−	−	−	+/−	−	−	N/D	−
LCS	−	−	+/−	−	−	+	++	+	−	−	−	−	−
IDC	−	−	+/−	−	−	++	−	−	++	−	−	+/−	−
FCS	−	−	+/−	−	−	+/−	−	−	+/−	++	++	++	−
JXGS	−	++	++	++	−	−	−	−	+	−	−	N/D	+

[a] Histiocytic sarcomas can be designated as macrophage-type or dendritic cell type, largely on their S100/fascin content.
Abbreviations: HS, histiocytic sarcoma; LCS, Langerhans cell sarcoma; IDC, interdigitating cell sarcoma; FCS, follicular cell sarcoma; JXGS, histiocytic sarcoma, juvenile xanthogranuloma phenotype; N/D, not done.

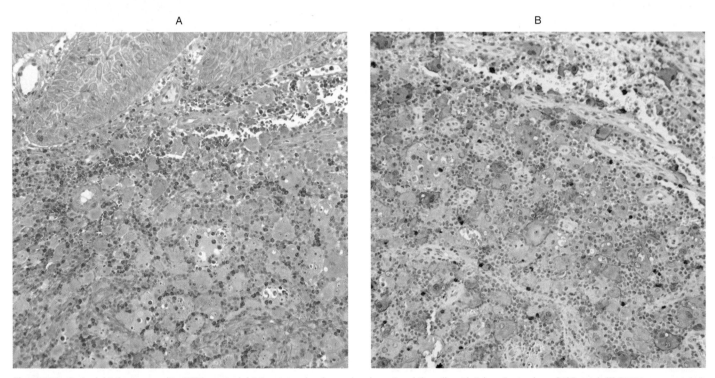

Fig. 25.21. Reticulohistiocytoma, skin. (A) The reticulohistiocytoma has large, deeply eosinophilic cells with "glassy" cytoplasm (H&E stain). (B) S100 immunostain is very sparse, unlike Rosai–Dorfman disease.

not required for diagnosis if the phenotypic criteria are met (Fig. 25.23). CD21 and CD35, the dendritic follicular cell markers, are negative, excluding the major differential consideration. The immunohistochemical features of the histiocytic/dendritic sarcomas are summarized in Table 25.7.

Interdigitating dendritic cell sarcoma

Like the Langerhans cell sarcoma, these lesions can occur in children and present as nodal or extranodal soft-tissue masses in the nasopharynx, intestine, retroperitoneum, or mesentery [108, 167]. The lesions have few distinguishing features to their short, spindle-cell appearance, with fascicles or whorls of cells that can indicate their affiliation if the paracortex of a lymph node is selectively involved.

Occasionally there is also a component of rounded, more eosinophilic cells, and even epithelioid features. The nucleolus can be prominent. Ultrastructure will demonstrate the complex cytoplasmic interdigitations, rare tight junctions without true desmosomes, and no Birbeck granules. The phenotype is generally that of an interdigitating dendritic cell, with high expression of S100, high fascin levels, and surface staining for HLA-DR. In common with other dendritic cells, there is paranuclear CD68 but no staining for CD163, CD1a, CD21, or CD35 (Fig. 25.24). Because of the S100 positivity, malignant melanoma can enter the differential consideration, but HMB45 is absent.

Biologic behavior and the degree of cytologic anaplasia can vary widely from minimal to high grade, and low clinical stage is associated with better outcome.

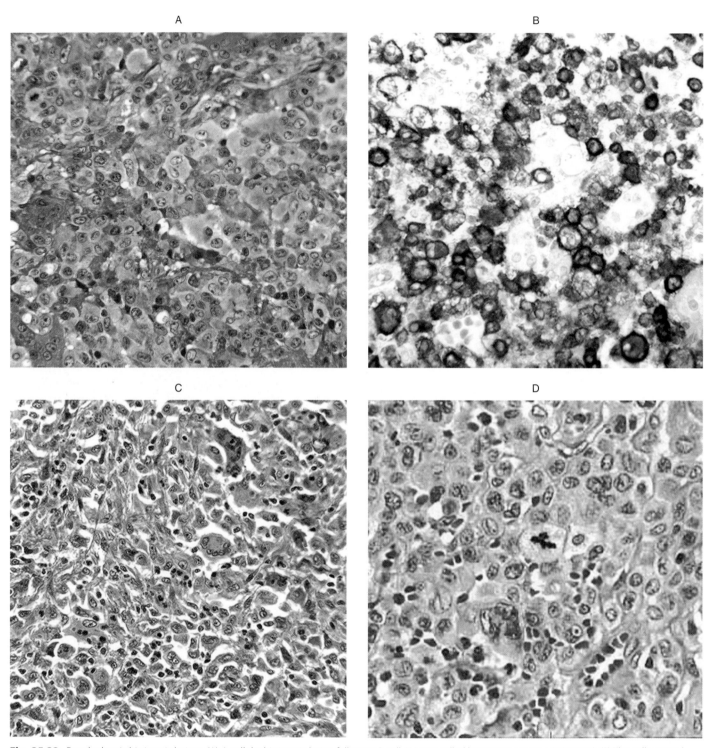

Fig. 25.22. Post-leukemic histiocytic lesions. (A) A cellular histiocytic lesion following B-cell ALL was called histiocytic sarcoma (H&E stain). (B) The cells stained diffusely for CD163 (and CD68). (C) A soft tissue lesion following B-cell ALL recurred. The histologic and phenotypic features were those of an "atypical" JXG (H&E stain). (D) A multiple recurring tumor following T-cell ALL had the cytologic and phenotypic features of a Langerhans cell lesion (sarcoma).

Follicular dendritic tumors and sarcomas

Nodal and extranodal follicular dendritic cell lesions are rare in children [168–171]. Lymph nodes are the primary site in the head and neck or mediastinum, though extranodal disease is found in the oropharyngeal and gastrointestinal tracts, spleen, liver, and lung. Although, like the other dendritic cell sarcomas, there are few clues to be gleaned from histopathology, the nodal growth pattern can be quite distinctive with a tight, whorled pattern of the spindled cells. Pleomorphism, like the biologic

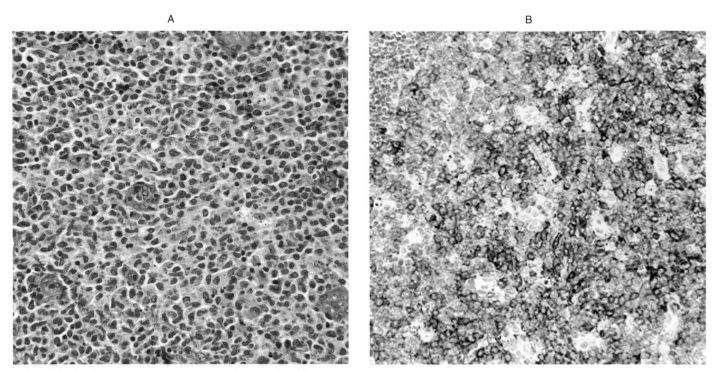

Fig. 25.23. Langerhans cell sarcoma, soft tissue. (A) The lesion, while reminiscent of LCH, was more cellular and pleomorphic (H&E stain). (B) CD1a (and Langerin) were present on lesional cells.

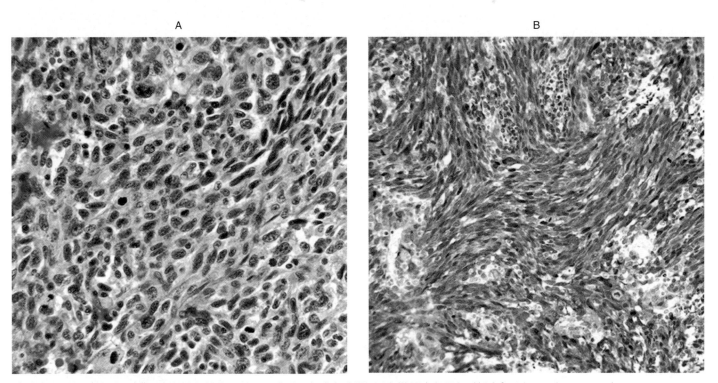

Fig. 25.24. Interdigitating cell sarcoma. (A) The lesion is spindled and cellular (H&E stain). (B) High S100 (and high fascin) were demonstrated.

A

B

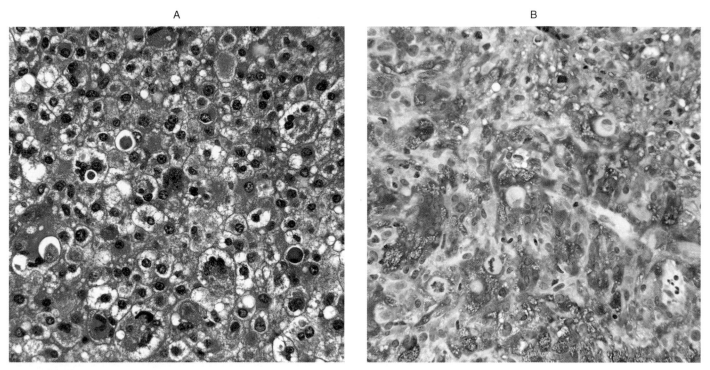

Fig. 25.25. Sarcoma, juvenile xanthogranuloma phenotype. (A) An intradural lesion had Touton-type appearance (H&E stain). (B) A similar lesion reveals the Factor 13a in the cytoplasm.

A

B

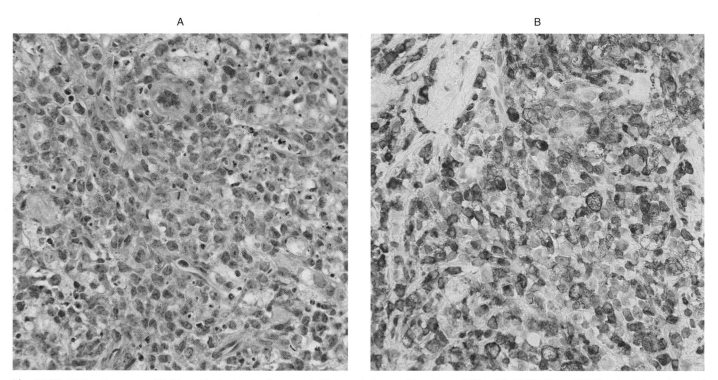

Fig. 25.26. Histiocytic sarcoma. (A) A breast lesion has the features of a high-grade, large cell lymphoma (H&E stain). (B) CD163 (and CD68) stained the surface and cytoplasm of the cells.

behavior, can vary widely, with greater aggression being associated with worse outcome. In general though, the malignancy is low, with local recurrences in about half, and distant metastases in less than a third [108].

The diagnosis is made by demonstrating the typical phenotype of the follicular dendritic cells that have fascin, CD21, CD23, CD35, and clusterin. CD1a, actins, and cytokeratins are absent.

Sarcoma, juvenile xanthogranuloma phenotype

The aggressive JXG lesion that follows ALL has been described. There are examples too of a high-grade lesion with pleomorphism and atypical mitoses that has the morphologic and phenotypic features of the JXG: CD14, CD68, CD163, Factor XIIIa, and fascin reactivity with little or no staining for S100 (Fig. 25.25). Some have been in the brain [172, 173], though soft tissue tumors are encountered.

Histiocytic sarcoma

This is a malignant tumor that has the features of a large cell lymphoma, commonly epithelioid, that has the pheno-type of a macrophage histiocyte or a dendritic cell [108, 174–176]. Although more common in adults, pediatric cases are described, mostly of lymph nodes, but extranodal and gastrointestinal tumors are encountered.

The epithelioid large cells have eosinophilic cytoplasm, but hemophagocytic activity is not a feature. Nuclei are generally large and oval with a prominent nucleolus. The cells stain for LCA and CD45RO, with granular cytoplasmic staining for CD68 and membrane staining for CD14. CD163 has a membrane and cytoplasmic pattern, and lysozyme is demonstrable in a paranuclear cytoplasmic pattern. S100 is high in the dendritic phenotype [177], CD1a is absent, and CD30 is not detected (Fig. 25.26). The differential diagnosis includes the other large cell lymphomas, so that all lineage-specific markers for T-, B- and granulocytic cells, melanoma, and carcinomas should be absent. The biologic behavior is that of a high-grade lymphoma.

References

1. **Cline MJ**. Histiocytes and histiocytosis. *Blood*. 1994;**84**:2840–2853.

2. **Onciu M**. Histiocytic proliferations in childhood. *American Journal of Clinical Pathology*. 2004;**122**(Suppl 1):S128–S136.

3. **Fedeel B, Henter JI**. Langerhans-cell histiocytosis: neoplasia or unbridled inflammation? *Trends in Immunology*. 2003;**24**:409–410.

4. **Laman JD, Leenen PJ, Annels NE,** *et al.* Langerhans-cell histiocytosis 'insight into DC biology'. *Trends in Immunology*. 2003;**24**:190–196.

5. **Reid CD, Fryer PR, Clifford C,** *et al.* Identification of hematopoietic progenitors of macrophages and dendritic Langerhans cells (DL-CFU) in human bone marrow and peripheral blood. *Blood*. 1990;**76**:1139–1149.

6. **Ishikawa F, Niiro H, Iino T,** *et al.* The developmental program of human dendritic cells is operated independently of conventional myeloid and lymphoid pathways. *Blood*. 2007; **110**:3591–3600.

7. **Hume DA**. The mononuclear phagocyte system. *Current Opinion in Immunology*. 2006;**18**:49–53.

8. **Hume DA**. Differentiation and heterogeneity in the mononuclear phagocyte system. *Mucosal Immunology*. 2008;**6**:432–441.

9. **Wu L, Liu YJ**. Development of dendritic-cell lineages. *Immunity*. 2007;**26**:741–750.

10. **Savina A, Amigorena S**. Phagocytosis and antigen presentation in dendritic cells. *Immunological Reviews*. 2007;**219**: 143–156.

11. **Gordon S, Taylor PR**. Monocyte and macrophage heterogeneity. *Nature Reviews. Immunology*. 2005;**5**:953–964.

12. **Stout RD, Jiang C, Matta B,** *et al.* Macrophages sequentially change their functional phenotype in response to changes in microenvironmental influences. *Journal of Immunology*. 2005;**175**:342–349.

13. **Nestle FO, Nickoloff BJ**. Deepening our understanding of immune sentinels in the skin. *Journal of Clinical Investigation*. 2007;**117**:2382–2385.

14. **Ginhoux F, Tacke F, Angeli V,** *et al.* Langerhans cells arise from monocytes in vivo. *Nature Immunology*. 2006;**7**: 265–273.

15. **Merad M, Manz MG, Karsunky H,** *et al.* Langerhans cells renew in the skin throughout life under steady-state conditions. *Nature Immunology*. 2002;**3**:1135–1141.

16. **Merad M, Ginhoux F, Collin M.** Origin, homeostasis and function of Langerhans cells and other Langerin-expressing dendritic cells. *Nature Reviews. Immunology*. 2008;**8**: 935–947.

17. **Martinez FO, Gordon S, Locati M,** *et al.* Transcriptional profiling of the human monocyte-to-macrophage differentiation and polarization: new molecules and patterns of gene expression. *Journal of Immunology*. 2006;**177**:7303–7311.

18. **Geissmann F, Dieu-Nosjean MC, Dezutter C,** *et al.* Accumulation of immature Langerhans cells in human lymph nodes draining chronically inflamed skin. *Journal of Experimental Medicine*. 2002;**196**:417–430.

19. **Valladeau J, Saeland S**. Cutaneous dendritic cells. *Seminars in Immunology*. 2005;**17**:273–283.

20. **van Nierop K, de Groot C**. Human follicular dendritic cells: function, origin and development. *Seminars in Immunology*. 2002;**14**:251–257.

21. **Liu YJ**. IPC: professional type 1 interferon-producing cells and plasmacytoid dendritic cell precursors. *Annual Review of Immunology*. 2005; **23**:275–306.

22. **Gretz JE, Kaldjian EP, Anderson AO,** *et al.* Sophisticated strategies for

information encounter in the lymph node: the reticular network as a conduit of soluble information and a highway for cell traffic. *Journal of Immunology.* 1996;**157**:495–499.

23. Jaffe R. Disorders of histiocytes. In Hsi ED, ed. *Hematopathology.* Philadelphia, PA: Churchill Livingstone Elsevier; 2007, 513–550.

24. Cruz PD Jr., East C, Bergstresser PR. Dermal, subcutaneous, and tendon xanthomas: diagnostic markers for specific lipoprotein disorders. *Journal of the American Academy of Dermatology.* 1988;**19**:95–111.

25. Lynch JM, Barrett TL. Collagenolytic (necrobiotic) granulomas: part II – the 'red' granulomas. *Journal of Cutaneous Pathology.* 2004;**31**:409–418.

26. Doffinger R, Patel S, Kumararatne DS. Human immunodeficiencies that predispose to intracellular bacterial infections. *Current Opinion in Rheumatology.* 2005;**17**:440–446.

27. Landing BH, Shirkey HS. A syndrome of recurrent infection and infiltration of viscera by pigmented lipid histiocytes. *Pediatrics.* 1957;**20**:431–447.

28. Yousef GM, Naghibi B. Malakoplakia outside the urinary tract. *Archives of Pathology & Laboratory Medicine.* 2007;**131**:297–300.

29. Lewis JT, Candelora JN, Hogan RB, *et al.* Crystal-storing histiocytosis due to massive accumulation of Charcot-Leyden crystals: a unique association producing colonic polyposis in a 78-year-old woman with eosinophilic colitis. *The American Journal of Surgical Pathology.* 2007;**31**:481–485.

30. Schaefer HE. Gammopathy-related crystal-storing histiocytosis, pseudo- and pseudo-pseudo-Gaucher cells. Critical commentary and mini-review. *Pathology, Research and Practice.* 1996;**192**:1152–1162.

31. Parizhskaya M, Youssef NN, DiLorenzo C, *et al.* Clofazimine enteropathy in a pediatric bone marrow transplant recipient. *Journal of Pediatrics.* 2001;**138**:574–576.

32. Turk JL. The mononuclear phagocyte system in granulomas. *The British Journal of Dermatology.* 1985; **113**(Suppl 28):49–54.

33. Morimoto Y, Routes JM. Granulomatous disease in common variable immunodeficiency. *Current Allergy and Asthma Reports.* 2005;**5**: 370–375.

34. Schaffer JV, Chandra P, Keegan BR, *et al.* Widespread granulomatous dermatitis of infancy: an early sign of Blau syndrome. *Archives of Dermatology.* 2007;**143**:386–391.

35. Pileri S, Falini B, Delsol G, *et al.* Lymphohistiocytic T-cell lymphoma (anaplastic large cell lymphoma CD30+/Ki-1+ with a high content of reactive histiocytes). *Histopathology.* 1990;**16**:383–391.

36. Applegarth DA, Dimmick JE, Hall JG. *Organelle Diseases.* London: Chapman & Hall Medical; 1999.

37. Schibler KR, Georgelas A, Rigaa A. Developmental biology of the dendritic cell system. *Acta Paediatrica. Supplement.* 2002;**91**:9–16.

38. Luscieti P, Hubschmid T, Cottier H, *et al.* Human lymph node morphology as a function of age and site. *Journal of Clinical Pathology.* 1980;**33**:454–461.

39. Muretto P. An immunohistochemical study on fetuses' and newborns' lymph nodes with emphasis on follicular dendritic reticulum cells. *European Journal of Histochemistry.* 1995;**39**:301–308.

40. Imal Y, Yamakawa M. Morphology, function and pathology of follicular dendritic cells. *Pathology International.* 1996;**46**:807–833.

41. McClain KL, Natkunam Y, Swerdlow SH. Atypical cellular disorders. *Hematology/the Education Program of the American Society of Hematology.* 2004:283–296.

42. Taylor GB, Smeeton IW. Cytologic demonstration of "dysplastic" follicular dendritic cells in a case of hyaline-vascular Castleman's disease. *Diagnostic Cytopathology.* 2000;**22**: 230–234.

43. Alavaikko MJ, Blanco G, Aine R, *et al.* Follicular dendritic cells have prognostic relevance in Hodgkin's disease. *American Journal of Clinical Pathology.* 1994;**101**:761–767.

44. Deguchi M, Aiba S, Ohtani H, *et al.* Comparison of the distribution and numbers of antigen-presenting cells among T-lymphocyte-mediated dermatoses: CD1a+, factor XIIIa+, and CD68+ cells in eczematous dermitis, psoriasis, lichen planus and graft-versus-host disease. *Archives for Dermatological Research.* 2002;**294**: 297–302.

45. Pigozzi B, Bordignon M, Belloni Fortina A, *et al.* Expression of the CD1a molecule in B- and T-lymphoproliferative skin conditions. *Oncology Reports.* 2006;**15**:347–351.

46. Gilcrease MZ, Rajan B, Ostrowski ML, *et al.* Localized thymic Langerhans cell histiocytosis and its relationship with myasthenia gravis. Immunohistochemical, ultrastructural, and cytometric studies. *Archives of Pathology & Laboratory Medicine.* 1997;**121**:134–138.

47. Christie LJ, Evans AT, Bray SE, *et al.* Lesions resembling Langerhans cell histiocytosis in association with other lymphoproliferative disorders: a reactive or neoplastic phenomenon? *Human Pathology.* 2006;**37**:32–39.

48. Yousem SA, Colby TV, Chen YY, *et al.* Pulmonary Langerhans' cell histiocytosis: molecular analysis of clonality. *The American Journal of Surgical Pathology.* 2001;**25**:630–636.

49. Facchetti F, Blanzuoli L, Ungar M, *et al.* Lymph node pathology in primary combined immunodeficiency diseases. *Springer Seminars in Immunopathology.* 1998;**19**:459–478.

50. Jouan H, LeDeist F, Nezelof C. Omenn's syndrome – pathologic arguments in favor of a graft versus host pathogenesis: a report of nine cases. *Human Pathology.* 1987;**18**:1101–1108.

51. Vossbeck S, Friedrich W, Heymer B. Pathogenesis and histomorphology of the so-called Omenn syndrome. *Verhandlungen der Deutschen Gesellschaft für Pathologie.* 1991;**75**: 121–125.

52. Jegalian AG, Facchetti F, Jaffe ES. Plasmacytoid dendritic cells. Physiologic roles and pathologic states. *Advances in Anatomic Pathology.* 2009;**16**:392–404.

53. Mantovani A, Sica A, Locati M. Macrophage polarization comes of age. *Immunity.* 2005;**23**:344–346.

54. Mosser DM. The many faces of macrophage activation. *Journal of Leukocyte Biology.* 2003;**73**:209–212.

55. Kzhyshkowska J, Gratchev A, Goerdt S. Stabilin-1, a homeostatic scavenger receptor with multiple functions. *Journal of Cellular and Molecular Medicine.* 2006;**10**:635–649.

56. **Moestrup SK, Møller HJ.** CD163: a regulated hemoglobin scavenger receptor with a role in the anti-inflammatory response. *Annals of Medicine.* 2004;**36**:347–354.

57. **Auffray C, Sieweke MH, Geissmann F.** Blood monocytes; development, heterogeneity, and relationship with dendritic cells. *Annual Review of Immunology.* 2009;**27**:669–692.

58. **Strauss-Ayali D, Conraf SM, Mosser DM.** Monocyte subpopulations and their differentiation patterns during infection. *Journal of Leukocyte Biology.* 2007;**82**:244–252.

59. **Newman KC, Riley EM.** Whatever turns you on: accessory-cell-dependent activation of NK cells by pathogens. *Nature Reviews. Immunology.* 2007;**7**:279–291.

60. **Menasche G, Feldmann J, Fischer A,** *et al.* Primary hemophagocytic syndromes point to a direct link between lymphocyte cytotoxicity and homeostasis. *Immunological Reviews.* 2005;**203**:165–179.

61. **Filipovich A, McClain K, Grom A.** Histiocytic disorders: recent insights into pathophysiology and practical guidelines. *Biology of Blood and Marrow Transplantation.* 2010;**16**(1 Suppl):S82–S89.

62. **Favara BE, Jaffe R, Egeler RM.** Macrophage activation and hemophagocytic syndrome in Langerhans' cell histiocytosis: report of 30 cases. *Pediatric and Developmental Pathology.* 2002;**5**:130–140.

63. **Ishii E, Imashuku S, Yarukawa M,** *et al.* Nationwide survey of hemophagocytic lymphohistiocytosis in Japan. *International Journal of Hematology.* 2007;**86**:58–65.

64. **Stabile A, Bertoni B, Ansuini V,** *et al.* The clinical spectrum and treatment options of macrophages activation syndrome in the pediatric age. *European Review for Medical and Pharmacological Sciences.* 2006;**10**:53–59.

65. **Katano H, Cohen JI.** Perforin and lymphohistiocytic proliferative disorders. *British Journal of Haematology.* 2005;**128**:739–750.

66. **Trapani JA, Voskoboinik I.** Infective, neoplastic, and homeostatic sequelae of the loss of perforin function in humans. *Advances in Experimental Medicine and Biology.* 2007;**601**:235–242.

67. **Fischer A, Latour S, de Saint Basile G.** Genetic defects affecting lymphocyte cytotoxicity. *Current Opinion in Immunology.* 2007:**19**:348–353.

68. **Janka GE.** Familial and acquired hemophagocytic lymphohistiocytosis. *European Journal of Pediatrics.* 2007;**166**:95–109.

69. **Allen CE, Yu X, Kozinetz CA,** *et al.* High elevated ferritin levels and the diagnosis of hemophagocytic lymphohistiocytosis. *Pediatric Blood & Cancer.* 2007;**50**:1227–1235.

70. **Henter JI, Horne A, Arico M,** *et al.* HLH-2004: diagnostic and therapeutic guidelines for hemophagocytic lymphohistiocytosis. *Pediatric Blood and Cancer.* 2007;**48**:124–131.

71. **Schneider EM, Lorenz I, Muller-Rosenberger M,** *et al.* Hemophagocytic lymphohistiocytosis is associated with deficiencies of cellular cytolysis but normal expression of transcripts relevant to killer-cell-induced apoptosis. *Blood.* 2002;**100**:2891–2898.

72. **Verbsky JW, Grossman WJ.** Hemophagocytic lymphohistiocytosis: diagnosis, pathophysiology, treatment and future perpectives. *Annals of Medicine.* 2006;**38**:20–31.

73. **Chen HH, Kuo HC, Wang L,** *et al.* Childhood macrophage activation syndrome differs from infection-associated hemophagocytosis syndrome in etiology and outcome in Taiwan. *Journal of Microbiology, Immunology, and Infection.* 2007;**40**:265–271.

74. **Jaffe R.** The histopathology of hemophagocytic lymphohistiocytosis. In Weitzman S, Egeler RM, eds. *Histiocytic Disorders of Children and Adults. Basic Science, Clinical Features and Therapy.* Cambridge: Cambridge University Press; 2005, 321–336.

75. **Henter JI, Elinder G, Ost A.** Diagnostic guidelines for hemophagocytic lymphohistiocytosis. The FHL Study Group of the Histiocyte Society. *Seminars in Oncology.* 1991;**18**:29–33.

76. **Macheta M, Will AM, Houghton JB,** *et al.* Prominent dyserythropoiesis in four cases of haemophagocytic lymphohistiocytosis. *Journal of Clinical Pathology.* 2001;**54**:961–963.

77. **Ost A, Nilsson-Ardnor S, Henter JI.** Autopsy findings in 27 children with haemophagocytic lymphohistiocytosis. *Histopathology.* 1998;**32**:310–316.

78. **Jaffe ES.** Histiocytoses of lymph nodes: biology and differential diagnosis. *Seminars in Diagnostic Pathology.* 1988;**5**:376–390.

79. **Arico M, Janka G, Fischer A,** *et al.* Hemophagocytic lymphohistiocytosis. Report of 122 children from the International Registry. FHL Study Group of the Histiocyte Society. *Leukemia.* 1996;**10**:197–203.

80. **Favara BE.** Histopathology of the liver in histiocytosis syndromes. *Pediatric Pathology and Laboratory Medicine.* 1996;**16**:413–433.

81. **De Kerguenec C, Hillaire S, Molinie V,** *et al.* Hepatic manifestations of hemophagocytic syndrome: a study of 30 cases. *The American Journal of Gastroenterology.* 2001;**96**:852–857.

82. **Jaffe R.** Liver involvement in the histiocytic disorders of childhood. *Pediatric and Developmental Pathology.* 2004;**7**:214–215.

83. **Kapelari K, Fruehwirth M, Heitger A,** *et al.* Loss of intrahepatic bile ducts: an important feature of familial hemophagocytic lymphohistiocytosis. *Virchows Archiv.* 2005;**446**:619–625.

84. **Parizhskaya M, Reyes J, Jaffe R.** Hemophagocytic syndrome presenting as acute hepatic failure in two infants: clinical overlap with neonatal hemochromatosis. *Pediatric and Developmental Pathology.* 1999;**2**:360–366.

85. **Stapp J, Wilkerson S, Stewart D,** *et al.* Fulminant neonatal liver failure in siblings: probable congenital hemophagocytic lymphohistiocytosis. *Pediatric and Developmental Pathology.* 2006;**9**:239–244.

86. **Draper NL, Morgan MB.** Dermatologic perivascular hemophagocytosis: a report of two cases. *The American Journal of Dermatopathology.* 2007;**29**:467–469.

87. **Haddad E, Sulis ML, Jabado N,** *et al.* Frequency and severity of central nervous system lesions in hemophagocytic lymphohistiocytosis. *Blood.* 1997;**89**:794–800.

88. **Horne A, Trottestam H, Arico M,** *et al.* Frequency and spectrum of central nervous system involvement in 193 children with haemophagocytic lymphohistiocytosis. *British Journal of Haematology.* 2007;**140**:327–335.

89. **Henter JI, Nennesmo I.** Neuropathologic findings and neurologic symptoms in twenty-three children with hemophagocytic lymphohistiocytosis. *Journal of Pediatrics.* 1997;**130**:358–365.

90. **Henter JI, Elinder G.** Cerebromeningeal haemophagocytic lymphohistiocytosis. *Lancet.* 1992; **339**:104–107.

91. **Rostasy K, Kolb R, Pohl D**, *et al.* CNS disease as the main manifestation of hemophagocytic lymphohistiocytosis in two children. *Neuropediatrics.* 2004;**35**:45–49.

92. **Jaffe R, Weiss LM, Facchetti F.** Tumours derived from Langerhans cells. In Swerdlow SH, Campo E, Harris NL, *et al.*, eds. *WHO Classification of Tumours of Haematopoietic and Lymphoid Tissues* (4th edn.). Lyon: IARC Press; 2008, 358–360.

93. **Steiner M, Matthes-Martin S, Attarbaschi A**, *et al.* Improved outcome of treatment-resistant high-risk Langerhans' cell histiocytosis after allogenic stem cell transplantation with reduced-intensity conditioning. *Bone Marrow Transplant.* 2005;**36**:215–225.

94. **Jaffe R.** The diagnostic histopathology of Langerhans' cell histiocytosis. In Weitzman S, Egeler RM, eds. *Histiocytic Disorders of Children and Adults. Basic Science, Clinical Features and Therapy.* Cambridge: Cambridge University Press; 2005, 14–39.

95. **Geissmann F, Lepelletier Y, Fraitag S**, *et al.* Differentiation of Langerhans' cells in Langerhans' cell histiocytosis. *Blood.* 2001;**97**:1241–1248.

96. **Bechan GI, Meeker AK, DeMarzo AM**, *et al.* Telomere length shortening in Langerhans cell histiocytosis. *British Journal of Haematology.* 2008;**140**:420–428.

97. **Chikwava K, Hunt JL, Mantha GS**, *et al.* Analysis of loss of heterozygosity in single-system and multisystem Langerhans cell histiocytosis. *Pediatric and Developmental Pathology.* 2007;**10**: 18–24.

98. **Willman CL, Busque L, Griffith BB**, *et al.* Langerhans' cell histiocytosis (histiocytosis X) – a clonal proliferative disease. *New England Journal of Medicine.* 1994;**331**:154–160.

99. **Egeler RM, Willman CL.** Is Langerhans' cell histiocytosis a myeloid dendritic stem cell disorder related to myelodysplastic disorders? *Medical and Pediatric Oncology.* 2000;**35**:426–427.

100. **Kaste SC, Rodriguez-Galindo C, McCarville ME**, *et al.* PET-CT in pediatric Langerhans cell histiocytosis. *Pediatric Radiology.* 2007;**37**:615–622.

101. **Meyer JS, DeCamargo B.** The role of radiology in the diagnosis and follow-up of Langerhans' cell histiocytosis. *Hematology/Oncology Clinics of North America.* 1998;**12**: 307–326.

102. **Kapur P, Erickson C, Rakheja D**, *et al.* Congenital self-healing reticulohistiocytosis (Hashimoto-Pritzker disease): ten-year experience at Dallas Children's Medical Center. *Journal of the American Academy of Dermatology.* 2007;**56**:290–294.

103. **Lau L, Krafchik B, Trebo MM**, *et al.* Cutaneous Langerhans' cell histiocytosis in children under one year. *Pediatric Blood and Cancer.* 2006;**46**:66–71.

104. **Minkov M, Prosch H, Steiner M**, *et al.* Langerhans' cell histiocytosis in neonates. *Pediatric Blood and Cancer.* 2005;**45**:802–807.

105. **Aterman K, Krause VW, Ross JB.** Scabies masquerading as Letterer-Siwe's disease. *Canadian Medical Association Journal.* 1976;**115**:443–444.

106. **Bhattacharjee P, Glusac EJ.** Langerhans cell hyperplasia in scabies: a mimic of Langerhans cell histiocytosis. *Journal of Cutaneous Pathology.* 2007;**34**:716–720.

107. **Burch JM, Krol A, Weston WL.** *Sarcoptes scabiei* infestation misdiagnosed and treated as Langerhans cell histiocytosis. *Pediatric Dermatology.* 2004;**21**:58–62.

108. **Pileri SA, Grogan TM, Harris NL**, *et al.* Tumours of histiocytes and accessory dendritic cells: an immunohistochemical approach to classification from the International Lymphoma Study Group based on 61 cases. *Histopathology.* 2002;**41**: 1–29.

109. **Billings SD, Hans CP, Schapiro BL**, *et al.* Langerhans' cell histiocytosis associated with myelodysplastic syndrome in adults. *Journal of Cutaneous Pathology.* 2006;**33**:171–174.

110. **Edelweiss M, Medeiros LJ, Suster S**, *et al.* Lymph node involvement by Langerhans' cell histiocytosis: a clinicopathologic and immunohistochemical study of 20 cases. *Human Pathology.* 2007;**38**: 1463–1469.

111. **Favara BE, Steele A.** Langerhans' cell histiocytosis of lymph nodes: a morphological assessment of 43 biopsies. *Pediatric Pathology and Laboratory Medicine.* 1997;**17**:769–787.

112. **Nezelof C.** Histiocytosis X: a histological and histogenetic study. *Perspectives in Pediatric Pathology.* 1979;**5**:153–178.

113. **Chikwava K, Jaffe R.** Langerin (CD207) staining in normal pediatric tissues, reactive lymph nodes, and childhood histiocytic disorders. *Pediatric and Developmental Pathology.* 2004;**7**:607–614.

114. **Lee JS, Lee MC, Park CS**, *et al.* Fine needle aspiration cytology of Langerhans' cell histiocytosis confined to lymph nodes. A case report. *Acta Cytologica.* 1997;**41**:1793–1796.

115. **Braier J, Ciocca M, Latella A**, *et al.* Cholestasis, sclerosing cholangitis, and liver transplantation in Langerhans' cell histiocytosis. *Medical and Pediatric Oncology.* 2002;**38**:178–182.

116. **Haas S, Theuerkauf I, Kuhnen A**, *et al.* Langerhans' cell histiocytosis of the liver. Differential diagnosis of a rare chronic destructive sclerosing cholangitis. *Der Pathologe.* 2003;**24**: 119–123.

117. **Kaplan KJ, Goodman ZD, Ishak KG.** Liver involvement in Langerhans' cell histiocytosis: a study of nine cases. *Modern Pathology.* 1999;**12**:370–378.

118. **Minkov M, Potschger U, Grois N**, *et al.* Bone marrow assessment in Langerhans' cell histiocytosis. *Pediatric Blood and Cancer.* 2007;**49**:694–698.

119. **Caminati A, Harari S.** Smoking-related interstitial pneumonias and pulmonary Langerhans' cell histiocytosis. *Proceedings of the American Thoracic Society.* 2006;**3**:299–306.

120. **Al-Trabolsi HA, Alshehri M, Al-Shomrani A**, *et al.* "Primary" pulmonary Langerhans' cell histiocytosis in a two-year-old child: case report and literature review. *Journal of Pediatric Hematology/Oncology.* 2006;**28**:79–81.

121. **Refabert L, Rambaud C, Mamou-Mani T,** *et al.* CD1a-positive cells in bronchoalveolar lavage samples from children with Langerhans' cell histiocytosis. *Journal of Pediatrics.* 1996;**129**:913–915.

122. **Smetana K Jr., Mericka O, Saeland S.** Diagnostic relevance of Langerin detection in cells from bronchoalveolar lavage of patients with pulmonary Langerhans cell histiocytosis, sarcoidosis and idiopathic pulmonary fibrosis. *Virchows Archiv.* 2004;**444**: 171–174.

123. **Tazi A.** Adult pulmonary Langerhans' cell histiocytosis. *The European Respiratory Journal.* 2006;**27**:1272–1285.

124. **Grois NG, Favara BE, Mostbeck GH,** *et al.* Central nervous system disease in Langerhans' cell histiocytosis. *Hematology/Oncology Clinics of North America.* 1998;**12**:287–305.

125. **Grois N, Prayer D, Prosch H,** *et al.* Neuropathology of CNS disease in Langerhans' cell histiocytosis. *Brain.* 2005;**128**:829–838.

126. **Prosch H, Grois N, Wnorowski M,** *et al.* Long-term MR imaging course of neurodegenerative Langerhans' cell histiocytosis. *American Journal of Neuroradiology.* 2007;**28**:1022–1028.

127. **Geissmann F, Thomas C, Emile JF,** *et al.* Digestive tract involvement in Langerhans' cell histiocytosis. The French Langerhans' Cell Histiocytosis Study Group. *Journal of Pediatrics.* 1996;**129**:836–845.

128. **Hait E, Liang M, Degar B,** *et al.* Gastrointestinal tract involvement in Langerhans' cell histiocytosis: case report and literature review. *Pediatrics.* 2006;**118**:e1593–e1599.

129. **Boccon-Gibod LA, Krichen HA, Carlier-Mercier LM,** *et al.* Digestive tract involvement with exudative enteropathy in Langerhans' cell histiocytosis. *Pediatric Pathology.* 1992;**12**:515–524.

130. **Junewick JJ, Fitzgerald NE.** The thymus in Langerhans' cell histiocytosis. *Pediatric Radiology.* 1999;**29**:904–907.

131. **Thompson LD, Wenig BM, Adair CF,** *et al.* Langerhans' cell histiocytosis of the thyroid: a series of seven cases and a review of the literature. *Modern Pathology.* 1996;**9**:145–149.

132. **Jaffe R, Favara BE.** Non-Langerhans' dendritic cell histiocytosis (abstract). *Pediatric and Developmental Pathology.* 2002;**5**:99.

133. **Martin Flores-Stadler E, Gonzalez-Crussi F, Greene M.** Indeterminate-cell histiocytosis: immunophenotypic and cytogenetic findings in an infant. *Medical and Pediatric Oncology.* 1999;**32**:250–254.

134. **Zelger BW, Cerio R.** Xanthogranuloma is the archetype of non-Langerhans' cell histiocytosis. *The British Journal of Dermatology.* 2001;**145**:369–371.

135. **Janssen D, Harms D.** Juvenile xanthogranuloma in childhood and adolescence: a clinicopathologic study of 129 patients from the Kiel pediatric tumor registry. *The American Journal of Surgical Pathology.* 2005;**29**: 21–28.

136. **Jaffe R, Fletcher CDM, Burgdorf W.** Disseminated juvenile xanthogranuloma. In Swerdlow SH, Campo E, Harris NL, *et al.*, eds. *WHO Classification of Tumours of Haematopoietic and Lymphoid Tissues* (4th edn.). Lyon: IARC Press; 2008, 366–367.

137. **Dehner JP.** Juvenile xanthogranulomas in the first two decades of life: a clinicopathologic study of 174 cases with cutaneous and extracutaneous manifestations. *The American Journal of Surgical Pathology.* 2003;**27**:579–593.

138. **Freyer DR, Kennedy R, Bostrom BC,** *et al.* Juvenile xanthogranulomas: forms of systemic disease and their clinical implications. *Journal of Pediatrics.* 1996;**129**:227–237.

139. **Isaacs H Jr.** Fetal and neonatal histiocytoses. *Pediatric Blood and Cancer.* 2006;**47**:123–129.

140. **Vendal Z, Walton D, Chen T.** Glaucoma in juvenile xanthogranuloma. *Seminars in Ophthalmology.* 2006;**21**:191–194.

141. **Caputo R, Veraldi S, Grimalt R,** *et al.* The various clinical patterns of xanthoma disseminatum. Consideration on seven cases and review of the literature. *Dermatology.* 1995;**190**:19–24.

142. **Sheu SY, Wenzel RR, Kersting C,** *et al.* Erdheim-Chester disease: case report with multisystemic manifestations including testes, thyroid, and lymph nodes, and a review of literature. *Journal of Clinical Pathology.* 2004; **57**:1225–1228.

143. **Veyssier-Belot C, Cacoub P, Caparros-Lefebvre D,** *et al.* Erdheim-Chester disease. Clinical and radiologic characteristics of 59 cases. *Medicine.* 1996;**75**:157–169.

144. **Barroca H, Farinha NJ, Lobo A,** *et al.* Deep-seated congenital juvenile xanthogranuloma: report of a case with emphasis on cytologic features. *Acta Cytologica.* 2007;**51**:473–476.

145. **Sidwell RU, Francis N, Slater DN,** *et al.* Is disseminated juvenile xanthogranulomatosis benign cephalic histiocytosis? *Pediatric Dermatology.* 2005;**22**:40–43.

146. **Caputo R, Marzano AV, Passoni E, Berti E.** Unusual variants of non-Langerhans cell histiocytoses. *Journal of the American Academy of Dermatology.* 2007;**57**:1031–1045.

147. **Lüftl M, Seybold H, Simon M Jr., Burgdorf W.** Progressive nodular histiocytosis – rare variant of cutaneous non-Langerhans cell histiocytosis. *Journal der Deutschen Dermatologischen Gesellschaft.* 2006;**4**:236–238.

148. **Jang KA, Lee HJ, Choi JH,** *et al.* Generalized eruptive histiocytoma of childhood. *The British Journal of Dermatology.* 1999;**140**:174–176.

149. **Hu WK, Gilliam AC, Wiersma SR,** *et al.* Fatal congenital systemic juvenile xanthogranuloma with liver failure. *Pediatric and Developmental Pathology.* 2004;**7**:71–76.

150. **Bostrom J, Janssen G, Messing-Junger M,** *et al.* Multiple intracranial juvenile xanthogranulomas. Case report. *Journal of Neurosurgery.* 2000;**93**: 335–341.

151. **Schultz KD Jr., Petronio J, Narad C,** *et al.* Solitary intracerebral juvenile xanthogranumola. Case report and review of the literature. *Pediatric Neurosurgery.* 1997;**26**:315–321.

152. **Chan JK, Lamant L, Algar E,** *et al.* ALK+ histiocytosis: a novel type of systemic histiocytic proliferative disorder of early infancy. *Blood.* 2008;**112**:2965–2968.

153. **Gaitonde S.** Multifocal, extranodal sinus histiocytosis with massive lymphadenopathy: an overview. *Archives of Pathology & Laboratory Medicine.* 2007;**131**:1117–1121.

154. **Foucar E, Rosai J, Dorfman R**. Sinus histiocytosis with massive lymphadenopathy (Rosai-Dorfman disease): review of the entity. *Seminars in Diagnostic Pathology*. 1990;**7**:19–73.

155. **Maric I, Pittaluga S, Dale JK**, *et al.* Histologic features of sinus histiocytosis with massive lymphadenopathy in patients with autoimmune lymphoproliferative syndrome. *The American Journal of Surgical Pathology*. 2005;**29**:903–911.

156. **Sachdev R, Shyama J**. Co-existent Langerhans cell histiocytosis and Rosai-Dorfman disease: a diagnostic rarity. *Cytopathology*. 2008;**19**:55–58.

157. **Zelger BW, Cerio R, Soyer HP**, *et al.* Reticulohistiocytoma and multicentric reticulohistiocytosis. Histopathologic and immunophenotypic distinct entities. *The American Journal of Dermatopathology*. 1994;**16**:577–584.

158. **Miettinen M, Fetsch JF**. Reticulohistiocytoma (solitary epithelioid histiocytoma): a clinicopathologic and immunohistochemical study of 44 cases. *The American Journal of Surgical Pathology*. 2006;**30**:521–528.

159. **Outland JD, Keiran SJ, Schikler KN**, *et al.* Multicentric reticulohistiocytosis in a 14-year-old girl. *Pediatric Dermatology*. 2002;**19**:527–531.

160. **Tajirian AL, Malik MK, Robinson-Bostom L**, *et al.* Multicentric reticulohistiocytosis. *Clinics in Dermatology*. 2006;**24**:486–492.

161. **Bouabdallah R, Abena P, Chetaille B**, *et al.* True histiocytic lymphoma following B-acute lymphoblastic leukemia: case report with evidence for a common clonal origin in both neoplasms. *British Journal of Haematology*. 2001;**113**:1047–1050.

162. **Feldman AL, Minniti C, Santi M**, *et al.* Histiocytic sarcoma after acute lymphoblastic leukaemia: a common clonal origin. *Lancet*. 2004;**5**:248–250.

163. **Rasaiyaah J, Yong K, Katz DR**, *et al.* Dendritic cells and myeloid leukaemias: plasticity and commitment in cell differentiation. *British Journal of Haematology*. 2007;**138**:281–290.

164. **Rodig SJ, Payne EG, Degar BA**, *et al.* Aggressive Langerhans cell histiocytosis following T-ALL: clonally related neoplasms with persistent expression of constitutively active NOTCH1. *American Journal of Hematology*. 2008;**83**:116–121.

165. **Costa da Cunha Castro E, Blazquez C, Boyd J**, *et al.* Clinicopathologic features of histiocytic lesions following ALL, with a review of the literature. *Pediatric and Developmental Pathology*. 2010;**13**:225–237.

166. **Ben-Ezra J, Bailey A, Azumi N**, *et al.* Malignant histiocytosis X. A distinct clinicopathologic entity. *Cancer*. 1991;**68**(5):1050–1060.

167. **Pillay K, Solomon R, Daubenton JD**, *et al.* Interdigitating dendritic cell sarcoma: a report of four paediatric cases and review of the literature. *Histopathology*. 2004;**44**:283–291.

168. **Bradshaw EJ, Wood KM, Hodgkinson P**, *et al.* Follicular dendritic cell tumour in a 9-year-old child. *Pediatric Blood and Cancer*. 2005;**45**:725–727.

169. **Chan JK, Fletcher CD, Nayler SJ**, *et al.* Follicular dendritic cell sarcoma. Clinicopathologic analysis of 17 cases suggesting a malignant potential higher than currently recognized. *Cancer*. 1997;**79**:294–313.

170. **Fonseca R, Yamakawa M, Nakamura S**, *et al.* Follicular dendritic cell sarcoma and interdigitating reticulum cell sarcoma: a review. *American Journal of Hematology*. 1998;**59**:161–167.

171. **Shia J, Chen W, Tang LH**, *et al.* Extranodal follicular dendritic cell sarcoma: clinical, pathologic, and histogenetic characteristics of an under-recognized disease entity. *Virchows Archiv*. 2006;**449**:148–158.

172. **Ernemann U, Skalej M, Hermisson M**, *et al.* Primary cerebral non-Langerhans cell histiocytosis: MRI and differential diagnosis. *Neuroradiology*. 2002;**44**:759–763.

173. **Orsey A, Paessler M, Lange BJ**, *et al.* Central nervous system juvenile xanthogranuloma with malignant transformation. *Pediatric Blood and Cancer*. 2008;**50**(4):927–930.

174. **Copie-Bergman C, Wotherspoon AC, Norton AJ**, *et al.* True histiocytic lymphoma: a morphologic, immunohistochemical, and molecular genetic study of 13 cases. *The American Journal of Surgical Pathology*. 1998;**22**:1386–1392.

175. **Hornick JL, Jaffe ES, Fletcher CD**. Extranodal histiocytic sarcoma: clinicopathologic analysis of 14 cases of a rare epithelioid malignancy. *The American Journal of Surgical Pathology*. 2004;**28**:1133–1144.

176. **Vos JA, Abbondanzo SL, Barekman CL**, *et al.* Histiocytic sarcoma: a study of five cases including the histiocytic marker CD163. *Modern Pathology*. 2005;**18**:693–704.

177. **Porter DW, Gupte GL, Brown RM**, *et al.* Histiocytic sarcoma with interdigitating dendritic cell differentiation. *Journal of Pediatric Hematology/Oncology*. 2004;**26**:827–830.

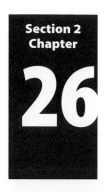

26 Cutaneous and subcutaneous lymphomas in children

Kenneth Chang, Elena Pope, and Glenn Taylor

Introduction

Classification of cutaneous lymphomas

The skin is the second most common site of extranodal lymphoma after the gastrointestinal tract [1]. The term *primary cutaneous lymphoma* refers to cutaneous lymphomas that present in the skin with no evidence of extracutaneous disease at the time of diagnosis [2].

This chapter adopts the 2005 WHO/EORTC classification (Table 26.1) for cutaneous lymphomas [2, 3]. Prior to its publication, the two classification schemes most widely used were the 2001 World Health Organization (WHO) classification [4] and the 1997 European Organization for the Research and Treatment of Cancer (EORTC) classification [5].

The 2005 WHO/EORTC classification is a consensus system based on the premise that primary cutaneous lymphomas often have a completely different clinical behavior and prognosis from histologically similar nodal lymphomas: therefore, they require different management strategies and treatment. This new classification is validated by clinical follow-up data on 1905 patients from the Dutch and Austrian registries for primary cutaneous lymphomas [6].

Epidemiology in the pediatric age group

Primary cutaneous lymphomas are extremely rare, with an incidence of approximately 0.36 per 100 000 [7] persons per year. Cutaneous T-cell lymphomas (CTCLs) account for approximately 75% of all cutaneous lymphomas in Europe [5] and >90% in North America. Although typically considered a disease of adulthood (approximately 75% of patients are diagnosed after 50 years of age [8]), pediatric cases make up from 4 to 11% of CTCL cases, and many adult patients report initial onset in childhood [8–10]. In both adults and children, there seems to have been an increase in the incidence of CTCL over the past 20 years [8]. The rate of childhood CTCL is currently estimated at 0.1 per million in the 0–9 years of age group, and 0.3 per million in the 10–19 years of age group [11]. Whether this is due to a true rise in the incidence, or an increased diagnostic aware-

ness and recognition of CTCL, is still debated. Primary B-cell lymphomas in children are extremely rare. In the largest pediatric cutaneous lymphoma series to date, only 8 of 62 cases were of B-cell lineage (one follicle center cell lymphoma, and seven marginal zone B-cell lymphomas) [12].

Cutaneous T-cell and NK-cell lymphomas

Mycosis fungoides

Introduction/definition

Mycosis fungoides (MF) is a peripheral, epidermotropic T-cell lymphoma of mature T-cells of small to medium size with characteristic cerebriform nuclei [1, 2].

Epidemiology

Mycosis fungoides is the most common form of cutaneous T-cell lymphoma in both the adult and pediatric population. While MF most frequently affects adults in the fifth and sixth decades of life, it is also seen in younger persons including adolescents and children [9, 10, 12–17]. It can be seen in children as young as three years of age [12, 18]. The male : female preponderance in the pediatric age group is approximately equal [10, 13, 15, 19]. The incidence and mortality rates of MF are increasing across all age groups [7, 11].

Clinical features

The clinical diagnosis for early cutaneous lymphoma is difficult, as many of its clinical and pathologic features are also seen in benign inflammatory diseases. The label "the great imitator" was attached to CTCL [20], and illustrates the protean clinical manifestations of the disease. This fact, in addition to its rarity, accounts for the lack of a timely diagnosis in childhood years. Other diagnostic entities, such as psoriasis, tinea corporis, pityriasis lichenoides chronica, lichen aureus, atopic dermatitis, post-inflammatory hypopigmentation, and vitiligo, are common labels given to children with CTCL. One feature that helps distinguish CTCL from these other diseases is its

Diagnostic Pediatric Hematopathology, ed. Maria A. Proytcheva. Published by Cambridge University Press.
© Cambridge University Press 2011.

Table 26.1. WHO/EORTC classification of cutaneous lymphomas [2].

Cutaneous T-cell and NK-cell lymphomas
Mycosis fungoides
Mycosis fungoides variants and subtypes
    Folliculotropic mycosis fungoides
    Pagetoid reticulosis
    Granulomatous slack skin
Sézary syndrome
Adult T-cell leukemia/lymphoma
    Primary cutaneous CD30+ lymphoproliferative disorders
    Primary cutaneous anaplastic large cell lymphoma
Lymphomatoid papulosis
Subcutaneous panniculitis-like T-cell lymphoma
Extranodal NK/T-cell lymphoma, nasal type
Primary cutaneous peripheral T-cell lymphoma, unspecified
    Primary cutaneous aggressive epidermotropic CD8+ T-cell
      lymphoma[a]
    Cutaneous $\gamma\delta$ T-cell lymphoma[a]
    Primary cutaneous CD4+ small/medium-sized pleomorphic T-cell
lymphoma[a]

Cutaneous B-cell lymphomas
Primary cutaneous marginal zone B-cell lymphoma
Primary cutaneous follicle center lymphoma
Primary cutaneous diffuse large B-cell lymphoma, leg type
Primary cutaneous diffuse large B-cell lymphoma, other
    Intravascular large B-cell lymphoma

Precursor hematologic neoplasm
CD4+/CD56+ hematodermic neoplasm (blastic NK-cell lymphoma)

[a] Provisional entities.

persistent nature, despite therapy. The suspicion for B-cell lymphoma is even less often entertained due to its rarity in the pediatric population.

Cutaneous T-cell lymphoma can present with a number of different morphologies including patches, plaques, tumors, and Sézary syndrome (widespread erythroderma and scaling) (SS), which is a rare leukemic manifestation of cutaneous T-cell lymphoma. Other rare variants include poikiloderma (reticulate dyspigmentation, follicular atrophy, and telangiectasias), and granulomatous slack skin syndrome (abnormal tissue that has lost elastic recoil, leading to sagging, pendulous skin).

The earliest form and the most common presentation of CTCL is the patch stage, which consists of sharply demarcated, erythematous scaly lesions [21]. The scale is typically less thick than in psoriasis and covers the entire affected area. Skin atrophy is also present, giving the "cigarette paper" wrinkling appearance. With disease progression, patches may evolve into the plaque stage, in which the lesions are infiltrated and more palpable. The tumor stage is characterized by raised nodules or tumors with epidermal change in the form of erythema, scaling, and/or ulceration. Lesions may appear anywhere, but there is a predilection for non-sun-exposed areas, such as the trunk below the waistline, buttocks, flanks, breasts, inner thighs, inner arms, and periaxillary areas. Rarely, CTCL may also present with lesions on the scalp, palms, and soles [22].

There are certain clinical features that differentiate pediatric CTCL from adult CTCL. In children, studies have consistently shown presentation in early stage disease. In one study of 10 patients, all presented at stage IIB or less and included 2 patients with unilesional disease [23]. An interesting feature of pediatric CTCL is an over-representation of hypopigmented and poikilodermic appearance [9, 12, 19]. The hypopigmented lesions present as non-atrophic white patches, with minimal scaling [24, 25]. In a study by Wain *et al.*, 24% and 26% of patients had hypopigmented and poikilodermic CTCL, respectively [9]. The incidence is as high as 70% in one pediatric study, with 43% presenting in light-skinned individuals [23]. Recent results from an international registry of pediatric CTCL patients confirmed the over-representation of early stage disease and hypopigmented CTCL in pediatric patients [26]. More common conditions such as pityriasis alba and vitiligo can be misdiagnosed as hypopigmented MF [27].

Histopathology

Mycosis fungoides in children is histologically and immunophenotypically indistinguishable from that seen in adults [28].

The patch stage is characterized by a superficial band-like or lichenoid infiltrate. There is epidermotropism, taking the form of a haphazard colonization of the basal aspects of the epidermis by atypical lymphocytes which may be in linear groups or singly dispersed [29]. The atypical lymphocytes manifest hyperchromatic nuclei with cerebriform nuclear contours. The intraepidermal cells are typically larger and more atypical compared to their dermal counterparts. The epidermis may be variably hyperplastic, but typically, spongiosis is minimal, and keratinocyte necrosis is not prominent. Distinctive halo-like lacunar spaces may be seen to surround the intraepidermal cells [30], imparting to them a quiescent disposition amid vacuous spaces within the intact epidermis. Such haloed lymphocytes are a discriminating diagnostic feature of MF (Fig. 26.1A). A variable admixture of plasma cells, eosinophils, and histiocytes may be present, but these are not prominent, and may be minimal in early lesions. The dermis may show edema or fibrosis. In early stages of MF, architectural abnormalities are often more helpful in establishing the diagnosis than cytologic features, which may not be highly atypical [31–33]. Early lesions have protean histologic features, and it is not unusual for multiple biopsies to be required for diagnosis in some cases [32]. The International Society for Cutaneous Lymphomas (ISCL) has proposed a diagnostic algorithm for early MF [22].

The plaque stage features a denser infiltrate with more easily identified atypical lymphocytes. There is more prominent epidermotropism. Pautrier microabscesses (sharply marginated clusters of lymphocytes within the epidermis) may be present (Fig. 26.1B). The tumor stage shows diffuse dermal infiltrates, and loss of epidermotropism and Pautrier microabscesses. The infiltrate is monomorphous and dominated by large atypical cells [34]. Mitoses are generally numerous. The infiltrate may extend into the subcutis. Large cell transformation, defined as a biopsy specimen showing large cells at least four-times the size of a small lymphocyte in 25% or more of the dermal infiltrate, may occur [35–37]. This may be either CD30 negative or positive, and is associated with a poor prognosis [38].

A

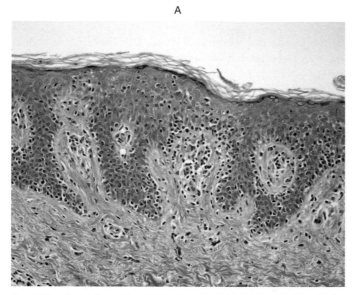

B

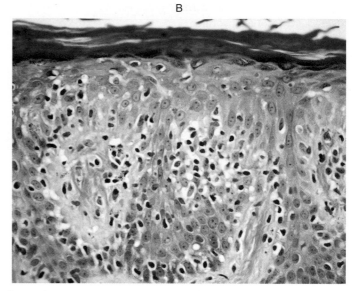

Fig. 26.1. Mycosis fungoides. (A) Patch stage. A relatively sparse dermal infiltrate of atypical lymphocytes is present. Atypical lymphocytes surrounded by clear halos are present in the basal aspect of the epidermis. Note the absence of epidermal spongiosis (H&E stain). (B) A collection of atypical lymphocytes within the epidermis, forming a Pautrier microabscess (H&E stain).

The International Society for Cutaneous Lymphomas (ISCL) and the Cutaneous Lymphoma Task Force of the EORTC have recently proposed certain revisions to the staging and classification of MF and Sézary syndrome [39].

Immunophenotype

The neoplastic cells in MF have a mature T-cell phenotype, usually of helper T-cells, and the most common immuno-histochemical profile is CD2+, CD3+, CD4+, CD5+, and CD45RO+. During progression of the disease, loss of CD2, CD5, and CD7 may be seen, particularly in the epidermotropic cerebriform cells.

Variant immunophenotypic profiles described in the literature include the following:

(1) Cases with a CD4−, CD8+ mature T-cell phenotype [40–43]. Such CD4−, CD8+ cases appear to be over-represented in childhood [23, 42] and in hypopigmented variants [9, 44]. They have the same clinical behavior and prognosis as CD4+ cases.

(2) Cases with a CD4−, CD8− phenotype [45]. A series of 18 cases reported from the Middle East included 6 which presented in the pediatric age group. The clinical course was not different [45].

(3) Cases with a CD56+ phenotype [46–48]; one reported case with such a phenotype is that of a six-year-old boy who presented at age three years [48]. The clinical course is felt to be similar [48], although experience of this rare immunophenotypic variant is limited.

Genetics

Genetic features in pediatric MF do not appear different from those in adult cases. Although childhood disease should be sim-

ilar to its adult counterpart, clonal T-cell rearrangements are found less commonly in childhood MF, possibly related to the reluctance on the patients' and physicians' part to perform large or repeated biopsies and/or to the early stage presentation with relatively low infiltrate load. Various structural and numeric chromosomal abnormalities are described, but recurrent, MF-specific chromosomal translocations have not been identified [29, 49].

Prognosis and predictive factors

Although the earlier literature suggested that pediatric MF has a more aggressive disease course and association with other forms of lymphomas [14], more recent and larger case series indicate that the natural history is stage dependent [9, 10, 15, 19, 23, 24]. When matched for stage, the prognosis is similar to that in adults, although the onset of lesions of MF in childhood may increase the probability of disease progression during the lifetime of the patient [12]. Hypopigmented or poikiloderma-tous lesions, and those with associated lymphomatoid papulosis, showed improved disease-specific survival and reduced disease progression [9].

Therapy

The ideal treatment for pediatric CTCL is still unclear. To date, there are no controlled trials delineating a survival benefit from any of the therapies currently used [50]. It is always important to balance between achieving disease control in order to alleviate symptoms, decrease tumor load, and chances of large cell transformation, and preventing long-term damage from the therapy used, particularly in a growing child.

Accepted methods of treating patch and plaque stage include: topical steroids, topical mechlorethamine (chlormethine), topical carmustine (BCNU), and topical bexarotene, PUVA (psoralen chemotherapy with ultraviolet light radiation), UVA1, UVB1, localized electron beam therapy, and topical nitrogen mustard [51–57].

In a recent consensus statement from Europe, emollients with or without moderate topical steroids for localized disease was an acceptable therapeutic choice, given that life expectancy is not adversely affected [9].

Pediatric usefulness of other topical options, such as mechlorethamine hydrochloride 0.01% or 0.02%, carmustine (BCNU), imiquimod, tazarotene, and a novel retinoid, 1% bexarotene, is limited due to the high rate of severe irritant dermatitis. For more advanced disease, stem cell therapy, extracorporeal photopheresis, systemic steroids, interferon-α, methotrexate, and multimodal chemotherapy have all been used with varying success. Our institutional practice is to treat patients with stage IA disease with topical steroids, retinoids, and/or imiquimod, and to use UVB1/PUVA for stage IB or IIA disease (Elena Pope, personal communication).

Mycosis fungoides variants and subtypes

Folliculotropic mycosis fungoides

Folliculotropic MF is a variant of MF characterized by the presence of folliculotropic lymphoid infiltrates. Most cases show mucinous degeneration of the hair follicles (follicular mucinosis) which is, by itself, of no clinical significance; this has been previously [4] referred to as MF-associated follicular mucinosis. The clinical significance of this disease is the deep, follicular and perifollicular localization of the neoplastic infiltrates, which renders the disease more refractory to skin-targeted therapies [58]. Folliculotropic MF occurs mostly in adults, and is extremely rare in children and adolescents [58–61].

Pagetoid reticulosis

Pagetoid reticulosis (PR) is a distinct variant of MF characterized clinically by localized patches or plaques with an indolent behavior, and histologically by an exclusively intraepidermal infiltrate of neoplastic T-cells. The term PR as used in the 2005 WHO/EORTC classification [2] refers to the localized form (Woringer–Kolopp disease). The disseminated form (Ketron–Goodman disease) would, in the scheme of this classification, be reclassified as one of the following: tumor-stage MF, aggressive epidermotropic CD8-positive cutaneous T-cell lymphoma, or cutaneous gamma delta-positive T-cell lymphoma. This disease entity was first described by Woringer and Kolopp in 1939 with reference to a 13-year-old boy who presented with a solitary, polycyclic, and infiltrated 7 cm plaque-like lesion on the left forearm [62]. Pagetoid reticulosis is seen in both pediatric [62–65] and adult populations with a male to female ratio of 2 : 1 [65]. Clinically, patients present with a large, solitary, erythematous, scaly or verrucous patch or plaque, usually on the distal part of a limb. The disease is slowly progressive, and extracutaneous dissemination is not seen.

Histologically, the epidermis is irregularly acanthotic with overlying hyperkeratosis and spotty parakeratosis [65]. There is epidermal infiltration by singly dispersed or clustered medium-sized to large atypical lymphoid cells with pale eosinophilic or vacuolated cytoplasm [65]. Accompanying Langerhans cells and histiocytes are also present [66]. These atypical cells are present at all levels of the epidermis, but are more numerous in the lower third, with a predisposition for the tips of the rete ridges [65]. The basement membrane remains intact [65]. Degenerating tumor cells may be seen in the upper epidermis [67]. In contrast to MF, the infiltrate is exclusively epidermal; the dermis contains no neoplastic cells, only a mixed infiltrate of non-neoplastic lymphocytes and histiocytes [67]. The neoplastic epidermal lymphoid infiltrate is composed of T-cells which may have a CD4-positive T-helper phenotype, CD8-positive T-cytotoxic/suppressor phenotype, or a CD4/CD8 double-negative phenotype [68–70]. CD30 expression is variable [68, 71]. The exquisite epidermotropism of this lesion may be explained by the expression of skin-homing receptors and epithelial cell adhesion molecules by the neoplastic cells [72].

Granulomatous slack skin

Granulomatous slack skin (GSS) is a very rare subtype of CTCL. It is a clinicopathologic entity characterized by development of areas of pendulous, lax skin in the major skin folds (especially axillae and groins) [73]. Males are predominantly affected [74]. While the majority of cases have been reported in adults, cases in adolescents/younger adults aged 14 to 20 years have also been reported [75–79], with similar clinical behavior and histological appearance.

Histology reveals a dense granulomatous dermal infiltrate containing atypical T-cells with variably cerebriform nuclei, macrophages, and numerous multinucleated giant cells containing a large number of nuclei [74]. The atypical T-cells have a CD3-positive, CD4-positive, and CD8-negative immunophenotype [78]. The multinucleated giant cells are reactive for lysozyme, CD68, and S100 [79]. Destruction of elastic fibers is characteristic and accounts for the formation of the pendulous skin folds. Most cases have an indolent course with long survival. However, there is an association with Hodgkin lymphoma in one-third of patients [73, 75, 80]. The pendulous skin folds tend to recur after surgical excision [81].

Sézary syndrome

Sézary syndrome (SS) is a distinctive erythrodermic cutaneous T-cell lymphoma characterized by pruritic erythroderma, generalized lymphadenopathy, and circulating malignant T-cells in the peripheral blood. Other useful diagnostic criteria include: (1) an absolute Sézary cell count of 1000 cells/mm^3 or more; (2) a CD4/CD8 ratio of 10 or higher caused by an increase in circulating T-cells, and/or an aberrant loss or expression of pan-T-cell markers by flow cytometry; (3) increased lymphocyte counts with evidence of a T-cell clone in the blood by the

Southern blot or polymerase chain reaction technique; or (4) a chromosomally abnormal T-cell clone [82].

Sézary syndrome is a rare condition that occurs almost exclusively in adults. Only occasional case reports describe its occurrence in children [83, 84]. Meister *et al.* describe an 11-year-old girl who had generalized exfoliative erythroderma, intense pruritus, peripheral lymphadenopathy, mycosis cells in the skin and lymph nodes, and Sézary cells in the peripheral blood [83]. LeBoit *et al.* report a 12-year-old girl who had erythrodermic follicular mucinosis, hypereosinophilia, circulating Sézary cells, and both immunophenotypic and genotypic evidence of T-cell neoplasia, commenting that erythrodermic follicular mucinosis may represent an unusual variant of the Sézary syndrome [84]. The ISCL and the Cutaneous Lymphoma Task Force of the EORTC have recently proposed revisions to the staging and classification of mycosis fungoides and Sézary syndrome, which take into account recent advances related to tumor cell biology and diagnostic techniques in relation to these disorders [39].

Adult T-cell leukemia/lymphoma

Adult T-cell leukemia/lymphoma is a T-cell neoplasm etiologically associated with the type C retrovirus, human T-cell leukemia virus 1 (HTLV-1). Although the condition is seen predominantly in adults [85–89], cases occurring in children have been reported [90, 91]. It is endemic in areas with a high prevalence of HTLV-1 in the population, such as Japan, the Caribbean Islands, South America, and parts of Central Africa. It develops in 1–5% of seropositive individuals after more than two decades of viral persistence. Skin lesions may resemble those of mycosis fungoides clinically (papules, plaques, and tumors) [86] and histologically. There is a superficial band-like infiltrate of medium-sized to large T-lymphoid cells, with prominent epidermotropism, and intraepidermal Pautrier-like microabscesses [86, 88]. The tumor cells contain polylobated and hyperchromatic nuclei. Skin lesions in the smoldering variant may contain only sparse neoplastic cells with mild atypia. The neoplastic T-cells have a CD3+, CD4+, and CD8− phenotype with expression of CD25 [85, 92]. Adult T-cell leukemia/lymphoma is an aggressive malignant disease associated with regulatory T-cells. FOXP3 is a key molecule of regulatory T-cells, and its expression has been found to be associated with a clinically and pathologically immunodeficient state [93].

Primary cutaneous CD30+ lymphoproliferative disorders

Primary cutaneous CD30-positive lymphoproliferative disorders are the second most common group of cutaneous T-cell lymphomas [2]. However, in children under 20 years of age, equal numbers of MF and primary cutaneous CD30+ lymphoproliferative disorders were noted [12]. Primary cutaneous CD30-positive lymphoproliferative disorders comprise a clinical and morphologic spectrum of diseases which include lym-

phomatoid papulosis (LyP) and primary cutaneous anaplastic large cell lymphoma (C-ALCL) at two ends of the spectrum. Despite good clinicopathological correlation, some cases cannot be easily classified into one of the two [94]. Other disease entities falling into this spectrum include Hodgkin lymphoma, MF with large cell transformation, CD30-positive large B-cell lymphoma, and CD30-positive lymphomatoid drug reactions [95]. The common feature to all is the expression of CD30, which is a cytokine receptor belonging to the tumor necrosis factor receptor superfamily [96].

Lymphomatoid papulosis
Definition

Lymphomatoid papulosis (LyP) was first described by Macaulay [97] in 1968 as an enigmatic recurring self-healing eruption which was clinically benign but histologically malignant. It is a chronic recurrent lymphoproliferative skin disease with a generally indolent clinical course, characterized by self-regressing papulonodular skin lesions, that have histological features of CD30-positive lymphomatous cells with a variable admixed inflammatory background.

Epidemiology

The prevalence of LyP is estimated at 1.2 to 1.9 cases per 1 000 000 people [98]. Although uncommon, the reported pediatric cases of childhood LyP do not represent the true incidence of the disease. Boys are reported to have an earlier onset of LyP compared to girls [99].

Clinical features

Lymphomatoid papulosis is characterized by recurrent crops of lesions that last between three and eight weeks. The number of lesions per crop varies from patient to patient. In some, the number of lesions decreases after the initial crop. Morphologically, the LyP lesions consist of a red papule/nodule that becomes hemorrhagic/necrotic after a few days from the eruption and resolves with a varioliform scar on a dyspigmented background [99]. The common sites of involvement are the trunk and extremities [100], although other locations have also been documented [101]. The literature suggests that cases of regional LyP featuring clusters of lesions localized to one anatomic region are more often found in the pediatric age group than in adults [101–103].

Histopathology

The histological features of LyP are variable, and depend in part on the age of the biopsied cutaneous lesions. Three histological subtypes (A, B, and C) are described, and these represent a spectrum of diseases with overlapping features.

LyP type A (histiocytic type) is the most common histologic manifestation, accounting for approximately 75% of LyP cases [102, 104]. A similar proportion was seen in a series of pediatric patients [99]. In fully developed cases, a wedge-shaped dermal infiltrate is seen. This consists of medium-sized to large pleomorphic or anaplastic lymphoid cells which may be scattered

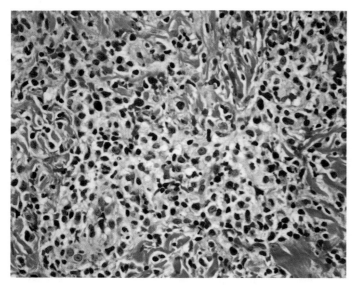

Fig. 26.2. Lymphomatoid papulosis, type A. Scattered or small clusters of large cells are intermingled with numerous mixed inflammatory cells (H&E stain).

or grouped in small clusters (Fig. 26.2). These tumor cells are of a large size and have irregular nuclei; multinucleated and Reed–Sternberg-like cells may be seen. Mitoses are usually numerous. Epidermotropism does not exclude the diagnosis. Numerous admixed inflammatory cells (neutrophils, eosinophils, lymphocytes, and histiocytes) are present. Cases with ulceration may display vasculitic changes and prominent upper dermal edema [105].

LyP type B (lymphocytic or mycosis-fungoides-like type) is least common (less than 10%), and features an epidermotropic infiltrate of small to medium-sized lymphoid cells with cerebriform nuclei reminiscent of those seen in MF.

LyP type C (ALCL-like type) consists of a nodular infiltrate of large, atypical lymphoid cells arranged in large cohesive sheets with only small numbers of admixed reactive inflammatory cells present. Differentiating LyP type C from primary cutaneous ALCL may be exceedingly difficult, with the diagnosis of the former becoming clear only after follow-up reveals spontaneous resolution of skin lesions.

It should be noted that various histologic manifestations of LyP lesions can be seen at the same time in the same patient. The most common association is between LyP types A and C [102].

Immunophenotype

The tumor cells of LyP types A and C share the same immunophenotype as tumor cells of C-ALCL in their reactivity for CD30 [106, 107]. The tumor cells represent a proliferation of activated mature T-helper cells, and usually display reactivity for CD3 and CD4. Activation markers such as HLA-DR [108] and CD25 (interleukin-2 receptor) [109] are also positive. CD7 [108], CD8 [109], and CD56 [110] are negative. Most

cases appear to lack CD15 expression, but express cytotoxic molecules such as TIA-1 and granzyme B [109].

In contrast to the expression of CD30 in LyP type A and C cases, the small to medium-sized mycosis-fungoides-like tumor cells of LyP type B are usually negative for CD30.

Prognosis and predictive factors

The duration of the disease is variable; most patients have chronic, recurrent crops of lesions for months to years. The significance of this condition is the potential for development of non-lymphoid malignancies (relative risk 3.11) and malignant lymphomas (relative risk 13.33) [111]. Nijsten's study of 35 childhood cases of LyP also showed a significantly increased risk of developing non-Hodgkin lymphoma as compared to the general population [99]. These data support the practice of life-long monitoring of these patients, even in the absence of skin lesions.

Therapy

The treatment options for LyP depend on the degree of skin involvement. Patients with few localized lesions could be clinically observed or treated with topical corticosteroids or immunomodulators. Diffuse lesions may require a more aggressive approach such as PUVA light therapy [112] or systemic medication with low-dose methotrexate [113]. These modalities are not curative, but helpful in achieving remission; recurrences are noted shortly after therapy discontinuation in most patients.

Primary cutaneous anaplastic large cell lymphoma
Introduction/definition

Primary cutaneous anaplastic large cell lymphoma (C-ALCL) is a lymphoid neoplasm composed of large cells with an anaplastic, pleomorphic, or immunoblastic cytomorphology, with expression of CD30 by the majority (greater than 75%) of the tumor cells [94]. There should be no evidence of prior or concurrent lymphomatoid papulosis, MF, or any other form of a cutaneous lymphoma [94]. Cutaneous-ALCL is different clinically and biologically from systemic anaplastic large cell lymphoma (S-ALCL), from which it must be distinguished [114, 115].

Epidemiology

Cutaneous ALCL generally occurs in adults, and is rare in the pediatric age group [104, 114, 116–121]. In contrast, S-ALCL is a relatively common lymphoma in this age group, and has a propensity for cutaneous involvement. Cutaneous ALCL may be seen in HIV-infected individuals [114].

Clinical features

Patients have a history of rapidly growing, asymptomatic, solitary or multiple skin nodules/tumors with a violaceous color. Most lesions have a tendency to ulcerate [117].

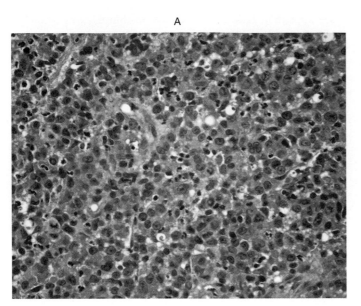
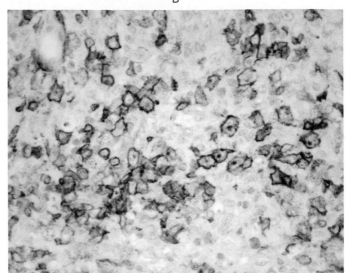

Fig. 26.3. Primary cutaneous anaplastic large cell lymphoma. (A) Cohesive sheets of large, anaplastic cells with admixed inflammatory cells (H&E stain). (B) CD30 is expressed by the majority of the tumor cells. In addition to membranous staining, some cells display a dot-like paranuclear Golgi staining pattern (immunoperoxidase stain for CD30).

Histopathology

The tumor consists of a diffuse, cohesive, and sheet-like infiltrate of large lymphoid cells which are CD30 positive. The infiltrate is dense, and usually extends through all levels of the dermis and often into the subcutis. In most cases, the tumor cells appear anaplastic, displaying eccentric, round/oval, or irregularly shaped nuclei and prominent nucleoli (Fig. 26.3A). The cytoplasm is abundant and eosinophilic, and prominent inclusion-like Golgi accentuation may be seen [114]. The background contains a scant inflammatory cell infiltrate. Less commonly, the tumor cells have a non-anaplastic (pleomorphic or immunoblastic) appearance [104, 122].

Immunophenotype

By definition, CD30 must be expressed by at least 75% of the large lymphoid tumor cells [2]. This is usually strong and diffuse, with a membranous and Golgi pattern of staining [114] (Fig. 26.3B). The tumor cells usually show an activated CD4-positive T-cell phenotype, with frequent expression of cytotoxic proteins (granzyme B, TIA-1, and perforin) [109, 123]. There may be variable loss of CD2, CD3, or CD5 expression [115]. Unlike S-ALCL, most C-ALCLs do not express epithelial membrane antigen (EMA) [115] or anaplastic lymphoma kinase (ALK-1) [124]. Clusterin may be expressed, but does not help to distinguish C-ALCL from S-ALCL [125, 126]. CD99 staining may be positive [114]. Unlike Reed–Sternberg cells of classical Hodgkin lymphoma, staining for CD15 is usually negative [120]. CD56 expression may be observed, but does not appear to have any prognostic significance [119, 127].

Genetics

The t(2;5)(p23;q35) translocation, characteristically seen in S-ALCL, is not usually found in C-ALCL [128], although a case report to the contrary exists [119].

Prognosis and predictive factors

The prognosis is very favorable, with an estimated survival of >90% at five years. A large number of pediatric cases resolve spontaneously without any intervention [129]. Skin manifestation only without extracutaneous spread is considered to be associated with better prognosis.

Therapy

When intervention is warranted, topical or intralesional corticosteroids, local excision and/or radiotherapy may be employed [104].

Subcutaneous panniculitis-like T-cell lymphoma

Introduction/definition

Subcutaneous panniculitis-like T-cell lymphoma (SPTCL) is a T-cell lymphoma which preferentially involves the subcutaneous tissue. The category of SPTCL in the 2005 WHO/EORTC classification refers specifically to cases with an αβ T-cell phenotype; cases with a γδ T-cell phenotype are excluded from this category and included instead in the category of cutaneous γδ T-cell lymphomas [2] (see below).

A

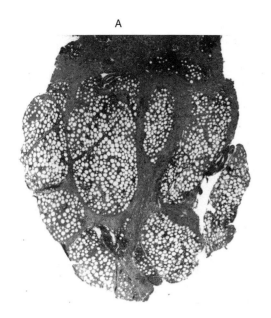

B

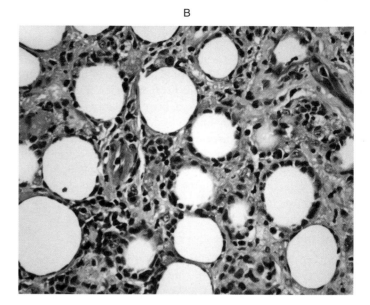

C

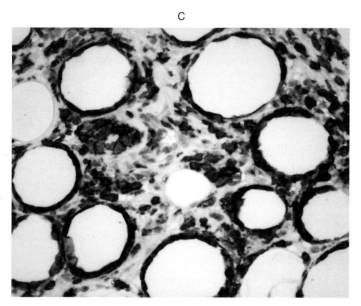

Fig. 26.4. Subcutaneous panniculitis-like T-cell lymphoma. (A) The lymphomatoid infiltrate predominantly involves the adipose lobules of the subcutis (H&E stain). (B) Neoplastic lymphoid cells rim the adipocytes in a lace-like pattern (H&E stain). (C) CD8 is usually positive in cases with an αβ+ phenotype (immunoperoxidase stain for CD8).

Epidemiology

Due to the evolving classification of this condition, it is difficult to estimate the exact incidence of the condition.

Clinical features

Patients present with acute or recurrent episodes of red-violaceous, deep and tender skin nodules, primarily on the lower extremities or the trunk [130]. The first episode is clinically indistinguishable from other panniculitides. Occasionally, individual nodules may ulcerate. Mild constitutional symptoms may accompany the skin lesions. The episodes last for a few weeks and resolve either spontaneously or with therapy.

Histopathology

It is characterized by a lobular subcutaneous infiltrate composed of an admixture of pleomorphic small, medium, to large lymphoid cells (Fig. 26.4A). The individual lymphoid cells have rounded nuclei with variably irregular nuclear contours, inconspicuous nucleoli, and a moderate amount of pale-staining eosinophilic cytoplasm. The neoplastic lymphoid cells characteristically rim individual adipocytes (Fig. 26.4B), but this feature is not specific and may be seen in other lymphoproliferative disorders involving the skin [131]. Karyorrhexis and necrosis, including fat necrosis, are common. Admixed reactive histiocytes with vacuolated cytoplasm are frequently present, may form a granulomatous reaction, and often contain phagocytosed red blood cells and other cellular debris [132]. These histiocytes are often referred to as "bean bag histiocytes" [133]. Vasculopathic changes range from a pauci-inflammatory thrombogenic vasculopathy to a lymphomatoid vasculitis featuring prominent lymphocytic angioinvasion with mural and luminal fibrin [134]. The lymphoid infiltrate is usually confined to the subcutaneous tissue; focal extension into the overlying lower dermis may be present, but should not be extensive. The epidermis is typically uninvolved. The lymphoid infiltrate in early phases of the disease may be mild, with corresponding absence of significant cytologic atypia, phagocytosis, and fat necrosis, and may be deemed to be an atypical lymphocytic lobular panniculitis representing a preneoplastic subcutaneous lymphoid dyscrasia [135, 136].

Immunophenotype

The neoplastic lymphoid cells are derived from mature post-thymic cytotoxic T-cells of the adaptive immune system, and hence are usually CD3 and CD8 positive (Fig. 26.4C), with expression of cytotoxic molecules including granzyme B, perforin, and T-cell intracellular antigen (TIA-1) [132, 137]. CD4 is negative, and there may be aberrant loss of expression of CD5, CD7, and CD3 [46, 138, 139]. CD30, CD56, and CD57 are negative.

Genetic features

The neoplastic T-cells show clonal T-cell receptor gene rearrangements. They are, in the vast majority of cases, negative for Epstein–Barr virus (EBV) sequences [132, 137], although EBV genetic material has been found in some cases [140].

Prognosis and predictive factors

Dissemination to lymph nodes and other organs is uncommon, and occurs late in the clinical course of the disease. Patients generally have an indolent, waxing and waning clinical course, and may achieve remission with combination chemotherapy [141]. A hemophagocytic syndrome may be a complication, and usually precipitates a fulminant downhill clinical course.

Therapy

The need for therapy is difficult to assess from the existing literature. Although, traditionally, various combination systemic chemotherapeutic agents have been used, most patients probably do not require aggressive intervention. Systemic corticosteroids have been used successfully to alleviate symptoms. More recently, the use of cyclosporine led to long-term remission in two children [142].

Extranodal NK/T-cell lymphoma, nasal type

Extranodal NK/T-cell lymphoma, nasal type, is an EBV-positive lymphoma of small, medium-sized or large cells usually with an NK-cell, or more rarely a cytotoxic T-cell, phenotype [143]. Skin is the second most common site of involvement after the nasal cavity/nasopharynx, and skin involvement may be a primary or secondary manifestation of the disease [144]. This entity occurs predominantly in adults [145, 146], with a male–female ratio of 3 : 2 [143]. The literature contains a small number of possible cases occurring in the pediatric age group [147–149]. Histologically, there is a dense dermal infiltrate of usually medium-sized tumor cells, with prominent angiocentricity and angiodestruction with zonal necrosis. Subcutaneous extension is common. Most cases demonstrate a NK-cell lineage with expression of CD2, CD7, cytoplasmic CD3 and CD56, and absence of surface CD3 and CD5, and no evidence of clonal TCR gene rearrangements. There is expression of cytotoxic granule proteins (TIA-1, granzyme B, and perforin). LMP-1 is inconsistently expressed, and EBER-ISH is preferred for diagnosis.

Hydroa vacciniforme-like cutaneous T-cell lymphoma

Introduction/definition

Hydroa vacciniforme-like cutaneous T-cell lymphoma (HV-like CTCL) is a rare pediatric EBV-associated lymphoma of CD8-positive cytotoxic T-cells clinically resembling hydroa vacciniforme, seen predominantly in Asia and Latin America [150–153]. In the 2005 WHO/EORTC classification, this entity is regarded as a variant of extranodal NK/T-cell lymphoma.

Epidemiology

In contrast to the nasal type, extranodal NK/T-cell lymphoma, HV-like CTCL affects children and teenagers. Virtually all reported cases originate from Asia [152] and Latin America [150, 153]. Boys and girls are affected in equal numbers [154].

Clinical features

Presentation is with impressive cutaneous vesiculopapular eruptions. There is an evolutionary course characterized by erythema, edema, blisters, ulcers, necrosis, crusts, and scars, with lesions seen mainly on the face and sometimes on the extremities [150]. There may be extensive tissue loss, resulting in severe scarring and disfigurement [153]. Fever, wasting, hepatosplenomegaly, and hypersensitivity to insect bites are common. Accompanying lymphadenopathy, which may be generalized, and visceral involvement may be present [150]. Some cases are accompanied by a hemophagocytic syndrome.

Histopathology

Histologically, there is a dense and diffuse infiltrate within the dermis, composed of atypical medium-sized lymphocytes. The depth of the lymphomatoid infiltrate corresponds to the evolution of the disease [150]. Advanced lesions may show deep subcutaneous involvement resembling that of lobular panniculitis [150]. Angiotropism and angioinvasion may be seen, and the infiltrate may also be seen to be perineural and periadnexal [153]. Ulceration is common.

Immunophenotype

The lymphomatous cells are cytotoxic T-cells which are most commonly positive for CD2, CD3, and CD8, and negative for CD4 [150]. Cytotoxic molecules are expressed. Aberrant loss of CD5 and CD7 is common. CD56 is variably positive. Expression of CD30 may be seen in a subset of activated cells. *In situ* hybridization for EBV-encoded RNA is positive [150, 154].

Prognosis

The prognosis is poor, with a two-year survival rate of 36% [150].

Therapy

Treatment of HV-like CTCL is unsatisfactory. Systemic corticosteroids used alone or in combination with other chemotherapeutic agents do not often lead to long-term remission [155].

Primary cutaneous peripheral T-cell lymphoma

Primary cutaneous aggressive epidermotropic CD8+ T-cell lymphoma

This is a provisional entity in the 2005 WHO/EORTC classification, and is characterized clinically by an aggressive course, and histologically by an infiltrate of epidermotropic CD8-positive cytotoxic T-cells [2]. Other well-defined CTCLs (more than half the cases of pagetoid reticulosis, and in rare cases of MF, LyP, and C-ALCL) may also have a CD8-positive cytotoxic T-cell phenotype; this entity is differentiated on the basis of clinical presentation and clinical behavior alone [40]. This entity is rare, and thus far, described largely in the adult population [40, 41].

Cutaneous γδ T-cell lymphoma

This is a provisional entity in the 2005 WHO/EORTC classification, and is defined as an EBV-negative lymphoma composed of a clonal proliferation of mature, activated cytotoxic gamma delta T-cells [2]. It includes a subset of entities, previously lumped under the category of SPTCLs, which have a gamma delta phenotype. Distinction between primary and secondary cutaneous cases is not useful as the prognosis is grim in both groups. Clinical presentation is similar to SPTCL, with large violaceous nodules/tumors or plaques with a tendency for ulceration. Diffuse involvement, including the mucosal membranes, rapid progression and deterioration, and hemophagocytosis as the final event, are clinical distinguishing features from SPTCL.

Primary cutaneous CD4+ small/medium-sized pleomorphic T-cell lymphoma

This is a provisional entity in the 2005 WHO/EORTC classification, and is defined by a predominance of small to medium-sized CD4-positive and CD30-negative pleomorphic T-cells, in patients without a clinical history of patches and plaques typical of MF [2]. The vast majority of cases are reported in adults [156–159], with a possible pediatric case of a 16-year-old female presenting with a localized tumor; however, no immunohistochemical details are provided on this case [158]. These lymphomas present with either solitary or multiple plaques or tumors on the head and neck or trunk. Histologically, there is a dense nodular or diffuse lymphomatoid infiltrate within the dermis, which may be perivascular or periadnexal. The individual lymphoid cells are small to medium-sized, pleomorphic, and have irregular, hyperchromatic nuclei and pale, scanty cytoplasm [156, 159]. The clinical course is favorable [156–159].

Primary cutaneous peripheral T-cell lymphoma, unspecified

This category is maintained for all other CTCLs which do not fall into any of the above categories. Like the three above provisional entities, pediatric cases are extremely rare.

Cutaneous B-cell lymphomas

Primary cutaneous marginal zone B-cell lymphoma

Introduction/definition

Primary cutaneous marginal zone B-cell lymphoma (PCMZL) is an indolent lymphoma composed of small B-cells, comprising marginal zone (centrocyte-like) cells, lymphoplasmacytoid cells, and plasma cells [1, 2]. PCMZL forms part of the broad category of extranodal marginal zone B-cell lymphomas involving mucosal sites, referred to as mucosa-associated lymphoid tissue (MALT) lymphomas.

Epidemiology

Most cases of PCMZL occur in adults. Only a few cases have been documented in the pediatric age group [160]. An association with *Borrelia burgdorferi* infection has been reported in some European cases of PCMZL [161, 162], but not in cases from Asia [163] and the United States [164]. The association between PCMZL and various microbial agents suggests a role of chronic and sustained stimulation of the immune system in the lymphoproliferative transformation [165]. A case of PCMZL in a 15-year-old atopic male with a history of chronic antihistamine use has been documented [166].

Clinical features

Patients present with solitary or multiple erythematous or violaceous papules, plaques, or tumors on the extremities and trunk.

Histopathology

Pathologically, PCMZL consists of a nodular to diffuse dermal lymphoid infiltrate which spares the epidermis. The infiltrate is composed of small lymphocytes, marginal zone (centrocyte-like) B-cells, lymphoplasmacytoid cells, and plasma cells, with admixed centroblast- or immunoblast-like cells and reactive T-cells. Reactive germinal centers are seen in early lesions, but become colonized by tumor cells as the disease progresses. Such germinal centers are usually surrounded by an interfollicular population of marginal zone B-cells [167] which feature irregular nuclei, inconspicuous nucleoli, and abundant, pale cytoplasm. The periphery of the infiltrates and the subepidermal region show the presence of lymphoplasmacytoid cells and plasma cells which are monotypic and may contain PAS-positive intranuclear pseudoinclusions, known as Dutcher bodies [167]. The presence of clusters of epithelioid histiocytes and occasional multinucleate giant cells has been described in a case report of an 11-year-old boy [168].

Immunophenotype

The neoplastic marginal zone B-cells express CD20, CD79a, CD19, and CD22 [1, 169]. CD43 may be positive [167]. CD5, CD10, BCL6, and CD23 are negative. The tumor cells are positive for BCL2 and negative for germinal center-associated antigens BCL6 and CD10, and this combination is useful in the diagnostic distinction from cutaneous follicle center lymphoma [170]. Native reactive germinal centers are composed of uniformly BCL6-positive, CD10-positive, and BCL2-negative centrocytes and centroblasts, with interspersed CD21-positive follicular dendritic cells. As the follicles are colonized in the course of disease progression, BCL6-negative and BCL2-positive neoplastic cells are seen to intermix with the native population of germinal center cells with an opposite BCL6 and BCL2 reactivity [170]. Further and more extensive neoplastic colonization leads to large and irregular aggregates of CD21-positive follicle dendritic cells, which correspond to histologic features of large, vague nodules or diffuse areas [170]. The lymphoplasmacytoid cells and plasma cells show monotypic expression of immunoglobulin light chains, and express CD138 and CD79a [2]. IRTA1 (immunoglobulin superfamily receptor translocation-associated 1) has been used as a diagnostic marker for extranodal marginal zone lymphomas [171].

Genetic features

Immunoglobulin heavy chain genes are clonally rearranged. Various cytogenetic abnormalities have been found in PCMZL, such as chromosomal translocations t(14;18)(q32;q21) [172] and t(3;14)(p14.1;q32) [173]. The most common translocation seen in gastric marginal zone B-cell lymphomas [t(11;18)(q21;q21) [174–176]] has not been identified in PCMZL [177]. *Fas* gene mutations are seen in a minority of cases [177]. *BCL10* mutations are not seen [177].

Prognosis and predictive factors

Data for the pediatric age group are scarce. Adult PCMZL has a favorable prognosis, with five-year survival rates of between 90 and 100% [169].

Therapy

Local excision of solitary lesions is usually curative. Multiple lesions can be treated with systemic corticosteroids, interferon-α or anti-CD20 antibodies [178, 179].

Primary cutaneous follicle centre lymphoma

Introduction/definition

Primary cutaneous follicle centre lymphoma (PCFCL) is a tumor of neoplastic follicle centre cells, usually a mixture of centrocytes (small and large cleaved cells) and centroblasts (large non-cleaved cells with prominent nucleoli). The growth pattern may be follicular, follicular and diffuse, or diffuse.

Epidemiology

It presents predominantly in middle-aged adults with no gender predominance. Much of the literature on PCFCL relates to adult disease. Only rare reports of cases in the pediatric age group exist [12, 180].

Clinical features

Patients typically present with red papules on the head and neck region or on the back. Extension of the lesions can be seen around the primary one in a centrifugal pattern [181]. Ulceration is uncommon.

Histopathology

PCFCL consists of a dermal infiltrate with epidermal sparing and variable subcutaneous extension. The architecture is follicular, follicular and diffuse, or diffuse. Neoplastic cells consist of centrocytes (small or large) and centroblasts. Small and early lesions more frequently consist of small centrocytes with a predominantly follicular architecture, and reactive T-lymphocytes may be numerous. More advanced lesions more frequently consist of large centrocytes (which may be multilobated) and centroblasts.

Immunophenotype

The neoplastic cells express CD20 and CD79a. There is consistent expression of BCL6 [170, 182]. CD5 and CD43 are negative. In contrast to nodal and secondary cutaneous follicular lymphomas, expression of BCL2 is negative or very focal and faint [181, 183]. In contrast to leg-type primary cutaneous large B-cell lymphoma, staining for MUM-1 is negative [184]. In cases where follicular structures are present, CD21-positive and CD35-positive follicular dendritic cells may be seen.

Genetic features

Clonally rearranged immunoglobulin genes are present. *BCL2* gene rearrangement and t(14;18) chromosomal translocation are absent in most but not all cases [185, 186].

Prognosis and predictive factors

Information pertaining to the pediatric age group is scant. The literature indicates a favorable prognosis in adult cases [187]. Cytologic grade and architecture do not appear to affect the prognosis.

Therapy

Excision or local radiotherapy is recommended. Systemic therapy is rarely necessary [5].

Primary cutaneous diffuse large B-cell lymphoma

Primary cutaneous diffuse large B-cell lymphoma (PCDL-BCL) characteristically presents with skin lesions on the legs [188–191], hence the designation "*leg type*" in the 2005 WHO/EORTC classification. These lesions are not seen in the pediatric population.

Intravascular large B-cell lymphoma

Intravascular large B-cell lymphoma is a subtype of large B-cell lymphoma which is defined by the accumulation of large, neoplastic B-lymphoid cells only within the lumina of blood vessels, mainly capillaries [192]. There is preferential involvement of the central nervous system, lungs, and skin. These lesions almost exclusively affect adult patients [192–197]. The youngest patient reported was a 19-year-old female with indurated erythematous-violaceous plaques on the left shoulder and mammary regions, who had a rapidly fatal clinical course [198].

Precursor hematologic neoplasm

CD4+/CD56+ hematodermic neoplasm (blastic NK-cell lymphoma)

Introduction/definition

CD4+/CD56+ hematodermic neoplasm (HDN) is a rare but distinct and clinically aggressive hematologic malignancy, with a high incidence of cutaneous involvement and high risk of leukemic dissemination. Although the blastic cytomorphology and CD56 positivity was previously thought to suggest an NK-precursor origin [199], more recent studies point towards derivation from a plasmacytoid dendritic cell precursor [200–202].

Epidemiology

Around 150 well-documented cases of HDN have been reported in the literature [201]. It primarily affects elderly patients, but a few cases have been reported in childhood and young adulthood [146, 201, 203, 204]. The male–female ratio is 3 : 1 [201].

Clinical features

Cutaneous lesions are present in over 90% of the cases before the hematologic spread, and consist of single or multiple papules/tumors or plaques with a violaceous or bruise-like appearance. Ulceration is not common. Mucosal lesions have been reported.

Histopathology

Hematodermic neoplasm forms a diffusely dermal, non-epidermotropic, dense, monotonous infiltrate of medium-sized, blast-like cells with finely dispersed powdery chromatin, indistinct nucleoli, and sparse cytoplasm [202, 205, 206]. Mitotic figures are numerous. Inflammatory cells do not accompany the neoplastic cells, and there is usually absence of necrosis and angioinvasion. In contrast to many NK- and NK-like T-cell disorders, azurophilic cytoplasmic granules are absent or inconspicuous [205].

Immunophenotype

The tumor cells of HDN are characterized by the expression of CD4 and CD56 in the absence of lineage-specific markers of T-cells, B-cells, or myelomonocytic cells. Expression of EBV antigens, myeloperoxidase, lysozyme, CD20, CD22, PAX-5, and T-cell receptor protein exclude a diagnosis of HDN [201]. CD43, HLA-DR, and CD45RA, also expressed by B-cells and naïve T-cells, are expressed in most cases [201]. Expression of CD123 and TCL1 (T-cell leukemia 1) by the tumor cells of HDN support a relationship to dendritic cells [207, 208]. There is variable expression of TdT, CD7, CD33, CD36, CD68, CD94, and CD99 [201].

Genetic features

T-cell receptor genes are in germline configuration [1, 2]. There is no association with EBV [1, 2]. Karyotypic analysis often shows complex aberrations, with the most frequently observed being deletion of 5q. Other less common aberrations are alterations of 13q, 12p, and 6q, and losses of chromosomes 15 and 9 [205, 206, 209, 210].

Prognosis and predictive factors

The prognosis for patients with HDN is grim, with an overall median survival of a year. Long-lasting remissions have rarely been reported in younger patients receiving acute leukemia-type induction therapy followed by allogeneic stem cell transplantation [201, 211, 212]. A majority of patients across all age groups show an initial response to multiagent chemotherapy but relapse within the first year. Patients with single isolated skin lesions may have a better prognosis.

A

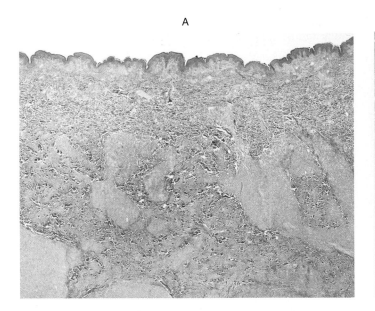

B

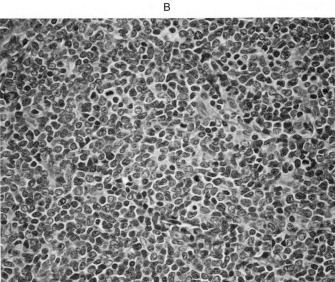

C

Fig. 26.5. Precursor lymphoblastic leukemia/lymphoma. (A) The neoplastic infiltrate involves the dermis and subcutis with sparing of the epidermis (H&E stain). (B) There is a diffuse infiltrate of monomorphic medium-sized lymphoid cells with fine chromatin. Mitoses are numerous (H&E stain). (C) The majority of cells display nuclear staining for TdT (immunoperoxidase stain for terminal deoxynucleotidyl transferase).

Therapy

Affected patients require treatment with combination chemotherapy.

Other lymphomas with frequent cutaneous involvement

Precursor T- and B-lymphoblastic leukemia/lymphoma

Introduction/definition

Precursor lymphoblastic leukemia/lymphoma is a malignancy derived from precursor cells of either T-cell or B-cell lineage in which tumor cells show expression of terminal deoxy-nucleotidyl transferase (TdT). Patients may present with disease primarily in the bone marrow and peripheral blood (leukemia) or in solid tissues (lymphoma).

Epidemiology

Skin is the most common site of extranodal involvement [213]. Precursor B-cell lymphoblastic malignancies are more common in skin than those of precursor T-cell origin [214–216], which more commonly involve lymph nodes and mediastinum.

Clinical features

The head and neck region is the most commonly involved site [215, 217]. The cutaneous lesions take the form of soft erythematous or violaceous papules or nodules. Ulceration is uncommon.

Histopathology

The neoplastic infiltrate is composed of a dense, diffuse, monomorphous infiltrate located in the entire dermis and subcutaneous fat, which may dissect through collagen and skeletal muscle fibers [213] (Fig. 26.5A). The epidermis is usually not involved, and a Grenz zone may be apparent. A "starry sky" pattern is common, and the tumor cells have been described as being aligned in a "mosaic-like" fashion [215]. Cytologically, the tumor cells are blastic [213] and medium-sized, with round or convoluted nuclei, fine chromatin, inconspicuous nucleoli, and scant cytoplasm [215] (Fig. 26.5B). Mitoses, including atypical forms, are characteristically numerous. Crush artifact and the Azzopardi effect may be common in biopsies [213].

Immunophenotype

T-cell lymphoblastic leukemia/lymphoma

The tumor cells are positive for TdT (Fig. 26.5C), CD43, BCL2, and CD99 [215]. CD7 is nearly always positive [218]. There is variable expression of CD1a, CD2, CD3, CD4, CD5, CD8, and CD10 [215].

B-cell lymphoblastic leukemia/lymphoma

The tumor cells are positive for TdT, CD43, BCL2, and CD99 [215, 219]. CD79a is more useful than CD20 for delineating the B-cell phenotype [215]. An erroneous diagnosis of Ewing sarcoma should not be made on the basis of this tumor's positivity for CD99 and negativity for leukocyte common antigen (LCA) [220]. Indeed, CD99 positivity is useful for distinguishing this tumor from other B-cell lymphomas.

The clinical approach to diagnosis

All pediatric patients with suspected cutaneous lymphoma should undergo a thorough history, physical examination, and investigations to confirm the diagnosis and to rule out systemic involvement [221]. Whenever possible, at least two skin biopsies should be collected; one for standard hematoxylin and eosin, and the other for specific markers and clonality. It is important, whenever possible, to collect specimens from skin lesions that received no therapy for at least two weeks. Clonal expansion studies are more reliable if a generous number of cells are analyzed. In children where large-sized biopsies are not feasible, shave biopsies may be a useful alternative (the shave consists of removing an elongated, $\sim 1 \times 0.2$ cm thin piece of the skin with a blade). If morphological evaluation is suggestive of T-cell lymphoma, the immunohistochemistry panel should include staining for CD2, CD3, CD4, CD5, CD7, CD8, CD20, CD30, and CD45. Further studies with ALK-1, CD56, TIA-1, and granzyme B are dictated by the previous positive stains. Dermal infiltrates beneath the Grenz zone suggest a B-cell morphology. Additional staining for HTLV-1, myeloperoxidase, kappa, lambda, BCL2, BCL6, CD10, MUM-1, and EBER-1 may need to be performed to further delineate the diagnosis.

Blood investigations consist of a complete blood count, blood smear for Sézary syndrome, a general chemistry panel, and lactic dehydrogenase. A chest X-ray, and ultrasound examinations of the abdomen and pelvis will screen for systemic involvement of patients with no clinical lymphadenopathy or organomegaly. When clinically indicated (organomegaly or lymphadenopathy), or in cases of abnormal screening investigations, additional staging examinations should be performed that include bone marrow biopsy, a CT/MRI, and lymph node dissection. Etiological investigations such as EBV, HIV, HTLV-1, and HTLV-2 serology are also recommended.

References

1. LeBoit PE, Burg G, Weedon D, et al. (eds.). *World Health Organization Classification of Tumours: Pathology and Genetics of Skin Tumours*. Lyon: IARC Press; 2006.

2. Willemze R, Jaffe ES, Burg G, et al. WHO-EORTC classification for cutaneous lymphomas. *Blood*. 2005;**105**:3768–3785.

3. Burg G, Kempf W, Cozzio A, et al. WHO/EORTC classification of cutaneous lymphomas 2005: histological and molecular aspects. *Journal of Cutaneous Pathology*. 2005;**32**:647–674.

4. Jaffe ES, Harris NL, Stein H, Vardiman JW. *Pathology and Genetics of Tumours of Haematopoietic and Lymphoid Tissues*. Lyon: IARC Press; 2001.

5. Willemze R, Kerl H, Sterry W, et al. EORTC classification for primary cutaneous lymphomas: a proposal from the Cutaneous Lymphoma Study Group of the European Organization for Research and Treatment of Cancer. *Blood*.1997;**90**:354–371.

6. Kadin ME. Latest lymphoma classification is skin deep. *Blood*. 2005;**105**:3759.

7. Weinstock MA, Horm JW. Population-based estimate of survival and determinants of prognosis in patients with mycosis fungoides. *Cancer*. 1988;**62**:1658–1661.

8. Weinstock MA, Gardstein B. Twenty-year trends in the reported incidence of mycosis fungoides and associated mortality. *American Journal of Public Health*. 1999;**89**:1240–1244.

9. Wain EM, Orchard GE, Whittaker SJ, Spittle M, Russell-Jones R. Outcome in 34 patients with juvenile-onset mycosis fungoides: a clinical, immunophenotypic, and molecular study. *Cancer*. 2003;**98**:2282–2290.

10. Crowley JJ, Nikko A, Varghese A, Hoppe RT, Kim YH. Mycosis fungoides in young patients: clinical characteristics and outcome. *Journal of the American Academy of Dermatology*. 1998;**38**:696–701.

11. Criscione VD, Weinstock MA. Incidence of cutaneous T-cell lymphoma in the United States, 1973–2002. *Archives of Dermatology*. 2007;**143**:854–859.

12. Fink-Puches R, Chott A, Ardigo M, et al. The spectrum of cutaneous lymphomas in patients less than

20 years of age. *Pediatric Dermatology.* 2004;**21**:525–533.

13. Koch SE, Zackheim HS, Williams ML, Fletcher V, LeBoit PE. Mycosis fungoides beginning in childhood and adolescence. *Journal of the American Academy of Dermatology.* 1987;**17**: 563–570.

14. Peters MS, Thibodeau SN, White JW. Jr., Winkelmann RK. Mycosis fungoides in children and adolescents. *Journal of the American Academy of Dermatology.* 1990;**22**:1011–1018.

15. Zackheim HS, McCalmont TH, Deanovic FW, Odom RB. Mycosis fungoides with onset before 20 years of age. *Journal of the American Academy of Dermatology.* 1997;**36**:557–562.

16. van Doorn R, Van Haselen CW, van Voorst Vader PC, *et al.* Mycosis fungoides: disease evolution and prognosis of 309 Dutch patients. *Archives of Dermatology.* 2000;**136**: 504–510.

17. Zackheim HS, Amin S, Kashani-Sabet M, McMillan A. Prognosis in cutaneous T-cell lymphoma by skin stage: long-term survival in 489 patients. *Journal of the American Academy of Dermatology.* 1999;**40**: 418–425.

18. Tan ES, Tang MB, Tan SH. Retrospective 5-year review of 131 patients with mycosis fungoides and Sezary syndrome seen at the National Skin Centre, Singapore. *The Australasian Journal of Dermatology.* 2006;**47**:248–252.

19. Tan E, Tay YK, Giam YC. Profile and outcome of childhood mycosis fungoides in Singapore. *Pediatric Dermatology.* 2000;**17**:352–356.

20. Zackheim HS, McCalmont TH. Mycosis fungoides: the great imitator. *Journal of the American Academy of Dermatology.* 2002;**47**:914–918.

21. Zackheim HS. Treatment of mycosis fungoides/Sezary syndrome: the University of California, San Francisco (UCSF) approach. *International Journal of Dermatology.* 2003;**42**:53–56.

22. Pimpinelli N, Olsen EA, Santucci M, *et al.* Defining early mycosis fungoides. *Journal of the American Academy of Dermatology.* 2005;**53**:1053–1063.

23. Ben-Amitai D, Michael D, Feinmesser M, Hodak E. Juvenile mycosis fungoides diagnosed before 18 years of age. *Acta Dermato-Venereologica.* 2003; **83**:451–456.

24. Quaglino P, Zaccagna A, Verrone A, Dardano F, Bernengo MG. Mycosis fungoides in patients under 20 years of age: report of 7 cases, review of the literature and study of the clinical course. *Dermatology.* 1999;**199**:8–14.

25. Neuhaus IM, Ramos-Caro FA, Hassanein AM. Hypopigmented mycosis fungoides in childhood and adolescence. *Pediatric Dermatology.* 2000;**17**:403–406.

26. Abha G, Lam J, Weitzman S, Pope E. Cutaneous T-cell lymphoma (CTCL) in children: report from an international registry (abstract). *Pediatric Blood and Cancer.* 2006;**46**:846 (A37).

27. Werner B, Brown S, Ackerman AB. "Hypopigmented mycosis fungoides" is not always mycosis fungoides! *The American Journal of Dermatopathology.* 2005;**27**:56–67.

28. Liu V, McKee PH. Cutaneous T-cell lymphoproliferative disorders: approach for the surgical pathologist: recent advances and clarification of confused issues. *Advances in Anatomic Pathology.* 2002;**9**:79–100.

29. Smoller BR, Santucci M, Wood G, Whittaker SJ. Histopathology and genetics of cutaneous T-cell lymphoma. *Hematology/Oncology Clinics of North America.* 2003;**17**:1277–1311.

30. Smoller BR, Detwiler SP, Kohler S, Hoppe RT, Kim YH. Role of histology in providing prognostic information in mycosis fungoides. *Journal of Cutaneous Pathology.* 1998;**25**:311–315.

31. Sanchez JL, Ackerman AB. The patch stage of mycosis fungoides. Criteria for histologic diagnosis. *The American Journal of Dermatopathology.* 1979;**1**: 5–26.

32. Massone C, Kodama K, Kerl H, Cerroni L. Histopathologic features of early (patch) lesions of mycosis fungoides: a morphologic study on 745 biopsy specimens from 427 patients. *The American Journal of Surgical Pathology.* 2005;**29**:550–560.

33. Nickoloff BJ. Light-microscopic assessment of 100 patients with patch/plaque-stage mycosis fungoides. *The American Journal of Dermatopathology.* 1988;**10**:469–477.

34. Horiuchi Y, Tone T, Umezawa A, Takezaki S. Large cell mycosis fungoides at the tumor stage. Unusual T8, T4, T6 phenotypic expression. *The American Journal of Dermatopathology.* 1988;**10**:54–58.

35. Cerroni L, Rieger E, Hodl S, Kerl H. Clinicopathologic and immunologic features associated with transformation of mycosis fungoides to large-cell lymphoma. *American Journal of Surgical Pathology.* 1992;**16**:543–552.

36. Salhany KE, Cousar JB, Greer JP, *et al.* Transformation of cutaneous T cell lymphoma to large cell lymphoma. A clinicopathologic and immunologic study. *American Journal of Pathology.* 1988;**132**:265–277.

37. Vergier B, de Muret A, Beylot-Barry M, *et al.* Transformation of mycosis fungoides: clinicopathological and prognostic features of 45 cases. French Study Group of Cutaneous Lymphomas. *Blood.* 2000;**95**:2212–2218.

38. Diamandidou E, Colome-Grimmer M, Fayad L, Duvic M, Kurzrock R. Transformation of mycosis fungoides/ Sezary syndrome: clinical characteristics and prognosis. *Blood.* 1998;**92**:1150–1159.

39. Olsen E, Vonderheid E, Pimpinelli N, *et al.* Revisions to the staging and classification of mycosis fungoides and Sezary syndrome: a proposal of the International Society for Cutaneous Lymphomas (ISCL) and the Cutaneous Lymphoma Task Force of the European Organization of Research and Treatment of Cancer (EORTC). *Blood.* 2007;**110**:1713–1722.

40. Agnarsson BA, Vonderheid EC, Kadin ME. Cutaneous T cell lymphoma with suppressor/cytotoxic (CD8) phenotype: identification of rapidly progressive and chronic subtypes. *Journal of the American Academy of Dermatology.* 1990;**22**:569–577.

41. Berti E, Tomasini D, Vermeer MH, *et al.* Primary cutaneous CD8-positive epidermotropic cytotoxic T cell lymphomas. A distinct clinicopathological entity with an aggressive clinical behavior. *The American Journal of Pathology.* 1999; **155**:483–492.

42. Whittam LR, Calonje E, Orchard G, *et al.* CD8-positive juvenile onset mycosis fungoides: an immunohistochemical and genotypic analysis of six cases. *The British Journal of Dermatology.* 2000;**143**:1199–1204.

43. **Lu D, Patel KA, Duvic M, Jones D.** Clinical and pathological spectrum of CD8-positive cutaneous T-cell lymphomas. *Journal of Cutaneous Pathology.* 2002;**29**:465–472.

44. **El-Shabrawi-Caelen L, Cerroni L, Medeiros LJ, McCalmont TH.** Hypopigmented mycosis fungoides: frequent expression of a CD8+ T-cell phenotype. *The American Journal of Surgical Pathology.* 2002;**26**:450–457.

45. **Hodak E, David M, Maron L,** *et al.* CD4/CD8 double-negative epidermotropic cutaneous T-cell lymphoma: an immunohistochemical variant of mycosis fungoides. *Journal of the American Academy of Dermatology.* 2006;**55**:276–284.

46. **Santucci M, Pimpinelli N, Massi D,** *et al.* Cytotoxic/natural killer cell cutaneous lymphomas. Report of EORTC Cutaneous Lymphoma Task Force Workshop. *Cancer.* 2003;**97**: 610–627.

47. **Ohshima A, Tokura Y, Misawa J, Yagi H, Takigawa M.** Erythrodermic cutaneous T-cell lymphoma with CD8+CD56+ leukaemic T cells in a young woman. *The British Journal of Dermatology.* 2003;**149**:891–893.

48. **Wain EM, Orchard GE, Mayou S,** *et al.* Mycosis fungoides with a CD56+ immunophenotype. *Journal of the American Academy of Dermatology.* 2005;**53**:158–163.

49. **Karenko L, Hyytinen E, Sarna S, Ranki A.** Chromosomal abnormalities in cutaneous T-cell lymphoma and in its premalignant conditions as detected by G-banding and interphase cytogenetic methods. *The Journal of Investigative Dermatology.* 1997;**108**:22–29.

50. **Fung MA, Murphy MJ, Hoss DM, Grant-Kels JM.** Practical evaluation and management of cutaneous lymphoma. *Journal of the American Academy of Dermatology.* 2002;**46**: 325–357; quiz, 58–60.

51. **Apisarnthanarax N, Talpur R, Ward S,** *et al.* Tazarotene 0.1% gel for refractory mycosis fungoides lesions: an open-label pilot study. *Journal of the American Academy of Dermatology.* 2004;**50**:600–607.

52. **de Quatrebarbes J, Esteve E, Bagot M,** *et al.* Treatment of early-stage mycosis fungoides with twice-weekly applications of mechlorethamine and topical corticosteroids: a prospective study. *Archives of Dermatology.* 2005; **141**:1117–1120.

53. **Deeths MJ, Chapman JT, Dellavalle RP, Zeng C, Aeling JL.** Treatment of patch and plaque stage mycosis fungoides with imiquimod 5% cream. *Journal of the American Academy of Dermatology.* 2005;**52**:275–280.

54. **Ramsay DL, Meller JA, Zackheim HS.** Topical treatment of early cutaneous T-cell lymphoma. *Hematology/ Oncology Clinics of North America.* 1995;**9**:1031–1056.

55. **Zackheim HS.** Topical carmustine (BCNU) for patch/plaque mycosis fungoides. *Seminars in Dermatology.* 1994;**13**:202–206.

56. **Zackheim HS.** Cutaneous T cell lymphoma: update of treatment. *Dermatology.* 1999;**199**:102– 105.

57. **Zackheim HS, Kashani-Sabet M, Amin S.** Topical corticosteroids for mycosis fungoides. Experience in 79 patients. *Archives of Dermatology.* 1998;**134**:949–954.

58. **van Doorn R, Scheffer E, Willemze R.** Follicular mycosis fungoides, a distinct disease entity with or without associated follicular mucinosis: a clinicopathologic and follow-up study of 51 patients. *Archives of Dermatology.* 2002;**138**:191–198.

59. **Hess Schmid M, Dummer R, Kempf W, Hilty N, Burg G.** Mycosis fungoides with mucinosis follicularis in childhood. *Dermatology.* 1999;**198**: 284–287.

60. **Gibson LE, Muller SA, Peters MS.** Follicular mucinosis of childhood and adolescence. *Pediatric Dermatology.* 1988;**5**:231–235.

61. **Gerami P, Rosen S, Kuzel T, Boone SL, Guitart J.** Folliculotropic mycosis fungoides: an aggressive variant of cutaneous T-cell lymphoma. *Archives of Dermatology.* 2008;**144**:738–746.

62. **Woringer F, Kolopp P.** Lésion érythémato-squameuse polyclique de l'avant-bras évoluant depuis 6 ans chez un garçonnet de 13 an: Histologiquement infiltrat intra-épidermique d'apparence tumorale. *Annales de Dermatologie et de Vénéréologie.*1939;**10**:945–958.

63. **Cohen EL.** Woringer–Kolopp disease (pagetoid reticulosis). *Clinical and Experimental Dermatology.* 1978; **3**:447–450.

64. **Jones RR, Chu A.** Pagetoid reticulosis and solitary mycosis fungoides. Distinct clinicopathological entities. *Journal of Cutaneous Pathology.* 1981;**8**:40–51.

65. **Mandojana RM, Helwig EB.** Localized epidermotropic reticulosis (Woringer-Kolopp disease). *Journal of the American Academy of Dermatology.* 1983;**8**:813–829.

66. **MacDonald DM.** Pagetoid reticulosis – is it a disease entity? *The British Journal of Dermatology.* 1982;**107**:603–604.

67. **Wood WS, Killby VA, Stewart WD.** Pagetoid reticulosis (Woringer-Kolopp disease). *Journal of Cutaneous Pathology.* 1979;**6**:113–123.

68. **Haghighi B, Smoller BR, LeBoit PE,** *et al.* Pagetoid reticulosis (Woringer-Kolopp disease): an immunophenotypic, molecular, and clinicopathologic study. *Modern Pathology.* 2000;**13**:502–510.

69. **Mielke V, Wolff HH, Winzer M, Sterry W.** Localized and disseminated pagetoid reticulosis. Diagnostic immunophenotypical findings. *Archives of Dermatology.* 1989;**125**:402–406.

70. **Burns MK, Chan LS, Cooper KD.** Woringer-Kolopp disease (localized pagetoid reticulosis) or unilesional mycosis fungoides? An analysis of eight cases with benign disease. *Archives of Dermatology.* 1995;**131**:325–329.

71. **Smoller BR, Stewart M, Warnke R.** A case of Woringer-Kolopp disease with Ki-1 (CD30)+ cytotoxic/suppressor cells. *Archives of Dermatology.* 1992; **128**:526–529.

72. **Drillenburg P, Bronkhorst CM, Van Der Wal AC,** *et al.* Expression of adhesion molecules in pagetoid reticulosis (Woringer-Kolopp disease). *The British Journal of Dermatology.*1997;**136**:613–616.

73. **LeBoit PE.** Granulomatous slack skin. *Dermatologic Clinics.* 1994; **12**:375–389.

74. **Tsang WY, Chan JK, Loo KT, Wong KF, Lee AW.** Granulomatous slack skin. *Histopathology.* 1994;**25**:49–55.

75. **Noto G, Pravata G, Miceli S, Arico M.** Granulomatous slack skin: report of a case associated with Hodgkin's disease and a review of the literature. *The British Journal of Dermatology.* 1994;**131**:275–279.

76. **LeBoit PE, Beckstead JH, Bond B,** *et al.* Granulomatous slack skin: clonal

rearrangement of the T-cell receptor beta gene is evidence for the lymphoproliferative nature of a cutaneous elastolytic disorder. *The Journal of Investigative Dermatology.* 1987;**89**:183–186.

77. **Convit J, Kerdel F, Goihman M, Rondon AJ, Soto JM.** Progressive, atrophying, chronic granulomatous dermohypodermitis. Autoimmune disease? *Archives of Dermatology.* 1973;**107**:271–274.

78. **Helm KF, Cerio R, Winkelmann RK.** Granulomatous slack skin: a clinicopathological and immunohistochemical study of three cases. *The British Journal of Dermatology.* 1992;**126**:142–147.

79. **Camacho FM, Burg G, Moreno JC, Campora RG, Villar JL.** Granulomatous slack skin in childhood. *Pediatric Dermatology.* 1997;**14**:204–208.

80. **DeGregorio R, Fenske NA, Glass LF.** Granulomatous slack skin: a possible precursor of Hodgkin's disease. *Journal of the American Academy of Dermatology.* 1995;**33**:1044–1047.

81. **Clarijs M, Poot F, Laka A, Pirard C, Bourlond A.** Granulomatous slack skin: treatment with extensive surgery and review of the literature. *Dermatology.* 2003;**206**:393–397.

82. **Vonderheid EC, Bernengo MG, Burg G,** *et al.* Update on erythrodermic cutaneous T-cell lymphoma: report of the International Society for Cutaneous Lymphomas. *Journal of the American Academy of Dermatology.* 2002;**46**: 95–106.

83. **Meister L, Duarte AM, Davis J, Perez JL, Schachner LA.** Sezary syndrome in an 11-year-old girl. *Journal of the American Academy of Dermatology.* 1993;**28**:93–95.

84. **LeBoit PE, Abel EA, Cleary ML,** *et al.* Clonal rearrangement of the T cell receptor beta gene in the circulating lymphocytes of erythrodermic follicular mucinosis. *Blood.* 1988;**71**: 1329–1333.

85. **Setoyama M, Katahira Y, Kanzaki T.** Clinicopathologic analysis of 124 cases of adult T-cell leukemia/lymphoma with cutaneous manifestations: the smouldering type with skin manifestations has a poorer prognosis than previously thought. *The Journal of Dermatology.* 1999;**26**:785–790.

86. **DiCaudo DJ, Perniciaro C, Worrell JT, White JW Jr., Cockerell CJ.** Clinical and histologic spectrum of human T-cell lymphotropic virus type I-associated lymphoma involving the skin. *Journal of the American Academy of Dermatology.* 1996;**34**:69–76.

87. **Nicot C.** Current views in HTLV-I-associated adult T-cell leukemia/ lymphoma. *American Journal of Hematology.* 2005;**78**:232– 239.

88. **Yamaguchi T, Ohshima K, Karube K,** *et al.* Clinicopathological features of cutaneous lesions of adult T-cell leukaemia/lymphoma. *The British Journal of Dermatology.* 2005;**152**: 76–81.

89. **Uchiyama T, Yodoi J, Sagawa K, Takatsuki K, Uchino H.** Adult T-cell leukemia: clinical and hematologic features of 16 cases. *Blood.* 1977;**50**: 481–492.

90. **Lin BT, Musset M, Szekely AM,** *et al.* Human T-cell lymphotropic virus-1-positive T-cell leukemia/lymphoma in a child. Report of a case and review of the literature. *Archives of Pathology & Laboratory Medicine.* 1997;**121**:1282– 1286.

91. **Bittencourt AL, Primo J, de Oliveira MF.** Manifestations of the human T-cell lymphotropic virus type I infection in childhood and adolescence. *Jornal de Pediatria.* 2006;**82**:411–420.

92. **Shimoyama M.** Diagnostic criteria and classification of clinical subtypes of adult T-cell leukaemia-lymphoma. A report from the Lymphoma Study Group (1984–87). *British Journal of Haematology.* 1991;**79**:428–437.

93. **Gerami P, Guitart J.** The spectrum of histopathologic and immunohistochemical findings in folliculotropic mycosis fungoides. *The American Journal of Surgical Pathology.* 2007;**31**:1430–1438.

94. **Willemze R, Beljaards RC.** Spectrum of primary cutaneous CD30 (Ki-1)-positive lymphoproliferative disorders. A proposal for classification and guidelines for management and treatment. *Journal of the American Academy of Dermatology.* 1993;**28**: 973–980.

95. **Magro CM, Crowson AN, Kovatich AJ, Burns F.** Drug-induced reversible lymphoid dyscrasia: a clonal lymphomatoid dermatitis of memory and activated T cells. *Human Pathology.* 2003;**34**:119–129.

96. **Kennedy MK, Willis CR, Armitage RJ.** Deciphering CD30 ligand biology and its role in humoral immunity. *Immunology.* 2006;**118**:143–152.

97. **Macaulay WL.** Lymphomatoid papulosis. A continuing self-healing eruption, clinically benign – histologically malignant. *Archives of Dermatology.* 1968;**97**:23–30.

98. **Wang HH, Lach L, Kadin ME.** Epidemiology of lymphomatoid papulosis. *Cancer.* 1992;**70**:2951–2957.

99. **Nijsten T, Curiel-Lewandrowski C, Kadin ME.** Lymphomatoid papulosis in children: a retrospective cohort study of 35 cases. *Archives of Dermatology.* 2004;**140**:306–312.

100. **Thomsen K, Wantzin GL.** Lymphomatoid papulosis. A follow-up study of 30 patients. *Journal of the American Academy of Dermatology.* 1987;**17**:632–636.

101. **Thomas GJ, Conejo-Mir JS, Ruiz AP,** *et al.* Lymphomatoid papulosis in childhood with exclusive acral involvement. *Pediatric Dermatology.* 1998;**15**:146–147.

102. **El Shabrawi-Caelen L, Kerl H, Cerroni L.** Lymphomatoid papulosis: reappraisal of clinicopathologic presentation and classification into subtypes A, B, and C. *Archives of Dermatology.* 2004;**140**:441–447.

103. **Scarisbrick JJ, Evans AV, Woolford AJ, Black MM, Russell-Jones R.** Regional lymphomatoid papulosis: a report of four cases. *The British Journal of Dermatology.* 1999;**141**:1125–1128.

104. **Bekkenk MW, Geelen FA, van Voorst Vader PC,** *et al.* Primary and secondary cutaneous CD30(+) lymphoproliferative disorders: a report from the Dutch Cutaneous Lymphoma Group on the long-term follow-up data of 219 patients and guidelines for diagnosis and treatment. *Blood.* 2000; **95**:3653–3661.

105. **Kempf W.** CD30+ lymphoproliferative disorders: histopathology, differential diagnosis, new variants, and simulators. *Journal of Cutaneous Pathology.* 2006; **33**(Suppl 1):58–70.

106. **Kadin ME.** Common activated helper-T-cell origin for lymphomatoid papulosis, mycosis fungoides, and some types of Hodgkin's disease. *Lancet.* 1985;**2**:864–865.

107. **Kaudewitz P, Burg G, Stein H**, *et al.* Monoclonal antibody patterns in lymphomatoid papulosis. *Dermatologic Clinics.* 1985;**3**:749–757.

108. **Varga FJ, Vonderheid EC, Olbricht SM, Kadin ME.** Immunohistochemical distinction of lymphomatoid papulosis and pityriasis lichenoides et varioliformis acuta. *The American Journal of Pathology.* 1990;**136**:979–987.

109. **Kummer JA, Vermeer MH, Dukers D, Meijer CJ, Willemze R.** Most primary cutaneous CD30-positive lymphoproliferative disorders have a CD4-positive cytotoxic T-cell phenotype. *The Journal of Investigative Dermatology.* 1997;**109**:636–640.

110. **Harvell J, Vaseghi M, Natkunam Y, Kohler S, Kim Y.** Large atypical cells of lymphomatoid papulosis are CD56-negative: a study of 18 cases. *Journal of Cutaneous Pathology.* 2002;**29**:88–92.

111. **Wang HH, Myers T, Lach LJ, Hsieh CC, Kadin ME.** Increased risk of lymphoid and nonlymphoid malignancies in patients with lymphomatoid papulosis. *Cancer.* 1999;**86**:1240–1245.

112. **Wantzin GL, Thomsen K.** PUVA-treatment in lymphomatoid papulosis. *The British Journal of Dermatology.* 1982;**107**:687–690.

113. **Lynch PJ, Saied NK.** Methotrexate treatment of pityriasis lichenoides and lymphomatoid papulosis. *Cutis.* 1979;**23**:634–636.

114. **Kumar S, Pittaluga S, Raffeld M**, *et al.* Primary cutaneous CD30-positive anaplastic large cell lymphoma in childhood: report of 4 cases and review of the literature. *Pediatric and Developmental Pathology.* 2005;**8**:52–60.

115. **de Bruin PC, Beljaards RC, van Heerde P**, *et al.* Differences in clinical behaviour and immunophenotype between primary cutaneous and primary nodal anaplastic large cell lymphoma of T-cell or null cell phenotype. *Histopathology.* 1993;**23**:127–135.

116. **Hazneci E, Aydin NE, Dogan G, Turhan IO.** Primary cutaneous anaplastic large cell lymphoma in a young girl. *Journal of the European Academy of Dermatology and Venereology.* 2001;**15**:366–367.

117. **Tomaszewski MM, Moad JC, Lupton GP.** Primary cutaneous Ki-1(CD30) positive anaplastic large cell lymphoma in childhood. *Journal of the American Academy of Dermatology.* 1999;**40**:857–861.

118. **Beljaards RC, Kaudewitz P, Berti E,** *et al.* Primary cutaneous CD30-positive large cell lymphoma: definition of a new type of cutaneous lymphoma with a favorable prognosis. A European Multicenter Study of 47 patients. *Cancer.* 1993;**71**:2097–2104.

119. **Gould JW, Eppes RB, Gilliam AC,** *et al.* Solitary primary cutaneous CD30+ large cell lymphoma of natural killer cell phenotype bearing the t(2;5)(p23;q35) translocation and presenting in a child. *The American Journal of Dermatopathology.* 2000;**22**:422–428.

120. **Kadin ME, Sako D, Berliner N,** *et al.* Childhood Ki-1 lymphoma presenting with skin lesions and peripheral lymphadenopathy. *Blood.* 1986;**68**:1042–1049.

121. **Nakamura S, Takagi N, Kojima M,** *et al.* Clinicopathologic study of large cell anaplastic lymphoma (Ki-1-positive large cell lymphoma) among the Japanese. *Cancer.* 1991;**68**:118–129.

122. **Paulli M, Berti E, Rosso R,** *et al.* CD30/Ki-1-positive lymphoproliferative disorders of the skin – clinicopathologic correlation and statistical analysis of 86 cases: a multicentric study from the European Organization for Research and Treatment of Cancer Cutaneous Lymphoma Project Group. *Journal of Clinical Oncology.* 1995;**13**:1343–1354.

123. **Kaudewitz P, Stein H, Dallenbach F,** *et al.* Primary and secondary cutaneous Ki-1+ (CD30+) anaplastic large cell lymphomas. Morphologic, immunohistologic, and clinical-characteristics. *The American Journal of Pathology.* 1989;**135**:359–367.

124. **Wood GS, Hardman DL, Boni R,** *et al.* Lack of the t(2;5) or other mutations resulting in expression of anaplastic lymphoma kinase catalytic domain in CD30+ primary cutaneous lymphoproliferative disorders and Hodgkin's disease. *Blood.* 1996;**88**:1765–1770.

125. **Lae ME, Ahmed I, Macon WR.** Clusterin is widely expressed in systemic anaplastic large cell lymphoma but fails to differentiate primary from secondary cutaneous anaplastic large cell lymphoma. *American Journal of Clinical Pathology.* 2002;**118**:773–779.

126. **Saffer H, Wahed A, Rassidakis GZ, Medeiros LJ.** Clusterin expression in malignant lymphomas: a survey of 266 cases. *Modern Pathology.* 2002;**15**:1221–1226.

127. **Natkunam Y, Warnke RA, Haghighi B**, *et al.* Co-expression of CD56 and CD30 in lymphomas with primary presentation in the skin: clinicopathologic, immunohistochemical and molecular analyses of seven cases. *Journal of Cutaneous Pathology.* 2000;**27**:392–399.

128. **DeCoteau JF, Butmarc JR, Kinney MC, Kadin ME.** The t(2;5) chromosomal translocation is not a common feature of primary cutaneous CD30+ lymphoproliferative disorders: comparison with anaplastic large-cell lymphoma of nodal origin. *Blood.* 1996;**87**:3437–3441.

129. **Liu HL, Hoppe RT, Kohler S,** *et al.* CD30+ cutaneous lymphoproliferative disorders: the Stanford experience in lymphomatoid papulosis and primary cutaneous anaplastic large cell lymphoma. *Journal of the American Academy of Dermatology.* 2003;**49**:1049–1058.

130. **Jaffe ES, Ralfkier E.** Subcutaneous panniculitis-like T cell lymphoma. In Jaffe ES, Harris NL, Stein H, Vardiman J. (eds.). *World Health Organization Classification of Tumours: Pathology and Genetics of Tumours of Haematopoietic and Lymphoid Tissues.* Lyon: IARC Press; 2001, 212–215.

131. **Lozzi GP, Massone C, Citarella L, Kerl H, Cerroni L.** Rimming of adipocytes by neoplastic lymphocytes: a histopathologic feature not restricted to subcutaneous T-cell lymphoma. *The American Journal of Dermatopathology.* 2006;**28**:9–12.

132. **Salhany KE, Macon WR, Choi JK,** *et al.* Subcutaneous panniculitis-like T-cell lymphoma: clinicopathologic, immunophenotypic, and genotypic analysis of alpha/beta and gamma/delta subtypes. *The American Journal of Surgical Pathology.* 1998;**22**:881–893.

133. **Ikeda E, Endo M, Uchigasaki S**, *et al.* Phagocytized apoptotic cells in subcutaneous panniculitis-like T-cell lymphoma. *Journal of the European Academy of Dermatology and Venereology.* 2001;**15**:159–162.

134. **Magro CM, Crowson AN, Mihm MCJ.** *The Cutaneous Lymphoid Proliferations: A Comprehensive Textbook of Lymphocytic Infiltrates of the Skin.* Hoboken, NJ: John Wiley & Sons, Inc.; 2007.

135. **Magro CM, Crowson AN, Byrd JC, Soleymani AD, Shendrik I.** Atypical lymphocytic lobular panniculitis. *Journal of Cutaneous Pathology.* 2004;**31**:300–306.

136. **Guitart J, Magro C.** Cutaneous T-cell lymphoid dyscrasia: a unifying term for idiopathic chronic dermatoses with persistent T-cell clones. *Archives of Dermatology.* 2007;**143**:921–932.

137. **Kumar S, Krenacs L, Medeiros J**, *et al.* Subcutaneous panniculitic T-cell lymphoma is a tumor of cytotoxic T lymphocytes. *Human Pathology.* 1998;**29**:397–403.

138. **Hoque SR, Child FJ, Whittaker SJ,** *et al.* Subcutaneous panniculitis-like T-cell lymphoma: a clinicopathological, immunophenotypic and molecular analysis of six patients. *The British Journal of Dermatology.* 2003;**148**:516–525.

139. **Massone C, Chott A, Metze D**, *et al.* Subcutaneous, blastic natural killer (NK), NK/T-cell, and other cytotoxic lymphomas of the skin: a morphologic, immunophenotypic, and molecular study of 50 patients. *The American Journal of Surgical Pathology.* 2004;**28**:719–735.

140. **Harada H, Iwatsuki K, Kaneko F.** Detection of Epstein-Barr virus genes in malignant lymphoma with clinical and histologic features of cytophagic histiocytic panniculitis. *Journal of the American Academy of Dermatology.* 1994;**31**:379–383.

141. **Go RS, Wester SM.** Immunophenotypic and molecular features, clinical outcomes, treatments, and prognostic factors associated with subcutaneous panniculitis-like T-cell lymphoma: a systematic analysis of 156 patients reported in the literature. *Cancer.* 2004;**101**:1404–1413.

142. **Shani-Adir A, Lucky AW, Prendiville J**, *et al.* Subcutaneous panniculitic T-cell lymphoma in children: response to combination therapy with cyclosporine and chemotherapy. *Journal of the American Academy of Dermatology.* 2004;**50**:S18–S22.

143. **Mraz-Gernhard S, Natkunam Y, Hoppe RT**, *et al.* Natural killer/natural killer-like T-cell lymphoma, CD56+, presenting in the skin: an increasingly recognized entity with an aggressive course. *Journal of Clinical Oncology.* 2001;**19**:2179–2188.

144. **Gniadecki R, Rossen K, Ralfkier E,** *et al.* CD56+ lymphoma with skin involvement: clinicopathologic features and classification. *Archives of Dermatology.* 2004;**140**:427–436.

145. **Stokkermans-Dubois J, Jouary T, Vergier B, Delaunay MM, Taieb A.** A case of primary cutaneous nasal type NK/T-cell lymphoma and review of the literature. *Dermatology.* 2006;**213**:345–349.

146. **Chan JK, Sin VC, Wong KF**, *et al.* Nonnasal lymphoma expressing the natural killer cell marker CD56: a clinicopathologic study of 49 cases of an uncommon aggressive neoplasm. *Blood.* 1997;**89**:4501–4513.

147. **Ko YH, Cho EY, Kim JE**, *et al.* NK and NK-like T-cell lymphoma in extranasal sites: a comparative clinicopathological study according to site and EBV status. *Histopathology.* 2004;**44**:480–489.

148. **Pol-Rodriguez MM, Fox LP, Sulis ML, Miller IJ, Garzon MC.** Extranodal nasal-type natural killer T-cell lymphoma in an adolescent from Bangladesh. *Journal of the American Academy of Dermatology.* 2006;**54**:S192–S197.

149. **Shaw PH, Cohn SL, Morgan ER**, *et al.* Natural killer cell lymphoma: report of two pediatric cases, therapeutic options, and review of the literature. *Cancer.* 2001;**91**:642–646.

150. **Barrionuevo C, Anderson VM, Zevallos-Giampietri E**, *et al.* Hydroa-like cutaneous T-cell lymphoma: a clinicopathologic and molecular genetic study of 16 pediatric cases from Peru. *Applied Immunohistochemistry & Molecular Morphology.* 2002;**10**:7–14.

151. **Chen HH, Hsiao CH, Chiu HC.** Hydroa vacciniforme-like primary cutaneous CD8-positive T-cell lymphoma. *The British Journal of Dermatology.* 2002;**147**:587–591.

152. **Iwatsuki K, Satoh M, Yamamoto T,** *et al.* Pathogenic link between hydroa vacciniforme and Epstein-Barr virus-associated hematologic disorders. *Archives of Dermatology.* 2006;**142**:587–595.

153. **Magana M, Sangueza P, Gil-Beristain J**, *et al.* Angiocentric cutaneous T-cell lymphoma of childhood (hydroa-like lymphoma): a distinctive type of cutaneous T-cell lymphoma. *Journal of the American Academy of Dermatology.* 1998;**38**:574–579.

154. **Cho KH, Kim CW, Lee DY**, *et al.* An Epstein-Barr virus-associated lymphoproliferative lesion of the skin presenting as recurrent necrotic papulovesicles of the face. *The British Journal of Dermatology.* 1996;**134**:791–796.

155. **Wu YH, Chen HC, Hsiao PF**, *et al.* Hydroa vacciniforme-like Epstein-Barr virus-associated monoclonal T-lymphoproliferative disorder in a child. *International Journal of Dermatology.* 2007;**46**:1081–1086.

156. **Friedmann D, Wechsler J, Delfau MH,** *et al.* Primary cutaneous pleomorphic small T-cell lymphoma. A review of 11 cases. The French Study Group on Cutaneous Lymphomas. *Archives of Dermatology.* 1995;**131**:1009–1015.

157. **Beljaards RC, Meijer CJ, Van Der Putte SC**, *et al.* Primary cutaneous T-cell lymphoma: clinicopathological features and prognostic parameters of 35 cases other than mycosis fungoides and CD30-positive large cell lymphoma. *The Journal of Pathology.* 1994;**172**:53–60.

158. **Sterry W, Siebel A, Mielke V.** HTLV-1-negative pleomorphic T-cell lymphoma of the skin: the clinicopathological correlations and natural history of 15 patients. *The British Journal of Dermatology.* 1992;**126**:456–462.

159. **von den Driesch P, Coors EA.** Localized cutaneous small to medium-sized pleomorphic T-cell lymphoma: a report of 3 cases stable for years. *Journal of the American Academy of Dermatology.* 2002;**46**:531–535.

160. **Taddesse-Heath L, Pittaluga S, Sorbara L**, *et al.* Marginal zone B-cell lymphoma in children and young adults. *The American Journal of Surgical Pathology.* 2003;**27**:522–531.

161. Cerroni L, Zochling N, Putz B, Kerl H. Infection by *Borrelia burgdorferi* and cutaneous B-cell lymphoma. *Journal of Cutaneous Pathology*. 1997;**24**:457–461.

162. Goodlad JR, Davidson MM, Hollowood K, *et al.* Primary cutaneous B-cell lymphoma and *Borrelia burgdorferi* infection in patients from the Highlands of Scotland. *The American Journal of Surgical Pathology*. 2000;**24**:1279–1285.

163. Li C, Inagaki H, Kuo TT, *et al.* Primary cutaneous marginal zone B-cell lymphoma: a molecular and clinicopathologic study of 24 asian cases. *The American Journal of Surgical Pathology*. 2003;**27**:1061–1069.

164. Wood GS, Kamath NV, Guitart J, *et al.* Absence of *Borrelia burgdorferi* DNA in cutaneous B-cell lymphomas from the United States. *Journal of Cutaneous Pathology*. 2001;**28**:502–507.

165. Suarez F, Lortholary O, Hermine O, Lecuit M. Infection-associated lymphomas derived from marginal zone B-cells: a model of antigen-driven lymphoproliferation. *Blood*. 2006;**107**:3034–3044.

166. Sroa N, Magro CM. Pediatric primary cutaneous marginal zone lymphoma: in association with chronic antihistamine use. *Journal of Cutaneous Pathology*. 2006;**33**(Suppl 2):1–5.

167. Baldassano MF, Bailey EM, Ferry JA, Harris NL, Duncan LM. Cutaneous lymphoid hyperplasia and cutaneous marginal zone lymphoma: comparison of morphologic and immunophenotypic features. *The American Journal of Surgical Pathology*. 1999;**23**:88–96.

168. Dargent JL, Devalck C, De Mey A, *et al.* Primary cutaneous marginal zone B-cell lymphoma of MALT type in a child. *Pediatric and Developmental Pathology*. 2006;**9**:468–473.

169. Cerroni L, Signoretti S, Hofler G, *et al.* Primary cutaneous marginal zone B-cell lymphoma: a recently described entity of low-grade malignant cutaneous B-cell lymphoma. *The American Journal of Surgical Pathology*. 1997;**21**:1307–1315.

170. de Leval L, Harris NL, Longtine J, Ferry JA, Duncan LM. Cutaneous b-cell lymphomas of follicular and marginal zone types: use of Bcl-6, CD10, Bcl-2, and CD21 in differential diagnosis and classification. *The American Journal of Surgical Pathology*. 2001;**25**:732–741.

171. Falini B, Tiacci E, Pucciarini A, *et al.* Expression of the IRTA1 receptor identifies intraepithelial and subepithelial marginal zone B-cells of the mucosa-associated lymphoid tissue (MALT). *Blood*. 2003;**102**:3684–3692.

172. Streubel B, Lamprecht A, Dierlamm J, *et al.* t(14;18)(q32;q21) involving IGH and MALT1 is a frequent chromosomal aberration in MALT lymphoma. *Blood*. 2003;**101**:2335–2339.

173. Streubel B, Vinatzer U, Lamprecht A, Raderer M, Chott A. t(3;14)(p14.1;q32) involving IGH and FOXP1 is a novel recurrent chromosomal aberration in MALT lymphoma. *Leukemia*. 2005;**19**:652–658.

174. Akagi T, Motegi M, Tamura A, *et al.* A novel gene, MALT1 at 18q21, is involved in t(11;18)(q21;q21) found in low-grade B-cell lymphoma of mucosa-associated lymphoid tissue. *Oncogene*. 1999;**18**:5785–5794.

175. Dierlamm J, Baens M, Wlodarska I, *et al.* The apoptosis inhibitor gene API2 and a novel 18q gene, MLT, are recurrently rearranged in the t(11;18)(q21;q21) associated with mucosa-associated lymphoid tissue lymphomas. *Blood*. 1999;**93**:3601–3609.

176. Morgan JA, Yin Y, Borowsky AD, *et al.* Breakpoints of the t(11;18)(q21;q21) in mucosa-associated lymphoid tissue (MALT) lymphoma lie within or near the previously undescribed gene MALT1 in chromosome 18. *Cancer Research*. 1999;**59**:6205–6213.

177. Gronbaek K, Ralfkiaer E, Kalla J, Skovgaard GL, Guldberg P. Infrequent somatic Fas mutations but no evidence of Bcl10 mutations or t(11;18) in primary cutaneous MALT-type lymphoma. *The Journal of Pathology*. 2003;**201**:134–140.

178. Soda R, Costanzo A, Cantonetti M, *et al.* Systemic therapy of primary cutaneous B-cell lymphoma, marginal zone type, with rituximab, a chimeric anti-CD20 monoclonal antibody. *Acta Dermato-Venereologica*. 2001;**81**:207–208.

179. Wollina U, Hahnfeld S, Kosmehl H. Primary cutaneous marginal center lymphoma – complete remission induced by interferon alpha2a. *Journal of Cancer Research and Clinical Oncology*. 1999;**125**:305–308.

180. Ghislanzoni M, Gambini D, Perrone T, Alessi E, Berti E. Primary cutaneous follicular center cell lymphoma of the nose with maxillary sinus involvement in a pediatric patient. *Journal of the American Academy of Dermatology*. 2005;**52**:S73–S75.

181. Cerroni L, Arzberger E, Putz B, *et al.* Primary cutaneous follicle center cell lymphoma with follicular growth pattern. *Blood*. 2000;**95**:3922–3928.

182. Hoefnagel JJ, Vermeer MH, Jansen PM, *et al.* Bcl-2, Bcl-6 and CD10 expression in cutaneous B-cell lymphoma: further support for a follicle centre cell origin and differential diagnostic significance. *The British Journal of Dermatology*. 2003;**149**:1183–1191.

183. Cerroni L, Volkenandt M, Rieger E, Soyer HP, Kerl H. bcl-2 protein expression and correlation with the interchromosomal 14;18 translocation in cutaneous lymphomas and pseudolymphomas. *The Journal of Investigative Dermatology*. 1994;**102**:231–235.

184. Hoefnagel JJ, Dijkman R, Basso K, *et al.* Distinct types of primary cutaneous large B-cell lymphoma identified by gene expression profiling. *Blood*. 2005;**105**:3671–3678.

185. Bergman R, Kurtin PJ, Gibson LE, *et al.* Clinicopathologic, immunophenotypic, and molecular characterization of primary cutaneous follicular B-cell lymphoma. *Archives of Dermatology*. 2001;**137**:432–439.

186. Streubel B, Scheucher B, Valencak J, *et al.* Molecular cytogenetic evidence of t(14;18)(IGH;BCL2) in a substantial proportion of primary cutaneous follicle center lymphomas. *The American Journal of Surgical Pathology*. 2006;**30**:529–536.

187. Aguilera NS, Tomaszewski MM, Moad JC, *et al.* Cutaneous follicle center lymphoma: a clinicopathologic study of 19 cases. *Modern Pathology*. 2001;**14**:828–835.

188. Vermeer MH, Geelen FA, van Haselen CW, *et al.* Primary cutaneous large B-cell lymphomas of the legs. A distinct type of cutaneous B-cell lymphoma with an intermediate prognosis. Dutch Cutaneous Lymphoma Working Group.

Archives of Dermatology. 1996;**132**: 1304–1308.

189. **Hallermann C, Niermann C, Fischer RJ, Schulze HJ.** New prognostic relevant factors in primary cutaneous diffuse large B-cell lymphomas. *Journal of the American Academy of Dermatology.* 2007;**56**:588–597.

190. **Kodama K, Massone C, Chott A,** *et al.* Primary cutaneous large B-cell lymphomas: clinicopathologic features, classification, and prognostic factors in a large series of patients. *Blood.* 2005; **106**:2491–2497.

191. **Goodlad JR, Krajewski AS, Batstone PJ,** *et al.* Primary cutaneous diffuse large B-cell lymphoma: prognostic significance of clinicopathological subtypes. *The American Journal of Surgical Pathology.* 2003;**27**:1538–1545.

192. **Ponzoni M, Ferreri AJ, Campo E,** *et al.* Definition, diagnosis, and management of intravascular large B-cell lymphoma: proposals and perspectives from an international consensus meeting. *Journal of Clinical Oncology.* 2007;**25**: 3168–3173.

193. **Nakamura S, Murase T, Kinoshita T.** Intravascular large B-cell lymphoma: the heterogeneous clinical manifestations of its classical and hemophagocytosis-related forms. *Haematologica.* 2007;**92**:434–436.

194. **Ferreri AJ, Campo E, Seymour JF,** *et al.* Intravascular lymphoma: clinical presentation, natural history, management and prognostic factors in a series of 38 cases, with special emphasis on the 'cutaneous variant'. *British Journal of Haematology.* 2004; **127**:173–183.

195. **Murase T, Yamaguchi M, Suzuki R,** *et al.* Intravascular large B-cell lymphoma (IVLBCL): a clinicopathologic study of 96 cases with special reference to the immunophenotypic heterogeneity of CD5. *Blood.* 2007;**109**:478–485.

196. **Stroup RM, Sheibani K, Moncada A, Purdy LJ, Battifora H.** Angiotropic (intravascular) large cell lymphoma. A clinicopathologic study of seven cases with unique clinical presentations. *Cancer.* 1990;**66**:1781–1788.

197. **Glass J, Hochberg FH, Miller DC.** Intravascular lymphomatosis. A systemic disease with neurologic manifestations. *Cancer.* 1993;**71**: 3156–3164.

198. **Reyes-Castro M, Vega-Memije E.** Intravascular large cell lymphoma. *International Journal of Dermatology.* 2007;**46**:619–621.

199. **Chan JKC, Jaffe ES, Ralfkiaer E.** Blastic NK-cell lymphoma. In Jaffe ES, Harris NL, Stein H, Vardiman J. (eds.). *World Health Organization Classification of Tumours: Pathology and Genetics of Tumours of Haematopoietic and Lymphoid Tissues.* Lyon: IARC Press; 2001, 214–215.

200. **Grouard G, Rissoan MC, Filgueira L,** *et al.* The enigmatic plasmacytoid T cells develop into dendritic cells with interleukin (IL)-3 and CD40-ligand. *Journal of Experimental Medicine.* 1997;**185**:1101–1111.

201. **Herling M, Jones D.** CD4+/CD56+ hematodermic tumor: the features of an evolving entity and its relationship to dendritic cells. *American Journal of Clinical Pathology.* 2007;**127**:687–700.

202. **Petrella T, Comeau MR, Maynadie M,** *et al.* 'Agranular CD4+ CD56+ hematodermic neoplasm' (blastic NK-cell lymphoma) originates from a population of CD56+ precursor cells related to plasmacytoid monocytes. *The American Journal of Surgical Pathology.* 2002;**26**:852–862.

203. **Chang SE, Choi HJ, Huh J,** *et al.* A case of primary cutaneous CD56+, TdT+, CD4+, blastic NK-cell lymphoma in a 19-year-old woman. *The American Journal of Dermatopathology.* 2002;**24**: 72–75.

204. **Ruggiero A, Maurizi P, Larocca LM, Arlotta A, Riccardi R.** Childhood CD4+/CD56+ hematodermic neoplasm: case report and review of the literature. *Haematologica.* 2006; **91**(12 Suppl):ECR48.

205. **DiGiuseppe JA, Louie DC, Williams JE,** *et al.* Blastic natural killer cell leukemia/lymphoma: a clinicopathologic study. *The American Journal of Surgical Pathology.* 1997; **21**:1223–1230.

206. **Petrella T, Dalac S, Maynadie M,** *et al.* CD4+ CD56+ cutaneous neoplasms: a distinct hematological entity? Groupe Francais d'Etude des Lymphomes Cutanes (GFELC). *The American Journal of Surgical Pathology.* 1999; **23**:137–146.

207. **Chaperot L, Bendriss N, Manches O,** *et al.* Identification of a leukemic counterpart of the plasmacytoid dendritic cells. *Blood.* 2001;**97**: 3210–3217.

208. **Herling M, Teitell MA, Shen RR, Medeiros LJ, Jones D.** TCL1 expression in plasmacytoid dendritic cells (DC2s) and the related CD4+ CD56+ blastic tumors of skin. *Blood.* 2003;**101**: 5007–5009.

209. **Brody JP, Allen S, Schulman P,** *et al.* Acute agranular CD4-positive natural killer cell leukemia. Comprehensive clinicopathologic studies including virologic and in vitro culture with inducing agents. *Cancer.* 1995;**75**: 2474–2483.

210. **Hallermann C, Middel P, Griesinger F,** *et al.* CD4+ CD56+ blastic tumor of the skin: cytogenetic observations and further evidence of an origin from plasmocytoid dendritic cells. *European Journal of Dermatology.* 2004;**14**:317–322.

211. **Feuillard J, Jacob MC, Valensi F,** *et al.* Clinical and biologic features of CD4(+)CD56(+) malignancies. *Blood.* 2002;**99**:1556–1563.

212. **Rossi JG, Felice MS, Bernasconi AR,** *et al.* Acute leukemia of dendritic cell lineage in childhood: incidence, biological characteristics and outcome. *Leukemia & Lymphoma.* 2006;**47**: 715–725.

213. **Lin P, Jones D, Dorfman DM, Medeiros LJ.** Precursor B-cell lymphoblastic lymphoma: a predominantly extranodal tumor with low propensity for leukemic involvement. *The American Journal of Surgical Pathology.* 2000;**24**:1480–1490.

214. **Sander CA, Medeiros LJ, Abruzzo LV, Horak ID, Jaffe ES.** Lymphoblastic lymphoma presenting in cutaneous sites. A clinicopathologic analysis of six cases. *Journal of the American Academy of Dermatology.* 1991;**25**:1023–1031.

215. **Chimenti S, Fink-Puches R, Peris K,** *et al.* Cutaneous involvement in lymphoblastic lymphoma. *Journal of Cutaneous Pathology.* 1999;**26**:379–385.

216. **Link MP, Roper M, Dorfman RF,** *et al.* Cutaneous lymphoblastic lymphoma with pre-B markers. *Blood.* 1983;**61**: 838–841.

217. **Kahwash SB, Qualman SJ**. Cutaneous lymphoblastic lymphoma in children: report of six cases with precursor B-cell lineage. *Pediatric and Developmental Pathology*. 2002;**5**:45–53.

218. **Pittaluga S, Raffeld M, Lipford EH, Cossman J**. 3A1 (CD7) expression precedes T beta gene rearrangements in precursor T (lymphoblastic) neoplasms. *Blood*. 1986;**68**:134–139.

219. **Maitra A, McKenna RW, Weinberg AG, Schneider NR, Kroft SH**. Precursor B-cell lymphoblastic lymphoma. A study of nine cases lacking blood and bone marrow involvement and review of the literature. *American Journal of Clinical Pathology*. 2001;**115**:868–875.

220. **Hsiao CH, Su IJ**. Primary cutaneous pre-B lymphoblastic lymphoma immunohistologically mimics Ewing's sarcoma/primitive neuroectodermal tumor. *Journal of the Formosan Medical Association*. 2003;**102**:193–197.

221. **Ko CJ**. The new World Health Organization-European Organization for Research and Treatment of Cancer classification of cutaneous lymphomas. *Advances in Dermatology*. 2006;**22**: 259–277.

Index